ENDOCRINOLOGY
AND METABOLISM

ENDOCRINOLOGY AND METABOLISM

Editor-in-Chief
ALDO PINCHERA
Professor of Endocrinology
Department of Endocrinology
University of Pisa
University Hospital
Pisa – Italy

Editors
XAVIER Y. BERTAGNA
Professor of Endocrinology
Department of Endocrinology
University of Paris V René Descartes
Cochin University Hospital
Paris - France

JAN A. FISCHER
Associate Professor of Internal Medicine
Department of Orthopedic Surgery and Medicine
University of Zürich
Zürich - Switzerland

LEIF GROOP
Professor of Endocrinology
Department of Endocrinology
Lund University
University Hospital MAS
Malmö - Sweden

JOOP SCHOEMAKER
Emeritus Professor of Pathophysiology of Reproduction
Department of Obstetrics and Gynaecology
Vrije Universiteit Medical Center
Amsterdam - The Netherlands

MARIO SERIO
Professor of Endocrinology
Department of Clinical Physiopathology
University of Florence
Azienda Careggi Hospital
Firenze - Italy

JOHN A.H. WASS
Professor of Endocrinology
Department of Endocrinology
University of Oxford
Radcliffe Infirmary
Oxford - United Kingdom

Consulting Editor
LEWIS E. BRAVERMAN
Professor of Medicine
Section of Endocrinology, Diabetes, and Nutrition
Boston University School of Medicine
Boston Medical Center
Boston, Massachussets - USA 111

McGraw-Hill International (UK) Ltd.

London • New York • San Francisco • St. Louis • Auckland • Bogotá • Caracas • Lisbon • Madrid • Mexico City • Milan • Montréal • New Delhi • San Juan • Singapore • Sydney • Tokyo • Toronto

ENDOCRINOLOGY AND METABOLISM

Copyright © 2001 by
McGraw-Hill International (UK) Ltd.
Shoppenhangers Road
Maidenhead, Berkshire
SL6-2QL England

McGraw-Hill

A Division of The McGraw·Hill Companies

Editors-in-Chief: J. Dereck Jeffers, Fulvio Bruno
Acquisition Editor: Sandra Fabiani
Production Manager: Gino La Rosa
Copyediting and proof-reading: Lorenza Dainese, Laurie Vandermolen
Preparation of index: Marji Toensing
Typesetting: Linotipo srl, Parma, Italy
Printing and binding: CPM, Casarile (MI), Italy

Cover and page XXI illustration courtesy of: Pascoli Perugino A. *Il Corpo Umano*, Fidenza: Casa Editrice Mattioli, 1991; edition published exclusively for Master Pharma (Parma, Italy), plate II, page 21.

ISBN 007-709520-0
Printed in Italy

CONTENTS

CONTRIBUTORS

Numbers in brackets refer to chapters written or co-written by the contributor

MARC J. ABRAMOWICZ, MD, PhD
Associate Professor of Medical Genetics
Department of Medical Genetics
Free University of Brussels
Erasme University Hospital
Brussels – Belgium [3]

CARL-DAVID AGARDH, MD, PhD
Professor of Diabetes Research
Department of Endocrinology
University of Lund
University Hospital MAS
Malmö – Sweden [56, 61]

ELISABET AGARDH, MD, PhD
Associate Professor of Ophthalmology
Department of Ophthalmology
University of Lund
Malmö University Hospital
Malmö – Sweden [59]

BO AHRÉN, MD, PhD
Professor of Clinical Metabolism
Department of Medicine
University of Lund
Lund – Sweden [65]

JAN M. APELQVIST, MD, PhD
Associate Professor of Internal Medicine
Department of Endocrinology
University of Lund
Malmö University Hospital
Malmö – Sweden [59]

PETER ARNER, MD, PhD
Professor of Medicine
Department of Medicine
Huddinge University Hospital
Stockholm – Sweden [63]

LUIGI BARTALENA, MD
Professor of Endocrinology
Department of Endocrinology
University of Insubria
Circolo Hospital
Varese – Italy [12, app 2]

ANTONINO BELFIORE, MD
Associate Professor of Endocrinology
Department of Experimental and Clinical Medicine
University of Catanzaro
Policlinico Mater Domini Hospital
Catanzaro – Italy [2]

KERSTIN E. BERNTORP, MD, PhD
Associate Professor of Endocrinology
Department of Endocrinology
Malmö University Hospital
Malmö – Sweden [60]

XAVIER Y. BERTAGNA, MD
Professor of Endocrinology
Department of Endocrinology
University of Paris V René Descartes
Cochin University Hospital
Paris – France [29]

ANGELO RAFFAELE BIANCO, MD, PhD
Professor of Medical Oncology
Department of Molecular and Clinical Endocrinology,
    and Oncology
Federico II University
Nuovo Policlinico Hospital
Napoli – Italy [68]

ROBERTO BIANCO, MD
Doctor
Department of Molecular and Clinical Endocrinology,
    and Oncology
Federico II University
Nuovo Policlinico Hospital
Napoli – Italy [68]

KAARE I. BIRKELAND, MD, PhD
Doctor
Hormone Laboratory
University of Oslo
Aker Hospital
Oslo – Norway [73]

GEREMIA B. BOLLI, MD
Professor of Internal Medicine
Department of Internal Medicine
University of Perugia
Policlinico Monteluce Hospital
Perugia – Italy [62]

LEWIS E. BRAVERMAN, MD
Professor of Medicine
Section of Endocrinology, Diabetes, and Nutrition
Boston University School of Medicine
Boston Medical Center
Boston, Massachussets – USA [1]

EMMANUEL L. BRAVO, MD
Professor of Internal Medicine
Department of Nephrology and Hypertension
Cleveland Clinic Foundation
Cleveland – USA [32, 33]

MICHAEL BUCHFELDER, MD, PHD
Associate Professor of Neurosurgery
Department of Neurosurgery
University of Erlangen-Nürnberg
Erlangen – Germany [7]

ALBERT G. BURGER, MD
Associate Professor of Endocrinology
Department of Medicine
University of Geneva
Hôpital Cantonal Universitaire
Geneva – Switzerland [11]

HENRY BURGER, AO, MD, BS, FRCP, FRACP
Director
Prince Henry's Institute of Medical Research
Monash Medical Center
Melbourne – Australia [47]

SILVANO G. CELLA, MD
Doctor
Department of Medical Pharmacology
University of Milan
Milano – Italy [app 1]

LUCA CHIOVATO, MD, PHD
Assistant Professor of Endocrinology
Department of Endocrinology
University of Pisa
University Hospital
Pisa – Italy [15, app 2]

ANNIE CLAVIER, MD
Doctor
Department of Medicine
University of Montreal
CHUM Hospital
Montreal – Canada [26]

CYRUS COOPER, MA, MBBS, DM, FRCP
Professor of Rheumatology
MRC Environmental Epidemiology Unit
University of Southampton
Southampton General Hospital
Southampton – United Kingdom [25]

PIERRE CORVOL, MD
Professor of Experimental Medicine
Department of Hypertension
University of Paris IV
Broussais Hospital
Paris – France [35]

ALESSANDRA DE BELLIS, MD
Doctor
Department of Diabetology and Metabolic Diseases
University of Pistoia
University Hospital
Pistoia – Italy [38]

HENRIETTE A. DELEMARRE-VAN DE WAAL, MD, PHD
Professor of Pediatric Endocrinology
Department of Pediatrics
Vrije Universiteit
Vrije Universiteit Medical Center
Amsterdam – The Netherlands [43, 44]

ELAINE DENNISON, MA, MBBS, MRCP
Doctor
MRC Environmental Epidemiology Unit
University of Southampton
Southampton General Hospital
Southampton – United Kingdom [25]

PAUL P. DEVROEY, MD, PHD
Professor of Gynaecology
Department of Reproductive Medicine
Dutch-speaking Brussels Free University
University Hospital
Brussels – Belgium [50]

DOUGLAS B. EVANS, MD
Associate Professor of Surgery
Department of Surgical Oncology
University of Texas
M.D. Anderson Cancer Center
Houston, Texas – USA [71]

GIOVANNI FAGLIA, MD
Professor of Endocrinology
Institute of Endocrine Sciences
University of Milan
Ospedale Maggiore IRCCS
Milano – Italy [6]

ALAN P. FARWELL, MD
Associate Professor of Medicine
Division of Endocrinology
University of Massachussets Medical Center
University of Massachussets Memorial Health Care
Worcester, Massachussets – USA [1]

BART C.J.M. FAUSER, MD, PHD
Professor of Reproductive Endocrinology
Department of Obstetrics and Gynaecology
Erasmus University Medical Center Rotterdam
Rotterdam – The Netherlands [46]

GIANFRANCO FENZI, MD, PHD
Professor of Endocrinology
Department of Endocrinology
 and Oncology
Federico II University of Napoli
Napoli – Italy [14]

JOCK K. FINDLAY, MD, PHD, DSc
Professor of Reproductive Biology
Prince Henry's Institute of Medical Research
Clayton, Victoria – Australia [43]

JAN A. FISCHER, MD
Associate Professor of Internal Medicine
Department of Orthopedic Surgery and Medicine
University of Zürich
Zürich – Switzerland [18]

GIOVANNI FORTI, MD, PhD
Professor of Andrology
Department of Clinical Physiopathology
University of Firenze
Firenze – Italy [41]

ANDERS H. FRID, MD, PhD
Doctor
Department of Medicine
Malmö University Hospital
Malmö – Sweden [60]

ROBERT F. GAGEL, MD
Professor of Medicine
Department of Internal Medicine
University of Texas
M.D. Anderson Cancer Center
Houston, Texas – USA [71]

FRANCIS H. GLORIEUX, MD, PhD
Professor of Surgery and Pediatrics
McGill University
Shriners Hospital for Children
Montreal – Canada [22]

DAVID GOLTZMAN, MD
Professor of Medicine
Department of Medicine
McGill University
Royal Victoria Hospital
Montreal, Quebec – Canada [21]

GRIGORIS F. GRIMBIZIS, MD, PhD
Doctor
Department of Obstetrics and Gynaecology
Aristotle University of Thessaloniki
Hippokration General Hospital
Thessaloniki – Greece [50]

LEIF GROOP, MD, PhD
Professor of Endocrinology
Department of Endocrinology
Lund University
University Hospital MAS
Malmö – Sweden [55, 57]

KRISTIAN F. HANSSEN, MD, PhD
Professor of Endocrinology
Department of Endocrinology
University of Oslo
Aker University Hospital
Oslo – Norway [56, 58]

EGIL HAUG, MD
Professor of Endocrinology
Hormone Laboratory
University of Oslo
Aker Hospital
Oslo – Norway [73]

GEOFFREY N. HENDY, MD, PhD
Professor of Medicine
Department of Medicine
McGill University
Royal Victoria Hospital
Montreal, Quebec – Canada [21]

DOUWE J. HEMRIKA, MD, PhD
Doctor
Department of Obstetrics, Gynaecology
   and Reproductive Medicine
Onze Lieve Vrouwe Gasthuis Hospital
Amsterdam – The Netherlands [52]

JOHANNES HENSEN, MD, PhD
Professor of Medicine
Department of Medicine I
University of Erlangen-Nürnberg
Erlangen – Germany [7]

PETER C. HINDMARSH, MD, BSc, FRCP, FRCPCH
Doctor
Cobbold Laboratories
University College London
Middlesex Hospital
London – United Kingdom [8]

MICHAEL G.R. HULL †, MD, FRCOG
Professor of Reproductive Medicine and Surgery
Department of Obstetrics and Gynaecology
University of Bristol
Bristol – United Kingdom [48]

ALLAN E. KARLSEN, MD, PhD
Doctor
Steno Diabetes Center
Gentofte – Denmark [56]

JEAN-MARC KAUFMAN, MD, PhD
Professor of Internal Medicine
Department of Endocrinology
University Hospital of Gent
Gent – Belgium [42]

PETER KENEMANS, MD, PhD
Professor of Obstetrics and Ginecology
Department of Obstetrics and Ginecology
Vrije Universiteit
Vrije Universiteit Medical Center
Amsterdam – The Netherlands [43, 49]

ALLAN KOFOED-ENEVOLDSEN, MD, DMSC
Doctor
Department of Endocrinology and Internal Medicine
University of Copenhagen
Herlev Hospital
Herlev – Denmark [59]

MARKKU LAAKSO, MD
Professor of Medicine
Department of Medicine
University of Kuopio
Kuopio – Finland [59]

FERNAND LABRIE, MD, PhD, OC, OQ
Professor of Medicine
Department of Oncology and Molecular Endocrinology
Laval University
Chul Research Center
Sainte-Foy, Quebec – Canada [68]

ANDRÉ LACROIX, MD
Professor of Medicine
Department of Medicine
University of Montreal
CHUM Hospital
Montreal – Canada [26]

CORNELIS B. LAMBALK, MD, PhD
Doctor
Department of Obstetrics and Gynaecology
Vrije Universiteit
Vrije Universiteit Medical Center
Amsterdam – The Netherlands [43]

JOHN H. LAZARUS, MD, FRCP
Doctor
Department of Medicine
University of Wales College of Medicine
Cardiff, Wales – United Kingdom [13]

JEFFREY E. LEE, MD
Associate Professor of Surgery
Department of Surgical Oncology
University of Texas
M.D. Anderson Cancer Center
Houston, Texas – USA [71]

ANDREW LEVY, MD, PhD, FRCP
Doctor
Research Center for Neuroendocrinology
University of Bristol
Bristol Royal Infirmary
Bristol – United Kingdom [4]

STAFFORD L. LIGHTMAN, MD, PhD, MB, BCHIR, FCRP, EMEDSCI
Professor of Medicine
Department of Clinical Medicine
University of Bristol
Bristol Royal Infirmary
Bristol – United Kingdom [4]

DAVID G. LOWE, MD, FRCS, FRCPATH, FIBIOL
Professor of Surgical Pathology
Department of Histopathology
Queen Mary University of London
St Bartholomew's Hospital
London – United Kingdom [5]

JEAN-PIERRE LUTON, MD, PhD
Professor of Medicine
Department of Endocrinology
Cochin University Hospital
Paris – France [29, 30]

PAOLO E. MACCHIA, MD, PhD
Doctor
Department of Endocrinology and Oncology
Federico II University of Napoli
Napoli – Italy [14]

MARIO MAGGI, MD
Professor of Endocrinology
Department of Clinical Physiopathology
University of Firenze
Firenze – Italy [39]

THOMAS R. MANDRUP-POULSEN, MD, DMSc
Professor of Immunodiabetology
Steno Diabetes Center
Gentofte – Denmark [56]

FRANCO MANTERO, MD, PhD
Professor of Endocrinology
Department of Medical and Surgical Sciences
Division of Endocrinology
University of Padova
Padova – Italy [34, 37, 67]

STEFANO MARIOTTI, MD
Professor of Endocrinology
Department of Medical Sciences M. Aresu
University of Cagliari
Cagliari – Italy [70]

ENIO MARTINO, MD
Professor of Endocrinology
Department of Endocrinology
University of Pisa
University Hospital
Pisa – Italy [15]

T. JOSEPH MCKENNA, MD
Professor of Investigative Endocrinology
Department of Medicine
University College Dublin
St. Vincent's Hospital
Dublin – Ireland [31]

ROBERTA MINELLI, MD
Doctor
Department of Endocrinology
University of Parma
Parma – Italy [17]

HELEN MOSNIER-PUDAR, MD
Doctor
Cochin University Hospital
Paris – France [30]

EUGENIO E. MÜLLER, MD
Professor of Pharmacology
Department of Pharmacology, Chemoterapy and Tossicology
University Hospital of Milan
Milano – Italy [app 1]

MARIA I. NEW, MD
Professor of Pediatric Endocrinology
Department of Pediatrics
Weill Medical College of Cornell University
New York Presbyterian Hospital
New York, New York – USA [28]

GUIDO NORBIATO, MD
Professor of Endocrinology
Department of Endocrinology
L. Sacco University Hospital
Milano – Italy [74]

GIUSEPPE OPOCHER, MD
Doctor
Department of Medical and Surgical Sciences
University of Padova
Padova – Italy [67]

JEFFREY L.H. O'RIORDAN, MD, FRCP
Emeritus Professor of Metabolic Medicine
Department of Medicine
University College London
The Middlesex Hospital
London – United Kingdom [19]

FURIO PACINI, MD
Professor of Endocrinology
Department of Endocrinology
University of Pisa
University Hospital
Pisa – Italy [16]

SOCRATES E. PAPAPOULOS, MD, PhD
Professor of Medicine
Department of Endocrinology and Metabolic Diseases
Leiden University Medical Center
Leiden – The Netherlands [23, 24]

CARLO PATRONO, MD
Professor of Pharmacology
Department of Medicine and Ageing
University of Chieti G. D'Annunzio
Chieti – Italy [66]

FELICE PETRAGLIA, MD
Professor of Obstetrics and Gynaecology
Department of Paediatrics, Obstetrics and Gynaecology
University of Siena
Le Scotte Hospital
Siena – Italy [51]

ALDO PINCHERA, MD, PhD
Professor of Endocrinology
Department of Endocrinology
University of Pisa
University Hospital
Pisa – Italy

HORACIO PLOTKIN, MD
Doctor
Department of Genetics
McGill University
Shriners Hospital
Montreal – Canada [20]

PIERRE-FRANÇOIS PLOUIN, MD
Professor of Internal Medicine
Department of Hypertension
University of Paris IV
Broussais Hospital
Paris – France [35]

FLEMMING POCIOT, MD, PhD
Doctor
Steno Diabetes Center
Gentofte – Denmark [56]

BIANCA ROCCA, MD
Doctor
Department of Internal Medicine
Catholic University School of Medicine
Roma – Italy [66]

ROBERTO ROCCHI, MD
Doctor
Department of Endocrinology
University of Pisa
University Hospital
Pisa – Italy [app 2]

WINFRIED G. ROSSMANITH, MD, PhD
Professor of Gynaecology and Obstetrics
Department of Obstetrics and Gynaecology
University of Freiburg
Diakonissen Hospital
Karlsruhe – Germany [45]

ELIO ROTI, MD
Associate Professor of Endocrinology
Institute of Endocrinology
University of Milano
Milano – Italy [17]

MARIO SALVI, MD
Doctor
Department of Endocrinolgy
University of Parma
University Hospital
Parma – Italy [17]

LEONARDO SAMMARTANO, MD
Doctor
Department of Medical Sciences M. Aresu
University of Cagliari
University Hospital
Cagliari – Italy [70]

CLARK T. SAWIN, MD
Professor of Medicine
Department of Medicine
Boston University School of Medicine
Boston Veterans Administration Medical Center
Boston, MA – USA [54]

MARTIN J. SCHLUMBERGER, MD
Professor of Oncology
Department of Nuclear Medicine and Endocrine Tumors
University of Paris Sud
Institute Gustave Roussy
Villejuif – France [16]

JOOP SCHOEMAKER, MD, PhD
Emeritus Professor of Pathophysiology of Reproduction
Department of Obstetrics and Gynaecology
Vrije Universiteit
Vrije Universiteit Medical Center
Amsterdam – The Netherlands [46, 53]

MARIO SERIO, MD
Professor of Endocrinology
Department of Clinical Physiopathology
University of Firenze
Azienda Careggi Hospital
Firenze – Italy [38, 39]

PIERRE C. SIZONENKO, MD, MSc
Emeritus Professor of Pediatrics
Hôpital de la Tour
Meyrin – Switzerland [9]

ANDREW F. STEWART, MD
Professor of Medicine and Endocrinology
Department of Medicine
University of Pittsburgh School of Medicine
Pittsburgh, Pennsylvania – USA [20]

GÖRAN SUNDKVIST, MD, PhD
Associate Professor of Internal Medicine
Department of Endocrinology
University of Lund
Malmö University Hospital
Malmö – Sweden [59]

MARJA-RIITTA TASKINEN, MD, PhD
Professor of Medicine
Department of Medicine
Helsinki University Hospital
Helsinki – Finland [64]

PIERRE THOMOPOULOS, MD
Professor of Endocrinology
Department of Endocrinology
University of Paris V René Descartes
Cochin University Hospital
Paris – France [27]

MICHEL B. VALLOTTON, MD
Professor of Medicine
Department of Medicine
Division of Endocrinology and Diabetology
University of Geneva
University Hospital
Geneva – Switzerland [36]

GILBERT VASSART, MD, PhD
Professor of Genetics
Institute of Interdisciplinary Research
University of Brussels
Erasme Hospital
Brussels – Belgium [3]

ALEX VERMEULEN, MD, PhD
Professor of Internal Medicine
Department of Endocrinology
University Hospital of Gent
Gent – Belgium [42]

RICCARDO VIGNERI, MD
Professor of Endocrinology
Department of Internal Medicine, Endocrinology
  and Metabolic Diseases
University of Catania
Garibaldi Hospital
Catania – Italy [2]

AARON I. VINIK, MD, PhD, FCP, FACP
Professor of Medicine
Diabetes Research Institutes
Eastern Virginia Medical School
Norfolk, Virginia – USA [69]

PAOLO VITTI, MD
Associate Professor of Endocrinology
Department of Endocrinology
University of Pisa
University Hospital
Pisa – Italy [12]

**BEVERLEY VOLLENHOVEN, MD, PhD, MBBS,
  FRACOG, CREI**
Doctor
Department of Obstetrics and Gynaecology
University of Monash
Monash Medical Center
Melbourne – Australia [47]

JOHN A.H. WASS, MD, MA, FRCP
Professor of Endocrinology
Department of Endocrinology
University of Oxford
Radcliffe Infirmary
Oxford – United Kingdom

ANTHONY P. WEETMAN, MD, DSc
Professor of Medicine
Division of Clinical Sciences
University of Sheffield
Northern General Hospital
Sheffield – United Kingdom [72]

WILMAR M. WIERSINGA, MD, PhD
Professor of Endocrinology
Department of Endocrinology and Metabolism
University of Amsterdam
Academic Medical Center
Amsterdam – The Netherlands [10]

STEPHEN J. WINTERS, MD
Professor of Medicine
Department of Internal Medicine
University of Pittsburgh
University Medical Center
Pittsburgh, Pennsylvania – USA [40]

FOREWORD

This textbook of general endocrinology is intended primarily for the clinical endocrinologist and primary care physician, yet should also be widely applicable to academic endocrinologists and basic scientists. There are 74 chapters divided into 15 organ systems and two appendix chapters.

Professor Pinchera has chosen many outstanding contributors, the vast majority being from Europe and including ten authors from the United States.

Following a section dealing with general principles of endocrinology, the text covers neuroendocrinology and the pituitary, including growth and development and disorders during puberty. Each endocrine organ is then treated in great detail, with an emphasis on clinical diagnosis and management following an introduction of basic concepts.

The sections on the endocrinology of hypertension; lipid disorders; the gastrointestinal hormones; the endocrinology of the kidney, lung, and heart; hormones and cancer; the female reproductive system including dysfunctional uterine bleeding, management of menopause, and assisted reproduction; and special topics including endocrine immunology and the endocrinology of AIDS will be of great help to the clinician in fostering the awareness and management of these varied and complex disorders.

Finally, the more recently elucidated characteristics of the molecular biology and genetic defects of endocrine disorders, including genetic defects leading to under- and overproduction of specific hormones and cancer, are extremely well covered throughout the book.

We hope that this textbook will be widely used by our clinical colleagues and students and that it will provide them with a comprehensive approach to the diagnosis and management of a wide variety of endocrine disorders.

Lewis S. Braverman
Boston, Massachusetts, USA

PREFACE

The continuous and rapid growth of molecular and cell biology and other fields of basic science that have occurred in the last two decades is having a profound impact on the field of endocrinology. The understanding of endocrine physiology and the mechanism of hormone action has improved to the point that many pathophysiologic mechanisms of endocrine diseases, once obscure, are now unraveled.

A large body of evidence obtained from clinical and epidemiological studies is now available and provides invaluable help for the everyday decision making of the endocrinologist and of the physician at large. In fact, the high prevalence of many endocrine and metabolic disorders in the general population implies that every physician is challenged with endocrine-related problems on a regular basis.

This clinically oriented textbook endeavors to furnish an updated view of clinical endocrinology that is based upon the understanding of the basic mechanisms responsible for endocrine diseases and upon recent evidence derived from clinical studies. Each chapter has been prepared by recognized experts in the various areas of endocrinology, in a way that is accessible both to the endocrinologist and to the general physician faced with managing endocrine disorders. Accordingly, the book is simple and thorough at the same time, with a straightforward approach to the basic concepts in endocrinology, the pathophysiology of endocrine glands, the clinical features of endocrine diseases, and updated guidelines for therapeutic procedures.

This textbook is published by the European section of McGraw-Hill and edited by European scientists, although chapters have also been contributed by overseas authors.

The editors would like to thank all the colleagues who contributed to this book for their dedication and for the excellence of their efforts.

We are particularly grateful to Dr. L. Braverman for his help and continuous support as a consulting editor.

Finally we would like to express our gratitude to Sabrina Venturini (whose sudden loss was deeply felt), Sandra Fabiani, Anita Franchi and Eleonora Cardelli for their invaluable help, and to Dereck Jeffers in San Francisco for his enthusiastic support.

We believe that this textbook will find a relevant place in the medical literature, providing a useful source of information for inquiring clinicians and students, and a source of stimulation for basic scientists as well.

Aldo Pinchera
Pisa, Italy

Hormones secreted by endocrine glands have a central role in the economy of the body, because they influence multiple functions and are essential for growth, reproduction and homeostasis.

In addition to measurement of circulating hormones, recently developed imaging techniques, such as octreoscan, CT scan, MRI, echo-color doppler sonography, have greatly improved diagnostic sensitivity in endocrine disorders.

Application of modern molecular biology techniques to endocrinology has in recent years allowed to unravel the genetic basis of several endocrine disorders and, in some instances, to treat them earlier than in the past.

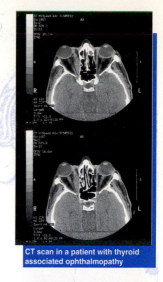

CT scan in a patient with thyroid associated ophthalmopathy

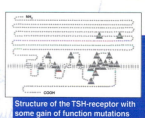

Octreoscan demonstrating a pituitary GH-secreting adenoma

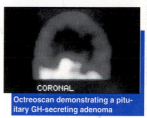

Structure of the TSH-receptor with some gain of function mutations

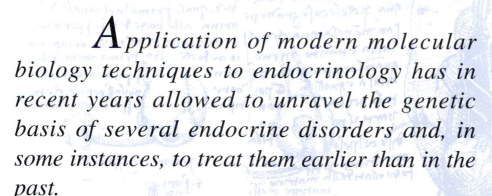

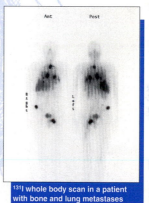

131I whole body scan in a patient with bone and lung metastases of a papillary thyroid cancer

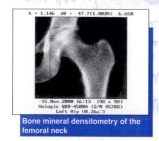

Bone mineral densitometry of the femoral neck

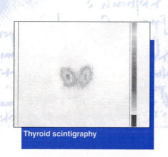

Thyroid scintigraphy

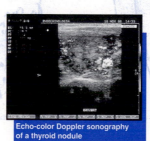

Echo-color Doppler sonography of a thyroid nodule

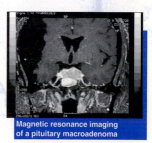

Magnetic resonance imaging of a pituitary macroadenoma

General principles

1

Introduction to the endocrine system

Alan P. Farwell, Lewis E. Braverman

The development of a means of communication between cells and organs was essential for the possibility of single cell organisms to evolve into complex multicellular species. The endocrine system provides a mechanism for such communication. The term *endocrine* is defined as the secretion of biologically active compounds from a ductless gland into the body. *Endocrinology* is, thus, the science dealing with internal secretions and their physiologic and pathologic relations. In humans, the endocrine system regulates growth and development, reproduction, homeostasis, energy production, utilization and storage, and responses to alterations in the internal and external environment.

In general, the substances that endocrine glands secrete are termed *hormones*, which is derived from the Greek verb "to rouse or set in motion". A hormone is classically defined as a chemical substance produced in one organ or cell that is carried by the bloodstream to act upon another organ or cell (Fig. 1.1). In order to act, hormones must interact with proteins known as receptors on or inside the target cell. Hormone receptors have two essential qualities: (1) the receptor must be able to recognize a unique binding site within the hormone in order to discriminate between the hormone and all other proteins, and (2) the receptor must be able to transmit the information gained from binding to the hormone into a cellular response. Thus, transport proteins that tightly bind hormones in the circulation and/or within the cell do not elicit a cellular response and are not receptors. Hormone receptors may be either intracellular, requiring entry of the hormone into the cell to elicit its action, or located on the cell surface, allowing interactions with hormones that are restricted from the intracellular compartment.

These definitions are adequate to define hormones and receptors in most cases. However, recent advances have broadened the concepts of what constitutes a hormone. Regulatory molecules that mainly act as neurotransmitters may also act as classic hormones. Examples of these com-

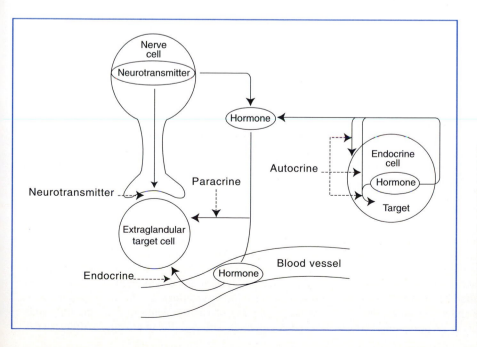

Figure 1.1 Interrelationships between various types of hormone action in the endocrine and nervous systems. Regulatory molecules may act as hormones, neurotransmitters, or both, with endocrine, paracrine, or autocrine actions. Similarly, endocrine cells may function as nerve cells and nerve cells as endocrine cells. (From Felig P, Baxter JD, Frohman LA [eds]. Endocrinology and metabolism. New York: McGraw-Hill, 1995.)

pounds are catecholamines and acetylcholine. Conversely, small peptides, such as thyrotropin-releasing hormone (TRH) – which is produced in the hypothalamus and acts on the anterior pituitary to release thyrotropin and prolactin – are also found distributed in neurons throughout the body, where they presumably function as neurotransmitters.

The concept of a hormone produced by a single endocrine gland must also be broadened. The classical endocrine glands, whose primary function is hormone production, include the thyroid, pituitary, adrenal, and parathyroid glands, and the pancreatic islets. However, the brain is a major source for some peptide hormones, including: pro-opiomelanocortin (POMC), the precursor molecule for corticotropin (adrenocorticotropic hormone, ACTH); endorphins; melanocyte-stimulating hormone (MSH); and β-lipotropin, which is also synthesized in the anterior pituitary, placenta, and the gastrointestinal tract. The ovary and testes, which produce the sex hormones, also produce oocytes and sperm. Other organs that produce hormones while serving other primary functions include: the heart (atrial natriuretic factor), the liver (insulin-like growth factor-1, angiotensinogen, and the conversion of thyroxine into the metabolically active 3,3',5'-triiodothyronine [T_3]), the kidney (erythropoietin and the active form of vitamin D), and the gastrointestinal tract (gastrin, cholecystokinin, somatostatin, and others).

Finally, it is clear that hormones do not have to travel through the circulation to act (*endocrine actions*) (Fig. 1.1). Locally-secreted hormones can act upon adjacent or surrounding cells (*paracrine actions*). Examples of this include the release of growth factors in bone; and the release of somatostatin by the delta cells of the pancreatic islets, which inhibits secretion of insulin from the beta cells and glucagon from the alpha cells. A hormone can also act on its own cell of origin (*autocrine actions*). For example, insulin has an inhibitory effect on its own secretion by the pancreatic beta cells.

INTERRELATIONSHIPS WITH OTHER SYSTEMS

The functions and actions of the endocrine system overlap considerably with the two other systems involved in extracellular communication: the nervous system and the immune system. Like the endocrine system, the nervous system has evolved to release regulatory substances from nerve cells that act across synaptic junctions to transmit a signal to adjacent cells. As noted above, these neurotransmitters may also function as true circulating hormones, while some hormones also function as neurogenic mediators in the central nervous system. Thus, if a regulatory molecule is released into the circulation to act, it is considered a hormone; if it is released from a nerve terminal to act locally, it is a neurotransmitter. The same regulatory molecule may be both a hormone and a neurotransmitter.

The hypothalamus serves as a direct connection

between the nervous and endocrine systems as the source of both hormones that are stored in the posterior pituitary, and releasing peptides that regulate hormone secretion from the anterior pituitary. The autonomic nervous system often exerts control over the function of endocrine tissues. The pituitary, pancreatic islets, renal juxtaglomerular cells, and the adrenal gland all respond to neural stimulation. Thus, the same cell can function as both an endocrine and a neural cell.

The immune system, initially thought to function autonomously, is now known to be subject to both neural and endocrine regulation. The cytokine regulators of the immune system are not usually considered hormones, but they clearly fit the definition as regulatory molecules that are secreted by one cell and influence another cell. The actions of cytokines are not limited to immunomodulation, as interleukins, interferons, and tumor necrosis factor produced by the immune system during systemic illness exert a major influence on hormone metabolism, especially that of thyroid hormone. Similarly, corticosteroids are major immunomodulators, as are the metabolic derangements produced by endocrine dysfunction, such as hyperglycemia in uncontrolled diabetes mellitus. Thus, while the central focus of endocrinology is on hormones, it is clear that not all hormones belong to the endocrine system and that there is considerable blurring between the boundaries of the endocrine, nervous, and immune systems.

CLASSES OF HORMONES

Hormones fall into three general categories based upon the mechanism of synthesis: peptide hormones, amino acid analogues, and steroid hormones (Tab. 1.1). The *peptide hormones* are the most abundant and most diverse and vary in size, composition, number of chains, modification of groups, and mechanisms of production. The peptide hormones are synthesized after transcription of specific genes, followed by translation and processing through the endoplasmic reticulum and the Golgi apparatus. Single chain peptides vary from the 191-amino acid growth hormone (GH) to the cyclic tripeptide TRH. The anterior pituitary hormones thyrotropin (thyroid-stimulating hormone, TSH), follicle-stimulating hormone (FSH), and luteinizing hormone (LH) consist of two chains, one of which is common to all three hormones (α chain), while the other is unique (β chain); in addition, these three hormones are glycosylated. Insulin has two chains that are derived from a single gene product (preproinsulin), which is post-translationally cleaved; while ACTH, MSH, and β-endorphin are single-chain proteolytic products of a large precursor molecule (pro-opiomelanocortin).

The *amino acid analogues* include the *iodothyronines* and the *amines*. The precursor of the iodothyronines is thyroglobulin, a 660 000-dalton glycoprotein synthesized by the thyroid follicular cell containing >100 tyrosine residues. The iodothyronines are formed by iodination and the coupling of two tyrosines and are the only iodinated compounds with significant biologic activity. In cat-

Table 1.1 Classes of hormones

Peptide hormones

Small peptides
Vasopressin (ADH)
Oxytocin
Melanocyte-stimulating hormone (MSH)
Thyrotropin-releasing hormone (TRH)
Gonadotropin-releasing hormone (GnRH)

Intermediate peptides
Insulin
Glucagon
Growth hormone (GH)
Prolactin (PRL)
Parathyroid hormone (PTH)
Calcitonin
Corticotropin (ACTH)
Corticotropin-releasing hormone (CRH)
β-Endorphin
Gastrointestinal peptides
Cytokines
Growth factors

Glycoproteins
Pro-opiomelanocortin (POMC)
Follicle-stimulating hormone (FSH)
Luteinizing hormone (LH)
Thyrotropin (TSH)
Chorionic gonadotropin (CG)

Amino acid analogues

Iodothyronines
Thyroxine (T_4)
3,5,3'-Triiodothyronine (T_3)
3,3',5'-Triiodothyronine (rT_3)

Amines
Dopamine
Epinephrine
Norepinephrine
Melatonin
Serotonin

Steroid hormones

Estrogens (E_2, E_3)
Progesterone (P)
Testosterone (T)
Dihydrotestosterone (DHT)
Cortisol
Aldosterone
Vitamin D
Retinoic acid
Prostaglandins

---

by the action of ultraviolet radiation on 7-dehydro-cholesterol; is transported to the liver, where it is converted to 25-hydroxy vitamin D; followed by transport to the kidney tubule, where it is converted to its most active form, 1,25-dihydroxy vitamin D [1,25(OH)$_2$D].

MECHANISM OF ACTION OF HORMONES

The mechanism of hormone action involves the interaction of a ligand (hormone) with a specific cellular receptor. The receptor serves two functions: (1) to recognize the hormone from all other substances, and (2) to activate a cellular response upon hormone binding. At the present time, two broad categories of hormone receptors are recognized: cell surface receptors and nuclear receptors.

Cell surface receptors

Cell surface receptors are glycoproteins that appear to be highly mobile within the plasma membrane. Hydrophilic portions of the receptor are exposed at the cell surface, while the hydrophobic portions of the molecule are buried within the lipid bilayer. Cell surface receptors bind water soluble hormones, including all the peptide hormones and the catecholamines. Since these water soluble hormones are not able to transverse the lipid bilayer to enter the cell, the cell surface receptor serves to transmit the hormonal "message" to the interior of the cell. The binding of the hormone to the cell surface receptor is reversible, allowing the receptor to be activated repeatedly. Alternatively, the hormone/receptor complex may be internalized, producing a single response from a single ligand/receptor interaction.

The binding of a hormone to a cell surface receptor stimulates a cascade of complex events (Fig. 1.2 A). Common to many of the intracellular pathways is the activation of protein kinases. Phosphorylations induced by these kinases alter the conformation of a diverse number of molecules, which then produce a diverse series of metabolic effects. Many pathways (peptides, neurotransmitters, prostaglandins) share the activation of adenyl cyclase by guanine nucleotide regulatory proteins (G-proteins). These in turn catalyze the conversion of ATP to cyclic AMP and activate serine and threonine kinases (A kinases). Other hormones (insulin, growth factors) activate tyrosine kinases directly. Still others (neurotransmitters, amino acids) increase calcium influx into the cells by altering the production or turnover of phospholipids (G-protein pathway) or by directly affecting calcium channels (ligand-gated calcium channels). The increase in intracellular calcium activates other protein kinases (C kinases), either directly or through the calcium-binding protein calmodulin. Thus, hormones may utilize a variety of intracellular mediators, and a given hormone may utilize one or more of these intracellular pathways. The metabolic events regulated by the activation of cell surface receptors may be rapid alterations in ion or substrate flux

echolamine-secreting cells, tyrosine is converted sequentially to dopamine, norepinephrine, and epinephrine. Serotonin (5-hydroxytryptamine) is derived from tryptophan.

Steroid hormones are derivatives of cholesterol, which have a similar core known as the cyclopentanohydrophenanthrene ring. Synthesis of the steroid hormones occurs as a result of enzymatically-induced changes to the cholesterol core, while prostaglandins are derivatives of arachidonic acid. Synthesis of the adrenal and sex steroids occurs in the adrenal cortex and testes or ovaries, respectively. Vitamin D differs in that it is produced in the skin

Figure 1.2 Mechanisms of hormone action. (**A**) *Cell surface receptors.* Three major classes of cell surface receptors exist for both hormones and neurotransmitters. Ligands may bind to receptors that directly activate tyrosine kinases, receptors (R) that are linked via G-proteins (G) to an effector (E) such as adenyl cyclase that activates protein kinases or receptors, which regulate ion channels and then activate protein kinases or other regulatory pathways. (From Kahn CR, Smith RJ, Chin WW. In: Wilson JD, Foster DW [eds]. Williams Textbook of endocrinology. Philadelphia: WB Saunders, 1992.) (**B**) *Nuclear receptors.* The steroids and thyroid hormones enter the cell and interact with nuclear receptors that bind to chromatin and alter the transcription of specific genes, which is then translated into proteins that result in altered cell function, constituting the hormone's effect. (From Clark JH, Schrader WT, O'Malley B. In: Wilson JD, Foster DW [eds]. Williams Textbook of endocrinology. Philadelphia: WB Saunders, 1992.)

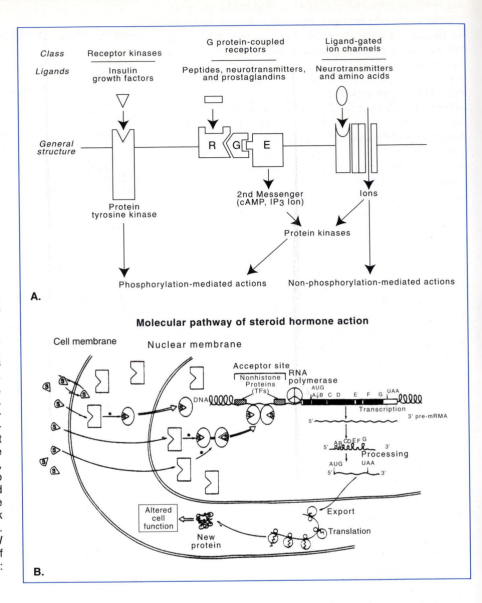

across the plasma membrane or slower alterations in protein levels by the modulation of gene transcription.

Nuclear receptors

Lipid soluble hormones such as thyroid hormone and the steroid-based hormones are able to penetrate the plasma membrane and interact with intracellular receptors (Fig. 1.2 B). Thyroid hormone receptors are bound to a hormone-response element on the chromatin in the presence and absence of the hormone. The hormone:receptor interaction alters the transcription of specific genes. Steroid receptors are either loosely associated or unassociated with chromatin. Steroid binding alters the conformation of the receptor so that the complex has a high affinity for nuclear chromatin or other nuclear transcription factors, which then alters the transcription of specific genes. The metabolic effects of these proteins are then produced by

the translation products of the steroid- or thyroid hormone-regulated mRNAs. Thus, the actions of these hormones are relatively slow.

ACTIONS OF HORMONES

Hormones have effects on and regulate many body processes. It is rare that only a single hormone controls a single process. Hormonal regulation of a particular system is characteristically the result of the coordinate action of several hormones, often acting by different mechanisms. By this means, the endocrine system regulates the body's response to a diverse variety of physiologic and pathologic perturbations.

The action of a hormone on a particular target tissue is possible because the cells comprising that tissue contain receptors capable of being activated by a particular hormone. The hormone in question is able to gain access to that tissue in sufficient quantities to bind to the receptors in order to evoke a response. In general, the principal target tissues for a particular hormone contain the largest complement of receptor molecules and are exposed to the highest concentration of hormone. For example, the liver is a major target tissue for insulin both because of its abundant insulin receptor content, and because of the delivery of high concentrations of insulin secreted directly into the hepatic-portal circulation. A similar example is the delivery of hypothalamic-releasing factors to the pituitary via the hypophyseal-portal system. Another mechanism to maximize the concentration of hormone within a tissue is by diffusion of the hormone from its site of secretion, as is the case with the delivery of testosterone from the Leydig cells of the testes to the adjacent spermatogenetic tubules. Finally, the local formation of the active hormone from a circulating hormone precursor can maximize the intracellular hormone concentration. This is demonstrated by the conversion of testosterone to dihydrotestosterone in androgen target tissues such as the prostate, and the production of T_3 from the deiodination of thyroxine in the thyrotrophs of the pituitary and within the brain and other tissues. While receptor content and hormone delivery define major sites of action for a particular hormone, there are likely gradations of hormone effects on tissues that contain less abundant receptors or where delivery of hormone is diminished or restricted.

The major processes regulated by hormones include energy production, utilization and storage (intermediary metabolism), growth, development, reproduction, and maintenance of the internal environment (mineral and water metabolism and cardiovascular effects).

Intermediary metabolism and growth

Hormones are the primary mediators of substrate flux and the conversion of food into energy production or storage. The mobilization of glucose and other fuels is regulated by a number of different hormones. Glucocorticoids, catecholamines, growth hormone, and glucagon promote lypolysis and hyperglycemia. In contrast, insulin and the insulin-like growth factors (IGFs) are anabolic, fuel-storing hormones. Many hormones are growth factors, including androgens, estrogens, growth hormone, prolactin, and thyroid hormone, while glucocorticoids, in excess, inhibit growth. Consistent with the occasional need for rapid mobilization of fuels, many of the catabolic hormones exert their actions by the activation of adenyl cyclase.

Developmental actions

Hormones are essential to normal growth and development. Thyroid hormone, growth hormone, the sex steroids, insulin, and other growth factors profoundly influence these processes. While growth hormone primarily regulates growth and the sex steroids mainly regulate sexual development, thyroid hormone affects both growth and development, especially in the central nervous system.

Reproductive functions

Hormones regulate both the production of ova and sperm and the dimorphic anatomical, functional, and behavioral development of males and females essential for sexual reproduction. Regulation of these reproductive processes is under absolute hormonal control, as seen by the lack of reproductive capacity in their absence. The gonadotropins in the pituitary are essential regulators of ovarian and testicular function and the subsequent secretion of the sex steroids. The sex steroids control functions crucial for pregnancy and for sexual differentiation and development.

Mineral and water metabolism

Aldosterone, parathyroid hormone, and vitamin D have primary functions in ion regulation, while vasopressin regulates water metabolism. The target tissue distribution for these hormones are restricted and their mechanism(s) of action are diverse. Several other hormones have secondary effects on water and electrolyte metabolism, including insulin, glucagon, catecholamines, thyroid hormone, and glucocorticoids.

Cardiovascular functions

While not usually considered an endocrine organ, the heart, specifically the atria, produces atrial natriuretic factor, which has extensive effects on the cardiovascular system. Many hormones affect cardiovascular function, including catecholamines, thyroid hormone, mineralocorticoids, and the sex steroids. The fact that many hormones regulate cardiovascular responses underscores the importance of the endocrine system in responding to physiologic and pathologic perturbations.

Tropic actions

During the evolution of the endocrine system, some hormones evolved to specifically regulate the production of other hormones. Many of these hormones are found in the anterior pituitary. Thyroid-stimulating hormone regulates thyroid hormone production, LH regulates estrogen production in the female and testosterone production in the male, and ACTH regulates glucocorticoid production in the adrenal gland. These hormones also share a similar mechanism by activating adenyl cyclase.

HORMONE SYNTHESIS, STORAGE AND SECRETION

Cells that synthesize peptide or amine hormones store the hormones in granules and, thus, have a readily releasable pool of hormone. Upon the appropriate stimulus, the storage granules are transported to the cell surface, fuse with the plasma membrane, and discharge their contents. In some cells, this process of exocytosis is dependent upon an influx of calcium into the cell. The stimulus for hormone release also induces synthesis of new hormone, resulting in a biphasic secretion pattern: early release of preformed hormone followed by release of newly synthesized hormone.

Steroid-producing cells store very little of their final product. The stimulus for release of steroid hormones is also the stimulus for increased synthesis of hormone. Secretion of steroid hormones follows simple bulk transfer down concentration gradients into the circulation.

Thyroid hormone is stored in the thyroid follicles in association with the precursor protein thyroglobulin. Stimulation of the thyroid follicular cell by TSH causes proteolysis of thyroglobulin and release of thyroid hormone into the circulation. However, despite a large amount of preformed hormone stored in the thyroid gland, secretion of thyroid hormone does not respond as quickly to a stimulus, which is in contrast to the peptide and amine hormones.

In general, only limited quantities of hormones are stored within the body, and even stores of peptide hormones are depleted within hours to days. The rate of the release of hormone is determined ultimately by its rate of synthesis, of which the general rule is for continuous synthesis and degradation of hormones. Two exceptions are thyroid hormone and vitamin D. Both hormones are stored in large amounts, providing a safeguard against long periods of iodine deficiency or absence of sunlight, respectively.

Hormone secretion does not occur at a uniform rate. Most peptide hormones are secreted in episodic bursts at irregular intervals. The frequency of pulses of secretion of some of the tropic hormones, such as the gonadotropins, determines whether these hormones will be stimulatory or inhibitory. Sleep-related release occurs with many hormones, including growth hormone and prolactin from the anterior pituitary. Still others are subject to circadian variation, such as ACTH (and subsequent cortisol) secretion.

TRANSPORT OF HORMONES

For the most part, hormones must be transported at least some distance to their target organs. The primary transport medium is the plasma, although the lymphatic system and the cerebrospinal fluid are also important. Since delivery of the hormone to its target tissue is required before a hormone can exert its effects, the presence or absence of specific transport mechanisms play a major role in mediating hormonal action.

The water-soluble hormones (peptide hormones, catecholamines) are transported in plasma in solution and require no specific transport mechanism. Because of this, the water-soluble hormones are generally short-lived, circulating in the plasma in concentrations in the femtomolar range. These properties allow for rapid shifts in circulating hormone concentrations, which is necessary with the pulsatile tropic hormones or the catecholamines. This is consistent with the rapid onset of action of the water-soluble hormones.

The lipid-soluble hormones (thyroid hormone, steroids) circulate in the plasma bound to specific carrier proteins. Many of the proteins have a high affinity for a specific hormone, such as thyroxine-binding globulin (TBG), sex hormone-binding globulin (SHBG), and cortisol-binding globulin (CBG). Non-specific, low-affinity binding of these hormones to albumin also occurs. Carrier proteins act as reservoirs of hormone, resulting in picomolar to micromolar circulating hormone concentrations. Since it is generally believed that only the free hormone can enter cells, a dynamic equilibrium must exist between the bound and free hormone. Thus, alterations in the amount of binding protein available, or in the affinity of the hormone for the binding protein, can markedly alter the total circulating pool of hormone without affecting the free concentration of hormone.

Carrier proteins act as buffers to both blunt sudden increases in hormone concentration and to diminish degradation of the hormone once it is secreted. Thus, the half-life of hormones that utilize carrier proteins is longer than those that are not protein-bound. Indeed, carrier proteins have a profound effect on the clearance rate of hormones; the greater the capacity for high affinity binding of the hormone in the plasma, the slower the clearance rate. Also, the carrier proteins allow slow, tonic delivery of the hormone to its target tissue. This is consistent with the slower onset of action of the lipid-soluble hormones.

HORMONE METABOLISM

Clearance of hormones from the circulation plays a critical role in the modulation of hormone levels in response to varied physiologic and pathologic processes. The time required to reach a new steady-state concentration in response to changes in hormone release is dependent upon the half-life of the hormone in the serum. Thus, an increase in hormone release or administration will have a much more marked effect if the hormone is cleared rapidly from the circulation as opposed to one that is cleared more slowly. Hormone metabolism is also linked to the processes that they regulate. For example, insulin and catecholamines participate in rapid cellular responses, and their short half-lives facilitate the wide swings in the levels that are essential for their regulatory actions. Conversely, hormones that participate in transcriptional regulation control more long-term cellular responses, and their longer half-lives buffer rapid fluctuations in free hormone levels.

Most peptide hormones have a plasma half-life measured in minutes, consistent with the rapid actions and pulsatile nature of the secretion of these hormones. This rapid clearance is achieved by the lack of protein binding in the plasma, degradation or internalization of the hormone at its site of action, and ready clearance of the hormone by the kidney. Binding to serum proteins markedly decreases hormone clearance, as is observed with the steroid hormones and the iodothyronines. Metabolism of the steroid hormones occurs primarily in the liver by reductions, conjugations, oxidations, and hydroxylations, which serve to inactivate the hormone and increase their water-solubility, facilitating their excretion in the urine and the bile. Metabolic transformation also may serve to activate an inactive hormone precursor, such as the deiodination of thyroxine to form T_3 and the hydroxylation of vitamin D at the 1 and 25 positions.

Hormone metabolism is not as tightly regulated as is hormone synthesis and release. However, alterations in the metabolic pathways may be clinically important. Drugs that increase activity of the liver p450 enzymes, such as phenytoin, rifampin, tegretol, and large doses of barbiturates, also increase the turnover of steroid and thyroid hormones and may expose latent adrenal insufficiency or decreased thyroid reserve. More commonly, the administration of these drugs may require increases in the doses of steroids or thyroid hormone administered to achieve the same effect. Thus, large doses of barbiturates may decrease the effectiveness of oral contraceptives. Alterations in the binding capacity of serum transport proteins also alter the dynamic equilibrium between bound and free hormone, leading to changes in hormone release or replacement requirements. For example, the estrogen-induced increase in TBG may be one possible explanation for the frequently observed increase in the administered dose of L-thyroxine required in the pregnant patient with hypothyroidism. Finally, starvation and illness markedly inhibits the activity of the 5'-deiodinase in the liver. This results in decreased serum T_3 concentrations due to the impaired production of T_3 from thyroxine (T_4), and increased concentrations of the metabolically inactive 3,3',5'-triiodothyronine (reverse T_3) due to decreased clearance. This may be a physiologic response to conserve the body's energy stores.

REGULATION OF HORMONE SECRETION

A distinguishing characteristic of endocrine systems is the feedback regulation of hormone production. Two major influences that are essential to feedback control of hormone secretion are input from higher neural centers and changing plasma levels of hormone or other substances. These regulatory networks allow: (1) hormone levels, and subsequent hormone action, to be controlled within relatively narrow parameters in the basal state, (2) the establishment of circadian rhythms for hormonal secretion, and (3) the stimulation or inhibition of hormone secretion in response to a variety of sensory inputs.

The paradigm for feedback regulation is the hypothalamic-pituitary-target gland axis, where the gland is either the thyroid, adrenal, or gonads (Fig. 1.3). Neural input from higher centers lead to the secretion of a releasing factor from the hypothalamus that acts upon the pituitary to release a tropic hormone. The tropic hormone then stimulates hormone production and release from the target gland. The increase in circulating hormone levels then inhibits further production of the hypothalamic releasing factor, the tropic hormone, or both. Other factors that exert feedback regulation on hormone production include

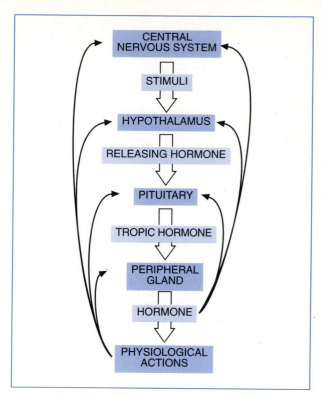

Figure 1.3 Feedback regulation of the endocrine system. Shown is the flow of information from higher cortical centers, activating releasing hormones in the hypothalamus, which then activate the tropic hormones of the pituitary that alter synthesis and release of hormones from an endocrine gland. These hormones then act upon their target cell as well as feedback to inhibit hormone release at multiple proximal loci. (From Baxter JD. In: Wyngaarden JB, Smith LH Jr [eds]. Cecil's Textbook of medicine. Philadelphia: WB Saunders, 1985.)

ions (calcium and parathyroid hormone secretion), metabolites (glucose, insulin, and glucagon), and osmolarity and fluid volume (vasopressin, renin, and aldosterone).

While most examples of feedback regulation are inhibitory, positive feedback systems also exist. Oxytocin release is stimulated by uterine contractions, which, in turn, stimulates more uterine contractions. The result of this positive feedback loop is the eventual expulsion of the newborn from the uterus. During the menstrual cycle, the gonadotropins are subject to both positive and negative control. In general, estradiol exerts a negative influence on gonadotropin secretion. However, during the late follicular phase, estradiol concentrations reach a critical level and trigger the LH/FSH surge leading to ovulation.

DISORDERS OF THE ENDOCRINE SYSTEM

The clinical consequences of dysfunction of the endocrine glands are primarily those associated with hormone deficiency or excess. The disorders that produce these clinical syndromes are diverse and occur by a variety of mechanisms. These include abnormalities with the endocrine glands themselves, including genetic defects, ectopic production of hormones, abnormal conversion of prohormones to their active form, diminished or enhanced response of target tissues to hormones, and iatrogenic factors. The few disorders of the endocrine glands that do not involve altered hormone secretion include simple goiter, non-functioning adenomas, and carcinomas.

Hormone deficiency syndromes

Gland dysfunction

The most common cause of hormone deficiency is the autoimmune destruction of endocrine tissue. All endocrine glands are susceptible to autoimmune involvement, and some syndromes include dysfunction of more than a single gland. Endocrine glands also may be injured or destroyed by infectious agents (tuberculosis of the adrenals), infection or hemorrhage (post-partum necrosis of the pituitary, adrenal hemorrhage), chemical or radiation exposure (testicular damage with chemotherapy, hypothyroidism after mantle irradiation for lymphoma, and, less commonly, hypopituitarism after brain irradiation), space-occupying lesions (hypopituitarism due to craniopharyngioma), primary or secondary neoplasia, or surgical removal. Defects in embryogenesis can lead to the absence or malformation of the endocrine glands, as seen with thyroid agenesis, sublingual thyroid, and chromosomal abnormalities leading to gonadal dysgenesis or agenesis (Turner's syndrome), or hyalinization of the seminiferous tubules and decreased testosterone production (Kleinfelter's syndrome). Alternatively, gland development may be normal, but an enzyme necessary for hormone production may be absent, as in most forms of congenital adrenal hyperplasia and some forms of congenital goiter. Finally, hormone production may be diminished or absent due to lack of a nutrient or an environmental factor, such as iodine-deficient goiter, or vitamin D deficiency due to lack of exposure to sunlight or malabsorbtion.

Extraglandular dysfunction

Extraglandular disorders resulting in hormone deficiency include defective conversion of a prohormone to the active form, and enhanced degradation of the hormone. These disorders also result from an inability of a target tissue to respond to a particular hormone – due to dysfunction or absence of hormone receptors – or from the production of substances that block access of the hormone to its receptor (hormone resistance). Examples of the impaired conversion of hormones include the impaired conversion of 25-vitamin D to 1,25-vitamin D, leading to vitamin D deficiency in vitamin D-dependent rickets and chronic renal failure and androgen deficiency due to an absent or dysfunctional 5α-reductase, which converts testosterone to dihydrotestosterone. Enhanced degradation of hormone usually affects the response to exogenously administered hormone, as in a phenytoin-induced increase in the metabolism of steroid hormones in patients with adrenal insufficiency, L-thyroxine in patients with hypothyroidism, or the unmasking of Addison's disease by the administration of thyroid hormone in individuals with Hashimoto's thyroiditis (Schmidt's syndrome).

Hormone resistance

Hormone resistance produces a clinical picture of hormone deficiency in the presence of normal, or supernormal, hormone secretion or administration. The most common cause of hormone resistance is dysfunction or absence of hormone receptors. Albright and his colleagues first recognized hormone resistance in their characterization of pseudohypoparathyroidism in 1942. This disorder is now known to be the result of altered receptor signaling due to absent or subnormal amounts of a G-protein subunit, which couples hormone:receptor binding to the activation of the catalytic subunit of adenyl cyclase (Fig. 1.2 A). These individuals have hypocalcemia in the presence of high circulating levels of parathyroid hormone.

The most common disorder of hormone resistance occurs in obese patients with type II diabetes mellitus. The pathogenesis of this disorder is multifactorial and includes abnormal down-regulation of the insulin receptor as well as post-receptor defects. The absence of one or more of the thyroid hormone receptor isoforms has been described in patients with generalized thyroid hormone resistance. Familial resistance to TSH – due to point mutations in the TSH receptor, the production of biologically less-active TSH, or as yet undetermined abnormalities – may result in elevated serum TSH and normal or even low serum thyroid hormone concentrations. Finally, the absence of testosterone receptors results in a female phenotype despite a 46,XY karyotype and high circulating testosterone concentrations (testicular feminization). Rarely, receptor antibodies may produce clinical hormone deficiency in the presence of elevated hormone concentrations and normal hormone receptors – as in rare forms of diabetes mellitus due to antibodies to the insulin receptor, and hypothyroidism due to TSH-receptor blocking antibodies.

Hormone excess syndromes

Gland dysfunction

Endocrine cells that continually produce excessive amounts of hormone are either hyperplastic or neoplastic. Virtually all endocrine cells have the potential to lose responsiveness to normal regulatory mechanisms and undergo neoplastic change. Hyperfunctioning tumors of endocrine glands are usually well-differentiated adenomas, with their clinical impact due primarily to the excess hormone production. Hormone-secreting carcinomas, while rare, can be lethal despite the presence of a hormone marker, as in adrenal and parathyroid carcinoma.

Despite their benign histopathology, endocrine adenomas can cause serious morbidity and mortality due to their hormone secretion. A pheochromocytoma may cause death due to a catecholamine-induced hypertensive crisis. Acromegly (growth hormone) and Cushing's disease (cortisol) may cause physical deformity, organ damage, and potentially lethal cardiovascular and metabolic perturbations. On the other hand, a pituitary macroadenoma may cause visual loss due to damage to the optic chiasm caused by suprasellar extension.

While an autonomously functioning tumor is made up of a subset of cells in an endocrine gland, hyperplasia involves all of the cells. A potential mechanism for hyperplasia is an abnormal setpoint for the negative feedback control of hormone secretion. This results in excess secretion of the tropic hormone and leads to hyperplasia and excess production of target gland hormones. Examples of hyperplasia are hyperparathyroidism secondary to the chronically low serum calcium concentrations seen in end stage renal disease, and bilateral adrenal hyperplasia secondary to excess ACTH stimulation (Cushing's disease). The clinical syndromes caused by excess hormone production due to an autonomously functioning adenoma is often indistinguishable from that caused by gland hyperplasia.

Extraglandular dysfunction

Non-endocrine tumors, mainly carcinomas, can occasionally produce hormones in excess and present as an endocrine disorder. In most cases, the hormones produced ectopically are those that arise from a single gene, such as ACTH, parathyroid hormone, erythropoietin, growth hormone, and serotonin. While a large number of non-endocrine cells can produce hormones, ectopic hormone production is primarily associated with APUD (amine precursor uptake and decarboxylation) cells. These cells are found in small cell lung carcinomas, carcinoid tumors, thymomas, and hormone-secreting tumors of the gastrointestinal system, among others.

Gland hyperplasia can occur in the absence of intrinsic glandular dysfunction if the hyperfunctioning gland is reacting appropriately to another stimulus. In Graves' disease, the hypersecretion of thyroid hormone is caused by an antibody that binds to and activates the TSH receptor on the thyroid follicular cells. The chronic stimulation of the thyroid leads to follicular cell hyperplasia and thyrotoxicosis. While hormone resistance usually produces a clinical picture of hormone deficiency in the setting of hormone hypersecretion, thyrotoxicosis due to pituitary thyroid hormone resistance has been described. The only abnormal or deficient T_3 receptors are located in the pituitary in this disorder, making the pituitary resistant to the inhibitory feedback inhibition of T_3.

Not all causes of hormone excess syndromes are due to hyperfunctioning glands or tumors. Leakage of thyroid hormone into the circulation following acute destruction of thyroid follicles, whether due to a virus (subacute thyroiditis) or autoimmune-mediated (post-partum thyroiditis), may produce thyrotoxicosis. In contrast to autonomous adenomas and hyperplasia, these disorders are transient.

Hormone excess states can occur by the administration of supraphysiologic doses of hormones, both as over-replacement of a primary hormone-deficient disorder and as treatment of a non-endocrine disorder. Cushing's syndrome due to pituitary or adrenal dysfunction is relatively rare, while iatrogenic Cushing's syndrome is exceedingly common due to the widespread use of corticosteroids as therapeutic agents. Rarely, the administration of a non-hormonal substance can have hormonal effects, as in the case of licorice ingestion producing a syndrome indistinguishable from primary hyperaldosteronism.

EVALUATION OF THE ENDOCRINE SYSTEM

Clinical evaluation

The evaluation of the endocrine patient, as with any medical patient, begins with the history and physical exam. Consistent with the systemic nature of endocrine disorders, all organ systems may be affected, some to a greater degree than others. Many signs and symptoms of hormone excess or deficiency, especially in long-standing or advanced cases, are readily apparent at the time of initial presentation. More often, the clinical presentation is subtle, and the use of laboratory testing is necessary to make a diagnosis. Finally, with the advent of sensitive hormone assays, the concept of subclinical disease, defined as abnormal hormone levels in the absence of clinical symptoms or signs, relies exclusively upon the laboratory to establish a diagnosis. The presenting signs and symptoms of many endocrine disorders are sufficiently vague as to include endocrine dysfunction in the differential diagnosis of many common problems, such as weakness, fatigue, weight loss or gain, hypertension, and diarrhea or constipation. Further, endocrine disorders may be secondary to other primary medical disorders that dominate the clinical presentation.

Laboratory evaluation

The laboratory is an integral part of the evaluation of the endocrine patient. Indeed, screening laboratory tests have identified some endocrine disorders before clinical symptoms arise. For example, the routine measurement of serum calcium has all but eliminated the presentation of the patient with advanced hyperparathyroidism, while identifying a large asymptomatic population, some of whom will never manifest clinical symptoms.

Assays are currently available to measure most, if not all, of the clinically important hormones. Immunoassays are the dominant techniques utilized. Hormones are measured by assessing the ability of the hormone in the sample to compete with a known amount of labeled hormone for binding to a hormone-specific antibody. The initial assays utilized radioactive labeling of hormones for quantification, but recently non-radioactive labels are being used that increase the sensitivity of the assay. The other technique utilized for measurement of hormones is high-performance liquid chromatography (HPLC).

Concentrations of free hormones can be measured or estimated by several methods. The most accurate method is by physically separating the free from the bound hormone, as is done by equilibrium dialysis, and measuring the free hormone directly. However, this is not routinely done due to the time-consuming, labor-intensive process required. Alternatively, measurement of the serum binding proteins will allow an estimate of free hormone. This may be done by direct measurement of the serum binding proteins or an indirect measurement by assessing the saturation of the binding proteins. The latter approach is used frequently in the determination of free thyroid hormone concentrations. Finally, measurement of urinary hormones or metabolites may give an assessment of overall hormone production, particularly with hormones whose plasma levels are subject to frequent variations, such as catecholamines and cortisol.

In hormone excess disorders where there is potentially more than one site of excess hormone secretion, plasma measurements of the specific hormone(s) do not define the site(s) of the excess production and are of limited utility. Measurement of hormone levels in samples obtained by cannulation of the venous outflow of a gland allows the determination of the site of hormone secretion. This is useful, for example, in evaluating adenoma vs. hyperplasia as the cause of hyperaldosteronism, and in differentiating between Cushing's disease (pituitary ACTH secre-

tion) and ectopic ACTH secretion. The use of imaging techniques such as magnetic resonance imaging (MRI), computerized tomography (CT), and specific isotope localization studies are often helpful in defining the tumor site.

Provocative testing

Provocative testing is a means to assess the ability of an endocrine gland to dynamically respond to regulatory factors. It is especially useful when the static plasma or urinary levels are borderline. In the case of suspected hypofunction or decreased hormonal reserve, an agent is administered to stimulate hormone production and release. The Cosyntropin© stimulation test measures the cortisol response to an intravenous administration of a synthetic fragment of ACTH. It is helpful in the evaluation of adrenal insufficiency, particularly when due to ACTH deficiency. Insulin-induced hypoglycemia, intravenous arginine infusion and exercise are provocative tests for growth hormone reserve. Gonadotropin-releasing hormone and thyrotropin-releasing hormone administration assess pituitary reserve for gonadotropin and thyrotropin secretion, respectively. In the case of excess hormone production, agents that suppress hormone secretion are employed. The oral glucose tolerance test is useful in suppressing growth hormone secretion in the evaluation of acromegaly. Variations on the dexamethasone suppression test are used to determine the etiology of Cushing's syndrome (pituitary-hypothalamic vs. adrenal adenoma, rarely ectopic ACTH production).

Mechanisms of hormone secretion, action, and response

Riccardo Vigneri, Antonino Belfiore

In multicellular organisms, cells need to communicate in order to regulate their function and development in a coordinated manner. Three major systems provide cell-to-cell communication: (1) *The endocrine system*, which signals via chemicals (hormones) secreted from one cell that are recognized by complementary structures (receptors) in another cell. This remote signaling by secreted molecules is relatively slow (seconds to minutes) because it requires time to transfer the hormone from the secreting cell to the bloodstream and then to the interstitial fluid surrounding the receiving cell. Target cells may be distributed in different organs and may respond differently to the same hormone according to the number and type of their receptors, and also according to their specific intracellular machinery. (2) *The nervous system*, which signals via electric impulses that move from one cell to the adjacent cell either by direct contact or by neurotransmitter intermediates. This signaling is more rapid (milliseconds to seconds) than the endocrine system signaling and is usually restricted to more limited areas or functions. (3) There is also another form of cell-to-cell communication, which is via plasma membrane-bound signaling molecules. This *contact-dependent signaling* is restricted to adjacent cells and is important in immune responses.

Cells use an enormous variety of interconnected chemicals in order to regulate the intensity and quality of the message for cell-to-cell communication.

One classification for the different forms of cell communication is based on the distance over which the signal must act (Fig. 2.1). The typical *endocrine signaling* is one in which cells (usually grouped in endocrine organs or glands) release hormones into the bloodstream that act on distant target cells, distributed in several target tissues and organs. A diffuse and complex response is elicited by this signal. In *paracrine signaling*, the target cell is close to the cell producing the hormone. Under these conditions, the hormone is bound (and possibly inactivated) only by cells that are adjacent to the cell sending the message: a

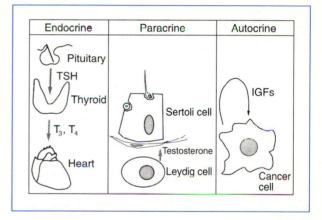

Figure 2.1 Endocrine, paracrine, and autocrine modes of intercellular communications. Hormones may be released in the bloodstream and interact with cells of distant target organs (endocrine). They may also interact with neighboring cells without entering the circulation (paracrine), or act directly on the same cell where they are produced (autocrine).

response limited to the local environment will follow. This situation is typical of neurotransmitters and locally produced growth factors. In *autocrine signaling*, cells respond to hormones that they themselves produce. Sometimes this situation occurs in pathological conditions. For instance, malignant cells may produce growth factors that are needed for their proliferation. When these factors happen to be active inside the same cell they are produced in (before being secreted) by interacting with and activating intracellular receptor proteins, the term *intracrine signaling* is used.

By these mechanisms, hormones regulate the activity of different cells, their metabolism, their specialized functions, and their proliferation. Complex feedback loops involving several hormones or hormones plus other chemicals (such as ions and metabolic substrates) coordinate the hormone-regulated metabolic and mitogenic responses of cells in a multicellular organism.

Feedback regulation of hormone secretion

The feedback control of hormone secretion is a typical feature of the endocrine system. This complex mechanism aims to maintain the body homeostasis when environmental conditions change. To obtain this response, serum hormone levels are finely controlled by both positive and negative stimuli. These stimuli include hormones – and also chemicals such as cations (e.g., calcium, potassium) and metabolites (e.g., glucose) conditions change. To obtain this response, serum hormone levels are finely controlled. The major regulation system involves two controllers, the hypothalamus and the pituitary gland. The hypothalamus regulates pituitary hormone secretion by either releasing or inhibiting factors produced by neuroendocrine cells. The pituitary hormones then regulate hormone secretion in the peripheral target endocrine glands and organs, and these in turn inhibit or stimulate back either the hypothalamus or the pituitary or both. For example, the hypothalamus produces corticotropin-releasing hormone (CRH), which stimulates the release of adrenocorticotropic hormone (ACTH) by the pituitary. ACTH stimulates the adrenals to produce cortisol which, in turn, inhibits both CRH and ACTH.

This mechanism maintains hormone concentration in serum and in the extracellular fluids within a physiological range that is appropriate for the specific situation. Changes in the feedback set-point may occur in physiological conditions. For instance, the gonadotropin set-point increases at puberty to allow for a change of sex steroid regulation. Furthermore, a feedback regulation may switch from negative to positive: this is the case of gonadotropin regulation by estrogens during the menstrual cycle. Estrogens normally elicit a negative feedback on gonadotropins, but at midcycle they stimulate the ovulatory surge of luteinizing hormone (LH) and follicle-stimulating hormone (FSH).

These regulatory loops imply that the measurement of both the effector and the stimulator hormone is often needed for a correct interpretation of the endocrine status. For instance, low serum thyrotropin (or thyroid-stimulating hormone, TSH), which may be caused by thyroid hormone excess but may also occur because of a pituitary deficit, requires thyroid hormone measurement for a correct interpretation. Similarly, circulating insulin levels should be interpreted in relation to plasma glucose levels. Finally, the knowledge of the feedback mechanism has allowed for the development of provocative tests that assess the ability of a gland to respond to stimuli, or to verify the integrity of the normal feedback loop.

Classification of hormones

Traditionally, hormones are classified according to their chemical structure and mechanism of action in two major classes. (1) *Peptide hormones* are water soluble, bind to receptors on the cell surface, and mainly induce rapid, metabolic responses. This group includes most hormones from the hypothalamus, the pituitary, and the gastrointestinal tract, including the pancreas. Catecholamines, although different in structure, are associated with this class of hormones. (2) The second class is the *lipid soluble hormones*, which are able to pass freely across the plasma membrane and interact with intracellular receptors. These hormones primarily induce slower, longer-acting changes in the pattern of a cell's gene expression. Steroids, vitamin D-related hormones, and thyroid hormones belong to this class.

PEPTIDE HORMONES AND GROWTH FACTORS

Biosynthesis of peptide hormones and growth factors

Peptide hormones and growth factors are secretory proteins. Their biosynthesis includes all of the steps followed by other proteins.

Gene transcription and post-transcriptional processes

Protein-encoding genes contain coding sequences (*exons*) interrupted by stretches of noncoding sequences (*introns*) (Fig. 2.2). The time and the extent of DNA transcription into RNA are finely regulated by regulatory regions that

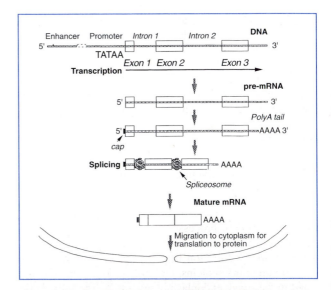

Figure 2.2 Gene structure and RNA transcription and processing. The structural DNA sequences of a gene include exons and introns. Regulatory sequences include the promoter and the TATAA box, which are close to the transcription site, and enhancer sequences that can be found at variable distances from the codification sequence. The primary transcript (pre-mRNA) includes both exon and intron sequences. The process of pre-mRNA maturation starts with a modification at the two ends of the transcript with the addition of a special nucleotide cap at the 5'-end and of a polyA tail at the 3'-end. Next, intronic sequences are removed by the splicing process with the aid of spliceosomes. Finally, the mature mRNA migrates to the cytoplasm for translation to protein.

include the promoter and enhancer regions. The *promoter* region is located upstream of the transcription start site and includes sequences that have binding sites for the complex enzyme RNA polymerase and for transcription factors (TFs). Often a sequence motif rich in adenine and thymidine (the TATAA box) is also present. *Enhancer* regions are regulatory elements that, like promoters, bind to transcription factors; however, in contrast with promoters, they can be located at a considerable distance from the start site, either upstream or downstream (Fig. 2.2).

The transcription start site is usually 20 to 30 base pairs downstream from the TATAA box. A number of basal transcription factors (TBP or TATAA box binding protein, TFIIA, TFIIB, and TFIIE) form a complex at the TATAA box level and facilitate the binding of RNA polymerase II. Together, these proteins form the transcription-initiation complex.

Gene transcription may be either positively or negatively regulated by a number of different cell signals, among which are hormones, cytokines, cell contact, temperature, and so on. Examples of regulated transcription factors are the nuclear receptors for steroid and thyroid hormones and the cAMP response element binder (CREB).

Once a gene has been transcribed into RNA, the primary transcript (for example, the RNA for the hormone precursor sequence) undergoes post-transcriptional processes. First, both ends of this primary transcript (pre-mRNA) are modified. At the 5'-end a special nucleotide structure (cap) is added that stabilizes the RNA and facilitates its translation into ribosomes. The 3'-end is also modified by the addition of a stretch of up to 200 adenines (polyA tail). The polyA tail may also serve to stabilize the RNA.

To form the mature mRNA, the sequences corresponding to introns must be eliminated. This process is called splicing and is a highly regulated and accurate process since the erroneous deletion of a single nucleotide would alter the reading frame. Once the introns have been removed, the mRNA transcript (mature RNA) can leave the nucleus and migrate into the cytoplasm through the nuclear pores.

mRNA translation and post-translational processing and modifications

Polypeptide hormones are synthesized as larger precursors that are then processed to smaller peptides. These smaller peptides in turn undergo modifications as glycosylation and/or sulfation to yield the final hormone. As they are secretory proteins, their mRNA needs to be translated in the rough endoplasmic reticulum. The same basic process is followed by membrane-bound hormone receptors with the difference that, at variance with hormones, receptor proteins are not secreted but inserted into the cell membrane (cell surface receptors) or released in the cell cytoplasm (nuclear receptors). mRNA translation starts at the AUG codon, downstream from the cap. A common feature of these mRNAs is a sequence coding for 15 to 25 amino acids (the leader sequence) that, as it is emerging by the ribosomes, is recognized by a signal recognition particle, a complex constituted by six proteins and a 7-S RNA, that stops the translation process. The process

resumes when the signal recognition sequence binds to a specific receptor on the cytoplasmic face of the endoplasmic reticular membrane. The forming peptide is then transported through a membrane channel to reach the cisternal space of the reticulum. Membrane-bound hormone receptors possess stop signals that block the peptide transport at a certain stage so that they remain inserted at the membrane level.

When synthesis is complete, the ribosomes detach from the reticular membrane and the membrane channel closes. Post-translational processing of the hormone precursor (*pre-pro-hormone*) begins in the reticulum with the clipping of the leader sequence by a peptidase. The resulting *pro-hormone* is then variously and specifically processed by proteases to form the mature and correctly folded hormone. For instance, insulin is obtained from pro-insulin by deletion of the connecting-peptide (C-peptide), which results in a correct folding of the insulin molecule (Fig. 2.3). Pro-hormone processing may also give rise to several hormonal peptides, as in the case of the ACTH precursor, POMC (pro-opiomelanocortin). This pro-hormone is cleaved into three sequences, corresponding respectively to ACTH, γ-lipotropin (γ-LPH), and γ-endorphin (Fig. 2.4). In some cases pro-hormone processing is tissue-specific. Pro-opiomelanocortin is processed to form ACTH in the anterior lobe and the related hor-

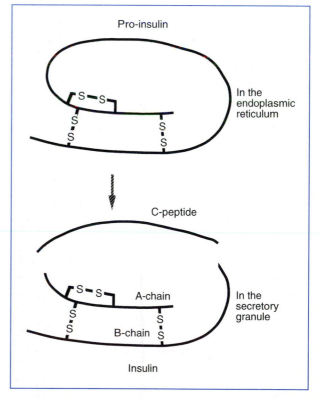

Figure 2.3 Structure of pro-insulin, insulin, and C-peptide. Insulin is obtained from pro-insulin by cleavage of the connecting-peptide (C-peptide) in the secretory granule.

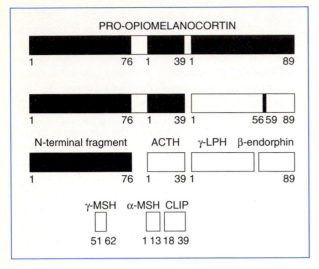

PRO-OPIOMELANOCORTIN

N-terminal fragment   ACTH   γ-LPH   β-endorphin

γ-MSH   α-MSH   CLIP

Figure 2.4 The processing of pro-opiomelanocortin. The cleavage of the ACTH precursor, pro-opiomelanocortin, gives rise to several biologically active peptides.

mone α-melanocyte-stimulating hormone (α-MSH) in the intermediate lobe of the pituitary. After processing, peptide hormones as well as membrane receptors are transported to the Golgi apparatus via transport vesicles that fuse with the Golgi cisternae. During this transport (and also in the Golgi apparatus), glycosylation, sulfation, acetylation, phosphorylation, disulfide bonding, and correct folding take place. Glycosylation is the major modification both for peptide hormones and their receptors. Since sugars add stability to the protein structure and shape its folding and surface, glycosylation has an important role in determining the specificity of receptor binding and in prolonging the plasma half-life of the hormone. Glycosylation more frequently occurs via nitrogen linkage (N-linked) at the level of asparagine residues and less frequently via oxygen linkage (O-linked) at the level of serine, threonine, or hydroxylysine. The initial glycosylation core is added in the endoplasmic reticulum, while complex carbohydrates are attached in the Golgi apparatus.

Synthesized hormones may be of different size and conformation. Their quaternary structure may result from the combination of separately synthesized subunits, as in the case of the glycoprotein hormones thyrotropin (TSH), LH, FSH, and human chorionic gonadotropin (hCG). Glycoprotein hormones share an identical α-subunit and specificity for each single hormone is obtained by the combination of the common α-subunit to another subunit (the β-subunit), which is different for either TSH, LH, FSH, or hCG.

Hormones may also be secreted in different variants: although coming from the same DNA sequence and the same mRNA, a variety of *isoforms*, due to the alternative splicing of mRNA or to the cleavage of the polypeptide chain, may be produced. For example, there are multiple copies of the GH (growth hormone) gene, but only one

gene is expressed in the pituitary and is responsible for GH production. However, many different forms of GH can be identified in human serum. The typical GH (22K molecular weight) represents approximately 80% of GH in serum. Other hormone variants are present, the most prominent being 20K-GH, lacking 14 of the 191-amino acid residues of the typical GH. In addition, GH may circulate both in the monomeric form as well as in the dimeric and polymeric forms (big-GH and big-big-GH), each having slightly different biological potency in relation to both affinity for the receptor and stability in the circulation.

Secretion, transport, and degradation of peptide hormones

Secretion of peptide hormones and growth factors

Following post-translational modifications within the Golgi apparatus, mature hormonal peptides are packaged into vesicles that lose water and form secretory granules where hormones are highly concentrated. Secretion occurs by fusing the vesicle membrane with the apical part of the cell membrane. The process of secretion may either be constitutive, as in the case of most growth factors, or regulated, as in the case of classical peptide hormones.

Regulatory stimuli include other hormones (e.g., pituitary tropins), changes in the plasma levels of electrolytes (e.g., sodium for antidiuretic hormone [ADH], calcium for parathyroid hormone [PTH]), glucose and amino acids (positive stimuli for insulin and negative for glucagon), and pH (for gastric hormones). Stimuli for secretion act on two distinct secretory pools: the first is rapidly released and is formed by the secretory granules accumulated inside the cell, and the second is slowly released and is formed by the hormone that is being synthesized by the cell.

Transport and binding proteins

Because they are water soluble, peptide hormones, in contrast to steroid or thyroid hormones, in most cases are not bound to transport proteins. Exceptions are GH, insulin-like growth factors I and II (IGFs), and vasopressin. As occurs with cytokines, GH may circulate bound to a truncated form of its own receptor.

There is a very complex network of binding proteins related to IGF-I and IGF-II. IGFs are partially homologous with insulin (the three peptides share approximately 50% of amino acid homology). However, their structure is more similar to proinsulin since they retain the C-peptide. IGFs are potent growth factors, and their action is dependent on the level of free IGF available for binding to the specific receptor. Whereas insulin circulates as free hormone, IGFs bind to at least six binding proteins (IGF-BP-1 to IGF-BP-6), which bind IGFs with an affinity higher than the affinity they have for their specific receptor. More than 90% of IGF-I and IGF-II circulate in a ternary complex formed by the hormone IGF-BP-3 and a glycoprotein called acid labile subunit. Both IGF-BP-3 and the acid labile subunit are mainly produced by the liver, and both are under the stimulatory regulation of GH. Less than 10% of the IGFs circulate bound to other IGF-BPs, and only small amounts circulate as free hormones. The main function of IGF-BPs is to regulate the local avail-ability of free hormones, and possibly also to regulate the IGFs' interaction with their receptor. In fact, at the level of the different tissues, IGFs are variously released by proteolytic digestion or phosphorylation of the IGF-BPs. Other functions of IGF-BP-3 include the extension of IGFs' half-life by the formation of a pool of slowly-released IGFs. Finally, IGF-BPs may have a more com-plex role since, under certain circumstances (e.g., wound healing), IGF-BP-1 and IGF-BP-3 may potentiate IGFs' effects.

Degradation of peptide hormones

Degradation of peptide hormones occurs either in the extracellular fluids (including the vascular compartment) or inside target cells. After their release in the blood-stream, hormones are degraded by circulating proteases. After receptor binding, the hormone degradation is car-ried out by enzymes present on the cell membrane and/or within the cells. When hormones bind to their receptors, the hormone/receptor complexes often aggregate into spe-cific areas ("coated pits") and then internalize inside the cell in the form of coated vesicles. Lysosomes, cell organelles carrying proteolytic enzymes, fuse with these vesicles. pH changes cause hormone dissociation from the receptor at this point. The hormone is then degraded by the lysosomal enzymes, while receptors, inserted in the vesicle membrane, are often recycled to the cell surface.

Non-glycosylated peptide hormones have a very short life in the circulation, in the range of minutes. Glycosylated peptide hormones have a longer half-life, up to hours.

CATECHOLAMINES

The catecholamines epinephrine, norepinephrine, and dopamine are amines derived from the amino acid tyrosine and characterized by a 3,4-dihydroxyphenyl (catechol) nucleus. Catecholamines are produced by nervous tissue cells. Neurons that synthesize and use epinephrine and norepinephrine for synaptic transmission are called adren-ergic neurons and constitute the sympathetic autonomous nervous system. Epinephrine and norepinephrine, in addi-tion to being neurotransmitters for the sympathetic ner-vous system, are also systemic hormones. Epinephrine is also produced and secreted by the adrenal medulla, an endocrine organ that is derived from precursor cells of the neural crest of the embryo but, unlike neurons, does not develop the typical nervous cell characteristics like axons and dendrites. In the adult subject, these adrenal medulla catecholamine-producing cells are located in the central part of the adrenal gland (adrenal medulla) and are sur-rounded by steroid-producing cells (adrenal cortex).

Different cells may express different receptors for the same catecholamine and, therefore, they may respond in a different way to the same type of stimulation (see below for receptors).

Catecholamine biosynthesis

The biosynthesis of catecholamines starts from the amino acid tyrosine, which is sequentially transformed to L-dopa, to dopamine, and then to norepinephrine and epinephrine (Fig. 2.5). Tyrosine hydroxylase, a cytosolic enzyme that converts tyrosine to L-dopa, is the rate limiting step in the biosynthetic pathway and is inhibited by the accumulation of end products. Dopamine β-hydroxylase (the enzyme converting dopamine to epinephrine) is localized inside the chromaffin granules where catecholamines are stored. Hence, dopamine must enter the granules in order to be converted into norepinephrine. Phenylethanolamine N-methyltransferase (PNMT), the enzyme that converts nor-epinephrine to epinephrine, is a cytosolic enzyme. Therefore, norepinephrine must leave the granule, be con-verted to epinephrine, and then be re-uptaken. PNMT is positively regulated by glucocorticoids, which play an important role in maintaining high levels of the enzyme in the adrenal medulla. Only the adrenal medulla and chro-maffin tissues have the enzyme necessary to convert nor-epinephrine to epinephrine. In all other catecholamine-producing tissues, the synthesis is arrested at the level of dopamine or norepinephrine because of a lack of either PNMT or both dopamine β-hydroxylase and PNMT.

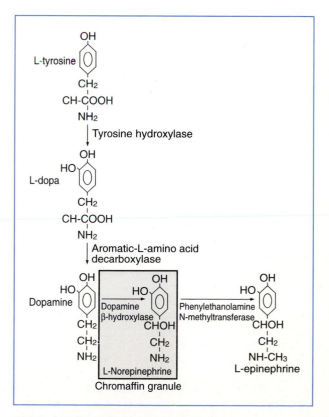

Figure 2.5 Biosynthesis of catecholamines.

Catecholamine storage, release, and inactivation

Within the cell, catecholamines are stored in vesicles called chromaffin granules. These granules contain high catecholamine concentrations (approximately 0.5 mmol/l) complexed to ATP and proteins called chromogranins. Ascorbic acid is also present at a high concentration and functions as an antioxidant. Catecholamine uptake into the granule is an active process; it is mediated by a stereospecific monoamine transporter coupled to an inwardly directed ATP-dependent proton pump, which uptakes catecholamines using a proton-catecholamine antiport system. This carrier is inhibited by reserpine. Storage of catecholamines is similar in the adrenal medulla and in sympathetic nerve endings. The level of catecholamines in granules is kept relatively constant by the feedback regulation of tyrosine hydroxylase activity and by re-uptake of released catecholamines.

The release of catecholamines involves a process of exocytosis: chromaffin granules first fuse with the plasma membrane and then the granule content is extruded in the extracellular space while the granule membrane is recycled. In the adrenal medulla, the release process is triggered by acetylcholine from the preganglionic sympathetic nerve endings and involves an increase of cytosolic calcium. This increase induces polymerization of a protein, synexin, that causes the aggregation of chromaffin granules, their transport to the cell surface, and their interaction with the cell membrane.

Once in the circulation, the catecholamine half-life is very short, at 1 to 2 minutes. The major routes of catecholamine inactivation are: (1) re-uptake by sympathetic nerves, (2) oxidative deamination, and (3) meta-O-methylation. Axonal re-uptake of norepinephrine is an important mechanism that is involved both in the maintenance of constant norepinephrine stores and in norepinephrine extracellular fluid clearance. Intraneural catabolism of catecholamines involves oxidative deamination by the enzyme monoamine oxidase, which is also present in extraneural tissues, although at low concentrations. Circulating catecholamines and their deaminated metabolites are mainly metabolized by catechol-O-methyltransferase, which is present in the liver and kidney but not in neurons. Catecholamines are also metabolized by monoamine oxidase in the liver. The catecholamine conjugation process, primarily sulfation, occurs in the liver and gut; it is also an important pathway for active catecholamine disposal.

RECEPTORS FOR PEPTIDE HORMONES AND CATECHOLAMINES (CELL SURFACE RECEPTORS)

Many hormones are not soluble in lipids and therefore cannot diffuse across the cell membrane to deliver their message to the cell. Large polypeptide hormones (insulin, GH, gonadotropins, etc.) and small charged hormones such as catecholamines must interact with specific cell surface proteins, the membrane receptors. These receptors are specialized proteins, present in target cells, and are able to recognize and bind the signaling molecule (the hormone). They initiate the cell response by causing conformational and chemical changes in the receptor molecule itself and in other cell molecules. Once the receptor has bound the hormone and has been modified by this binding, the changes occurring in its structure and/or function make it able to recruit, bind, and modify other molecules, thus initiating the cascade of chemical responses that will change the cell functions. Membrane receptors are glycosylated proteins that span the cell membrane and connect the cell external environment to the cell internal machinery. These receptors contain multiple functional domains that are specialized for the different functions of recognizing the ligand, binding it, and transferring its message inside the cell. These receptors have an NH$_2$-terminus that is usually *extracellular*, and it contains the hormone-binding site with a high affinity and specificity for a particular signaling substance (i.e., hormone, neurotransmitter). The *transmembrane* domain may be single or multiple and anchors the receptor to the membrane, and it may have a regulatory role in the hormone interaction and/or intracellular signal transduction. The *intracellular* domain transmits the signal produced by the hormone-receptor interaction to intracellular mediators that amplify the signal and generate multiple cell responses.

The binding of the hormone to its receptor initiates a sequence of actions that begin with changes in the receptor molecule itself, which then stimulates other molecules and induces changes in cell function. The effects of this hormone/receptor interaction are usually immediate (milliseconds to seconds) and, in most cases, of short term.

Abnormal receptor number, function, or regulation is the cause of diseases that are identified as *hormone resistance diseases* when the final hormone effects are decreased. When receptors are not completely absent or their function not completely impaired, an increase in the hormone concentration, up to a certain point, can overcome the receptor (functional) deficiency and cause normal, rather than excessive, hormone-induced responses. A typical example of this kind of disease is type II or non-insulin-dependent diabetes mellitus, the most common form of diabetes (over 90% of diabetic patients). The abnormal regulation of receptor function may, in contrast, result in excessive hormone effects even if the hormone concentration is normal or decreased. These diseases may cause hyperplasia or contribute to the malignant transformation of the affected cells. They may also result in increased hormone action, because the unregulated, ligand-independent and long-lasting receptor activation may mimic the condition of increased hormone secretion.

Membrane receptors are subdivided into different classes on the basis of the mechanisms they use for transducing the signal from the receptor molecule to other intracellular proteins. Receptors of the same class are related by evolution; they share structure homology and signal via similar pathways. The largest class of membrane receptors are the *G protein-linked receptors*: these receptors use trimeric G proteins to transduce the hormone signal to intracellular messengers (pituitary glyco-proteins, hypothalamic-releasing factors, PTH, etc.) (Tab. 2.1). Other membrane receptors are the *catalytic* receptors, which operate directly as enzymes. Most of these receptors use tyrosine phosphorylation and function like tyrosine protein kinases (insulin, IGF-I receptors, etc.). Receptors that do not have intrinsic tyrosine kinase activity but bind and activate intracellular tyrosine kinases (prolactin, GH, etc.) must be included in this group. Finally, the last class of hormone receptors are the *channel-linked receptors*. These receptors control the function of specific cell membrane ion channels and are present mainly in electrically excitable cells.

G protein-coupled receptors

In G protein-coupled membrane receptors, the interaction between the receptor molecule and the intracellular mediators located at the inner part of the cell membrane, such as enzymes (adenylate cyclase, phospholipase C) or ion channels, is mediated by a third protein, the *heterotrimeric G (guanine nucleotide)-binding regulatory protein (G proteins)*. The G protein-coupled receptors include approximately 150 members that are receptors, not only for peptide hormones but also for neurotransmitters, odorants, and photons.

Table 2.1 Principal G protein-coupled hormone receptors

Adenylyl cyclase-linked

Activation
  Corticotropin releasing hormone (CRH)
  Growth hormone releasing hormone (GHRH)
  Thyroid stimulating hormone (TSH)
  Luteinizing hormone (LH)
  Follicle stimulating hormone (FSH)
  Human chorionic gonadotropin (HCG)
  Adrenocorticotropic hormone (ACTH)
  Melanocyte stimulating hormone (MSH)
  Parathyroid hormone (PTH)
  Calcitonin
  Glucagon
  Beta-adrenergic (β1-β3)
  Dopamine D1
  Serotonin $5HT_3$

Inhibition
  Alpha-2-adrenergic (α2A-α2C)
  Somatostatin
  Opiate
  Angiotensin II
  Serotonin $5HT_1$

Guanylyl cyclase-linked
  Atrial natriuretic peptide

Phospholipase C and calcium flux-linked
  TSH releasing hormone (TRH)
  Gonadotropin releasing hormone (GnRH)
  Thyroid stimulating hormone (TSH)
  Alpha-1-adrenergic (α1A-α1D)
  Vasopressin V1
  Angiotensin II
  Serotonin $5HT_2$

General structure

These receptors are characterized by transmembrane α-helices with a serpentine structure spanning sevenfold the cell membrane ("seven-pass transmembrane glycoproteins"). This structure serves to anchor the receptor molecule to the membrane and to maintain the receptor conformation. The extracellular domain is variable in length in different receptors. While the serpentine portion is encoded by a single exon, the extracellular domain is encoded by a variable number of exons. The receptor interacts with G proteins primarily at the level of the third intracellular loop (which may have a variable length) and, in some cases, also at the level of the carboxy-terminal tail.

The specificity of ligand binding is determined by a pocket formed by the seven transmembrane domains in the case of small size agonists (epinephrine, nor-epinephrine, etc.), while it is determined by the extracellular domain in the case of the larger glycoprotein hormones (TSH, LH, FSH). The receptors for these glycoprotein hormones are characterized by a signal peptide and by a long extracellular domain with leucine-rich motifs. Further, these receptors have a strong homology (approximately 70%) in the serpentine domain and a lower homology (approximately 40%) in the extracellular domain. The serpentine domain has conserved amino acid residues that are important for ligand binding, receptor activation, and G protein binding.

In the absence of ligand binding, the receptor is in an inactive state. The interaction with the ligand releases the receptor from its inactive state and increases its affinity for the G proteins.

Heterotrimeric G proteins

Heterotrimeric G proteins consist of three protein subunits (α, β, and γ) that are interposed between the receptors and intracellular mediators (second messengers) and behave like an on-off switch. Hence, the function of the G proteins critically depends on their subunit structure. In the basal state (the "off" position), the three subunits are strongly noncovalently associated with GDP bound to the α-subunit; while the β- and γ-subunits, which are tightly bound to each other, anchor the G protein to the internal surface of the plasma membrane. The G proteins do not interact with the receptor in this condition (Fig. 2.6). When the receptor is activated by the ligand binding, its affinity for the G protein is increased. The interaction between the receptor and the G protein causes dissociation of guanosine diphosphate (GDP) and its substitution with guanosine triphosphate (GTP) (the "on" position). In this condition, the GTP-bound α-subunit dissociates from the other two subunits and binds and activates the second messenger (for instance, adenylate cyclase produces cAMP, a ubiquitous intracellular messenger in animal cells, from ATP). However, since the α-subunit has intrinsic GTPase activity, GTP is quickly hydrolyzed to GDP, making the α-subunit dissociate from the effector and reassociate with the $\beta\gamma$-complex. Although the α-subunit

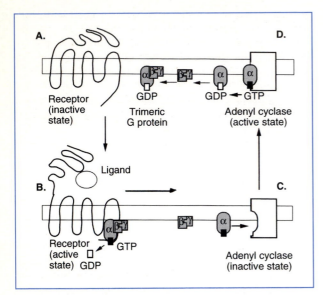

A. Receptor (inactive state) — Trimeric G protein — **D.** Adenyl cyclase (active state) — α β γ GDP — β γ — α GDP ← GTP — α

Ligand

B. Receptor (active state) GDP — α β γ GTP — β γ — α — **C.** Adenyl cyclase (inactive state)

Figure 2.6 Mechanism of activation and action of G protein-coupled membrane receptors. Heterotrimeric G proteins consist of three subunits (α, β, and γ) that are interposed between the receptors and intracellular mediators (second messengers) and behave like an on-off switch. (**A**) In "off" condition, the G proteins do not interact with the receptor. (**B**) Upon ligand binding, the receptor affinity for the trimeric G protein is increased. The interaction between the receptor and the G protein causes dissociation of GDP and its substitution with GTP (the "on" position). (**C**) In this condition the α-subunit dissociates from the other two subunits and binds and activates the second messenger. (**D**) The system returns to the "off" condition once GTP is hydrolyzed to GDP by intrinsic GTPase activity of the α-subunit.

has a crucial role in activating the receptor signaling pathway, in recent years specific actions for the βγ-complex have been recognized, including stimulation of phospholipase A2, Cβ2, and Cβ3, inhibition of K^+ channels, and stimulation of certain forms of adenylate cyclase (Tab. 2.2). Approximately 20 different species of G proteins are known. Since G proteins transduce the signals of approximately 150 receptors, each G protein couples to more than one receptor. G proteins that are involved in enzyme activation are called *stimulatory G proteins (Gs)*. G proteins that cause a decrease of the second messenger are called *inhibitory G proteins (Gi)*. The two types of G proteins have similar β- and γ-subunits but different α-subunits.

Second messengers

After ligand binding to the receptor, G proteins interact with and activate intracellular mediators to second messengers. The most important second messengers are cAMP and Ca^{++}, which are produced by the activation of adenylate cyclase and phospholipase C, respectively. The majority of hormone receptors belonging to this family activate both second messenger pathways.

Table 2.2 Characteristics and signaling functions of heterotrimeric G protein subunits

α-subunits	39-52 kDa (at least 16 genes) specific for each G protein binds to: - guanine nucleotides - receptors - βγ complex with intrinsic GTPase activity
β-subunits	35-36 kDa (at least 4 genes) binds strongly to the γ-subunit
γ-subunits	6-10 kDa (at least 8 genes) binds strongly to the β-subunit
βγ complex	binds to the α-subunit essential for activation of the α-subunit stimulates: - phospholipase A2 - phospholipase Cβ2 and Cβ3 - certain forms of adenylate cyclase inhibits: - activity of K^+ channels

Adenylate cyclase is a membrane-bound enzyme characterized by six membrane-spanning domains and by cytoplasmic N^- and COOH-terminal regions. Adenylate cyclase may be either stimulated or inhibited by G protein-coupled hormone receptors. In the first case, the α-subunit of the Gs-protein (αs) binds to and activates the enzyme. In the second case, the α-subunit (αi) is believed to bind GTP instead of GDP in the quiescent state and to directly inhibit the cyclase. In this condition, the β- and γ-subunits of the Gi protein, once free, bind the available adenylate cyclase, further preventing cyclase activation by Gs proteins.

Intracellular production of micromolar concentrations of cAMP activates specific cytoplasmic cAMP-dependent protein kinases that, in turn, activate or inactivate several enzymes by transferring a phosphate group to specific serine and threonine residues. cAMP-dependent protein-kinases are tetramers composed of two regulatory and two catalytic subunits. The regulatory regions have a consensus region termed the autoinhibitory domain that, in the absence of cAMP, interacts with the regulatory region and maintains the enzyme inactive. cAMP binding to the regulatory region causes the enzyme to dissociate into cAMP-bound regulatory subunits and free catalytic subunits, which are therefore fully active (Fig. 2.7). The cAMP produced is rapidly inactivated (it is degraded to 5'-AMP by phosphodiesterases), however, making its hormonal stimulation short-lasting.

The other dominant and ubiquitous intracellular second messenger is Ca^{++}. The concentration of free calcium in the cell cytosol is over 1000-fold lower than in the extracellular fluid and in the intracellular organelles where Ca^{++} is sequestered. This elevated chemical gradient is maintained by specialized Ca^{++} pumps that pump Ca^{++} out of the cytosol. Hormone/receptor interactions may cause the transient opening of the Ca^{++} channels. The activation of phospholipase C, in fact, induces the production of inositol 1,4,5-triphosphate and diacylglycerol from

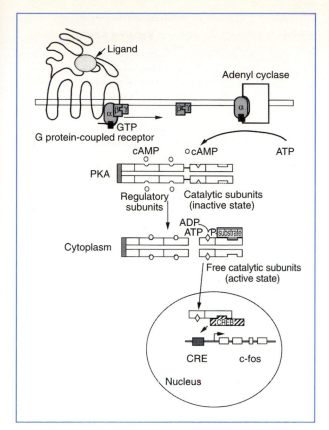

Figure 2.7 G protein-coupled membrane receptors signaling in the cytoplasm and in the nucleus. Ligand-activated membrane receptor activates adenylate cyclase via the α-subunit of the G protein. cAMP binds to the regulatory subunit of cytoplasmic protein kinase A (PKA), thus allowing the catalytic subunit to phosphorylate cytosolic substrates (enzymes). Free catalytic subunits enter the nucleus and activate the cAMP response element-binding protein (CREB), which binds to the consensus response element (CRE) on DNA.

plasma membrane phospholipids. These compounds increase the cytoplasmic content of Ca++ by inducing Ca++ influx from both intracellular organelles and from outside of the cell. The increase of cytoplasmic Ca++ activates the calcium/calmodulin-dependent kinases and the protein kinase C (calcium-dependent or C-kinase), which phosphorylates and activates other proteins, including the plasma membrane Na+/H+ exchanger. Ca++ also regulates the activity of adenylate cyclase, thus also affecting the cAMP pathway.

Hormonal regulation of gene transcription

In addition to activating or inactivating enzymatic processes, peptide hormone stimulation may also induce long-lasting responses, such as cell proliferation, by stimulating gene transcription. In fact, both protein kinase A and calcium/calmodulin-dependent kinases phosphorylate the transcription factor CREB (cAMP Response Element-Binding protein). When CREB is phosphorylated it activates the transcription of the c-fos proto-oncogene, which

in turn interacts with elements of the jun protein; this forms a heterodimer complex that is an important component of the AP-1 complex. The AP-1 complex is a transcription factor for a variety of hormones, receptors, and enzymes that binds to a cis-acting regulatory consensus sequence (Fig. 2.7).

Protein kinase C, via activation of the transcription factor SRF (serum response factor), is also able to activate c-fos.

Disorders associated with molecular abnormalities of G proteins and G protein-coupled receptors

A growing list of disorders has now being categorized as associated with either activating or inactivating mutations of G proteins or G protein-coupled receptors (Tab. 2.3). Since a single G protein may be involved in the function of several receptors, germline mutations of G proteins result in a generalized form of either hormone resistance (as in Albright's syndrome) or hyperfunction of more than one endocrine gland (as in McCune-Albright syndrome) (Tab. 2.3), depending on the type of G protein involved and on the type of mutation (activating or inhibiting). In contrast, when the mutation occurs in a hormone receptor

Table 2.3 Disorders caused by mutations of the G protein or G protein-coupled receptors

G protein

Somatic activating mutations
GH-producing cells	Acromegalia
Thyrocytes	Autonomously functioning thyroid adenomas

Germline activating mutations
Generalized	McCune-Albright syndrome

Germline inactivating mutations
Generalized	Albright syndrome

Receptors

Somatic activating mutations
TSH-R	Autonomously functioning thyroid adenomas
LH-R	Male pseudo-precocious puberty

Somatic inactivating mutations
V2 Vasopressin	Nephrogenic diabetes mellitus
GRF-R	Dwarfism

Germline activating mutations
TSH-R	Familial nonautoimmune hyperthyroidism
LH-R	Familial male pseudo-precocious puberty
Ca-R	Familial hypocalciuric hypercalcemia

Germline inactivating mutations
TSH-R	Familial resistance to TSH
ACTH-R	Familial resistance to ACTH
Ca-R	Familial hypoparathyroidism

gene, the abnormality (hyper- or hypofunction) involves a single endocrine gland. Generally speaking, mutations that occur in the serpentine portion of the receptor are activating, while those occurring in the hormone-binding domain are inactivating. When mutations are in the germinal line familial syndromes occur, and when they involve somatic cells, tumors often result.

In this context, one well-recognized example is found in the TSH receptor (TSH-R). Since the cDNA encoding for the TSH-R has been sequenced and its primary structure clarified, this receptor has been the object of intensive investigation. At low TSH concentrations, the TSH-R binds to Gs proteins and activates the adenylate cyclase, and consequently the cAMP pathway. At significantly higher concentrations, TSH induces TSH-R to bind a Gp protein (called Gp because it binds to phospholipase) that in turn activates phospholipase C and, subsequently, the inositol-1,4,5,triphosphate and diacylglycerol pathways. Several thyroid disorders have been described due to specific mutations of the TSH receptor. Germline mutations may be either activating or inactivating. Activating germline mutations have been described in the transmembrane segments and cause familial cases of congenital hyperthyroidism, which may range from subclinical to severe and may develop either in the newborn or in the adult. The thyroid is uniformly enlarged, but the goiter size is variable. Inactivating mutations of the TSH receptor involve the extracellular domain or the fourth transmembrane loop and cause decreased or abolished TSH binding, with consequent subclinical or overt hypothyroidism. Somatic activating mutations are scattered through the serpentine part of the receptor. They have a major role in the pathogenesis of autonomously hyperfunctioning thyroid nodules (15 to 80% of these nodules harbor activating TSH-R mutations) or, occasionally, in some nodules present in toxic multinodular goiter. Activating mutations of the TSH receptor have also been described in a subtype of thyroid carcinomas, which are therefore not responsive to TSH suppression with L-thyroxine (L-T$_4$) therapy and may show an aggressive phenotype.

Catalytic receptors

Catalytic receptors operate like enzymes that are normally in the quiescent, inactive form. When hormones bind to these receptors, their enzymatic kinase is activated and they phosphorylate the tyrosine residues, which are on the receptor protein itself (autophosphorylation) and also on a number of proteins recruited in the cell cytoplasm (heterophosphorylation). These receptors may be subdivided into two major groups: the tyrosine kinase receptors that have intrinsic enzymatic activity inside the molecule and receptors that do not have such intrinsic activity. The latter function as membrane-connecting proteins between the hormone and a specific cytoplasmic kinase bound to the receptor once it has been conformationally modified by the ligand binding.

Membrane receptors with intrinsic tyrosine kinase activity

Receptors of insulin, IGF-I, and most growth factors belong to the class of membrane receptors with intrinsic tyrosine kinase activity (Tab. 2.4). They are characterized by a cytoplasmic domain containing a ligand-dependent tyrosine kinase and an ATP-binding site. After ligand binding to the extracellular domain, the receptor undergoes conformational changes that activate the cytoplasmic tyrosine kinase domain. Receptor activation causes receptor autophosphorylation on tyrosine residues. Activation of the receptor tyrosine kinase is essential for subsequent signal transduction to intracellular mediators. Besides being activated by ligand binding, the kinase also undergoes regulation by regulatory domains that are located at the COOH-terminus or at the juxtamembrane region and regulate the accessibility and/or recognition of substrates.

At least two different mechanisms are used by receptor tyrosine kinases to transduce the hormonal signal. One mechanism is to directly bind and activate a variety of cytoplasmic enzymes containing sequences that are homologues to those present in the src oncogene, hence called src homology (SH2).

The second mechanism is to bind molecules containing SH2 domains that are devoid of enzymatic activity but that in turn bind to enzymes (docking or adapter proteins). Other important docking proteins are those in the insulin receptor substrate (IRS) family. These are named insulin receptor substrate proteins because they were first described as proteins phosphorylated by the insulin receptor, although it is known today that they bind to a variety of receptors. The biological response to these hormones and growth factors results from the different receptor affinity for each of these SH2 enzymes and adapters and thus also from the combination of the mediators activated, the relative amount of activation, and the duration of activation.

Membrane tyrosine kinases are receptors of key hor-

Table 2.4 Principal catalytic hormone and cytokine receptors

With intrinsic tyrosine kinase activity

Insulin
Insulin-like growth factor-I (IGF-I)
Epidermal growth factor (EGF)
Platelet-derived growth factor (PDGF)
Fibroblast growth factor (FGF)
Hepatocyte growth factor (HGF)
Colony-stimulating factor 1

With activation of cytoplasmic tyrosine kinases

Growth hormone (GH)
Prolactin (PRL)
Erythropoietin
Hematopoietin
Granulocyte monocyte-colony stimulating factor (GM-CSF)
Granulocyte-colony stimulating factor (G-CSF)
Interleukins (IL2-IL7)
Interferons

mones and factors involved in cell growth and differentiation. Because of this, somatic or germ line abnormalities of these receptors cause either constitutive activation or impaired function and have important consequences in a variety of disorders, including endocrine hypo- or hyperfunction, defects in development, and cancer.

Among the best-characterized receptor tyrosine kinases are the following: the insulin receptor and the homologue IGF-I receptor, the epidermal growth factor (EGF) receptor, the HGF (hepatocyte growth factor or scatter factor) receptor (called c-Met), and the GDNF (glial-derived nerve growth factor) receptor called Ret. We will use the *insulin and the IGF-I receptors* as examples of the function of this family of receptors.

The complexity of insulin receptor and IGF-I receptor signaling networks The insulin receptor (IR) and the insulin like growth factor I receptor (IGF-I-R) are tetrameric glycoproteins composed of two extracellular α- and two transmembrane β-subunits linked by disulfide bonds. Each α-subunit is approximately 130 kDa, both for the IR and the IGF-I-R, and is heavily glycosylated. The β-subunits are approximately 95 kDa for the IR and 110 kDa for the IGF-I-R and are glycosylated in their extracellular region (Fig. 2.8). Both receptors share more than 50% overall amino acid sequence homology and 84% homology in their tyrosine kinase domains. The IR mediates the biological responses of insulin and the IGF-I-R the effects of IGFs (IGF-I and IGF-II), which are potent regulators of cell metabolism and proliferation. Both insulin and IGF-I bind to the extracellular α-subunit of their own receptor, but they also cross-react (with a much lower affinity of approximately 1/100) with the cognate receptor. After ligand binding, a conformational change of the receptor occurs and causes activation of the receptor tyrosine kinase and autophosphorylation of the receptor intracellular β-subunit at the level of three tyrosine residues. This is followed by the binding to the receptor of several intracellular substrates, which function as either docking proteins that undergo phosphorylation (IRS proteins) or adapters (Shc, GRAB-2) for other intracellular proteins that have specific SH2 recognition domains. SH2 domain-containing proteins include, among others: phosphatidylinositol-3 kinase (PI3-kinase); the enzyme that catalyzes the phosphorylation of PI, PI-4-P and PI-4,5-P_2 on the inositol ring; two phosphotyrosine-phosphatases (SHPTP1 and SHPTP2); and the GTPase activating protein (GAP) of Ras. Ras is a GTP-binding protein with a GTPase activity that cycles from the active (GTP-bound) to the inactive (GDP-bound) form, as regulated by a GTPase activating protein (GAP). Ras activates a cascade of serine-threonine kinases, Raf-1 kinase (a cytoplasmic serine-kinase), MAP (microtubule-associated or mitogen-activated protein) kinase kinase (an enzyme able to activate the MAP kinase), MAP kinase, and the ribosomal pp90 S6 kinase. The Ras pathway is under the control of several growth factors and plays a crucial role in the regulation of cell proliferation.

A variety of mechanisms act as negative regulators of the receptor kinase activity. Among these are enzymes that phosphorylate the receptor on serine and/or threonine residues, tumor necrosis factor-α (TNF-α) and PC-1, a class II membrane glycoprotein with several enzymatic activities. All of these factors reduce the receptor tyrosine kinase activity and thus reduce hormone signaling.

Some important characteristics of the signaling pathways of these receptors are that they are pleiotropic (cause a variety of different biological effects); are redundant (different receptors may activate the same pathways); and they are variably regulated by the type and the number of pathways activated, the level of activation and

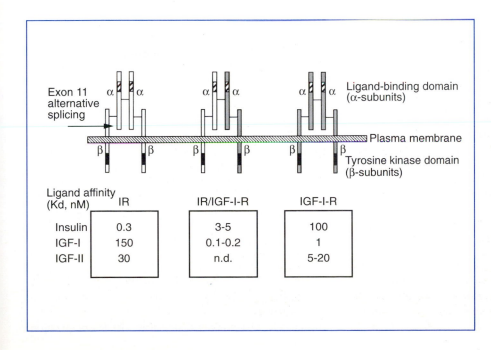

Ligand affinity (Kd, nM)	IR	IR/IGF-I-R	IGF-I-R
Insulin	0.3	3-5	100
IGF-I	150	0.1-0.2	1
IGF-II	30	n.d.	5-20

Figure 2.8 Structural schematics of different members of the insulin receptor family and respective affinities for the cognate ligands. Both the insulin receptor (IR) and its homologous IGF-I-receptor (IGF-I-R) are heterodimers. Hybrid receptors, IR/IGF-I-R – resulting from the assembly of one hemidimer α/β of IR and one hemidimer α/β from IGF-I-R – are present at various proportions in tissues expressing both the IR and the IGF-I-R. The human IR exists in two isoforms, which differ for 12 amino acids, resulting from the alternative splicing of exon 11 of the insulin receptor gene. At least three ligands bind to these receptors – insulin, insulin-like growth factor-I, and insulin-like growth factor-II – with the indicated affinities.

its duration. These mechanisms provide a very complex and very finely regulated cell response to hormone stimulation.

Receptor heterogeneity   Although the insulin receptor (IR) and the IGF-I receptor (IGF-I-R) are highly homologous receptors and activate similar intracellular signaling pathways, the IR stimulation by insulin is generally believed to predominantly elicit metabolic effect, while the IGF-I-R stimulation by IGF-I is believed to predominantly activate mitogenic effects. However, this concept is based on the fact that although the IR is expressed in virtually all tissues, high IR concentrations (more than 200000 receptors/cell) are present only in terminally differentiated, noncycling cells such as hepatocytes and adipocytes. Much lower IR levels and, conversely, higher IGF-I-R levels, are expressed by cells able to proliferate. This preferential expression of IRs on highly differentiated cells and IGF-I-R on cycling cells prevents cell proliferation from being activated by circulating insulin, and it allows for a fine modulation of cell proliferation control by the locally produced IGF-I, IGF-II, and IGF binding proteins. The complexity of the biological responses elicited by either insulin or IGFs is magnified by different IR isoforms, IR/IGF-R hybrids, and receptors with atypical binding characteristics.

As many other receptors, both IR and IGF-I-R may be present in cells in different *isoforms*. The human insulin receptor, for instance, is expressed in two natural isoforms differing by the absence (IR type A) or the presence (IR type B) of a 12-amino acid sequence corresponding to the C-terminal of the α-subunit. These two isoforms are produced by different splicing of the insulin receptor mRNA and have different functional characteristics: IR-A has a 2- to 3.5-fold higher ligand binding affinity and a dose-response curve for insulin-sensitive biological responses, including mitogenesis, shifted to the left compared to the IR-B isoform.

Another mechanism that adds complexity to the system is the formation of *IR/IGF-I R hybrids*. An IR dimer (α- and β-subunits) and an IGF-I-R dimer may combine to form IR/IGF-I-R hybrid receptors, which bind IGF-I with higher affinity than insulin (Fig. 2.8). Finally, cells may produce from the same gene and the same mRNA transcript a variety of receptors that are slightly different because during processing the protein is glycosylated in a different way before insertion into the plasma membrane. This mechanism will provide the formation of *atypical IRs and IGF-I Rs*. IRs with atypically high affinity for IGF-I and/or IGF-II have been described in certain tissues and cell lines, including human placenta, the nervous system, and human IM-9 lymphoblasts. Conversely, IGF-I-Rs with high affinity for insulin have been described in human breast cancer-cultivated MCF-7 cells.

Molecular abnormalities involving the insulin or the IGF-I signaling pathways, both at the receptorial or at the post-receptorial level, play an important role in human pathology. A very important example is the condition of insulin resistance (a condition of impaired insulin effect on glucose uptake and metabolism that mainly occurs at the level of muscle and adipose tissues) and that is associated with a variety of disorders, including non-insulin-dependent diabetes mellitus (NIDDM), obesity, functional ovarian hyperandrogenism, essential hypertension, dyslipidemia, and coronary artery disease. Insulin resistance is due to an impairment of insulin action because of defective receptorial or post-receptorial signaling of the insulin message.

Recent evidence suggests that the IGF-I-R has a key role in malignant cell transformation. In fact, IGF-I-R (1) is required for optimal growth both in vivo and in vitro, (2) is obligatory for the establishment and maintenance of the transformed phenotype and for tumorigenesis in several types of cells, and (3) protects cells from apoptosis. Because of these mechanisms, the IGF-I-R and its activation may become a target of choice for future therapeutic approaches to cancer.

Receptors that signal via nonreceptorial cytoplasmic tyrosine kinases

A family of receptors that signal via nonreceptorial cytoplasmic tyrosine kinases includes transmembrane receptors with no intrinsic tyrosine kinase activity but that associate with specific cytoplasmic tyrosine kinases to form a signaling complex. This family includes receptors for GH, prolactin, erythropoietin, granulocyte-macrophage colony-stimulating factor (GM-CSF), interferons, and other interleukins. All of these receptors are type I glycoproteins with an extracellular N-terminus and a single transmembrane domain. Most of these receptors are present in the serum as a truncated extracellular portion of the receptor (obtained by alternative splicing of the receptor gene) that serves as a hormone-binding protein. Although the intracellular domain is variable in length (from the 54 amino acids of the GM-CSF-R to the 568 amino acids of the IL-4-R), they share similar functions and two conserved regions, which are both located close to the transmembrane domain and are important for the proliferative response.

Although the ligands for this class of receptors do not share any homology in their primary structure (except for GH and prolactin), they have a similar tertiary structure composed of four antiparallel α helices. Ligand binding produces receptor dimerization and recruitment of the specific cytoplasmic tyrosine kinase and its activation. One of the best characterized receptor in this family is the *GH receptor*, which we will use as an example of the function of these receptors. The human GH-R is a single-chain polypeptide composed of an extracellular domain of 247 amino acids, a transmembrane domain of 24 amino acids, and an intracellular domain of 349 amino acids. The extracellular portion of the receptor is heavily glycosylated at asparagine residues. The extracellular domain of the GH-R contains three disulfide loops, the first of which is crucial for GH binding. One molecule of a monomeric form of GH first binds to one GH-R molecule and then binds, via a second binding site, to a second GH-R molecule. GH binding thus causes GH-R dimerization and activation. The activated GH-receptor complex recruits the cytoplasmic tyrosine kinase JAK2, a 130 kDa protein that belongs to the Janus kinase (JAK) family, which includes other tyrosine kinases such as JAK1 and tyk2. The association of the dimerized GH receptor with JAK2 will result in the tyrosine phosphorylation of both the receptor and JAK2. This will initiate the phosphorylation cascade that leads to the activation of MAP kinase, to the phosphorylation of the ribosomal protein S6 kinase, and to the expression of the early response genes, c-jun and c-fos.

As for other receptors of this family, a fragment of the extracellular domain is found in the serum and functions as GH-binding protein. In fact, approximately 50% of GH circulates associated with this binding protein. The measurement of the soluble GH receptor is of clinical value, as it allows for the identification of patients with one form of Laron dwarfism (short stature due to the lack of IGF-I that is not produced because the GH signal cannot be received by target cells in the absence of a functioning GH receptor). In these patients, characterized by a defective GH receptor due to deletions or mutations, GH binding activity is not present in the serum.

Channel-linked receptors

Channel-linked receptors are mainly involved in rapid synaptic signaling. Ion channels are membrane-spanning protein tunnels in which a small conformational change makes them change from closed to open, allowing the passage of millions of ions each second. Ion channels are classified according to the ion they allow to pass and may be activated by extracellular ligands, changes in the transmembrane potential, or intracellular mediators (Tab. 2.5).

Most ion channels are composed of subunits, each containing six transmembrane domains. However, the sodium and calcium channels are formed by a single subunit containing four repeats of the six transmembrane-spanning motifs.

The channel function can be regulated by receptors that are activated by neurotransmitters. Unlike a water-soluble hormone, the neurotransmitter acts upon a very close cell, a distance that is a fraction of a micrometer. The electrical stimulation of the pre-synaptic cell causes the release of the neurotransmitter, which then binds to the receptor on the post-synaptic cell. This is the receptor linked to an ion channel and, by changing its conformation, allows specific ions to cross the membrane and modify the membrane electrical potential. In this way, an electrical message (from the pre-synaptic cell) is first converted into a chemical message that may be finely regulated (neurotransmitter, synaptic level) and then transformed again into an electrical message (post-synaptic cell).

Ligand-activated ion channels include the acetylcholine receptor, the glutamate and gamma-aminobutyric acid (GABA) receptors, and the type I purinergic receptor. The muscarinic acetylcholine receptor is a hetero-multidimer consisting of two potassium ion channel subunits, GIRK1 and GIRK4, that is activated by binding the $\beta\gamma$-complex of the G protein. These channels, which have been only recently described, are called inwardly rectifying potassium-selective channels (Kir) to indicate that they are more efficient in conducting current inward than outward. However, the biologically important response is to allow an efflux of K^+ in response to acetylcholine.

Table 2.5 Principal hormone/neurotransmitter-gated ionic channels

Ligand-activated	
	Nicotinic acetylcholine (sodium)
	GABA (chloride)
	Bradykinin (potassium)
G protein-activated	
	Muscarinic 2, acetylcholine (potassium)
	Purinergic 1, adenosine (potassium)

Receptors of catecholamines

Receptors for catecholamines (adrenergic receptors) are members of the superfamily of G protein-linked receptors. Adrenergic receptors can be classified in two classes (α and β receptors) on the basis of their binding affinity for different agonists. Each class can be subdivided into two subclasses (α1 and α2; β1 and β2) on the basis of their pharmacological properties. The α1 receptors are the post-synaptic receptors on smooth muscle cells and mostly mediate vasoconstriction. The α2 receptors are located on pre-synaptic adrenergic neurons, cholinergic neurons, and blood vessels. These receptors also mediate vasoconstriction. The β receptors mediate cardiac stimulation, lipolysis (β1 receptors), and bronchodilatation, vasodilatation, and noradrenaline release from sympathetic neurons (β2 receptors). Recently, an additional β receptor (β3) has been identified, located in the brown fat adipocytes that provide energy expenditure for thermogenesis. This β3 receptor has raised much interest for possible application in the therapy of obesity.

Dopamine receptors are also subgrouped into D1 and D2 receptors on the basis of their ability to activate or inhibit adenylate cyclase and cAMP accumulation.

The tissue response to catecholamine stimulation depends on the relative expression of the different receptors in that specific tissue. Many physiologic (age, temperature) and pathologic states can contribute to the varying expression of catecholamine receptors in tissues and, thus, to the heterogeneity of the biological response to catecholamines.

At variance with receptors for pituitary glycoprotein, the extracellular domain of catecholamine receptors is much shorter and does not contain the hormone binding sites. Catecholamines, in fact, bind to the membrane-spanning domains of the receptor. However, as for other receptors in this family, ligand binding induces a conformational change, thus allowing the receptor to bind and activate a G protein. The size and structure of the third intracellular domain and the C-terminus domain are important to determine the specificity of the binding to individual G proteins. Each type of receptor is therefore preferentially coupled to a different G protein and activates a different intracellular pathway. Beta receptors via Gαs stimulate the adenylate cyclase and lead to cAMP accumulation, while α2 receptors, by coupling the Gαi, inhibit adenylate cyclase and decrease intracellular cAMP levels. Alpha1 receptors couple to Gαq and stimulate phospholipase C activating – throughout the phosphatidyl inositol cascade – the protein C kinase.

General mechanisms of hormone/receptor interaction

Spare receptors

Most hormones circulate in the serum at very low concentrations, ranging from 10^{-12} to 10^{-8} molar. This implies that the receptor must be able to recognize minute amounts of hormone with high specificity and bind them with high affinity. Membrane receptors may be uniformly distributed in the cell membrane but may also form clusters in limited regions, as happens in polarized cells. Receptor clustering positively affects hormone binding and, in some cases, clustering may be determined by hormone binding. In general, hormonal effects are linearly correlated with the extent of receptor occupancy. This is particularly true for very proximal effects (e.g., cAMP accumulation), whereas distal biological responses (e.g., insulin-induced glucose transport in adipocytes) may be maximally stimulated even when only a small fraction of cell receptors are activated. This phenomenon has led to the concept of spare receptors. However, it is important to point out that the proportion of receptors required to be activated to achieve a maximal biological response is variable in the different systems (e.g., from 1% for LH receptors in Leydig cells to almost 100% for angiotensin II receptors in adrenals). Furthermore, the fraction of activated receptors necessary to reach the maximal effect may also be different for the diverse effects elicited by a hormone in a single cell type (e.g., maximal glucose transport in adipocytes occur at 2% receptor occupancy whereas protein synthesis requires a higher proportion of receptor activation).

Since the velocity of the hormone/receptor interaction is determined by the concentration of both components (e.g., the hormone and the receptor), spare receptors determine a more rapid and a higher receptor occupancy at low hormone concentration. In a system with no spare receptors, a decrease in the number of receptors determines a parallel decrease in the biological response (Fig. 2.9); while in a system with many spare receptors, a decrease in the number of receptors determines only a small decrease in the biological response. Spare receptors may thus play an important role in pathophysiological states that are associated with a decrease in hormone receptors.

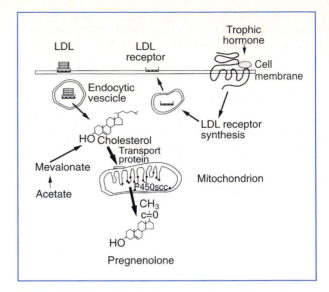

Figure 2.9 Biosynthesis of pregnenolone. The cyclopentanoperhydrophenatrene ring structure of steroid hormones is derived by modifications of the basic structure of cholesterol. Cholesterol can be provided by the diet or synthesized starting from acetate. Circulating LDL-cholesterol is taken up by the cells after binding to LDL receptors. The first step for conversion of cholesterol to steroids involves removal of the cholesterol side chain by cytochrome P450scc, which is located inside the mitochondria. This step produces pregnenolone, which is the common precursor for all steroids. Flow-back to mitochondrion of substrates is required in some subsequent steps of steroid biosynthesis.

Mechanisms of regulation of hormonal action at the receptorial level

Since most differentiated cells are specialized for one major function, they contain specific receptors that allow them to respond to hormones that regulate that particular function. A single hormone, on the other hand, may have different effects in different cells. This diversity is obtained either via receptors for the same hormone that have structural differences in different cells or via receptors that are identical but produce a different series of changes in different cells because of their specific intracellular signaling machinery.

Cells possess different mechanisms aimed at protecting against an excessive hormonal stimulation induced by continuous or repeated exposure to the specific ligand. Some of these mechanisms operate at the receptor level, others are active on post-receptor substrates. These mechanisms are part of the so-called "homologous desensitization". Receptors may also be regulated, either positively or negatively, by different ligands, a process called heterologous regulation or desensitization.

Homologous receptor desensitization and down-regulation In many systems, excessive exposure to the specific ligand induces an increase in the internalization and degradation rates of the receptor protein, ultimately leading to a down-regulation of the receptor number on the cell surface. This is a slow process, however, and it is not linearly related to the increase in hormone stimulation since even small increases of hormone concentration may significantly affect receptor number and, consequently, cell responsiveness.

Other, more rapid ligand-induced mechanisms that cause receptor modifications that impair receptor function may also be active. One example is the receptor phosphorylation at the level of serine and threonine residues in tyrosine kinase receptors. Receptor phosphorylation at serine and threonine residues (by still uncharacterized receptor-associated kinases) negatively regulate these receptors (e.g., the insulin receptor) by impairing their ability to phosphorylate other substrates in tyrosine residues. Another mechanism, active in G protein-linked receptors, is the uncoupling of the receptor and adenylate cyclase. At least six members of G protein-coupled receptor kinases are known and well-studied in the regulation of adrenergic receptors. These kinases translocate from the cytoplasm to the cell membrane upon ligand binding to the receptor and are activated by the βγ-complex of heterotrimeric G proteins. These kinases induce uncoupling of the receptor from adenylate cyclase activation by phosphorylating amino acid residues at the third intracellular loop of the receptor.

Heterologous receptor regulation Heterologous desensitization may result from receptor phosphorylation by heterologous activation of the protein kinase C or cAMP-dependent kinases. Increased phosphodiesterase activity which are caused by other, functionally connected hormones may also decrease the level of cAMP. The heterologous regulation, however, may also increase cell responsiveness to hormones. A number of examples exists of this positive heterologous receptor regulation. For example, estrogens increase the number of Oxytocin receptors in the uterus and of IGF-I receptors in the mammary gland. FSH induces an increase of LH receptors in the ovary.

STEROID AND THYROID HORMONES

Steroid and thyroid hormones are a class of signaling molecules that are water-insoluble and that are made soluble for transport in the blood by binding to specific carrier proteins. Hence, only a very small percentage of these hormones circulates in the free form. This free form is important, however, because it is responsible for the biological effects of these hormones. The lipid-soluble hormones can easily cross the cell plasma membrane and bind to specific receptors inside the target cell. These receptors are also called nuclear receptors because they are able to translocate inside the cell nucleus and bind to DNA. As soon as free hormone molecules enter target cells, their plasma (extracellular fluid) concentration decreases. At this point other hormone molecules are released from their carrier proteins, providing further biologically active signaling molecules and keeping the bound/free hormone concentration ratio constant. Once inside the target cell and bound to specific receptors, these hormones usually regulate long-lasting DNA functions.

Because of these mechanisms, that is, a longer persistence in the blood (extracellular) compartment with a half-life of hours to days and a longer intracellular mechanism of action, both steroid and thyroid hormones cause longer-lasting responses in target cells than peptide hormones.

Steroid hormones

Biosynthesis

Steroid hormones are members of a large family characterized by a basic common structure: the cyclopentanoperhydrophenatrene ring structure originating from cholesterol. Steroid hormones are synthesized in the adrenal cortex, the ovary, and the testis by specific enzymes that variously modify the basic structure of cholesterol. However, functional modifications of steroids synthesized in the endocrine glands occur inside the cells of several peripheral tissues (e.g., conversion from testosterone to dihydrotestosterone). Vitamin D is a signaling molecule that regulates mineral metabolism and whose basic steroid nucleus (the pro-hormone form) may be either synthesized or directly derived from the diet (and for this reason is regarded both as a "hormone" and as a "vitamin"); it is converted to active forms by hydroxylations that take place in the liver and the kidney.

Cholesterol is provided by the diet (70%) or can also be synthesized by the steroidogenic cells themselves, starting from acetyl coenzyme A (30%). Circulating LDL-cholesterol is taken up by the cells after binding to specific LDL receptors and internalized in coated pits by receptor-mediated endocytosis. LDL receptors are very numerous in steroidogenic cells. Their number is increased by stimulation with the specific tropic pituitary hormone, and they are down-regulated by LDL uptake. LDL uptake also down-regulates cholesterol synthesis by inhibiting the major synthesizing enzyme, hydroxymethylglutaryl-coenzyme A (HMG-CoA).

The conversion of cholesterol to steroids involves mono-oxygenations at different sites by cytochrome P450 enzymes. These enzymes have a substrate binding site and a heme-iron catalytic site. As a general scheme, cytochromes P450 bind the substrate and catalyze oxidation in the presence of molecular O_2 and of an electron provider system (NADPH, as a source of electrons) and the proteins, adrenoxin reductase and adrenoxin, as electron shuttles.

In all organs, the initial step in steroid biosynthesis is the cleavage of the side chain of cholesterol. This step is catalyzed by cytochrome P450scc, which is located inside the mitochondria and is rate limiting, and makes it necessary for cholesterol to have access to the inner side of mitochondria. This step is regulated by carrier proteins and may be important for steroid biosynthesis regulation. Removal of the cholesterol side chain produces pregnenolone, which is the common precursor for all steroids (except vitamin D) and moves out of the mitochondria into the cytosol, where it is variably modified in the different organs. Different steroids have specialized actions on target tissues and are subdivided into 6 major classes: *androgens, estrogens, progestins* (the three classes of sex steroid hormones), *glucocorticoids* (that have, among others, glucose-regulating properties), *mineralocorticoids* (regulating Na^+ and K^+ balance), and *vitamin D* (regulating Ca and P metabolism). Each class is primarily characterized by a specific molecular conformation, a consequence of the action of enzymes present in the different cells and involved in steroid biosynthesis. The steroid conformation causes the interaction with specific receptors in target cells. However, a certain degree of overlap may occur when a certain hormone is present at a high concentration (i.e., mineralocorticoid-like effects of glucocorticoids or androgen effects of progestins) and is due to the interaction with receptors for another class of steroids.

In the *adrenal cortex fasciculata and reticularis zone* cells, pregnenolone is first converted to 17OH-pregnenolone by cytochrome $P450_{17}$ and then to 17OH-progesterone by 3β-hydroxysteroid dehydrogenase-$\Delta^{4,5}$-isomerase, and to 11-deoxycortisol by cytochrome $P450_{21}$. 11-Deoxycortisol moves back into the mitochondria, where it is finally converted to cortisol, the most active glucocorticoid, by cytochrome $P450_{11\beta}$.

In the *adrenal cortex glomerulosa zone* cells, which lack cytochrome $P450_{17}$, pregnenolone is first converted to progesterone by 3β-hydroxysteroid dehydrogenase-$\Delta^{4,5}$-isomerase and then to 11-deoxycorticosterone by cytochrome $P450_{21}$. 11-Deoxycorticosterone then moves into the mitochondria where it is converted to aldosterone, the most active mineralocorticoid, by cytochrome $P450_{CMO}$, an enzyme that is specific of the adrenal glomerulosa cells.

In the *testis* and the *ovary*, 17OH-pregnenolone and 17OH-progesterone are also converted to dehydroepiandrosterone and to androstenedione, respectively, by removal of the C20,21 side chain by C17,20-lyase, an activity of the cytochrome $P450_{17}$. These weak androgens are produced by the Leydig cells and the theca cells of the ovary, and also by the adrenal cortex cells (reticularis and fasciculata zones). However, in the testicular Leydig cells and in the ovarian theca cells, which lack cytochrome $P450_{21}$ and cytochrome $P450_{11\beta}$ and the related synthesizing pathways, this pathway is predominant. In the Leydig cells, androstenedione is then converted to the final product testosterone. Testosterone is converted to dihydrotestosterone, the most potent androgen, inside target cells by the enzyme 5α-reductase.

Production of the two main steroids of the *ovary*, progesterone and 17β-estradiol, requires the interplay of two specialized sets of cells with different enzymatic sets: the theca cells that produce androgens and the granulosa cells that produce estrogens and progestins. Progesterone is the primary final product of cholesterol modifications in granulosa cells, as these cells have low levels of cytochrome $P450_{17}$ and C17,20-lyase and, like testis Leydig cells, lack cytochromes $P450_{21}$ and $P450_{11\beta}$. However, they have high levels of aromatase, an enzyme that converts androstenedione and testosterone to estrone and 17β-estradiol, respectively. As androstenedione is provided to the granulosa cells by diffusion from the adjacent theca cells, where it is the principal end product, the other major product of granulosa cells are the estrogens.

All the key steps of steroid hormones biosynthesis are positively regulated by the specific tropic pituitary hormones by stimulation of the synthesis of the specific enzymes involved. In addition, tropic hormones up-regulate receptors for peptide growth factors in the target cells, as well as the autocrine production of peptide growth factors that are involved in hypertrophy and hyperplasia of peripheral endocrine gland target cells.

Spontaneous rhythms of hormone secretion

Hormone secretion is not a continuous but rather an intermittent function, which causes the hormone concentration in serum to fluctuate according to complex biological rhythms. Most hormones are secreted in a pulsatile fashion that reflects the alternating prevalence of either releasing or inhibitory factors. For instance, hypothalamic GnRH is released in the pituitary portal system in an ultradian (shorter than 24 hours) pattern, which involves episodic secretory bursts. These bursts induce a pulsatile LH and FSH secretion with a periodicity of approximately 90 minutes that causes fluctuations in the serum levels of the two hormones. The hypothalamic pulse generator is modulated by the feedback effect of sex steroid hormones, primarily estradiol, that cross the blood-brain barrier and reach the hypothalamus. This feedback, usually negative, modulates the frequency and amplitude of GnRH pulses. At the same time at the pituitary level, sex steroids reduce the sensitivity of the gonadotrophs to hypothalamic GnRH. The continued effect of these multiple influences causes the *infradian* (longer than 24-hour) rhythmicity, in this case a 28-day rhythm of gonadotropin. The physiologic role of the pulsatile secretion of hormones is not entirely understood, although it is known that continuous hormone stimulation causes refractoriness and, therefore, intermittent stimulation is required to ensure optimal responsivity. The function of pulse generator is not exclusive to the hypothalamus: isolated pituitary or gonadal glands may also maintain autonomous episodic secretion, thus suggesting that episodic hormone secretion is a common mechanism that is in some way synchronized by a more complex system.

Hormone secretion may follow more than one rhythm at the same time. The *ultradian* (shorter than 24-hour) pulsatility pattern, for instance, may be combined with a *circadian* rhythm. The circadian rhythm (24-hour) is generated by an endogenous clock that resides in the CNS and is synchronized by dark-light shifts. In the absence of dark-light synchronization (e.g., complete blindness), this rhythm may have large variations (± 3 hours). The pineal gland is believed to be the mediator transforming a physical stimulation (dark-light) into an endocrine rhythm, at least for gonadotropins. Noradrenergic signals, which are higher at night, stimulate the pineal gland to secrete melatonin, which is released in the bloodstream and then acts on the pituitary and the CNS.

The best-known circadian rhythm is that of ACTH and cortisol, peaking at 4-6 a.m. and at 6-9 a.m., respectively. Both ACTH and cortisol are also secreted in pulses occurring every 30 to 120 minutes, but the frequency and amplitude of these pulses are increased in the morning. The mechanism leading to circadian rhythms involves not only an inherent rhythmicity in CRH activity secretion and the light/dark cycle, but also the inherent rhythmicity in gland activity (i.e., the adrenals). The CNS activity is mainly affected by the sleep-wake cycle, and most pituitary hormones are secreted in relation to the different sleep stages. For example, the main secretory bursts of ACTH occurs after 6 to 8 hours of sleep, and the cortisol peak follows, occurring after awakening. Provided that innervation is preserved, adrenals secrete cortisol with some circadian periodicity. Adrenal innervation may therefore modulate the sensitivity of adrenals to ACTH. The circadian rhythm of cortisol is not immediately affected by conditions such as sleep deprivation or prolonged bed rest. However, many stressful events, such as trauma, surgery, hypoglycemia, and exercise can temporarily affect cortisol secretion via signals of the CNS, resulting in either increased or reduced CRH production and, consequently, in a shift of the circadian rhythm of cortisol.

Secretion and production rates of steroid hormones

The biological effect of steroids at the target tissue level depends on several factors including: (1) the secretion rate of the steroid; (2) the hormone metabolic clearance; (3) the hormone conversion to a more active form; (4) the amount of steroid hormone in a biologically available form (i.e., not bound to plasma binding proteins); and (5) the transit time in the capillary bed and the permeability of the capillary bed in a specific organ, which can affect both hormone/protein dissociation and hormone diffusion to single cells.

The metabolic clearance rate of a steroid is an important parameter. Hormones with a high clearance rate in a certain organ may have a biological effectiveness lower than that predicted on the basis of the receptor's affinity because the hormone will be locally available only for a short time for receptor binding. Conversely, hormones with a low metabolic clearance rate will have high biological effectiveness. Another mechanism that significantly affects hormone biologic potency is the peripheral metabolic conversion of a steroid into another steroid with a different biological potency. We therefore must make a distinction between the amount of a steroid that is secreted by an endocrine tissue (*secretion rate*) and the total amount of the steroid that is produced. The latter includes, in addition to the secreted steroid, the aliquot produced by peripheral conversion from precursors (*production rate*). This mechanism applies to many steroid hormones, androgens, estrogens, progestins, and vitamin D. In addition, it also applies to thyroid hormones and some peptide hormones. Many examples can be mentioned in this regard. For instance, the intrinsic androgenic effect of adrenal androgens dehydroepiandrosterone (DHEA) and DHEA-sulfate (DHEAS) is low, but they can be convert-

ed into testosterone by peripheral tissues with a clear increase in biological potency. Furthermore, inside target cells, testosterone can be converted to 5α-dihydrotestosterone, a more potent androgen.

In the female, peripheral conversion of the androgen androstenedione to estrone contributes to the overall production of estrogens. This mechanism is responsible for only a small proportion of estrogen production in premenopausal women, but it becomes the major source of estrogens in postmenopausal women. Thyroid hormones are another example. In euthyroid subjects only 20% of circulating triiodothyronine (T_3) is directly secreted by the thyroid, while approximately 80% is produced by peripheral conversion of circulating thyroxine (T_4), which thus behaves as a T_3 precursor.

Transport and catabolism

Steroid hormones circulate primarily bound to carrier proteins produced by the liver and are inactive when bound to these proteins. Steroids bind to specific carrier proteins with high affinity and to serum albumin with a much lower affinity. Because of the large amount of albumin present in the extracellular fluids, steroid/albumin binding, although having a low affinity, has a large capacity. Three main steroid-specific carrier proteins are known: corticosteroid-binding globulin (CBG), sex hormone-binding globulin (SHBG), and vitamin D-binding globulin (DBG).

- *CBG* is a 59 000 m.w. glycoprotein that binds cortisol and progesterone with high affinity but low capacity. Since in nonpregnant women progesterone levels are much lower than cortisol levels, CBG is mainly occupied by cortisol. In normal conditions cortisol circulates as 90 to 95% protein-bound, mostly to CBG and far less so to albumin. Whenever the concentration of cortisol exceeds the capacity of CBG (25 µg/dl), the proportion of free cortisol rises. CBG very weakly binds aldosterone (only 20% is protein-bound). CBG is up-regulated by estrogens and thyroid hormones.
- *SHBG* is sometimes termed testosterone-binding globulin (TeBG) because it binds testosterone with a higher affinity than estrogens. SHBG is a 90 000 m.w. glycoprotein that is strongly related to the androgen binding protein produced by the Sertoli cells. SHBG is up-regulated by estrogens and thyroid hormones, whereas it is down-regulated by androgens.
- *DBG* is 56 000 m.w. and binds the 25-hydroxylated form of vitamin D with the highest affinity. Like CBG and SHBG, DBG is also up-regulated by estrogens.

The biological role of steroid hormone binding to carrier proteins is not completely clear. Protein binding is important for non-water-soluble steroid transport in the extracellular water environment. Furthermore, protein binding may serve as a reservoir of hormones, protecting hormones from catabolism and minimizing fluctuations of free hormone levels following episodic secretion of the relative tropines. A major function of steroid-binding proteins is that they allow for a uniform delivery of the hormone to cells in target tissues. However, subjects affected by carrier protein deficiency do not show major alterations of steroid hormone effects. Furthermore, potent synthetic steroids such as dexamethasone are weakly bound by plasma proteins.

The inactivation of steroid hormones involves the conversion of free hormones into inactive and more water-soluble compounds that are eliminated by the kidney through ultrafiltration. These metabolic steps take place mainly in the liver and include hydroxylation, conversion of ketone groups to more polar hydroxyl groups, and subsequent conjugation with glucuronide or sulfate. A variety of different metabolites and byproducts are therefore derived by steroid hormone degradation and processing. Since structural differences between different steroids are often eliminated during metabolism, the same metabolite may be generated by different steroid hormones. There are metabolites, however, that are mainly produced by one single class of hormones. Their measurements in urine may then provide specific information for that class of hormones. One example is the measurement of urinary 17-ketosteroids, which is used for evaluating the level of sex steroids.

Thyroid hormones

The unique characteristic of the thyroid hormones is that a major component of their chemical structure is iodine, a trace element that is provided with food and water but that is not always readily available in everyday diets. Thyroid hormones are very important in the organism economy, as they regulate normal development and intermediate metabolism, and almost all tissues are target tissues for them. The anatomy and the physiology of the thyroid gland is organized in such a manner that it provides an important reservoir of already-synthesized thyroid hormones. Therefore, day to day variations of iodine availability will not affect thyroid hormone levels and function.

Biosynthesis of thyroid hormones

Since thyroid hormones are iodinated tyrosine residues, the thyroid gland has efficient mechanisms to concentrate and store iodide that has reached the bloodstream after intestinal absorption. The thyroid gland has a follicular structure with polarized cells whose basal pole is exposed to the circulation and the apical pole faces the follicular lumen. Iodide is transported by an active mechanism from the bloodstream to the cell inside at the level of the baso-lateral membrane against both concentration and electro-chemical gradients. This mechanism is very efficient: iodide is concentrated in the thyroid more than 100-fold in respect to blood by a Na^+-I^- cotransporter (symporter), which was recently identified as a member of the same transmembrane proteins to which glucose transporters belong. TSH is the main regulator of thyroid cell func-

tions and is also a positive regulator of iodide transport. It is not entirely clear whether TSH stimulates iodide transport primarily via phospholipase A2 and intracellular Ca^{++} or via cAMP accumulation. Iodide itself, when in excess, inhibits iodide transport, perhaps through the formation of an iodinated form of arachidonic acid.

The thyroid cell iodide transporter is also able to transport other chemicals of similar size and charge than iodide, such as perchlorate and thiocyanate. All of these compounds may therefore act as competitive inhibitors of iodide transport and may aggravate iodide deficiency in the diet.

The iodine availability in the diet and thus iodine intake is variable. It is believed that 100 to 300 µg per day is the optimal iodine intake for an adult individuals. However, the thyroid may function normally in the presence of very different levels of iodine intake, ranging from 60 to 1000 or even 1500 µg/day. When iodine intake is low (below 60 µg/day), thyroid hormone synthesis becomes inadequate, and compensatory mechanisms (increased TSH, thyroid enlargement) take place in order to provide at least the minimum necessary amount of thyroid hormones (euthyroid goiter). Sufficient synthesis of thyroid hormones is not possible and hypothyroidism is common when iodine intake drops below 20 to 30 µg/day.

Mechanisms of iodination and release of thyroid hormones

The site of thyroid hormone formation is a large protein contained in the follicular lumen, thyroglobulin. Thyroglobulin is a 660 000 m.w. dimeric protein composed by two identical subunits and constitutes 70% of the thyroid protein content. Thyroglobulin in the thyroid lumen is highly concentrated (100 mg/ml) and present in part (about 30%) in nonsoluble form. Although other thyroid proteins may be iodinated, thyroglobulin represents the unique structure able to favor thyroid hormone biosynthesis.

In addition to thyroglobulin, the mechanism of thyroid hormone formation requires a system able to oxidize iodine to an effective iodinating agent. This system is composed of a thyroid-specific enzyme, thyroperoxidase, and by a generator of H_2O_2. Thyroperoxidase has been recently cloned and extensively studied.

Thyroperoxidase is a 90 000 m.w. glycoprotein with a 10% carbohydrate component and with a heme component in the form of protoporphyrin IX. Thyroperoxidase is a transmembrane protein located at the luminal pole of the thyroid cell and presents a small intracellular portion (56 residues) and a large extracellular domain (845 residues). The mechanism occurring in the thyroperoxidase-catalyzed iodination is not exactly known, although a few models have been proposed. One possibility is that oxidized thyroperoxidase interacts both with I- and with a tyrosine residue. Another model suggests that the I- bound to oxidized thyroperoxidase is in the form of ipoiodide.

The generation of H_2O_2 is essential for the process of iodination. H_2O_2 is formed at the apical membrane by the flavoprotein NADPH oxidase. It is not clear whether it involves the intermediate formation of O_2^-, which is then converted to H_2O_2 by superoxide dismutase. H_2O_2 generation is also stimulated by TSH via the Ca^{++} pathway. One possibility is that Ca^{++} converts NADPH oxidase from the inactive to the active form by blocking an inhibitor.

When only one iodine atom is covalently bound to the tyrosyl residue inside the thyroglobulin molecule, monoiodotyrosine is formed. When two iodine atoms are bound to the same tyrosyl residue, diiodotyrosine is formed (Fig. 2.10). This process is called organification and is the first step in thyroid hormone synthesis. It also prevents iodine from diffusing out of the thyroid cell into the blood compartment, as occurs in other tissues that also concentrate iodide, such as the salivary glands, the gastric mucosa, the choroid plexus, the breast, and the placenta.

Following the formation of monoiodotyrosine and diiodotyrosine, the following step is coupling either two diiodotyrosine residues to yield 3,5,3',5'-tetraiodothyronine or thyroxine (T_4) or one monoiodotyrosine with one diiodotyrosine residue to form 3,5,3'-triiodothyronine or T_3. T_3 thus has one less atom of iodine in the outer or phenylic ring as compared to T_4. When the iodine atom is absent in the inner or alanine side chain ring, the much less active "reverse" T_3 (3,3',5'-T_3) is formed. In the formation of T_4, two diiodotyrosine residues couple and form a quinol ether intermediate, which thereafter splits into a T_4 plus a dehydroalanine molecule. The enzyme required for the coupling reaction is again thyroperoxidase by acting at specific sites of thyroglobulin called "hormonogenic sites". Although one thyroglobulin molecule contains 134 tyrosyl residues, only about 18 are iodinated, and only two to four T_4 molecules are formed.

These synthesizing reactions occur in small vesicles that fuse with the thyroid cell apical membrane. As soon as thyroid hormones are synthesized, exocytosis occurs, and both thyroglobulin and thyroid hormones are released into the follicular lumen where they are stored (Fig. 2.10). Normal human thyroglobulin contains only 0.1 to 1.1% iodine, and one thyroglobulin molecule contains approximately 2 molecules of T_4, 0.3 of T_3, 6 of monoiodotyrosine, and 5 of diiodotyrosine.

The release of thyroid hormones in the circulation involves the reabsorption of thyroglobulin. Micropinocytosis is the major reabsorption process and is possibly a receptor-mediated endocytosis. In contrast, macropinocytosis, a nonspecific reabsorption of luminal material, is evident only after strong phasic TSH stimulation. Once internalized in the thyroid cell, the small vesicles containing thyroglobulin fuse with lysosomes and, thyroglobulin is degraded by a variety of lysosomal enzymes including cathepsins D, B, L, and H. Thyroid hormones are released at the cell basal membrane and enter the circulation.

Thyroid hormone transport

More than 99% of thyroid hormones circulate bound to plasma proteins. These proteins differ in structure and in their affinity for thyroid hormones and, therefore, for their ability to deliver thyroid hormones to the cells. Under normal conditions, approximately 70% of thyroid hormones are bound to thyroxine-binding globulin, 10 to 15% are bound to transthyretin or thyroxine-binding prealbumin, and the remaining 15 to 20% are bound to albumin. Very recently it has been reported that a small fraction of thyroid hormones circulates bound to lipoproteins by interacting with apolipoproteins.

Thyroxine-binding globulin is a globular α-globulin with only one binding site for thyroid hormones. It binds T_4 at very high affinity and T_3 with an affinity 10- to 20-fold lower.

Transthyretin is also a globular molecule with a tetrameric structure composed of four identical subunits that form a central channel with two symmetrical thyroid hormone-binding sites at both ends. However, a molecule of transthyretin binds only one molecule of T_3 or T_4 since the second site has a markedly lower affinity (negative cooperativity). Transthyretin circulates bound to the retinol-binding protein, the protein that binds vitamin A. The transthyretin affinity for T_3 is approximately tenfold lower than that for T_4. Because of their different affinity for the binding proteins, less than 0.1% of T_4 but less than 1% of T_3 circulate in the free form, the only biologically active form. Protein binding also affects the half-life of T_4 (approximately 7 days) much longer than that of T_3 (1 day).

Albumin is the thyroid hormone binding protein with the lowest affinity. However, its high concentration results in a relatively high proportion (15 to 20%) of both total T_3 and T_4 bound by albumin.

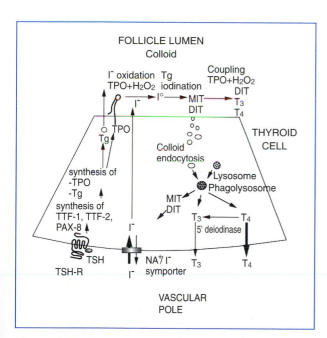

Figure 2.10 Synthesis, iodination, and processing of thyroglobulin with release of thyroid hormones. The synthesis, iodination, and processing of thyroglobulin occur at the level of the thyroid follicular cell. It is stimulated by TSH and requires tissue-specific transcription factors (TTF-1/2, PAX-8). Thyroglobulin (Tg) is then iodinated at tyrosyl residues by thyroperoxidase (TPO) and H_2O_2-forming monoiodotyrosine (MIT) and diiodotyrosine (DIT), which are then coupled to yield thyroxine (T_4) or triiodothyronine (T_3). The release of thyroid hormones in the circulation involves reabsorption and degradation of thyroglobulin by lysosomes.

Given the dissociation constants of these three binding proteins, it is calculated that the highest proportion of free thyroid hormones available for entering the cells derives from the albumin-bound thyroid hormone pool, with the thyroxine-binding globulin and the transthyretin-bound thyroid hormone pools contributing almost to the same extent.

Intracellular metabolism of thyroid hormones

Thyroxine is only produced by the thyroid gland and is the most abundant hormone secreted by the thyroid, 10- to 20-fold more than T_3. Triiodothyronine, in addition of being secreted by the thyroid (approximately 20% of circulating T_3) is also produced by deiodination of T_4 in peripheral tissues. Approximately 30 to 50% of the secreted T_4 is deiodinated to T_3 with the result that 70 to 90% of the daily production of T_3 originates from T_4 deiodination. Therefore, the extrathyroidal production of T_3 from T_4 contributes to maintaining a stable T_3 concentration and is an additional mechanism to regulate T_3 production in general and at the cellular level. It is not entirely clear whether T_4 represents a pro-hormone, with only T_3 being the active hormone that is either taken up from the circulation or produced inside the target cell by deiodination of the precursor T_4. It is believed that T_4 itself may also exert some hormonal effects. However, T_3 is much more potent than T_4 since it binds with a higher affinity than T_4 to the thyroid hormone nuclear receptors.

Two types of enzymes (5'-deiodinase and 5-deiodinase) with a different tissue distribution deiodinate T_4 and the other iodothyronines in a stepwise manner to produce either active (T_3), less active (rT_3), or inactive thyronines (3 forms of T_2 and 4 forms of T_1, according to the position of the iodine atom bound to the thyronine structure). Therefore, the metabolic status of thyroid hormone target tissues depends not only upon the circulating T_3 levels but also upon the amount of T_3 that is locally produced.

5'-Deiodinase removes an iodine atom from the phenylic ring of T_4 or rT_3. As this process generates T_3 from T_4, this enzyme activates thyroid hormones. 5'-Deiodinase is a membrane-bound enzyme that contains a selenocysteine at the catalytic site, which is essential for the activity of the enzyme. Two isoforms of 5'-deiodinase exist with a different tissue distribution.

Type I 5'-deiodinase is mostly expressed in the liver and the kidney. It is also present at lower concentrations in the central nervous system, in the adipose tissue, and in fibroblasts. Because of the high level of 5' deiodinase present in the liver and because of the liver size and ability to concentrate T_4, approximately 70% of the T_3 production originates from the liver. Therefore, a reduced functional liver mass, as occurs in cirrhosis, results in reduced hepatic T_3 production and a low T_3 syndrome. Other conditions (diabetes mellitus, caloric restriction, chronic heart failure) result in low T_3 syndrome and are associated with increased levels of nonesterified fatty acids that decrease T_4 uptake by the liver and, therefore, T_4 5'-deiodination to T_3.

Type II 5'-deiodinase differs from type I in tissue distribution, in different regulation in pathophysiological conditions, and in its resistance to inhibition by propylthiouracil. Type II 5'-deiodinase is specifically present in brain, pituitary, and brown adipose tissue and far less so in placenta. The brain possesses both 5'-deiodinase isoforms, and in the brain the majority of T_3 bound to nuclear receptors appears to derive from the intracellular deiodination of T_4, a potential protective mechanism against T_3 deficiency. The two isoforms are regulated differently. At the pituitary level, type II 5'-deiodinase is increased by thyrotropin-releasing hormone. Type II 5'-deiodinase is also increased in hypothyroidism, while the type I isoform increases in hyperthyroidism and may play a role in generating more circulating T_3. 5-Deiodinase, or type III, removes an iodine from the inner or alanine ring and generates the essentially inactive iodothyronine, rT_3. This deiodinase is probably also a selenoprotein and is present in high concentrations in the placenta and less so in other tissues.

Thyroid hormones may also be degraded by removal of the amino group and a methylene group from the alanine side chain, giving rise to tetraiodothyroacetic acid (TETRAC) from T_4 and triiodothyroacetic acid (TRIAC) from T_3.

RECEPTORS FOR STEROID AND THYROID HORMONES (NUCLEAR RECEPTORS)

General aspects

Steroid and thyroid hormones freely diffuse across the cell membrane and interact with intracellular proteins (receptors) that recognize the specific ligand (hormone). They then undergo complex modifications that make them able to interact with other intracellular components and activate the signaling pathway. This well-recognized mechanism of steroid and thyroid hormone action does not exclude other accessory effects of these hormones at the cell membrane level. Membrane effects have been described for both steroid and thyroid hormones.

The intracellular receptors for steroid and thyroid hormones behave as ligand-activated transcription factors and are encoded by genes that belong to a common superfamily and have possibly evolved by a common evolutionary precursor. Genes encoding the vitamin D receptor, retinoic acid receptors, and other transcription factors also belong to this superfamily.

The principal mechanism of action of nuclear receptors is to regulate, either positively or negatively, mRNA transcription. mRNA transcription requires the binding of polymerase II and additional auxiliary factors to the promoter region of the gene in order to form the pre-initiation complex. The activity of the promoter results from the interaction with many regulatory proteins that act in synergy. Positive regulation of mRNA transcription by nuclear receptors involves both binding with specific hormone response elements (HREs) and the contact with several proteins of the pre-initiation complex *via* the so-called "transactivation domains" and stabilization of the pre-initiation complex at the promoter region.

Nonexpressed genes are organized in chromatin structures containing histones and other proteins called nucleosomes that are resistant to nuclease digestion. Nuclear receptors have a higher affinity for nucleosome packaged DNA than for free DNA, while the opposite is true for other transcription factors. DNA binding of nuclear receptors causes disruption of the nucleosome structure (as can be evidenced by acquired nuclease sensitivity) and allows for the binding of different transcription factors.

Steroid and thyroid hormone receptors, however, differ in several aspects. In the absence of the ligand, the steroid receptors form complexes with chaperone proteins (such as the heat shock proteins) and are weakly bound to DNA but do not interact with HREs. In contrast, thyroid hormone receptors that do not bind heat shock proteins, also bind DNA in the absence of the ligand. Both types of receptors bind to DNA in the form of dimers, but while steroid receptors form homodimers, thyroid hormone receptors preferably form heterodimers with other proteins (mainly with the retinoid acid receptor). In the case of genetic mutations leading to a defective nuclear receptor, resistance to steroid hormones occurs only when both alleles are mutated. In contrast, in the case of thyroid hormone receptors, the mutation of a single allele leads to thyroid hormone resistance since the mutated receptor acts as dominant negative.

Steroid hormone receptors

Steroid receptors are proteins with a m.w. of approximately 90 000. Six classes of steroid receptor families are known: glucocorticoids, mineralocorticoids, estrogen, androgens, progesterone, and vitamin D (Fig. 2.11). Each of them is the product of a single gene and exists in one single form, with the exception of the progesterone receptor that it is produced in two isoforms (A and B) by RNA differential splicing.

The structure of a steroid receptor is organized into three functional domains. The amino-terminal region is called the transactivation domain and regulates the transcriptional activity of the receptor. This region is phosphorylated. The middle region contains the DNA-binding domains that recognize and bind HREs. The carboxy-terminal region contains the hormone-binding domain and the sites of interactions with heat shock proteins.

As lipophilic molecules, steroids freely diffuse through the plasma membrane and reach the receptors that are weakly associated to the cell nucleus. The plasma concentration of steroids is usually below that required to provide half maximal receptor saturation (Kd). This means that changes in the steroid plasma concentration parallel the receptor occupancy and hormone biological effects.

The steroid receptors are maintained in the inactive state by forming hetero-oligomeric complexes with other proteins (chaperone proteins), among which are the heat shock proteins hsp90 and hsp70 (Fig. 2.12). In the absence of the ligand, the receptors are probably weakly associated with the cell nucleus but are not able to interact with the HREs, most likely because the DNA-binding domains are masked. Chaperone proteins also maintain the receptors in the correct structure to bind the hormone with high affinity. Ligand binding induces a conformational change of the receptor hetero-oligomeric complex, causing the detachment of the receptor molecule from chaperone proteins and the assembly of receptor homodimers containing two molecules of the hormone. Receptor

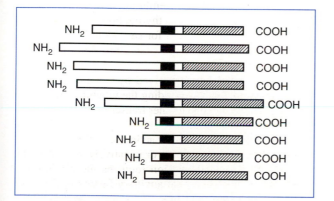

Figure 2.11 Primary structure of nuclear receptors for steroids, thyroid hormones, and vitamins. The primary structure of the different receptors for steroids is indicated with open bars and is proportional to the protein size. Receptors for thyroid hormones, vitamin D, and retinoic acid share structure similarities with steroid receptors. Conserved functional regions are indicated: DNA-binding regions by black bars and hormone-binding regions by dashed bars.

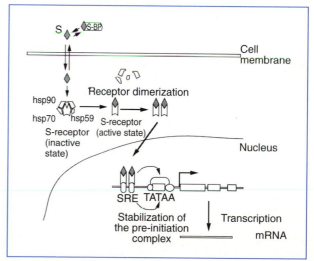

Figure 2.12 Intracellular signaling of steroid hormones. Free steroid hormones (S) are in a dynamic equilibrium with protein-bound steroids (S-BP). They enter the cell by diffusion and reach the steroid receptors that are maintained in an inactive state by chaperone proteins (heat shock proteins, hsp90 and hsp70, hsp59). Steroid binding to the receptor induces the detachment of chaperone proteins and receptor dimerization. Receptor homodimers then bind to steroid response elements (SRE) and promote transcription, causing a stabilization of the pre-initiation complex.

homodimers then bind with high affinity to HREs via the unmasked DNA-binding domains. It appears that the presence of the ligand is important mainly for homodimer formation and also affects the correct kinetics of DNA binding. Two classes of HREs have been characterized, one shared by glucocorticoids, progestins, mineralocorticoids, and androgens; and a second one common to estrogens, thyroid hormones, vitamin D, and retinoic acid. These HREs (of one or two classes) are usually clustered and integrated with other sites for different transcription factors. Interactions (sometime synergy) between different hormone receptors and between hormone receptors and other transcription factors are an important step in the regulation of mRNA transcription. In fact, ligand binding to the nuclear receptor is necessary but not sufficient for eliciting hormone effects. Recently, other widely distributed transcription factors have been shown to be required to allow the full action of steroid hormone receptors. Among these factors are NF1, SP1, Oct-1 and TFIID. In the case of negative regulation of transcription, it is speculated that steroid receptors compete for DNA binding at the level of the promoter region with factors necessary for mRNA transcription, although other less-known mechanisms are also likely to occur. For instance, glucocorticoid receptors have been shown to block the promoter activation by the AP1 complex by interacting with the components of the AP1 complex, Jun and Fos. The steroid receptor activity can be modulated by phosphorylation. Phosphorylation seems to be mainly induced by ligand binding but is also controlled by other mechanisms. For example, it has been demonstrated that protein kinase A can phosphorylate the progesterone receptor; by this mechanism the steroid receptor activity can be modulated by other signaling pathways.

Since specific steroids induce different effects in different target cells, an important problem is to understand how specificity occurs. Although much is still to be clarified, some mechanisms are well-established: (1) the presence and the level of specific hormone receptors; (2) the presence of chaperone proteins and/or additional transcription factors required by a specific receptor; (3) the particular location of HREs in the context of the promoter/enhancer region of the target gene and in relationship with other transcription sites; (4) the chromatin organization in a particular cell. In contrast with other transcription factors, the steroid receptors bind to chromatin organized in nucleosomes and may, therefore, regulate the access of other factors to DNA. In addition, the affinity of the receptor is higher in supercoiled than in relaxed DNA.

Steroid hormone antagonists

Several steroid antagonists have been synthesized. These antagonists may be more or less specific. For instance, antiandrogens such as cyproterone acetate also act as a progestin agonist, and RU-486 has both an antiglucocorticoid and antiprogestin effects. Steroid antagonists may act by competitive and also noncompetitive mechanisms. In fact, the synthetic antagonist ICI-164-384 impairs the dissociation of heat shock proteins and receptor dimerization, and RU-486 induces the receptor to bind DNA with a poor transactivation activity since it does not induce receptor phosphorylation.

Nuclear hormone receptors and cancer

Components of the steroid-thyroid hormone family have important effects on growth and development in a variety of tissues. Abnormal expression or expression of mutated receptors may, therefore, be relevant to the oncogenetic process. One of the two viral oncogenes of the avian erythroblast leukemia, v-erbA, is a mutated counterpart of thyroid hormone receptor (TR), which cannot bind the thyroid hormone and repress its differentiating effects by a dominant negative mechanism. The second oncogene of this virus, v-erbB, encodes a truncated form of the epidermal growth factor receptor with constitutive tyrosine kinase activity.

An example of the involvement in human oncogenesis of abnormal expression of this class of receptors is the presence of the receptors for estrogens and progesterone in approximately 50% of breast carcinomas. Both estrogens and progesterone play a key role in the development of the mammary gland and, when expressed in breast cancer cells, may increase the tumor proliferation rate. This is the basis for anti-estrogen therapy in receptor-positive breast cancer. Essentially the same concept applies to the use of anti-androgens as a therapy in prostate cancer. In a different malignancy, acute lymphoblastic leukemia, the abnormal expression of glucocorticoid receptors mediate growth inhibition, and thus glucocorticoids are used as therapeutic agents.

However, glucocorticoids stimulate the proliferation of at least two oncogenic viruses (mouse mammary tumor virus, MMTV, and mouse sarcoma virus, MSV), as these have glucocorticoid response elements within the long terminal repeat regions.

Thyroid hormone receptors

Specific nuclear binding of radiolabeled T_3 was first demonstrated in 1972, although only the recent cloning of the receptor cDNA has provided conclusive evidence of the existence of nuclear receptors, allowing for a better understanding of the mechanism of action of thyroid hormones at the DNA level.

The thyroid hormone receptor proteins (TRs) weigh 50 to 55 kDa. They are widely distributed in thyroid hormone target tissues such as the pituitary, liver, brown fat, kidney, and brain. The number of receptors per nucleus ranges from 2000 to 10000. They bind T_3 at high affinity (Kd ≈ 0.1 nM) and T_4 at an affinity approximately tenfold lower. T_3, therefore, is the major active thyroid hormone. Thyroid hormone receptors exist in various isoforms encoded by two separate genes (Fig. 2.13). One gene (gene β) is located on chromosome 3 and encodes the two isoforms, TR-β1 and TR-β2, originated by alternative splicing. The second gene (gene α) is located on chromosome 17 and encodes isoforms TR-α1, TR-α2, and TR-α3, also pro-

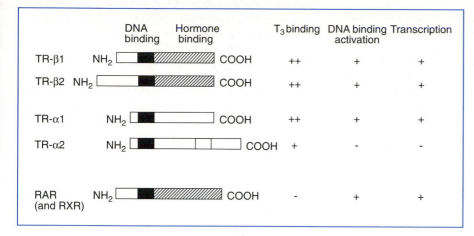

		DNA binding	Hormone binding	T_3 binding	DNA binding activation	Transcription
TR-β1	NH₂ ... COOH			++	+	+
TR-β2	NH₂ ... COOH			++	+	+
TR-α1	NH₂ ... COOH			++	+	+
TR-α2	NH₂ ... COOH			+	-	-
RAR (and RXR)	NH₂ ... COOH			-	+	+

Figure 2.13 Primary structure of nuclear receptors for thyroid hormones and retinoic acid. The primary structure of receptors for thyroid hormone (TR-α/β, Rev-ErbAα) and for retinoic acid (RAR) is indicated with open bars in proportion to the protein size. Similar patterns show areas of homology. The receptor ability to bind T_3, DNA, and to activate transcription is also indicated.

duced by alternative splicing. Isoforms TR-α2 and TR-α3 lack a functional T_3 binding domain, although they have a conserved DNA binding domain. Both the active and the inactive TR are variously distributed in the different tissues. For instance, the brain express the TR-β1 and the TR-α1 isoforms at approximately the same level, while the isoform TR-α2 is the most abundant. On the contrary, in liver the TR-β1 is the most abundant, and the isoform TR-α2 is nearly absent.

The thyroid receptors share with other receptors of this family at least two functional domains: a DNA-binding domain at the amino-terminus and a ligand-binding domain at the carboxy-terminus. The DNA-binding domain characteristically contains two zinc-finger motifs: the first contains the binding site specificity, while the second is involved in dimer formation. The ligand-binding domain also contains a motif primarily involved in receptor dimerization that is analogous to a "leucine zipper", a structure producing strong protein-to-protein interactions. The unliganded TR is located in the nucleus and binds to TR response elements (TREs), unlike the steroid receptor, which is complexed with chaperone proteins. The transcription of mRNA induced by thyroid hormone is repressed by the unliganded TR.

The transactivation capability of thyroid hormone receptors require receptor dimerization. In contrast with steroid receptors, although TR homodimers exist, the transactivation activity requires the formation of heterodimers between one receptor molecule and a different protein. Proteins able to dimerize with the TR are called auxiliary proteins or TRAPs and include the receptors for retinoic acid and 9-cis retinoic acid. The expression of different TRAPs is tissue-specific and, together with the different level of receptor isoform expression in the various tissues, determines the tissue specificity of thyroid hormone effects. The transactivation activity of thyroid hormone receptors depends on the DNA binding at the level of specific TREs at the promoter regions of target genes. Search for a consensus sequence of TREs indicates that the optimal binding motif consists of an octamer with a minimum 'core sequence' of six base pairs. Since TRs

acts as dimers, pairs of consensus sequences are necessary to elicit a biological response (Fig. 2.14).

Thyroid hormone receptors not only have positive but also regulatory effects on gene expression. The latter effect is mediated by the binding to negative TREs (nTREs). Negative TREs may contain a half site or may have specific orientation and spacing of the two half sites. Inhibition of mRNA transcription by nTREs binding may involve interference with basal transcription induced by

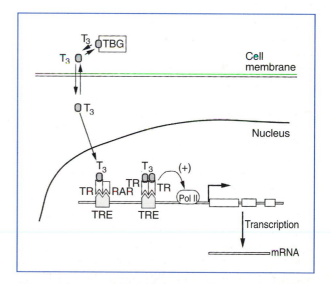

Figure 2.14 Intracellular signaling of T_3 by nuclear receptors. Free T_3 and T_4 diffuse inside the target cells (where T_3 may also be produced by T_4 deiodination) and bind to thyroid hormone receptors (TR) located in the nucleus. The unligated (TR) is located in the nucleus and, by binding to the TR response elements (TREs) on DNA, represses mRNA transcription, resulting in a decreased activity of RNA polymerase II (Pol II). Once bound to T_3, TRs dimerize and acquire transactivation capability. TRs frequently form heterodimers with proteins that include the receptors for retinoic acid (RAR) and 9-cis retinoic acid (RXR). Homo- and heterodimers then bind on the DNA at the level of specific TREs at the promoter regions of target genes.

other factors or blocking protein-to-protein interaction with other transcriptional factors such as c-fos and c-jun. In summary, the mechanisms through which TRs regulate gene expression are complex, finely tuned, and not fully understood. In general, TRs binding to TREs directly interferes with the initiation complex of the target gene or of genes that encode proteins that in turn regulate the expression of target genes. However, many questions remain unsolved such as: (1) the specific role of homo- and heterodimers; (2) the role of the different isoforms; and (3) the precise mechanisms of positive and negative regulation.

Resistance to thyroid hormones

The syndrome of resistance to thyroid hormones includes a heterogeneous group of disorders characterized by a reduced effect of thyroid hormones on one or more target tissues. The majority of these patients have a manifest hyposensitivity to thyroid hormones at the level of all target tissues (generalized tissue resistance to thyroid hormone, GRTH). GRTH, the most common form of thyroid hormone resistance, is mostly familial and appears to be transmitted by an autosomal dominant mechanism. It is characterized biochemically by elevated T_3 and T_4 with nonsuppressed TSH serum levels. It is characterized clinically by goiter (due to TSH stimulation), euthyroidism, or symptoms of hypothyroidism such as impaired mental function and delayed growth. However, symptoms suggesting hyperthyroidism (hyperactivity, tachycardia) may also be present. GRTH is caused by mutations in the T_3-binding domain of the TRβ that impair T_3 binding. Mutations of the TRβ may involve single amino acid deletions or substitutions or addition of new amino acids, as well as a complete deletion of the TRβ gene. Interestingly, to cause hormone resistance only one allele needs to be mutated; this allele will therefore interfere with the function of the normal receptor. This "dominant negative effect" is not fully understood. One hypothesis is the competition of the mutated receptor with the normal receptor for the interaction with TRs. Alternatively, it can be hypothesized that mutated receptors form homo- and heterodimers that block TREs since they can only scarcely be relieved from the TRE DNA sequence by binding T_3. Other forms of thyroid hormone resistance are more rare. Very few cases have been described in whom the resistance to thyroid hormone occurs only at the pituitary level (PRTH). As a consequence of nonsuppressed TSH, there is an increase of thyroid hormone levels that will cause clinical symptoms and signs of hyperthyroidism. PRTH may also be inherited but is sporadic in most cases.

The defect involved in PRTH is not known, although, at least some cases, it may be explained with the presence of a GRTH with predominant pituitary involvement.

Extranuclear actions of thyroid hormones

The thermogenic effects of thyroid hormones have suggested a possible direct effect of thyroid hormones at the mitochondrion level. Specific mitochondrion receptors for T_3 have been described, and the adenine nucleotide (ADP/ATP) translocase has been identified as a possible target of this action. Cell membrane Ca^{++}-ATPase activity has also been suggested as another target for non-nuclear effects of thyroid hormones. T_3 elicits rapid inotropic and vasodilatory effects on the heart that have been attributed to a direct stimulatory effect of sarcoplasmic reticulum Ca^{++}-ATPase activity. None of these effects is firmly demonstrated. They can be obtained in vitro only at T_3 concentrations well above the physiological range. Moreover, the biological effect of thyroid hormone analogues, which is observed in vivo, is not reproduced under these experimental conditions. To date, only the negative regulation of type II T_4 5'-deiodinase appears to be mediated by thyroid hormones via nontranscriptional mechanisms. Type II T_4 5'-deiodinase is selectively expressed in the brain and the pituitary and is finely regulated to locally maintain a constant production rate of T_3 in spite of consistent variations in the thyroid gland function. The enzyme production is induced by a decrease of T_4 concentration and declines shortly after T_4 administration. T_3 is less potent than T_4 in mediating this effect. The precise mechanism of this effect of T_4 is unknown, although it has been suggested that it may be related to the capacity of T_4 to regulate cellular actin cytoskeleton since an intact cytoskeleton is required for T_4 to produce this extranuclear effect.

Suggested readings

BROWN EM, POLLAK M, SEIDMAN CE, et al. Calcium-ion-sensing cell-surface receptors. N Engl J Med 1995;333:234-9.

DEFRANCO DB, RAMAKRISHNAN C, TANG Y. Molecular chaperones and subcellular trafficking of steroid receptors. J Steroid Biochem Mol Biol 1998;65:51-8.

DE NAYER P. The thyroid hormone receptors: molecular basis of thyroid hormone resistance. Horm Res 1992;38:57-61.

GETHER U, KOBILKA BK. G protein-coupled receptors. II. Mechanism of agonist activation. J Biol Chem 1998;273:979-82.

GLASS CK. Some new twists in the regulation of gene expression by thyroid hormone and retinoic acid receptors. J Endocrinol 1996;150:349-57.

GRADY EF, BOHM SK, BUNNETT NW. Turning off the signal: mechanisms that attenuate signaling by G protein-coupled receptors. Am J Physiol 1997;273:G586-G601.

GUTKIND JS. The pathways connecting G protein-coupled receptors to the nucleus through divergent mitogen-activated protein kinase cascades. J Biol Chem 1998;273:1839-42.

JI TH, GROSSMANN M, JI I. G protein-coupled receptors. I. Diversity of receptor-ligand interactions. J Biol Chem 1998;273:299-302.

KELLY PA, GOUJON L, SOTIROPOULOS A, et al. The GH receptor and signal transduction. Horm Res 1994;42:133-9.

LAZAR MA. Thyroid hormone receptors: multiple forms, multiple possibilities. Endocr Rev 1993;14:184-93.

LIU F, ROTH RA. Binding of SH2 containing proteins to the insulin receptor: a new way for modulating insulin signalling. Mol Cell Biochem 1998;182:73-8.

SPIEGEL AM. Mutations in G proteins and G protein-coupled receptors in endocrine disease. J Clin Endocrinol Metab 1996;81:2434-42.

TAGA T, KISHIMOTO T. Signaling mechanisms through cytokine receptors that share signal transducing receptor components. Curr Opin Immunol 1995;7:17-23.

ULLRICH A, SCHLESSINGER J. Signal transduction by receptors with tyrosine kinase activity. Cell 1990;61:203-12.

ZILLIACUS J, WRIGHT AP, CARLSTEDT-DUKE J, GUSTAFSSON JA. Structural determinants of DNA-binding specificity by steroid receptors. Mol Endocrinol 1995;9:389-400.

3

Molecular biology in endocrinology and metabolism

Marc J. Abramowicz, Gilbert Vassart

Living matter became amenable to study at the molecular level with the advent of gene cloning. The availability of virtually pure biomolecules in unlimited amounts, and of targeted modifications in vitro, made it possible to investigate discrete fundamental mechanisms of health and disease, such as hormone-receptor interactions or other steps of signal-transduction pathways. In the clinical setting, diagnostic techniques have been derived from these approaches and currently allow for the diagnoses of many hereditary disorders, such as Steinert's myotonic dystrophy, the multiple endocrine neoplasia syndromes, and the Prader-Willi syndrome.

The characterization of the genetic basis of human polymorphisms and the recognition of the normal variation among healthy individuals favor a novel approach of the patient that takes into account his or her unique biochemical identity when faced with disease. From the detailed study of many genetic disorders, it also appears that there is often no clear-cut limit between normal variation and disease-causing mutations. This parallels the identification of many genetic variants that are not sufficient to cause disease but predispose one to acquired disorders such as some cancers, ischemic heart disease, or diabetes. This progress should soon be translated into focused prevention. A few tests for genetic predisposition to specific health problems are already available as the so-called predictive medicine.

Cloning

A *clone* is a population of cells that arise from the successive divisions of one original cell and are therefore identical. By extension, a *molecular clone* is a population of molecules derived from one original molecule by successive replications. Clonal expansion of an *Escherichia coli* bacterium by binary fission implies the replication, if present, of a piece of extrachromosomal (episomal) deoxyribonucleic acid (DNA) called a *plasmid* into a population of identical plasmid molecules that can be readily isolated

to clonal purity. Modern molecular biology originated with the ability to manipulate plasmids as cloning vectors to integrate foreign, non-bacterial DNA (such as a piece of the human insulin gene) and yield *recombinant* DNA molecules; and to reintroduce them into bacteria in a process called artificial *transformation*; which then replicates to virtually unlimited amounts. Cloned genes can be artificially expressed in vitro into the corresponding pure protein product. After amplification by means of bacterial cultures, purified plasmids can be introduced into eukaryotic cells by *transfection*. Recombinant DNA can be processed to integrate into chromosomes in germinal or early embryonic mammalian cells, resulting in the production of transgenic animals after proper gestation.

Molecular genetics and molecular oncology

To produce molecules of clonal purity, one must first isolate the corresponding genes. Molecular genetics is the study of the gene in the organism and of its spontaneously occurring mutations, and it includes the study of its transmission to offspring or daughter cells. *Germ* cells give rise to gametes, ova and sperm. All other cell types are called *somatic*. Mutations in germ cells may be passed to children, while mutations in somatic cells cannot. Somatic mutations will, however, be inherited by daughter cells when the mutated cell divides. Tumorigenesis and malignant transformation results from somatic mutations that alter genes involved in the control of cell proliferation. These are classified as genes that normally promote cell proliferation (*cellular oncogenes, proto-oncogenes*) and genes that normally slow proliferation (*anti-oncogenes, tumor-suppressor genes*). Most cancers result from successive mutations of several proto-oncogenes or anti-oncogenes that confer a growth advantage to the cell and induce the mutated cell to proliferate over normal cells, forming malignant clones where successive mutations are selected for greater malignancy.

FUNCTIONAL ANATOMY OF DNA

The double helix

Deoxyribonucleic acid molecules are composed of two extended, linear polymers coiled into double helices. The monomeric units are called *nucleotides* and are made up of a phosphorylated sugar, deoxyribose, linked to a purine or a pyrimidine base. The sequence of the bases along the polymer constitutes the genetic message as a string of characters constitute a text. The nucleotides are covalently linked by phosphodiester bonds that involve the 3'-OH group of one sugar and the 5'-OH of the next. This defines a 3'-OH and a 5'-OH free extremity to the polymer strand, the 5' and 3' ends being the "left" and "right" ends of nucleic acids, respectively. Purines in one strand interact with pyrimidines in the other by means of hydrogen bonds, in such a manner that adenine (A) can only pair with thymine (T), and guanine (G) only with cytosine (C). Therefore, the sequence of any one strand contains all of the genetic information of the duplex. The two strands of one DNA molecule are said to be *complementary*, and are coiled together in opposite directions (5' → 3' facing 3' → 5'): hence, DNA *is an antiparallel double helix*.

Replication of DNA occurs during the S phase of the cell cycle, yielding two identical copies of the original double helix. In replication, the two strands separate and each serves as a template for the synthesis of complementary strands that reconstitute double helices. Replication is thus semi-conservative, as each daughter duplex will contain one of each original single strand. New strands are synthesized in the 5' → 3' direction.

Eukaryotic DNA polymerases can elongate strands but cannot start new ones. Short RNA molecules act as *primers* to DNA polymerization in vivo, and they are later removed from the mature molecule. Synthetic DNA oligomers (oligonucleotides) can prime DNA synthesis in vitro, as is widely exploited by the polymerase chain reaction methodology.

Synthesis of gene product

Like replication, *transcription* of DNA into RNA involves separation of the two DNA strands and synthesis of a new chain in the 5' → 3' direction. RNA is similar to DNA except that the backbone sugar is ribose, and uracil (U) faces adenine instead of thymine. Genes are transcribed into RNA in the nucleus of eukaryotic cells as colinear, short-lived *primary transcripts*. Genes contain non-coding intervening sequences called introns that are spliced out in a maturation process that further involves post-transcriptional modifications of both extremities of the primary transcript. The 5' extremity is capped specifically by a special nucleotide, 7-methyl guanosine, by a very stable 5'-5' phosphodiester bond. The 3' extremity is polyadenylated by a specific, DNA-independent enzymatic machinery that recognizes an AAUAAA motif (the polyadenylation signal) in the nearby sequence.

The mature transcript is exported to the cytoplasm and becomes a messenger RNA (mRNA), which can then be *translated* into protein by the ribosomal machinery. Secreted proteins begin with a signal peptide (the "pre" sequence) and are directed to the rough endoplasmic reticulum by means of a cytoplasmic complex that recognizes the signal peptide, which is later cleaved off in the cisternae of the rough endoplasmic reticulum. The sequence of the amino acids constitutes the primary structure of the protein and dictates its folding, disulfide bridging, and final conformation. Thus, the entire protein structure is essentially encoded at the genetic level by the sequence of DNA. Post-translational modifications include N- or O-glycosylation, which occurs in the Golgi apparatus, and the addition of prosthetic groups (like heme), as well as oligo- or multimerization into complexes that may include proteins encoded by other genes. For example, the alpha and beta chains of hemoglobin are encoded by genes that are located on different chromosomes. Of note, many protein complexes are made of subunits that are derived from the same gene, assembled after cleavage of the initial peptide into smaller ones, such as the insulin molecule.

Genes for ribosomal RNAs (rRNAs) or transfer RNAs (tRNAs) do not code for proteins, and RNA molecules with specific enzymic activities have been described.

RNA can be reverse-transcribed in vitro by the use of an RNA-dependent DNA polymerase enzyme (reverse transcriptase) of retroviral origin, which yields a complementary DNA (cDNA) molecule made double-stranded by further in vitro replication. Complementary DNA copies of mRNAs correspond to intron-free exonic sequences.

Genes constitute only a small fraction of the human genome, as approximately 70 to 90% of the DNA has no function known to date.

Regulation of gene expression

The portion of the gene that is effectively transcribed is called the structural gene. Transcription is regulated by *transcriptional factors* that bind precise DNA motifs found immediately upstream (5') from the structural gene in a region called the *promoter* region, or further upstream in a region(s) called distant promoter(s) or *enhancer* region(s). Together, the promoter region(s) and structural gene are called a *transcription unit*. Gene promoters can be active in all cell types, causing the gene to be expressed ubiquitously ("house-keeping" genes), or they can be active only in one or some cell types, yielding tissue-specific expression.

Alternative splicing is a well-known mechanism that produces different proteins (such as calcitonin and the calcitonin gene-related peptide) in the same or another cell type. Most genes spuriously generate alternatively spliced transcripts expressed at very low levels, whose biological relevance remains unclear. Similarly, spurious transcriptional activity generates very low levels of transcripts in illegitimate cell types from otherwise tissue-specific promoters.

For a promoter to be active, the chromosomal DNA in the gene area must first decondensate and separate from histones and other molecules that keep the chromatin compact. Conversely, condensation of DNA into compact chromatin (heterochromatin) silences the genes it bears;

virtually irreversible, tissue-specific DNA condensation is a major mechanism of cell differentiation. In a sequence of events that is still not completely understood, DNA methylation parallels DNA inactivation and condensation. Obviously, *epigenetic* (that is, not directly dependent on DNA sequence) mechanisms, such as DNA methylation, are involved in genetic expression.

Besides cell differentiation, epigenetic mechanisms are implicated in parental *imprinting*, a phenomenon by which some genes are expressed differently whether inherited from the father or the mother. In the offspring, the gonad resets the parental imprint and generates the new, gender-specific imprint at some point before the germ cell is passed to the next generation. It seems that only several (perhaps a dozen) regions of the human genome are imprinted, and that they are under the influence of a nearby *imprinting center*.

BASIC METHODS OF DNA ANALYSIS

DNA sampling

Biopsies of any tissue containing nucleated cells can be used as sources of genomic DNA. For practical purposes, most diagnostic techniques are performed on DNA extracted from circulating white blood cells, fibroblast cultures from skin biopsies, and biopsy samples of muscle, liver, or other organs. Properly extracted DNA is stable for days at room temperature and for months to years at 4 °C or lower temperatures.

Molecular hybridization

The double helix can be reversibly denatured, or *melted*, into its two complementary single strands by heat, alkaline pH, or low ionic strength. A labeled nucleic acid can then serve as a *molecular probe* to identify target nucleic acid molecules that contain an identical or closely related segment in terms of nucleotide sequence. The target usually consists of an immobilized mixture of nucleic acids. The probe may be prepared from cloned DNA or consist of a synthetic, single-stranded oligonucleotide. Probes can be labeled by a radioactive isotope or a non-isotopic tracer.

Hybridization with long (>200 bp) DNA probes may serve to identify complementary nucleic acid sequences in a target mix (*perfect match*), or, using less stringent hybridization and washing conditions, sequences that only share a certain degree of homology (*partial mismatch*), such as segments of other related genes. Low-stringency hybridization is exploited in *homology cloning*.

Hybridization with short oligonucleotide probes (about 20 bases long) is extremely accurate and can be used to identify single base differences in study samples, as experimental conditions can be found where a single base mismatch will make a 20-base pair duplex completely unstable. Hybridization with allele-specific oligonucleotides is a method based on the use of oligomers to detect known, single-base (point) mutations in patients with genetic disorders. Recently, a micromethod based on multiple allele-specific oligonucleotides was devised that scans long DNA targets for

mutations. Direct computer reading of these high-density DNA arrays on microchips (DNA chips) promise exciting clinical applications.

Restriction enzymes

Restriction enzymes, discovered and isolated from bacteria, recognize short segments of DNA – often 4, 5, or 6 base pairs of palindromic motifs – and cleave the double helix there with exquisite specificity. For example, restriction enzyme *Bam*H1 incubated in vitro with a solution of complex DNA will hydrolyze both strands each time it encounters the sequence GGATCC. The location of the GGATCC motifs in any piece of chromosomal DNA is precisely determined by the anatomy of the human genome. *Restriction mapping* (that is, locating respective restriction sites along chromosomal DNA) is a vast project that contributes to the global effort of deciphering the human genome (the Human Genome Project).

Restricted DNA fragments can be incorporated into plasmids cleaved by the same enzyme(s), and they can be cloned into bacteria after being sealed by a DNA ligase enzyme. Fragments from different sources can be manipulated to yield chimeric genes for research purposes, such as fusing the thyroglobulin gene promoter with the cDNA of an oncogene to study its targeted expression to thyroid cells.

Blotting

Blotting is a method of transferring deoxyribo- (Southern blotting) or ribo- (Northern blotting) nucleic acids from a gel onto a solid support after size fractionation by electrophoresis, prior to hybridization in aqueous solution.

Mixtures of DNA molecules can be easily and accurately sorted by size by means of electrophoresis in agarose or polyacrylamide gels. After chemical coloration, each DNA fragment will appear as a discrete band in the gel. Complex mixtures such as those obtained by restriction cleavage of total genomic DNA will result in smears instead of discrete bands. Molecular hybridization with a specific probe can then be used to reveal one band of interest after transfer and immobilization on a solid support such as a nylon or nitrocellulose membrane.

Similarly, the population of RNA molecules extracted from a tissue or a cell culture can be size-fractionated by electrophoresis, transferred on a membrane, and hybridized in solution to a specific probe (Northern blotting). This is a very efficient first-step method to study gene expression: once a new gene is cloned, it can be used as a probe to hybridize RNA preparations from various tissues after electrophoresis in parallel lanes. Results will show the range of cell types that express the gene, the relative intensity of expression, and the size of the full-length mRNA, which sometimes vary among cell types because of alternative splicing.

Polymerase chain reaction

The polymerase chain reaction (PCR) is an extremely sensitive method for detection and analysis of nucleic acids and is based on exponential in vitro (cell-free) replication of DNA that yields substantial amplification of a target sequence of interest. PCR is only possible if the target nucleic acid sequence is known and if it is of relatively short length (a few hundred bases, a few thousand at most).

Two synthetic (single-stranded) oligonucleotides are designed that are complementary to properly spaced segments of the target, with their 3'-OH extremities facing each other. Chemical amounts of the primers and four deoxynucleotides are mixed with minute amounts of target DNA and a special DNA-dependent DNA polymerase that resists very high temperatures. After denaturation of the reaction mix, the oligonucleotides are allowed to anneal to the target. Each oligo anneals to one strand and primes the synthesis of the complementary strand toward the other oligo, which produces two copies of the original target sequence. The three steps (melting of the target duplex, annealing of the primers, and elongation) are directed by the temperature of the reaction mix (e.g., circa 94 °C for denaturation, 55 °C for annealing, and 72 °C for elongation; the annealing temperature is very dependent on the sequence of the primer segment). The procedure is repeated about 30 to 40 times, which in theory will yield about 2^{30} to 2^{40} copies of the initial amount of target molecules, that is a 10^6 to 10^9 amplification factor. High specificity is provided by the sequences of the two primers and the convergent synthesis of each strand toward the other, which allows for annealing in the next cycle. Each cycle lasts about a few minutes, so the whole procedure takes a few hours. Automated thermal cyclers have been commercialized by several companies for more than a decade.

The PCR can be adjusted to target RNA molecules. This requires reverse transcription of RNA into complementary DNA (cDNA) prior to PCR amplification, which is referred to as reverse-transcription-PCR (RT-PCR).

Polymerase chain reaction may serve merely for the detection of nucleic acid, or it may be followed by analysis of the amplimer, such as a search for a mutation by use of restriction enzyme digestion, allele-specific oligonucleotide hybridization, or direct sequencing. Polymerase chain reaction is so sensitive that it can be used to detect and analyze a single target molecule, as in polar bodies or single blastomeres before the implantation of embryos. High sensitivity also allows RT-PCR to study illegitimate transcripts found in minute amounts in white blood cells, such as the thyroid-specific mRNA of the thyrotropin receptor.

High sensitivity is also a limitation of the method, as positive signals are often detected that have no physiological relevance. This method is also very liable to contamination within the laboratory.

Cloning vectors

A vector is a portion of bacterial or yeast genetic material made to accommodate a segment of foreign DNA, called an *insert*, such as a piece of DNA obtained from a tissue sample. The segment is obtained in order to multiply it and isolate it to clonal purity. Bacterial plasmid vectors are still widely used and allow for the cloning of relatively small (maximum size about 5-8 kb) DNA fragments in bacterial cells. Wild-type plasmids have been improved over the years to increase the number of copies per bacterial cell and to facilitate manipulation by restriction enzymes.

Vectors derived from bacteriophage viruses like the lambda phage can accommodate cosmid vectors of larger (15-20 kb) and still larger (30-50 kb) DNA fragments. More recently, artificial chromosomes of bacterial (BACs) and yeast (YACs) strains became available for cloning very large, gene-sized DNA fragments of about 100 kb and 300 to 1000 kb, respectively.

Library screening

A *library*, or *bank*, is a population of inserts covering a complex range, such as an entire mammalian genome (genomic library). *Screening* consists of identifying an insert of interest within the library such as one particular gene (or gene fragment) within the genome. A molecular probe generated from the extremity of a genomic insert can be used to screen genomic libraries for other clone(s). Repeating the operation several times (*chromosome walking*) yields an extended set of clones with overlapping inserts, called a *contig*, which encompasses a precise chromosomal segment. Technical short-cuts to this strategy are sometimes referred to as chromosome *jumping*. Contigs of large inserts in BAC or YAC vectors allow for the physical mapping of vast genomic areas.

A cDNA library is constructed from the population of mRNAs extracted from a particular tissue by use of a reverse transcriptase enzyme, followed by their insertion into a bacteriophage cloning vector. Infection of plated bacteria allows for the molecular probing of clone(s) of interest. In addition, some vectors are designed to express the protein product encoded by the cDNA insert, which allows for immunologic screening, provided the insert is cloned in the right coding triplet phase.

Sequencing

Sequencing refers to analyzing the primary structure of a biopolymer. Chemical techniques are effective on relatively small portions of polypeptides and somewhat larger polynucleotides, and enzymic DNA sequencing made it possible to decipher kb-sized fragments in relatively short periods of time. Current techniques use fluorescent dyes in sequencing reactions and can be coupled to semi-automated, computerized reading with a laser beam.

Fluorescent in situ hybridization

Fluorescent in situ hybridization (FISH) couples molecular and cytogenetic techniques to locate genes on chromosomes. Medium-sized probes, typically inserts from cosmid vectors, are denatured and hybridized directly on preparations of human (or rodent) chromosomes, deproteinized and denatured, and mounted on microscope slides. The hybridization signal is revealed under the microscope by means of a fluorescent label. Countercoloration provides identification of the chromosomal pair that produces a hybridization signal.

FISH has proven to be efficient for locating newly characterized genomic DNA fragments in the genome, and it can reveal chromosomal deletions or duplications that are too small for detection by conventional cytogenetics. Elaborate sets of probes that cover most of a chromosome length (painting probes) are now commercially available for each chromosome pair and can be used to reveal subtle translocations that escape conventional cytogenetics. Painting probes can be generated from a total genome of interest, to be competitively hybridized with painting probes form a normal, control genome labeled with another fluorescent marker (comparative genome hybridization, CGH). This approach is promising for the study of small chromosomal deletions, insertions, or duplications in cancer cells; and for the study of rare syndromes with multiple congenital anomalies presumed to be caused by submicroscopic chromosomal abnormalities.

Transfection

Cloned DNA can be artificially introduced into cultured cells by various transfection methods, upon which expression of the DNA product may be assayed. Expression assays can then be used to study the effects of mutations by comparing the functional properties of normal (wild type) and mutated molecules after transfection. Transfection can serve to study gene promoter sequences (sequences that regulate gene transcription) and the effects of mutations there. In such studies, the regulatory sequence of interest is fused to a reporter gene whose expression in a suitable cell line will directly reflect transcription.

Transfection does not require that the foreign DNA be integrated into the host genome. Integration, however, may be desirable in order to obtain a stable recombinant cell line.

Transgenics

Transgenesis is the introduction of forcing DNA into a whole animal, which allows for global in vivo analysis. The animal most often used is the mouse.

Random integration Cloned foreign DNA is introduced by physical methods into fertilized eggs, which are then placed in the uterus of a properly conditioned female mouse for gestation. After birth, pups are tested for the presence of the foreign DNA (the transgene), and the transgenic animals can be subjected to further study. In this approach, the foreign DNA may be fused to a tissue-specific promoter in order to target its expression to the tissue of interest.

Knock-out Transgenesis can target a particular gene at its locus in the host genome and disrupt its message, that is, "knock-out" (KO) the gene in question. A mutation is introduced artificially (site-directed mutagenesis) in a cloned copy of the murine gene or gene portion. The construct is then introduced in very early murine embryonic

cells. Immortalized, pluripotent embryonic stem cells have been developed for this purpose. In a proportion of cases, the mutated foreign DNA will pair with its wild-type counterpart at its chromosomal locus in the embryonic stem cell and be exchanged by a cellular machinery in a process called homologous recombination. The net result is the introduction of the site-directed mutation within the endogenous gene. The embryonic stem cells are introduced into blastocysts from a mouse strain and re-implanted into pseudogestant females. Successful gene targeting results in chimeric offspring with chimeric germlines. Further crossing of the chimeras produces two sorts of progeny: wild type and heterozygous knock-out transgenics. Homozygous transgenics are obtained by interbreeding. Knock-out mice are powerful tools to study precisely defined gene defects in vivo.

Knock-in Gene targeting can be refined to introduce another gene in lieu of the knock-out. For example, replacing the murine gene of the β^3-adrenergic receptor by the human gene produces humanized "knock-in" mice that allows for, among other things, the pharmacological analyses of selective β^3 agonists that are active on the human receptor that are not necessarily active on β^3-receptors in other mammals such as mice.

Conditional knock-out Permanent disruption of a gene product in all tissues may sometimes blunt the observable effect in the tissue of interest. For example, some genes are required for embryonic development, and unconditional knock-out simply results in miscarriage. Others are expressed in interplaying tissues, and the primary effect of their disruption is unclear. Therefore, the knock-out methodology has been further refined to depend on the conditional expression of another transgene, the latter being fused to a tissue-specific promoter that directs its expression to the organ of interest.

STRUCTURE OF THE GENOME

The nuclear genome Our genetic makeup consists of approximately 80 000 genes distributed over 23 chromosomes. The haploid genome is made of 3×10^9 base pairs of DNA, where genes represent about 10 to 30% of total DNA length, and the other 70 to 90% having no function known to date. Genes themselves contain introns, of which large portions have no apparent function either, so that most of the genome does not code for a product. Introns perhaps represent no more than a relic of evolution history.

Most expressed genes correspond to unique DNA sequences (*single copy genes*), but some genes are present in several copies. Duplicates of genes often escape selection pressure because of functional redundancy, and hence accumulate mutations, becoming inactive *pseudogenes*. Clustered pseudogenes may pose technical problems in cloning or in clinical diagnosis. On the other hand, gene duplication followed by divergence of sequence and function is a basic mechanism of evolution that can be traced over species. For example, thyroperoxidase and myeloperoxidase arose from the duplication of a common peroxidase ancestor, followed by the addition of exonic material that made thyroperoxidase membrane-bound. Thyroperoxidase and myeloperoxidase sequences share a significant similarity in the portion of cDNA or protein that is derived from their common ancestor. Of note, thyroperoxidase and myeloperoxidase are located on different chromosomes. Indeed, many large chromosomal segments have similar, *paralogous* counterparts in other chromosomes that are derived from an ancient duplication that is followed by complex chromosomal rearrangements frozen in speciation and functional divergence.

Duplications in tandem are found in countless places of the genome, giving rise to clusters of genes with related but different functions, such as the interleukin gene cluster on chromosome 2 that contains genes for IL-1 and related molecules. Large families of genes arose by both mechanisms of tandem duplication and chromosome shuffling, as illustrated by the superfamily of G protein-coupled receptors, whose thousand members or so share a common structure with seven transmembrane domains.

Pairs of chromosomes (one from each parent) contain the two *allelic* copies of each single copy gene. An exception stands for genes located on the XY pair, as human males are constitutively hemizygous for X-located genes. X and Y are called *gonosomes* (sexual chromosomes), the other pairs being *autosomes* (autosomal chromosomes). Microscopic examination of the chromosomes, or *cytogenetics*, allows, after appropriate staining, the unambiguous identification of each pair from its banding pattern. In a standard karyotype, the 23 chromosomes all together display about 450 to 550 bands. Thus, the smallest visible cytogenetic band contains a huge amount of DNA material, and each visible band, on average, represents over 5 Mb and 100 different genes. This order of magnitude corresponds to the limit of resolution of traditional cytogenetics. FISH methods address sizes that are intermediate between cytogenetic and molecular methods, which were once referred to as the "megabase gap."

The mitochondrial genome

Mitochondria also contain DNA, organized as a circular molecule of 16 kb and present in many copies per organelle. Mitochondrial DNA (mtDNA) is very dense in genetic information and has essentially no introns. It codes for specific mitochondrial rRNAs and tRNAs and for some of the polypeptide chains found in the respiratory complexes involved in oxidative phosphorylations. The other mitochondrial proteins are encoded by chromosomal genes, synthesized in the cytoplasm, and imported into the mitochondria.

Polymorphisms

Virtually any observable character exists in several normal versions. The first genetic polymorphisms studied consisted of protein markers such as blood groups, the HLA, and a few serum proteins. The DNA molecule itself is extremely polymorphic. In its non-coding (intergenic or intronic) portions, DNA is estimated to vary at 1/500 base pairs from one chromosomal copy to another. DNA polymorphisms are inherited. Segregation analysis enables one to draw a map of ordered polymorphic sites along each chromosome, with measures of genetic distances between them. Appropriately located polymorphic sites may in turn serve as markers to study the familial transmission of nearby genes. The more polymorphic a locus, the more informative its segregation analysis can be in a given family or population. *Heterozygosity* measures the mean probability for a polymorphic site to be represented by two different alleles in one individual.

By definition, a variation found in normal subjects will be called a polymorphism if its rarest allele has a frequency of at least 1% in the population. If less frequent, it is called a *rare normal variant*.

Single nucleotide polymorphisms and restriction fragment length polymorphisms

A single nucleotide polymorphism (SNP) is a harmless variation of one base pair found in the normal population that constitutes a marker locus with two or more alleles. The long-used technique of restriction fragment length polymorphism (RFLP) deals with those SNPs that by chance affect the site of a restriction endonuclease, thereby impeding DNA cleavage there. The presence or absence of cleavage may be denoted as a + or − sign. RFLPs are still widely used, but they show limited heterozygosity, and they have been gradually replaced by the more informative short tandem repeats. RFLPs, however, are but a fraction of SNPs, the majority of which will eventually be amenable to rapid and efficient routine analysis.

Short tandem repeat polymorphisms

Tandem repeats of very short sequences (2 to 6 bp) are found in innumerable places throughout the non-coding genome, and the number of repeats is frequently polymorphic. Short tandem repeat (STR) polymorphisms, or microsatellites, have a precise locus each and are inherited in a mendelian way, except for very occasional variations in size when transmitted to offspring. Short tandem repeats can readily be typed by PCR using primers that hybridize to flanking, invariant DNA sequences. The amplimers are size-fractionated by gel electrophoresis, and the number of repeats of each allele is computed from the fragment size.

Variable number of tandem repeats (VNTR) polymorphisms

This variant of Southern blot-coupled RFLPs is also called minisatellite polymorphism. It consists of somewhat longer stretches of nucleotides, usually 8 to 30 base pairs long, that are repeated up to several hundred times in tandem, with a number of repeats varying greatly from one allele to another. Detection is obtained by cleavage outside of the repeats with an appropriate restriction enzyme, size-fractionation by gel electrophoresis, Southern blotting, and hybridization with a locus-specific probe. Although usually quite informative, minisatellite VNTRs are cumbersome as compared to microsatellite STR polymorphisms.

Two loci on two different chromosomes will be transmitted together by chance to an offspring, or be separated, with equal 50% probability. By contrast, two loci that lie in the vicinity of each other on one chromosome will often be transmitted together, but not systematically because of meiotic recombinations (crossing overs) that occur randomly at least once per chromosomal arm in each normal meioses. Thus, the closer two loci are on a chromosome, the less often they will be separated by crossing over at meiosis, and the observed frequency of recombination is a measure of the *genetic distance* between them. The latter is measured in Morgan units: one centimorgan (1 cM) is the genetic distance between loci separated in 1% of gametes. Loci less than 50 cM apart are genetically linked. Regardless of linkage, the co-location of genes on the same chromosome is called *synteny*. Genetic and physical distances roughly correlate, with about 1 Mb for 1 cM. Thus, the whole genome (3 Mb) represents about 30 Morgans.

Segregation analysis is the study of the transmission, in families, of two or more characters. If one locus is known, loci of linked characters can be ordered around it, yielding a genetic map of the chromosome. The characters involved may be genetic disorders or harmless polymorphisms. The current map of the human genome includes several hundred genetic disorders and several thousand polymorphic loci, which provides an infra-centimorgan, infra-megabase resolution. Besides meiotic recombinations, the *radiation hybrids* approach has greatly increased mapping resolution. It takes advantage of experimental cell systems where irradiation-induced random chromosomal breakages are traceable, and it computes distances between loci from their probability of being separated by irradiation.

The genome project

An international effort aimed at deciphering the whole sequence of the human genome should be completed around the year 2005. The project includes mapping of known genetic traits and diseases as well as DNA polymorphic sites on each human chromosome. It should identify each of the estimated 80 000 human genes and characterize the genomic structures between them. The already cloned genes and DNA fragments provide sequence information but currently cover only a small portion of the genome. For any locus, the surrounding genome portion is physically available in the form of a large insert within a YAC or BAC vector and can be subjected to further study such as refined restriction mapping and systematic sequencing. Sequence-tagged sites are convenient markers for large genomic clones. A sequence-tagged site consists of any unique sequence readily amplifiable by PCR whose chromosomal locus can be mapped unambiguously.

Genetic databases that collect all of the information defined above are enhanced on a daily basis and made public on the Internet in nearly real-time by several organizations (such as the CEPH and the U.S. National Institutes of Health).

Cloning human genes

Functional cloning and positional cloning The biochemical and functional study of a genetic disorder can sometimes lead to the purification of the defective protein, and from there to gene isolation via partial protein sequencing and antibody or molecular probing. This functional ("traditional" or "direct") cloning approach has been almost completely supplanted by positional cloning, that is, cloning based solely on genetic data. This allows for gene characterization without prior knowledge of gene function. Positional cloning is based on linkage analysis in families with multiple affected members. A polymorphic marker locus is systematically searched for whose inheritance follows that of the disease, which locates the disease gene close to the marker locus. Further linkage studies delineate more precisely the chromosomal region that contains the gene until it is small enough for all transcripts from the region to be studied systematically. Several lines of evidence can be used to identify the actual transcript searched for, among which is the range of organs that express it, and the observation of mutations in patients that do not occur in control subjects. The isolation of the *CFTR* gene responsible for cystic fibrosis was one of the first demonstrations of how successful positional cloning can be. The biological function of the CFTR was thoroughly investigated after positional cloning of the gene. This dramatically improved the knowledge of the disease and the understanding of normal ion transport in epithelia.

Occasionally, positional cloning can be made much easier by the observation of a patient carrying a visible chromosomal rearrangement that disrupts the gene in search. Such patients, however, are rare.

Candidate gene approach Partial functional or biochemical data may allow investigators to determine what gene is defective in a particular disorder, thus enabling them to study it directly for disease-causing mutations in selected patients, provided the normal counterpart of the gene is already known.

Candidate gene testing can be fruitfully coupled with positional cloning. Linkage analysis is first used to map the gene of interest to a relatively small chromosomal region. Known genes that map to that region are then considered, and plausible candidates are further tested.

Animal models Genetic data in animals are often transposable to man, provided that the human gene has a counterpart in the model animal. For example, the study of genetically obese mice strains led to the identification of the murine genes for leptin and the leptin receptor, thereby opening a new field of investigation in human obesity. A great advantage in this is the possibility of experimental genetics in animals, such as inbreeding to obtain pure strains. Besides the usually strong conservation of gene function among mouse and man, large chromosomal portions retain the same general organization in mammals (conservation of synteny), which facilitates the identification of candidate genes in one species after mapping the locus in another.

In different species, genes encoding truly homologous products in terms of structure and function are called *orthologs*. It must be stressed, however, that not all genes are amenable to cross-species studies, and that structurally related genes may have different functions in different species. This caveat also applies to in vitro-created animal models, that is, transgenics.

DIAGNOSIS OF GENETIC DISEASE

Mutations

Strictly speaking, mutations are disease-causing, heritable alterations of the genetic make-up. Mutations are stable alterations, but exceptions do exist. Mutations may involve vast chromosomal regions (large-scale deletions, duplications, insertions, or rearrangements), or smaller ones. Mutations that affect a single (or a few) base pairs are called *point mutations*.

Mutations may affect germ cells or somatic cells. In the latter case, they will be heritable in daughter somatic cells only. The study of somatic mutations mostly concerns neoplasia and may take advantage of comparing genomic DNA extracted from the tumor with germ-line DNA (extracted from the patient's blood or non-neoplastic tissue). The differences reflect the tumorigenic pathway. Of note, the heterozygous loss of an anti-oncogene expressed in normal tissue, a frequent event in cancer, can often be traced via the loss of polymorphic markers closely linked to the anti-oncogene. Markers for which the patient is constitutively (i.e., germinally) heterozygous are informative, producing an image of *loss of heterozygosity* in the tumor.

Normal pluricellular organisms contain many mutations, as more than one replication error is expected in each cell cycle. The vast majority of somatic replication errors are clinically silent, either because they produce no functional effect or are lethal for the mutated cell, or because they remain confined to a very small clonal population. Significant exceptions are somatic mutations occurring in the embryo or fetus, which expand with normal growth and development to form a mosaic cell line; and mutations that confer a proliferation advantage to the mutated cell, which cause clonal expansion over normal cells and neoplasia.

Many germinally inherited mutations also have no functional consequence and represent harmless polymorphisms. The functional effect of a mutation may be classified as neutral, loss of function, or gain of function. The type of mutation – in other words, the molecular pathology of the gene – may sometimes help in functional interpretation.

Mendelian disorders (simply inherited disorders)

Some germinally inherited mutations are sufficient to cause disease. Accordingly, transmission of the mutation to the offspring will be accompanied by transmission of the disease as described by Mendel's laws of genetics. Such genetic disorders are called mendelian, or monogenic, or "stricto sensu" genetic disorders, or "simply inherited disorders".

Mendelian diseases are transmitted as autosomal dominant, autosomal recessive, or X-linked when caused by heterozygous, homozygous, or hemizygous (X chromosome in the male) mutations, respectively. This classification is oversimplified because most autosomal disorders show some clinical expression in both heterozygous and homozygous states, and most X-linked conditions show some expression in the heterozygous carrier female, but these distinctions nonetheless remain useful in diagnosis and genetic counseling.

It is important to realize that the familial nature of many diseases may not be apparent because of the small sizes of the sibships and of incomplete *penetrance*, which is defined as the percentage of mutation carriers that express the disease. Moreover, fresh mutations (neomutations) can cause autosomal dominant disorders and be absent from both parents. Nonetheless, it is essential to recognize familial expression and mode of inheritance when present.

Genetic heterogeneity refers to the observation that various mutations may cause the same clinical disorder. Various mutations of one gene represent *allelic* heterogeneity, such as the several mutations of the *RET* proto-oncogene encountered in families with indistinguishable syndromes of multiple endocrine neoplasia (MEN), type 2a. *Locus* (non-allelic) heterogeneity is exemplified by the MODY phenotype, which can result from mutations of the glucokinase gene on chromosome 7, the *HNF-1* gene on chromosome 12, the *HNF-4* gene on chromosome 20, or the *IPF1* gene on chromosome 13. Improved definition of associated phenotypes may sometimes resolve genetic heterogeneity, such as the identification of endocrine tumor sites in type 1 versus type 2 MEN, the corresponding genes being located on chromosome 11 and chromosome 10, respectively.

Direct and indirect genetic diagnoses

Direct genetic diagnosis means detecting a mutation of known pathogenic significance; it may be seen as anatomopathology at the molecular level. For example, detection in blood DNA of a *c-RET* proto-oncogene mutation that changes cysteine into tyrosine in position 634 of the polypeptide allows for the diagnosis of MEN2A, either already symptomatic or at the presymptomatic stage, and it mandates the prevention of specific neoplasia in the patient and presymptomatic diagnosis in unaffected, at-risk relatives.

In autosomal recessive disorders, patients with two different allelic mutations are referred to as *compound heterozygotes*, and they functionally behave like homozygotes. By contrast, *double heterozygosity* refers to normal carriers of two unrelated, non-allelic disorders.

In some disorders, a correlation exists between the type of mutation (genotype) and clinical severity (phenotype). The latter, however, usually depends on many other determinants, which make predictions in the individual patient uncertain. As a rule, mutation detection currently allows investigators to reach a final diagnosis but has variable predictive value on clinical outcome.

By contrast, indirect genetic diagnosis concerns families affected with a clinically diagnosed mendelian disorder. It consists of segregation analysis of the corresponding locus in order to deduce which alleles an at-risk relative has inherited. For example, when the MEN2 gene was mapped near polymorphic markers of the pericentromeric region of chromosome 10, and before its identity with proto-oncogene *c-RET* was known, segregation analysis in MEN2 families (at least two patients with clinically certain MEN2) allowed for the diagnosis in additional relatives by comparing the alleles of linked markers they had inherited. The use of intragenic or of very close polymorphic markers, or of markers flanking the gene locus, minimizes errors from meiotic recombinations. Locus heterogeneity remains a potential cause of error, and clinical misdiagnosis of MEN2 for MEN1 would have caused that type of error here. Despite these limitations, indirect diagnosis remains a basic tool in clinical genetics and molecular biology, especially when a great number of mutations of one single gene (allelic heterogeneity) makes direct diagnosis cumbersome. If many affected family members are available for DNA sampling, segregation analysis may help confirm linkage to the culprit gene prior to presymptomatic testing in additional family members.

Non-Mendelian inheritance

Fresh mutations (neomutations) A fresh mutation in one particular egg or sperm cell may produce an effect in the offspring though it is absent from the parents. Such DNA replication errors in germ-line cells are responsible for the new occurrence of autosomal dominant or X-linked disorders, which are not inherited from the parents but will be in the next generations, following Mendel's laws of genetics in the descendants. Neomutations contribute a significant proportion of mutations in very severe dominant or X-linked disorders where the patients are not fit enough to reproduce and transmit the mutated allele.

Fresh point mutations primarily result from the accumulation of DNA replication errors in the testis. Advanced paternal age is modestly but clearly associated with an increased incidence of new dominant disorders such as Marfan's syndrome and achondroplasia in children, and with an increased incidence of X-linked disorders such as hemophilia in male grandchildren.

Mosaicism Somatic mutations that occur early in embryogenesis may be present in a sizable proportion of the cells of an individual; this is referred to as carrying a mosaic cell line. Somatic mosaicism may explain, for example, focal neurofibromatosis type I from mutations of the gene that cause NF1 (Von Recklinghausen's disease) when germinally inherited. Individuals with mosaic cell lines are at risk of producing offspring with the full-blown disease because of germline mosaicism, that is, the presence of two populations of eggs or sperms, wild-type and mutated. Confined germ-line mosaicism is a mechanism by which an unaffected parent may produce several children

with the same autosomal dominant or X-linked genetic disorder, which is often initially attributed to a fresh mutation in the first affected child.

Mitochondrial disorders Mitochondrial DNA (mtDNA) is inherited exclusively through the female germline. Thus, mitochondrial mutations show maternal inheritance, and paternal inheritance of a genetic syndrome rules out mitochondrial origin. Maternal mtDNA mutations are transmitted to all children, and replication errors are frequent. With numerous mitochondria per cell and up to several hundred copies of mtDNA per organelle, new mutations often show heteroplasmy, that is, the presence of more than one mtDNA population per cell. Transmission through one ovum creates a bottleneck effect that drives toward homoplasmy for the original or mutated mtDNA in offspring.

Point mutations, usually homoplasmic, have been observed in association with well-described syndromes, and several lines of evidence have demonstrated a causal role for many of them. For example, a mutation of an adenine into guanosine in position 3243 of the mitochondrial genome, within the gene of the leucine-tRNA, causes a syndrome of progressive mitochondrial encephalopathy, lactic acidosis, and stroke-like episodes (MELAS), which may show maternal inheritance clinically. The same mutation has been associated with diabetes mellitus and perception deafness. Generally speaking, phenotypic expression is variable with mitochondrial mutations, and maternal inheritance may hence be difficult to recognize. As for mendelian diseases, environmental factors may be involved in phenotypic expression. This is obvious in the case of mitochondrial mutations causing susceptibility to hearing loss from aminoside antibiotics. The latter example also underscores the ill-defined boundary between mutations and polymorphisms in mitochondrial genetics.

Severe mtDNA alterations, such as mtDNA deletions, have not been described in the homoplasmic state, presumably because of lethality. Heteroplasmic deletions are found in several syndromes of multiorgan dysfunction that result from the progressive failure of cell respiration. Tissue mosaicism is usually superimposed on cell heteroplasmy, and the extent of tissue dysfunction correlates with the local ratio of mutated mtDNA on normal mtDNA.

Some mitochondrial diseases with mtDNA deletions or point mutations show mendelian inheritance, either autosomal dominant or recessive, which implies nuclear genes whose mutations eventually damage mtDNA. The Wolfram syndrome of diabetes insipidus, diabetes mellitus, optic atrophy, and deafness, shows multiple mtDNA deletions in affected tissues. It clearly follows autosomal recessive transmission, and positional cloning in affected families identified the responsible gene on the short arm of chromosome 4.

Imprinting Imprinting is an epigenetic mechanism by which an allele is expressed differently whether inherited from the father or the mother. It seems to involve only a marginal proportion of genes. Imprinting may blunt mendelian inheritance when a mutation is passed by a parent of the gender that physiologically silences the gene. If inherited by an offspring of the opposite gender, the mutation will produce its effects later when passed to the following generation. DNA methylation parallels gene inactivation at all imprinted loci known to date. For example, it appears that a submicroscopic region of chromosome 15q13 is imprinted during human oogenesis, with silencing of a particular gene(s), so that only the paternal copy is expressed in the offspring. Deletion of the q13 region of the paternally inherited chromosome 15 results in the Prader-Willi phenotype (hypotonia at birth, followed by hyperphagia, severe obesity, and moderate mental retardation). Interestingly, deletion of the maternal 15q13 segment results in another disease, Angelman's syndrome, which is associated with quite a different phenotype (profound mental retardation, ataxia, and paroxysmal laughter). This is due to the presence in the same genomic region of an additional gene with opposite imprinting (maternal copy active in offspring, paternal copy inactive). Inactivating mutations in the maternal copy of the Angelman gene also cause Angelman's syndrome and may show familial recurrence if transmitted by a normal woman carrying the mutation on her paternally inherited chromosome 15.

Mirror imprinting of unrelated, closely located genes has also been reported in chromosomal region 11p15, which is implicated in the Beckwith-Wiedemann syndrome (hyperinsulinism, disproportionate growth, malformations, and tumors).

Uniparental disomy In the absence of a point mutation or chromosomal deletion, genomic imprinting can, infrequently, cause disease via uniparental disomy, that is, inheritance of both copies of a particular chromosome (or part thereof) from one parent only. Uniparental disomy is subdivided into uniparental heterodisomy, that is, inheritance of both homologous chromosomes of one parental pair, and isodisomy, or inheritance of two copies of the same chromosome from one parent. Heterodisomy often results from age-related meiotic non-dysjunction during oogenesis. As an example, fecundation of an oocyte that is disomic for chromosome 15 will produce a zygote with trisomy 15, which is a condition not compatible with live birth. The pregnancy, however, may be rescued during embryonic life by the random loss of one chromosome 15, which restores disomy. Rescue loss of the paternal chromosome 15, however, results in the Prader-Willi phenotype. The standard karyotype of the fetus will appear normal (no numerical or structural anomaly), but maternal heterodisomy 15 will be evident on DNA analysis. With routine fetal karyotyping of pregnancies in women older than 35, a trace of the initial trisomy 15 is sometimes found as confined placental mosaicism.

Like heterodisomy, isodisomy may produce disease if it involves an imprinted gene(s). In addition, isodisomy is a rare cause of autosomal recessive disease by duplication to homozygosity of recessive parental mutations.

Although uniparental disomy seems a relatively rare event, cases have been discovered fortuitously in normal subjects that involved various portions of the genome, underscoring that imprinting is not a general phenomenon in the genome.

Multigenic/multifactorial disorders (complex traits)
Molecular genetics has proven effective in the mapping and eventual cloning of virtually any simply inherited (Mendelian) character. The entirely genetic strategy based on linkage and positional cloning can be adjusted to address complex traits, that is, characters that do not show strict dominant or recessive inheritance, such as diabetes, asthma, or hypertension. Complex heredity often arises from the involvement of several independent, unlinked genes (multigenic traits or disorders). Complexity can further result from non-genetic, environmental factors, such as allergen exposure, diet, or viral infection (multifactorial disorders). Diabetes type II (NIDDM) is an example of a multigenic disorder. Its genetic nature is evident from its very high concordance rate among monozygotic twins, even if separated at birth, in contrast to its otherwise small trend toward familial aggregation, including low concordance among dizygotic twins. Although essentially genetic in nature, NIDDM is not truly hereditary.

Sib pair analysis is a genome-wide linkage approach that aims at mapping genes involved in polygenic inheritance. In siblings, copies of the same parental allele of a gene or polymorphic marker are referred to as *identical by descent*. Statistically, for any locus, a common identical-by-descent allele is found in 50% of siblings. Analysis of a large number of pairs of siblings affected with the same multifactorial disorder can identify DNA markers found to be identical-by-descent with a frequency significantly different from 50%, pointing to the presence of a nearby gene involved in the pathogenesis of the disorder, and amenable to positional cloning. The latter step may pose a problem, as a vast contribution of missense mutations with only a partial effect on gene function – which is hard to demonstrate in experimental assays – are expected to be responsible for the modest genetic contribution of each locus, which can make the final identification of the culprit genes difficult. In recent years, analyses of pairs of siblings with IDDM confirmed the major implication of the genomic region bearing the HLA complex on chromosome 6, and pointed to other genomic regions, among which was the locus of the insulin gene on chromosome 11. Presumably, quantitative variations in insulin gene expression may increase or reduce the risk of developing IDDM, but this remains to be demonstrated, and the involvement of another, closely linked gene remains a possibility.

As in mendelian traits, the genome-wide strategy can be coupled with the candidate gene approach. Missense mutations in the extracellular domain of the TSHr that show little if any effect on receptor function in vitro have been reported as more frequent in Grave's disease patients than in the general population. While the rationale of a polymorphism in an epitope favoring an autoimmune response makes sense, a genome-wide approach such as sib pair analysis is needed to give a global, unbiased view of the respective importance of the loci involved.

PRINCIPLES OF GENE THERAPY

Gene therapy is a field of research with no established direct clinical applications as yet. Gene therapy may be defined as treatment based on the transfer of genetic material to the patient, whatever the nature of disease.

By definition, gene therapy does not only address genetic diseases stricto sensu, but also acquired metabolic, viral, neoplastic, or other disorders that can be cured or improved by the transfer of genetic material. Mendelian disorders are relatively simple models for research, but they should eventually represent only a limited field of application. The financial price of clinical gene therapy will probably be a major burden in coming years.

Safety considerations are of prime importance in gene therapy approaches. Among others, concerns about iatrogenic alteration of germ-line DNA have motivated a general ban on germinal gene therapy, and restricted research to gene transfer to somatic cells (somatic gene therapy).

Current efforts aim at improving vectors used to transduce genetic material to the target cells in terms of efficacy of expression of therapeutic insert DNA, and in terms of immunogenicity and infectious hazard, as many vectors derive from human viruses. Regarding possible iatrogenic germ-line alterations, it must be stressed that the question theoretically applies to any treatment that allows patients to transmit their genes to children they would not have produced without treatment. As an example, cystic fibrosis patients who previously died in childhood now fortunately reach adulthood and have children, to whom they transmit their genes, primarily due to the benefits of antibiotherapy and nutritional care. A final ban on germinal gene therapy should thus logically raise many questions in other fields of medicine.

While rightly raising great hope in the treatment of hereditary diseases, gene therapy is still far from representing an alternative to prevention by prenatal diagnosis. Clinical benefit seems closer in neoplastic disorders (by transducing anti-oncogenes and/or silencing oncogenes in tumors) and viral disorders (by silencing crucial viral genes and/or enhancing specific defense mechanisms).

Suggested readings

McKusick VA. Mendelian inheritance in man. Catalogs of human genes and genetic disorders. 12th ed. Baltimore: Johns Hopkins University Press, 1998 and Online Mendelian Inheritance in Man, OMIM (TM), Genetics, Johns Hopkins University (Baltimore, MD) and National Center for Biotechnology Information, National Library of Medicine (Bethesda, MD), 1999

World Wide Web URL: http://www.ncbi.nlm.nih.gov/omim/.

Rimoin DL, Connor JM, Pyeritz RE. Principles and practice of medical genetics. 3rd ed. New York: Churchill Livingstone, 1996.

Scriver CR, Beaudet AL, Sly WS, Valle D (eds). The metabolic and molecular bases of inherited disease. 7th ed. New York: McGraw-Hill, 1995.

Strachan T, Read AP. Human molecular genetics. Oxford: BIOS Scientific Publishers, 1999.

SECTION

2

Neuroendocrinology

CHAPTER 4

Neuroendocrinology

Andrew Levy, Stafford Lightman

ANATOMY AND PHYSIOLOGY OF THE HYPOTHALAMUS

Since the demonstration almost 90 years ago that hypothalamic damage produces gonadal deficiency in dogs, and the series of elegant transplantation experiments that followed Popa's identification of hypophyseal portal vessels, the hypothalamus has been recognized as the major, central integrator of the endocrine system. The generation of behavioral and hormonal rhythmicity, synthesis of vasopressin and oxytocin, regulation of hormone release from the anterior lobe of the pituitary gland, and response to feedback effects from distal endocrine organs are classical, well-recognized functions. There are also less well-known hypothalamus interfaces of considerable complexity through which limbic, autonomic, immune and higher cerebral functions are integrated with the endocrine system. Our understanding of these neuroendocrine relationships, and of the intricate interplay between the immune system, central nervous system, and endocrine system are still far from complete. Much of the work carried out to elucidate these relationships is descriptive, and in some cases considerable caution is required if results of anatomical and physiological studies carried out in rodents are to be directly extrapolated to man. This overview describes the main elements of the neuroendocrine system: the integration of higher brain function with the endocrine and immune systems via the hypothalamus.

Hypothalamic surface anatomy

The hypothalamus consists of two slightly wedge-shaped areas of tissue barely 15 mm in length, containing an extraordinary abundance of pathways, tracts, and cellular nuclei with unique functions (Figs. 4.1 in Color Atlas and 4.2). The surface markings of the free inferior surface of the hypothalamus approximate to the optic chiasm anteriorly and the optic tracts as they diverge from the chiasm on their way back to the midbrain. The most posterior extension of the hypothalamus is marked by the posterior poles of the mamillary bodies. Immediately behind the optic chiasm, the infundibulum, a region of the floor of the third ventricle, is pulled down into the median eminence, a

squat cone outside the blood brain barrier, at the tip of which, about 1 cm below the optic chiasm, is attached the pituitary gland. The two sides of the hypothalamus are separated by the slit-like third ventricle and joined anteriorly by the lamina terminalis, a thin sheet of tissue that crosses the midline and represents, embryologically, the most rostral extension of the neural tube. Between the optic chiasm below and the anterior commissure above lies a midline region of the lamina terminalis known as the organum vasculosum of the lamina terminalis. It separates the cerebrospinal fluid of the third ventricle from the cerebrospinal fluid of the prechiasmatic cistern and has its own blood supply distinct from that found in other circumventricular regions. Penetration of large molecules into the organum vasculosum of the lamina terminalis indicates that in this richly innervated region, the blood brain barrier is deficient. Anterior to the hypothalamus lies the cerebrospinal fluid in the prechiasmatic cistern.

Hypothalamic-limbic interactions

Dividing the hypothalamus arbitrarily into a medial and lateral segment along the plane of the fornix, the dominant feature of the lateral region, which merges imperceptibly with surrounding brain tissue, is the median forebrain bundle. This is a loose collection of longitudinal fibers interspersed with neuronal perikarya that links together the various hypothalamic nuclei with each other, with the midbrain, and with the limbic forebrain. The medial segment of the hypothalamus is extensively interconnected with the lateral division of the hypothalamus and contains a series of neuronal perikarya-rich nuclei, which project, amongst other locations, to the median eminence. The medial forebrain bundle, fornix and stria terminalis; by carrying hypothalamic afferents from the limbic forebrain, the hippocampus, and the amygdala, respectively; form a robust interface between the limbic and neuroendocrine systems. This interface allows higher brain areas implicated in the control of mood and emotions, hunger, libido, and the response to olfactory and gustatory information to directly impinge on the tuberoinfundibular system, which are the neurons that project down into the lateral zone of the median eminence.

Toward the upper pole of the lamina terminalis, a bulge marks the anterior commissure that carries the compact fiber bundles of the stria terminalis as they cross the midline. The stria terminalis arises in the amygdala, which are exposed superiorly and medially on the uncus of the temporal lobe, follows a C-shaped curve around the inferolateral margin of the lateral ventricle, and, after traversing the anterior commissure, divides into two loose bundles. These project to the ventromedial nucleus of the hypothalamus, which has rich connections with the arcuate nucleus, and to the bed nucleus of the stria terminalis, a large inferomedial nucleus positioned slightly anterolateral to the paraventricular nucleus of the hypothalamus. The superior surface of the hypothalamus is impaled by the fornix, a thick, curving fiber bundle carrying inhibitory afferents from the hippocampus – another limbic structure – to almost all areas of the hypothalamus before terminating in the mammillary bodies.

Hypothalamic-autonomic interactions

In addition to such close connections with the limbic system that the exclusion of the hypothalamus as a principal element of that system seems almost a taxonomic over-

sight, the hypothalamus receives extensive autonomic afferents from the brain stem, particularly the dorsomedial and ventrolateral medulla. Baroreceptor and atrial receptor afferents from the glossopharyngeal and vagus nerves reach the nucleus of the tractus solitarius in the dorsomedial medulla, from where they project principally to the parvocellular division of the paraventricular nucleus of the hypothalamus. Catecholaminergic fibers from the ventrolateral region of the caudal medulla oblongata also project to the hypothalamus via the ventral noradrenergic bundle, predominantly to the vasopressin-producing perikarya of the paraventricular nucleus and the supraoptic nucleus. The ventral noradrenergic bundle is part of the central tegmental tract in the dorsal brainstem that carries both noradrenergic and adrenergic fibers. In the caudal midbrain, a substantial proportion of the central tegmental tract runs dorsally to join axons from the locus ceruleus. The locus ceruleus receives afferent autonomic information from the heart and projects to the neocortex, hippocampus, and periventricular zone of the hypothalamus via the dorsal noradrenergic bundle. Direct electrical stimulation of the locus induces a pressor effect.

Peptidergic inputs to the hypothalamus

Many of the catecholaminergic neurons described above also contain neuropeptide Y (NPY), a peptide present in

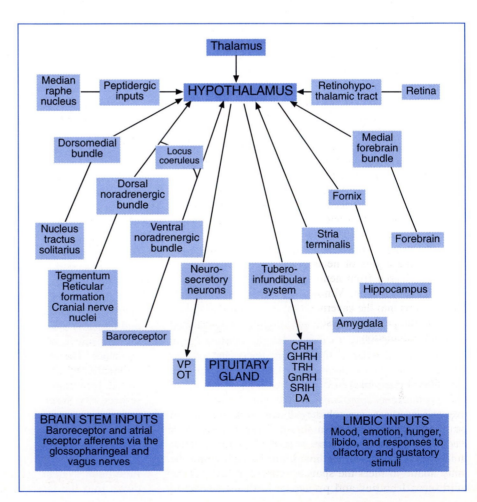

Figure 4.2 Schematic diagram of principal hypothalamic afferent and efferent pathways.

large amounts in the paraventricular nucleus, which also receives an NPY-ergic innervation from the arcuate nucleus. Anatomically closely related, the medial raphe nucleus of the brain stem projects serotonergic fibers to the suprachiasmatic nucleus, the anterior hypothalamus, and median eminence.

The suprachiasmatic nucleus, located above the optic chiasm in the same coronal plane as the paraventricular and supraoptic nuclei in the medial basal hypothalamus, receives serotonergic inputs from the medial raphe nucleus of the brainstem, as well as a direct input from the retina via the retinohypothalamic tract. The suprachiasmatic nucleus produces a diffusible substance that induces circadian rhythmicity, as suprachiasmatic cells grafted back into the rat hypothalamus in a semipermeable membrane restore circadian rhythm. Two distinct cellular populations undergo suprachiasmatic nucleus-induced circadian fluctuation: vasopressinergic somata that produce higher vasopressin levels in the morning than the evening, and vasoactive intestinal polypeptidergic neurons, which produce higher levels of vasoactive intestinal polypeptide in the evening.

Hypothalamic efferents

Hypothalamic efferents include ascending reciprocal projections to the limbic system (particularly the amygdala), the cortex, and the thalamus; and descending projections to the tegmentum, the reticular formation, and the cranial nerve nuclei. Cells in the paraventricular, supraoptic, periventricular, arcuate and medial pre-optic nuclei produce releasing- and release-inhibiting factors. These factors are transported first in the axons of the neurons that make them, often undergoing limited proteolytic cleavage to yield active peptides from pro-hormones in the maturing secretory vesicles, and are then released at the median eminence into the hypothalamo-hypophyseal portal system. Although the anterior lobe of the pituitary gland amplifies and modulates instructions passed down from the hypothalamus through neuropeptide release into the hypothalamo-hypophyseal portal system, there is no direct innervation between the hypothalamus and anterior pituitary. Vasopressin and oxytocin, synthesized in the paraventricular and supraoptic nuclei of the hypothalamus, are transported to the posterior lobe of the pituitary gland in the axons of neurosecretory neurons and are directly released from neurosecretory terminals into the systemic circulation. Venous blood from the pituitary gland drains into the cavernous sinuses on either side and then via the petrosal sinuses to the jugular veins and the systemic circulation.

NEUROTRANSMITTERS

Neurotransmitters are substances that induce target cell activity when released from the presynaptic terminals of "activated" or depolarized neurons. Many putative neurotransmitters have been identified (Tab. 4.1), but thus far, only about 40 meet the specific criteria of being found within cell bodies and presynaptic terminals, being released in response to stimulation of that neuron, and being shown to induce a response in target cells when the latter are exposed to the substance in question. The most familiar of these are the biogenic amines, such as acetylcholine, noradrenaline, adrenaline, dopamine and serotonin, and amino acid neurotransmitters such as glutamate, γ-aminobutyric acid and aspartate. There are also nucleotides such as adenosine and adenosine triphosphate (ATP), neuropeptides such as enkephalin and vasopressin, gut polypeptides such as cholecystokinin and somatostatin, and (probably) nitric oxide (Tab. 4.1).

Storage, release and mode of action

In most cases neurotransmitters or combinations of neurotransmitters are stored in small synaptic vesicles or large dense-cored vesicles near the site of eventual docking and membrane fusion following neuronal stimulation. Diffusion across the synaptic cleft is rapid, and the overall response time of postsynaptic neurons may take from several to several hundred microseconds, depending largely on whether the postsynaptic receptor is a ligand-gated ion channel or involves G protein-coupled mechanisms. Movement of sodium, potassium, calcium, and chloride ions through ligand-gated ion channels results in a rapid change in membrane potential and action potential generation. Ligand binding to G protein-coupled receptors, subsequent dissociation of the α from the βγ subunits, and

---

Table 4.1 Neurotransmitters

Small molecules	Pituitary peptides
Small molecules	**Pituitary peptides**
Biogenic amines	Vasopressin
Acetylcholine	Oxytocin
Monoamines	
Dopamine	**Tachykinins**
Noradrenaline	Substance P
Adrenaline	Neurokinins
Serotonin	Eledoisin
Histamine	
	Other polypeptides
Amino acids	Vasoactive intestinal
GABA	polypeptide
Glutamate	Glucagon
Glycine	Galanin
Aspartate	Secretin
Homocysteine	Growth hormone-releasing
Taurine	hormone
	Corticotropin-releasing
Nucleotides	hormone
Adenosine	Neuropeptide Y
ATP	Somatostatin
	Corticotropin-releasing
Neuropeptides	factor
Opioid peptides	Calcitonin gene-related
Enkephalins	peptide
β-endorphin	Cholecystokinin
Dynorphins	Angiotensin II
Propiomelanocortin	**Other**
	Nitric oxide

interaction of the various components with effector proteins such as adenylyl cyclase or ion channels is usually but not invariably a more prolonged affair. Once released, neurotransmitters are subjected to either rapid re-uptake or enzymatic degradation to limit the duration of effect. Substances that share the above characteristics but tend to remain in the synaptic cleft for longer periods and have more prolonged actions tend to be termed neuromodulators rather than neurotransmitters. Neurosecretion, as opposed to neurotransmission, refers to the release of hormone into the circulation from a nerve terminal and is typified by release of vasopressin or oxytocin from nerve terminals in the posterior lobe of the pituitary gland, or by adrenaline and noradrenaline release from the adrenal medulla directly into the circulation to influence distant organ systems.

Neurotransmitter functions

At present, our understanding of the specific functions of many of these neurotransmitters or neuromodulators in man is incomplete. Peptide neurotransmitters such as cholecystokinin, gastrin-releasing peptide, galanin, NPY, and substance P may modulate pituitary hormone secretion, particularly growth hormone (GH) and prolactin release. Corticotropin-releasing hormone, in addition to its complex hormonal roles, serves as a neurotransmitter at the level of the locus ceruleus, a small nucleus of almost entirely noradrenergic neurons near the dorsal surface of the rostral pons (see above).

HYPOTHALAMIC HORMONES

Corticotropin-releasing hormone

Identified in 1981, corticotropin-releasing hormone (CRH) is an essential modulator of the endocrine, metabolic, cardiovascular, and behavioral responses to stress. Synthesized in the paraventricular nucleus of the hypothalamus, CRH is released into the hypophyseal portal system from where it acts on type 1 receptors on pituitary corticotroph cells to exert a trophic effect and stimulate pro-opiomelanocortin (POMC) transcription and adrenocorticotropic hormone (ACTH) release. Exercise, acute stress, immobilization, systemic bacterial lipopolysaccharide, and treatment with interleukin 1β all stimulate CRH gene expression in the paraventricular nucleus, and the effects of CRH are restrained by adrenal cortical steroid feedback inhibition on type I mineralocorticoid and type II glucocorticoid receptors in the pituitary, hypothalamus, and hippocampus. Stress-induced CRH neuronal activity down-regulates the hypothalamo-pituitary-gonadal axis, indicating important cross-talk between CRH and gonadotropin-releasing hormone neuronal activity within the central nervous system.

CRH also functions as a classical neurotransmitter. CRH-ergic neurons in the central amygdala project to the lateral parts of the bed nucleus of the stria terminalis, the lateral hypothalamic area, the midbrain reticular formation, the medial and lateral parts of the parabrachial nucleus, the mesencephalic nucleus of the trigeminal nerve, and the dorsal vagal complex. CRH transcripts are found in the locus ceruleus and other noradrenergic cell groups in the brain stem, as well as the nucleus tractus solitarius and cerebral cortex. In this way the effects of CRH on the neuroendocrine response to stress are derived not only from CRH released into the median eminence, but also from the influence of CRH on ascending noradrenergic pathways in the brain stem.

Effects of CRH on mood

Since it was first reported that circulating cortisol levels are increased in depression, a number of studies have indicated a causal link between hypothalamo-pituitary-adrenal axis dysregulation and psychopathology. Major depressive episodes are characterized by enlargement of the zona fasciculata of the adrenal glands, an increase in the number of ACTH-secretory episodes and magnitude of cortisol-secretory episodes, elevation of circulating and urinary free cortisol, and an increase in the level of CRH in cerebrospinal fluid. Dexamethasone suppressibility of circulating cortisol levels is reduced in up to 50% of patients, and the ACTH response to CRH is blunted, probably through increased cortisol feedback. Persistence of many of these effects is associated with a worse prognosis, and successful treatment of depression tends to cause their resolution before the mood changes occur. Two-thirds of patients with Cushing's disease have major psychiatric pathology akin to depression, and as many as 10% attempt suicide. The related finding that antidepressants interfere not only with the production and release of catecholamines and indolamines, but also with the signal transduction of a number of neurotransmitters including CRH and with genes in the hypothalamo-pituitary-adrenal axis, further supports the concept that disturbed corticosteroid receptor function is closely related to the development of affective disorders.

CRH is highly expressed in human placenta at the end of gestation, and circulating levels are high enough (if unencumbered) to activate the pituitary adrenal axis. The association between maternal plasma CRH concentrations in the second trimester of pregnancy and the duration of pregnancy suggests that CRH is involved in regulating the timing of parturition. Central suppression of hypothalamic CRH secretion postpartum has been implicated in the vulnerability of women to affective disorders (postpartum "blues") during this time.

Vasopressin and oxytocin

Vasopressin, a nonapeptide first identified in 1954, is synthesized in the paraventricular and supraoptic nuclei of the hypothalamus and secreted from the terminals of neurosecretory nerve terminals that run from there to the neurohypophysis (the posterior lobe of the pituitary gland). The principal physiological role of vasopressin is to reduce the urinary excretion of water by enhancing its reabsorption from filtrate in the distal and collecting tubules of the kidney. In this respect the secretion of vasopressin is influenced principally by changes in plasma osmotic pressure, sensed by osmoreceptors situated near the lamina terminalis at the anterior hypothalamus. When osmolality falls below 280 mOsm/l or sodium falls below 135 mmol/l in healthy adults, plasma vasopressin falls to undetectable levels and urine reaches maximal dilution (<100 mOsm/kg). Only in exceptional circumstances such as psychiatric illness or potomania is it possible to drink enough to lower plasma osmolality below the normal range. At plasma osmolalities of about 295 mOsm/l and a sodium concentration of 145 mM, vasopressin reaches levels that produce maximum antidiuresis (urine osmolality >800 mOsm/l: urine flow <1 ml/min) and thirst is stimulated.

Changes in vasopressin secretion can also occur in response to acute changes in blood pressure and volume. These changes are mediated by pressure sensitive atrial and arterial receptors that communicate with the neurohypophysis by way of multisynaptic neuronal afferents in the cranial nerves, medulla, and pons.

Vasopressin is not only found in the magnocellular cells of the paraventricular and supraoptic nuclei of the hypothalamus that project to the posterior pituitary, but it is also expressed in parvocellular cells of the paraventricular nucleus, which are the same cells that contain CRH and project to the median eminence. Like CRH, vasopressin in the parvocellular division of the paraventricular nucleus is negatively regulated by circulating glucocorticoids and positively regulated during stress. Vasopressin released into portal blood causes ACTH release and has a synergistic action with CRH. In some chronic conditions it may even be the major ACTH secretogogue.

Oxytocin is the other peptide released by direct neurosecretion. It is synthesized in cell bodies in the magnocellular paraventricular nucleus and supraoptic nucleus and released from terminals of the same neurons that project to the posterior pituitary. In anticipation of and during suckling, oxytocin is released simultaneously from almost all of the oxytocin-secreting hypothalamo-neurohypophyseal neurons. The resulting pulse of oxytocin induces myoepithelial cell contraction and milk ejection. At the same time, oxytocin-induced myometrial contractions are thought to promote the return of the uterus to pregravid proportions.

Neurotransmitter functions

In addition to vasopressin and oxytocin release from magnocellular cells into the systemic circulation via the posterior pituitary, which are targeted predominantly to the kidneys, myometrium, and breast, various regions of the central nervous system also express vasopressin and oxytocin receptors. Vasopressin receptors are found in the hypothalamic arcuate nucleus as well as the suprachiasmatic nucleus, where neuronal excitation by endogenous vasopressin may well contribute to the circadian cycle of electrical activity in this structure. Oxytocin receptors have been identified toward the front of the hypothalamus in the area of the ventromedial nucleus and bed nucleus of the stria terminalis, one of the afferent targets of the amygdala. Oxytocin receptors, unlike vasopressin receptors, are induced by female sex hormones, and central administration of oxytocin produces sexual and maternal behavioral effects as well as the milk ejection reflex in rodents.

Thyrotropin releasing hormone

Thyrotropin-releasing hormone (TRH) is a cyclic tri-peptide, first characterized in 1970, that is widely distributed throughout the central nervous system. High levels of transcription are found in the hypothalamus, hippocampus, cerebral cortex, cerebellum, and spinal cord, as well as the gastrointestinal tract and retina. TRH-producing cells within the paraventricular nucleus of the hypothalamus are largely responsible for the TRH found in portal blood and therefore for the effect of the peptide on anterior pituitary mammotrophs and thyrotrophs. TRH stimulates thyrotropin (thyroid-stimulating hormone, TSH) production by anterior pituitary thyrotrophs and, in man, prolactin production by mammotrophs. Evidence for a direct trophic effect of TRH at the anterior pituitary is not as strong as that for CRH or growth hormone-releasing hormone (GHRH); nevertheless, modest pituitary enlargement in hypothyroidism is common and in some cases may be extensive enough for visual field defects to develop through compression of the optic chiasm. Under basal conditions hypothalamic TRH transcriptional activity is under tonic inhibition by hippocampal inputs via the fornix. Hypothalamic TRH production is also feedback-regulated by circulating and locally deiodinated thyroid hormones acting at triiodothyronine (T_3) receptors. Stress, starvation, and isolated protein deprivation centrally down-regulate TRH production and produce a biochemical state that mimics central hypothyroidism. This condition, the 'sick euthyroid' or sometimes 'euthyroid sick' syndrome, is often seen in patients on intensive care and is not thought to be an indication for exogenous thyroid hormone replacement.

Neurotransmitter functions

There is increasing evidence that TRH has a generally excitatory neurotransmitter or neuromodulatory role. TRH has been shown to potentiate the effect of 5-hydroxytryptamine (5HT), and also to increase autonomic nervous system activity and biogenic amine neurotransmitter turnover (i.e., adrenaline, acetylcholine, noradrenaline, and dopamine). Centrally administered TRH has a neurotropic effect, stimulates axonal growth and myelination in motor neurons, and, transiently at least, reduces axonal degeneration in spinocerebellar degeneration. It also increases heart rate and blood pressure when injected intracerebroventricularly or by microinjection into the suprachiasmatic nucleus, and it increases gastric acid output when microinjected into the dorsal motor nucleus of the vagus nerve in the brain stem.

Gonadotropin-releasing hormone

Gonadotropin-releasing hormone (GnRH), a decapeptide that stimulates the release of follicle-stimulating hormone

(FSH) and luteinizing hormone (LH) from pituitary gonadotrophs, was first isolated in 1984. During early development, GnRH-expressing neurons (numbering only 1500 to 2000 in primates) are found in the epithelia of the olfactory placode in the olfactory pit. They migrate back from there during embryogenesis and in man come to lie predominantly in the arcuate nucleus of the medial basal hypothalamus. From there, the GnRH-ergic neurons project principally to the primary portal blood vessels in the median eminence, from where pulsatile release of hypothalamic GnRH controls the menstrual cycle. Axons also project to the limbic system and circumventricular organs such as the organum vasculosum of the lamina terminalis and neural lobe of the pituitary. The neuroendocrine role of these projections is unclear.

From late in fetal development and for the first 6 to 12 months of life, GnRH is actively secreted from the hypothalamus at levels similar to those found in midpuberty. GnRH then drops to almost undetectable levels during childhood, with pulsatile GnRH secretion sufficient to stimulate pituitary gonadotrophs only reappearing at the onset of puberty. The interactions between noradrenaline, γ-aminobutyric acid (GABA), opiates, 5HT, and excitatory amino acids on GnRH neuronal activity are complex, and because of this the mechanisms that underlie the onset of puberty remain unknown. Pubertal activation of the gonadal axis can be delayed by low absolute body weight, psychosocial and environmental problems, weight loss, stress, and excessive exercise. The onset of any of these factors after the menarche can lead to hypothalamic amenorrhoea (see below), the resumption of a state that mimics prepuberty.

Growth hormone-releasing hormone

GHRH was first isolated from tumors producing the peptide ectopically in the early 1980s. Its two major forms, 40- and 44-amino acid peptides, are derived from a larger precursor peptide produced in quantity by neurons in the arcuate nucleus of the hypothalamus that project to the outer lamina of the median eminence. GHRH released into the hypothalamo-hypophyseal portal blood reaches anterior pituitary somatotroph cells expressing specific cell surface receptors coupled to the cyclic AMP second messenger system, where it produces trophic and GH-synthetic and secretory responses.

The regulation of GHRH transcription and secretion is complex and not fully understood. GH receptors have been found on cells in the arcuate nucleus of the hypothalamus, however, and transcription of GHRH in these cells is up-regulated by hypophysectomy and down-regulated by GH infusions. These findings, and observations of GH receptor prevalence after hypophysectomy and intracerebroventricular infusions of GH, suggest that despite limitations imposed by the blood brain barrier, direct GH feedback at the level of the hypothalamus is involved in the regulation of GHRH gene expression. Reciprocal connections between GHRH and somatostatin

(somatotropin release-inhibiting hormone, or SRIH)-producing neurons in the hypothalamus indicate that there is cross-talk between these neuronal groups, and dopaminergic and adrenergic modulatory inputs to GHRH neuronal activity have also been well-described.

Somatostatin

Somatostatin, or somatotropin release-inhibiting hormone (SRIH) or "GH-releasing inhibiting hormone", is a 14-amino acid neuropeptide that is widely distributed in the central nervous system, gastrointestinal system, and elsewhere. The main source of median eminence, SRIH is the periventricular region of the anterior hypothalamus, particularly the periventricular nuclei. SRIH-producing neurons are distributed in many other regions of the central nervous system including the amygdala, caudate, putamen, hippocampus, cell groups within cortical layers and the spinal cord, as well as the peripheral nervous system. SRIH has a very wide portfolio of inhibitory actions throughout the neuroendocrine system. The principal actions of SRIH that reach the pituitary in hypothalamo-hypophyseal portal blood are the inhibition of GH release from somatotrophs, and to a lesser extent the inhibition of TSH release from thyrotrophs. The release of SRIH is modified by paracrine and autocrine mechanisms, and it is almost certainly influenced by direct GHRH-ergic neuronal inputs as described above.

Long-acting somatostatin analogues

Somatostatin, acting through the inhibitory GTPase Gi, rapidly reduces growth hormone synthesis and secretion from normal somatotrophs. Adenomatous somatotrophs from between 50 and 94% of patients with somatotrophinomas causing clinical acromegaly respond similarly, and a minority of tumors are thought to show some slowing in growth or overall reduction in size during treatment. As SRIH is only active parenterally and has a half-life of several minutes, a number of long-acting analogues (with serum half lives of 1.5 to 3 hours) have been developed to allow the effects of SRIH to be exploited clinically. To extend the duration of effect still further, these long-acting analogues have been microencapsulated so that the dose interval is extended to weeks. A similar inhibition of secretion is seen in thyrotroph adenomas, although unlike somatotroph adenomas, escape usually occurs.

Neurotransmitter/neuroregulatory role

In the context of neuroendocrine modulation, reduced levels of SRIH in the brain and cerebrospinal fluid have been found in depression, schizophrenia, Parkinson's disease, and Alzheimer's disease, and levels tend to be increased in Huntington's disease. SRIH is also involved in central modulation of pain transmission in the brain and spinal cord. The periventricular region of the hypothalamus and periaqueductal gray matter of the midbrain communicate via an enkephalinergic pathway, and the descending projection from the periaqueductal region uses a number of neurotransmitters including neurotensin, glutamate, 5-hydroxytryptamine, and SRIH.

Most of the dopamine-containing fibers that control pituitary function arise from the arcuate nucleus of the medial, basal hypothalamus that projects to the median eminence, from where dopamine binds to the D2 class of dopaminergic receptors on the mammotroph cell membrane. Dopamine is the principal prolactin release inhibitory hormone found in portal blood, and its effects on the synthetic and trophic activity of neoplastic mammotrophs have been extensively exploited, since the prolactin radioimmunoassay and dopamine agonist bromocriptine became available almost simultaneously in the early 1970s. In addition to the dopaminergic system that modulates pituitary prolactin synthesis and release, the projection to the external layer of the median eminence may have a local modulatory role on the release of GnRH and thyrotropin-releasing hormone (TRH) from neurosecretory nerve terminals.

Neurotransmitter/neuroregulatory role

The projections of dopaminergic fibers to the median eminence account for a relatively minor proportion of the dopamine-mediated neuronal traffic that originates within the central nervous system. Most dopaminergic neurons project from the substantia nigra in the midbrain to the forebrain, but they are also directed from the ventral tegmental area medial to the substantia nigra to the cerebral cortex and limbic system. Degeneration of the nigrostriatal dopaminergic projection to the basal ganglia results in Parkinson's disease, and chemical destruction of the same pathway has been reported to interfere with drinking and appetitive behavior, although the mechanism may be indirect.

Dopamine receptor abnormalities are probably central to the pathogenesis of schizophrenia. An increase in the number and sensitivity of striatal D2 dopamine receptors has been implicated in the pathogenesis and symptomatology of schizophrenia, while reduced levels of D1-like dopamine receptors in the prefrontal cortex, irrespective of prior exposure to antipsychotic drugs, may be responsible for hallucinations and delusions as well as negative symptoms such as diminished volition and emotional blunting.

Dopamine has been shown to induce the release of GHRH and probably also SRIH from the rat hypothalamus, and dopamine itself has been shown to be co-localized with neurotensin and galanin in some cells of the arcuate nucleus of the hypothalamus. The level of D1-like receptor expression may also be important in the cellular basis of "working memory".

NEUROREGULATORS

More than twenty neuropeptides have been localized to the hypothalamus, and the parvocellular cells of the paraventricular nucleus of the hypothalamus are able to make no fewer than seven of these. Some of the hypothalamic neuropeptides influence the behavior of the pituitary directly, or they innervate other hypothalamic neurons or neurons in the median eminence or lower brain stem.

Although neuropeptidergic neurons show considerable anatomical and functional plasticity, they fall broadly into three groups: (1) the vasopressin- and oxytocin-ergic neurons that project to the posterior pituitary; (2) neuropeptidergic secretory neurons in the arcuate nucleus and surrounding regions that project to the median eminence; and (3) a group formed principally by the parvocellular cells in the paraventricular, periventricular, and medial preoptic nuclei that also project to the median eminence. The latter group synthesize and secrete GnRH, TRH, CRH, SRIH, cholecystokinin, galanin, dynorphin, enkephalins, ANP, and angiotensin II, whereas neuropeptidergic neurons of the arcuate nucleus synthesize and release GHRH, POMC, dynorphin, NPY, galanin, and substance P. The arcuate nucleus of the hypothalamus also hosts a large number of GABA-ergic neurons that project to the median eminence and account for the high concentrations of GABA in portal blood.

Current understanding of the integrated function of the neurotransmitters within the hypothalamus is far from complete, and the many published summaries that catalogue the location of neuropeptides and neurotransmitters and their putative functions are often not particularly helpful in establishing an overview of the range of functions that are likely to be modulated by each. Not only do many hypothalamic peptides have combined neurohormonal and neurotransmitter activity, but the effects of neuropeptidergic transmission may be qualitatively different under different physiological circumstances. NPY, for example, has been shown to stimulate LH release in estrogenized rodents but inhibit LH release when female sex hormones are absent, and SRIH and GHRH probably regulate the release of pituitary GH both at the hypothalamic level and within the pituitary itself. The function of the large numbers of GABA-ergic interneurons in the hypothalamus is not clearly understood at present.

Opioid peptides

Enkephalin and dynorphin are synthesized in hypothalamic neurons, and neuronal perikarya within the region of the hypothalamic arcuate nucleus transcribe POMC and project to other parts of the hypothalamus. The pre-proenkephalin gene is activated by estradiol in rat brain neurons in a tissue-specific and genetic sex-specific manner, and transcript levels in the ventromedial hypothalamus correlate strongly with estradiol-dependent reproductive behavior. Depending on the receptor subtype and the site of action in the brain, opioid peptides can inhibit or facilitate female sexual behaviors such as adoption of a lordotic posture in rats, and they have been shown to inhibit gonadotropin and oxytocin release and stimulate prolactin release.

Atrial natriuretic peptide

Atrial natriuretic peptide is found in many parts of the brain, including the amygdala and basal nucleus of the stria terminalis, medial habenular nucleus, mammillary nuclei, periaqueductal gray and nucleus of the tractus solitarius. In addition to the ascending pathways of the brain stem and the limbic system, atrial natriuretic peptide is also extensively distributed within the hypothalamus, with a dense cluster of cells at the organum vasculosum of the lamina terminalis, extending backwards in a broad band into the paraventricular, arcuate and ventromedial nuclei. In some of these somata, atrial natriuretic peptides are co-localized with oxytocin. A further separate group of atrial natriuretic peptidergic cells are found in the lateral hypothalamic area.

In addition to atrial natriuretic peptide, nerve fibers of the organum vasculosum of the lamina terminalis are rich in SRIH, GnRH, and other peptides. The paraventricular nucleus is responsible for about 90% of the atrial natriuretic peptidergic innervation of the median eminence. Functionally, the place of atrial natriuretic peptide is unclear, as the effect of central administration of the peptide on sodium intake and excretion are variable and depend on the model used. There is good evidence, however, that dehydration-induced drinking is diminished by central administration of atrial natriuretic peptide and enhanced by central administration of atrial natriuretic peptide antiserum. Brain natriuretic hormone and brain atrial natriuretic peptide are highly homologous, and it seems likely that the central actions of atrial natriuretic peptide are mediated by the former.

Other peptides

In addition to abundant cholinergic fibers within the hypothalamus, histamine and galanin are found in fairly large amounts in the median eminence. Galanin elevates GH after intracerebroventricular injection and in the median eminence is thought to augment the pituitary response to GHRH.

GABA inhibits prolactin secretion and secretin, and cholecystokinin and vasoactive intestinal polypeptide stimulate prolactin secretion. The effects of vasoactive intestinal polypeptide in stimulating prolactin release are additive to the effects of TRH, and both TRH and vasoactive intestinal polypeptidergic neuronal perikarya are present in the parvocellular paraventricular nucleus, which projects axons to the external zone of the median eminence. Cholecystokinin and motilin stimulate GH release, an effect that is modified by gastrin-releasing peptide.

IMMUNE NEUROENDOCRINE INTERACTIONS

Although the immunosuppressive actions of the glucocorticoid hormones have been known for a very long time, it has only been during the last two decades that we have been able to demonstrate more subtle bidirectional interactions between the endocrine and immune systems. Not only has there been a considerable increase in our understanding of how the neuroendocrine and autonomic nervous systems provide routes through which the central nervous system can modulate endocrine activity, but we now also realize that immunological activation can itself alter central nervous system activity.

Neuroendocrine regulation of the immune system

Macrophages and lymphocytes have now been shown to have receptors for a remarkable number of hormones and neuropeptides. These include receptors for glucocorticoids, sex steroids, thyroid hormones, hypothalamic-releasing factors, opioid peptides, substance P, and VIP. All of these have been shown to be able to increase or diminish immune responses, at least in vitro. Glucocorticoids are, of course, the most powerful immune modulators, and there is good evidence that the hypothalamic-pituitary-adrenal (HPA) response to stress is an important factor in limiting disease progression in autoimmune diseases such as inflammatory arthritis and encephalomyelitis. Immune cells can also produce hormones and neuropeptides including growth hormone, prolactin, TSH, LH, FSH, POMC-derived peptides, opioid peptides, CRH, and GHRH. The expression of these can alter in response to inflammation or infection, or even mild psychological stress. Although these are all tantalizing results, there is as yet no good evidence that secretion of these peptides by the immune system has significant paracrine, autocrine, or indeed endocrine effects.

Immunological regulation of the endocrine system

The clearest example of immunological regulation of the endocrine system is to be found in the response of the HPA axis to immunologically derived cytokines. Since the original observation that interleukin 1 and interleukin 6 could release ACTH from the AtT20 corticotroph cell line, cytokines have been shown to activate the HPA axis at hypothalamic, pituitary, and adrenal levels. Following injection of interleukin 1 there is a pattern of activation of the immediate early gene c-fos in the central nervous system similar to that seen after stressful stimuli. It is interesting to note that although the HPA response to acute immunological activation is largely mediated via increased hypothalamic CRF release, in more chronic immunological disorders, vasopressin becomes the dominant hypothalamic factor activating the pituitary adrenal axis. The HPA axis is not, of course, the only neuroendocrine system to be affected by cytokines that also seem to be, at least in part, responsible for the fall in TRH and TSH, as well as in the gonadotropins that occur in chronic disease. The significance of all these changes in man is uncertain, but diminished immune function is associated with marital separation and divorce, and stressful life events increase the infectivity of administered rhinoviruses. The susceptibility to infectious disease, autoimmune disease, and stress-related disorders are all potentially subject to neuroendocrine regulation, although good evidence of causality in man is still awaited.

Neuropeptidergic neurons project to the posterior pituitary from the supraoptic nucleus, the paraventricular nucleus, cells scattered in the perifornical and lateral hypothalamic areas, and the bed nucleus of the stria terminalis, toward the anterior end of the hypothalamus. In addition to vasopressin and oxytocin, these fibers also contain enkephalins, galanin, dynorphins, cholecystokinin, and angiotensin II. In the median eminence and in the posterior pituitary itself, stimulation evokes reversible retraction of glial processes and an increase in the contact area between neurosecretory terminals and the perivascular space.

Neurohypophyseal (posterior pituitary) secretion of vasopressin controls free water clearance by the kidneys through its actions on tubular reabsorption of water. The production and secretion of vasopressin is influenced by hypothalamic thirst mechanisms, probably located toward the front of the hypothalamus, which in turn are controlled by central osmoreceptors, peripheral blood volume sensors, and angiotensin II.

The principal components of the neural lobe of the pituitary (posterior lobe or neurohypophysis) are nerve tracts from the paraventricular and supraoptic nuclei that project down through the medial, ventral hypothalamus, infundibulum and pituitary stalk to terminate in the neural lobe. Further vasopressin and oxytocin somata are located in the suprachiasmatic nuclei, and in addition to the neural lobe, paraventricular vasopressinergic neurons project to the hippocampus, amygdala and the brain stem and spinal cord, from where they terminate on neurons of the glossopharyngeal and vagus nerves and neurons of origin of the autonomic system. Vasopressin and oxytocin synthesized in the hypothalamus are transported down to the neural lobe of the pituitary gland by axoplasmic flow and released from nerve terminals into fenestrated capillaries. In salt-loaded or water-deprived rats, vasopressin transcripts are also evident in the neural lobe. The precise source of these transcripts and whether they contribute to the neurosecretory peptide pool remains unknown. Vasopressin release is stimulated by decreased blood volume, increased osmolality, and, amongst other drugs, nicotine, and it is decreased by emotion, increased blood volume, and ethanol ingestion.

THE PINEAL GLAND

The pineal gland is a neurosecretory gland that contains glial cells and pinealocytes, formed as an evagination of the caudal portion of the diencephalic roofplate known as the epithalamus. It is about 5 mm x 7 mm in size and lies in the midline above the superior colliculi at the back of the midbrain, hence the propensity of pineal tumors to compress the dorsal midbrain and cause communicating hydrocephalus by obstructing the cerebral aqueduct. Pinealocytes do not have synaptic contacts with central nervous system neurons and are not true neurons themselves, but they receive extensive peptidergic afferents from vasoactive intestinal polypeptide, vasopressin, somatostatin, NPY, and thyrotropin-releasing hormone-producing neurons.

The pineal produces a number of biologically active peptides and is the only source of melatonin, which it secretes in an irregular, acyclic pulsatile pattern superimposed on a nyctohemeral rhythm (i.e., high at night and low during the day), independent of LH pulses. Melatonin falls throughout childhood, reaches adult levels at puberty, and continues to fall from adulthood to old age. There are no threshold changes in melatonin levels with any stage of puberty in normal children, neither is there a correlation in humans between LH levels and melatonin. Noradrenergic nerve input acting on β-adrenergic receptors determine the uptake of tryptophan and the synthesis of melatonin from serotonin.

Melatonin receptors are not present in the hypothalamus, but in rodents are present in the pars tuberalis, a rostral extension of the anterior pituitary that covers the pituitary stalk at the inferior tip of the median eminence. The two major physiological roles of melatonin are its subtle influence on circadian rhythmicity and the induction of seasonal responses to changes in day length. Oral melatonin has a slight stimulatory effect on circulating prolactin levels, but no effect on growth hormone, gonadotropins, testosterone, or thyrotropin secretion. The function of the pineal is not well-established in man, but in lower vertebrates the pineal is directly light sensitive and in some rodents, pinealectomy enhances gonadal axis activity and can modestly advance puberty. The association of pinealomas with premature puberty is almost certainly due to hypothalamic damage rather than to a direct effect of changes in pineal secretory activity. In man, the pathway for light entrainment is complex and involves the retina, suprachiasmatic nucleus, preganglionic neurons in the upper thoracic spinal cord and postganglionic sympathetic fibers from the superior cervical ganglia. Patients with autonomic neuropathy, such as diabetics, Shy-Drager syndrome, those with idiopathic orthostatic hypotension, or quadriplegia following cervical spinal cord transection, have significantly lower nocturnal peaks of melatonin. If the sympathetic nerve input to the pineal is cut, pineal rhythms persist but are no longer entrained.

Prolonged nocturnal melatonin secretion in long-day breeding animals is responsible, via inhibition of gonadotropin-releasing hormone secretion, for the winter regression in breeding activity. In short-day breeders such as sheep, prolonged melatonin exposure is stimulatory. In man, anecdotes have been published of pineal hyperplasia causing hypermelatoninemia and hypogonadotropic hypogonadism that resolve once melatonin levels returned to normal. Oral melatonin supplements are reputed to reduce the effect of jet lag. The use of melatonin as an oncostatic neurohormone or oral contraceptive is still being investigated, as is its place in seasonal affective disorder and sudden infant death syndrome.

HYPOTHALAMIC SYNDROMES

The considerable functional redundancy at a number of sites of peptide synthesis within the hypothalamus and the small, overall size of the structure means that a detailed understanding of the precise location of nerve tracts and regions of peptide synthesis within the hypothalamus is rarely critical from a clinical standpoint.

Broadly speaking, the more anterior nuclei are principally concerned with the production of vasopressin and oxytocin, and the sensation of thirst and fluid balance. Central nuclei are concerned with body temperature regulation and the more dorsal nuclei – the posterior hypothalamic nucleus, supramamillary, and mammillary nuclei – are mainly concerned with appetite, satiety, feeding reflexes, peristalsis, and to some extent the control of various secretions associated with eating and digestion. Lesions toward the posterior hypothalamus may change appetitive behavior, resulting in total loss of appetite or gross overeating. By modifying limbic inputs, lesions can produce more or less subtle changes in personality, either blunting responses, causing bad temper or hypersomnolence. Exaggerated autonomic effects such as shivering, pilo-erection, miosis, hypo- or hyperthermia, and hypotension are most unusual, and like alterations in temperature control are associated with acute hypothalamic injuries. Fortunately, altered thirst mechanism, particularly adipsia (loss of thirst), is rare. The three features that are most characteristic of a hypothalamic cause of hypopituitarism are mild hyperprolactinemia, diabetes insipidus, and visual changes. Diabetes insipidus, obesity and hyperphagia, psychiatric problems, and somnolence each occur in about 20% of patients with hypothalamic disease. Hypogonadism or precocious puberty together affect around 40% of patients with hypothalamic problems.

There is very little change in hypothalamic function with aging. In particular, and somewhat surprisingly, the activity of the hypothalamo-pituitary-adrenal axis shows no evidence of decline. The pituitary becomes slightly smaller, however, and the vasopressin response to changes in blood volume, osmolality, and pressure is greater. Particularly in men, secretion of thyrotropin in response to thyrotropin-releasing hormone is somewhat blunted.

Hypertension associated with increased cerebrospinal fluid pressure has long been attributed to sympathetic discharge from the medulla oblongata in response to ischemia. Electrical or mechanical stimulation of the rostral, ventrolateral medulla in the floor of the fourth ventricle has been shown to mimic raised cerebrospinal fluid pressure-induced hypertension. If, as has been proposed, compression of the left lateral medulla in the region of the emergence of the glossopharyngeal and vagus nerves – typically by loops of the vertebral artery or posterior inferior cerebellar artery – is responsible for some instances of 'essential' hypertension, it is possible that autonomic afferents routed through the anterior hypothalamus may be in part responsible for the changes in intravascular volume that are necessarily associated.

Trauma and irradiation

The hypothalamus is most typically damaged by tumors, or by surgery to remove tumors that arise immediately beneath it. Transcranial surgery to resect craniopharyngiomas is the most common cause. Head injuries, particularly head on, can cause rupture of the pituitary stalk with the onset of diabetes insipidus and, most characteristically, hyperprolactinemia. Hypothalamic ischemia during prolonged hypotension may also play a part in the syndrome.

The pituitary is more radioresistant than the hypothalamus and the rest of the brain, and again, a modest elevation of the prolactin level after external beam radiotherapy can occur. Progressive hormonal deficiencies can begin to appear as early as a year after radiotherapy, and although the maximum decline in pituitary function tends to occur with the first 2 years, pituitary hormone output continues to fall thereafter, with the proportion of irradiated patients requiring hormone replacement plateauing at around 33% after 8 to 10 years.

The hypothalamic amenorrhea syndrome

"Functional hypothalamic amenorrhea" is the reversible cessation of menstrual cycles in young women who do not have any clinically demonstrable abnormalities of the rest of the gonadal axis. This entity is almost certainly a collective term for a number of physiologically and pathophysiologically related events, including psychogenic (stress-induced) amenorrhea, exercise-induced amenorrhea, and amenorrhea associated with weight loss.

The reduction in activity of the GnRH pulse generator with which functional hypothalamic amenorrhea is associated appears to mimic regression to a prepubertal state, but the underlying mechanisms remain unclear. It may involve hypothalamic β-endorphin and/or dopamine, as these, and infusions of naloxone and metoclopramide, modulate the secretory activity of GnRH neurons. Hypercortisolemia and changes in GH and melatonin have also been considered to play a part as CRH tends to inhibit the hypothalamo-pituitary-gonadal axis (in primates), and the secretory pattern of GH and melatonin have been found to increase during the night in women with psychogenic amenorrhea, whereas 24-hour profiles of prolactin and serum thyroxine and triiodothyronine are reduced.

More recently, it has been suggested that leptin (see "Neuroendocrine mediators of appetite and satiety" below), a peptide isolated in 1994, may also be implicated in the control of GnRH secretion in response to changes in weight. It has been known for many years that menstruation only starts when fat stores reach a threshold level, and menarche is delayed by about 3 years in gymnasts and ballet dancers. Even in those who exercise much less, there is a direct relationship with exercise, so that even gentle jogging is associated with a reduction in the number of menstrual periods. Equally, women who are obese often have deranged menstrual cycles that are restored to normality by modest weight loss. Leptin, perhaps through its putative action in suppressing NPY expression, reduces food intake and signals to the hypothalamus that body fat stores are adequate for reproduction. Anovulation in response to suckling is mediated hypothalamically via reduced GnRH pulsatility. Contrary to much-published literature, this effect seems to be related to suckling itself, rather than the levels of prolactin.

Syndrome of inappropriate vasopressin secretion

The syndrome of inappropriate antidiuretic hormone secretion (SIADH) is diagnosed when there is an absence of intravascular volume depletion, edema-forming states, or renal, adrenal, and thyroid disease; and there is hyponatremia and hypotonicity of plasma, and a urine osmolality greater than that of plasma associated with excess renal sodium excretion. In general, both impaired urine dilution as well as excessive fluid intake are necessary for the clinical signs and symptoms of SIADH to develop. The condition is frequently asymptomatic or associated with mild lethargy, anorexia, nausea, and vomiting. More marked cases are associated with muscle cramps, and may eventually lead to coma, convulsions, and death.

An extensive list of diagnoses have been associate with SIADH. These fall predominantly into four main groups: respiratory, central nervous system, drug-related, and neoplastic disorders. Malignant tumors such as oat cell carcinomas of the lung can produce vasopressin themselves, but in many cases of tumor-associated SIADH, the excess vasopressin 'effect' is not due to ectopic vasopressin production, but rather from excessive and inconsistent vasopressin release from the hypothalamus. Mild, transient SIADH is probably fairly common and is often detected 3 to 5 days after surgery, particularly after partial hypophysectomy.

Once renal, thyroid, and adrenal insufficiency have been excluded, mild cases of SIADH do not often warrant specific treatment other than fluid restriction. If that is insufficient or the patient complains of excessive thirst, demeclocycline (the effects of which may take a week or two to develop) can be used to induce nephrogenic diabetes insipidus. The principal therapeutic danger is in rapid correction of hyponatremia that leads to dehydration and shrinking of brain cells, predisposing a patient to central pontine myelinolysis.

Kallmann's syndrome

Etiology

Kallmann's syndrome of hypogonadotropic hypogonadism associated with anosmia was first described in 1944 and is now believed to be due to deletion or translocation of the gene locus at Xp22.3. In early fetal life the GnRH neurons migrate back from the region of the olfactory placode at the front of the brain toward the anterior pole of the hypothalamus, following a trail of neural cell adhesion molecules. This 'chemical trail' is absent in Kallmann's syndrome, hence the association of absent GnRH secretion and anosmia in 85% of those with the condition.

The male to female ratio is about 5:1, and the incidence of Kallmann's syndrome of 1/7500 in males makes the condition considerably more common than Cushing's disease or acromegaly. The prominent manifestation of partial or complete agenesis of the olfactory apparatus in association with secondary hypogonadism and sexual infantilism is sometimes associated with a number of other problems such as color blindness, synkinesia, mental retardation, and congenital midline fusion defects. Incomplete forms in which LH levels are low but FSH levels and spermatogenesis are normal in the face of very low androgen levels have been described (the fertile eunuch syndrome), as have kindreds showing recessive, dominant, and sex-linked patterns of inheritance. In some cases, magnetic resonance imaging of the anterior cranial fossa can demonstrate the deficiency.

Differential diagnosis

The differential diagnosis of hypogonadotropic hypogonadism includes anatomic problems such as craniopharyngiomas (often associated with calcification within the sella turcica in children presenting with headaches, visual disturbance, and pituitary hormone deficiency), dysgerminomas (histologically similar to seminoma of the testis and dysgerminoma of the ovary), hamartomas, prolactinomas and the Langerhans-cell histiocytosis. Other pituitary adenomas and parasellar lesions such as meningiomas, optic nerve as well as hypothalamic tumors, and rarely other granulomatous conditions such as sarcoidosis, can cause hypogonadotropic hypogonadism.

The "empty sella syndrome"

In the empty sella syndrome, a fold of dura appears to herniate into the pituitary fossa. The pituitary gland becomes compressed to the rim of the fossa, and although different combinations of pituitary hormone hyposecretion may occur, hypothalamic-pituitary connections and pituitary function is frequently preserved. This condition may have a primarily mechanical etiology from transmitted cerebrospinal fluid pressure, or it may follow infarction of an occult pituitary adenoma. Magnetic resonance imaging or computed tomography demonstrate the cerebrospinal fluid-filled sella.

The condition is said to be more common in women and may be associated with obesity, benign intracranial hypertension, hydrocephalus, Pickwickian syndrome, and extrasellar tumors. Headache and hypertension are frequently associated, and visual symptoms have been attributed to herniation of the optic apparatus into the sella, but in many cases the condition is likely to remain occult or appear as an incidental finding.

Miscellaneous hypothalamic syndromes

Laurence-Moon-Biedle syndrome

In the autosomal recessive Laurence-Moon-Biedle syndrome, hypogonadotropic hypogonadism is associated with mental retardation, obesity, retinitis pigmentosa, and polydactyly. In many cases diabetes insipidus occurs, and in some kindreds nerve deafness and hyperlipidemia are also found. No gross chromosomal abnormalities are evident, and at postmortem examination the pituitary and hypothalamus are grossly intact.

Prader-Willi syndrome

The Prader-Willi syndrome is the association of mental retardation, small hands and feet, hypotonia at birth, short stature, non insulin-dependent diabetes mellitus, and cryptorchidism, with a series of symptoms thought to be related to an undefined hypothalamic deficit. Isolated hypogonadotropic hypogonadism is an almost invariable finding along with hyperphagia, which develops between the ages of 6 months and 2 years and leads to gross obesity. TSH, GH, and ACTH responses are all essentially normal. In a few cases, deletion of chromosome 15 has been found, but it is still unclear whether a perinatal insult is responsible for subtle cerebral and hypothalamic damage that causes the majority of cases.

Kleine-Levin syndrome

In the Kleine-Levin syndrome, recurrent episodes of hyperphagia, sexual overactivity, and somnolence lasting for 1 to 3 weeks followed by partial amnesia, occur in adolescent boys at intervals of 3 to 6 months. Although the syndrome suggests a hypothalamic etiology or hypothalamic involvement, proof of this is lacking.

NEUROENDOCRINE MEDIATORS OF APPETITE AND SATIETY

The rate at which energy is utilized is closely linked to the food-seeking drive, and in many cases the same neurotransmitters or hormones that lead to utilization of energy will also activate food-seeking behavior. The precision of the association between energy intake and expenditure is so remarkable that in population studies, the average excessive calorie intake between the ages of 20 and 40 as a proportion of total intake is less than 0.8% per year. Nevertheless, obesity is extremely common in Western society. In the obese population, damage to the ventromedial hypothalamus by tumors, trauma, inflammatory disease or neurosurgery; or genetic problems leading to hyperphagia, obesity and hyperinsulinemia (perhaps with the exception of polycystic ovarian disease); accounts for a very small minority of cases. It is thought that only about 5% of transmissible variance across generations for body mass index is genetic. NPY, glucagon-like polypeptide I, dynorphin (the endogenous k agonist), and melanin-concentrating hormone tend to increase appetite, whereas cholecystokinin-pancreozymin and the central administration of CRH decreases it. Central administration of NPY has a marked stimulatory effect on carbohy-

drate-rich food intake, and it will reverse the anorectic effects of lateral hypothalamic lesions. Central administration of GHRH enhances food intake, and injections of galanin directly into the paraventricular nucleus enhances appetitive behavior.

Leptin

The identification of leptin (after leptos, Gk. thin), a 167-amino acid peptide, in 1994 and cloning of the human homologue in 1995 provided a strong impetus to further research the control of appetite. Leptin is the human homologue of a gene, the absence of which is responsible for gross obesity in the homozygous obese (ob/ob) mouse. It is a circulating protein derived from a gene expressed exclusively in white adipose tissue. By acting through specific, high-affinity receptors in the hypothalamus and choroid plexus, leptin reduces food intake and increases energy expenditure, perhaps by reducing the concentrations of neuropeptide Y. Defects in the leptin receptor are responsible for the mutant diabetic (db/db) mouse phenotype, which is indistinguishable from the ob/ob mouse. In the ob/ob mouse but not the db/db mouse, exogenous leptin has been shown to reduce food intake, decrease blood glucose concentrations, reduce insulin concentrations, increase energy expenditure, and, importantly, restore fertility to homozygotes of this phenotype. Given daily leptin injections and free access to food, ob/ob mice lost one-third of their weight in 2 weeks. Normal mice who were fat through overeating, however, did not lose any weight in response to exogenous leptin supplementation.

Under normal circumstances leptin is decreased by fasting and increased by eating, in parallel with changes in insulin levels. Obese subjects tend to have high leptin levels, suggesting either that they are relatively insensitive to the hormone or that the hedonistic aspects of food consumption induce overeating despite peripheral signals to stop. A low leptin state induced by a reduction in body fat mass leads to a state in which food intake exceeds energy expenditure. A number of physiological aspects of this state, such as hypothermia, stunted linear growth, hormonal abnormalities in the gonadal, thyroid, and adrenal axes, and reduced physical activity are akin to those found in early starvation. Indeed, in starved, normal rats, exogenous leptin normalizes some of the above. Thus leptin appears to signal how much fat is in the body to the hypothalamus and appears to serve as a signal from white adipose tissue to the brain that fat stores are adequate for reproduction. This again emphasizes the close association between gonadal hormone production and body mass index.

In general the circulating levels of leptin are proportional to the degree of obesity, women tend to have higher leptin levels than men of equal body mass index, and voluntary reduction in food intake reduces the level of circulating leptin. Despite much early excitement about the possibility of exonerating obese and morbidly obese patients from accusations of voluntary excessive food intake, at the time of writing, a clinical example of an obese human subject lacking leptin or leptin receptor has not been found. Furthermore, the exact relationship between insulin resistance; "leptin resistance"; hunger;

and a possible satiety signal generated from brown fat that can override low leptin levels, weight gain, NPY, and fertility remains to be established.

Neuropeptide Y

Hypothalamic neuropeptide Y increases with starvation, and intracerebroventricular infusion of NPY activates the hypothalamo-pituitary-adrenal axis but down-regulates the gonadal axis, with reduced production of gonadotropins and sex steroids. The starvation-induced increase in NPY transcription in mice is partly corrected by concurrent leptin treatment, as is the starvation-induced down-regulation of the thyroid and gonadal axis, and up-regulation of the adrenal axis. NPY levels in ob/ob mice are much higher than normal, and they too decrease following leptin treatment. Injections of NPY into the brain increase food intake and weight gain, and inactivating mutations in the NPY gene lead to a reduction in obesity seen in ob/ob mice. Curiously, however, mice with NPY mutations alone (NPY-/- knockout mice) are surprisingly normal.

Other neuropeptides involved in food intake

A further group of neurons involved in the control of satiety has been identified using a murine model of obesity that results from ectopic expression of a peptide called agouti, normally found only in the skin of mice. The agouti peptide is a high-affinity antagonist of the melanocyte-stimulating hormone receptor in skin, but also antagonizes the melanocortin-4 receptor found in the hypothalamus. Intracerebroventricular administration of melanocortin-4 receptor agonists inhibited feeding in a number of mouse models of hyperphagia, including ob/ob mice and mice injected with NPY. Thus hypothalamic melanocorticotropic neurons appear to exert a tonic inhibitory effect on feeding.

In addition to the central components of body weight control that have been identified in mice, namely NPY, hypothalamic melanocortinergic neurons and leptin receptors, 5-hydroxytryptamine has also been implicated in appetitive behavior and body weight control. Indeed, the serotonergic drug dexfenfluramine, which reduces appetite and induces weight loss, is one of the few centrally acting appetite suppressors currently available for clinical use. At the present time, a potential clinical role for leptin or leptin analogues in this context has been reduced to a role in helping patients maintain weight loss after successful dieting.

Suggested readings

ASCHNER B. Uber die Funktion der Hypophyse. Pfleugers Arch Ges Physiol 1909;146:1-146.

GIBBONS JL. Cortisol secretion rate in depressive illness. Arch Gen Psychiatry 1964;10:572-5.

HARBUZ MS, LIGHTMAN SL. Signals from the hypothalamus to the pituitary during chronic immune responses. In: Rook GAW, Lightman SL (eds). Steroid hormones and the T-cell cytokine profile. London: Springer-Verlag, 1997.

HARRIS G. Neural control of the pituitary gland. Physiol Rev 1948;28:139-79.

KALLMANN FJ, SCHOENFELD WA, BARRERA SE. The genetic aspects of primary eunuchoidism. Am J Ment Defic 1944;48:203.

LIUZZI A, DALLABONZANA D, PETRONCINI MM, MARINONI T, OPPIZZI G. Growth hormone-releasing hormone. In: Motta M (eds). Brain endocrinology. New York: Raven Press, 1991;281-99.

MCLEAN M, BISITS A, DAVIES J, WOODS R, LOWRY P, SMITH R. A placental clock controlling the length of human pregnancy. Nature Medicine 1995;1:460-3.

MCNEILLY AS. Lactational amenorrhea. In: Veldhuis JD (ed). Endocrinology and metabolism clinics of North America. Philadelphia: WB Saunders, 1993;59-73.

NIKITOVITCH-WINER M, EVERETT JW. Functional restitution of pituitary grafts re-transplanted from kidney to median eminence. Endocrinol 1958;63:916-30.

POPA G, FIELDING U. A portal circulation from the pituitary to the hypothalamic region. J Anat 1930;65:88.

RIVIER J, SPIESS J, THORNER M, VALE W. Characterization of a growth hormone-releasing factor from a human pancreatic islet tumour. Nature 1982;300:276-8.

VALE W, SPIESS J, RIVIER C, RIVIER J. Characterization of a 41 residue ovine hypothalamic peptide that stimulates secretion of corticotropin and ß-endorphin. Science 1981; 213:1394-7.

WEIGENT DA, BLALOCK JE. Interactions between the neuroendocrine and immune systems: common hormones and receptors. Immunological Reviews 1987;100:79-108.

WOLOSKI BMRNJ, SMITH EM, JEYER II WJ, FULLER GM, BLALOCK JHE. Corticotropin releasing activity of monokines. Science 1995;230:1035-7.

5

Anatomy and physiology of the pituitary gland

David Lowe

The pituitary gland was named from the assumption that it controlled or contributed to nasal secretions. It was recognized very early in anatomic history that it was related to the hypothalamus, hence it is also known as the hypophysis. In the 1920s the neuronal link between the neurohypophysis and the hypothalamus was known, and shortly afterwards the portal link between the hypothalamus and the adenohypophysis was demonstrated.

Gross anatomy

The body of the pituitary gland lies in the sella turcica, a pocket in the sphenoid bone in the anterior cranial fossa. The sella is lined by dura, with the dura superiorly forming the diaphragma sellae, which is pierced by the pituitary stalk. In proximity to the pituitary gland are the tuberculum sellae and anterior clinoid processes anteriorly, which are immediately behind the sphenoid air sinus; the sphenoid sinus inferiorly; the dorsum sellae and posterior clinoid processes posteriorly; and the diaphragma sellae superiorly. The lateral walls of the sella are in contact with the cavernous sinuses, which connects with intercavernous sinuses inferior, posterior, and anterior to the pituitary. Immediately above the pituitary stalk as it leaves the sella is the optic chiasm. The base of the brain and pituitary stalk are covered by arachnoid mater and cerebrospinal fluid.

The normal weight of the pituitary is 600 mg and its volume is approximately $1.5 \times 1.0 \times 0.5$ cm^3. The gland enlarges in pregnancy due to the relative increase in lactotrophs, when its weight becomes about 1 g. After lactation, regression may be incomplete, and multiparous women may have pituitary glands of 700 mg or more. In old age the size of the pituitary decreases in both sexes: the somatotrophs decrease in number, but the number of the other anterior pituitary cell types remains much the same. The amount of interstitial fibrosis increases with age. Amyloid and hemosiderin deposition may be seen in post mortem pituitaries from elderly patients, but the significance of these is uncertain.

The pituitary is composed of an adenohypophysis anteriorly and a neurohypophysis posteriorly. The first is formed from the partes distalis, intermedia, and tuberalis. In human beings the pars intermedia is rudimentary and is called the zona intermedia; it has no significant endocrine activity. The pars tuberalis is similarly vestigial, though this does have functioning endocrine cells, principally gonadotrophs. Squamous metaplasia is common in the pars tuberalis, especially with increasing age. Only the pars distalis secretes appreciable amounts of hormones in adult human beings.

The anterior pituitary has no large direct arterial supply, unlike the posterior pituitary. The adenohypophysis receives only a small proportion of its blood supply (about 10%) from the internal carotid artery directly via the middle and inferior hypophyseal arteries. The superior hypophyseal artery provides the main supply to the hypothalamic nuclei and the median eminence, from where blood flows to the adenohypophysis via a long portal system of anterior veins that provides about 75% of the blood supply to the anterior pituitary. About one-quarter of the blood supply arrives via the short portal system of veins connecting the posterior pituitary to the anterior. The venous drainage of almost all of the gland goes into the cavernous sinus. The nerve supply to the anterior pituitary is adrenergic or noradrenergic, consists predominantly of sympathetic fibers to the muscle of vessel walls, and controls to some extent the secretion of adrenocorticotropic hormone (ACTH), prolactin, and thyroid-stimulating hormone (TSH, or thyrotropin). The posterior pituitary is smaller than the anterior and has a volume of only about 100 mm^3. The extension of the neurohypophysis into the pituitary stalk is principally posterior to the pars tuberalis of the anterior pituitary. The junction of the stalk with the posterior pituitary is called the "genu" and is composed of fibrovascular bundles in a loose stroma, which can be mistaken for edema of the area. The stalk therefore has two important components: the specialized vasculature that forms the portal system, and the large nerve tracts that terminate in the neurohypophysis.

At the top of the pituitary stalk lies the median eminence, a structure of great importance in the regulation of the pituitary gland as it is the common pathway of all of the regulatory hormones that pass down the portal system to the anterior pituitary. The tuberoinfundibular system of nerves that abut the median eminence produce over 30 trophic peptides, including vasoactive intestinal polypeptide (VIP), cholecystokinin, FSHRH, and GABA. In the median eminence and upper infundibulum lie the primary capillary beds of the portal system of blood flow supplying the anterior pituitary, which start as specialized vascular structures called gomitoli bodies. These coiled capillary structures measure 50 to 100 μm in diameter and are centered on arterioles that have a regulatory role in the blood flow to the anterior lobe. It has been demonstrated that corticotropin-releasing hormone (CRH) is present in the cells surrounding the gomitoli capillaries, but interestingly, immunohistochemistry for epithelial cells, endothelial cells, glial cells, and neuroendocrine cells in gomitoli is negative.

The hypothalamus developmentally forms part of the diencephalon. It lies superoposterior to the pituitary and is connected to it by the infundibulum. Its anatomic relations are the optic chiasm anteriorly, the optic tracts and temporal lobe laterally, the mammillary bodies posteriorly, and the anterior and posterior commissures superiorly. There are two distinct parts of the hypothalamus: a medial part rich in neurons and nuclear groups and a lateral part with relatively few neurons and nuclear groups.

The origin of the nerve fibers to the posterior pituitary is principally in the large neurons of the supraoptic and paraventricular nuclei. Vasopressin and oxytocin and their respective precursors are produced in separate neurons, with the great majority producing vasopressin and a peripheral cuff of neurons producing oxytocin. Other hormones are also produced, which are angiotensin II, glucagon, endorphins, and cholecystokinin. There are axons in the pituitary infundibulum and posterior pituitary that do not originate in the supraoptic and paraventricular nuclei and secrete a number of trophic substances, including thyrotropin-releasing hormone (TRH), luteinizing hormone-releasing hormone (LHRH), corticotropin-releasing hormone, somatostatin, and dopamine. Some of these, such as TRH and dopamine, may have a regulatory effect on vasopressin, but these and others might also reach the anterior pituitary via the short portal system that connects the anterior and posterior parts of the gland.

Developmental anatomy of the pituitary

The anterior pituitary is derived from Rathke's pouch or cleft, which is an outpouching of the roof of the stomatodeum that forms at about the third week of gestation. The pouch elongates, resulting in a bulbous proximal end from which the cells of the adenohypophysis are derived and a hollow process distally called the craniopharyngeal duct. This duct is lined by stratified squamous epithelium. At about 5 weeks gestation, the proximal end comes into contact with the descending process of the diencephalon, which will eventually form the infundibulum and neurohypophysis.

Corticotroph development is apparent on electron microscopy in the median aspect of the anterior pituitary at the age of about 6 weeks gestation, with ACTH demonstrable immunohistochemically shortly afterwards. Somatotrophs develop in the lateral aspects at about the 7th week. Development of the glycoprotein hormones begins with the common α-subunit at about this time, but the defining β-subunits of the glycoproteins (TSH and gonadotropins) are found later at about the 12th week. Lactotrophs are the last cells to become recognizable. Somatolactotrophs form at about the 12th week, containing both prolactin and human growth hormone (hGH), and discrete lactotrophs develop only at about the 24th week of gestation.

The posterior pituitary develops between about the 6th and 20th weeks of gestation. Posterior lobe hormones are demonstrable between 10 and 14 weeks in the paraventricular and supraoptic nuclei of the hypothalamus and descend to the bulbous axon terminations ("Herring bodies") in the posterior pituitary for secretion.

Microscopic anatomy and physiology

The normal anterior pituitary can be divided histologically into three areas: the median or mucoid wedge and the two anterolateral wings. Classically the cells in these areas can be classified as chromophobes, basophils and acidophils, but these chromatic terms have been superseded by the more precise terms somatotroph, lactotroph (or mammotroph), corticotroph, thyrotroph, gonadotroph, and null cells, which more precisely reflect the physiology of the cells.

Somatotrophs

Somatotrophs comprise about half of all anterior pituitary cells and are found principally in the acidophil anterolateral wings. Somatotrophs contain hGH, human placental lactogen, galanin, and bombesin, and some additionally contain the α-subunit of the glycoprotein hormones. The number of somatotrophs decreases with age and may be functionally suppressed in pregnancy, when they switch to prolactin production in a reactivation of their potential in the embryo; this state reverses at the end of pregnancy. Indeed, somatolactotrophs containing both hGH and prolactin can be found in normal pituitaries of adult patients.

Secretion of hGH is regulated by growth hormone-releasing hormone (GHRH), a 44-amino acid peptide made in the arcuate nucleus of the hypothalamus. When GHRH is given intravenously there is a rapid rise in hGH, which is pronounced in young adults and less so in people over 45 years of age. Growth hormone is normally released in a pulsatile, episodic fashion. Constant infusion of GHRH over several hours will result in a reduction of circulating hGH levels. Somatostatin release occurs out of phase with hGH, and it may be responsible for the trough levels of hGH by suppressing cAMP in somatotroph cells. Growth hormone release is stimulated by catecholamines, which may be the mechanism by which opioids also stimulate hGH release, and by thyroid hormones.

Lactotrophs

Lactotrophs are chromophobic, acidophilic, or very occasionally basophilic cells found in a similar distribution to somatotrophs, and they account for 10 to 30% of all adenohypophyseal cells (lowest in men; highest in multiparous, pregnant women). They are found throughout the gland but predominate in the lateral wings. Lactotrophs are often found in very close association with gonadotrophs, and it has been suggested that there may be some paracrine interaction between the two cell types. Ultrastructurally, lactotrophs can be shown to secrete granules both at the cell base and at the lateral margins away from the vascular pole, the so-called "misplaced exocytosis". Prolactin is the only hormone that is discharged by this type of visible granule exocytosis. The number and size of lactotrophs increase greatly during pregnancy under the stimulus of estrogen.

Lactotrophs contain prolactin, vasoactive intestinal polypeptide, galanin, and bombesin. The secretion of prolactin is regulated by both inhibitory and releasing factors, the most important of which is dopamine from the tuberoinfundibular neurons in the arcuate nucleus of the hypothalamus. Dopamine inhibits secretion of prolactin by the inhibition of cyclic adenosine monophosphate (cAMP), and phosphoinositol synthesis, both of which are necessary for dopamine secretion; dopamine inhibition is the basis of treatment with dopamine antagonists such as bromocriptine. Releasing factors for prolactin include TSH, vasoactive intestinal polypeptide, and peptide histidine isoleucine, which have a common precursor molecule that is formed in the parvocellular neurons of the paraventricular nucleus. The same neurons contain CRH, and it is postulated that the parallel release of prolactin and ACTH in stress may be explained by this. Serotonin has the double effect of suppressing dopamine release from neurons in the tuberoinfundibular area and stimulating prolactin releasing factors from the paraventricular nucleus. Other prolactin releasing factors include cholecystokinin, angiotensin II, vasopressin, oxytocin, TRH, and enkephalin.

Corticotrophs

Corticotroph cells are basophilic. This is because the precursor molecule pro-opiomelanocortin (POMC) is glycogenated rather than because ACTH itself is glycogenated. Corticotrophs account for about 20% of the cells in the anterior pituitary and contain ACTH, LPH, endorphins, enkephalins, and MSH (all of which are derived from the precursor POMC molecule). Corticotrophs may extend into the posterior pituitary, especially with advancing age, forming the so-called "basophil invasion", a feature of histological interest but of no known clinical significance. It may be that the cleavage of POMC is different in the zona intermedia and pars nervosa, as the amount of immunostaining for α-MSH is higher in these invading cells than would be expected by chance.

Corticotrophs contain ACTH, β-LPH, α-MSH, galanin, and bombesin. Secretion of the first two is stimulated by the 41-amino acid peptide CRH. CRH is secreted by the paraventricular nucleus of the hypothalamus and inhibited by circulating cortisol. CRH binds to receptors on the plasma membranes of corticotrophs and activates adenyl cyclase to produce increased amounts of cAMP. As a consequence, protein kinases are activated and stimulate ACTH secretion and the production of more ACTH. The effect of CRH is enhanced by cholecystokinin, vasopressin, and angiotensin II from the hypothalamus and by circulating adrenaline. The rise in ACTH in response to insulin hypoglycemia is mediated predominantly by the effect of vasopressin. Adrenal cortisol is the most important negative feedback hormone on the pituitary and the hypothalamus.

Excess of cortisol and related steroids causes a change in pituitary corticotrophs called "Crooke's hyaline change", after the pathologist working at the London Hospital in 1935 who first described it. These cells have an accumulation of intermediate filaments around or adjacent to the nucleus of the affected corticotrophs that immunostain positively for cytokeratins and ubiquitin. Crooke's change requires several months of hypercortisolemia to develop, and it can persist for more than a year after the cortisol levels have been corrected by pituitary adenomectomy (partial hypophysectomy) or adrenalectomy. It can also be found in the tumor cells of corticotroph adenomas of the pituitary.

Gonadotrophs and thyrotrophs

Gonadotrophs are about twice as common as thyrotrophs and are scattered throughout the pituitary gland. FSH and LH are produced by the same cell but the commitment of cells to each can vary. There is no difference between the sexes in the amount of production of FSH and LH in the adult, the amount of each being approximately equal. In the male fetus, conversely, the amount of LH produced is significantly higher than in the female fetus. Control of the secretion of gonadotrophs is under positive and negative control: the positive control is via the permissive effect of the decapeptide gonadotropin-releasing hormone (GnRH), and the negative via feedback from gonadal steroids.

Thyrotrophs are the least numerous cells in the anterior pituitary, accounting for only one in twenty. They are basophilic and PAS-positive, and they tend to predominate in the mucoid wedge. Secretion of TSH is primarily controlled by negative feedback by thyroid hormones, but the basal level is determined by TRH synthesized in the paraventricular nucleus. Noradrenaline stimulates secretion of TRH, as does melatonin.

Other cells regarded as normal constituents of the anterior pituitary

Stellate or folliculostellate cells form about 5% of anterior pituitary cells. They contain glial fibrillary acidic protein and immunostain positive for S100 protein. They have a close association with somatotrophs and gonadotrophs, possibly because they have a regulatory role via cytokine secretion. There is some evidence for a regulatory role for dendritic cells derived from circulating blood monocytes on anterior pituitary hormone-secreting cells.

Lymphocytes are commonly found in small numbers in the pituitary, especially at the junction of the anterior and posterior aspects. A diagnosis of lymphocytic hypophysitis should only be made when there is a severe lymphocyte infiltrate with evidence of destruction of anterior pituitary cells. Plasma cells are not seen in the normal pituitary.

Other hormones found in the anterior pituitary

Galanin was originally isolated from pig intestine and subsequently found in rats and human beings. Messenger RNA for galanin is found almost entirely in corticotrophs in the human pituitary, while in other species it is more widely distributed in corticotrophs, lactotrophs, somatotrophs, and thyrotrophs. It is likely that galanin has tonic inhibitory local effects on ACTH and potentiates the increase in prolactin and TSH secretion induced by TRH. Galanin has also been shown to increase GH.

Neuropeptide Y affects LHRH release from the hypothalamus and may amplify the degree of LH release caused by LHRH. In tissue cultures of anterior pituitary cells from postnatal rats, neuropeptide Y in physiological concentrations stimulates the development of corticotrophs and lactotrophs. Neurotensin is found in intestinal tissues and in the secretory granules of gonadotrophs, and small amounts are also demonstrable in thyrotrophs. Its main effects are on the release of prolactin and TSH: neurotensin increases prolactin secretion, an action that is additive to the effect of TRH increasing prolactin secretion. Its precise function in the anterior pituitary is unknown. Neuromedin N is a peptide closely related to neurotensin, which is coded for by very similar mRNA. Neuromedin is found in a similar distribution to neurotensin.

Bombesin is found in many human tissues and has a wide variety of actions. It increases the secretion of several pituitary, gut, and pancreatic hormones and causes smooth muscle contraction. Bombesin represents a family of peptides, which includes gastrin-releasing peptide and neuromedins B and C. Bombesin is present in many cells of the anterior pituitary, but mostly in corticotrophs, lactotrophs, and somatotrophs. Its effects are unknown, though there are some reports that bombesin augments secretion of prolactin and hGH. Bombesin also stimulates the secretion of ACTH and can potentiate the secretion of ACTH due to CRH stimulation. In addition, bombesin can be secreted ectopically by oat cell carcinomas and carcinoid tumors of the lung, and result in Cushing's syndrome by stimulating the release of ACTH from the anterior pituitary.

Cholecystokinin and gastrin are structurally related peptides found in anterior pituitary cells as well as hypothalamic neurons. Immunoreactivity for cholecystokinin and gastrin is found predominantly in corticotrophs. The propeptides are found in larger amounts than the peptides,

which suggests that processing into the active hormone may be inhibited in the pituitary. Both hormones have been shown to induce secretion of prolactin and hGH.

Vasoactive intestinal polypeptide is synthesized in the hypothalamus and anterior pituitary. It is increased following treatment with estrogen and after adrenalectomy. VIP stimulates prolactin secretion and is reduced in hyperprolactinemic states; growth hormone and vasopressin release are also stimulated.

Inhibin from the granulosa cells of the ovary and the Sertoli cells of the testis stimulates the synthesis and release of FSH from gonadotrophs by actions on the hypophysis and pituitary. Apparently paradoxically, FSH stimulates the secretion of inhibin. Both are inhibited by progesterone.

Pro-opiomelanocortin-derived peptides predominate in corticotrophs in the pars anterior and the zona intermedia. The POMC gene translates into the precursor protein for ACTH, lipotrophic hormones, α- and β-LPH, melanocyte stimulating hormones, α- and β-MSH, and α- and β-endorfins. Basal release of many POMC-derived peptides is stimulated by CRH and antidiuretic hormone and inhibited by somatostatin. Opioids and enkephalins principally affect LH and FSH release in vivo, though ACTH, prolactin, and hGH are affected as well. β-endorphin has a complex range of actions, including stimulating TSH release, inhibiting prolactin release, and increasing LH release. Interestingly, pro-opiomelanocortin is quite a ubiquitous molecule: it is found in epidermal keratinocytes and melanocytes, and it modulates immunocompetent cells and cytokines in the skin and other tissues.

Atrial natriuretic peptide (ANP) has hypotensive, diuretic, and natriuretic effects when infused into healthy volunteers. ANP is predominantly limited to gonadotrophs, though corticotrophs and lactotrophs may contain small amounts, and ANP receptors are found on the plasma membranes of these cell types.

Renin, angiotensin II, and angiotensin-converting enzyme (ACE) are found in lactotrophs in the anterior pituitary and in the pituicytes of the neurohypophysis. These hormones are related to the pituitary response of prolactin to stress: no significant changes in ACTH or GH appear to occur.

The neurohypophysis

The posterior pituitary is the effector organ of the neurosecretory units that begin in the supraoptic and paraventricular nuclei of the hypothalamus. The infundibular nerves passing into the posterior lobe are non-myelinated and terminate in bulbs from which vasopressin, oxytocin, neurophysin, and other peptides are secreted. These are surrounded by specialized glial cells called pituicytes, which are considered to affect the release of oxytocin and vasopressin into the bloodstream.

Vasopressin is a nonapeptide that takes the arginine form in human beings (some animals produce lysine vasopressin). It acts on the renal tubules to retain water and causes contraction of smooth muscle, glycogenolysis, and prostaglandin synthesis. Oxytocin is also a nonapeptide, primarily bringing about contraction of the uterus during labor. Experiments in animals have shown that oxytocin is important in affiliation, mating, bonding, parental behavior, and in the response to stress. More minor actions are inducing contraction of the mammary ducts to express milk during lactation and causing a mild sodium-losing effect on the kidney.

Other tissues found in the pituitary

Remnants of Rathke's pouch are quite often found in the zona intermedia as glands and clefts. The lining cells may be low cuboidal or columnar and are rarely ciliated. They may secrete hormones but usually do not, and they are usually positive for low molecular weight cytokeratins. It is thought that Rathke's cleft cysts arise from these developmental remnants. Salivary gland tissue is occasionally found on the surface of the pituitary and probably accounts for the very rare occurrence in the pituitary of neoplasms that are identical to salivary gland tumors.

Suggested readings

ASA SL, KOVACS K, LASZLO FA, DOMOKOS I, EZRIN C. Human fetal adenohypophysis: histologic and immunocytochemical analysis. Neuroendocrinology 1986;43:308-16.

CROOKE AC. A change in the basophil cells of the pituitary gland common to conditions which exhibit the syndrome attributed to basophil adenoma. J Pathol Bacteriol 1935;40:339-49.

DUBOIS PM, EL AMRAOUI A. Embryology of the pituitary gland. Trend Endocrinol Metab 1995;6:1-7.

HALLIDAY WC, ASA SL, KOVACS K, SCHEITHAUER BW. Intermediate filaments in the human pituitary gland: an immunohistochemical study. Canadian Journal of Neurosciences 1990;17:131-6.

HOEK A, ALLAERTS W, LEENEN PJ, SCHOEMAKER J, DREXHAGE HA. Dendritic cells and macrophages in the pituitary and the gonads. Evidence for their role in the fine regulation of the reproductive endocrine response. Eur J Endocrinol 1997;136:8-24.

PRAGER D, BRAUNSTEIN GD. Pituitary disorders during pregnancy. Endocrinol Metab Clin North Am 1995;24:1-14.

Clinical aspects of the anterior pituitary gland

Giovanni Faglia

◼ KEY POINTS ◼

- Growth hormone defect in adults increases the mortality rate for cardiovascular diseases.
- The mortality rate for cardiovascular diseases is also increased in the presence of growth hormone excess (acromegaly).
- Prolactin, contrary to all other anterior pituitary gland hormones, is primarily regulated by the inhibitory control of dopamine. As a consequence, hypothalamic disconnection causes prolactin to rise and other pituitary hormones to decrease.
- In patients with prolactinoma, serum prolactin levels are related to tumor size. The finding of only moderately high prolactin levels in patients with a pituitary macroadenoma is suggestive of nonprolactinoma.
- Thyrotropin-releasing hormone not only stimulates thyroid-stimulating hormone secretion, but also its biological activity.
- Thyroid-stimulating hormone-secreting pituitary tumors secondary to primary thyroid failure usually regress after L-thyroxine replacement therapy.
- Magnetic resonance imaging with paramagnetic contrast medium infusion is the best way to visualize pituitary microadenomas. However, minute lesions are detected in about 15 to 25% of normal subjects. Thus, MRI should be interpreted in the light of hormonal and clinical data.
- Pituitary apoplexy has been described after gonadotropin-releasing hormone and thyrotropin-releasing hormone tests in patients with extremely large adenomas.
- Hypothalamic pituitary sarcoid lesions usually regress after corticosteroid treatment.
- The first-choice treatment for pituitary tumors is surgery for growth hormone, ACTH, thyroid-stimulating hormone, luteinizing hormone/follicle-stimulating hormone and non-secreting tumors, while it is dopamine agonist administration for prolactinomas. Medical treatment with slow-release somatostatin analogs may also be the first choice treatment in responsive acromegalic patients with large infiltrating pituitary adenoma.
- In hypopituitary patients, L-thyroxine replacement therapy should be started after cortisol treatment institution.

In vertebrates, some of the most important physiological functions, such as reproduction, growth, metabolism, energy balance, maintenance of internal milieu equilibri-um, and adaptive responses to environmental stimuli are regulated by the pituitary gland, which represents an intermediate control station between the central nervous system (CNS) and the peripheral glands. Pituitary activity is controlled by the feedback of peripheral hormones and by the stimulating and inhibiting hypothalamic neurohormones that reach the gland through the portal vessels. In turn, pituitary hormones may modulate hypothalamic activity via short loop feedback mechanisms. The pituitary forms a functional unit with the hypothalamus.

Anterior pituitary hormones

Anterior pituitary hormones are either polypeptides or glycoproteins and require specific receptors on their target cell plasma membrane for hormone signal transduction. Growth hormone (GH) and prolactin (PRL) act directly on peripheral tissues, while thyroid-stimulating hormone (TSH), adrenocorticotropic hormone (ACTH), follicle-stimulating hormone (FSH), and luteinizing hormone (LH) stimulate hormone synthesis and secretion from their respective peripheral glands. As anterior pituitary hormones also exert a trophic function on the target cells, they are commonly termed "tropins". In addition to tropins, the pituitary gland produces growth factors, interleukins, and neurohormones that are locally active.

Growth hormone or somatotropin

Growth hormone is a 191-amino acid polypeptide (MW 21.5 kDa, half-life 20 to 25 minutes), derived from a larger precursor (pre-GH), and is synthesized and secreted by somatotrophs. A variant lacking residues 32 to 46 is produced through alternative splicing, but it is secreted at a low rate. Circulating GH also includes a "big GH" variant that is likely to be a dimer. The GH gene (5 exons and 4 introns) is located on the long arm of chromosome 17. A factor denominated PIT-1 facilitates GH gene transcription. GH circulates in blood partly bound to a transport protein that, interestingly, is identical to the extracellular portion of the GH receptor.

Regulation GH secretion is dually regulated by growth hormone-releasing hormone (GHRH) and somatostatin (somatotropin-release inhibiting hormone, or SRIH). These are in turn under complex neural, metabolic, and hormonal influences. These influences result in a finely pulsating GH secretion to which are superimposed episodic peaks associated to meals, physical exercise, and psycho-physical stresses, and characteristic nocturnal sleep-related bursts occurring during the sleep stages III and IV. A negative feedback is exerted by insulin-like growth factor I (IGF-I) by increasing SRIH gene expression (Fig. 6.1). Novel peptidyl and nonpeptidyl GH secretagogues able to exert a potent GH releasing activity by binding specific receptors at both hypothalamic and pituitary level have been synthetized. A putative 28 aminoacid physiological ligand for these receptors has been isolated from the stomach and termed *Ghrelin*. Its role in the physiological GH regulation is still under investigation.

Action The primary role of GH is to promote linear bone growth. This action is mostly mediated by IGF-I (or somatomedin C; MW 7.5 kDa; coding gene on the long arm of chromosome 12), and the synthesis, mainly by the liver, is GH-dependent. IGF-I causes the epiphysial cartilage to grow. GH also has general metabolic effects that result in a positive protein balance. This increases lipolysis, which causes the release of free fatty acids from the adipose tissue. The availability of this alternative fuel allows for the utilization of the spared proteins for growth. Carbohydrate metabolism is affected through the stimulation of neoglycogenesis. However, while acute increases in serum GH concentration improves glucose utilization, chronic GH excess reduces glucose uptake and utilization and causes insulin resistance.

The GH receptor is a monomeric transmembrane protein that transduces GH signals in a very complex manner.

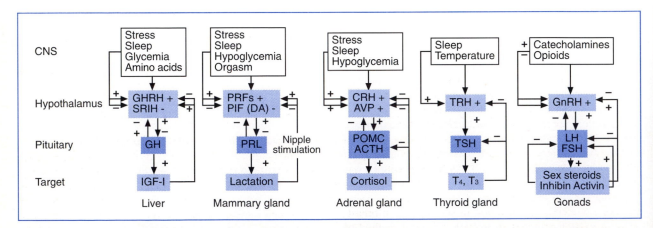

Figure 6.1 Hypothalamic-pituitary-target axes. (CNS = central nervous system; GHRH = growth hormone-releasing hormone; SRIH = somatotropin release-inhibiting hormone; GH = growth hormone; IGF-I = insulin-like growth factor I; PRFs = prolactin-releasing factor(s); PIF = prolactin-inhibiting factor; DA = dopamine; PRL = prolactin; CRH = corticotropin-releasing hormone; AVP = arginine-vasopressin; POMC = pro-opiomelanocortin; ACTH = adrenocorticotropin; TRH = thyrotropin-releasing hormone; TSH = thyroid-stimulating hormone; T_4 = thyroxine; T_3 = 3,3',5-triiodothyronine; GnRH = gonadotropin-releasing hormone; LH = luteinizing hormone; FSH = follicle-stimulating hormone.)

Each GH molecule binds two receptors, forming a dimer that is either directly translocated to the nucleus or primes a cascade of intracellular phosphorylations. In addition, GH receptor occupancy activates phospholipase C that, by hydrolyzing phosphatidylinositol, causes the generation of inositol-triphosphate (IP_3) that mobilizes intracellular Ca^{2+} stores, and of diacylglycerol (DAG) that activates the protein kinase C cascade.

Prolactin

Prolactin is a 198-amino acid polypeptide (MW 22 kDa; half-life 30 minutes) that is synthesized and secreted by lactotrophs. It is derived from a 40 to 50 kDa precursor (pre-PRL). The PRL gene is located on chromosome 6 and is made up of 5 exons and 4 introns; gene transcription requires PIT-1.

Regulation   Prolactin secretion is mainly under hypothalamic inhibitory control exerted by dopamine, which reaches lactotrophs through the hypothalamic-pituitary portal vessels and binds plasma membrane D2 receptors. Dopamine signal transduction is negatively coupled with adenylyl cyclase. Gamma-aminobutyric acid (GABA) and acetylcholine also have inhibitory effects on PRL secretion. A stimulatory action is exerted by thyrotropin-releasing hormone (TRH), vasoactive intestinal polypeptide (VIP), pituitary adenylil-cyclase activating peptide (PACAP), and endogenous opioids, although their physiological role is still debated (Fig. 6.1).

PRL is secreted in a pulsatile fashion. Serum PRL concentration increases during sleep until the first morning hours. Due to the inhibitory nature of the hypothalamic control of PRL secretion, experimentally induced or naturally occurring lesions of the pituitary stalk, median eminence, or hypothalamus can cause PRL hypersecretion. Similarly, antidopaminergic drugs cause serum PRL to rise. PRL secretion is also enhanced by physical and psychological stresses, hypoglycemia, and nipple stimulation. Serotoninergic agents, estrogens, and opioids also have stimulatory effects, while glucocorticoids exert a weak inhibition.

Action   In mammalians, the main physiological role of PRL is to stimulate lactation in the puerperium. During pregnancy, PRL concurs – along with estrogens, progesterone, placental lactogen (hPL), insulin, and cortisol – to prepare breast for milk production. However, its lactogenic action becomes patent only after parturition when the levels of circulating estrogens fall. Subsequently, lactation is maintained by breast suckling via a peripheral nervous loop. It is likely that PRL is also implicated in so-called "maternal behavior". As PRL inhibits ovulation by blocking the pulsatile secretion of gonadotropin-releasing hormone (GnRH), the elevation in serum PRL in breast-feeding women provides them with a natural method of contraception. PRL also influences several metabolic functions, and its excess is associated with reduced glucose tolerance and hyperinsulinemia.

PRL receptors belong to the same superfamily as GH receptors and work in a similar manner.

Corticotropin

ACTH is a 39-amino acid polypeptide (MW 4.5 kDa; half-life 7 to 15 minutes) that originates from the cleavage of a bigger molecule, pro-opiomelanocortin (POMC, MW 28.5 kDa), which also generates β-LPH, β-MSH, α-MSH, β-endorphin, and an N-terminal fragment. The POMC gene (3 exons and 2 introns) is located on chromosome 2.

Regulation   ACTH secretion is stimulated by corticotropin-releasing hormone (CRH) and arginine-vasopressin (AVP). CRH binds specific receptors that utilize cAMP as a second messenger, while AVP binds V3 type receptors that utilize intracellular $[Ca^{2+}]$ for signal transduction. ACTH is secreted in a pulsatile manner. Its plasma concentration varies according to a characteristic circadian rhythm (nadir at 23:00 to 24:00, and zenith in the first morning hours). ACTH and other POMC derivatives are secreted in response to stressful events. The inhibitory control is exerted by negative cortisol feedback through two different modalities: "fast feedback", in response to brisk variations in circulating cortisol concentrations, and "slow feedback", which is sensitive to absolute cortisol levels (Fig. 6.1).

Action   ACTH stimulates adrenal steroidogenesis and exerts a trophic action on the adrenal cortex. As α- and β-MSH do not exist as separate hormones in man, ACTH also stimulates the expansion of skin melanophores. β-LPH and N-terminal peptide functions have not been fully elucidated in man, while it is well known that β-endorphin participates in the central control of pain.

The ACTH receptor, on the plasma membrane of the adrenocortical cells, utilizes cAMP as a second messenger.

Thyrotropin

TSH is a glycoprotein (MW 28 kDa, 15% carbohydrates; half-life about 50 minutes) produced and secreted by thyrotrophs. It is composed of 2 subunits, α and β, and encoded by genes mapped to chromosomes 6 and 19, respectively. The α-subunit is common to luteinizing hormone (LH), follicle-stimulating hormone (FSH), and chorionic gonadotropin (GC), whereas the β-subunit confers functional and immunological specificities. The biological activity is possessed by the whole molecule and is influenced by the degree of glycosylation.

Regulation   TSH secretion is pulsatile and shows a circadian rhythm (zenith at 22:00 to 02:00). Although TSH secretion is centrally regulated by the stimulatory action of thyrotropin-releasing hormone (TRH) and by the inhibitory effect of somatostatin and dopamine, the most important regulatory mechanism is the negative feedback by thyroid hormone at both the pituitary and hypothalamic levels. At the pituitary level, the inhibitory effect is mainly exerted by triiodothyronine (T_3), which is generated from thyroxine inside the thyrotrophs. This inhibits TSH β-subunit gene transcription. At the hypothalamic level, T_3 also inhibits TRH gene transcription (Fig. 6.1).

Action   After binding the receptor, TSH activates all the steps of synthesis and secretion of thyroid hormones, and it maintains the trophism of the thyroid gland. TSH receptors utilize cAMP as a second messenger.

Gonadotropins

Luteinizing hormone (MW 30 kDa; carbohydrates 16%; half-life about 30 to 60 minutes) and follicle-stimulating hormone (MW 30 kDa; carbohydrates 30%; half-life about 180 to 240 minutes) are glycoproteins composed of α- and β-subunits and are secreted by gonadotrophs. Specificity and bioactivity are conferred by the β-subunits. Genes coding for β-subunits are located on chromosomes 19 for LH and 11 for FSH.

Regulation   LH and FSH secretion are both stimulated by GnRH, which peaks every 90 to 120 minutes. This causes gonadotropins to be secreted in the pulsatile fashion necessary for appropriate gonadal stimulation.

Estrogens exert a *positive feedback* that starts 12 to 24 hours after the midcycle estrogen increase and causes the preovulatory LH surge. The estrogen signal is amplified by progesterone. Estrogens and testosterone also exert a *negative feedback* that inhibits gonadotropin secretion.

A selective inhibition of FSH secretion is exerted by *inhibin*, a heterodimeric protein (MW 32 kDa) formed by 2 subunits (α and β) that is produced by ovarian follicles and seminiferous tubules. Low levels of inhibin are responsible for the more marked FSH increase, with respect to LH, during menopause in women, or following seminiferous tubule lesions in men. The inhibin α-subunit is present in two isoforms that may form homodimers called *activins*, as they possess FSH-stimulatory properties (Fig. 6.1). Another FSH-inhibiting protein, *follistatin*, has recently been isolated, but its physiological role is not yet clarified.

Action   In men LH stimulates testosterone synthesis and secretion from the interstitial cells of the testis (Leydig cells), while FSH stimulates the tubular component and Sertoli cells to produce an androgen-binding protein that sustains the locally elevated concentration of testosterone necessary for gamete maturation.

In women, FSH provides for the recruitment and development of ovarian follicles, and in concert with LH, it stimulates the secretion of estrogens, progesterone, and ovarian androgens. At midcycle, a secretory peak of LH causes follicle rupture and ovulation. Corpus luteum formation and activity is sustained by LH.

LH and FSH receptors utilize cAMP as a second messenger.

Investigation of hypothalamic-pituitary function

The availability of extremely specific and sensitive immunometric methods has made it possible for their measurement in basal conditions and in response to neu-rohormonal and pharmacological manipulations, which allows for the assessment of hypothalamic-pituitary function. Of the many proposed tests, we describe here only those currently used for diagnostic purposes.

Hypothalamic-GH-IGF-I axis

The investigation of the hypothalamic-GH-IGF-I axis is based on the evaluation of circulating GH and IGF-I levels.

In normal subjects, mean serum GH levels over 24-hours do not exceed 7.5 mU/l (1 mU = 0.33 μg = 15.5 pmol). However, most of the samples show very low or undetectable levels, whereas samples corresponding to episodic bursts may show GH concentrations as high as 120 to 150 mU/l. For this reason, GH determination on one single sample is of poor diagnostic value. Plasma IGF-I measurement is a more reliable index of GH function, as it reflects GH activity over time and does not show wide spontaneous fluctuations. Normal IGF-I levels vary with age, sex, and nutritional status and should be interpreted accordingly.

Recently, the evaluation of IGF-binding proteins has been introduced. It has been demonstrated that the levels of the type 3 IGF-binding protein (IGFBP3) are directly proportionate to GH and IGF-I concentrations. Thus, IGFBP3 measurement may be taken as an index of GH-IGF-I activity, provided the nutritional status is normal.

In the presence of suspected GH deficiency, the evaluation of serum GH levels on multiple samples over 24-hours, or overnight, is the most reliable diagnostic test (although costly and cumbersome), as the absence of the sleep-related peak is of absolute value. Low levels of IGF-I and IGFBP3 are also indicative of GH deficiency. In adult-onset type GH deficiency, IGF-I and IGFBP3 are not considered reliable, as their levels spontaneously decline with age.

Insulin-induced hypoglycemia (ITT) (regular insulin 0.05-0.1 U/kg iv; blood sampling every 15 to 30 minutes from −30 to +60 minutes), arginine infusion (0.50 g/kg iv up to maximum 30 g, over 30 minutes; sampling every 30 minutes for 2 hours), and clonidine (100-200 μg orally) are the most widely used. A GH increase <20 mU/l in children is conventionally considered indicative of GH deficiency. In adults, both arginine and clonidine give inconsistent results; GH increases <9 mU/l in response to ITT are considered diagnostic for GH deficiency. As ITT requires blood sugar to fall below 2.2 mmol/l, the test is contraindicated in patients with cardiovascular and/or cerebrovascular problems and in those with epileptic fits. The absence of a GH response to a single test should be confirmed by a second one. In order to evaluate the ability of the pituitary to produce GH and to ascertain the hypothalamic versus pituitary origin of GH deficiency, a GHRH test (1 μg/kg iv, sampling every 30 minutes from −30 to +120 minutes) may be performed. This test is sensitized by pyridostigmine preadministration (60 mg po) or by the simultaneous infusion of arginine, as both the maneuvers potentiate GH response to GHRH by removing the inhibitory somatostatinergic tone. GHRH + arginine test is well-tolerated and safe, and it gives reliable responses both in children and in adults, including the elderly (cut-off value <45 mU/l).

The interpretation of results requires attention, as the coexistence of nutritional or endocrine problems such as obesity, hypercortisolism, hypothyroidism, and hypogonadism may blunt GH responsiveness to stimulatory tests.

Basal serum GH >15 mU/l in at least three different samples accompanied by supranormal IGF-I levels are diagnostic for GH secretory excess (acromegaly, giantism) and do not require further investigation. However, dynamic testing is mandatory when GH and IGF-I are not clear-cut in spite of signs and symptoms of the disease, or when it is necessary to assess the effects of surgical or radiation therapy of a GH-secreting pituitary adenoma.

The most reliable inhibitory test is the oral glucose tolerance test (OGTT, 100 g glucose po; sampling every 30 minutes over 3 hours), which in normal subjects causes serum GH levels to fall below 0.3 mU/l within 60 to 90 minutes, followed by a late increase at 120 to 180 minutes. In 95% of patients with acromegaly, GH levels are not suppressed by OGTT that may even cause a paradoxical GH rise in about 15 to 20% of cases.

Inhibitory tests with the somatostatin analogue octreotide (100 µg iv; blood sampling every 30 minutes over 4 hours) and with bromocriptine (Brc, 2.5 mg po, blood sampling every 30 minutes over 240 minutes) are of no diagnostic value, although they may be useful to identify patients who could benefit from medical treatment.

In acromegalic patients, abnormal GH responses to the administration of nonspecific releasing hormones such as TRH (200 µg iv) and GnRH (100 µg iv) have been described in about 50 and 30% of patients, respectively, and demonstrated to be typical of the adenomatous tissue. These tests may be employed to assess the completeness of adenoma excision in preoperatively responsive patients. The interpretation of the results requires attention, as GH response to TRH may also occur in patients with hepatic, renal, or thyroid insufficiency, as well as in anorexia nervosa, diabetes, and depression. In all of the above-mentioned conditions, IGF-I levels are normal or low. Children with constitutionally tall stature may also occasionally show a serum GH increase after TRH administration.

Hypothalamic-prolactin axis

The investigation of the hypothalamic-prolactin axis is only required in patients with suspected hyperprolactinemia, as PRL deficiency does not have clinical importance. Measurement of serum PRL carried out on multiple samples obtained every 30 minutes during slow saline infusion is the best diagnostic test. Serum PRL levels (1 mU = 0.05 µg = 0.23 pmol) >400 mU/l in women and >300 mU/l in men, without any trend downward, are suggestive of hyperprolactinemia. Serum PRL levels >4000 mU/l are diagnostic for a PRL-secreting pituitary adenoma, whereas PRL levels between >400 and <4000 mU/l may be found in many different physiological (pregnancy, breast-feeding) and pathological conditions (microprolactinomas, hypothalamic disconnection, empty sella, antidopaminergic drug administration, hypothyroidism, and polycystic ovary syndrome). Attention should be paid to prolactin assay methods, as falsely low a high PRL levels may be found due to the so-called "hook effect" or the presence of PRL molecular aggregates (macroprolactinemia), respectively.

Several dynamic inhibitory and stimulatory tests were proposed with the aim of discriminating microprolactinomas from other conditions associated with hyperprolactinemia. However, the present availability of high resolution imaging procedures (Fig. 6.2) able to detect few millimeter lesions has rendered PRL testing obsolete.

Hypothalamic-pituitary-adrenal (HPA) axis

The functional study of the hypothalamic-pituitary-adrenal axis is based on the measurement of circulating levels of ACTH (1 ng = 0.22 pmol; normal values: 10-90 ng/l) and cortisol (1 µg = 2.76 nmol; normal values: 138-690 nmol/l), and of the excretion of urinary free cortisol (30-275 nmol per 24 hours).

In the presence of suspected adrenocortical failure, the evaluation of plasma cortisol levels on a single sample is of poor diagnostic value, while the estimation of urinary free cortisol is more reliable. Low urinary free cortisol levels support the diagnosis of adrenal insufficiency, while plasma ACTH measurement is helpful in discriminating a central versus adrenal origin of the disease.

A low-dose ACTH-stimulation test (1 µg synthetic 1-24 ACTH iv; cortisol peak >490 nmol/l at 30 to 40 minutes) may give further support to the diagnosis of adrenal insufficiency of central origin, as prolonged ACTH deficiency causes adrenal atrophy and blunts cortisol response to exogenous ACTH.

ITT may be utilized to assess the integrity of the entire HPA axis (cortisol net increase at peak >165 nmol/l, ACTH net increase at peak >4.5 pmol/l). In cases of suspected adrenal insufficiency, insulin should be given at reduced doses (0.05 U/kg body weight). The administration of CRH (1.0 µg/kg body weight iv; blood sampling every 15 minutes for 2 hours; normal cortisol net increase

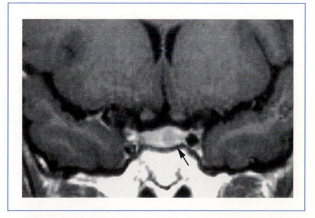

Figure 6.2 Magnetic resonance image of a pituitary microprolactinoma (arrow, coronal view, T1). The adenoma appears as a hypodense area in a slightly thickened pituitary with a convex superior margin.

>165 nmol/l) assesses the ACTH pituitary reserve. An absent response is indicative of corticotroph insufficiency. Normal or even exaggerated ACTH responses may be found in hypothalamic hypoadrenocorticism.

ACTH hypersecretion from the pituitary is the cause of Cushing's disease. More rarely, ACTH hypersecretion originates either from the pituitary overstimulated by ectopic CRH or from ectopic ACTH secretion.

The finding of ACTH plasma levels inappropriately high with respect to urinary free cortisol or plasma cortisol levels is suggestive of ACTH-dependent hypercortisolism, while suppressed ACTH levels favor adrenal autonomy.

The discrimination between central and adrenal origin of hypercortisolism is based upon inhibitory tests. The absence of cortisol suppression after the "overnight suppression test" (dexamethasone 1 mg at 11 p.m., plasma cortisol evaluation the following morning at 8 a.m.; cortisol suppression below 138 nmol/l) is widely utilized as a first-line screening test. This test may also fail to suppress cortisol (false positive) in patients with obesity, hyperestrogenism, psychiatric diseases, alcoholism, or on dintoin or barbituric treatment. The "low-dose dexamethasone test" (0.5 mg dexamethasone every 6 hours over 2 days) is more reliable. In normal subjects, but not in Cushing's syndrome independent of its origin, urinary free cortisol excretion measured on the second day is reduced by at least 50% with respect to the basal levels. The "high-dose dexamethasone test" (dexamethasone 2 mg every 6 hours over 2 days) allows for the discrimination of patients affected with adrenocortical hyperfunction of central origin whose urinary free cortisol excretion on the second day is suppressed by at least 50%, from those with adrenocortical hyperfunction due to adrenal autonomy, ectopic ACTH, or CRH overproduction, whose urinary free cortisol excretion is not suppressed. The same information may be obtained by the overnight "high-dose dexamethasone test" (dexamethasone 8 mg at 11 p.m., plasma cortisol evaluation the following morning at 8 a.m.). About 95% of patients with adrenocortical hyperfunction of central origin suppress plasma cortisol by al least 50%, while those with ectopic ACTH syndrome or cortisol-producing adrenal tumors do not.

A CRH-stimulation test may be useful to differentiate patients with adrenocortical hyperfunction of hypothalamic or pituitary (usually responsive) from those with ectopic ACTH/CRH syndrome (usually unresponsive). Also useful for this purpose (although not of absolute value) is the administration of desmopressin (DDAVP, 10 µg iv, blood sampling every 30 minutes over 2 hours), which increases serum ACTH and cortisol in patients with adrenocortical hyperfunction of pituitary origin, while it does not in normal subjects and in those with ectopic ACTH/CRH.

Hypothalamic-pituitary-thyroid (HPT) axis

The measurement of basal serum TSH concentration should be carried out utilizing ultrasensitive TSH immunometric methods able to distinguish normal from suppressed TSH levels, and it should always be accompanied by the evaluation of free thyroid hormones. Normal levels vary from 0.2 to 4 mU/l.

Low thyroid hormone and high TSH levels are indicative of primary thyroid failure, while high thyroid hormone and suppressed TSH levels are typical of classical hyperthyroidism. Both conditions do not require more extensive investigations of HPA function. On the contrary, these are mandatory when hypo- or hyperthyroidism are of central origin.

Thyroid failure secondary to TSH deficiency is characterized by low serum free thyroid hormone and TSH levels. However, in some cases of hypothalamic origin, basal serum TSH levels may be slightly elevated, but with reduced biological activity. The TRH test (TRH 200 µg iv; blood sampling every 30 minutes over 3 hours) assesses the TSH pituitary reserve, allowing for the distinction between the pituitary (absent or impaired TSH response) or hypothalamic (positive TSH response, frequently delayed and/or exaggerated and prolonged) origin of TSH deficiency. When a positive TSH response is not accompanied by an adequate increase in serum free thyroid hormones, the secretion of TSH with reduced biological activity should be suspected.

Unsuppressed TSH levels in patients with high levels of free thyroid hormones are suggestive of inappropriate secretion of TSH, a condition that may be due to either a TSH-secreting pituitary adenoma or pituitary resistance to thyroid hormone (PRTH). The TRH test distinguishes patients with thyrotropinomas (unresponsive in 95% of cases) from those with PRTH (100% responsive). A T_3 suppression test (L-triiodothyronine, 80-100 µg/die po over 10 days) is also useful, as serum TSH levels are lowered in 100% of patients with PRTH, while they are not in 98% of those with thyrotropinoma. The measurement of alpha-subunit (α-SU) may also help, as the α-SU/TSH molar ratio (MR) is high in patients with thyrotropinoma with respect to normal subjects matched for age and sex, while it is normal in those with PRTH.

Hypothalamic-pituitary-gonadal (HPG) axis

The study of the hypothalamic-pituitary-gonadal (HPG) axis requires the simultaneous estimation of LH, FSH, and sex hormone levels. In women, the interpretation of the data should take into consideration the physiological wide fluctuations of these parameters throughout the menstrual cycle and lifespan.

Low or low-normal nonpulsatile gonadotropin levels are typical of hypothalamic-pituitary dysfunction. Gonadotropin pulsatility may be assessed by multiple sampling (every 10 minutes over 24 hours), with pulsatory episodes being detectable every 90 to 120 minutes in normal subjects.

The GnRH test (100 µg iv, blood sampling every 30 minutes from –60 to +120 minutes) is used for the evaluation of pituitary gonadotropin reserve. Patients with pituitary failure show absent or impaired gonadotropin response, whereas those with hypothalamic disorders usually respond to a single or repeated GnRH boli and often show a higher FSH than LH increase. Patients should be carefully monitored, as pituitary apoplexy has been reported in some patients with extremely large primary or metastatic pituitary tumors.

The clomiphene test (100 mg per day po over 5 days in women, or 10 to 14 days in men) is used to evaluate the ability of the entire hypothalamic-pituitary-gonadal axis to react to the feedback mechanism elicited by the administration of this antiestrogenic compound. In responsive woman, a clear elevation in serum LH levels occurs within 5 to 10 days, which is accompanied by modifications in basal body temperature profile and followed 10 to 15 days later by a menstrual cycle.

The estrogen test (1 mg estradiol benzoate im) is used to investigate the positive feedback mechanism of estrogen. In normal women an elevation in serum LH levels occurs within 48 to 72 hours. Unresponsiveness to clomiphene and estrogen test in the presence of a normal response to GnRH suggests a hypothalamic disorder.

Gonadotropin hypersecretion is present in postmenopausal women and in patients with primary gonadal failure. Inappropriately high gonadotropin levels for age and sex hormones are found in patients with central precocious puberty. High levels of circulating gonadotropins in the absence of hypogonadism are suggestive of an inappropriate secretion that is usually caused by a pituitary tumor. Conceptually, a suppression test with gonadal steroids would be useful to distinguish tumoral from non-tumoral hypersecretion, however the tests proposed so far do not give reliable results. As gonadotropinomas frequently show positive FSH/LH responses to TRH administration, a TRH test could be utilized to confirm the origin of gonadotropin hypersecretion from a pituitary tumor.

Pituitary multifunction test

Pituitary function could be investigated by the simultaneous administration of several stimuli (e.g., GHRH, CRH, TRH, and GnRH; or ITT, TRH, and GnRH) and the evaluation of the corresponding pituitary and peripheral gland hormones. Although some minor interferences have been described, the combined tests are still used. Attention should be paid to the reported occurrence of pituitary apoplexy in patients with large pituitary tumors.

Imaging techniques

In a suspected hypothalamic pituitary disorder, an imaging study of the sellar region is mandatory. However, caution should be used in the interpretation of neuroradiological studies, which should always be additionally based on endocrinological criteria. In fact, minute, asymptomatic pituitary lesions have been reported in about 10 to 20% of the healthy population, while sometimes extremely small functioning microadenomas may go undetected.

Standard X-ray A standard X-ray film is recommended as the first-line, low-cost investigation that allows for the detection or exclusion of gross lesions. Antero-posterior projection visualizes the sella floor, while a lateral view allows for the study of the sella shape and morphology and for the measurement of diameters. Moreover, the presence of intra-, para-, or suprasellar calcifications can be seen.

Computed tomography (CT) CT carried out with contrast medium and dynamic study, thin coronal sections (1.5-2 mm), and sagittal reconstruction allows for the detection of focal lesions as small as 2 to 3 mm in diameter. A pituitary microadenoma usually appears as a hypodense, well-circumscribed lesion in a slightly thick pituitary with a convex superior profile; the sella floor is thinned in correspondence to the lesion, and the pituitary stalk is deviated toward the side opposite the adenoma. Macroadenomas are easily detectable, and a CT will reveal their size, expansion, and invasiveness. CT can also show the presence of liquoral hypodensity within the sella (empty sella), or nonadenomatous expansive lesions of the pituitary or surrounding structures.

Magnetic resonance imaging (MRI) MRI is the procedure of choice for the neuroradiological investigation of the hypothalamic-pituitary region. Although it does not allow for the study of bone alterations, it offers a better spatial definition and imaging resolution than CT when it is carried out with the use of the paramagnetic contrast agent gadolinium. Moreover, MRI directly visualizes the stalk, the optic chiasm, the chiasmatic cisternae and the third ventricle, and the posterior pituitary, which appears as a bright spot.

Scintigraphy The use of labeled ligands has allowed for the visualization of the pituitary by scintigraphy. These procedures generally do not have diagnostic applications, but they give information about the presence of specific receptors for a given ligand. The most widely used is ^{111}In-pentetreotide, which allows for the detection of tumors with somatostatin receptors. It is likely that in the near future radiolabeled compounds for radiobiological therapy of pituitary tumors will be developed.

Ophthalmological evaluation Careful ophthalmoscopic examination is mandatory for suspected expanding pituitary lesions impinging on the optic pathways. Optic fibers may exhibit axonic degeneration of various degrees up to optic atrophy. Papilledema due to impaired liquoral circulation rarely occurs.

The visual field perimetry defect most commonly encountered is bitemporal hemianopsia, which is indicated by a compression of the median portion of the optic chiasm. A rapidly developing impairment of visual field, up to complete amaurosis, indicates a fast growing lesion, while a mono-ocular visual field defects suggest an asymmetric growth. Binasal defects are typical of lesions that involve noncrossing fibers or the optic nerves.

Functional integrity of the entire optic pathways can be evaluated by the study of the pattern of visual evoked potentials (PVEP), which detects even initial minimal lesions.

HYPOTHALAMIC-PITUITARY DISEASES

Very similar clinical pictures may result from organic lesions involving either the pituitary or the hypothalamus or both, or from functional alterations without any detectable lesion. Organic lesions may be subdivided into non-neoplastic and neoplastic, the latter (mostly benign adenomas) being predominant. A clinical-etiological classification is outlined in Table 6.1.

In general, the clinical endocrine picture is that of impaired (hypopituitarism) or excessive (hyperpituitarism) functioning of the pituitary gland. However, as the pituitary is a multifunctional organ, sometimes hyper- and hypofunction of different tropins may coexist. This is typical of patients with hyperfunctioning pituitary tumors, who may show the clinical manifestations caused by the oversecreted hormone associated with those of other anterior pituitary hormone failure. Ophthalmological, neurological, and behavioral disturbances may be associated.

Hypopituitarism

We define hypopituitarism as the clinical picture of pituitary insufficiency. Hypopituitarism may be *total* (panhypopituitarism), *partial*, or even *unitropic*. It may also be subdivided into *acute* when it is the consequence of a lesion that causes a sudden and dramatic impairment of trophic hormone secretion; *chronic* when it is the consequence of a slowly evolving or permanent lesion; into *overt* when it is clinically evident; and *latent* when it becomes manifest only under particular conditions (stress) or when revealed by clinical laboratory tests.

Defects in peripheral hormone secretion caused by hypopituitarism are termed *central*, and they are distinguished into *secondary* or *tertiary* according to the pituitary or hypothalamic origin of the underlying disorder, respectively.

Clinical findings

The clinical manifestations of pituitary insufficiency vary according to the presence of one or multiple hormone defects, the age of onset, and the severity and type of the underlying lesion.

Acute anterior pituitary failure is usually caused by lesions that rapidly destroy the pituitary tissue, such as pituitary apoplexy or hemorrhage, or by stressful events (fever, acute diseases, exhaustive exercise, prolonged cold exposure, etc.) precipitating or aggravating a pre-existing mild or latent pituitary insufficiency. In the classical form, signs and symptoms of acute adrenal failure predominate (hypotension, shock). Rapidly expanding lesions, such as hemorrhage, are associated with progressively worsening headache and visual defects, with sign and symptoms of endocranial hypertension and mental confusion progressing to coma and death.

In chronic hypopituitarism, the development of the clinical picture is usually slow and insidious. Central

Table 6.1 Clinical-etiological classification of the hypothalamic-pituitary diseases

Non-neoplastic lesions

Malformations
  Agenesia, hypoplasia
  Primary empty sella

Genetic disorders (associated with neurological defects)
  Kallmann's syndrome
  Laurence-Moon-(Bardet-Biedl)'s syndrome
  Alström's syndrome
  Prader-Willi's syndrome

Genetic and idiopathic disorders
  Growth hormone deficiency
  Idiopathic hypoprolactinemia
  Idiopathic central hypothyroidism
  Idiopathic central hypogonadism
  Idiopathic central hypoadrenalism
  Idiopathic hyperprolactinemia
  Idiopathic central precocious puberty
  Non neoplastic inappropriate secretion of TSH (pituitary resistance to thyroid hormone, PRTH)

Vascular lesions
  Aneurisms
  Pituitary apoplexy
  Ischemic pituitary necrosis

Inflammatory and granulomatous lesions
  Bacterial hypophysitis
  Lymphocitic hypophysitis
  Sarcoidosis
  Histiocytosis X

Metabolic disorders
  Hemochromatosis
  Amiloidosis
  Mucopolysaccharidosis
  Chronic renal failure, chronic liver failure, malnutrition

Head injuries

Psychogenic disorders
  Psychiatric diseases
  Psychogenic amenorrhea
  Psychosocial dwarfism
  Pseudociesis
  Eating disorders (bulimia-anorexia)

Iatrogenic disorders
  Postsurgical hypopituitarism
  Radiant therapy
  Hormones and drugs

Neoplastic lesions

Secreting pituitary adenomas
  Somatotropinomas
  Prolactinomas
  Corticotropinomas
  Thyrotropinoma
  Gonadotropinomas
  Plurohormonal mixed adenomas

Clinically nonfunctioning pituitary adenomas
  Nonsecreting adenomas
  Alpha-subunit-secreting adenomas
  Silent adenomas

Pituitary adenocarcinomas

Non-pituitary tumors
  Craniopharyngiomas
  Meningiomas
  Gliomas
  Hamartomas
  Choristomas
  Deposits from malignant tumors
  Leukemic infiltrates

chronic unitropic defects cause signs and symptoms similar to but milder than those caused by the respective peripheral gland insufficiency. There are no clear-cut clinical differences between secondary and tertiary defects, which are sometimes difficult to be differentiated.

In prepubertal children, growth hormone defect causes dwarfism, while the clinical picture of GH deficiency in adults has only been recently delineated (Tab. 6.2). Signs and symptoms are not specific. The condition must be suspected in patients who had been previously treated with hGH, in those with other anterior pituitary hormone defects, or who had had pituitary surgery or radiation. The GH secretory capacity should be carefully investigated.

Prolactin defect is generally asymptomatic, except for patients presenting with the inability to lactate.

Patients with panhypopituitarism are usually slightly overweight and also have thinner muscular masses than normal. Their skin is pale and thin, and they have a fine wrinkle facial network that confers an aged appearance that, in patients in whom the hormone defect arose in the prepubertal age, may be characteristically associated with short stature. Sun tanning is impaired. Hair is thin and nails are fragile. In adult patients of both sexes, axillary and pubic hair are scanty. In males, the beard is scarce, and the volume of the testes, prostate, and seminal vesicles is low; libido and potency may be severely reduced, and there is hypo-oligospermia. In females, the breast and the external genitalia are poorly developed, the nipples, mammary areolas, and the genital skin are depigmented. Patients complain of disorders of menstrual cycles from hypo-oligomenorrhea to amenorrhea and infertility. Children show pubertal delay.

Muscular strength is reduced and patients complain of weakness and fatigue, symptoms that recognize a multifactorial origin such as GH deficiency, sex hormone defect, adrenocortical, and thyroid failure. Moreover, hypopituitaric patients show a tendency toward hypo-

glycemia due to glucocorticoid and GH defects. Patients may also show psychological changes, such as depression, abulia, reduced self-confidence and esteem, irritability, and difficulty in socializing and doing teamwork. In rare instances, if the causal lesion involves the hypothalamus and/or the pituitary stalk, vasopressin secretion is also impaired, resulting in diabetes insipidus.

Diagnosis

Appropriate hormonal investigations enable the confirmation of the patient clinically suspected of hypopituitarism. The basal levels of both the anterior pituitary and target gland hormones are low. The administration of hypothalamic-releasing hormones causes the corresponding tropin to increase if the pituitary insufficiency recognizes a defective hypothalamic stimulation. In this condition, high basal PRL levels are frequently seen due to the defective inhibition. All patients with hypopituitarism should have their hypothalamic-pituitary region imaged and their visual function investigated.

Treatment

As acute pituitary failure is a fulminant clinical syndrome in which adrenocortical failure predominates, immediate treatment with high doses of iv corticosteroids is mandatory. Emergency transsphenoidal surgery may be necessary in order to decompress the pituitary fossa and reduce visual damage and intracranial hypertension.

Treatment of chronic hypopituitarism is essentially aimed at the compensation of endocrine defect(s). ACTH and TSH deficiencies are generally treated with the administration of cortisol and thyroxine, as this modality is better accepted and far less expensive than the administration of the defective trophic hormone(s). The administration of hydrocortisone (20-25 mg, orally, in the morning + 10-12.5 mg in the afternoon) does not require accompaniment with mineralocorticosteroids, as their secretion, being HPA-independent, is usually not impaired.

The administration of L-thyroxine (1.4-1.8 µg/kg body weight, orally) should not be initiated before the compensation of adrenal insufficiency, and it should be instituted very gradually up to the optimal dose.

Gonadotropin deficiency may be compensated either by sex hormone replacement therapy, or if the patient is in the reproductive age and wants children, it can also be treated with appropriate FSH/hCG treatment or pulsatile injection of GnRH by portable pump in order to restore fertility.

The treatment of GH deficiency with recombinant human GH (rhGH) is mandatory in prepubertal hypopituitary dwarfism, at least until epiphysial fusion. There is accumulating evidence that rhGH therapy may also be useful in adult patients with GH deficiency in restoring well-being, muscular strength, cardiac function, and bone mineral mass. In several countries, due to the high cost,

---

Table 6.2 Main clinical features of growth hormone deficiency in adults (in alphabetical order)

Anxiety
Depression
Doubled cardiovascular risk
Hypercholesterolemia
Other anterior pituitary hormone deficiencies
Previous GH treatment for pituitary dwarfism
Previous pituitary surgery or irradiation
Reduced bone mineral content
Reduced glomerular filtration rate
Reduced lean/fat mass ratio
Reduced muscular size and strength
Reduced oxygen consumption
Reduced physical energy
Reduced quality of life
Reduced self-confidence
Reduced self-control
Skin: thin, dry, pale, cool
Sleep disturbances
Tendency to dehydration
Tendency to hypoglycemia

rhGH treatment in adults is only reimbursed by their national health service in patients with severe GH deficiency. The optimal therapeutical regimen in adults is not firmly established yet, but it is recommended that the doses should be lower than those in children and not exceeding those able to normalize IGF-I levels (i.e., 0.04-0.07 mg/kg per week).

Patients in whom diabetes insipidus is associated should be treated with vasopressin analogue desmopressin by nasal spray (5 µg at bedtime, and 2.5-5 µg in the morning) or orally (100 µg at bedtime and 50-100 µg in the morning).

Hyperpituitarism

The clinical picture of anterior pituitary hormone excess is generally sustained by functioning pituitary tumors or by the defective action of inhibitory neurohormones, or, more rarely, by excessive stimulation from releasing hormones eutopically or ectopically overproduced. Diseases causing anterior pituitary hormone hypersecretion will be described in the appropriate sections.

NON-NEOPLASTIC DISEASES

Genetic and idiopathic disorders

Rare hypothalamic-pituitary disorders are genetic in origin, generally caused by recessive autosomal or X-linked inheritance and may be present in a familial setting or as sporadic manifestations. They may be part of more complex syndromes involving the central nervous system, sometimes accompanied with intellective defects and/or with other somatic malformations. The recent advances in the knowledge about the genetic and molecular bases of pituitary embryogenesis and pituitary cell differentiation and committment from a unique progenitor have allowed to recognize also the molecular genetic bases of several of these rare syndromes previously defined as "idiopathic". Alterations of genes coding for transcription factors involved in early pituitary embryogenesis, or in the Rathke's pouch formation, such as Pax6, Six3 and Rpx, may cause pituitary agenesia or extreme hypoplasia. Mutations of Ptx-1, a gene coding for a factor acting on the transcription of all pituitary hormone genes, may cause panhypopituitarism. Mutations of Prop-1 (prophet of Pit-1) result in familial LH/FSH, TSH, GH and PRL deficiency, while mutations of Pit-1 gene are associated with deficiency of GH, PRL and TSH but not gonadotropins.

These diseases should be distinguished from disorders caused by hypothalamic pituitary disconnection following a breech delivery.

Idiopathic isolated GH deficiency

Idiopathic isolated GH deficiency is a sporadic, or more rarely familial, disorder causing the characteristic clinical picture of pituitary dwarfism. The prevalence of idiopathic GH deficiency is estimated to be about 1:3000 to 1:10 000. In about 70% of patients GH deficiency is of hypothalamic origin, as patients are able to release GH upon exogenous GHRH administration. In the remaining 30% of patients, GH deficiency is of pituitary origin. Defects of the gene coding for GH have been described.

Clinical findings

Patients with congenital GH deficiency are normal length at birth, but they exhibit reduced growth velocity by 1 to 2 years of age. The growth rate is usually <2.5 to 3 cm per year and the stature is below the 3rd centile. Patients are well-proportioned, although they have relatively small hands and feet, an immature facial appearance, and a high-pitched voice. Occasionally male patients may have a microphallus. Bone age is delayed by 2 to 3 years. Growth hormone deficiency is accompanied by a tendency toward hypoglycemia that could become symptomatic and cause seizures. Intelligence is usually normal. About 10 to 30% of patients show midline anatomic defects that may be seen on MRI (absence of the septum pellucidum and/or dislocation of posterior pituitary). Puberty is delayed, and in some patients it may spontaneously appear when patients are treated with GH.

Diagnosis

The clinical suspicion of GH deficiency should be substantiated by the evaluation of subjects' GH profile over 24 hours, or by GH stimulatory tests and IGF-I and/or IGFBP-3 levels. The hypothalamic or pituitary origin of the secretory defect may be tested by administering a GHRH test. The secretion of anterior pituitary hormones other than GH should be appropriately investigated in order to exclude other defects. An MRI is mandatory to rule out expanding lesions. Congenital GH deficiency should be differentiated from congenital resistance to GH (Laron's dwarfism), which is characterized by high levels of circulating GH and low levels of IGF-I not stimulated by the administration of exogenous GH.

Treatment

Treatment of GH-deficient children requires the administration of rhGH, at least until epiphysial fusion. rhGH should be administered at doses of 0.18-0.30 mg/kg per week, subdivided in daily doses. An increased tendency to develop slipped capital femoral epiphyses has been described. The claimed increased risk for leukemia or recurrence of pre-existing tumors has not been confirmed.

Idiopathic ACTH deficiency

This is a rare disease causing adrenocortical failure. Hypocortisolism is often latent and may be precipitated by acute stressful events. The absence of skin hyperpigmentation and the low concentrations of plasma ACTH associated with low levels of circulating or urinary free cortisol are distinctive with respect to primary adrenocortical insufficiency. Repeated ACTH stimulation with ACTH restores cortisol secretion, while ACTH and cortisol responses to CRH administration allow for the discrimination between ACTH deficiency of hypothalamic or pituitary origin. Treatment is based on hydrocortisone administration.

Idiopathic TSH deficiency

Idiopathic TSH deficiency is a rare disease of either genetic or acquired origin. Mutations of the gene coding for TSH-β have been described that lead either to truncated forms unable to couple with α-SU to form the complete molecule of TSH, or unable to bind the TSH receptor. Mutations in the TRH receptor gene resulting in TSH deficiency have been reported. Acquired forms are usually of hypothalamic origin. TRH defects are presumed to alter TSH glycosylation, which causes diminution of its bioactivity. Circulating levels of free thyroid hormones are low and antithyroid antibodies are absent. TSH levels are generally low, but they may be slightly elevated in patients secreting TSH with reduced biological activity. TSH response to TRH is absent or impaired if central hypothyroidism is of pituitary origin, while the response can be positive and frequently delayed, prolonged, and sometimes exaggerated if the disease is of hypothalamic origin. Therapy is based on L-thyroxine administration.

Idiopathic gonadotropin deficiency

Idiopathic gonadotropin deficiency is the term used for a group of diseases of either genetic or acquired origin. Mutations of the genes coding for β-subunits of LH or FSH may cause the defect. Acquired forms are generally due to alterations of GnRH secretion. Patients demonstrate eunuchoidism. Women present with primary or secondary amenorrhea and breast hypoplasia; and men with testicular hypoplasia or retention, a small-sized penis, poor sexual hair, altered sperm counts, and reduced muscular masses. In younger patients the clinical picture should be differentiated from delayed puberty, which usually remits spontaneously. Serum LH and FSH levels are low and the physiological pulsatile secretion pattern is lost. Repeated administration of chorionic gonadotropin elicits an adequate increase in plasma sex hormones. Repeated GnRH-stimulation tests cause gonadotropins to rise if the disease is of hypothalamic origin. Isolated LH deficiency results in the rare "fertile eunuch syndrome." In rare instances gonadotropin deficiency is part of more complex syndromes.

Kallmann's syndrome is an isolated gonadotropin deficiency syndrome associated with hypo- or anosmia. In about 20% of cases the syndrome is inherited as an X-linked dominant trait due to the deletion of a region in the short arm of the X chromosome (usually Xp 22.3), which contains a gene (Kal) encoding for an adhesion protein (KAL) involved in the migration of GnRH neurons from the olfactory placode to the medio-basal hypothalamus.

The loss of genetic material also causes other somatic alterations such as chondroplasia punctata, daltonism, palatoschisis, bone and kidney malformations, and ichthyosis. Undescended testes, gynecomastia, and mental retardation are also frequent. Syncinetic bimanual "mirror movements" are typical of the X-linked syndrome. The endocrinological picture is characterized by hypogonadotropic hypogonadisms and by an absent or reduced sense of smell. Apart from gonadotropin secretion, the pituitary function is otherwise normal.

Laurence-Moon-(Bardet-Biedl)'s syndrome is a disorder characterized by hypogonadotropic hypogonadism, obesity, retinitis pigmentosa, mental retardation, poly- and syndactylia, and, occasionally, short stature. Retinitis may progress to blindness. Nystagmus, ataxia, and paraplegia may coexist (Laurence-Moon's variant), as well as heart and kidney malformations. Hypogonadotropic hypogonadism is due to a GnRH defect.

Alström's syndrome is a recessive autosomal inherited hypogonadotropic hypogonadism due to a GnRH defect associated with vasopressin-resistant diabetes insipidus and obesity, reduced tolerance to carbohydrates, and degenerative retinitis that may progress to blindness. Deafness, chronic aminoaciduric nephropathy, and other defects may also be associated.

Prader-Willi's syndrome is characterized by hypogonadotropic hypogonadism, obesity, short stature, acromicry, severe mental retardation, emotional instability, and hypotonic musculature. It affects both sexes equally. Cryptorchidism and micropenis are frequently present in males. The genetic basis is uniparental maternal disomy of chromosome 15.

Idiopathic central precocious puberty

The anticipated activation of GnRH pulsatile secretion in the absence of organic lesions is classified as idiopathic central precocious puberty. The etiology of the disease is unknown, although in rare instances autosomal or X-linked dominant traits have been reported. The clinical picture may start in the first few years of life, with an equal frequency in both sexes. Patients have an anticipated onset-time of puberty accompanied with a faster bone maturation, which results in an initial height gain due to accelerated growth velocity and in a final short stature due to premature epiphysial fusion. Some patients may show electro-encephalographic abnormalities and epileptic equivalents. Serum gonadotropin and sexual hormone levels are high for age. This permits the distinction from precocious puberty of nonhypothalamic-pituitary origin, where gonadotropin levels are suppressed. MRI allows for the distinction from central precocious puberty, which is associated with organic lesions of the CNS.

The therapy of choice is the administration of GnRH superagonists that, by desensitizing pituitary GnRH receptors, block gonadotropin secretion. hrGH treatment may be associated to obtain a higher final stature.

Empty sella

Empty sella is the most common cause of sella enlargement. Autopsy series have revealed that in 5 to 20% of individuals the subarachnoid space extends into the sella turcica, which causes symmetrical enlargement of the sellar cavity and flattening of the pituitary on the sella floor. This is caused either by the absence or incompleteness of the *diafragma selle* due to developmental malformations (primary empty sella), by augmented intracranial pressure, or by destructive processes of a pre-existing expanding lesion of the pituitary (secondary empty sella).

Clinical findings

In the majority of cases primary empty sella is an incidental finding, as signs and symptoms are scarce and not very specific. About half of the patients are middle-aged obese women complaining of headache. Visual field defects are limited to those patients in whom the chiasm or optic tracts herniate into the sella. Hypopituitarism, sometimes associated with hyperprolactinemia, is seldom clinically overt; it is revealed at functional testing in about one-fourth of patients. In secondary empty sella, pituitary insufficiency, headache, and visual disturbances are more frequent and severe.

The diagnosis of empty sella is based on CT or MRI that show liquoral density images within the sella.

Treatment

Neurosurgical reduction of the arachnoid herniation and reconstruction of the diaphragma selle is needed only in the presence of impaired visual function and/or intolerable headache. Hypopituitarism should be managed as described above.

Vascular lesions

Aneurysms Aneurysms of the anterior communicant cerebral artery may cause sellar enlargement and pituitary lesions. The prominent clinical manifestations are the progressive loss of pituitary function and the visual loss due to the compression of optic nerves. The insufficiency of the HPA axis is common and may be associated with an inappropriate secretion of antidiuretic hormone from the hypothalamus. CT and eventually angiography allow for differentiation from pituitary adenomas.

Pituitary apoplexy Intrapituitary hemorrhage is almost invariably a complication that will occur with pituitary tumors. Radiation therapy of the adenoma, head traumatic lesions, GnRH testing, or concomitant anticoagulant treatment may favor its occurrence. The rupture of the tumor capsule may cause the dispersion of necrotic pituitary cells and blood into the chiasmatic cistern. The clinical picture is characterized by dramatically worsening headache, meningism, visual disturbances, ophthalmoplegia, mental confusion, and signs and symptoms of acute adrenocortical failure. Sometimes clinical manifestations are modest (e.g., silent pituitary apoplexy). Partial or total hypopituitarism and the radiological picture of secondary empty sella are late consequences.

Ischemic pituitary necrosis The brisk diminution of blood supply can cause pituitary ischemic necrosis. The most common cause is postpartum hemorrhage (Sheehan's syndrome). Diabetes mellitus, hypovolemic shock, and head trauma may also cause the disease. Pituitary necrosis results in hypopituitarism. In women with Sheehan's syndrome, the presenting symptoms may be the inability to breast-feed and postpartum amenorrhea.

Inflammatory and granulomatous diseases

Bacterial hypophysitis Bacterial hypophysitis has become extremely rare due to the wide use of antibiotics. Its clinical picture is characterized by symptoms of sepsis, meningism, and adrenocortical failure.

Lymphocytic hypophysitis Lymphocytic hypophysitis is a rarely recognized autoimmune disease. It is most prevalent in women, occurring during pregnancy or puerperium, isolated or in association with other autoimmune diseases. Presenting symptoms and radiological features resemble those of nonfunctioning pituitary adenoma: visual disturbances and hypopituitarism, frequently associated with hyperprolactinemia, in the presence of pituitary enlargement with suprasellar expansion. The clinical diagnosis is difficult and requires histopathological confirmation. Pituitary parenchyma and stalk show lymphocytic and plasma cellular infiltration.

Histiocytosis X Anterior pituitary insufficiency is often associated with diabetes insipidus and may occur in histiocytosis X due to hypothalamic infiltration. Hyperprolactinemia secondary to hypothalamic-pituitary disconnection is common. The association with exophthalmos is the consequence of orbital infiltration by histiocytotic granulomata.

Sarcoidosis The most frequent intracranial sarcoid lesions are in the hypothalamic-pituitary region. Thus, sarcoidosis may cause diabetes insipidus, hyperprolactinemia, and hypopituitarism. It is frequently associated with visual defects and involvement of other cranial nerves, according to the extent of the sarcoid lesions. The diagnosis is facilitated by the detection of other classical localizations of the disease (lung, lymph nodes, etc.). Corticosteroid treatment usually causes the lesions to shrink and visual and neurological defects to improve.

Metabolic diseases

Metabolic diseases may cause intrapituitary accumulation of different substances that result in an impaired pituitary function. A typical example is *hemochromatosis*, which causes hemosiderin deposits within the pituitary cells, in particular gonadotrophs. *Amyloidosis* and *mucopolysaccharidosis* may also cause hypopituitarism.

Head injuries

Head injuries may cause lesions of the stalk that result in anterior hypopituitarism, which is frequently associated with diabetes insipidus. Secretory defects are generally transitory.

Psychogenic diseases

Psychogenic amenorrhea Irregularities of menstrual cycles – ranging from hypo/oligomenorrhea to amenorrhea – are frequently encountered in young women with psychoaffective disturbances, as well as alterations of eating behavior, and physical overactivity in the absence of organic lesions. Serum gonadotropin levels are low-normal, but they have a low LH/FSH ratio and are nonpulsatile, and there may be moderate hyperprolactinemia. The disruption of GnRH pulsatile secretion is likely due to an increased central opioergic tone and/or CRH hypersecretion in response to stressful situations. Gonadotropin response to a GnRH test may show an exaggerated FSH response.

Psychosocial dwarfism Psychosocial deprivation may induce reduced GH secretion and slow down growth. These patients are difficult to distinguish from those with true pituitary dwarfism. Linear growth restarts upon favorable changes of psychoaffective and environmental conditions.

Iatrogenic hypopituitarism

Pituitary surgery may cause hypopituitarism related to the extent of pituitary tissue ablation and to possible damage of the pituitary stalk.

The hypopituitarism that develops in patients undergoing radiotherapy directed to the pituitary or other intracranial tumors or to the skull is a slowly evolving and insidious disease that may require years to become fully manifest. Gonadotropin secretion is usually the first impaired, followed by GH, TSH, and ACTH secretion. Hyperprolactinemia is often associated. Pituitary function tests show that in the majority of cases hypopituitarism is of hypothalamic origin.

Long-term treatment with corticosteroids may cause permanent inhibition of the hypothalamic-pituitary-adrenal axis. The brisk withdrawal of corticosteroid therapy is still in the present age the main cause of acute adrenal failure. In children, corticosteroid treatment may cause GH deficiency leading to growth impairment. Transient defects of thyrotropin and gonadotropin secretion may follow long-term treatment with L-thyroxine or sexual steroids, respectively. High-dose estrogen treatment (as in male to female transsexuals) may induce hyperprolactinemia. Neuroactive drugs interfering with dopamine action may cause hyperprolactinemia.

PITUITARY TUMORS

Pituitary tumors are generally primary, originating from hypophyseal cells, or much more rarely are metastatic deposits from other tumors. Primary pituitary tumors are usually benign adenomas and are only rarely carcinomas. They may be classified according to different criteria: as for *size*, as microadenomas (diameter <10 mm) and macroadenomas (diameter >10 mm); as for *extension*, as intrasellar and extrasellar; and finally, as for the *invasiveness* of adjacent structures, such as dura, bone and cavernous sinuses, as non-invasive and invasive (Fig. 6.3). There is no strict correlation between size and invasiveness. Pituitary tumors may also be classified according to their *function* as nonsecreting and secreting, and among the latter as mono- and plurihormonal.

Histologically, pituitary adenomas are classified according to cytofunctional criteria through the identification of intracellular secretory granules by means of optic or electron microscopy immunocytochemistry.

Epidemiology

The prevalence of clinically manifest pituitary tumors in the general population is about 0.02%, while autopsy series have revealed a prevalence of about 1000-fold higher (16 to 23%). About 40 to 50% of pituitary tumors are prolactinomas, 20 to 25% somatotropinomas, 8 to 10% corticotropinomas, 1 to 2% gonadotropinomas and thyrotropinomas, and about 25% are clinically nonfunctioning adenomas.

Etiopathogenesis

Whether the formation of pituitary adenomas is the consequence of a primary pituitary lesion or of a hypothalamic derangement leading to pituitary hyperplasia subsequently progressing to tumor has long been a debate. The recent discovery that, similar to most other tumors, pituitary ade-

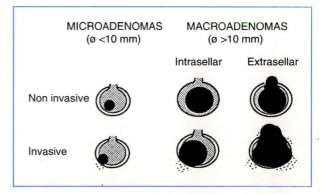

Figure 6.3 Classification of pituitary tumors according to size, invasiveness, and expansion.

nomas are monoclonal in origin (i.e., they originate from one single transformed cell) has led to the concept that the general rules of tumorigenesis also apply to pituitary tumors. In this view, pituitary tumor formation may be considered the result of a multistep process involving "initiating" and "promoting" events. Initiating events may be either oncogenic mutations or loss of tumor-suppressor genes, while either hypothalamic dysfunctions or locally produced growth factors may act as promoting events. This view is supported by the recent discovery of oncogenic mutations of the α-subunit of the Gs protein (*gsp*) in about 40% of somatotropinomas, and of the loss of heterozygosity in 11q13 (suggestive of loss of tumor-suppressor genes) in about 25% of pituitary adenomas. Recently, estrogen-inducible gene sequences with transforming properties (pituitary tumor transforming gene, PTTG) have been identified in human pituitary and found overexpressed in most pituitary tumors. hPTTG appears involved both in early pituitary tumorigenesis, as it causes *in vitro* and *in vivo* transformation acting as a transcription activator, and in tumor progression, as it regulates the production of basic fibroblast growth factor (bFGF), a potent activator of angiogenesis and mitogenesis. Alterations of hypothalamic regulation and the intrapituitary production of growth factors have also been demonstrated.

Clinical findings

Irrespective of their nature and secretory activity, space-occupying lesions of the hypothalamic-pituitary region may cause the same presenting symptoms. Retro-orbital, frontotemporal or frontoparietal headache due to the pressure on meningeal structures, and visual defects due to the compression of optic chiasm or optic pathways are the most frequent clinical manifestations. Tumor expansion in the cavernous sinus may cause palsy of the III, IV, and VI cranial nerves. Suprasellar expansion may obliterate Monro's foramina, resulting in hydrocephalus that may cause signs and symptoms of endocranial hypertension, such as generalized headache, vomiting, diabetes insipidus, bulimia or anorexia, somnolence, dysthermia, dysphoria, mental confusion, and psychosis.

Treatment

The aims of the treatment of pituitary adenomas are to remove or reduce the tumor mass, to normalize hormonal hypersecretion if any, to restore or preserve the pituitary function, and to correct the residual endocrine defects with an appropriate hormone replacement therapy. Treatment may be surgical, radiant, or medical. A combination of different approaches is often necessary.

Surgery Transsphenoidal surgery is the most widely used approach to selectively remove the tiny adenomas and to debulk the enormous ones. In noninvasive microadeno-

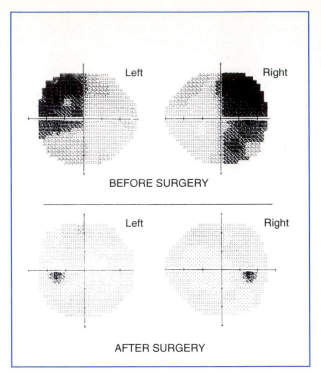

Figure 6.4 Computer-assisted visual field perimetry showing bitemporal hemianopsia (upper panel) that fully regressed after complete excision of a pituitary nonfunctioning adenoma (lower panel).

mas, the success rate is very high, approaching 80 to 90%, while it is about 40 to 50% in invasive microadenomas, and 30 to 40% in invasive macroadenomas. Anterior pituitary function is preserved or even improved in most cases, while additional defects may arise according to the extent of the excision or the surgical lesion of the pituitary stalk. Visual field defects improve or completely regress in most patients (Fig. 6.4).

Mortality is nearly null, and major complications such as hemorrhage, rhinoliquorrhea, and meningitis are very rare. About 10% of cases suffer from transient postoperative diabetes insipidus.

Transcranial surgery may be necessary to remove tumors with ample extrasellar expansion. This approach is followed by a higher mortality (about 3 to 6%) and complication rate.

In several centers, patients are given corticosteroids during and immediately after surgery in order to prevent acute adrenocortical failure.

Radiotherapy Radiotherapy is currently only considered the first-choice treatment in inoperable patients, while it is widely used as a valid complementary treatment in patients not radically operated on. Several techniques may be used, such as the conventional telecobalt radiation, linear accelerator, α-particles, stereotaxic radiosurgery (γ-knife) and adrontherapy. According to the procedures utilized, the time necessary for the achievement of full therapeutic effect may vary from a few months with the γ-knife to 8 to 10 years with the traditional two-field telecobalt radiation technique.

Drug The availability of neuroactive drugs and long-acting analogues of neurohormones (such as dopaminergic drugs and somatostatin analogues) has made an effective medical treatment of prolactinomas and somatotropinomas possible by controlling hormonal hypersecretion and reducing the tumor size. As for hormone replacement therapy, see the "Hypopituitarism" section above.

Acromegaly

Growth hormone overproduction by a GH-secreting pituitary adenoma (somatotropinoma) is the most frequent cause of GH excess syndromes (>99%). GH hypersecretion arising before epiphysial fusion causes giantism, while GH excess arising later induces acromegaly.

Epidemiology

Acromegaly is a rare disease (prevalence about 0.005%) that affects both sexes (female/male ratio 1.4), particularly in the third to fifth decade of life.

Etiopathogenesis

In more than 99% of cases, acromegaly and giantism are caused by a GH-secreting pituitary adenoma. Recently it has been demonstrated that about 40% of GH-secreting pituitary adenomas carry mutations (Cys or His for 201 Arg, or Arg or Leu for 227 Gln) in the α-subunit of the Gs protein, coupled with the GHRH receptor, that keep the protein constitutively activated and sustain GH secretion and cell proliferation. No other activating mutations have been discovered so far. The clinical phenotype of patients with *gsp-* mutated adenomas (*gsp*+ve) do not show clear-cut differences from patients with *gsp*-ve tumors. Acromegaly may be one of the components of the McCune Albright's syndrome (precocious puberty, osseous fibrous dysplasia, cutaneous *café au lait* spots, pituitary tumor) that is also caused by *gsp* mutations expressed in different tissues. A GH-secreting pituitary adenoma may be part of multiple endocrine neoplasia type I (MEN-I). However, no inactivating mutations of *menin* (the oncosuppressor gene that causes MEN-I syndromes) have been found in MEN-I non associated somatotropinomas.

In very rare cases GH hypersecretion is caused by excessive stimulation of somatotrophs by GHRH either overproduced eutopically by hypothalamic gangliocytomas or ectopically by pancreatic tumors, carcinoids, lung oat cell cancers, or other neoplasias. Ectopic secretion of GH has been appropriately documented in only a few cases.

Pathology

Twenty to 30% of GH-secreting adenomas are microadenomas, and 70 to 80% are macroadenomas. About 70 to 80% are monohormonal and can be subdivided into two main histological types: densely and sparsely granulated. Densely granulated adenomas are composed of well-differentiated monomorphic somatotrophs, are acidophilic at light microscopy, and have abundant GH secretory granules of 300 to 500 nm in size. Sparsely granulated adenomas are composed of pleomorphic cells that resemble cells of nonfunctioning tumors, are chromophobic at light microscopy, and have rare secretory granules of 100 to 250 nm in size. Sparsely granulated adenomas are usually more aggressive and tend to grow larger. Multihormonal adenomas show an associated secretion of PRL or TSH or α-subunit of glycoprotein hormones (α-SU). A variant is composed of mammosomatotrophic cells. Very rarely, GH-secreting pituitary carcinomas that can produce distant deposits have been reported.

Pathophysiology

GH excess causes bones and soft tissues to grow, induces resistance to insulin, and reduces carbohydrate tolerance.

GH secretion shows an increased number of pulsatile episodes with peaks that also appear wider than normal. Conversely, the sleep-induced nocturnal GH peak is abolished. The secretory responses to stimuli acting through hypothalamic activation, such as ITT or arginine infusion, are blunted in about 50% of cases, while the inhibitory effect of glucose is abolished in 95% of patients. Most patients reduce serum GH levels in response to exogenous somatostatin, while the secretory response to exogenous GHRH is highly variable. Typical is the secretory response to releasing hormones not specific for GH, such as TRH (50-60% of cases) and GnRH (20-30% of cases). Dopamine or dopamine agonists, such as bromocriptine, that in normal subjects stimulates GH release, induce a paradoxical GH inhibition in about 50% of patients.

Clinical findings

The clinical effects of GH excess vary according to the pubertal stage at the time of onset of the disease. The prominent signs and symptoms of acromegaly are listed in Table 6.3. The somatic changes induced by GH excess evolve slowly, such that they only became clinically manifest 5 to 15 years after the presumable onset of the disease. They consist of the enlargement of extremities (hands, feet, nose, mandible, supraorbital ridges), compelling patients to enlarge the size of their rings, gloves, and shoes; and it modifies his/her physiognomy (Fig. 6.5, see Color Atlas.) In children, growth velocity is increased and leads to giantism.

The skin is thickened, seborrheic, moist, and oily. Sebaceous cysts are frequent, as well as cutaneous small fibroepithelial tags. Axillary and neck acanthosis nigricans and (in women) hypertrichosis may be present. Teeth are widely spaced as a consequence of the downward and forward growth of the jaws. Visceromegaly is also present in most patients. Enlargement of the tongue, salivary glands, thyroid, and liver are particularly frequent and easily detectable. Overgrowth of bones and cartilages causes degenerative arthritis of the spine, hips, and knees, leading to arthralgias and paresthesias. Paresthesias of the

Table 6.3 Clinical features of acromegaly (in descending order of frequency)	
Enlargements of extremities	99%
Facial coarsening	97%
Visceromegaly	92%
Necessity to increase the shoe size	88%
Necessity to increase ring size	87%
Sella enlargement	83%
Acroparesthesias	82%
Arthralgias	80%
Hyperhidrosis, seborrhea	78%
Arthrosis	76%
Frontal bossing	72%
Oily skin	70%
Malocclusion and overbite	65%
Teeth separation	65%
Prognathism	62%
Headache	52%
Sleep apnea	52%
High blood pressure	45%
Impaired glucose tolerance	40%
Skin tags	38%
Goiter	38%
Menstrual abnormalities	36%
Asthenia	35%
Sexual disturbances	34%
Carpal tunnel syndrome	28%
Visual field defects	27%
Overt diabetes	25%
Galactorrhea	4%
Cranial nerve palsy	3%

fingers are present in the majority of patients and are sustained by the compression of the median nerve in the carpal tunnel. Polyneuropathy may occur, along with impaired tactile and pain sensation, and diminished motor function. Patients frequently complain of fatigue, hyperhidrosis, headache, somnolence, diminution of libido, and potency or menstrual disturbances.

Acromegaly is not only a disfiguring disease, but it is also the cause of increased morbidity and mortality. The expected risk of death for cardiovascular diseases, cerebrovascular stroke, respiratory insufficiency, and malignancy is increased by two- to fourfold in acromegalic patients with respect to the normal population. Cardiac insufficiency may be secondary to the hypertension that occurs in approximately 25% of patients, or to atherosclerotic disease or the so-called acromegalic cardiomyopathy. The latter is characterized by an increased left ventricular mass, which is caused by fibrous connectival hyperplasia and then by diminished left ventricular function and arrhythmias. Cardiac insufficiency may be worsened by the concomitant impairment of the respiratory function due to obstruction of the upper respiratory tract by hyperplastic mucosa and to the deformation and rigidity of the thoracic cage. An increased frequency of malignancy has been suspected in acromegalic patients, but never confirmed by controlled studies, while an increased frequency of benign lesions such as uterine leiomyomata and hyperplastic colonic polyps has been reported. About 10% of patients are suffering from nephrolithiasis secondary to increased calcium urinary excretion. Overt diabetes mellitus occurs in a minority of patients, while glucose intolerance and hyperinsulinism due to GH-induced insulin resistance are found in about one-half to three-quarters of patients, respectively.

Secondary hypogonadism occurs in about 60% of female and 40% of male patients. The origin of gonadal insufficiency is multifactorial. In fact, gonadotropin secretion may be impaired because of tumor growth, by the associated hyperprolactinemia, or by a prolactin-like effect of GH excess. Hyperprolactinemia is present in about 30% of patients and may be caused by either a pituitary adenoma with a mixed population of somatotrophs and lactotrophs or the co-secretion of GH and PRL by the same cell. Moreover, in adenomas with suprasellar expansion, hyperprolactinemia may be caused by hypothalamic disconnection. Galactorrhea is present in about 15% of patients, and gynecomastia occurs in about 10% of men. Secondary hypothyroidism is found in 15 to 25% of patients, while hyperthyroidism due to mixed GH/TSH-secreting adenomas is far less frequent (<1%). The frequency of multinodular goiter is increased.

Secondary adrenal insufficiency is rare (<5%). In relation to the adenoma size and expansion are the symptoms and signs due to the tumor mass. Nowadays these are reported in a lower percentage of patients with respect to the older series due to earlier diagnosis.

Diagnosis

In the majority of cases, a medical history and careful physical examination provide enough evidence to suspect acromegaly. The evaluation of basal serum levels of GH and IGF-I is usually sufficient to confirm the diagnosis. However, in about 5% of patients, serum GH levels are <15 mU/l and IGF-I only borderline high. In these cases an appropriate testing is mandatory (Fig. 6.6). The absence of serum GH suppressibility after OGTT is the best confirmation. In contrast, the evaluation of GH modifications after bromocriptine or somatostatin is indicated only on the basis of the intention to treat patients with these agents. The integrity of the hypothalamic-pituitary-peripheral gland axes other than GH-IGF-I should be assessed in order to exclude either secretory defects or associated hypersecretion of other anterior pituitary hormones (PRL: 30-35% of cases; α-SU: 10-20%; TSH <1%).

Imaging of the sella region with MRI or CT after contrast media and visual perimetry are mandatory.

Acromegaly, although very rarely (<1%), may be secondary to GHRH overproduction. This possibility should be considered in patients in whom MRI or CT imaging is suggestive of pituitary hyperplasia rather than adenoma, or who show a suprasellar hamartoma or rapid regrowth of the pituitary mass after apparently successful pituitary surgery. A reliable diagnostic index is the finding of GHRH circulating levels >300 pg/ml. The localization of the GHRH-producing tumor requires CT of the pancreas and the gastroduodenal region, as well as of the lungs and thymus. As GHRH-secreting tumors express somatostatin receptors, the use of ^{111}In-pentetreotide scintigraphy has revealed a very reliable tool for their localization.

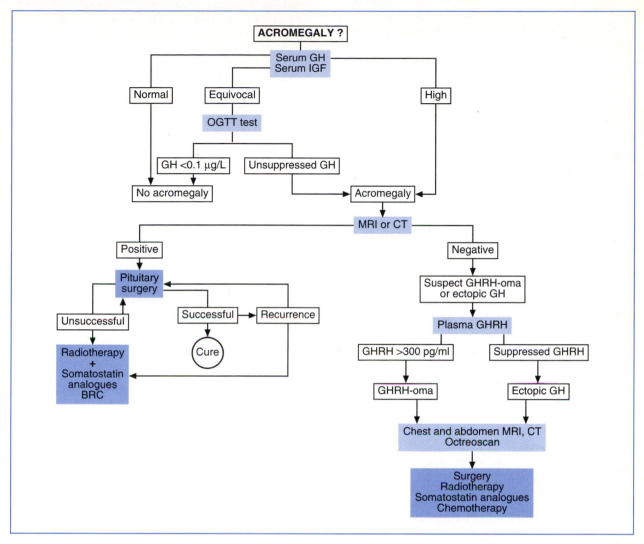

Figure 6.6 Pathways to the diagnosis and treatment of acromegaly. (GH = growth hormone; IGF-I = insulin-like growth factor 1; OGTT = oral glucose tolerance test; MRI = magnetic resonance imaging; CT = computed tomography; BRC = bromocriptine; GHRH-oma = GHRH-secreting neuroendocrine tumor.)

In about 20% of patients with multiple endocrine neoplasia type 1 (MEN-1), acromegaly is part of the syndrome and large study series have shown that MEN-1 is present in about 2.5 to 4% of acromegalic patients. This justifies the evaluation of serum ionized calcium and parathormone concentration. Differential diagnosis with acromegaloidism and pachydermoperiostosis, two rare diseases causing clinical features resembling those of acromegaly, is rarely a problem, as patients affected with either diseases show normal serum GH and IGF-I levels.

The radiological study of bones may help in confirming the diagnosis in very nascent cases showing thickening of the skull, enlargement of frontal and maxillary sinuses, and augmentation of the amplitude of the mandibular angle. Radiography of extremities show increased thickness of the soft tissues, which is particular-

ly evident at the heel pad; tufting of the phalanges; and cystic changes of the carpal and tarsal bones.

Although not useful for the primary diagnosis, glucose-insulin homeostasis and lipid pattern should be investigated. Cardiac function should also be carefully studied, particularly in patients with high blood pressure. Echocardiography shows an increased left ventricular mass associated with reduced left ventricular function.

Colonoscopy is recommended for patients over 50 years of age, particularly in those with skin tags.

Treatment

The criteria for the "cure" of acromegaly are still debated. At the present time, most clinicians agree that acromegalic patients may be considered "cured" when there is a stable reduction of serum GH levels below 7.5 mU/l, an IGF-I concentration within the normal range, and a normal GH suppressibility by OGTT. The disappearance of GH responses to TRH or GnRH in preoperatively responsive patients is also a reliable index of cure. Selective adenomectomy is the first-choice treatment, with the cure being obtained in about 80% of micro- and 40% of macroadenomas. Recurrences happen in about 6% of patients. In the case of surgical failure, reoperation is successful in about 30% of intrasellar tumors. Whether or not preoperative treatment with somatostatin analogues improves surgical success rate is still debated. Radiotherapy is indicated as adjuvant treatment. However, as the effects of radiotherapy may require even years to be manifest, medical treatment is recommended in the intervening period. Dopamine agonists (bromocriptine 10-30 mg per day or cabergoline 1-3 mg per week) have been proven able to reduce serum GH levels by 50% in about 50% of patients and to below 7.5 mU/l in about 20% of cases. The recent introduction of slow-release somatostatin analogues, such as octreotide and lanreotide, has made available an effective and safe tool for the control of GH hypersecretion. Treatment with somatostatin analogues reduces serum GH below 50% in 70 to 80% of patients and normalizes IGF-I levels in 40 to 50%. Pituitary tumor shrinkage by 20 to 50% occurs in about 30% of patients. Recently, slow-release somatostatin analogues have been proposed as first choice therapy for acromegalic patients with large and invasive adenomas that have few changes to be surgically cured. The diminution of soft tissue swelling, the improvement of headache, joint pain, and sensorimotor disturbances are impressive. However, after drug withdrawal the tumor rapidly re-expands, and serum GH and IGF-I levels return toward the pretreatment values. Somatostatin analogues are generally well-tolerated. Gallstone formation is the most important adverse event. Flatulence and loose stools are generally transitory side effects. Recently, a GH hormone antagonist that blocks GH effects by preventing GH receptor dimerization has been introduced. The compound, that has no effect on GH-secreting tumor mass, has very rapid effects on the relief of clinical symptoms of GH excess.

Prolactinomas and hyperprolactinemia

Hyperprolactinemia is a widely diffuse disorder (25-30% of women with alterations of the menstrual cycle). It is due to a host of causes, resulting in a clinical syndrome characterized by menstrual disorders, anovularity and galactorrhea in women, and by loss of libido and potency in men.

Epidemiology

Prolactinomas make up 40 to 50% of pituitary adenomas, and their prevalence is estimated to be about 0.008 to 0.012%. Microprolactinomas represent more than 70% of PRL-secreting adenomas and are more frequently diagnosed in women than in men (female/male: 20/1). The frequency of macroprolactinomas is the same in both sexes (female/male: 1.04/1). The median age at the time of diagnosis is 21 to 30 years for micro- and 41 to 50 for macroprolactinomas.

Other causes of hyperprolactinemia are listed in Table 6.4; these include the use of neuroactive drugs able to block dopamine receptors and to reduce dopamine synthesis or release, high-dose estrogen treatment, expanding lesions of the hypothalamic pituitary region able to impair dopamine secretion and transport, and irritating lesions of the nipple, thoracic wall or spine able to activate the neural pathways of the "suction reflex". Several other diseases such as chronic renal failure, liver cirrhosis, primary hypothyroidism, and polycystic ovary syndrome may be associated with hyperprolactinemia.

Table 6.4 Causes of hyperprolactinemia

Physiological

Sleep
Stress
Pregnancy
Nursing
Nipple stimulation
Orgasm
Neonate

Pharmacological

Dopamine receptor blockers
Phenothiazines: chlorpromazine, perphenazine, etc.
Butyrophenones: haloperidol
Tiaprides: sulpiride, metoclopramide, domperidone
Dopamine synthesis inhibitors
α-Methyldopa
Catecholamine depletors
Resepin, opioids, morphine
H_2 antagonists
Cimetidine, ranitidine
Imipramine
Estrogens

Pathological

Lesions of the hypothalamus or pituitary stalk
Hypothalamic tumors
Inflammatory or granulomatous diseases
Other expanding lesions
Pituitary lesions
Prolactinomas
Plurihormonal adenomas
Tumors deconnecting pituitary from hypothalamus
Empty sella
Primary hypothyroidism
Polycystic ovary syndrome
Lesions of the mammary region
Spinal cord lesions
Chronic renal failure
Liver cirrhosis
Paraneoplastic syndromes
Idiopathic (?)

As PRL secretion is primarily under inhibitory hypothalamic control, the pathogenetic role of either reduced central dopaminergic tone or primary alterations of lactotroph dopaminergic receptors in prolactinoma formation has long been debated. As of now, no specific mutation has been discovered except for an H-ras mutation in one single malignant prolactinoma. Loss of heterozygosity in 11q13 has been reported in some familial cases or in association with MEN-1. It is still debated whether the so-called idiopathic hyperprolactinemia represents a distinct disease sustained by neurosecretory dysfunction of the tubero-infundibular dopaminergic system or rather is due to microadenomas so minuscule that they go radiologically undetected.

Pathology

Prolactinomas usually originate in the lateral wings of the anterior pituitary. They appear weakly acidophilic or chromophobic with light microscopy. With electron microscopy, adenomatous lactotrophs appear as small monomorphic cells with well-developed Golgi complexes and prominent rough endoplasmic reticulum (RER). Secretory granules, 100 to 500 nm in size, immunostain for PRL.

Pathophysiology

Prolactin excess impairs reproductive function by acting both at the hypothalamic and gonadal level. The pulsatile episodes of GnRH are reduced or abolished. In women, LH and FSH secretions are not pulsatile, estrogen positive feedback upon LH is blunted, and the ovulatory LH peak does not occur. Moreover, at the gonadal level hyperprolactinemia inhibits the synthesis of 17β-estradiol and progesterone, impairing follicle development. In men, LH pulsatile secretion is also altered, and there is evidence that testicular steroidogenesis, as well as the peripheral conversion of testosterone into 5α-dihydrotestosterone, are affected by PRL excess.

Clinical findings

In women, the most early and frequent symptom is the alteration of menstrual cycles, which may range from hypo-oligomenorrhea to secondary or, rarely, primary amenorrhea. In rare cases there may be hyperpolymenorrhea due to a shortened luteal phase. Amenorrhea is usually secondary and may appear following pregnancy or oral contraceptive use. Almost invariably, menstrual disorders are associated with anovulation and infertility. Galactorrhea, either spontaneous or provoked by gentle breast expression, occurs in about 30 to 60% of women. Frequently the patients complain of dyspareunia, which is due to reduced vaginal secretion caused by hypoestrogenism. Long-standing exposure to low estrogen levels causes osteopenia. Moderate hir-

sutism may be present, accompanied by elevated levels of dehydroepiandrosterone sulphate.

In men, the most common clinical manifestations are the progressive loss of libido and potency, and the diminution of the ejaculate volume that may be associated with oligospermia. Galactorrhea is present in less than 5% of patients.

Patients with macroadenoma may present with signs and symptoms typical of expanding lesions of the hypothalamic-pituitary region. Hyperprolactinemic patients may suffer from anxiety, depression, fatigue, and irritability.

Diagnosis

There are three diagnostic problems frequently encountered in hyperprolactinemic patients: (1) Is the patient really affected with pathological hyperprolactinemia? (2) If so, does she/he harbor a pituitary tumor? and (3) If so, is that tumor a prolactinoma?

Many patients present with marginally elevated serum PRL when measured on a single sample if it is taken under stressful conditions or during a period of drug consumption. To address the first question, serum PRL levels should be measured with multiple samples taken during a slow saline infusion to avoid multiple venipuncture; it should be performed in the absence of any stress in patients resting in bed and off any drug known to affect PRL secretion. Serum PRL levels <2000 mU/l that progressively drop to within the normal limits exclude the diagnosis of hyperprolactinemia. Serum PRL levels >4000 mU/l are distinctive of prolactinoma. To address the second and third questions, all patients with confirmed hyperprolactinemia should undergo pituitary imaging, which could help to distinguish pituitary adenomas from other conditions associated to PRL elevations. In patients with pituitary macroadenomas and serum PRL levels <4000 mU/l, the diagnosis of nonprolactinoma (generally a nonfunctioning pituitary adenoma) is most likely. In patients with negative imaging, hypothyroidism, chronic renal failure, liver cirrhosis, and other diseases associated with increased serum PRL levels should be excluded by routine tests. Figure 6.7 shows the pathway to the diagnosis and treatment of prolactinomas.

Treatment

The poor success rate of pituitary surgery in macroprolactinomas (30-40%), the relatively high recurrence rate in microprolactinomas (16-50%), and the availability of effective and generally well-tolerated dopamine agonists has rendered medical treatment of prolactinomas to be the first-choice therapy. Dopaminergic agents inhibit PRL synthesis and release and are able to reduce the tumor volume in the vast majority of patients (Fig. 6.8). The widest experience has been accumulated with bromocriptine (2.5-20 mg/day po) and cabergoline (0.25-1.5

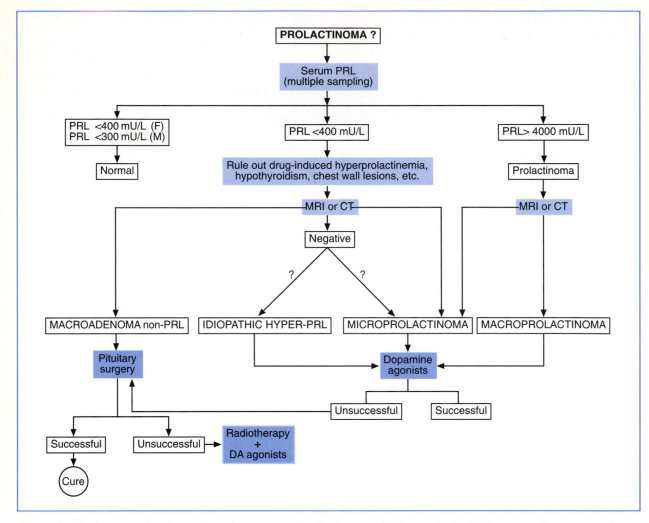

Figure 6.7 Pathways to the diagnosis and treatment of prolactinomas. (PRL = prolactin; MRI = magnetic resonance imaging; CT = computed tomography; TRH = thyrotropin-releasing hormone; DA = dopamine.)

mg/twice a week po). Dopamine agonists cause a prompt reduction of serum PRL levels (to within the normal range in 70 to 80% of cases), followed by the clinical remission of the hyperprolactinemic syndrome. Women resume regular ovulatory menses, and galactorrhea disappears after 1 to 3 months of treatment. Restored fertility requires precise patient counseling: (1) oral contraceptives are allowed; (2) in patients with microprolactinoma who desire children, pregnancies are easily obtained, and the risk of tumor expansion is less than 5%, while it is as high as 15 to 25% in macroprolactinomas; (3) pregnancies are generally uneventful and deliveries occur normally; the frequency of miscarriages, premature births, or congenital malformations is not different from that in healthy women; (4) dopamine agonist administration should be stopped as soon as pregnancy is diagnosed and eventually re-instituted if tumor expansion occurs; (5) serum PRL levels and visual field perimetry should be monitored; and (6) in patients with extremely large adenomas, pregnancy

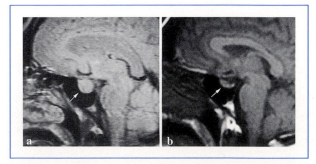

Figure 6.8 MRI showing the impressive reduction in size of a macroprolactinoma treated with the dopaminergic agent cabergoline.

is not advisable unless there is previous tumor debulking.

In men, libido, potency, and normal sperm counts are promptly restored in the majority of cases by dopamine agonists.

Side effects, such as nausea, vomiting, dizziness, drowsiness, and orthostatic hypotension are generally mild, and they tend to disappear after the first weeks of treatment; thus, only a minority of patients need to discontinue treatment. Tumor shrinkage is usually evident after 2 to 3 months of therapy and may be massive in macroprolactinomas (Fig. 6.8), permitting a rapid improvement of visual field defects. After drug withdrawal, the large majority of patients show a gradual, progressive return of PRL levels, tumor size, and signs and symptoms toward the pretreatment pattern. A minority (10-25%) of patients are partially or totally resistant to bromocriptine, although it is difficult to clearly distinguish refractoriness from intolerance to doses of dopamine agonists high enough to produce clinical effects.

With the aim of improving tolerability and overcoming the resistance to treatment, new dopaminergic agents have been developed. Among them are cabergoline, a naturally long-acting ergot derivative (0.25-1.5 mg twice a week), and quinagolide, a non-ergot compound (0.15-0.75 mg/day), which seem to meet these goals.

Pituitary surgery (eventually followed by radiation therapy) is recommended in patients (1) who are refractory or intolerant to dopamine agonists, (2) who do not want to be medically treated life-long, (3) in whom medical treatment is unable to shrink the adenoma, or (4) who are bearing cystic or rapidly expanding tumors. In patients with microprolactinoma, pituitary surgery results in a definitive cure in about 80% of cases. Therefore, the surgical option should be discussed with patients. Radiotherapy is indicated in the case of surgical failure and intolerance or resistance to dopamine agonists.

In hyperprolactinemic patients with space-occupying masses of the hypothalamic-pituitary region, the ideal treatment is the removal of the lesions in association with dopaminergic drugs. Sarcoid granulomas may be reduced by corticosteroid treatment. Adequate L-thyroxine replacement therapy usually normalizes PRL excess in hypothyroid patients. In patients with drug-induced hyperprolactinemia, the discontinuation of the drug may be necessary. Renal transplantation normalizes serum PRL levels in patients with chronic renal failure.

Corticotropinomas

Pituitary ACTH-secreting adenomas are the most frequent cause of hyperadrenocorticism (Cushing's syndrome). Bilateral adrenalectomy may cause the rapid expansion of the pre-existing pituitary tumor (Nelson's syndrome) in these patients.

Cushing's disease The clinical picture and the metabolic consequences of chronic exposure to high levels of glucocorticosteroids (Cushing's syndrome) are described in the Chapter 29. The term "Cushing's disease" refers only to hypercortisolism due to pituitary ACTH hypersecretion.

Epidemiology

Cushing's disease is responsible for 60 to 70% of Cushing's syndrome cases. Its prevalence is estimated to be about 0.001%. The disease occurs more frequently in young women (20 to 40 years) than in men (female/male ratio: 4.1).

Etiopathogenesis

Corticotropinomas, generally microadenomas of less than 5 mm in diameter, are present in about 90% of patients with Cushing's disease. Local microinvasiveness is frequent. Rarely, ACTH-secreting adenomas will progress to macroadenomas, altering sellar morphology and invading adjacent structures. The adenomatous corticotrophs appear basophilic under light microscopy. With electron microscopy they appear monomorphous, well-granulated, and often with perinuclear jalinized areas. Immunocytochemistry reveals strong reactivity for ACTH, β-LPH, and other POMC-derivatives. In 10% of the pituitaries removed from patients with Cushing's disease, no definite adenoma is found in the anterior pituitary, but areas or small nests of hyperplasia or tiny adenomas may be present in the intermediate lobe.

Clinical findings

Patients with Cushing's disease present with typical signs and symptoms of glucocorticoid excess (see Chap. 29). The onset of the disease is insidious, as it usually takes 2 to 5 years to become fully manifest. In rare cases, clinical and hormonal manifestations of the disease appear cyclically alternated with asymptomatic phases (so-called periodic Cushing's disease).

Diagnosis

On clinical grounds, there are no absolute criteria that allow for the distinction of Cushing's disease from other forms of Cushing's syndrome. Therefore, the diagnosis is largely based on hypothalamic-pituitary function tests (Fig. 6.9). Unsuppressed plasma ACTH rules out ACTH-independent Cushing's syndrome (i.e., functioning adrenal tumors and corticosteroid treatment). The distinction from the various forms of ACTH-dependent Cushing's syndrome is not always easy. Extremely high plasma ACTH levels suggest an ectopic source of ACTH secretion, since plasma ACTH is usually moderately high in Cushing's disease. In Cushing's disease, plasma cortisol and ACTH levels are not inhibited by the low-dose dexamethasone suppression test, while they are inhibited by the high-dose test; they are also responsive to CRH and desmopressin administration. This is not the case in most but not all patients with Cushing's syndrome due to CRH-secreting tumors or ectopic ACTH production. In 10 to 20% of patients with Cushing's disease, plasma ACTH

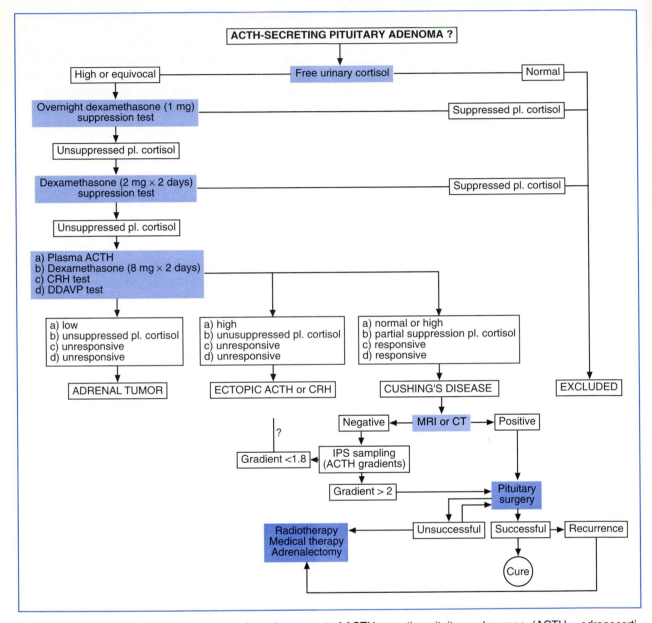

Figure 6.9 Pathways leading to the diagnosis and treatment of ACTH-secreting pituitary adenomas. (ACTH = adrenocorticotropic hormone; CRH = corticotropin-releasing hormone; DDAVP = desmopressin; MRI = magnetic resonance imaging; CT = computed tomography; IPS = inferior petrosal sinus; pl = plasma.)

and cortisol increase following the administration of nonspecific neurohormones such as TRH, GnRH, and VIP, thus allowing the diagnosis in responsive patients. Pituitary imaging permits the detection of microadenomas in about two-thirds of patients. In those with negative pituitary imaging, the presumptive tumor localization may be suggested by the evaluation of basal and CRH-stimulated ACTH gradients on blood obtained from inferior petrosal sinus sampling. A gradient for inferior petrosal sinuses versus peripheral blood >2 is consistent with a pituitary ACTH-secreting adenoma, while a gradient <1.8 favors the diagnosis of ectopic ACTH.

Treatment

If untreated, Cushing's disease can be lethal in 5 to 7 years. Every effort should therefore be done to control glucocorticoid excess. Selective adenomectomy is the treatment of choice in patients in whom ACTH-secreting pituitary adenoma is clearly localized by imaging techniques. In patients with negative pituitary imaging, if the neurosurgeon is unable to localize the adenoma intraoperatively, hemihypophysectomy is recommended on the basis of the gradient of ACTH concentration previously obtained after inferior petrosal sinus catheterism.

Transsphenoidal surgery is effective in about 75 to 90% of patients with microadenoma (Fig. 6.10, see Color Atlas), but in only 50 to 60% of those in whom microadenoma is not seen, and in 25 to 30% of those with macroadenomas. Secondary transient hypoadrenalism occurring after pituitary surgery and requiring cortisol replacement therapy is the best criterion of cure. Recurrences are frequent (10 to 20% at 5 years).

Conventional radiation therapy is of limited efficacy in adults (25 to 30%), while it is effective in 80% of children. The recently introduced use of γ-knife radiosurgery is more effective.

Medical treatment with adrenolytic drugs such as mitotane, ethomidate, aminogluthetimide, ketoconazole, or glucocorticoid receptor antagonists (e.g., mifepristone) (see Chap. 29) for details) is indicated only in preparation of surgery or while waiting for the effects of radiation therapy. Medical treatment with neuroactive drugs such as cyproheptadine, bromocriptine, and valproic acid, aimed to suppress ACTH secretion, has proven effective only episodically. Total bilateral adrenalectomy is indicated in patients unresponsive to any other treatment, as it causes permanent hypoadrenalism and may induce pituitary tumor expansion (see below).

Nelson's syndrome In about one-third of patients with Cushing's disease who undergo total bilateral adrenalectomy, the pituitary adenoma may rapidly expand up to the size of a giant adenoma. This expansion is thought to be due to the abolition of negative feedback by cortisol. Plasma ACTH levels markedly increase (up to 1000-10000 pg/ml), and patients show skin and mucosal hyperpigmentation and signs and symptoms of pituitary tumor expansion. The tumor is aggressive, not only invading locally, but sometimes causing intracranial deposits. The rapid increase in size may not be accompanied by an adequate increase of the vascular bed, which results in a diminution of blood supply and ischemic pituitary necrosis.

Due to patients' typical medical history, the diagnosis of Nelson's syndrome is easy. Tumor size and extension should be radiologically documented and the function of other pituitary axes investigated.

Treatment consists of surgical removal of the pituitary tumor followed by radiation therapy.

Thyrotropinomas

Primary TSH-secreting pituitary tumors are rare. TSH hypersecretion causes unrestrained thyroid overstimulation, which results in hyperthyroidism. In contrast, patients with long-standing hypothyroidism may develop enormous pituitary gland growth (so-called TSH feedback tumor or Furth's tumor).

Pathology

Primary TSH-secreting pituitary tumors are composed of monomorphous cells with well-developed RER and Golgi complexes. The secretory granules are small and typically aligned along the plasma membrane. Immunocytoche-

mistry reveals that TSH-secreting adenomas are frequently mixed tumors that may co-secrete α-SU (90%), GH (20-25%), PRL (15%), and, rarely, gonadotropins.

The so-called feedback tumors are enormous masses, more resembling extreme grade hyperplasia, that may reach Monro's foramina and cause hydrocephalus.

Clinical findings

Patients with pituitary TSH-secreting adenomas usually show mild hyperthyroidism characterized by uniform diffuse goiter. The goiter typically tends to expand during antithyroid drug administration and to recur after partial thyroidectomy or radiometabolic treatment. Graves' ophthalmopathy is typically absent. Due to the frequent mixed nature of TSH-secreting adenomas, the association with acromegaly and hyperprolactinemia is not rare. In some of these cases the mild hyperthyroidism may be overshadowed by the prominent features of acromegaly or hyperprolactinemia.

Diagnosis

The typical hormonal pattern is represented by elevated free thyroid hormone levels associated with unsuppressed TSH and absent antithyroid antibodies (Fig. 6.11). Serum TSH concentrations are clearly above the normal range in about two-thirds of patients, while in the remaining patients they are within the normal range, which is different than classical hyperthyroidism where serum TSH is invariably suppressed. The serum levels of α-SU and the α-SU/TSH molar ratio are elevated with respect to those found in healthy people matched for age and sex. Serum TSH and α-SU are not stimulated by TRH in 95% of cases and typically not suppressed by T_3 administration. Pituitary imaging reveals the presence of pituitary adenoma, which is a macroadenoma in more than 90% of cases. Thyroidal ^{131}I uptake is elevated and the tracer accumulation is uniform.

TSH-induced hyperthyroidism sustained by a TSH-secreting adenoma should be distinguished from that due to pituitary resistance to thyroid hormone (PRTH); which is characterized by the absence of pituitary lesions on CT or MRI, the normality of α-SU/TSH molar ratio, the preserved TSH suppressibility after T_3 administration, and TSH responsiveness to TRH stimulation. Moreover, PRTH is often present in a familial setting of generalized resistance to thyroid hormone.

Primary TSH-secreting tumors are easily distinguishable from feedback adenomas, as both the clinical history and picture are those of long-term primary, often congenital, hypothyroidism.

Treatment

Pituitary surgery followed by radiation therapy is the treatment of choice in primary TSH-secreting tumors. The

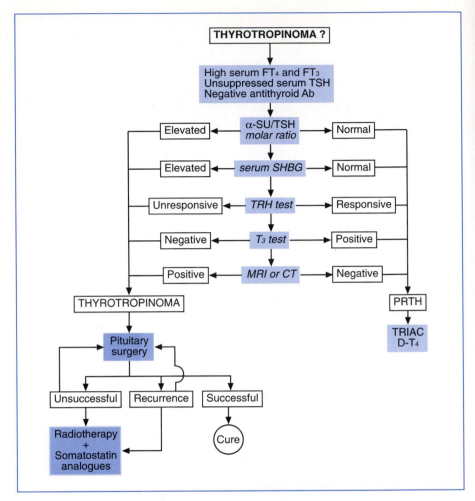

Figure 6.11 Pathways to the diagnosis and treatment of TSH-secreting pituitary tumors and pituitary resistance to thyroid hormones. (FT_3 = free triiodothyronine; FT_4 = free thyroxine; Ab = antibodies; α-SU = alpha-subunit of glycoprotein hormones; TSH = thyroid-stimulating hormone; SHBG = sex hormone-binding globulin; TRH = thyrotropin-releasing hormone; T_3 = triiodothyronine; MRI = magnetic resonance imaging; CT = computed tomography; PRTH = pituitary resistance to thyroid hormone; TRIAC = triiodothyroacetic acid; D-T_4 = D-thyroxine.)

success rate of surgery is around 50%. Bromocriptine, which has been suggested as adjuvant therapy, has been effective in a minority of cases. Somatostatin analogues, however, are effective and well-tolerated in the large majority of cases. Total thyroid ablation either by surgery or radioiodine is indicated only in the case of failure of the above approaches.

In patients with PRTH, treatment should be aimed to reduce TSH hypersecretion, avoiding, if possible, thyroid-directed therapy that further increases TSH secretion. Serum TSH and free T_4 (FT_4) normalization have been reported by using thyroid hormone derivatives able to inhibit TSH secretion without exerting a comparable metabolic effect, such as triiodothyroacetic acid (TRIAC, 2-3 mg per day) or D-thyroxine (2-3 mg per day). PRTH tends to escape from the inhibitory effect of somatostatin analogues, which are therefore not indicated.

The first-line approach to TSH feedback adenomas is replacement therapy with L-thyroxine, which has been shown to be effective in controlling the metabolic status and in dramatically reducing pituitary tumor volume in the vast majority of cases.

Gonadotropin-secreting adenomas

Although a number of clinically nonfunctioning pituitary adenomas contain gonadotropin immunoreactive cells and are able to release gonadotropins in vitro, with the term gonadotropin-secreting adenomas we classify those adenomas that actively release FSH and/or LH in vivo and thus enhance their concentration in the peripheral blood.

Gonadotropin-secreting adenomas are rare. About 50% of them secrete both LH and FSH, while the remaining secrete FSH only. Most patients are 40- to 60-year-old males (70%). The prevalence of the disease is likely underestimated in women due to the physiological gonadotropin elevation in menopausal age. Rare cases of gonadotropin-secreting adenomas resulting in precocious puberty have been described in children.

They are usually macroadenomas that stain chromophobes with traditional histology. At electron microscopy, cells are large and poorly granulated and immunostain for FSH, LH, and/or the common α-SU.

In most patients the pituitary tumor is discovered because of visual field defects. About 30% of men complain of libido loss and impotence that are usually not accompanied by diminution of the testicular volume. In women in fertile age, menstrual irregularities and infertility are the most frequent presenting symptoms.

Inappropriately elevated FSH and/or LH levels with respect to sex hormone concentrations is typical of these adenomas. Gonadotropin pulsatile secretory episodes are generally maintained, and after GnRH administration they have a normal or even exaggerated response. TRH administration causes serum LH-β, LH, FSH, and/or α-subunit to increase in most cases.

Diagnosing gonadotropin-secreting adenomas is difficult and always requires immunohistochemical confirmation.

The treatment of choice is pituitary surgery followed by radiation therapy. In some individual cases bromocriptine has been effective. The use of GnRH superagonists, with the aim of reducing gonadotropin secretion, has been elusive. GnRH antagonists have been shown to lower gonadotropin secretion, but therapeutical trials are still lacking.

Clinically nonfunctioning pituitary adenomas

The term "nonfunctioning pituitary adenomas" encompasses different biological entities that share the common characteristic of not releasing in vivo any bioactive pituitary hormone in sufficient amount to produce specific clinical signs, although they are able to secrete minute amounts of FSH, LH, α-SU, or POMC derivatives *in vitro*. Nonfunctioning pituitary adenomas, as a whole, represent about 25% of pituitary tumors. Their prevalence is about 0.005 to 0.006%, and they are evenly distributed among sexes. Nonfunctioning pituitary adenomas are generally diagnosed between 40 and 60 years of age. They are usually macroadenomas that stain chromophobes with traditional histology. Some of them may undergo oncocytic change, and the cells may appear to be filled of mitochondria. At electron microscopy, cells are large with poorly developed RER and Golgi complexes and have very few secretory granules. Rare immunoreactive cells (mainly for FSH, LH, and α-SU) are scattered within the tumor.

Alpha-SU-secreting adenomas and the so-called silent adenomas are also classified among nonfunctioning pituitary adenomas. Alpha-subunit-secreting adenomas are usually macroadenomas. Since the routine estimation of α-SU has become available, it was shown that about 15 to 20% of nonfunctioning pituitary adenomas were actually pure α-SU-secreting adenomas. Thus, the evaluation of serum α-SU levels has become important as a tumor marker. Silent adenomas are tumors that are able to synthesize GH, PRL, or ACTH without causing the corresponding clinical picture, as secretory processes may be impaired or the secretory products bioinactive.

Patients usually arrive for medical investigation with signs and symptoms of a space-occupying lesion and partial or total hypopituitarism (Tab. 6.5). In a minority of patients the adenoma is incidentally found at X-ray of the skull or visual perimetry carried out for other indications (pituitary incidentaloma).

The diagnosis in based on imaging of the hypothalamic pituitary region, visual field perimetry, and the presence of clinical and hormonal signs of hypopituitarism. About one-third of patients show mildly elevated serum PRL levels (generally <4000 mμ/l) due to hypothalamic disconnection, 15 to 20% show high levels of serum α-SU, and about 30 to 40% increase gonadotropin(s) after TRH administration.

Pituitary surgery followed by radiotherapy is the treatment of choice. Only 15 to 25% of patients may be considered cured (disappearance of pathological tissue at pituitary imaging and normalization of pituitary function), but in most of the remaining patients satisfactory results are obtained (improvement of visual function and disappearance of other "mass" symptoms and signs). In about 75% of patients, uni- or plurihormonal replacement therapy is needed. Medical therapy with dopamine agonists or somatostatin analogues has not proven to be effective.

Table 6.5 Frequency of presenting symptoms as compared with that of corresponding documented defects in a series of 214 patients with clinically nonfunctioning pituitary adenomas

Presenting symptoms	%	Documented defects	%
Visual disturbances	57	Visual perimetry defects	72
Symptoms suggestive of adrenocortical insufficiency	18	Low urinary free cortisol	31
		Impaired cortisol response to 1μg ACTH	46
		Impaired response to ITT	44
Symptoms suggestive of thyroid insufficiency	24	Low serum FT$_4$ levels	36
		Altered TSH responses to TRH	45
Symptoms suggestive of gonadal insufficiency	46	Low basal gonadotropin level	32
		Low basal sex hormone levels	64
		Impaired LH response to GnRH	54
Gynecomastia and/or galactorrhea	21	Elevated serum PRL levels	56
Symptoms suggestive of somatotropin deficiency	76	GH response to ITT <3.0 μg/l	67

HYPOTHALAMIC TUMORS

Hypothalamic tumors may originate from nervous, glial, and meningeal structures or from embryonal remnants.

Meningiomas

Meningiomas may develop from intrasellar meningeal structures and cause enlargement or even destruction of the sella walls, which occurs in a manner very similar to that of extremely large pituitary adenomas. Presenting symptoms are headache, visual disturbances, and hypopituitarism. The diagnosis is based on the radiological picture; generally the distinction from nonfunctioning pituitary adenomas is possible only on a histopathological basis. Treatment is surgical.

Craniopharyngiomas

Craniopharyngiomas originate from epithelial rests of the Rathke's pouch and easily show cystic transformation. They most frequently occur in children, showing an incidence peak between 6 and 14 years. Patients present with ophthalmologic and neurological signs accompanied by panhypopituitarism. In children, growth and pubertal delay predominate, but in some patients, in spite of documented GH deficiency, stature is not affected (Fig. 6.12). Diabetes insipidus, caused by hypothalamic and posterior pituitary involvement, is often associated. Some children present with the clinical picture of Frölich's syndrome (obesity, short stature, hypogonadism). The diagnosis is generally suggested by the onset of neurological signs in an overweight child with short stature and delayed puberty. Standard X-rays of the skull often show sellar enlargement with erosion of the posterior wall and clinoids. More rarely, the sella profile may appear normal as the tumor develops upwards. Fine calcifications spread inside the tumor are typical although not constant. CT or MRI allow for the delimitation of the tumor expansion. Ophthalmologic examination is mandatory, as well as hormonal investigation of the anterior pituitary function. Transfrontal surgery followed by radiotherapy is recommended. Recurrence rate is high. Most patients need appropriate hormone replacement therapy.

Other hypothalamic tumors

Gangliocytomas, choristomas, and hamartomas are

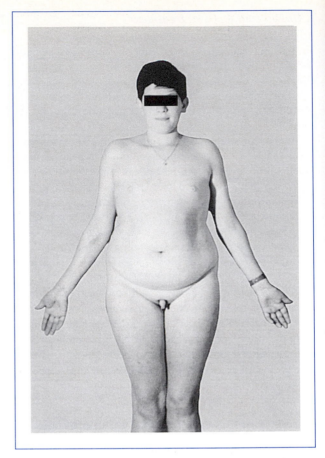

Figure 6.12 A 14-year-old boy affected with craniopharyngioma and panhypopituitarism. Linear growth was normal despite the patient being GH deficient.

extremely rare. However, they may produce hypothalamic neurohormones, in particular GHRH or GnRH, that may cause giantism/acromegaly or precocious puberty, respectively. Precocious puberty may also be caused by the secretion of chorionic gonadotropin or by the destruction of the pineal gland. The diagnosis is based on imaging of the hypothalamus by MR. Ophthalmological and hormonal investigations are mandatory. Transcranial surgery is the treatment of choice. Adjunctive radiotherapy is not very effective. The use of somatostatin analogues and GnRH superagonists may allow for the control of GH and gonadotropin excess, respectively.

Suggested readings

BARTYNSKI WS, LIN L. Dynamic and conventional spin-echo MR of pituitary microlesions. Am J Neuroradiol 1997;18:965-72.

BATES AS, VANTHOFF W, JONES PJ, CLAYTON RN. The effect of hypopituitarism on life expectancy. J Clin Endocrinol Metab 1996;81:1169-72.

EZZAT S, JOSSE RG. Autoimmune hypophysitis. Trends Endocrinol Metab 1997;8:74-80.

FAGIN JA. Pituitary tumors. Ballière's Clinical Endocrinology and Metabolism 1995;9:2.

IMURA H. The pituitary gland. 2nd ed. New York: Raven Press, 1994.

LANDOLT AM, VANCE ML, REILLY PL. Pituitary adenomas. New York: Churchill Livingstone, 1996.

MELMED S. The pituitary. Cambridge, Mass: Blackwell Science, 1995.

RAY D, MELMED S. Pituitary cytokine and growth factor expression and action. Endocr Rev 1997;18:206-28.

SHEAVES R, JENKINS PJ, WASS JAH. Clinical endocrine oncology. Section 3. Oxford: Blackwell Science, 1997;147-280.

The posterior pituitary and its diseases

Johannes Hensen, Michael Buchfelder

PHYSIOLOGY

The human body constantly loses water via urine (u), feces, skin, and lungs. Salt concentrations in plasma (p) and tissues would rapidly increase if not for a compensatory water intake, hence a system exists that adjusts water intake as well as renal water excretion according to requirements (Fig. 7.1). Osmosensitive cells located intracranially measure the tonicity of plasma and react upon an increase in (p) osmolality by stimulating thirst, which animates drinking, and by releasing the antidiuretic hormone (ADH) from the posterior pituitary lobe. This hormone *conserves body water* by acting on the principal cells of the renal collecting ducts, into which up to 20 liters of primary watery urine passes per day. The collecting tubules will become water-permeable under the influence of ADH, and up to some 19 liters of water will then flow back passively into the hypertonic renal medulla, where it is reabsorbed and returned to the bloodstream.

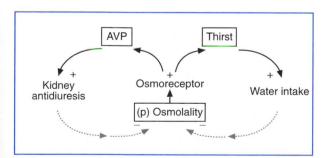

Figure 7.1 Osmoregulatory system. Intracranial osmoreceptors continuously sense plasma (p) osmolality. An increase in (p) osmolality is followed by an increase in AVP secretion and thirst. Water intake and renal antidiuresis decrease (p) osmolality, representing a double negative feedback system.

Antidiuretic hormone (vasopressin)

The name vasopressin arises from the vasoconstrictive and thus pressor effects of the hormone. Besides its vasopressor and antidiuretic effects, vasopressin has further actions that are beyond the scope of this chapter. The human antidiuretic hormone is the nonapeptide arginine-8-vasopressin (AVP). The molecular weight of AVP is 1084 g/mol, and it has a biological activity of about 400 U/mg. One mU corresponds to about 2.5 pg or 2.3 pmol. The normal (p) AVP strongly depends on the (p) osmolality, which again is mainly determined by (p) sodium concentration. Furthermore, (p) AVP exhibits a circadian rhythm with the highest levels around midnight and in the morning and lowest levels in the early afternoon. With normal (p) osmolality or normal (p) sodium concentrations, (p) AVP ranges between 0.5 and 3 ng/l. The normal range also varies whether platelet fraction AVP is included or not. The metabolic half-life of AVP only lasts about 10 to 20 minutes. Therefore, for the determination of (p) AVP, blood should be withdrawn into a cooled tube, followed by iced transport, quick separation of plasma (20 minutes at 1000 g), and storage at –70 °C. The determination of AVP is performed by radioimmunoassay and mandatory extraction procedures, such as using Sephadex C18 cartridges.

Oxytocin

The second hypothalamic hormone, also stored in the posterior pituitary lobe, is oxytocin. The molecular weight of oxytocin is 1007 g/mol. Its main effects are to induce milk ejection and uterine contraction. Oxytocin and vasopressin are formed in different neurons and transported in different axons. The antidiuretic and the pressor effects of oxytocin and AVP are approximately related in the ratio 5:400 IU/mg. As in the case of AVP, psychic effects have been described for oxytocin.

Neurohypophysis

The classic magnocellular neurosecretory system consists of the paired supraoptic and paraventricular nuclei and the supraoptic-neurohypophysial tract, which leads some 70 000 mostly unmyelinated axons of the magnocellular neurons down to the posterior pituitary lobe, where AVP and oxytocin are stored. The number of magnocellular neurons in the supraoptic nucleus is higher than in the paraventricular nucleus, and the ratio of vasopressin/oxytocin neurons in the supraoptic nucleus is 4:1 and in the paraventricular nucleus 4:3. Of anatomic and physiologic importance is the funnel-shaped reduction from hypothalamus to the hypophysial stalk (infundibulum), where one also finds the median eminence, a small medially located swelling at the bottom of the third ventricle. Magnocellular neurons from the supraoptic nucleus and the paraventricular nucleus that project to the posterior pituitary pass the internal zone of the median eminence. Other axons from paraventricular neurons (mostly parvocellular) project to the portal circulation via the external zone of the median eminence. Here AVP participates, together with corticotropin-releasing hormone (CRH), in the release of adrenocorticotropic hormone (ACTH). The pituitary gland and the infundibulum are vascularized by branches of carotid arteries, and the posterior pituitary lobe is fed mainly by the inferior hypophysial artery. The venous outflow takes place via veins to dural sinuses. The adult neurohypophysis weighs on average 120 mg, with the weight increasing slightly with age.

Measurement of osmolality in vivo and in vitro

An increased (p) osmolality results in a reduced osmoreceptor cell volume, as the plasma membrane of the osmosensitive neurons is impermeable to most solutes. The increased firing activity of the neurons is followed by induction of thirst, as well as by stimulation of the synthesis and release of AVP.

Osmolality measured in vitro by means of freezing point depression usually correlates well with the tonicity that is the effective osmotic pressure, which the solutes actually exercise upon the plasma cell membrane of the osmosensitive cells. However, while tonicity and osmolality of sodium and other electrolytes are identical, urea and glucose show large differences between the osmotic pressure ascertained by freezing point depression and the effective osmolality in vivo. The accuracy of measurement of (p) osmolality by routine hospital laboratories and by freezing point depression is usually not high enough to fulfill the quality criteria required (coefficient of variation of 1% or less at 290 mosmol/kg), especially when osmolality is determined in serum or frozen plasma. An alternative and possibly better approach is to relate (p) AVP directly to (p) sodium when urea and glucose are normal and constant during the test period. Sodium is measured more accurately by most clinical laboratories with sodium-selective electrodes. The latter method also excludes the false low sodium levels in cases where flame photometry is used (pseudohyponatremia with protein or lipid-rich blood).

REGULATION OF AVP

Osmotically induced AVP release

With low or low-normal (p) osmolality or (p) sodium, the currently used radioimmunoassays measure (p) AVP low or below the detection limit if nonosmotic stimulation of AVP is not active (Tab. 7.1). From an osmotic threshold concentration of about 284 mosmol/kg and a (p) sodium of about 138 mmol/l, a linear increase in (p) AVP occurs.

Table 7.1 Concentration of plasma (p) AVP that corresponds to a (p) osmolality and a urinary (u) osmolality in normal persons

(p) Sodium[1] [mmol/l]	(p) Osmolality [mosmol/kg]	(p) AVP[2,3] [ng/l]	(u) Osmolality [mosmol/kg][4]
131	270	<0.2	<50
132	272	<0.2	<50
133	274	<0.2	50
134	276	<0.2 - 0.3	50 - 100
135	278	<0.2 - 0.5	50 - 100
136	280	0.2 - 0.6	100 - 150
137	282	0.3 - 1	100 - 200
138	284	0.3 - 0.8 - 2	100 - 400
139	286	0.5 - 2.0 - 3	200 - 500
140	288	1.0 - 3.0 - 4	400 - 1000
141	290	1.5 - 3.5 - 6	700 - 1100
142	292	1.5 - 4.0 - 7	700 - 1200
143	294	1.5 - 5.0 - 7.5	800 - 1200
144	296	2 - 5.5 - 8	800 - 1200
145	298	2 - 6 - 9	>1000
146	300	3 - 7 - 11	1200
147	302	4 - 8 - 12	1200
148	304	4.5 - 9 - 14	1200

[1] Sodium is calculated by the formula:
(p) osm [mmol/kg] = 2 x (p) Na$^+$ [mmol/l] + (p) glucose [mmol/l] + (p) BUN [mmol/l] x [mmol/l].
[2] It is strongly recommended for each laboratory to acquire its own normal range. Commercially available AVP assays may not always be suitable.
[3] Plasma (p) AVP is influenced by many factors. There is a strong interindividual variance, but the relation of (p) AVP and (p) osmolality and (p) sodium is remarkably stable in a given individual. In a given normal individual, a rise in serum sodium by 1 mmol/l may increase (p) AVP by about 0.75 pg/ml. According to different authors, the mean threshold osmolality for AVP release is 280 mosmol/kg, 284 mosmol/kg, and 288.5 mosmol/kg.
[4] In normal persons without polyuria, the rise in (p) AVP by 1 ng/ml may further increase urine osmolality by about 250 mosmol/kg, up to a maximum of 1200 mosmol/kg. In patients, the urinary concentrating mechanism is strongly influenced by the degree of polyuria. With a polyuria of 6 l, the renal washout effect may only allow a maximum urinary concentration of 600 mosmol/kg, up from a (p) AVP of 2 ng/l. Urinary (u) osmolality may not further increase even with highest dosages of exogenous desmopressin. With hypothalamic diabetes insipidus, very little AVP is already needed for a maximal concentrating effect, however, with a polyuria of 6 l, the maximum urinary concentration may also be reduced to 600 mosmol/kg.

The sensitivity of the system is high. Thus, a further increase in (p) osmolality by 1% will further raise (p) AVP (Fig. 7.2). After 18 to 24 hours of water deprivation, (p) sodium in healthy individuals hardly rises above 145 mmol/l.

Nonosmotic AVP release

AVP is also released by baro- and volume-receptor-induced stimuli (hypovolemia, hypotension), as well as by pharmacological, neural, and other stimuli (Tab. 7.2). The AVP release induced by baro- and volume receptors is not as sensitive as the AVP release induced by osmoreceptors. The fall in blood pressure after blood losses, however, is the most potent stimulus and can lead to extremely high AVP levels (>100 ng/l). In cases of these high concentrations of AVP, vasoconstriction results. A decrease in arterial blood volume is sensed by volume receptors in the left atrium and will decrease tonic inhibitory inputs on magnocellular neurons, which also leads to the release of AVP. This plays a role in cases of hemorrhage, and to a minor extent, in an upright position, vasodilation, and positive pressure respiration. On the other hand, supine position, head-out water immersion, abolition of gravitation, and respiration with negative pressure as well as cold can inhibit the AVP release through an increased intrathoracal arterial volume.

Neural and pharmacological influences

A number of hypothalamic neurotransmitters and neuropeptides have an influence on AVP release as well. Stress and pain are strong stimuli of AVP, possibly indirectly via vasovagal reactions in connection with hypotension and nausea. Nicotine, morphine, vincristine, cyclophosphamide, chlorpropamide, narcotics, carbamazepine, neuroleptics, as well as antidepressants, also belong to the stimulatory substances. Lithium also leads to a slightly increased release of AVP, possibly secondary on account of the renal AVP resistance. Hypoxia and hypercapnia also seem to be related to a nonosmotic AVP stimulation, presumably also indirectly via evocation of

Table 7.2 Important variables that influence the secretion of vasopressin

Osmotic
Plasma osmolality
Infusion of hypertonic or hypotonic solution
Changes in water balance
Hyperglycemia (in diabetes mellitus)

Emetic
Nausea
Drugs (nicotine, apomorphine, morphine)
Motion sickness

Glucopenic
Intracellular hypoglycemia
Drugs (insulin, 2-deoxyglucose)

Hemodynamic
Posture
Orthostatic hypotension
Vasovagal reaction
Blood pressure
Blood volume (total or effective)
Hemorrhage
Aldosterone deficiency or excess
Gastroenteritis
Positive pressure breathing
Diuretics
Drugs (morphine, isoproterenol, norepinephrine, nicotine, nitroprusside, trimethaphan, histamine, bradykinin)
Congestive failure
Cirrhosis
Nephrosis
Pregnancy

Other
Angiotensin
Glucocorticoids
Drugs
pCO_2
pO_2
pH
Stress, temperature (see text)

nausea via vasovagal reactions. Alcohol can inhibit AVP release, as well as phenytoin and chlorpromazine. The modulating factors can be differentiated as to whether they preferably influence the sensitivity (slope) of the relation between (p) osmolality and (p) AVP or the threshold osmolality for AVP release.

Natriuretic hormones, angiotensin II, aldosterone, glucocorticoids

Natriuretic hormones are a family of structurally related peptides that share a common ring of 17 amino acids closed by a disulfide bridge. Atrial natriuretic peptide (-ANP[99-126]; -ANP) is a weak inhibitor of AVP release and also of AVP effects at the collecting tubules. High pressor dosages of angiotensin II, intravenously administered, result in the

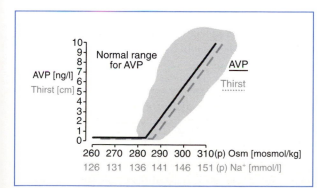

Figure 7.2 Schematic representation of plasma (p) AVP and thirst in relation to changes in (p) osmolality. Up from a threshold osmolality, AVP is secreted linearly. The threshold osmolality for thirst is a few osmols higher than the threshold for AVP secretion.

stimulation of AVP. The effect is modulated by the (p) osmolality. Glucocorticoids exercise a tonic inhibitory effect upon AVP secretion within the negative feedback regulation. Aldosterone leads to an increase in the osmotic threshold for the AVP release, as (p) volume expansion.

Interactions between osmotic and nonosmotic AVP regulation

The two major regulatory inputs for AVP release can complement each other synergistically, but they may also have an unfavorable competitive effect. Water deprivation, as well as water loading, influences (p) volume and (p) osmolality reciprocally, leading to a synergistic reinforcement of the AVP increase. Under other conditions, AVP stimulation by hypovolemia and AVP inhibition by low (p) sodium compete with each other. One example is hypovolemia caused by blood loss, which leads to extremely high levels of (p) AVP. The resulting AVP-induced water retention causes hyponatremia when fluid intake exceeds water losses. Thus, in the latter situation, osmoregulation is sacrificed in favor of volume regulation. Teleologically, this may make sense, as the loss of blood or volume, respectively, is acutely more life-threatening than the constancy of (p) sodium. A further example is the fall in effective arterial blood volume that may occur in edematous disorders such as congestive heart failure or decompensated liver cirrhosis. Hyponatremia in this condition is primarily due to an increased nonosmotic release of AVP.

Age

With progressing age the urinary concentration capacity of the kidneys declines. AVP release and also the response to an increase in (p) osmolality become augmented. Thirst sensation diminishes, which makes elderly patients more prone to hypernatremia.

Thirst

The increase in plasma tonicity results in thirst animating water intake. Thirst is quantified by visual assessment on a linear analogous scale; as in the case of AVP secretion, a linear correlation is found between thirst and (p) osmolality from a threshold (p) osmolality of about 285 mosmol/kg. The threshold (p) osmolality for thirst stimulation is only a few osmoles higher than the threshold (p) osmolality of AVP secretion (Fig. 7.2). There are, however, considerable individual variations in threshold (p) osmolality for thirst. A higher set threshold osmolality for thirst seems useful, as it may exert relief from unnecessary thirst if an antidiuresis alone could initially be sufficient for preventing a further rapid increase in osmolality. As in the case of AVP, thirst sensation can be stimulated nonosmotically. Important nonosmotic stimuli are oropharyngeal stimuli (dry throat) and volume deficiency, such as after salt loss or after bleeding.

Drinking is stopped before (p) osmolality has normal-ized, which points to the participation of complex oral, pharyngeal, and intestinal factors in thirst saturation. Thermal and chemical factors (iced sour or bitter drinks) and social aspects also have an influence on ending drinking. A complete satisfaction of thirst, however, only occurs when the total amount of fluid is sufficient to normalize the tonicity of the plasma.

INFLUENCE ON THE TARGET CELL

AVP receptors

The effects of AVP are mediated through three types of receptors: V_1, V_2, and V_3. The first step of the antidiuretic action of AVP is binding to the renal V_2-AVP receptors located on the basolateral principal cell membrane of collecting ducts. Adenylate cyclase is activated via stimulating G proteins and its product; the second messenger cAMP will lead to activation of protein kinase A with subsequent phosphorylation of proteins not yet identified in detail. Finally, the process leads to exocytosis and insertion of water channels into the luminal (apical) cell membrane recently identified as aquaporin-2 (AQP-2). AQP-2 is only expressed in principal cells of collecting tubules of the inner medulla. After exogenous administration of AVP, AQP-2 molecules accumulate in the luminal (apical) cell membrane, making possible the passive inflow of water into the collecting tubule cell transcellularly along the osmotic gradient. Aquaporin-3 and aquaporin-4 are responsible for the water flow through the basolateral membrane.

AVP DEFICIENCY (HYPOTHALAMIC DIABETES INSIPIDUS)

When more than 80% of the AVP-secreting hypothalamic neurons are destroyed or are nonfunctioning, increased polyuria occurs. The disorder is referred to as hypothalamic, cranial, or neurogenic diabetes insipidus (DI). It is characterized by the excretion of abnormally large volumes (>30 ml/kg per 24 h) of a dilute urine (less than 250 mosmol/kg). It is a rare illness with a prevalence of about 1:25 000. The incidence is the same in both females and males.

AVP deficiency can be complete or partial; that is, there may be a completely or partially reduced response to the appropriate stimuli. Three types of central diabetes insipidus can be differentiated when examining the increase in (u) osmolality or the increase in (p) AVP during thirsting or infusion of hypertonic saline (Fig. 7.3). Patients with complete diabetes insipidus centralis have an absolute AVP deficiency. Even at a very high (p) osmolality, no increase in AVP or (u) osmolality occurs. This type is the most frequent and also the most easy to identify. Other patients also show no increase in (p) AVP during hypertonic saline infusion, but they will show a sudden increase in (u) osmolality after long-term thirsting when hypertonic dehydration has also developed. These patients suffer from an osmoreceptor defect, as nonosmotic release of AVP induced by hypovolemia still functions. Another group of patients brings out a slight increase in (u) osmo-

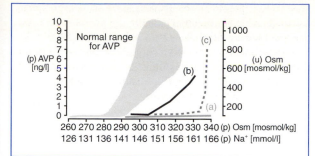

Figure 7.3 Three major types of central diabetes insipidus (DI) can be differentiated when examining the increase in urinary (u) osmolality or plasma (p) AVP during water deprivation and hypertonic saline infusion (schematic view). Patients with the first type (a) show no AVP secretion at all. Patients with the second type (b) have an elevated osmotic threshold for AVP release and/or a decreased AVP reserve. Patients with the third type (c) of DI show an abrupt increase in (p) AVP during water deprivation when becoming hypovolemic (nonosmotic AVP release), but they will not release AVP during hypertonic saline infusion.

Table 7.3 Etiology of hypothalamic diabetes insipidus

Familial
  Hereditary (usually autosomal dominant)
  Association of diabetes insipidus with diabetes mellitus, optic atrophy, nerve deafness (DIDMOAD)

Acquired
  Head trauma
  Neurosurgery
  Tumors (craniopharyngioma, germinoma, glioma, hypothalamic metastases)

Granulomatous disease
  Tuberculosis
  Histiocytosis
  Sarcoidosis
  Wegener granulomatosis

Infections
  Encephalitis
  Meningitis

Vascular disorders
  Sheehan syndrome
  Cerebral aneurysms
  Thrombotic thrombocytopenic purpura
  Embolism

Autoimmunity
  Circulating antibodies to vasopressin (e.g., secondary to Pitressin injection)
  Idiopathic

lality with increasing (p) osmolality, however, with a distinct rise of the threshold (p) osmolality. A high-set osmoreceptor (upward setting) may be responsible for this phenomenon. The neurosecretory capacity may also be decreased in these patients (diminished AVP reserve).

Etiopathogenesis

Diabetes insipidus is usually acquired and is predominantly secondary to disturbances in the sella region or hypothalamus. Frequently, diabetes insipidus is an early symptom that leads to the detection of sellar and suprasellar masses. The causes of diabetes insipidus may be divided into posttraumatic or postoperative disturbances; benign or malignant diseases including craniopharyngioma, metastasis and leukemias; inflammatory or granulomatous diseases (lymphocytic infundibuloneurohypophysitis, encephalitis, sarcoidosis, Langerhans cell granulomatosis [histiocytosis X]); and vascular diseases (aneurysm, emboli, infarction) (Tab. 7.3). Other rare causes of central diabetes insipidus are germinoma, pinealoma, and AIDS; in the latter case, infections of the central nervous system with *toxoplasma gondii*, cytomegaly, herpes simplex, or lymphocytic infiltrations of the CNS have been described. Brain death patients will also develop diabetes insipidus and need replacement when destined for organ donation. In one-third of the patients with the very rare Wolfram syndrome, diabetes insipidus is also present. Wolfram syndrome is an autosomal recessive hereditary disorder consisting of diabetes insipidus (DI), diabetes mellitus (DM), nervous opticus atrophy (OA) and deafness (D) (DIDMOAD syndrome). Recently, a mitochondrial DNA defect has been identified as responsible for this syndrome. In about one-third of diabetes insipidus patients, the cause remains unknown (idiopathic diabetes insipidus). Whether circulating antibodies against hypo-

thalamic nuclei play a role is not yet clear. In some patients, small hitherto undetectable lesions may grow and be detected during follow-up by magnetic resonance image (MRI) at intermediate intervals (3 to 12 months). Neurohypophysial familial diabetes insipidus is a very rare autosomal dominant hereditary disease with 100% penetration. The presenting manifestation is the delayed polyuria in early infancy. The AVP deficiency is never 100%, although the disease's complete picture does not differ from acquired hypothalamic diabetes insipidus. The autopsies of five patients from different families showed small posterior pituitary lobes with gliosis and a degeneration of magnocellular neurons in the supraoptic nucleus, as well as (less distinctly) in the paraventricular nucleus. A loss of the typical hyperintensity of the posterior pituitary lobe (hot spot) is shown in the T_1-weighted magnetic resonance image. During the last several years, about two dozen different heterozygous mutations in the polypeptide precursor gene for AVP-NP II have been detected that result in the exchange or deletion of one or more amino acids in the pre-pro-hormone. Despite the great number of different mutations, the clinical picture produced by the mutations is relatively consistent. These mutations seem to uniformly disturb the transport process or the folding and self-association of the pre-hormone. Incorrectly folded proteins cannot be correctly transported and will remain in the endoplasmic reticulum, where they accumulate to large aggregates and probably thereby induce the cellular decay. This mechanism explains the dominance of the heterozygous mutations (dominant negative effect), the delayed manifestation of diabetes insipidus, as well as the post mortem findings of degenerated magnocellular neurons. During pregnancy, a partial, thus-far compensated diabetes insipidus may become manifest on account of an increased (p) vasopressinase release from the placenta. The patients are resistant to native AVP, which is rapidly degraded, though they can be treated favorably with desmopressin. A mild diabetes insipidus in the case of Simmonds-Sheehan syndrome can deteriorate or even become manifest after replacement of the cortisol deficit. Removal of the posterior pituitary does not lead to complete diabetes insipidus, as some axons of AVP-secreting neurons end proximal to the posterior pituitary, such as in the median eminence. Diabetes insipidus only occurs when less than 10 to 20% of the magnocellular neurons remain after surgery. The lower the remaining amount of magnocellular neurons below this threshold, the more severe the diabetes insipidus would be. The degree of polyuria is thus only dependent from the remaining number of AVP-secreting neurons. After transsection of the hypophysial stalk, a build-up of AVP takes place at the proximal end of the section while the proximally located axons slowly empty. This is followed by a retrograded ascending degeneration of the magnocellular neurons (Fig. 7.4). The nearer the lesion lies to the ganglia cells, the more neurons that degenerate.

Pituitary adenomas do not cause diabetes insipidus, even with suprasellar expansion, as enough AVP-secreting neurons will remain. After transsphenoidal surgery for pituitary adenomas, about one-third of the patients develop transient hypotonic polyuria (>2500 ml, specific gravidity <1005 g/l) for some days, which is attributed to a secretional arrest of AVP release. After 3 months the prevalence of diabetes insipidus decreases to 0.9%, and

after 1 year the prevalence of permanent diabetes insipidus is 0.25%. After transcranial surgery, the prevalence of permanent diabetes insipidus is somewhat higher (2%).

The polyuric phase after surgery in the sella region may be interrupted by an oliguric interphase one week after surgery (Fig. 7.4). During this period, which usually lasts only a few days, AVP is released uncontrolled from the damaged axons in the posterior pituitary and also from retrogradely degenerating hypothalamic AVP-secreting neurons.

Course of hypothalamic diabetes insipidus

Idiopathic hypothalamic diabetes insipidus almost never recedes. On the other hand, posttraumatic or postoperative DI is often transient, presumably because destroyed axons in the pituitary gland's stalk regenerate. The probability of permanent DI becomes higher with increasing severity of the underlying head trauma or skull base fracture. The longer the DI exists, the less likely is a remission.

Anterior pituitary function in diabetes insipidus

Anterior pituitary function is mostly normal in patients with idiopathic DI with normal MRI of the sella region and the hypothalamus. In secondary DI, however, an accompanying insufficiency of anterior pituitary hormones is frequently observed. Also, visus diminishments, visual field deficiency, and ocular muscle paralysis depending on the size and extension of the lesion, occur. Mild hyperprolactinemia can be a first indication of a suprasellar lesion.

Clinical findings

History and physical examination will reveal important clues, such as age of onset, and will identify possible causes for hypothalamic DI, such as trauma, tumor, bleeding, metastasis, former surgery or radiation, inflammatory

Figure 7.4 Damage of the supraoptic-neurohypophysial tract during surgery for a pituitary adenoma may initially lead to secretional-AVP arrest. After several days (maximum day-7 postoperative), this may be followed by an unregulated release of AVP from the posterior pituitary and from retrogradely degenerating magnocellular neurons (vide infra: SIADH). The nearer the lesion lies to the ganglia cells, the more neurons that degenerate. With depletion of the storage capacity, AVP becomes normal again or hypotonic polyuria may persist (see text).

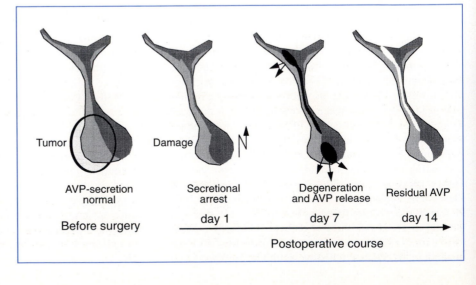

Tumor — AVP-secretion normal — Before surgery

Damage — Secretional arrest — day 1

Degeneration and AVP release — day 7

Residual AVP — day 14

Postoperative course

or infiltrative disorders of the hypothalamus, or skin lesions in cases of histiocytosis.

Symptoms and signs

Leading symptoms of DI are *persistent polyuria* and *polydipsia*. Thirst following dehydration is compulsory, which is also termed imperative thirst. Polyuria and subsequent polydipsia can develop slowly, but they frequently appear suddenly. In complete DI, night rest is always disturbed by frequent *nocturia*. In children, a newly appeared *enuresis* can point to the disease. Polyuria and water losses that cannot always be totally compensated for by drinking can cause some indirect symptoms such as dry skin and dry mucosae, constipation, sleep disturbed by thirst, and irritability. Non-compensated water deficits in children may cause thirst fever, typically reaching its peak in the morning. Severe hypertonic dehydration can cause a decrease in cerebral function, especially in patients with congenital nephrogenic DI. Polyuria over years can lead to dilatation of the urinary tract accompanied by hydronephrosis, especially in patients with nephrogenic DI. Memory tests have shown no deficits in patients with DI. Whether and how often an oxytocin deficiency accompanies DI is not known. Women with DI can give birth normally. Whether and to what extent oxytocin administration is required if milk ejection does not occur is not known.

Diagnostic procedures

The approach to determining the cause of diabetes insipidus should be safe, pragmatic, reliable, and inexpensive. Before a detailed diagnostic procedure is initiated, it is advised to measure urinary volume and fluid intake during one or two 24-hour periods after any diuretic medication has been discontinued for 2 days or more under conditions of ad libitum water intake. Diagnosis of diabetes insipidus requires a urinary output of more than 30 ml/kg/24 h and a (u) osmolality of less than 250 mosmol/kg. Also, (p) osmolality and (p) Na$^+$ should be determined once or twice in the morning under conditions of ad libitum water intake. In cases of DI, (p) Na$^+$ and (p) osmolality are shifted to upper normal concentrations in the morning, but this is not at all diagnostic. However, for practical purposes, a (p) osmolality above 296 mosmol/kg or a (p) sodium of 144 mmol/l or more excludes primary polydipsia.

If polyuria is present and there are no other obvious explanations for polyuria-like hyperglycemia, hypokalemia, hypercalcemia, chronic renal disease, or the polyuric phase of an acute renal failure, and so on, then a further diagnostic procedure should be initiated.

Dehydration test An indirect test of AVP release and function is fluid deprivation (dehydration test) followed by the administration of desmopressin (DDAVP: 1-deamino-8-D-arginine-vasopressin, Minirin®). The major advantage of this test is that it is easily performed in every hospital. The thirsting stimulates endogenous AVP as

osmolality rises, and only very late nonosmotic AVP stimulation by volume deficiency is added. The decrease in urine excretion and the increase in (u) osmolality are the main parameters that must be ascertained accurately during the test (Fig. 7.5). Generally the concentration test is begun at 6 a.m. During the test urine excretion, (u) osmolality, body weight, blood pressure, and heart rate is measured every 2 hours. In addition, in the beginning and at the end of the test, blood is drawn for (p) osmolality, (p) Na$^+$, and possibly (p) AVP. Constant supervision of the patient during the test is necessary, as patients with DI could rapidly develop considerable fluid deficiency, and also to ensure that he or she does not drink during the test. Thirsting must be discontinued if patients lose more than 3 to 4% of their body weight or become hypotensive. After 16 hours of dehydration, normal persons concentrate their urine to about 900 to 1200 mosmol/kg, whereas patients with complete central diabetes insipidus concentrate their urine to less than 250 mosmol/kg. Patients with primary psychogenic polydipsia, however, also show a distinct reduction of their maximum urine concentration capacity to about 450 to 700 mosmol/kg. A decline of the medullary tonicity, probably due to an increase in the medullary perfusion and wash-out, is responsible for this loss of urine concentration capacity. However, only patients with hypothalamic diabetes insipidus will show a further increase in (u) osmolality after fluid deprivation subsequent to the injection of 4 μg desmopressin iv (Fig. 7.5). This proves indirectly that the DI patient has not yet secreted maximum quantities of endogenous AVP. Defective AVP secretion can be assumed if exogenous AVP stimulates (u) osmolality by more than 10% after prolonged thirsting. Patients with complete hypothalamic diabetes insipidus show a medium increase from 168 ± 13 mosmol/kg to 445 ± 52 mosmol/kg (increase by 183 ±

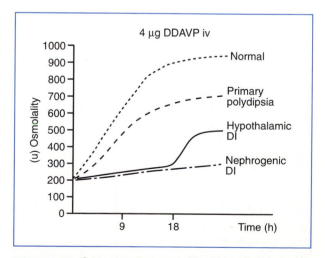

Figure 7.5 Concentration test. The decrease in urine excretion during the test and the increase in (u) osmolality before and after injection of desmopressin are the main parameters that must be ascertained accurately during the test.

41%); patients with psychogenic polydipsia and normal persons show no further increase at the end of the concentration test after AVP.

Unfortunately, the indirect test to differentiate between the three forms of polyuria does not always succeed. Indirect tests are reliable only in patients with severe defects in AVP secretion or action. The reasons for misdiagnosis in indirect tests include a residual AVP secretion in patients with hypothalamic DI. More important, however, are abnormalities in renal responsiveness caused by the renal "washout" effect, by an incomplete AVP resistance in acquired nephrogenic DI, and finally, by dilatations in the urinary tract and an increased residual capacity of the bladder in DI, making changes in (u) osmolality during the test difficult to ascertain.

The direct measurement of AVP in plasma or urine after a suitable period of fluid deprivation provides a reliable way of differentiating polyuria, providing the AVP levels are interpreted in conjunction with (p) osmolality or (p) Na⁺, respectively. Low AVP concentrations are evidence of central DI if demonstrated at the end of a thirst test when (p) osmolality is higher than 300 mosmol/kg or 146 mmol/kg. Care should be taken to guard against interference by nonosmotic AVP stimuli, such as nausea and hypotension, that can cause a significant increase in (p) AVP levels even in some patients with severe hypothalamic DI.

Hypertonic NaCl Hypertonic saline infusion is of invaluable assistance in ambiguous cases, especially when the distinction between primary polydipsia partial central DI or partial nephrogenic DI is not clear. It is to be considered as the golden standard of the differential diagnostics of polyuria. The infusion of hypertonic saline represents a strong osmotic AVP stimulation. Five percent saline (855 mmol/l) is infused into a large vein, preferably centrally, at a speed of 0.06 ml/kg/min over 2 hours. If a sufficiently strong vein is not accessible, a 3% saline infusion (513 mmol/l) may be infused during 3 hours at the same speed. Sodium concentration may rise by about 10 mmol/l, and care should be taken to avoid any hypertonic state, which could lead to severe headaches with (p) sodium of 155 mmol/l and more. The dose of saline must be reduced significantly if (p) sodium is already higher than 145 mmol/l before the test.

During the test, thirst may be registered on a linear thirst scale. Whereas (p) sodium baseline lies around 140 mmol/l, and (p) AVP between 0.3 to 0.8 ng/l, with hypertonic saline the (p) sodium may increase to 150 mol/l or more depending on the starting point, and (p) AVP to about 2 to 8 ng/l (Fig. 7.5). In cases of complete hypothalamic DI, no increase takes place, and in partial DI a subnormal or delayed increase is registered. In primary polydipsia, basal (p) sodium often lies in the lower normal range. Most patients with nephrogenic diabetes insipidus already have a high normal or (p) sodium with elevated AVP and show a further strong increase in (p) AVP after hypertonic saline.

Therapeutic trial A therapeutic trial with desmopressin at night and also later in the morning in patients with hypothalamic DI has demonstrated an immediate positive effect. The patients instantly feel relief of polyuria and are extremely pleased because thirst and nocturia have disappeared and an undisturbed night rest is possible again. Patients with primary polydipsia, however, do not feel any or little relief and may become hyponatremic because of water retention. Therefore, a therapeutic experiment must be carefully supervised, preferably on the ward with daily assessment of water intake, weight, urine output, and (p) Na⁺.

Imaging studies T₁-weighted coronal and sagittal magnetic resonance imaging (MRI) is most appropriate for visualizing the pituitary gland, stalk, hypothalamus and adjacent areas since it may depict space-occupying intracranial lesions that cause diabetes insipidus, such as craniopharyngioma, germinoma or metastasis to the pituitary gland. The AVP-containing posterior lobe is hyperintense in the T₁-weighted sequence, probably reflecting the presence of neurosecretory granules. After hypophysectomy or pituitary stalk rupture, a regenerated posterior pituitary containing functioning AVP secreting neurosecretory granules can occasionally be demonstrated ectopically in the median eminence or pituitary stalk as a bright spot in the T₁-weighted image.

Differential diagnosis

Polydipsia

Primary polydipsia due to organic hypothalamic lesions such as sarcoidosis is very rare. A selective defect in osmoregulation by thirst was described by Robertson (dipsogenic DI). These patients had normal AVP secretion although the threshold for thirst was abnormally low.

More important is the differential diagnosis of psychogenic primary polydipsia (dipsomania, potomania). It may be accompanied by other neurotic disturbances. Women seem to be affected more often. Patients sometimes report drinking for a definite reason, such as to cleanse or to wash out the body. Whereas DI patients always have nocturia, patients with neurotic polydipsia often do not. While untreated DI patients are slightly dehydrated in the morning and (p) sodium is in the upper normal range, polydipsia patients will show lower normal range or slightly lowered (p) sodium. Psychogenic polydipsia is treated by psychotherapy and the prognosis is favorable.

Essential hypernatremia

In patients with hypernatremia, diabetes insipidus with adipsia (essential hypernatremia) is a rare, but important differential. The disease is caused by an osmoreceptor lesion. In such a case, the osmotically stimulated AVP secretion, as well as the protecting thirst sensation, fail. Extended hypothalamic masses, neurosurgery, or aneurysmal bleeding from the anterior communicans artery may cause the disease. Untreated patients continue to excrete a hypotonic urine resulting in significant hypernatremia up to 190 mmol/l and dehydration, which can eventually lead to an AVP increase and hypertonic urine. In addition, there may be a sensitizing against small remaining AVP quantities or against oxytocin. The hypernatremia causes shrinkage of the brain cells with neurologic symptoms and signs (somnolence, confusion, myospasms, collapse, and thirst fever in babies).

Treatment

Conservative approaches

The treatment of DI must be orientated toward its etiology and the intensity of symptoms. Patients with mild (partial) and long-standing disease do not always need to be treated with drugs. Many patients, especially with familial hypothalamic diabetes insipidus, have become accustomed to the increased fluid intake and to the necessity of getting up once or twice during the night.

Medical treatment

The natural AVP is obtainable in two parenteral forms: a suspension of peanut oil with depot effect (Pitressin Tannat®, 5 IU/ml, dosage 0.3-1 ml per day IM or SC) and an aqueous preparation with short duration (Pitressin®, 1 ml containing 20 IU). Intravenous AVP, however, has a short half-life and may have side effects due to its pressor effects (hypertension, angina).

Desmopressin (DDAVP: 1-deamino-8-D-arginine-vasopressin, Minirin®) is a synthetic AVP analogue with high affinity for the V_2-AVP receptor and low affinity for the V_{1a}-AVP receptor (antidiuretic/pressure ratio of 4000:1). Desmopressin has no pressor side effects and is the treatment of choice in patients with hypothalamic diabetes insipidus. Its half-time and its duration of effect is significantly prolonged when compared to AVP because of the lack of the α-amino group (about 2 to 4 hours, and 6 to 24 hours after 20 µg intranasally, respectively). The bioavailability of desmopressin is about 10% intranasally and 1% orally. On average, 20 µg desmopressin intranasally and 400 to 600 µg orally may be therapeutically equivalent. However, considerable individual variation exists, which makes it difficult to predict the required dose and essential to adapt the dosage and timing of desmopressin individually. The duration of effect can be ascertained by recurrence of hypotonic polyuria and polydipsia. Fortunately, in a given patient, the effect of desmopressin is quite reproducible.

Initiating therapy with desmopressin In adult patients we generally start desmopressin at a low dosage, such as 1 puff or 0.1 ml intranasally at bedtime (10 µg). Some patients only need desmopressin to enable undisturbed sleep through the night. Depending on the effect and the daily activities, a second puff (or 0.05 to 0.1 ml) can be prescribed for the morning or at noon. At the beginning of treatment with desmopressin, hyponatremia with headaches and nausea, abdominal cramps, and local reactions at the nasal mucous membrane (perfusion increase) might occur. As a precaution for water intoxication, we recommend initially daily measurements of body weight and also a weekly control of (p) Na+ during the first weeks of therapy. Furthermore, the patient is advised not to drink large quantities of fluid (such as beer) during the first 4 hours after administration of desmopressin.

Desmopressin is available in many countries in various preparations (100 µg/ml) and also in tablets of 100 and 200 mg. The spray lasts for a maximum of 25 days when 2 × 1 puff per day is administered. The Rhinyle® has the advantage of more exact administration of small doses (0.025 or 0.05 ml, respectively, corresponding to 2.5 or 5 µg). For treatment of children and babies, desmopressin can be diluted in normal saline. DI in parenterally fed patients or postoperative or posttraumatic DI can be treated with 2 µg desmopressin IM 1 to 2 times a day. Pregnancy and lactation are no contraindication for a therapeutic replacement therapy of desmopressin.

Side effects and therapy controls When thirst sensation is maintained, it is not necessary to precisely control fluid intake or weight every day in chronic treatment of DI. When the patients are properly adjusted to their dose and also educated during the initial phase of therapy, the control of (p) sodium every 3 to 6 months is sufficient. Sometimes, however, it may be that patients are not sure whether they really still feel thirsty. In such cases, the desmopressin dose should be temporarily reduced.

Diabetes insipidus with inadequate thirst (essential hypernatremia) is more difficult to manage. Afflicted patients must be advised to ensure regular water intake with documentation of input, output, and weight in addition to desmopressin. We recommend a constant drinking quantity of 1.5 to 2 l per day and a daily weight control with daily documentation (as in diabetes mellitus) so that hyperhydration and dehydration can be detected early. Frequent regular controls of (p) Na+ cannot be avoided in such patients.

Treatment with non-AVP derivatives Carbamazepine (400-600 mg per day), clofibrate (4 × 500 mg per day), or chlorpropamide (200-500 mg per day) have been used in the treatment of partial hypothalamic DI. These drugs have become obsolete since the introduction of desmopressin. In the case of the antidiabetic drug chlorpropamide, which may also increase thirst, the risk of developing hypoglycemia is increased.

Emergency The treatment of hypertonic dehydration consists of the careful supply of free water, such as by infusion of 5% glucose. If volume depletion is also present (orthostatic hypotension), isotonic saline should be added until the hemodynamic situation has been stabilized. Correction of hypernatremia should be performed slowly. If extracellular hypertonicity is corrected too rapidly, for example with simultaneously administrating desmopressin and infusion of free water, an intracellular inflow of water will occur, with the consequence of cerebral edema. To avoid this, a correction up to only the upper limits of normal of (p) Na$^+$ and a maximum speed of 0.5 to 1 mmol/l/h is recommended. The approximate quantity of water that is required for the correction, assuming a constant total body water (TBW) of 60%, can be estimated by using the formula:

$$\text{water required for correction} = (TBW \times \text{actual (p) Na}^+ / \text{desired (p) Na}^+) - TBW$$

Consequently, in a patient with a body weight of 70 kg and a (p) Na$^+$ of 165 mmol/l, about 3.8 liters of free water must be administered for the correction to 150 mmol/l. Aiming for a correction rate of below 0.75 mmol/h, the 3.8 l should be infused in 20 hours minimum.

RENAL AVP RESISTANCE (NEPHROGENIC DIABETES INSIPIDUS)

Nephrogenic DI can be congenital or acquired, the latter being much more frequent. Currently, two different forms of congenital nephrogenic DI are described: X-linked and non-X-linked.

X-linked congenital nephrogenic diabetes insipidus

Numerous mutations in the V$_2$-AVP receptor gene have been identified that lead to X-linked nephrogenic DI. The disease only affects males. Female carriers can occasionally show mild polyuria and polydipsia, which is attributed to an increased (unbalanced) X-chromosomal inactivation of the healthy allele. The untreated disease in young children leads to hypernatremia and hyperthermia. Some mental retardation is detectable in many adult patients, and it is probably caused by repeated episodes of undiscovered dehydration in early childhood before the diagnosis has been established. Typically, thirst fever will reach its maximum in the morning, in contrast to fever caused by inflammation. Some children may develop subdural hematoma or intraventricular hemorrhage during dehydration. When the disease is diagnosed and treated at an early stage, mental development will be normal. Whether this also applies to the dilatation of the urinary tract (hydronephrosis) is not known.

Extrarenal V$_2$-AVP receptors are also affected by the mutations. Injection of 4 μg desmopressin normally leads to extrarenal effects, such as vasodilation in forearm vessels, an increase in plasma renin activity, and an increase in coagulation factors such as factor VIIIc, the von Willebrand Jürgens factor (vWJF), and tissue type plasminogen activator. These peripheral effects are considerably weakened or completely omitted in cases of mutations.

Non-X-linked congenital nephrogenic diabetes insipidus

Few families with nephrogenic DI have been described who show a normal vWJF- and vasodilation response to desmopressin. Both women and men are affected by the disease, indicating an autosomal recessive etiology. Recent studies on the AQP-2 gene identified a "compound heterozygosity" for two missense mutations in these families.

Acquired nephrogenic diabetes insipidus

Acquired nephrogenic DI is much more common than the congenital forms (Tab. 7.4). The polyuria is usually mild (3-4 l/day). One of the most frequently observed forms is lithium-induced nephrogenic DI, which is present in about 50% of patients on chronic lithium therapy. A reduced AVP-induced insertion of AQP-2 into the luminal cell

Table 7.4 Etiology of acquired nephrogenic diabetes insipidus

Electrolyte disorders
Hypokalemia
Hypercalcemia

Chronic renal disease
Polycystic disease
Medullary cystic disease
Pyelonephritis
Ureteral obstruction
Far-advanced renal failure

Dietary abnormalities
Excessive water intake
Decreased sodium chloride intake
Decreased protein intake

Drugs
Alcohol
Angiographic dyes
Phenytoin
Lithium
Demeclocycline
Osmotic diuretics
Furosemide and ethacrynic acid
Acetohexamide
Glyburide
Propoxyphene
Amphotericin
Methoxyflurane
Norepinephrine
Vinblastine
Colchicine
Gentamicin
Methicillin
Isophosphamide

Miscellaneous
Multiple myeloma
Amyloidosis
Sjogren's disease
Sarcoidosis
Sickle cell disease

membrane of principal cells was recently found to be responsible for lithium-induced nephrogenic DI. Hypo kalemia- and hypercalcemia-induced nephrogenic DI are also associated with a reduced number of AQP-2 water channels. A therapeutic option, besides omitting the triggering noxae, has not yet resulted from this perception. Some drugs may also cause acquired nephrogenic DI, such as demeclocycline, which is an inhibitor of the AVP-induced adenylate cyclase activity. This drug has been used in the treatment of chronic hyponatremia in the syndrome of inappropriate ADH secretion (SIADH) (vide infra).

Treatment

The main goal of treatment is to reduce urinary output. Strict sodium restriction and diuretics of the thiazide type or amiloride or a combination of both substances are of some effectiveness. Diuretics will initially decrease Na^+ reabsorption in the cortical water-impermeable dilution segments, leading to an increased sodium excretion and to a decrease in extracellular volume. This accomplishes a decrease in glomerular filtration rate and an increase in proximal reabsorption of salt and water so that the distal water delivery is reduced. As a consequence, less water streams into the collecting tubules controlled by AVP, and the total amount of urine declines. Prostaglandin E_2 impairs the antidiuretic action of AVP by inhibiting baseline and AVP-induced cAMP synthesis. It also inhibits reabsorption of sodium in the thick ascending part of the Henle's loop and thereby impairs the urinary concentrating mechanism. As a potent vasodilator, it increases renal blood flow, particularly the medullary blood flow, and attenuates the vasoconstrictive actions of angiotensin II. Thus, the actions of prostaglandins on blood flow and glomerular filtration rate are dependent on activation of the renin angiotensin system.

In nephrogenic DI, the raised AVP levels result in an increased renal PGE_2 synthesis via activation of renal V_1-AVP receptors. Prostaglandin inhibitors have proved to be therapeutically effective, such as 50 mg indomethacin every 8 hours, but not aspirin. Side effects that can result are headaches, gastrointestinal ulcers, and a decreased glomerular filtration rate.

Unfortunately, none of the therapeutic methods accomplishes a (u) osmolality exceeding (p) osmolality. However, even a small rise in (u) osmolality from 50 to 200 mosmol/kg can reduce the amount of urine needed for excretion of the 24-hour urine solute load of 600 mmol from 10 to 12 l/day to a tolerable 3 to 4 l/day, thus helping to avoid the dilatation of the urinary tract.

SYNDROME OF INAPPROPRIATE ADH SECRETION (SIADH)

The classical syndrome of inappropriate ADH secretion (SIADH) has basically been defined as an exclusion diagnosis when other causes for hyponatremia can be excluded, that is, when there is (1) no hypovolemia; (2) no disease accompanied by edema; (3) no endocrine dysfunc-

tion, including primary or secondary adrenal insufficiency and hypothyroidism; (4) no renal failure; and (5) no drug taken that can influence water excretion. Inappropriate AVP secretion in an extended sense may be defined as an absence of appropriate AVP suppression despite low (p) osmolality and hyponatremia in the presence of euvolemia or even arterial hypervolemia. This extended definition puts the joint and typical clinical and laboratory findings of SIADH to the forefront. This must, however, not lead to therapeutic water restriction in cases where hormone replacement or discontinuation of drugs would have been more suitable.

Pathophysiology

An inappropriate secretion of AVP, referred to (p) osmolality, results in antidiuresis and excretion of a concentrated urine, followed by volume expansion and an increase in weight. As a consequence of water retention and unadapted high fluid intake, hyponatremia will develop. The development of hyponatremia is further augmented by hypervolemia-induced activation of natriuretic mechanisms, including a suppression of renin and aldosterone, a decrease in renal proximal tubular absorption of sodium, and an increase in atrial natriuretic hormone secretion from the heart. In summary, the basic features of SIADH are hyponatremia and natriuresis in the presence of euvolemia or slight hypervolemia. The AVP escape phenomenon describes a decrease in the antidiuretic action of AVP, which might occur in chronic severe SIADH after some time, probably due to a decrease in AQP-2 water channels.

Excretion of sodium results only in correction of the extracellular fluid volume, although the intracellular fluid volume will initially remain elevated. Subsequently the cell volume regulation leads to an excretion of intracellular potassium and intracellular organic osmolytes. It may require about 48 hours of sustained hyponatremia to initiate intracellular fluid volume accomodation. When the intracellular osmolytes are lost, the cells are less able to buffer sudden increases in osmolality. This may become of particular importance to intracranial brain cells.

The elevation of AVP in SIADH may follow different patterns. Some 40% of the patients present with an absolutely unregulated fluctuation of elevated (p) AVP levels independent of osmotic (and nonosmotic) stimuli. A second group of patients shows a normal pattern, but a lowered osmotic threshold for AVP release. These patients can dilute their urine maximally if they are sufficiently hyponatremic. A third group of patients (about 20%) shows a constant baseline AVP secretion despite low (p) osmolality (AVP leak). Finally, in a small number of patients, the relation between AVP and (p) osmolality is normal, with the cause for the limited urine dilution capacity of the kidneys being unknown. However, the discrimination in different types of SIADH is not of very much clinical value since the patterns are not related to the underlying etiology of the disease.

In adrenal insufficiency, large differences in volume status exist depending on whether its genesis is primary or of pituitary origin. Patients with primary adrenal insufficiency lack cortisol and also severely lack aldosterone. They will develop hypovolemic hyponatremia as a consequence of salt and volume losses. In addition, a certain renal component (impairment of renal dilution capacity without cortisol) may participate in the development of hyponatremia. On the other hand, in secondary adrenal insufficiency, mineralocorticoid deficiency and salt loss do not play a major role. Indeed, in contrast to primary adrenal failure, the patients are euvolemic or mildly hypervolemic, resembling the typical pattern of SIADH. The patients are not always hyponatremic but will easily become so in certain situations, such as when nauseous. This has been attributed to a lack of negative feedback inhibition of cortisol on its releasing hormone, AVP.

Epidemiology

Syndrome of inappropriate ADH secretion in the restricted sense is a rare disease, but in the extended sense, it occurs more often. The overall incidence of hyponatremia of less than 130 to 131 mmol/l ranges from 1 to 4%, wherefrom a third of cases might represent SIADH. Thus, in larger hospitals, SIADH can be anticipated on a daily basis.

Etiology

Syndrome of inappropriate ADH secretion is almost always the consequence of an underlying disease (tumor, central nervous system disorder, pulmonary disease) or of a medical therapy (Tab. 7.5). A primary overproduction of AVP secondary to a genetic defect is not known. Excess AVP may come from the ectopic secretion of a tumor or, more frequently, from the normal source of AVP in the hypothalamus. In the latter, AVP is probably released by nonosmotic pathways. It is supposed that this is due to disruptions of the baro- and volume regulatory system of AVP, which is anatomically much more diffuse compared to the osmotic control of AVP. Signals of the baro- and volume receptors are carried over a long distance by the 9th and 10th cranial nerves from the chest to the brain stem and are subsequently transmitted to the magnocellular neurons, where the input is primarily inhibitory. Any disruption of this system in the chest or in the central nervous system may lead to a decrease in inhibition and thus, to an increased secretion of AVP. This assumption is supported by the fact that a variety of drugs and tumors in the central nervous system and intrathoracal diseases cause SIADH. Recently, a pulmonary peptide, pneumadin, was isolated that might stimulate AVP release directly.

Table 7.5 Disorders associated with the syndrome of inappropriate secretion of the antidiuretic hormone (SIADH)

Tumors

Pulmonary/mediastinal tumors
Small-cell carcinoma of the lung
Other bronchogenic carcinomas
Mesothelioma
Thymoma
Hodgkin's lymphoma

Brain tumors

Other tumors
Nasopharyngeal carcinoma
Duodenal carcinoma
Pancreatic carcinoma
Ureteral/prostatic carcinoma
Bladder carcinoma
Uterine carcinoma
Leukemia

Central nervous system disorders

Demyelinative/Degenerative
Guillain-Barre syndrome
Peripheral autonomic neuropathy
Spinal cord lesions
Cerebellar and cerebral atrophy

Infectious/Inflammatory
Encephalitis
Meningitis
Systemic lupus erythematodes
Acute intermittent porphyria
Human immunodeficiency virus
Brain abscess

Miscellaneous
Subarachnoid hemorrhage
Subdural hematoma
Cavernous sinus thrombosis
Neonatal hypoxia
Head trauma
Pituitary stalk section (interphase)
Acute psychosis
Delirium tremens
Hydrocephalus

Drugs

Stimulation of AVP release
Nicotine
Tricyclic antidepressants
Phenothiazines

Direct renal effect and/or potentiation of AVP action
Desmopressin (DDAVP)
Oxytocin
Prostaglandin inhibitors (salicylates, nonsteroidal anti-inflammatory agents)
Chlorpropamide

Others
Colchicine
Vincristine
Cyclophosphamide
Clofibrate
Carbamazepine, oxcarbazepine
Lisinopril
Clozapine

Pulmonary affections

Pulmonary infections
Pneumonia (bacterial, viral, mycoplasma)
Aspergillosis
Tuberculosis
Empyema

Pulmonary ventilatory problems
Acute respiratory failure (pneumothorax, asthma, bronchiolitis, cystic fibrosis)
Chronic obstructive pulmonary disease
Positive pressure ventilation

A patient's history very frequently provides important clues about the underlying disease, such as: (1) heart, lung, and kidney diseases or endocrine disturbances (menstruation history); (2) use of drugs such as diuretics, laxatives, desmopressin, alcohol, or nicotine; (3) weight changes, nausea, vomiting, polydipsia, or diarrhea; (4) septic bacterial infections, AIDS (cytomegaly virus-induced adrenalitis, etc.); and (5) subarachnoidal hemorrhage, or conditions after neurosurgery or other operations.

One of the most important purposes of the physical examination is to correctly assess volume state in the hyponatremic patients. In SIADH, in contrast to most other forms of hyponatremia, clinical signs of dehydration are absent. Patients with SIADH are euvolemic or slightly hypervolemic without peripheral edema appearing. Jugular veins are filled, blood pressure and heart rate in the supine and ambulatory position are normal, and central venous pressure, if accessible, is also normal or high-normal. Attention must also be directed at endocrine stigmata such as the absence of axillary and pubic hair.

Symptoms and signs

Syndrome of inappropriate ADH secretion manifests symptoms of hyponatremia that are secondary to encephalopathy and due to cerebral edema. The symptoms vary and depend upon the severity and duration of hyponatremia, as well as on the speed at which hyponatremia has developed. Initially, weight increase by water retention may occur, although, peripheral edema is rarely present. The patients will be anorectic, and nausea and vomiting may follow. Patients appear irritable, later uncooperative, lethargic, and confused. Finally, extrapyramidal disturbances, convulsions, coma, and/or apnea may occur in acute hyponatremia.

In chronic hyponatremia, on account of a normalization of the brain volume, a regression of the clinical signs and symptoms occurs. Patients with considerable but chronic hyponatremia can, therefore, be surprisingly asymptomatic. This will also be the case if hyponatremia has developed very slowly.

Diagnostic procedures

Good evidence for the assessment of arterial blood volume is available from (p) creatinine, (p) uric acid, and (p) urea. In SIADH, all three parameters are normal-low or decreased. Urinary sodium excretion is increased (>20 mmol/l). If, however, SIADH patients have been on a low sodium diet or are hypovolemic, the (u) sodium excretion may also be lower. The (u) osmolality in SIADH is always higher than 100 mosmol/kg, indicating that urine is not maximally diluted, as would be appropriate after the administration of excess water in healthy subjects. Although it is written so in various textbooks, it is not necessary for (u) osmolality to exceed (p) osmolality to fulfill the criteria for SIADH. Moreover, measurement of (u) osmolality is usually of no help in the differential

diagnosis of SIADH, because in each of the categories of hyponatremia, urine osmolality will be elevated. AQP-2 has also been studied in hyponatremia and also appears to have little value in the diagnosis. AQP-2 is elevated in SIADH but also in other forms of hyponatremia, such as in liver cirrhosis or congestive heart failure.

Water loading

Water loading is rarely necessary for a diagnosis of SIADH. The test is based upon measurement of urine excretion after oral water load (20 ml water per kg body weight in 15 to 20 minutes orally). Normally, in the supine position, 80% of the water load is excreted within 5 hours. The (u) osmolality of at least one sample, mostly that of the second hour, falls under 100 mosmol/kg (specific weight 1.005 g/l or less). Patients with SIADH often excrete only 40% of the water load. The test is, however, of low specificity, as patients with hyponatremia and elevated (p) AVP of another genesis (liver cirrhosis, heart failure, hypovolemia) also show an impaired water excretion. Another disadvantage of this test is that (p) sodium could fall by about 4 mmol/l after water loading, which could aggravate symptoms of hyponatremia. Therefore, it is recommended to increase (p) Na^+ to about 125 mmol/l by water restriction or another adequate therapy before performing water loading. Finally, patients who have a low-set osmoreceptor or a "downward resetting" of the osmostat are nevertheless able to adequately dilute the urine at low (p) Na^+. The latter disturbance (frequent in SIADH) can be detected by a saline infusion test with synchronous measuring of the AVP concentration.

Differential diagnosis _____

The differential diagnosis of SIADH is the same differential diagnosis as hyponatremia (Fig. 7.6). After exclusion of pseudohyponatremia, the following two questions must be answered: (1) Is the effective arterial blood volume decreased? and (2) Is venous blood volume increased? A correct and quick answer can usually be given on the basis of history, physical examination, and the above-mentioned laboratory parameters. Important evidence for a decrease of the effective arterial blood volume are previous salt or volume losses, such as by vomiting or diuretics (the latter case may be accompanied by low potassium values), dry mucous membranes, thirst, and a fall in blood pressure and an acceleration in heart rate in recumbency. With low effective arterial blood volume, (p) creatinine, (p) urea, and (p) uric acid are somewhat increased. The sodium concentration in urine will be low (<10 mmol/l). The most important practical indication of a decrease in effective arterial blood volume is a fall in blood pressure and an increase in heart rate in recumbency. The decrease in arterial blood volume can be accompanied by venous and interstitial volume excess, such as in heart failure, liver cirrhosis, and nephrotic syndrome. The most impor-

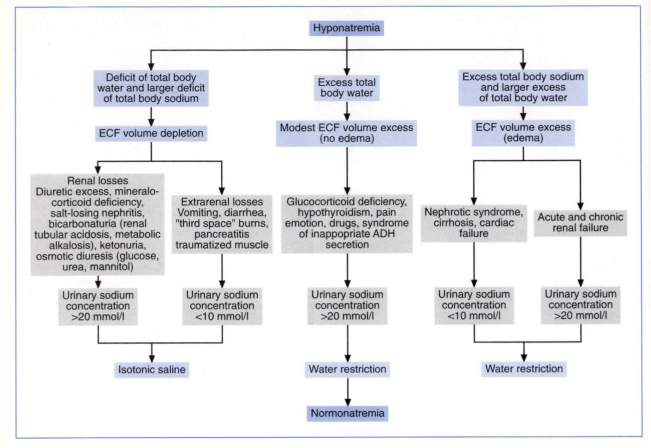

Figure 7.6 Diagnostic and therapeutic flow-chart for the hyponatremic patient. (ECF = extracellular fluid; ADH = antidiuretic hormone.)

tant clinical indication of venous volume excess are peripheral edema and filled jugular veins.

In some cases of hyponatremia in the elderly, it may be difficult to determine the state of hydration. A urine sodium of 50 mmol/l may be elevated, but it may have been due to a recent administration of diuretics or to an underlying intrinsic renal disease. In such patients, a cautious diagnostic trial of normal saline for 5 to 6 hours may be indicated, while following serum sodium, (u) sodium, and (u) osmolality or specific gravity. If there is a dilution of the urine and an increase in serum sodium within a few hours with the administration of normal saline, this would confirm that the patient was dehydrated and that normal saline should be continued. If, however, the urine sodium increased and the serum sodium remained the same or even decreased with the administration of normal saline, this would suggest the diagnosis of SIADH.

Cerebral salt wasting syndrome

The cerebral salt-wasting syndrome was first described by Peters and colleagues in 1950. It describes the concerted occurrence of hyponatremia and natriuresis in patients with cerebral diseases, such as in patients with subarachnoid hemorrhage or after head injury. The pathogenesis of this

syndrome has not yet been determined, and it is not clear whether the syndrome represents a clinically distinct entity. It may present mixed clinical pictures of SIADH associated with renal tubular dysfunction resulting in salt loss. Interestingly, despite hypovolemia, the release of brain natriuretic peptide and atrial natriuretic peptide are (inappropriately) increased, which may be a partial cause of the natriuresis. The decreased concentrations of (p) renin and (p) aldosterone in cases of cerebral salt-wasting syndrome were also attributed to the increased (p) natriuretic peptides. The knowledge of this syndrome is necessary for the differential therapy of hyponatremia in the neurosurgical intensive care unit. In contrast to SIADH, patients with cerebral salt-wasting syndrome are hypovolemic (central vein pressure <5 cm H$_2$O) and do not require water restriction but an isotonic or hypertonic saline infusion, preferably guided by central venous pressure.

Polydipsia-hyponatremia

The polydipsia-hyponatremia syndrome described in the psychiatric literature is characterized by excessive fluid intake and intermittent dilutional hyponatremia. It has all the features of SIADH, but it also has disturbances of osmoregulation, including alteration in osmoreceptor function and increased thirst, which are not completely understood. Polydipsia-hyponatremia syndrome is most commonly found in chronic schizophrenic patients, but it is seen in other psychiatric conditions as well. Most, if not all, patients develop hyponatremia while under treatment with neuroleptics or tricyclics. Thus, SIADH in this condition is most frequently regarded as at least partly drug-related.

Treatment

The therapy should be orientated towards the underlying disease and the severity and speed at which symptoms have developed (Tab. 7.6). A causal therapy of SIADH is possible in only a few cases, such as chemotherapy in cases of bronchogenic carcinoma or in patients with central nervous inflammatory diseases. If possible, drugs

---

Table 7.6 Recommendations for treatment of hyponatremia in SIADH

General recommendations
- Hyponatremic patients with SIADH are primarily treated by water restriction and a salt-rich diet
- Employment of an additional treatment with hypertonic saline must be guided by *neurological symptoms*
- Patients with long-standing hyponatremia are especially prone to the risks of rapid correction of hyponatremia (central pontine myelinolysis) and require a lower rate of correction of plasma (p) sodium
- Patients with symptomatic hyponatremia of unknown duration should be treated like patients with chronic hyponatremia

Asymptomatic hyponatremia
- Essentially always of chronic duration
- Treat with water restriction and a salt-rich diet in case of SIADH

Acute symptomatic hyponatremia (hyponatremic encephalopathy)
- The risk of the further complications of brain edema (incarceration, brain death) exceeds the risk for demyelination
- Plasma (p) Na^+ must rapidly be increased by hypertonic saline infusion until symptoms (convulsions) lessen (limited and controlled)
- Patients with postoperative symptomatic hyponatremia occurring immediately after surgery (<24-48 h) should be treated without delay by 3% saline with an initial correction rate of 2 mmol/l/h

Symptomatic hyponatremia (chronic or of unknown duration)
- Increase plasma (p) Na^+ rapidly by hypertonic saline infusion until symptoms lessen; restrict water intake in case of SIADH
- A maximal correction rate of 2 mmol/l/h must never be exceeded
- Limit the end-point of correction to 120-125 mmol/h. After serum sodium is raised by 10%, recheck neurological symptoms for the necessity of further saline infusion
- Serum sodium must not be increased by more than 20 mmol/l in total

---

potentiating AVP action or stimulating AVP release (such as neuroleptics or tricyclics) should be discontinued. The replacement of carbamazepine by phenytoin and a change in ventilation parameters to less positive pressure breathing may be considered.

The basic therapy for SIADH is fluid restriction. We restrict fluid to 0.5 to 1 l/day, always in conjunction with a high-sodium diet (10 g/day orally). The patient should be clearly advised to restrict all fluids, not only water. If successful, this will lead to a negative water balance followed by a slow increase of (p) Na^+ of about 1 to 2% per day. Administration of normal saline will not correct hyponatremia in SIADH, and it may even lead to a further increase in hypervolemia, natriuresis, and to a further lowering of (p) sodium. Thus, the infusion of saline can only correct the hyponatremia if (p) volume is first normalized by fluid restriction. It is important to notice that patients with SIADH are potentially volume-depleted because of their negative total sodium balance. Thus, after successful therapy by water restriction, patients may end up with normal (p) sodium but are slightly hypovolemic, that is, the decrease in total body sodium may become evident after successful therapy. This is the reason for instituting a salt-rich diet in conjunction with water restriction. If patients with hyponatremia do not respond to water restriction despite some weight loss, the extracellular fluid (ECF) volume status and the diagnosis of SIADH should be reassessed carefully, and eventually isotonic saline should be infused.

Drug therapy in chronic hyponatremia of SIADH

Patients with chronic hyponatremia are often remarkably asymptomatic and may not need treatment besides water restriction. It may be difficult, however, to comply with water restriction in all patients, and some patients may complain of extreme thirst despite efforts to reduce this being made (e.g., ice chips). A relapse of symptomatic hyponatremia may also occur. In these patients, an additional drug therapy could prove useful. Possible drugs are lithium carbonate (in antidepressant doses of $3-4 \times 300$ mg/day), and demeclocycline 300 mg 2 to 4 times a day. The effect of lithium is uncertain and may be connected with some toxicity. Better results have been achieved with demeclocycline, which induces a state of nephrogenic DI. Urea (30-60 g in 100 ml orange juice once a day) increases the free-water-clearance and decreases urinary sodium excretion. Side effects are its poor taste and the possibility of azotemia. Furosemide (40 mg/day) has also been employed, combined with a very salt-rich diet (e.g., 200 mmol/kg/day).

Treatment of symptomatic hyponatremia (chronic or unknown duration) in patients with SIADH

Hyponatremia in SIADH usually develops slowly. Severe and dangerous symptoms requiring rapid and drastic interventions are rare. However, if a patient with SIADH develops symptomatic hyponatremia (such as convulsions), hypertonic saline (3%) should be infused without delay, but always in a *limited and controlled* matter to avoid severe complications of rapid correction (demyelination syndrome, see below). Treatment is best carried out at an intensive care unit where input and output, as well as sodium in serum and urine (initially every 3 to 4 hours), can be controlled. To avoid complications of rapid correction (see below), it is important to limit the increase in (p) sodium to 120 mmol/l, or until the patientsí symptoms are abolished, or when a total magnitude of correction of 20 mmol/l is reached. An initial *rapid* placement may be desirable in severely symptomatic patients to correct any cerebral edema. The brain can only enlarge about 10% in the rigid skull, and a rapid correction of 5 to 10% of the measured serum sodium may be desirable to decrease brain edema. After an initial rapid correction, a slower rate of correction described above may be continued. The initial speed of correction should not exceed 2 mmol/l/h in severely symptomatic patients, whereas in less symptomatic patients 0.5 mmol/l/h may be sufficient.

The *initial infusion rate* in ml 3% saline per hour may be estimated from the formula:

$$body\ weight\ [kg] \times desired\ initial\ correction\ rate\ [mmol/l/h]$$

For example, if the sodium concentration is intended to increase by 1 mmol/l within one hour, 3% saline should be infused initially at a rate of 70 ml/h. The total amount of sodium, which is necessary to correct (p) Na^+ to about 120 mmol/l (in case) of a symptomatic patient, may be estimated from the formula:

$$amount\ of\ sodium\ required\ for\ correction\ [mmol] =$$
$$= (120 - actual\ (p)\ Na^+) \times TBW\ (total\ body\ water)$$

Thus, a symptomatic patient with a (p) Na^+ of 110 mmol/l weighing 70 kg (about 42 l of total body water) may require a total of 420 mmol of sodium, corresponding to 800 ml 3% saline (520 mmol Na^+/l). With an aimed correction rate of 0.5 mmol/l/h, these 800 ml may be infused in 30 h minimum, that is, 40 ml/h. However, very importantly, these are only estimates for infusion speed and

sodium requirements. The actual flow rate must be adjusted to the actual development of (p) sodium, which cannot always be predicted. A spontaneous occurrence of polyuria can be by chance, for example. Consequently, thorough supervision in the intensive care unit is always necessary.

Central pontine myelinolysis

Central pontine and extrapontine myelinolysis are severe complications that typically occur 1 to 2 days after rapid correction of severe hyponatremia of more than 48-hour duration. After this time, cell volume regulatory processes have already largely normalized the enlarged brain volume by excreting intracellular solutes (potassium and organic osmolytes). Correcting hyponatremia too rapidly by hypertonic saline infusion in this situation will cause further shrinking of the brain, followed by disruption of the blood brain barrier in certain regions. This causes a predominantly pontine demyelination via mechanisms that are not completely understood. Severe symptoms such as dysphagia, dysarthria, para- or tetraplegia, coma, and/or apnea may follow. If the patient survives, the syndrome may be partly reversible. Risk factors are the severity of hyponatremia, the speed of its development, the duration of hyponatremia (>48 hours), and the speed and extension of chronic hyponatremia correction. It will never occur in acute hyponatremia. Undernourished alcoholics with accompanying hypokalemia seem to be particularly at risk. The diagnosis can be confirmed by MRI imaging. In order to avoid the syndrome, hyponatremia must always be treated according to the guidelines given above.

Outlook on future possibilities

At the present time, highly specific non-peptide V_2-AVP-receptor antagonists (so-called aquaretics) are being clinically tested for their usefulness in treating hyponatremia of SIADH. In preliminary experiments, dosage-dependent "diabetes insipidus" was induced, leading to the desired normalization of (p) sodium. Moreover, as AVP is elevated in nearly all forms of hyponatremia, the aquaretics could be helpful. In addition to being effective in treating hyponatremia in SIADH, they could also be helpful in treating hyponatremia in cases of decompensated heart failure, liver cirrhosis, and nephrotic syndrome.

Suggested readings

BICHET DG. The posterior pituitary. In: Melmed S (ed). The pituitary. Cambridge: Blackwell Science, 1995;227-306.

BICHET DG, LONERGAN M, ARTHUS M-F, FUJIWARA TM, MORGAN K. Nephrogenic diabetes insipidus due to mutations in AVPR2 and AQP2. In: Saito T, Kurokawa K, Yoshida S (eds). Neurohypophysis - Recent progress of vasopressin and oxytocin research, 1995;605-14.

BOEHNERT M, BUCHFELDER M, FAHLBUSCH R, HENSEN J. Hyponatremia in the ICU. Kidney Int 1998;S64:2.

DÜRR J, HOFFMAN WH, HENSEN J, SKLAR AH, EL-GAMMAL T, STEINHART CM. Osmoregulation of vasopressin in diabetic ketoacidosis. Am J Physiol 1990;259:E723-28.

GREGER NG, KIRKLAND RT, CLAYTON GW, KIRKLAND JL. Central diabetes insipidus: 22 years' experience. Am J Dis Child 1986;140:551-4.

HENSEN J, DOLZ M, OELKERS W. Transiente Polyurie in der Schwangerschaft bei Diabetes insipidus und Gestationsdiabetes [Transient diabetes insipidus and diabetes mellitus in pregnancy]. Med Klin 1991;86:623-8.

HENSEN J, SEUFFERLEIN T, OELKERS W. Atherosclerosis, aortic stenosis and sudden onset central diabetes insipidus. Exp Clin Endocrinol Diabetes 1997;105:227-33.

HONEGGER J, FAHLBUSCH R, BORNEMANN A, et al. Lymphocytic and granulomatous hypophysitis: experience with nine cases. Neurosurgery 1997;40:713-22.

MOSES AM, BLUMENTHAL SA, STREETEN DHP. Acid-base and

electrolyte disorders associated with endocrine disease:pituitary and thyroid. In: Arieff AI, de Fronzo RA (eds). Fluid, electrolyte, and acid-base disorders. New York: Churchill Livingstone, 1985;851-92.

OELKERS W. Hyponatremia and inappropriate secretion of vasopressin (antidiuretic hormone) in patients with hypopituitarism. N Engl J Med 1989;321:492-6.

RAFF H. Glucocorticoid inhibition of neurohypophyseal vasopressin secretion. Am J Physiol 1987;252:R635-44.

RITTIG S, ROBERTSON GL, SIGGAARD C, et al. Identification of 13 new mutations in the vasopressin-neurophysin II gene in 17 kindreds with familial autosomal dominant neurohypophyseal diabetes insipidus. Am J Hum Genet 1996;58:107-17.

ROBERTSON GL. Diagnosis of diabetes Insipidus. In: Czernicho P, Robinson AG (eds). Diabetes insipidus in man (International Symposium on Diabetes Insipidus in Man). Front Horm Res, vol 13 (Series editor: van Wimersma Greidanus TJB). Basel: S. Karger, 1985;176-89.

VERBALIS JG, ROBINSON AG, MOSES AM. Postoperative and post-traumatic diabetes insipidus. In: Czernichow P, Robinson AG (eds). Diabetes insipidus in man (International Symposium on Diabetes Insipidus in Man) Front Horm Res, vol 13 (Series editor: van Wimersma Greidanus TJB). Basel: S. Karger, 1985;247-66.

ZERBE RL, ROBERTSON GL. Osmoregulation of thirst and vasopressin secretion in human subjects: effects of various solutes. Am J Physiol 1983;244:E607-14.

Disorders of growth

Peter Hindmarsh

Failure of physical growth is an important sign of systemic disease. It is also the hallmark of endocrine disease, since pituitary, thyroid, adrenal, and gonadal hormones are all involved in the growth process. Extremes of stature may signal a disease process, as well as be a source of disability and cause of emotional distress. This chapter discusses the endocrine causes of short and tall stature. In a text dedicated to endocrinology, it is especially important to be clear that the categorization of an individual child depends upon growth assessment and clinical examination. It does not depend, at least not initially, on laboratory investigations, which should not be employed unless auxological data indicate them to be necessary.

SHORT STATURE

The definition of shortness is arbitrary. The general rule has been that any child whose height falls below the 3rd centile for his or her community should be considered short. This immediately raises problems over the definition of the term and the most appropriate standards for the assessment of height. It is important to realize that height standards are only a statistical description of the general population. Three percent of children will have heights below the 3rd centile regardless of whether or not there is anything wrong with them. Different ethnic groups have different growth standards. Secular trends in heights are well-documented and are more marked in certain groups, and up-to-date growth charts need to be used to account for such changes. In the United Kingdom there is still a secular trend in height such that each generation tends to be 1 to 1.5 cm taller than the previous one.

GROWTH ASSESSMENT

There is a tendency with height charts to simply look at stature as a static process rather than a dynamic one. This has led to the use of height velocity charts to assist in decision-making. However, because of the cyclical nature of growth, constructing simple decision models on the basis of these charts was difficult.

The British 1990 Growth Reference Standards for boys allows for decision-making to be made more easily using one single chart. It utilizes equi-spacing of the new centiles, which more adequately define standard deviations about the mean, coupled with the introduction of two new centiles, 0.4 and 99.6.

Parental heights provide an estimate of the genetic height potential of their child, which is a useful measure against which to judge the current height of the individual. Adjustments need to be made to parental heights depending upon whether the subject is a boy or a girl. Males are taller than females by about 14 cm, so if a boy's height is being considered, the father's height can be plotted on the "Boys Chart" directly, but the mother's height must be adjusted by adding 14 cm and this derived value entered on the chart. The mid-parental height can be derived (in this case: [paternal height + corrected maternal height]/2), as well as the target height (mid-parental height ± 1 standard deviation approximately 3 cm), and plotted. When the father's height is plotted on a "Girls Chart", 14 cm must be deducted from his current height before plotting.

Unless the current height falls above or below a centile trigger point, it is likely that further measurements will be required. The time interval between these measurements will be determined by the precision of height measurement, but the minimum time interval will be about 3 months, and at least 6 to 12 months will need to elapse before a growth pattern can be established.

Making decisions using new charts has been simplified. Using the old cut-off of the 3rd height centile means that in each year in the United Kingdom 24 000 individuals (the vast majority of whom will be normal) might require further monitoring or investigation. Introduction of the 0.4th centile is important, because the likelihood that in this situation the individual is considered normal is markedly diminished. The diagnostic return on investigating individuals whose heights are below the 0.4th centile is actually quite high, and it is much higher than the 2 per 1000 return when the cut-off value was around the 3rd height centile. Identification of the short child is, therefore, based on diagnostic return, not on an arbitrary height centile.

The charts also allow for decisions to be made about

individuals whose height may be normal but whose growth pattern is crossing centile bands. The correlation between heights measured at different ages is extremely high. For example, a height measured at the age of 3 years has a correlation coefficient associated with another measurement made at 6 years of 0.91. Taking this type of correlation into account, 2% of children might be expected to fall half a centile band or more between 5 and 6 years; a similar percentage should rise by half a centile band. More conservative changes of 1 centile or more over a similar time period are extremely rare, with a rate well below 1 per 1000 individuals. Simple rules can be constructed for referral and/or investigation (Tab. 8.1). Less stringent criteria can be applied if there are more than two measurements, as the chances of two successive growth rates being low is very small.

One final point worth considering relates to when growth problems may evolve. Congenital abnormalities, such as growth hormone gene deletion, will present early in life. As a general rule, any period of fast growth (e.g., infancy and puberty) may unmask a growth disorder. In the totality of growth disorders, however, there is a law of diminishing returns with the age of a child. For example, by school entry, 60 to 70% of growth disorders should have presented and/or been identified, with pubertal growth disorders contributing a further 15 to 20%. Growth surveillance programs are best concentrated, therefore, in the preschool and early school years.

Classifications on growth assessment

Using the above approaches, small children can be classified into three groups. A flow chart for the differential diagnoses of short stature is shown in Figure 8.1.

Table 8.1 Recommendations for growth surveillance and referral

Single measurements

Children whose heights are below the 0.4 or above the 99.6 centile
Refer if height is outside the range of parental target height

Two measurements 1-2 years apart

Refer if the fall in height centile exceeds the width of 1 centile band (up to 5 years of age) or 2/3 of a centile band (over 5). If the centile falls by at least 2/3 of this amount (e.g., 2/3 of a band for under-5s, or half a band for over-5s), flag the individual for recall 1-2 years later

Three or more measurements, at least 9 months apart, covering 2 or more years

Refer if the cumulative height centile fall exceeds the width of 1 centile band (up to 5 years of age) or 2/3 of centile band (over 5). Check that all the measurements are consistent, with no obvious outliers

Generally

Respond to parental concern about growth, irrespective of the current centile, by monitoring height over a period of at least 9 months

---

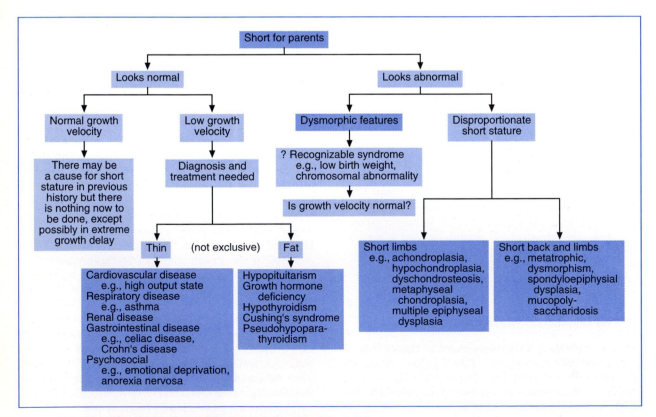

Figure 8.1 Flow chart for use in the differential diagnosis of short stature.

Short normal children

This group of children contains at least two subgroups. The first are characterized by a height close to the 3rd centile and a normal growth velocity. The height of one or both of the parents is likely to be close to the 3rd height centile. The second group, which may include some children from the first, consists of children whose stature may be anywhere between the 3rd and 25th centiles and whose growth rate is normal during the childhood years, but who lost ground because of the late onset of puberty and a delayed pubertal growth spurt. Skeletal maturation becomes delayed in children toward the end of the first decade of life, and a final height appropriate for the parents is likely to ensue.

Short stature due to an early event

In most cases children with a syndrome who are short have been of low birth weight. The problem is not just confined to intrauterine growth retardation. Poor nutritional support of pre-term infants will produce similar effects. It is important to remember that growth in the first 6 months of life is independent of growth hormone and is largely dependent on nutrition, so poor nutritional intake during this period of rapid growth can have profound and long-lasting effects. Once growth hormone (GH)-dependent growth becomes established, normal growth follows, but stature lost at this stage is not easily recovered.

Two syndromes deserve mention. First is the association of low birth weight and its resultant short stature with dysmorphic characteristics, the Silver-Russell syndrome. The clinical features are a triangular-shaped facies, body symmetry, thinness, and clinodactyly of the fifth fingers. However, the most characteristic feature is the formidable difficulty encountered by the parents in feeding such children in infancy. Postnatal growth beyond 12 months of age is characteristically normal in these children. Most cases are sporadic, but familial cases have been described. Evidence from mice and humans suggests that uniparental disomy may be an important explanation of many cases of intrauterine growth retardation. Knockout experiments in mice of the insulin-like growth factor (IGF) family also lead to low birth weight, and evidence for a human parallel has recently been presented.

The second syndrome of note is that of Turner's syndrome, which results from abnormalities – absence, mosaicism, rings, or isochromosomes – of the X chromosome. Mosaicism is common, but the effect of Turner's syndrome on growth is to add persistent low-growth velocity to a prenatal growth deficit. Growth over the first 3 years of life tends to be relatively normal in terms of growth velocity, but thereafter a decline in growth rate can be discerned with no obvious pubertal growth spurt. The condition is common (1 in 3000 female births), and the well-known dysmorphic features may not necessarily appear. Short stature is common, but the major implication of diagnosis relates to pubertal development and reproductive capacity.

Short stature with a remedial condition

These children may or may not be short; more importantly, their growth velocity is slow. This group includes a wide spectrum of disease. An explanation for the poor growth rate must be found and appropriate treatment recommended. A careful history and examination may point to a remediable cause. Full investigation encompassing the renal, gastrointestinal, cardiac, respiratory, hematological, and neurological systems is often required. Finally, careful attention must be paid to the social and family history. Psychological deprivation can take forms ranging from emotional deprivation to anorexia-by-proxy, as well as extremes of physical and sexual abuse.

Classification of growth hormone secretory disorders

The characteristic clinical picture of severe GH insufficiency is of a very short, rather plump child with a round, immature face. Birth weight is usually normal, and poor growth is apparent from about 6 months of age. The insufficiency may be isolated or associated with other pituitary hormone deficiencies. Small genitalia are especially characteristic of associated gonadotropin deficiency. Hypoglycemia in the newborn period is often a feature of adrenocorticotropic hormone (ACTH) deficiency. Prolonged neonatal jaundice, particularly conjugated hyperbilirubinemia, raises the question of thyroxine or cortisol deficiency.

Pituitary gland

The term GH deficiency should be applied only to children with deletion of the GH gene. Onset of GH deficiency in children with gene deletion is extremely early, and poor growth can be detected as early as the 6th month of postnatal life. The genetic causes of GH deficiency, in isolation or in association with multiple pituitary hormone deficiency, have been described, and they are summarized in Table 8.2. As there is a cascade of genes regulating anterior pituitary development, this list is likely to expand considerably in the future.

Pituitary aplasia is commonly associated with multiple pituitary hormone deficiency. Growth failure occurs early, although the effects of hypoglycemia, hypothyroidism, and the consequent persistent conjugated hyperbilirubinemia brings the disorder to the attention of the clinician at an earlier stage. Failure of the migration of the anterior pituitary, derived embryologically from Rathke's pouch, leads to characteristic high resolution computed tomographic (CT) scan or magnetic resonance image (MRI) appearances in children with this disorder. The pituitary fossa is very small and the neurohypophysis does not descend, remaining at the base of the infundibulum. This may be evident on CT and MRI as a small enhancing nodule.

Hypoplastic pituitary glands are often seen on both computed tomography and magnetic resonance imaging

Table 8.2 Disorders of growth hormone synthesis

	Type	Inheritance	GH
Primary defect: growth hormone	IA	Autosomal recessive	Absent
	IB	Autosomal recessive	Reduced
	II	Autosomal dominant	Reduced
	III	X-linked	Reduced
Multiple pituitary hormones	I (pit-1 gene deletion, PROP-1 abnormalities)	Autosomal recessive	Reduced
	II	X-linked	Reduced
GHRH receptor abnormalities		Autosomal recessive	Reduced

(GHRH = growth hormone-releasing hormone.)

in children with GH secretory abnormalities. The understanding of these morphological changes has been helped tremendously by the molecular and cellular findings in the studies of the growth hormone-releasing hormone (GHRH) receptor in the *little* mouse and the earlier identification of the role of GHRH in the stimulation of GH gene transcription and induction of somatotrope cell proliferation.

The clinical and auxological features of GH deficiency are also manifest in a situation where abnormal polymers of GH are secreted from the pituitary gland. Such material is bioinactive, but it is measurable by immunoassay. The phenotypic features of absent GH with severe growth failure is also seen in individuals who have mutations of the GH receptor that cause GH insensitivity syndromes. Individuals with this disorder, which is inherited in an autosomal recessive pattern, have high plasma levels of GH but low levels of IGF-1.

Acquired destruction of the anterior pituitary gland is most often associated with the presence of a craniopharyngioma. Visual disturbances or headaches may be the first signs. Infiltration of the pituitary gland in histiocytosis X may result in growth hormone deficiency, as could transection of the pituitary stalk as a result of severe head injury.

The hypothalamus and disturbances of pulsatile GH secretion

GH secretion is characterized by secretory bursts that raise the serum concentration from undetectable (by current assay) values to peak values. Secretion then ceases, and plasma values return to undetectable values. This process is regulated mainly by two hypothalamic peptides: GHRH and somatostatin. In addition, a complex set of neurotransmitter pathways, as well as various peripheral metabolic and hormonal factors, influence growth hormone secretion, though their exact role in terms of the physiological control of GH secretory bursts is uncertain. In humans, and in many animal species, GH-dependent growth appears to be a pulse amplitude-modulated phenomenon. The frequency of GH-secretion is relatively fixed, with a periodicity of between 3 and 4 hours.

The vast majority of short children formerly labeled as GH deficient appear to have GH insufficiency on the basis of 24-hour GH secretory profiles. Disorders in secretion of GHRH would explain most of the GH pulse amplitude problems observed.

GH secretion and GH insufficiency

GH secretion is low during many hours of the day. As a result, provocative tests were designed to test the integrity of the hypothalamo-pituitary axis. The standard test, the insulin-induced hypoglycemia stimulation test (ITT), has been the mainstay of pharmacological assessment of GH secretion. Clonidine, L-dopa, glucagon, and arginine have also been used. The accepted criteria in the United Kingdom used to be to label a child as *severely insufficient* if the peak GH response to pharmacological stimuli was <7 mU/l and *partially insufficient* if the values lay between 7 and 15 mU/l. These values were based largely on the GH responses to pharmacological stimuli in adults. However, these cut-off values present many problems of interpretation: for example, a peak GH response of 25 mU/l in a 5-year-old child may be acceptable as a normal GH response, but such a value in a child at the height of the pubertal growth spurt is probably inadequate. Using strict cut-off values may seem to be inappropriate in view of the evidence that the peak serum GH concentration response to pharmacological stimuli is continuous in a large group of short children with varying growth rates. The wide range of methods now available for measuring serum GH concentrations makes comparison between laboratories difficult and the use of universal cut-off values impossible.

One of the main problems in pediatrics in interpreting the response to these tests is the lack of normal data; as standards would be needed for tall, normal, and short children, because their GH secretion differs. If age is an important determination of GH secretion, and puberty clearly is, then values for these would have to be included as well.

In general, there is little choice between the tests when compared with the ITT (Tab. 8.3). Such an analysis assumes that the ITT obtains a correct diagnosis in all cases. Where repeat ITTs have been performed, values of efficiency and sensitivity approach values given in Table 8.3. The cut-off chosen for the definition of GH deficiency/insufficiency depends on the sensitivity and specificity of the test. It will also depend, in part, on the type of assay used.

Although great emphasis has been placed on the physiological tests of GH secretion, neither sleep nor 24-hour profiles studies are easy to perform. Urinary GH measurements may be a step forward in this situation, but variabil-

Table 8.3 Performance characteristics of various tests of growth hormone (GH) secretion in the diagnosis of growth hormone insufficiency, compared with the insulin tolerance test, using a cut-off value of 15 mU/l

Test	Efficiency (%)	Sensitivity (%)	Specificity (%)
Sleep			
EEG monitored	88	86	95
Not monitored	79	67	82
Arginine	72	73	85
Clonidine	70	70	85
IGF-1	75	95	60
IGF-1 (field)	–	34	72
IGFBP-3	96	97	95
IGFBP-3	93	83	44
IGFBP-3 (field)	–	22	92

(EEG = electroencephalogram; IGF-1 = insulin-like growth factor-1; IGFBP-3 = insulin-like growth factor binding protein-3; Field = field studies.)
(From: Hindmarsh PC, Brook CGD. Clin Endocrinol 1995;43:133-42.)

ity is high, and two or three overnight collections must be performed to overcome this problem. An alternative approach might be to measure the serum levels of insulin-like growth factor and/or their binding proteins. The advantages of a single blood test are obvious. Serum IGF-1 is low in growth hormone insufficiency but, because normal IGF-1 values are also low in early childhood, poor discrimination ensues. IGF-1 binding protein 3 (IGFBP-3) is largely regulated by circulating levels of GH and could be used to reflect GH status. These observations, coupled with recent "field studies" suggest that these measures may be overestimated in terms of specificity and sensitivity, particularly following cranial irradiation.

It is unlikely that any test will improve on the 80 to 90% sensitivity and specificity reported. The reasons for the false-negative results are easier to understand than false-positives. Growth velocity of necessity is measured over a long period of time, between 6 and 12 months. The pharmacological and even the physiological tests are performed over a very short period of time, a day at the most. This must mean, in view of our knowledge of seasonal growth, that some stimulatory tests are performed in the period of relatively good growth but of necessity would have to be compared with the overall growth period of 6 months to 1 year. Explaining the false-positive results is more difficult. It is a well-recognized phenomenon that when a stimulation test is performed and the 0-min specimen is high, any further elevation in response to the stimulus is unlikely to occur during the period of the test. This has widely been ascribed to the effects of stress resulting from the insertion of the intravenous cannula. A more likely explanation is that the stimulation test has been performed upon a background of endogenous GH secretory activity. ITT was devised for performance in adult patients in whom GH secretory episodes are unlikely to occur during the morning. This is not the case in children, where GH secretory episodes between the hours of 9 a.m. and 12 a.m. hours are commonplace, particularly if the individual

is in puberty. GH secretory bursts probably take place due to a withdrawal of somatostatin inhibitory tone with or without concomitant stimulation of GHRH. It is quite likely, therefore, that endogenous secretory bursts in some individuals are followed by an increase in somatostatin tone, preventing further release in GH.

Treatment

Growth hormone

Growth hormone insufficiency Exogenous human GH promotes rapid growth in the short-term, with the most dramatic response seen over the first 6 months. Subsequently, this growth rate slowly returns to normal values.

In general, long-term effects have not been as dramatic as the short-term studies might have suggested. Although final height has been increased compared with what would have happened if no treatment had been given to the patients, most groups found that patients with isolated GH insufficiency were still some 2 standard deviation scores (SDS) from the mean at the end of treatment. Selection of patients on the basis of height achieved rather than on height velocity must have contributed a great deal, as one of the original criteria was a height of -2 SDS from the mean. However, the dose of GH administered and the frequency of administration may have been additional important factors.

Treatment of short children without GH insufficiency The initial studies of Tanner and his colleagues included children who were short but growing normally. These children showed an improvement in growth velocity that was less than that seen in their GH-insufficient peers, but there was nonetheless an improvement on the rate at which they had been growing previously.

Short-term studies have demonstrated acceleration of growth in short children following the administration of exogenous GH. The promising short-term response of many studies of short, normal children has been disappointing longer-term. The net gain in stature has ranged between 2.5 to 8 cm.

Turner's syndrome Children with Turner's syndrome have a classical growth pattern as described above and illustrated in Figure 8.2. Long-term studies have demonstrated that treatment with GH alone or with oxandrolone results in an increase in height relative to Turner's standards, with net gains ranging from 2 to 8 cm.

Silver-Russell syndrome: intrauterine growth retardation Children with Silver-Russell syndrome display poor growth in utero yet normal growth once they escape from that environment. On conventional pharmacological testing they have normal GH secretion, but recent work has clearly demonstrated that the pattern of GH secretion is anything but normal. Treatment of these children with GH

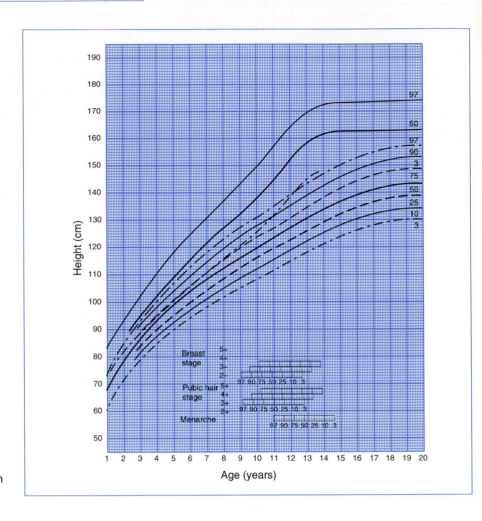

Figure 8.2 Growth of children with Turner's syndrome.

increases their height velocity in the short-term, however there are no data to show long-term improvement in height.

PUBERTAL DELAY

A common problem encountered by pediatricians and adult endocrinologists is the child with delayed puberty. Centile band crossing occurs with an increasing delay in skeletal maturation due to delay in the onset of puberty. If the onset of the pubertal growth spurt is significantly delayed, then growth can slow considerably and almost come to a stop. In such situations, many clinicians move to investigate these individuals for GH insufficiency/deficiency. In fact, the problem lies more with deficiency of sex steroids than GH. Testing these individuals for GH sufficiency will show evidence of low GH secretion in response to the usual provocative stimuli, but once sex steroid concentrations, particulalry estradiol, start to rise, GH production returns to normal and the ultimate prognosis is good. Investigation of these individuals is largely unwarranted. As a rule of thumb, the growth rate of such individuals decreases from a mean of 5 cm per year (± 1 cm per year)

at 12 years of age, decreasing by 1 cm per year (± 1 cm per year) for every year thereafter that the individual does not undergo their pubertal growth spurt. Deviations beyond these values do require further evaluation.

In children with constitutional delay of growth and development, oxandrolone or very low doses of testosterone produce growth acceleration that is not at the expense of an inappropriate advance in skeletal maturity.

TALL STATURE

The problems encountered in defining short stature apply equally to tall stature. The height that may be acceptable in adult life is for the most part a matter of opinion. For boys, heights of up to 2 meters are probably acceptable, whereas, girls find a height in excess of 180 cm difficult to accommodate. Cultural background is an important factor in determining who is going to require treatment.

Tall stature is a familiar characteristic in the majority of cases. The diagnoses with which tall stature may be associated, although rare, are in several respects more sinister than those associated with short stature. Figure 8.3 shows a clinical algorithm for the management of tall stature. The principles of assessment differ little from that practiced for the individual with short stature. Growth assessment is the key, and the height of the child should be compared with the measured height of the parents in exactly the same way as it would be for short stature. Clinical examination will reveal answers to the question as to whether there is an underlying syndrome to be diagnosed, and additional clues may come from the child showing signs of puberty. Caution must be exercised with children who are growing fast and in whom there are no signs of puberty. GH excess and hyperthyroidism are suggested diagnoses in the algorithm, but it is important to realize that although adrenal disease usually presents with the appearance of pubic hair and growth of the phallus, increased growth velocity may be the only complaint initially. Precocious puberty, either gonadotropin-dependent or gonadotropin-independent, is also an important diagnosis to consider.

Gigantism

Clinical and endocrinolgical investigations in gigantism reveal features characteristic of acromegaly, elevated unstimulated serum GH concentrations, paradoxical GH responses to exogenous administration of thyrotropin-releasing hormone (TRH), and failure to suppress serum GH concentrations with oral glucose loading. The 24-hour GH secretion in such individuals is very similar to that seen in acromegaly can be a most helpful investigation, particularly when the child is in the pubertal years.

Endocrinology of tall stature

The investigation of children growing rapidly requires answers to the question of whether the hypothalamo-pituitary-adrenal, -thyroid, or -GH axis is involved. Hyperthyroidism is easily identified by measuring free levels of 3,5,3'-triiodothyronine (T_3), and thyroxine (T_4). Adrenal disorders, such as congenital or acquired adrenal

hyperplasia, a functioning adrenal tumor, or Cushing's syndrome must be excluded. A useful screening test is the analysis of a 24-hour urine sample for steroid metabolites. The tall stature and rapid growth of precocious puberty will require separate consideration in conjunction with a pediatric endocrinologist.

Childhood growth is GH-dependent, and during this period, tall children grow with a height velocity greater than their peers by secreting a greater concentration of GH over a 24-hour period. The majority of this secretion occurs during the night, but as age advances, secretory episodes can be observed during the day. Daytime GH secretion is more marked in tall than in small children.

It has been observed that some constitutionally tall children have biochemical findings reminiscent of acromegaly. In tall children who have frequent daytime GH pulses, it is difficult to separate abnormal responses from their normal endogenous secretory patterns. It is therefore likely that the paradoxical GH response to TRH is not a pathological disturbance in tall adolescents. In fact, this abnormality lacks specificity: it is seen in acromegaly, anorexia nervosa, chronic renal failure, and diabetes mellitus, which are all conditions associated with elevated GH concentrations. Paradoxical responses can be predicted from the simple analysis of the patient's own endogenous hormonal secretion.

Treatment

There are several reasons to treat tall stature. Psychological problems expressed by tall children include difficulty with self image and rejection by peer group. From a medical point of view, a common problem in tall children is that of kyphoscoliosis. Since the pubertal growth spurt is likely to make kyphoscoliosis worse,

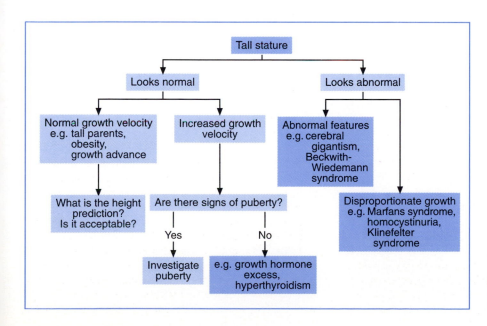

Figure 8.3 Flow chart for use in the differential diagnosis of tall stature.

these children deserve consideration for medical treatment.

Height prediction

The measurement of skeletal maturity to predict height is important in the management of tall stature. It bears on the decision of whether to or when to embark on therapy, and how to assess the effects. The prediction depends on the adequacy of the assessment of skeletal maturation. Overall, there is no superiority in any method.

The accuracy of height prediction is judged by the size of the residual standard deviation. The standard deviation for a height prediction of girls at bone age 12 years is approximately 2.5 cm according to the methods of Bayley and Pinneau. The Tanner-Whitehouse method has a standard deviation of 3.5 cm for a 12-year-old boy, and of 2.7 cm for a premenarcheal and 2.1 cm for a post-menarcheal 12-year-old girl. The newer Tanner-Whitehouse mark 2 method includes bone age assessment and height predictions of tall and very short individuals, reducing the error in the case of a 12-year-old boy to 3.2 and in the post-menarcheal girl to 1.1 cm. These findings are important to take into account when assessing treatment regimens.

Once height prediction is known, it can be used to determine the timing of pubertal induction. The gain in height during puberty is relatively fixed at 20 to 30 cm. Hence, if a final height of 180 cm is wanted, puberty needs to be induced at 150 cm.

Sex steroids

Estrogen therapy for tall girls was based on the observation that children with precocious puberty did not become tall adults because premature epiphyseal closure occurred. This therapy aims to superimpose the pubertal growth spurt by inducing puberty at an earlier chronological age. Standard induction regimens are used and high dose estrogen therapy is not necessary. The earlier treatment is started, the greater the reduction in final height.

Experience with testosterone therapy in boys is limited because fewer boys complain of tall stature than girls. The principle, induction of puberty, is the same.

Neurotransmitters and somatostatin

The aim of these therapies is to reduce GH secretion while allowing sex steroids to continue the process of bone maturation. Neither bromocriptine nor anticholinergic therapy have been shown to have any effect.

The development of octreotide, a long-acting analogue of somatostatin, has made possible the administration of this medication as a subcutaneous injection that suppresses GH secretion with no rebound secretion. Octreotide treatment of tall children has led to some reaction in height prediction.

Suggested readings

AMSELEM S, DUQUESNOY P, GOOSSENS M. Molecular basis of Laron dwarfism. Trends Endocrin metab 1991;2:35-40.

DATTANI MT, PRINGLE PJ, HINDMARSH PC, BROOK CGD. What is a normal stimulated growth hormone concentration? J Endocrinol 1992;133:447-50.

DE ZEGHER F, MAES M, GARGOSKY SE, et al. High-dose growth hormone treatment of short children born small for gestational age. J Clin Endocrinol Metab 1996;81:1887-92.

FREEMAN JV, COLE TJ, CHINN S, JONES PRM, WHITE EM, PREECE MA. Cross sectional stature and weight reference curves for the UK. Arch Dis Child 1990;73:17-24.

ROSENFELD RG, FRANE J, ATTIE KM, et al. Six year results of a randomised, prospective trial of human growth hormone and oxandrolone in Turner syndrome. J Pediatr 1992;121:49-55.

THALANGE NKS, FOSTER PJ, GILL MS, PRICE DA, CLAYTON PE. Model of normal prepubertal growth. Arch Dis Child 1996;5:427-31.

TILLMAN V, BUCKLER JM, KIBIRIGE MS, et al. Biochemical tests in the diagnosis of childhood growth hormone deficiency. J Clin Endocrinol and Metab 1997;82:531-5.

Disorders of pubertal development

Pierre C. Sizonenko

Puberty is defined as the period of life during which sexual maturation occurs, that is, when the growth and maturation of the gonads (named *gonadarche*) and the internal sex organs and external genitalia take place, as well as when sexual secondary characteristics develop. In addition to these changes, growth velocity is increased in relation to the growth and maturation of the bones and cartilage. Ages at which such changes are seen are presented in Tables 9.1

and 9.2. In boys, puberty onset is characterized by a testicular volume of above 4. In girls, the main sign of gonadarche is the breasts budding. Modifications of uterine and ovarian volumes have been well-characterized by ultrasonography as well. Simultaneously, psychological and behavioral changes are observed during this period, also referred to as adolescence. Maturation of the adrenal cortex with increased secretion of adrenal androgens (named *adrenarche*) occurs between the age of 6 and 8 years in girls and 7 and 9 years in boys. A major increase of bone mineral density occurs during the critical growth

Table 9.1 Stages of development of the breast and peak height velocity in girls in relation to chronological and bone ages[1]

Development of the breast	Chronological age	Bone age
B1 prepubertal		
B2 first budding enlargement of the areola	8.5 - *10.9* - 13.3	8.5 - *10.5* - 13.2
B3 enlargement of the breast palpable mammary gland	9.8 - *12.2* - 14.6	10.2 - *12.0* - 14.0
B4 additional enlargement of the breast and of the areola	11.4 - *13.2* - 15.0	11.5 - *13.5* - 15.0
B5 adult breast	11.6 - *14.0* - 16.4	12.5 - *15.0* - 16.0
Menarche	9.9 - *12.9* - 14.9	11.3 - *12.8* - 13.6
Peak height velocity	10.2 - *12.2* - 14.2	10.0 - *12.4* - 14.5

[1] 95% Confidence limits and means (in italics) of chronological and bone ages are expressed in years.
(Adapted from Sempe M. et al. Croissance et développement. In: Sizonenko PC, Griscelli C [eds]. Précis de pédiatrie. Lausanne: Editions Payot, 1996;64-65).

Table 9.2 Stages of development of testicular volume and peak height velocity in boys in relation to chronological and bone ages[1]

Testicular volume[2]	Chronological age	Bone age
G1 prepubertal testes (TVI <4)		
G2 pubertal testes (TVI between 4 and 5)	9.2 - *11.2* - 14.2	9.0 - *11.5* - 14.2
G3 TVI between 7 and 11	10.5 - *12.9* - 15.4	10.5 - *13.2* - 15.0
G4 TVI between 9 and 17	11.6 - *13.8* - 16.0	12.5 - *14.5* - 16.0
G5 adult testes	12.5 - *14.7* - 16.9	
Peak height velocity	12.3 - *13.9* - 15.5	12.5 - *14.5* - 16.0

[1] 95% Confidence limits and means (in italics) of chronological and bone ages are expressed in years.
[2] Testicular volume is expressed by the testicular volume index (TVI), representing the sum of the length width of the right side and the length × width of the left side, divided by 2.
(Adapted from Sempe M. et al. Croissance et développement. In: Sizonenko PC, Griscelli C [eds]. Précis de pédiatrie. Lausanne: Editions Payot, 1996;64-65).

phase of puberty in boys and girls, with a plateau reached at the end of puberty. A possible relationship between the bone density accretion during puberty and osteoporosis in later life has been questioned, particularly in delay of puberty and hypogonadism. Many factors – such as genetic, racial, nutritional, and psychological – affect the onset of puberty.

PRECOCIOUS PUBERTY

Sex characteristics before the age of 8 years in the girl and 10 years in the boy are considered to be precocious development. Three conditions are to be considered. (1) Partial precocious puberty. (2) True precocious puberty due to the precocious activation of the hypothalamo-pituitary-gonadal axis, or the ectopic secretion of gonadotropins (principally human chorionic gonadotropin by a tumor). In this case the puberty is isosexual, meaning in the same direction as the child's genetic sex. In girls, the main clinical symptom is development of the breasts; in boys it is an increase in size of the phallus, associated or not with frequent erections, and a presence of pubic hair. In both sexes, an increase of height velocity is observed. (3) Pseudoprecocious puberty due to a gonadal or adrenal tumor. Puberty can be either isosexual or heterosexual (in the opposite direction to the child sex: feminization of the boy or virilization of the girl). Clinically, in heterosexual pseudoprecocious puberty, girls present with pubic (and axillary) hair with possible clitoromegaly, accelerated growth, and acne; boys consult for gynecomastia.

Partial precocious puberty

Two conditions are usually described (Tab. 9.3). In addition, gynecomastia seen in boys has been included in this section as part of a normal variant of pubertal development, although it may be the first sign of pseudoprecocious puberty (see below and Tab. 9.4). They consist in the occurrence of: (1) premature isolated breast development (*premature thelarche*); (2) premature pubic and/or axillary hair (*premature adrenarche*); and (3) gynecomastia.

Premature thelarche is observed in girls between the ages of 1 and 3 years. This condition is not associated with maturational changes of the vulvae (i.e., development of labia minora), with vaginal maturation and with an increase in the volume of the uterus at the echographic examination of the pelvis. Ovaries are of prepubertal size. Plasma follicle-stimulating hormone (FSH) is sometimes elevated, but estradiol is low. This condition lasts for 6 to 18 months and resolves spontaneously without any treatment. These girls usually have normal pubertal development, menarche at the normal age, and normal fertility. In some cases, ovarian cysts have been noted. Recurrence of these cysts have been rarely observed, but in some cases they may progress in several years to true precocious puberty. They usually disappear spontaneously, but they

Table 9.3 Management of premature thelarche and adrenarche

Early development of breasts in girls (premature thelarche)

Age: 18 to 36 months
No other signs of pubertal development
No increase of growth velocity
Normal bone age for chronological age
Pelvic ultrasonogram can show an ovarian cyst
Plasma FSH may be high, estradiol is low
Spontaneous disappearance
No therapy is available
Need for regular 6-month follow-ups

Early development of pubic (and axillary) hair (premature adrenarche)

Before the age of 7 yr in girls and 8 yr in boys
No other signs of pubertal development
No breast development, no increase in testicular size
Possible slight increase in growth velocity
Possible slight increase in bone age
Adrenal androgens slightly elevated for age
Measure plasma 17OH-progesterone to rule out congenital virilizing adrenal hyperplasia

may also be the first sign of precocious puberty due to McCune-Albright syndrome.

Premature adrenarche consists of the premature and isolated development of pubic and/or axillary hair before the age of 7 years in girls and 8 years in boys, in relation either with the premature and excessive activation of the adrenal cortex and/or a change in the sensitivity of the hair follicle receptors to androgens. A slight increase in growth velocity with advancement of bone age can be observed. Slight clitoromegaly is rarely observed. In boys, testes are prepubertal. Adrenal androgens are usually slightly above the normal range for age, in relation with the slightly advanced bone age. Plasma 17α-hydroxyprogesterone and adrenal androgens should be measured in order to rule out late-onset congenital adrenal hyperplasia due to 21-hydroxylase deficiency. Partial forms of non salt-losing 3β-hydroxysteroid dehydrogenase deficiency with slightly elevated plasma 17-hydroxy-Δ5-pregnenolone have been also suggested. No therapy is required and gonadarche occurs normally. However, long-term follow-up have shown that polycystic ovary syndrome may appear more frequently later in life in this population of girls as compared to normal girls.

Pubertal gynecomastia represents a condition that is frequently seen during puberty in 38 to 64% of boys. It generates concerns in the adolescent boy as well as in his parents. Generally, no etiology is found, but the administration of neuroleptics or estrogens, chronic liver disease, and estrogen-secreting adrenal or testicular tumors should be ruled out (Tab. 9.4). In the presence of small testes, a measurement of plasma FSH, a buccal smear, and a karyotype should be performed in order to rule out Klinefelter's syndrome (see below). In most cases no cause is found, though it is hypothesized that a disequilib-

Table 9.4 Etiology of pubertal gynecomastia

Pubertal idiopathic gynecomastia

Gynecomastia without sexual ambiguity

Klinefelter's syndrome
Testicular estrogen-secreting tumor
hCG-secreting tumor (chorioepithelioma or hepatoma)
Hypothyroidism
Adrenal cortex estrogen-secreting tumor

Gynecomastia with sexual ambiguity

Male pseudohermaphroditism
Virilizing and non virilizing congenital adrenal virilizing
    hyperplasia
        11β-hydroxylase deficiency
        17α-hydroxylase deficiency
        17-ketoreductase deficiency

Drug-induced gynecomastia

Estrogens	Testosterone
Cyproterone acetate	op'DDD
Phenothiazine	Reserpine
Chlorpromazine	Meprobamate
Hydroxyzine	Sulpiride
Spironolactone	Ketoconazole
d-Penicillamine	Cimetidine

(Adapted from Sizonenko PC. Gynecomastia. In: Grossman A
[ed]. Clinical gynecomastia. Oxford: Blackwell Scientific
Publications, 1992;713-20.)

rium between the androgen and estrogen secretion is present, or that there is an increased sensitivity of the breast tissue to estrogens. Idiopathic pubertal gynecomastia disappears spontaneously in 1 to 2 years. In some cases (1 out of 10), gynecomastia persists, and surgery is required in view of the psychological difficulties encountered by the adolescent boy. Such surgery should be performed by an experienced surgeon, as it could leave very unsightly post-surgery scars.

True precocious puberty

At the present time, two types of true precocious puberty are described: the first one (called central) is gonadotropin-dependent and is responsive to therapy by gonadotropin-releasing hormone (GnRH) agonist; the second type does not respond to GnRH agonist therapy and is referred to as gonadotropin-independent. These conditions should be differentiated from other forms of pseudo-precocious puberty (Tabs. 9.5 and 9.6).

GONADOTROPIN-DEPENDENT TRUE PRECOCIOUS PUBERTY

Central true precocious puberty is due to an increased secretion of pituitary gonadotropins, with a pubertal amplitude and frequency of luteinizing hormone (LH) pulses during the night. The development of a child with this condition is isosexual (i.e., in accordance with his or her sex).

Etiology

The etiology varies according to the sex of the child (Tab. 9.7). Brain tumors such as dysgerminoma, glioma of the optic chiasma are frequently encountered in boys. In girls, a tumor is rarely found, and usually no etiology is found. True precocious puberty is referred to as idiopathic. Hamartomas are currently found by magnetic resonance imaging in many patients of both sexes. Hamartomas of the *tuber cinereum* are congenital tumors containing GnRH neurosecretory neurons, which are often associated with gelastic crises that represent a particular form of epilepsy. They are sessile or pedunculated benign masses attached to the posterior hypothalamus that project into the suprasellar cistern. They usually do not enlarge. They act as an ectopic GnRH pulse generator. Another group of tumors consists of tumors that secrete gonadotropins and often α-fetoprotein: hepatoblastoma (in the boy), germinoma located in the central nervous system, or chorioepithelioma.

In patients who have received cranial radiotherapy for leukemia or intracranial tumors, an increase in the prevalence of true precocious puberty has been observed, in particular in the case of gliomas of the optic nerves. The doses of radiation that may cause such precocious development are above 18 to 24 Gy. In combination with precocious puberty, growth hormone (GH) deficiency can be observed, although growth rate can be normal or even increased as a result of the increase in the secretion of sex steroids. A careful evaluation of the hypothalamopituitary axes should be made regularly (at least every year) in patients who have received radiation. Gonadotropin deficiency, thyrotropin deficiency, adrenocorticotropin deficiency, and hypoprolactinemia may occur with radiation doses above 40 Gy. Children who have received central nervous system irradiation (more than 25 Gy) for extrahypothalamopituitary tumors or total body irradiation should also be followed carefully for early pubertal development.

An increased incidence of true precocious puberty has been reported in several countries in children who have been adopted after the age of 3 years (with established birth dates) from countries with a high rate of malnutrition. The mechanism by which these children develop precocious sexual maturation is not known.

Clinical findings

Symptoms and signs

Clinical symptoms include precocious development of breasts in girls, and increased testes size (>4) is associated with increased height velocity (with advanced bone age) and increased somatic development in boys. In girls, menstruation may be observed, and isolated vaginal bleeding has also been observed. Bone age is advanced. Complete examination includes fundi of the eyes and evaluation of the visual fields. Psychological problems are usually present in the child as well as in the parents, who are concerned by the early development of secondary sex characteristics: tallness, development of breasts, and menstruation in the young girl; and increased size of the genitalia, erections, and masturbation in the boy. These problems should be thoroughly discussed with the parents and not underestimated. These children are often asked to behave like much older boys and girls because of their tallness.

Diagnostic procedures

Biological markers Plasma luteinizing hormone (LH) and FSH are usually in the pubertal range. In girls, the measurement of plasma estradiol is a poor indicator of pubertal development as it can be high (>25 pg/ml), but it can also frequently be normal for age. A vaginal smear demonstrating estrogenization of the vaginal epithelium can be helpful. In boys, plasma testosterone concentrations are elevated for age (>0.25 ng/ml). A pubertal response of LH and FSH after gonadotropin-releasing

hormone (GnRH, 50 to 100 μg iv) stimulation is observed, in particular in girls with an LH response much higher than the FSH response, similar to a normal pubertal response. Such a finding means that the hypothalamo-pituitary-gonadal axis is in its pubertal maturational phase. During prepuberty the converse is observed: the FSH response is much higher than the LH response. More recently, supersensitive assays of plasma LH allows for the diagnosis of true central precocious puberty based on a single serum sample measurement. Plasma insulin-growth factor I (IGF-I) as well as adrenal androgen levels are elevated for chronological age, but they are usually in the normal range for bone age.

Radiological findings Bone age is advanced. In girls, pelvic ultrasonography allows for the measurement of the volume of the uterus, which takes a mature shape, and it allows for the measurement of the ovaries and the observation of ovarian cysts, which are considered to be pathological if the diameter is greater than 2 cm. An X-ray of the skull and sella turcica is helpful in showing calcifications or erosion of the sella turcica, which would be suggestive of an intracranial tumor. Computerized tomography and magnetic resonance imaging of the brain permits

Table 9.5 Diagnosis and management of precocious and pseudopuberty in girls

Possible diagnosis	Specific tests	Gonadotropins	Estradiol (E_2) adrenal androgens
True precocious puberty			
Idiopathic	EEG	Moderately	Pubertal E_2
CNS tumors	Computed tomography Magnetic resonance Imaging	elevated	Pubertal E_2
Specific syndromes	(see Tab. 9.7)	Moderately	Pubertal E_2
Hypothyroidism	High TSH and low Thyroid hormones	elevated	Pubertal E_2
Pseudo-precocious puberty with feminization			
Ovarian tumor	Ultrasonography		
Ovarian cyst	or	Low	High E_2
Adrenal tumor	Computerized tomography		
Exogenous estrogen administration		Low	Usually low E_2
Pseudo-precocious puberty with virilization			
Congenital adrenal hyperplasia	High androgens and 17α-OH progesterone	Low	Prepubertal E_2 High androgens
Primary cortisol resistance	High ACTH, cortisol and androgens	Low	Prepubertal E_2 High androgens
Adrenal cortex tumor	Ultrasonography	Low	Prepubertal E_2 High androgens
Ovarian tumor	Ultrasonography	Low	Elevated E_2 High androgens
Exogenous androgen administration	Low		Low E_2

(ACTH = adrenocorticotropic hormone; TSH=thyroid-stimulating hormone.)
(Adapted from Sizonenko PC. Precocious puberty. In: Bertrand J, Rappaport R, Sizonenko PC [eds]. Pediatric endocrinology. Baltimore: Williams & Wilkins, 1993;387-403.)

the delineation and diagnosis of a tumor. X-rays of the skeleton are indicated when there is a suspicion of McCune-Albright syndrome.

In untreated patients, pubertal development continues, with an advanced bone age leading to reduced final height that is much below midparent height (145 to 155 cm below, for both sexes). Fertility has been reported in some cases, even at a young age.

Treatment

Therapy of central precocious puberty consists of the administration of GnRH agonist, intramuscularly daily or every 4 weeks with a depot preparation (Tab. 9.8). Such a long-acting agonist paradoxically provokes desensitization of the GnRH receptors at the pituitary level (due to its long half-life), resulting in a decrease of both LH and FSH secretions. Clinically, the therapy induces a regression of the pubertal signs, a decrease of the height velocity, and a reduction of the bone age advancement, which generally leads to an improved final adult height. Careful

clinical as well as laboratory monitoring of therapy is mandatory, following decreases of breasts in girls, the testicular volume in boys (which is usually incomplete and back to prepubertal volume), acne and erections in boys, the growth rate, advancement of bone age, plasma gonadotropins, and sex steroid concentrations in both sexes. Testosterone or estradiol plasma levels, less than 0.25 ng/ml or 15 pg/ml, respectively, indicate good suppression of the hypothalamopituitary-gonadal axis. Pelvic ultrasonograms should demonstrate a decrease in the size of the ovaries and uterus. Stimulation by GnRH should show the absence of response of both LH and FSH. The latter two investigations should not be performed on a regular monitoring schedule, but they are indicated in case of poor response to therapy. Long-term studies have clearly demonstrated the efficacy and the safety of the GnRH agonist therapy. Poor results in therapy come from inadequate doses, irregularity in the once-every-4-week injections, or from poor compliance. Discontinuation of

Table 9.6 Diagnosis and management of precocious and pseudoprecocious puberty in boys

Testes	Possible diagnosis	Pituitary gonadotropins	Testosterone	Additional tools
Both enlarged	True precocious puberty Idiopathic CNS tumors	Low or normal	Moderately elevated	
	Pseudo-precocious puberty Gonadotropin-secreting tumor	Low	Moderately elevated	High α-fetoprotein High β-hCG
	Overlap syndrome Hypothyroidism	Moderately elevated	Moderately elevated	TSH and thyroid hormones
	Congenital adrenal hyperplasia	Low	Moderately elevated	Elevated 17α-OH progesterone and androgens
One enlarged	Benign tumor Leydig cell tumor	Low	Elevated	Low FSH & LH
	Malignant tumor Chorioepitheloma	Low	Elevated	High hCG
Both small	Congenital adrenal hyperplasia	Low	Moderately elevated	Elevated 17α-OH progesterone and androgens
	Primary cortisol resistance	Low	Moderately elevated	High cortisol and ACTH Abnormal cortisol receptors (?)
	Adrenal tumor	Low	Moderately elevated	Elevated androgens
	Exogenous androgen administration	Low	Usually low	Personal history

(ACTH = adrenocorticotropic hormone.)
(Adapted from Sizonenko PC. Precocious puberty. In: Bertrand J, Rappaport R, Sizonenko PC [eds]. Pediatric endocrinology. Baltimore: Williams & Wilkins, 1993;387-403.)

Table 9.7 Etiology of true precocious puberty

Intracranial tumors

Hypothalamus
Dysgerminoma
Astrocytoma
Ganglioneuroma
Craniopharyngioma
Arachnoid cyst
Ependymoma
Mamilary body and tuber cinereum
Hamartoma
Pineal gland region
Teratoma, dysgerminoma
Chorioepithelioma
Pinealoma
Optic nerves
Glioma of the chiasma
Brain and cerebellum
Astrocytoma
Unknown origin

Congenital malformations

Stenosis of the aqueduct of Sylvius
Hydrocephaly
Microcephaly
Craniostenosis
Porencephaly

Post-trauma causes

Perinatal injuries
Craniocerebral trauma

Post-infectious causes

Meningitis
Tuberculosis
Bacterial
Encephalitis
Toxoplasmosis
Syphilis

Idiopathic forms

Sporadic
Familial

Other causes

McCune-Albright syndrome ?
van Recklinghausen neurofibromatosis
Tuberous sclerosis of Bourneville
Russell-Silver syndrome
Late-diagnosed congenital adrenal hyperplasia
Idiopathic epilepsy
Gelastic crisis with hamartoma

(Adapted from Sizonenko PC. Precocious puberty. In: Bertrand J, Rappaport R, Sizonenko PC [eds]. Pediatric endocrinology. Baltimore: Williams & Wilkins, 1993;387-403.)

Table 9.8 Drugs and dosages used for the therapy of precocious puberty

GnRH-dependent (central) precocious puberty

GnRH agonists		Desensitization of
in	800-1800 mg/d in 3 to 4 doses	gonadotropes
sc	4-50 m/kg/d	Blocks action of
im	(long-acting preparation)	endogenous
	60-300 mg/kg every 2-4 weeks[1]	GnRH

GnRH-independent precocious puberty

Medroxyprogesterone acetate		Inhibition of
po	100 mg/m^2/d	gonadal
im	(long-acting preparation)	steroidogenesis
	200-300 mg every 15 d	
	100-200 mg every 7 d	
Cyproterone acetate		Inhibition of FSH
po	70 to 150 mg/m^2/d	and LH secretion
im	100-200 mg/m^2, every 14/28 d	Anti-androgen
Ketoconazole		Inhibition of
po	30 µg/kg/d	P450c17α
		17,20-
		lyase activity)
Testolactone		Inhibition of
po	20-40 mg/kg/d	aromatase;
		blocks estrogen
		synthesis
Spironolactone		Anti-androgen;
po	50-100 mg/d	blocks sex
		steroids synthesis

(im = intramuscular; in = intranasal; po = oral; sc = subcutaneous routes).
[1] Dose depends upon the agonist used.
(Adapted from Sizonenko PC. Precocious puberty. In: Bertrand J, Rappaport R, Sizonenko PC [eds]. Pediatric endocrinology. Baltimore: Williams & Wilkins, 1993;387-403.)

therapy is decided when chronological age is in the mid-pubertal range (11 years in girls and 13 in boys). At the interruption of therapy, pubertal development resumes, with menstruation in girls occurring within 6 months to 2 years. Fertility does not seem to be affected. In the first published studies, the final height achieved with the therapy by GnRH analogues is below –1 SD for midparental height. However, recent studies seem to indicate that the final height is within the mean adult height and is much higher than the untreated control group. In some cases, ovarian cysts have been reported on the ultrasonograms after termination of therapy. In cases of central nervous system tumors, pathological diagnosis by biopsy sampling is required in order to assume the correct therapy: surgery and/or radiotherapy. However, in cases of hamartoma, there is no reason to perform neurosurgery, except in cases of intractable seizures or compression by the tumor inducing hydrocephalus.

Indications for such therapy are based on the rate of the patient's pubertal maturation and poor predicted adult height. In many patients, the progression of sexual maturation is often more rapid than the normal pattern of puberty. However, in some cases the progression is slow, and the bone age is slightly advanced with no loss of predicted adult height. In the latter cases, estradiol levels are usually slightly elevated (as well as IGF-I). If progression of the sexual maturation is slow and the height prediction within the limits of the familial target height, that is, not impaired, therapy is not indicated. However, a follow-up of these patients remains essential in order to evaluate the rate of sexual development and bone age advancement. The rate of sexual development should be clearly established 6 months after the diagnosis has been made, as the best response to therapy comes from the more severely and progressively affected patients. In cases of associated GH deficiency, GH therapy is added to the treatment of the precocious puberty.

GONADOTROPIN-INDEPENDENT PRECOCIOUS PUBERTY

Two particular forms of gonadotropin-independent isosexual precocious puberty have been described, which are considered to be separate from gonadotropin-dependent precocious puberty because of a lack of response to GnRH agonist therapy. The conditions correspond to mutations in the gonadotropin receptors: (1) the first one is the McCune-Albright syndrome in girls; (2) the second one is testitoxicosis in boys.

McCune-Albright syndrome is characterized by the association of polyostotic fibrous dysplasia of the bone that is slowly evoluting, skin pigmentation (café-au-lait spots) that is often unilateral and limited on one side by the trunk midline, and isosexual precocious puberty. The bone disease can affect any bone, and it is frequently associated with facial asymmetry and hyperostosis of the base of the skull. The disease is sporadic. Mutations of the gene coding for the α-subunit of the stimulatory Gs-protein of the adenyl cyclase, linked to the LH receptor, have been described. The single base substitution of arginine to histidine at position 201 of the Gs gene is responsible for the constitutive activation of the Gs protein at the ovarian receptor, which leads to increased sex steroid synthesis. Plasma LH and FSH are low and do not respond to GnRH stimulation. The mutations are somatic and not in the germ line, and only one allele needs to be affected since the mutations are dominant. There is a segmental distribution of the mutation in the individual. Therefore, autonomous activation of other hormonal receptors may involve the thyroid gland (nodular hyperplasia with or without thyrotoxicosis), adrenal gland (Cushing's syndrome due to multiple hyperplastic nodules), pituitary (gigantism or acromegaly due to GH-secreting adenoma, frequently with hyperprolactinemia), and parathyroid glands (hyperparathyroidism due to an adenoma or a hyperplasia). In addition, pseudo-hypophosphatemic rickets and osteomalacia, which are resistant to vitamin D, have been described.

Follicular cysts are found in the ovaries, which are enlarged. The LH and FSH responses to GnRH stimulation are blunted. The night profile of LH demonstrates the absence of pulses at the onset of sexual development. Later, after completion of puberty, the LH pulses appear and ovulatory cycles are observed, as well as fertility. This suggests that the girls, by an unknown phenomenon, shift from a GnRH-independent puberty to a GnRH-dependent cyclicity. Therapy consists of the administration of ovarian steroid synthesis blockers or of anti-estro-gens. In the rapidly progressing cases, it consists of the use of a progestational agent, medroxyprogesterone; an anti-androgen, cyproterone acetate; blockers of steroid synthesis; ketoconazole; spironolactone; or of an aromatase inhibitor, testolactone (Tab. 9.8). These drugs usually block the pubertal development, but their effects do not last very long.

Cases of McCune-Albright syndrome have been observed in boys, though rarely. Clinically, asymmetrical enlargement of the testes may be noticed, and testosterone levels are in the pubertal range, with low plasma LH and FSH levels and an absent response of gonadotropins to GnRH stimulation.

Testitoxicosis is considered to be an autonomous activation of the LH receptor of the Leydig cells due to mutations of the LH receptor gene. It can be familial and is a sex-limited autosomal dominant disorder, with premature Leydig cell and germ cell maturation. The volume of the testes and the penis are increased, testosterone levels are in the pubertal or adult range, basal plasma LH and FSH concentrations are low, and night pulses of LH and FSH are absent. An absent response of gonadotropins to GnRH stimulation is part of the disease. Testicular biopsies demonstrate Leydig cell and Sertoli cell maturation with spermatogenesis. At adulthood, fertility is present, and pulsatility of LH and FSH are restored. Several mutations of the LH receptor have been described. This condition does not respond to GnRH agonist administration. Therapy consists of the administration of blockers of testicular steroid synthesis such as ketoconazole (which may have side effects and cause hepatic or kidney injury) or of anti-androgens such as cyproterone acetate (Tab. 9.8).

Precocious pseudopuberty

Abnormal secretion of sex steroids are responsible for the condition of precocious pseudopuberty (Tabs. 9.5 and 9.6). Gonadal tumors are present in children but are rare. Congenital adrenal hyperplasia and adrenal tumors are more frequent causes of precocious puberty (Tab. 9.9).

Signs of puberty can be isosexual or heterosexual (i.e., feminization of the boy with gynecomastia; virilization of the girl with pubic and/or axillary hair, hypertrophy of the clitoris). Bone age is advanced and plasma sex steroid levels are increased. In girls, a tumor of the ovary or the adrenal gland should be ruled out by palpation of the abdomen and by ultrasonography of the abdomen and pelvis. Boys should be examined for testicular and adrenal tumors.

Autonomous cysts can be observed in an ultrasonogram of the pelvis, suggesting either true precocious puberty or isosexual pseudoprecocious puberty. In the latter case, the cysts are much bigger, usually above 5 cm in diameter.

Therapy depends on the etiology of the condition.

Table 9.9 Etiology of precocious pseudopuberty (P.P.P.)

Girls	Boys
Isosexual P.P.P.	**Isosexual P.P.P.**

Ovarian tumors
  granulosa cell tumor
  theca cell tumor
  teratoma
Autonomous functional
  cyst of the ovary
Adrenal tumor
Administration of estrogens
	Congenital adrenal
	  virilizing hyperplasia
	Adrenal cortex tumor
	Leydig cell tumor
	Teratoma (with adrenal tissue)
	Administration of estrogens

Heterosexual P.P.P. **(virilization)**	**Heterosexual P.P.P.** **(feminization)**

Congenital adrenal virilizing
  hyperplasia
Adrenal cortex tumor
Ectopic adrenal tissue of
  the ovary
Administration of androgens
	Adrenal cortex tumor
	Administration of estrogens

(Adapted from Sizonenko PC. Precocious puberty. In: Bertrand J, Rappaport R, Sizonenko PC [eds]. Pediatric endocrinology. Baltimore: Williams & Wilkins, 1993;387-403.)

DELAYED PUBERTY AND HYPOGONADISM

Delayed puberty is defined by the absence of any sign of gonadal puberty (gonadarche) after the age of 13 years in girls (no breast development) and 14 years in boys (no increase in testicular size). Delayed sexual maturation may represent deficient gonadotropin secretion due to a lesion of the central nervous system, or variants of normal puberty (particularly in boys), or a lesion of the gonads. The two former conditions are often difficult to differentiate from each other.

Above these age limits, the condition should be investigated in order to diagnose any pathological condition or, by exclusion of any recognized disease, simple delay of puberty (or delayed adolescence), which is of good prognosis. In the latter case, reassurance of the adolescent is necessary.

Girls are referred for an absence of development of the mammary glands, usually with short stature; boys, for an infantile aspect of the genitalia, frequent short stature with decreased growth rate, frequently associated with some weight excess. Pubic hair and axillary hair are often present. Testicular volume under 4 will confirm the prepubertal stage of the adolescent boy. Testicular volume above 4 indicates that pubertal development has started.

Clinical findings

In both sexes, a family history of delayed puberty, in particular in the father, should be noted. Bone age should be determined, and a radiogram of the sella turcica per-

formed. In girls a karyotype rules out the possibility of Turner syndrome, for which clinical symptoms such as short stature, small triangular nails, cubitus valgus, webbed neck, and so on, should be looked for. Basal plasma gonadotropins will differentiate between *hypergonadotropic* and *hypogonadotropic* conditions. In hypogonadotropic conditions, further investigation may include a GnRH stimulation test, in boys an hCG stimulation test and eventually a testicular biopsy, and in girls an ultrasonogram of the pelvis in order to evaluate the development of the uterus and the ovaries.

Etiological causes of hypogonadism can therefore be classified into two categories (Tabs. 9.10 and 9.11): *hypergonadotropic hypogonadism* (high basal LH and FSH, primary gonadal lesions), and *hypogonadotropic hypogonadism* (low or normal LH and FSH, primary hypothalamo-pituitary lesions). High basal concentrations of gonadotropins are usually observed only after a bone age of 11 years in girls and 13 years in boys.

Hypergonadotropic hypogonadism

In boys: Klinefelter's syndrome is described among the causes of hypergonadotropic hypogonadism, although no delay of puberty is observed in these patients. The main clinical features are the small size of the testes, eunuchoid body proportions, and the frequently observed gynecomastia. Bilateral congenital anorchidia is less frequently diagnosed. Rarely, anorchidia is secondary to orchidopexia. Due to the current high rate of survival of children with malignant tumors or hematological diseases, testicular lesions after chemotherapy and/or testicular radiotherapy are frequently observed: azoospermia with high plasma levels of FSH due to lesions of the tubules. Doses of 15 Gy may cause oligospermia, whereas 35 Gy are likely to cause azoospermia, which may still be reversible. Higher doses cause permanent damage to the germ cells. Leydig cell function may be affected at high radiation doses (20 Gy), with decreased secretion of testosterone.

In girls: Turner syndrome is the most frequent cause of hypogonadism and short stature. In some cases, the reason for consulting is primary amenorrhea, which is considered to be pathological after the age of 15 years (Tab. 9.12). Acquired lesions after chemotherapy and/or radiotherapy are often seen after survival of oncologic diseases. Ovaries of prepubertal and pubertal girls are more resistant to chemotherapy than adult ovaries. Permanent damage is observed above a cumulative dose of 5 g of cyclophosphamide and at a radiation dose higher than 8 Gy.

Hypogonadotropic hypogonadism

In both sexes, the differential diagnosis between hypogonadotropic hypogonadism and simple delay of puberty is often difficult. Affected hypogonadotropic boys present with tall stature and eunuchoid body proportions, small testes, and some pubic hair. In girls, pubic and axillary hair are often present. In case of panhypopituitarism, the

Table 9.10 Etiology of hypogonadism and delayed puberty in girls

Hypergonadotropic hypogonadism

Congenital
Turner syndrome (XO and its variants)
Other forms of gonadal dysgenesis (XO/XY, XY)
Ovarian agenesis (XX)
Noonan syndrome (XX)
Precocious ovarian insufficiency

Acquired
Traumatic or surgical bilateral castration
Post-chemotherapy and/or radiotherapy
Autoimmune ovaritis associated to Addison's disease, thyroiditis, etc.
Chronic infections (tuberculosis)

Hypogonadotropic hypogonadism

Hypothalamus
Sporadic or familial GnRH insufficiency
Gonadotropic insufficiency with anosmia (Kallmann's syndrome)
Isolated LH insufficiency
Isolated FSH insufficiency?
Suprasellar tumors
Interrupted pituitary stalk syndrome with ectopic posterior pituitary
Prader-Willi-Labhardt syndrome; Laurence-Moon-Biedl syndrome
Post-trauma

Pituitary
Panhypopituitarism
Pituitary tumor (prolactinoma?)
Association to growth hormone insufficiency
Post-trauma

Simple delay of puberty

Sporadic
Familial (+++)

Delayed puberty associated with chronic disease

Same etiology as in the boy
Anorexia nervosa

(Adapted from Sizonenko PC. Endocrinologie et diabétologie. In: Sizonenko PC, Griscelli C [eds]. Précis de pédiatrie. Lausanne: Editions Payot, 1996;1034-5.)

Table 9.11 Etiology of hypogonadism and delayed puberty in boys

Hypergonadotropic hypogonadism

Congenital
Klinefelter's syndrome
Chromatine-negative gonadal dysgenesis
Anorchidia
Noonan syndrome (male Turner syndrome)
Abnormal testosterone synthesis
Agenesis of Leydig cells
Sertoli cell syndrome
Smith-Lemli-Opitz syndrome, Steinert myotonia, Bloom's syndrome, etc.

Acquired
Traumatic or surgical bilateral castration
Syndrome of rudimentary testes
Bilateral orchitis
Abnormal Leydig cells
Post-chemotherapy
Post-radiotherapy
Deficiency of spermatogenesis
Post-chemotherapy
Post-radiotherapy

Hypogonadotropic hypogonadism

Hypothalamus
Sporadic or familial GnRH insufficiency
Gonadotropic insufficiency with anosmia (Kallmann's syndrome)
Isolated LH insufficiency
Isolated FSH insufficiency?
Suprasellar tumors
Interrupted pituitary stalk syndrome with ectopic posterior pituitary
Prader-Willi-Labhardt syndrome; Laurence-Moon-Biedl syndrome; association to congenital ichtyosis, etc.
Post-trauma

Pituitary
Panhypopituitarism
Pituitary tumor (prolactinoma?)
Association to growth hormone insufficiency
Post-trauma

Simple delay of puberty

Sporadic
Familial (+++)

Delayed puberty associated with chronic disease

Celiac disease
Cystic fibrosis
Chronic renal failure
Crohn's disease

(Adapted from Sizonenko PC. Endocrinologie et diabétologie. In: Sizonenko PC, Griscelli C [eds]. Précis de pédiatrie. Lausanne: Editions Payot, 1996;1034-5.)

diagnosis is easy, because it is associated with other pituitary deficiencies, such as growth hormone, adrenocorticotropin or thyroid-stimulating hormone, or diabetes insipidus. It is more difficult if the hypogonadotropic hypogonadism is isolated. A tumor or a congenital defect of the hypothalamopituitary region will be excluded by magnetic resonance imaging of the brain.

Isolated hypogonadotropic hypogonadism can be associated with an impaired sense of smell (Kallmann's syndrome) and with frequent unilateral or bilateral cryptorchidism. This condition represents a permanent absence of sexual development due to an abnormal migration of the GnRH neurons, which normally originate from the olfactory placode to the hypothalamus. An abnormal KAL gene present on the short arm of the chromosome X at location p22.3 codes for abnormal adhesion molecules.

The disease is either sporadic or familial and much more frequent in boys than in girls. Basal plasma gonadotropins and sex steroids are low. Urinary gonadotropin determinations may be useful, but they are not conclusive for the diagnosis of hypogonadotropic

Table 9.12 Etiology of primary amenorrhea

Rule out abnormalities of the genital tract
  Imperforate hymen
  Absence of uterus (Rokitansky's syndrome)

Gonadal abnormalities
Congenital
  Gonadal dysgenesis (XO, and variants)
  Pure gonadal dysgenesis (46,XX)
  Enzymatic defects of testosterone synthesis

Acquired
  Primary ovarian insufficiency
  Polycystic ovarian syndrome
  Resistant ovarian syndrome
  Androgens excess from ovarian or adrenal origin

Hypothalamo-pituitary abnormalities
Anatomical
  Suprasellar tumor or pituitary adenoma
  Sheehan syndrome
  Interrupted pituitary stalk syndrome with ectopic
    posterior pituitary

Functional
  Loss of weight (anorexia nervosa, fear of overweight,
    dieting)
  Psychogenic, stress
  Intensive physical exercise (marathon, gymnastics)
  Chronic diseases
  Hyperprolactinemia
  Drugs

(Adapted from Bourguignon JP. Delayed puberty and hypogo-nadism. In: Bertrand J, Rappaport R, Sizonenko PC [eds]. Pediatric endocrinology. Baltimore: Williams & Wilkins, 1993;404-19.)

hypogonadism. Responses of LH and FSH to GnRH or GnRH agonist stimulation are low or of prepubertal type. Gonadotropin profiles during sleep have not been proven to be differential in many cases. In boys, the response of testosterone to hCG administration is usually low (less than 2.5 ng/ml, after an injection of hCG, 5000 U/m^2, twice a week during 2 weeks, i.e., a total of four injections). More recently superactive GnRH agonists have been used to differentiate between hypogonadotropic hypogonadism, in which the response is low, and constitutionally delayed puberty, in which the response is higher. Suggestions have also been made that new supersensitive immunoassays for measurements of basal plasma FSH and LH would differentiate the two conditions. However, presently most of the routine tests used in routine are usually not helpful in the differential diagnosis between these two conditions. After 1 to 2 years of treatment with sex steroids, discontinuing the therapy is advised during 6 months in order to evaluate whether puberty can develop spontaneously or not. This will indicate the final diagnosis, which sometimes cannot be made

definitively before 16 or 17 years of age. Adrenal androgens are normal and bone age is only slightly delayed. Follow-up of the patient will indicate whether the condition is permanent or not. In girls, delayed puberty can be due to anorexia nervosa with their underweight due to undernutrition and particular psychological behavior towards the food.

Simple delay of puberty

Simple delay of puberty should be considered in the absence of any recognized cause of hypogonadism. It represents a variant of normal development in which somatic and endocrine markers are delayed for chronological age and are usually normal for bone age, which is usually markedly delayed. It is associated with short stature and relatively low levels of adrenal androgens. A familial history of delay of growth and puberty is found in 50% of the cases. Evolution is benign, puberty develops and growth catches up, leading to a normal final height in relation to the familial target height. Psychological disturbances should be evaluated, as short stature and the absence of development of the genitalia can impact the behavior of an adolescent.

Treatment

Therapy in the *hypogonadic* adolescent boy consists of the substitution of long-acting preparations (50 mg/month during the first year of therapy, 100 mg/month the second year, and thereafter 250 mg/month), or percutaneous preparations of testosterone (Tab. 9.13). In the hypogonadic adolescent girl, therapy consists of the administration of low-doses of estrogens given orally (Ethinyl-estradiol 0.1 µg/kg/day, Equigyne 10 µg/kg/day), or percutaneously during over 6 to 12 months; sequential estroprogestative therapy is then initiated in order to induce regular menstruation. As indicated above, a window in the therapy is advised for the final diagnosis of the condition. Later in adulthood, gonadotropins or pulsatile GnRH administration are required to achieve spermatogenesis or ovulation in these patients when fertility is desired.

In *simple delayed puberty*, indications for hormonal therapy are essentially based on psychological disturbances (Tab. 9.13). In the boy, long-acting preparations of testosterone (50 mg/month during over 3 to 6 months) can be of great help, as it stimulates growth velocity and further development of the genitalia. Such short-term therapy appears to be safe, does not seem to decrease the final height, and brings some psychological satisfaction to the delayed adolescent boy with enhanced growth and increased muscle mass. In some countries, anabolic steroids are prescribed and are of benefit. In girls, though rarely, estrogens are prescribed in low doses (Ethinyl-estradiol 0.1 µg/kg/day, Equigyne 10 µg/kg/day) during over 3 to 6 months. In all cases, psychological reassurance of the good prognosis of a simple delay in puberty, and follow-up of growth and bone age, are helpful to the adolescent patient.

Table 9.13 Therapy of hypogonadism and delayed puberty

Hormone	Galenic forms	Routes of administration	Dosage	Frequency
Androgens	Long-acting esters of testosterone	im	50-200 mg	Every 3 to 4 weeks
Estrogens	Ethinyl-estradiol	po	0.1-0.3 mg/kg	Once a day
	Conjugated estrogens	po	0.1-0.3 mg/kg	Once a day
Anabolic steroids	Oxandrolone	po	0.05-0.1 mg/kg	Once a day
GnRH	Synthetic decapeptide	iv/sc (pump)	25-250 ng	90-120 min
hCG	Urinary gonadotropin	im	1500-2000 U	Once a week
hMG	Urinary gonadotropin	im	75-150 U	Twice a week
FSH	Recombinant gonadotropin	im	75-150 U	Twice a week
LH	Recombinant gonadotropin	im	75-150 U	Twice a week

(GnRH = gonadotropin-releasing hormone; hCG = human chorionic gonadotropin; hMG = human menopausal gonadotropins; im = intramuscular; iv = intravenous; po = oral; sc = subcutaneous routes.)
(Adapted from Bourguignon JP. Delayed puberty and hypogonadism. In: Bertrand J, Rappaport R, Sizonenko PC [eds]. Pediatric endocrinology. Baltimore: Williams & Wilkins, 1993;404-19.)

Suggested readings

BLIZZARD RM, ROGOL AD. Variations and disorders of pubertal development. In: Kappy MS, Blizzard RM, Migeon CJ (eds). The diagnosis and treatment of endocrine disorders in childhood and adolescence. Springfield: Charles C Thomas, 1994;857-918.

BOURGUIGNON JP. Delayed puberty and hypogonadism. In: Bertrand J, Rappaport R, Sizonenko PC (eds). Pediatric endocrinology. Baltimore: Williams & Wilkins 1993;404-19.

GRUMBACH MM, STYNE DM. Puberty. Ontogeny, neuroendocrinology, physiology, and disorders. In: Wilson JD, Foster DW (eds). Williams Textbook of endocrinology. 9th ed.

Philadelphia: WB Saunders, 1998;1509-1675.

SIZONENKO PC. The adrenal gland and sexual maturation. In: Delemarre-van der Waal HA, Plant TM, van Rees GP, Schoemaker J (eds). Control of onset of puberty III. Amsterdam: Excerpta Medica, 1989;375-387.

SIZONENKO PC. Gynecomastia. In: Grossman A (ed). Clinical gynecomastia. Oxford: Blackwell Scientific Publications, 1992;713-720.

SIZONENKO PC. Precocious puberty. In: Bertrand J, Rappaport R, Sizonenko PC (eds). Pediatric endocrinology. Baltimore: Williams & Wilkins, 1993;387-403.

STYNE DM. New aspects in the diagnosis and treatment of pubertal disorders. Ped Clin North Am 1997;44:506.

The thyroid gland

10

Functional anatomy, physiology and pathophysiology

Wilmar M. Wiersinga

The thyroid gland in the human embryo starts to develop during the fourth week as a midline structure extending caudally from the foramen cecum. It migrates anteriorly and inferiorly to the hyoid bone and laryngeal cartilages. The original hollow stalk connecting it to the pharyngeal floor (the thyroglossal duct) atrophies and breaks by the fifth week. Shortly thereafter the thyroid anlage fuses with ultimobranchial bodies developing from the fourth pharyngeal pouches. By the seventh week the thyroid diverticulum has reached its adult position anterior to the trachea. It forms a bilobed gland, with a small isthmus connecting the two lobes; often some thyroid tissue extends superiorly from the isthmus, known as the pyramidal lobe. Follicles are present by the tenth week, and the thyroid accumulates iodide by the eleventh or twelfth week; thyroid hormone production begins by the end of the first trimester.

The mean weight of the adult thyroid gland in non-iodine deficient areas is 11 g with a range of about 5 to 19 g; the thyroid of males is larger than of females. The length of the lateral lobes is usually 4 cm, their breadth 1.5 to 2 cm, and their thickness 2 to 3.5 cm. The thyroid has an abundant blood supply provided from two superior and two inferior thyroid arteries, and the normal flow rate is ~5 ml/g thyroid/minute. Innervation of the gland is by sympathetic and parasympathetic fibers, which are mainly involved in regulating blood flow.

The thyroid gland is composed of follicles, the structural and functional units of the organ. The spheroidal follicles vary considerably in size. The walls consist of one layer of follicular epithelial cells (the thyrocytes or thyroid parenchyma), and they are usually cuboidal in shape. The lumen of the follicles is filled with homogeneous gelatinous material known as colloid, containing mainly thyroglobulin. The interfollicular space contains connective tissue, blood vessels, and the calcitonin-secreting parafollicular or C cells, which are derived from the neural crest by the ultimobranchial bodies.

Abnormal development of the thyroid gland adversely affects the descent of the gland to its normal position.

Consequently, an ectopic thyroid (usually associated with hypothyroidism) may be located anywhere between the foramen cecum at the base of the tongue and the normal position in the neck. Along the path of migration a thyroglossal duct remnant or cyst can be encountered.

Goiter is defined as an enlarged thyroid gland, diffuse or nodular in nature. Thyroid size is usually assessed by inspection and palpation, but a more precise method is the measurement of thyroid volume by ultrasound: a gland larger than 20 ml represents a goiter. Palpation of a single thyroid nodule, however, also qualifies as a goiter even if total thyroid volume is less than 20 ml.

The histological appearance of thyroid follicles reflects their metabolic activity. The follicular epithelial cells become flatter in the resting gland, but columnar epithelium develops under thyroid-stimulating hormone (TSH) stimulation: the height of the epithelium is inversely related to the diameter of the follicle lumen.

THYROID HORMONE BIOSYNTHESIS

The primary function of the thyroid gland is to synthesize and secrete thyroxine (3,5,3',5'-tetraiodothyronine or T_4). Approximately 150 µg of inorganic iodide is required daily for normal thyroid hormone biosynthesis. Iodine is an essential but rare element; it is mainly provided with nutrition, either naturally (especially in seafish) or artificially by the iodination of salt, bread, or milk. The thyroid gland accumulates iodide by an active energy-requiring transport mechanism: the recently cloned Na^+/I^- symporter (NIS) is able to concentrate iodide from the serum against a large concentration gradient. Other proteins involved in thyroid hormone biosynthesis (schematically represented in Figure 10.1) are thyroid peroxidase (TPO) and thyroglobulin; characteristics are given in Table 10.1. Thyroid peroxidase (carbohydrate content 10%) contains four glycosylation sites that are important for the tertiary structure at the active site, and a prosthetic (heme) group; its main form is TPO-1 (103 kD), but alternative splicing (by which exon 10 is spliced out) gives rise to the variant TPO-2 of 97 kD, which is inactive with respect to iodination. Thyroglobulin is a large homodimeric glycoprotein (carbohydrate content 10%) containing 134 tyrosyl residues, of which 40 are available for iodination. Tyrosine residues 5, 1290, 2533 and 2746 are located in the amino-terminus of the thyroglobulin molecule and are preferentially iodinated, which are known as the hormonogenic sites.

Once iodide is taken up in the thyrocyte, it rapidly moves to the apical surface and into the lumen. Thyroid hormone biosynthesis occurs within the thyroglobulin molecule at the apical surface. It involves two oxidative reactions, both catalyzed by TPO located in the apical plasma membrane. The first is iodination of the tyrosyl residues in thyroglobulin, resulting in monoiodotyrosine and diiodotyrosine. The iodination requires prior peroxidation of I^- to form its more reactive form I^+ (or hypoiodite). The second is the coupling of iodotyrosines in the thyroglobulin: coupling of a donor diiodotyrosine residue to an acceptor diiodotyrosine results in T_4, and that of a donor monoiodotyrosine to an acceptor diiodotyrosine in

3,5,3'-triiodothyronine (T_3) (Fig. 10.2). The hormonogenic sites are only partially used in the biosynthesis: under normal circumstances (at an iodine content of thyroglobulin of 0.5%, i.e., 26 atoms iodine per 660 kD molecule of thyroglobulin), each thyroglobulin molecule contains 5 monoiodotyrosine, 4.5 diiodotyrosine, 2.5 T_4 and 0.7 T_3 molecules. The thyroglobulin is stored in the colloid.

Release of T_4 and T_3 from the thyroid gland firstly involves resorption of stored thyroglobulin from the colloid. In a process called micropinocytosis, or coated-vesicle-dependent endocytosis, there is an invagination of the apical plasma membrane into small vesicles, producing colloid droplets. The vesicles are transported to the basolateral surface of the thyrocyte via endosomes; internalized thyroglobulin that is poorly iodinated is, however, recycled back to the follicular lumen. Colloid droplets with highly iodinated thyroglobulin fuse with lysosomes. Intralysomal peptidases catalyze the degradation of thyroglobulin, releasing T_4, T_3, monoiodotyrosine and diiodotyrosine. Monoiodotyrosine and diiodotyrosine are deiodinated by an NADPH-dependent dehalogenase, and the liberated iodide is largely re-utilized for hormone synthesis, being only partly lost from the thyroid gland. The thyrocyte also contains 5'-deiodinase activity (type I), converting a small amount of hydrolyzed T_4 into T_3.

Figure 10.1 Schematic diagram of thyroid hormone biosynthesis and release. Subsequent metabolic steps are: *a)* iodide transport via the Na$^+$/I$^-$ symporter (NIS), inhibited by ClO$_4^-$ and SCN$^-$; *b)* oxidation of I$^-$ to I$^+$ and iodination of tyrosine residues in thyroglobulin (Tg), and coupling of monoiodotyrosine (MIT) and diiodotyrosine (DIT) to thyroxine (T_4) or triiodothyronine (T_3), catalyzed by thyroid peroxidase (TPO) and inhibited by propylthiouracil and methimazole; *c)* colloid resorption, inhibited by lithium and I$^-$; *d)* proteolysis of Tg, inhibited by I$^-$; *e)* deiodination of MIT and DIT; *f)* deiodination of T_4, inhibited by propylthiouracil.

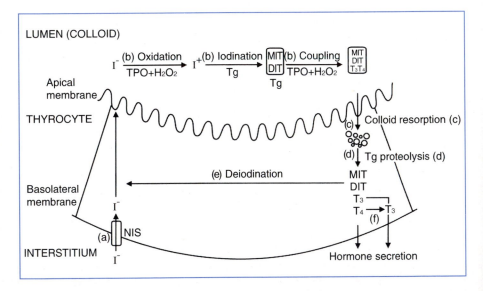

Table 10.1 Characteristics of some important thyroid proteins

		NIS	TPO	Tg[1]	TSH-R
Protein	Size (kD)	69	103	660	84.5
	No. of amino acids	643	933	5496	744
	Localization	Basolateral membrane	Apical membrane	Mainly colloid	Basolateral membrane
Gene	Chromosome	19	2	8	14

(NIS = Na$^+$/I$^-$ symporter; TPO = thyroid peroxidase; Tg = thyroglobulin; TSH-R = thyroid-stimulating hormone receptor.)
[1] Tg is a homodimer of two 330 kD units of ~2700 amino acids.

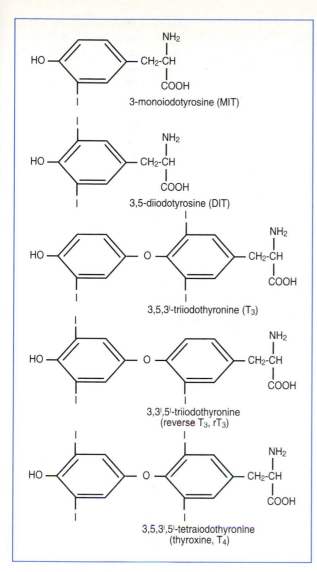

HO—〈 〉—CH₂-CH(NH₂)COOH

3-monoiodotyrosine (MIT)

3,5-diiodotyrosine (DIT)

3,5,3ᴵ-triiodothyronine (T₃)

3,3ᴵ,5ᴵ-triiodothyronine
(reverse T₃, rT₃)

3,5,3ᴵ,5ᴵ-tetraiodothyronine
(thyroxine, T₄)

Figure 10.2 Structure of some iodotyrosines and iodothyronines.

Table 10.2 Thyroid hormone kinetics in a 70 kg healthy human

	T_4	T_3	rT_3
Serum concentration (nmol/l)	103	2	0.4
Distribution volume (l)	10	38	90
Metabolic clearance rate (l/kg)	1.2	24	110
Production rate (mol/day)	130	49	43
thyroidal production (%)	100	20	5
extrathyroidal production (%)	80	80	95
Serum half-life (days)	7	1	0.16

transactivation expression of these genes, but they may also play a role in ontogenesis: during embryonic development TTF-1 is expressed before thyroglobulin and TPO, and mutant mice lacking TTF-1 do not develop a thyroid gland.

Clinical relevance

Iodine deficiency understandably may result in hypothyroidism, the most prevalent thyroid disease in the world. When iodine supply is sufficient, diiodotyrosine is the iodotyrosine preferentially formed, leading to the production of T_4. A lack of iodine, however, will favor the formation of monoiodotyrosine, causing a shift in thyroid hormone biosynthesis towards the production of T_3. Furthermore, the conversion of T_4 into T_3 in the thyroid gland may be enhanced by a TSH-induced increase of 5'-deiodinase activity. Iodine deficiency thus results in a preferential secretion of T_3 by the thyroid gland.

Similar mechanisms operate in the preferential T_3 secretion observed in patients with either primary hypothyroidism (due to loss of functional thyroid parenchyma) or hyperthyroidism. In primary hypothyroidism the increase of TSH stimulates thyroidal 5'-deiodinase activity, which results in an overproduction of T_3. Indeed, in the transition from the euthyroid to the hypothyroid state, plasma T_3 concentrations remain within the normal reference range until an advanced stage of the disease. However, the fall of plasma T_4 is an early phenomenon. It follows that plasma T_3 is not a sensitive test for the diagnosis of hypothyroidism. In Graves' hyperthyroidism, thyroid-stimulating immunoglobulins (mimicking the effect of TSH) contribute to the preferential T_3 secretion by the thyroid. This is also encountered in non-Graves' hyperthyroidism with a suppressed TSH, however. This is explained by the development of relative intrathyroidal iodine deficiency, which is caused by the consumption of large quantities of iodine in the presence of excessive thyroid hormone production. In the transition from the euthyroid to the hyperthyroid state, plasma T_3 concentration indeed rises prior to plasma T_4.

Thyroid hormone (and a small amount of thyroglobulin) are secreted from the basolateral surface of the thyrocyte into the circulation. Thyroxine is the main secretory product of the thyroid gland (~130 mol/day). Thyroidal T_3 secretion is much lower (~10 mol/day), providing only 20% of the daily T_3 production (Tab. 10.2). Secretion of the inactive iodothyronine rT_3 (reverse triiodothyronine) is still smaller, because the conditions for its formation within the thyroglobulin molecule (requiring coupling of a donor diiodotyrosine residue to an acceptor monoiodotyrosine) are less favorable.

The iodide uptake in the thyrocyte, the iodide organification (i.e., the incorporation of iodine in tyrosines) and the formation of iodothyronines, the resorption of colloid, and the release of T_4 and T_3 are all stimulated by thyroid-stimulating hormone. Recently specific transcription factors have been identified that bind to the promoter region of thyroglobulin and TPO genes: thyroid-transcription factors TTF-1 and TTF-2, and PAX-8. They induce via

Autoimmune thyroid disease is also prevalent. Each of the four thyroid proteins listed in Table 10.1 serves as an antigen against which an autoimmune reaction may develop. Antibodies directed against thyroglobulin (TgAb) and TPO (TPOAb) are useful serum markers for the presence of thyroid autoimmunity. TgAb probably plays no role in the pathogenesis of autoimmune thyroid disease, but TPOAb contributes to destruction of thyrocytes that result in hypothyroidism (Hashimoto's disease). Antibodies directed against the TSH receptor are the hallmark of Graves' hyperthyroidism. The clinical relevance of antibodies against the sodium-iodide transporter is presently unknown.

The uptake of iodide in the thyrocyte and its subsequent organification, the resorption of colloid, the proteolysis of thyroglobulin, the intrathyroidal deiodination of T_4, and the release of thyroid hormones provide multiple sites for pharmacological interference (as depicted in Figure 10.1), which find wide application in the treatment of hyperthyroid patients. The main action of the classical antithyroid drugs propylthiouracil and methimazole is inhibition of TPO activity, which results in a marked decrease of thyroid hormone biosynthesis.

Mutations in the genes encoding the transcription factors TTF-1, TTF-2 and PAX-8 that regulate the expression of the thyroid-specific proteins thyroglobulin and TPO might in theory be involved in thyroid agenesis or ectopy. No mutations of TTF-1, however, have been found in such cases; only one patient with thyroid ectopy had a point mutation in the PAX-8 gene, which resulted in a stop codon. Mutations in the genes encoding thyroglobulin and TPO, in contrast, have provided the molecular basis to explain part of the rare dyshormonogenesis disorders that usually present as congenital hypothyroidism. Eight different mutations in the TPO gene cosegregating with total iodide organification defects have been detected in the genomic DNA of patients from 13 unrelated families: three were frame-shifting mutations, and five single nucleotide substitutions. Partial iodide organification defects may have still other causes (such as defects in the TPO heme or substrate binding site, or the presence of an inhibitor), and its occurrence in the setting of Pendred's syndrome (goitrous hypothyroidism and sensorineural hearing impairment) remains unexplained. Three even rarer defects in thyroglobulin synthesis in humans have been reported: in the first one, exon 4 of thyroglobulin mRNA is missing, in another a single base mutation in the thyroglobulin gene leads to a truncated thyroglobulin molecule, and in the third a low expression of TTF-1 resulted in poor thyroglobulin synthesis. The abnormal thyroglobulin structure of the first two defects preclude effective coupling of iodotyrosines into T_4 and T_3.

REGULATION OF THYROID FUNCTION

The main regulator of thyroid function is thyroid-stimulating hormone (TSH, or thyrotropin), produced in the thyrotrophs of the anterior pituitary. TSH stimulates thyroid hormone biosynthesis and release by the thyroid gland. Circulating thyroid hormones control TSH synthesis and release via a classical negative feedback mechanism: a decrease in T_4 and T_3 is followed by an increase of TSH, and vice versa. TSH synthesis and release is further regulated by hypothalamic TSH-releasing hormone (TRH) via a feed-forward mechanism; TRH itself is also subject to negative feedback by thyroid hormones (Fig. 10.3).

TSH-releasing hormone is a weakly basic tripeptide (pyroglutamyl-histidyl-proline amide) derived from post-translational cleavage of a larger precursor molecule. TRH produced in peptidergic neurons of the hypothalamic paraventricular nuclei is transported along their axons to specialized nerve terminals in the median eminence, where it is released into hypophyseal portal blood, thus reaching the anterior pituitary. TRH mRNA in the paraventricular nuclei increases in hypothyroidism, and it decreases with thyroid hormone treatment. Lesions of the paraventricular nuclei or pituitary stalk transection decrease pituitary synthesis and release of TSH. TRH is also produced in other brain areas and outside the central nervous system (e.g., in the pancreas), acting as a neurotransmitter.

The pituitary *TRH receptor* belongs to the family of seven transmembrane domain, G-protein-coupled receptors; it consists of 393 amino acids. Binding of TRH to the TRH receptor stimulates TSH synthesis by enhancing transcription of the TSH subunit genes, actions that involve calcium influx and the activation of phosphatidylinositol pathways and protein kinase C. These actions are modulated by cAMP and the pituitary-specific transcription factor Pit-1. TRH also influences the biological activity of TSH by affecting its glycosylation.

Thyroid-stimulating hormone belongs to the glycoprotein hormone family together with luteinizing hormone, follicle-stimulating hormone, and chorionic gonadotropin. These hormones are heterodimers comprised of a common α-subunit and a hormone-specific β-subunit. The α-subunit consists of 92 amino acids with two glycosylation sites; its gene is located on chromosome 6. The TSH β-subunit has 118 amino acids (six can be cleaved at the C-terminal end), one glycosylation site, and its gene is on chromosome 1. The molecular weight of TSH is 28-30 kD; its carbohydrate moiety is 15 to 35% by weight. A sulfated and sialylated asparagine (N)-linked oligosaccharide is found in pituitary human TSH. A specific hepatic receptor for oligosaccharides is likely involved in the rapid clearance of TSH. Terminal sialylation of the glycoprotein, however, bypasses this clearance mechanism. Glycosylation and terminal sialylation thus greatly affect plasma levels and thereby bioactivity of TSH. The plasma half-life of TSH is ~15 to 30 minutes.

Regulation of TSH synthesis and release is mainly exerted through negative feedback control of thyroid hormones. In the thyrotroph, T_3 bound to the β_2 thyroid hormone receptor is derived half from serum T_3 and half from local conversion of T_4 catalyzed by type II deiodinase (see "Peripheral thyroid hormone metabolism", below). Receptor occupancy with T_3 decreases transcription of the gene encoding for TSHβ, and eventually also

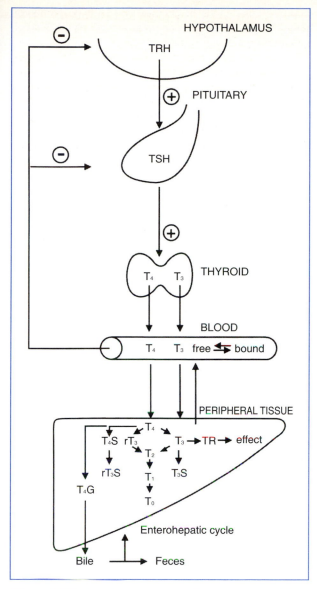

Figure 10.3 Regulation and metabolism of thyroid hormone.

Thyroid-stimulating hormone is secreted in a pulsatile manner with increases in pulse amplitude and pulse frequency at night, probably at least partially mediated by signals from the hypothalamic suprachiasmatic nuclei. The significance of the nocturnal increase of TSH is not known. Cold exposure increases serum TSH, via an α-adrenergic mediated release of TRH; a slight seasonal variation in TSH has been described with higher levels in the winter. Both aged and fasting individuals exhibit decreased TSH secretion, which is associated with a reduced nocturnal TSH surge (due to a decrease in pulse amplitude but not in pulse frequency).

The *TSH receptor* is a member of the large family of G protein-coupled receptors. The TSH receptor gene is located on chromosome 14, is comprised of 10 exons, and encodes a single chain glycoprotein of 744 amino acids of approximately 80 to 100 kD. The extracellular amino terminal domain of the TSH receptor consists of 398 amino acids encoded largely by exons 1 to 9 and for one-third by exon 10; it contains the TSH binding site. The seven transmembrane segments connected by three intracellular and three extracellular loops (hence the term serpentine receptor) and the short intracellular domain of 76 amino acids are encoded by exon 10. The TSH receptor controls the on/off rate of trimeric G proteins (Gαβγ) by stimulating the exchange of GDP for GTP on the α-subunit (Gα). Binding of TSH to the TSH receptor induces dissociation of the trimer and activation of adenyl cyclase via Gsα, generating cAMP. TSH at higher concentrations may also activate the phosphatidylinositol pathways via the TSH receptor. The expression of the TSH receptor protein in the basolateral membrane of the thyrocyte is rather robust: it decreases only upon marked dedifferentiation of thyroid parenchyma, such as in anaplastic thyroid carcinoma. The TSH receptor is also expressed in extrathyroidal tissues, notably in adipocytes, fibroblasts, and lymphocytes. The expression of TSH receptor mRNA is controlled by transcription factors binding to specific regions of its promotor, such as TTF-1 and CREBs (proteins binding to a cAMP response element or CRE).

Regulation of thyroid hormone biosynthesis and release is accomplished mainly via TSH and iodide. TSH stimulates all steps in thyroid hormone biosynthesis and release depicted in Figure 10.1. The TSH mediated rise of intracellular cAMP increases the enzymatic activity of TPO and the transcription of thyroglobulin and TPO genes (possibly by induction of TTF-2 binding to the promoter). Autoregulation by iodide serves to maintain a normal thyroid hormone secretion despite wide variations in daily dietary iodide intake. Excess iodide acutely inhibits thyroidal organification of iodine (known as the Wolff-Chaikoff effect) and the secretion of thyroid hormones. The Wolff-Chaikoff effect is presumably mediated by iodinated lipids (which may down-regulate iodide uptake into the thyroid gland), relatively independent of TSH: organic iodine content and iodide-transport activity are inversely related, even in hypophysectomized rats. Eventually, however, the thyroid gland escapes from these acute inhibitory effects.

of the α-subunit gene; this is mediated by binding of the receptor to DNA sequences (remarkably located entirely within the first exon of the TSHβ gene. See Thyroid Hormone Receptors and Biological Effects section). TRH stimulates transcription of the TSH subunit genes three- to fivefold, presumably mediated via upstream DNA sequences that bind Pit-1. Secondary modulators of the neuroendocrine regulation of TSH are somatostatin and dopamine, which inhibit the function of thyrotrophs (likely by decreasing intracellular cAMP), whereas α-adrenergic pathways are in general stimulatory. Still other modulators include glucocorticoids (possibly decreasing TSH subunit synthesis at a posttranslational level) and various cytokines like IL-1β (which reduces TRH gene expression in the paraventricular nucleus, but may also act in an autocrine or paracrine manner in view of its colocalization with TSH in the thyrotrophs).

Regulation of thyroid cell proliferation is accomplished via TSH and a number of other growth factors, including epidermal growth factor, insulin-like growth factor type 1, transforming growth factor β, and fibroblast growth factor. Growth-stimulating cascades activated by binding of TSH to the TSH receptor are both the Gs-protein-linked adenylyl cyclase pathway and the Gq-protein-linked phospholipase C pathway. TSH also modulates the effects of other growth factors on the thyrocyte. Low iodine levels directly enhance the thyroid sensitivity to growth stimuli.

Clinical relevance

The secretion of TSH is very sensitive to changes in serum thyroid hormone concentrations. The assay of serum TSH has proven to be an accurate test for the diagnosis of thyroid function disorders, which are almost excluded by the finding of a normal TSH value. A suppressed TSH indicates thyrotoxicosis and an elevated TSH hypothyroidism, the rare exceptions being a raised TSH in hyperthyroidism due to a TSH-producing pituitary adenoma and a low or slightly high TSH in hypothyroidism due to hypothalamic/pituitary lesions (see Chap. 11). Secreted TSH in central hypothyroidism is usually less bioactive due to loss of glycosylation. Pharmacological doses of glucocorticoids and dopamine suppress serum TSH. The finding of a high serum TSH is seldom due to the pulsatility of TSH release, which is limited in magnitude.

TRH has found diagnostic application. Intravenous administration of TRH results in an increase of serum TSH and prolactin, but not of α-subunits. The TSH response to TRH is flattened in thyrotoxicosis and increased in primary hypothyroidism. The prolactin response to TRH is inhibited in many patients with prolactinomas, and an increase of α-subunits after TRH is observed in patients with TSH-producing adenomas. The long-acting somatostatin analogue octreotide, as well as the dopamine agonist bromocriptine, are applied in the treatment of TSH-producing adenomas. Pharmacological doses of iodide are used to acutely inhibit thyroid hormone synthesis and release, such as in the treatment of thyrotoxic storm or in the preparation for thyroidectomy (as advocated by Plummer). Failure to escape from the Wolff-Chaikoff effect may explain the development of hypothyroidism upon chronic exposure to iodide excess.

Mutations in regulatory genes have elucidated the molecular mechanisms of a number of thyroid diseases in the last few years. A loss-of-function mutation in the TRH receptor gene is described in central hypothyroidism. Mutations in the α-subunit gene have not been reported, but three types of mutations in the TSHβ gene (missense, nonsense, and frameshift mutations) are known to cause secondary familial hypothyroidism. Somatic gain-of-function mutations in the TSH receptor gene (all located in the transmembrane domain of the protein encoded by exon 10) or in the Gsα gene are responsible for constitutive activation of the adenylyl cyclase pathway, which results

in intracellular cAMP accumulation; a large proportion of thyroid toxic adenomas develop as a result of this kind of mutation. Interestingly, gain-of-function mutations in the TSH receptor gene have also been found in the genomic DNA of some newborns presenting with congenital hyperthyroidism and of patients with familial non-autoimmune hyperthyroidism (which mimics Graves hyperthyroidism but is characterized by the lack of TSH receptor antibodies). Genomic loss-of-function mutations in the TSH receptor gene (located in the extracellular domain) result in partial resistance to TSH, probably due to a reduced binding affinity for TSH; a high TSH may prevent the development of hypothyroidism.

'Specificity spillover' at the TSH receptor by excessive amounts of chorionic gonadotropin explains the thyrotoxic state of some patients with hyperemesis gravidarum or trophoblast tumors. Goitrogenesis in many instances can be explained from the growth-stimulatory effect of high TSH levels (as in iodine-deficient goiter) or of high IGF-1 levels (as in acromegaly).

SERUM THYROID HORMONE-BINDING PROTEINS

Thyroid hormone circulates predominantly bound to serum binding proteins (Tab. 10.3), such that only 0.03% of T_4 and 0.3% of T_3 is unbound or free. The hormone binding to these proteins follows the law of mass action. Any change in binding protein concentrations will acutely alter the free hormone concentration, but eventually a new equilibrium will be reached with a return of the free hormone concentration to its original level. The dissociation constant K_d (the reciprocal of the association constant K_a) defines the free hormone concentration at which a particular binding site is half occupied; together with the number of binding sites it determines the proportion of hormone carried on each of the binding proteins at equilibrium.

Thyroxine-binding globulin is a 54 kD glycoprotein synthesized by the liver; its gene resides on the long arm of the X chromosome. It consists of a polypeptide chain of 359 amino acids, and four polysaccharide units each composed of five to nine sialic acid residues. Thyroxine-binding globulin has a single thyroid hormone-binding site that has a tenfold greater affinity for T_4 than for T_3; under normal circumstances, only one-third of the binding sites are occupied with thyroid hormone. It is the major carrier of thyroid hormone in serum: although its serum concentration is 20-fold less than that of transthyretin, its affinity for T_4 is 100-fold greater.

Transthyretin is a 55 kD protein synthesized by the liver and to some extent in the chorioid plexus. It is a tetramer of four identical polypeptide chains of 125 amino acids, without carbohydrate moieties. The tetramer structure is symmetrical about a central cavity; the two hormone binding sites are located at each end of the cavity, occupancy by T_4 is <1%.

Albumin is a 66.5 kD, 585-amino acid protein synthesized by the liver, with a carbohydrate content of <0.05%. It binds many hormones and substances, albeit in a weak and rather nonspecific manner. It has numerous low-affinity thyroid hormone binding sites, occupied by T_4 less than 0.01%. A small amount of serum T_4 and T_3 is bound to apolipoproteins A-1 and B-100; its significance is unclear.

The serum binding proteins may serve as a buffer store of thyroid hormone in order to maintain a rather constant free hormone centration. According to the free hormone hypothesis, the hormone delivery to tissues is a function of the free hormone concentration at equilibrium. Because the various bound moieties are in rapid equilibrium with the free hormone, any drop in the free hormone concentration as a result of tissue uptake or clearance is "buffered" by dissociation. During tissue transit, free hormone is rapidly cleared from the capillaries, which may give rise to a non-steady-state condition. The dissociation rate (off rate expressed as $t^{1/2}$ in s) is then relevant, which is the rate of unidirectional dissociation, or delivery, of hormone from a particular binding site. Under these circumstances the bound hormone may contribute to some extent to the quantity of hormone that is taken up by the tissues, especially the albumin-bound fraction in view of its rapid off rate. Indeed, labeled T_4 is more evenly distributed within perfused liver in the presence of binding proteins than in buffer alone. Nevertheless, serum binding proteins are not absolutely necessary, as individuals with a congenital absence of these proteins are euthyroid with a normal free thyroid hormone concentration. This occurs, however, at the expense of increased hormone turnover and iodide requirements.

Clinical relevance

Hereditary or drug-induced changes in the affinity and capacity of serum binding proteins for thyroid hormones will affect the results of T_4 and T_3 assays that measure total thyroid hormone content in serum (determined for more than 99% by the protein-bound hormone fraction). Hereditary variants of each of the three major binding proteins exist. Very prevalent are partial or complete thyroxine-binding globulin deficiency due to X-linked thy-roxine-binding globulin mutants (affecting 1 in 2000 males), and familial dysalbuminemic hyperthyroxinemia (0.01-1.8% of the Caucasian population) which results from a variant albumin with increased affinity for T_4 due to an Arg218His mutation. Serum T_4 concentration will be decreased in the former and increased in the latter condition; serum free T_4 and TSH, however, are normal in both instances. Of the many drug effects on serum binding proteins, the most familial one is the increase of serum thyroxine-binding globulin by estrogens largely due to a reduced degradation rate of thyroxine-binding globulin; androgens conversely decrease serum thyroxine-binding globulin. Consequently, estrogens increase and androgens decrease serum T_4 and T_3, but free T_4 and free T_3 concentrations remain constant. Effects on serum binding proteins may jeopardize a correct assessment of thyroid function if one relies on the assay of total T_4 and T_3 rather than on free T_4 and free T_3.

PERIPHERAL THYROID HORMONE METABOLISM

Upon arrival at the peripheral (extrathyroidal) tissues with the blood stream, thyroid hormones have to pass the plasma membrane of target cells. It has long been assumed that tissue uptake through the plasma membrane is accomplished by simple diffusion in view of the lipophilic properties of thyroid hormone. Evidence, however, has been obtained for a carrier-mediated, mostly energy- and Na^+-dependent uptake of thyroid hormones into target cells, in humans as well as in other species. Uptake into many cell types is mediated by saturable high-affinity binding sites, and the transport is stereospecific and temperature-dependent. The putative transporter protein has not yet been cloned. Transport of thyroid hormones into target cells

---

Table 10.3 Characteristics of thyroid hormone-binding proteins in normal human serum at 37 °C

	TBG	TTR	Albumin
Serum concentration			
μmol/l	0.27	4.6	640
mg/dl	1.5	25	4200
K_a of major binding site (L/M)			
T_4	1×10^{10}	7×10^7	7×10^5
T_3	5×10^8	1.4×10^7	1×10^5
Off rate ($t_{1/2}$ sec)			
T_4	20-40	8	<2
T_3	5-10	<2	<1
Hormone distribution (%/protein)			
T_4	68	11	20
T_3	80	9	11

(TBG = thyroxine-binding globulin; TTR = transthyretin.)

might well be rate-limiting upon subsequent metabolism of thyroid hormones. An example of its pathophysiological significance is the reduction of T_4 uptake in the liver during fasting, resulting in a proportional decrease of hepatic T_3 production out of T_4; a decrease in liver ATP content is presumably the mediating factor, compatible with the energy-dependency of the plasma membrane transport mechanism.

Once inside the cell, thyroid hormones undergo a variety of metabolic reactions (Fig. 10.4). Most important in both quantitative and qualitative terms is *deiodination*: T_4 is converted by 5'-deiodination (outer ring deiodination) into the biologically active hormone T_3, and by 5-deiodination (inner ring deiodination) into the inactive metabolite reverse T_3 (rT_3). Further sequential deiodination results in the formation of diiodothyronines (T_2), monoiodothyronines (T_1), and ultimately thyronine (T_0) devoid of iodine. Outer ring deiodination of the prohormone T_4 can thus be seen as an activating pathway, and inner ring deiodination as inactivating. Deiodination is catalyzed by three iodothyronine deiodinase isoenzymes, which are homologous, integral membrane proteins all requiring thiols as cofactor. They have distinct tissue distributions, catalytic specificities, physiological functions and regulatory aspects (Tab. 10.4). The cDNA of all three isoenzymes have recently been obtained, apparently encoding proteins of about 250 amino acids with a molecular weight of ~27 kD. This is lower than the kD of the native proteins extracted from membranes, suggesting that the deiodinases are dimers or multimers. Another interesting feature is that all three deiodinases are selenoproteins, that is, they contain selenocysteine residues that probably form the catalytic center of type I.

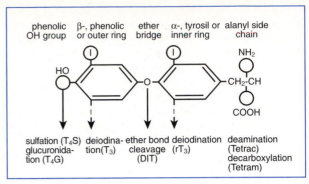

Figure 10.4 The molecular constitution of thyroxine (3,5,3',5'-tetraiodothyronine) and its metabolic pathways.

The *Type I deiodinase* catalyzes both outer and inner ring deiodination, with high K_m and V_{max} values. Reverse T_3 is by far the preferred substrate; its outer ring deiodination is orders of magnitude faster than the deiodination of any other iodothyronine. Consequently type I is likely the primary site for clearance of plasma rT_3. Although it catalyzes the outer ring deiodination of T_4 into T_3 less effectively, type I activity is apparently the main source of plasma T_3. The liver is thus the main site for the metabolic clearance of rT_3 and the production of T_3. It is remarkable to note that at least 80% of the daily production of T_3 is generated outside the thyroid gland by the peripheral conversion of T_4 into T_3. Type I is under positive control by T_3 at the transcriptional level.

The *Type II deiodinase* catalyzes only outer ring deiodination, exhibiting low K_m and V_{max} values. T_4 is slightly preferred over rT_3 as a substrate. Tissues expressing type II deiodinase derive their T_3 largely from local conversion of T_4 and less from plasma T_3. Type II is under negative

Table 10.4 Characteristics of iodothyronine deiodinase isoenzymes

	Type I	Type II	Type III
Molecular weight (kD)	55 (dimer of ~27)	200 (multimer of ~29)	Unknown
Tissue distribution	Liver, kidney, thyroid	Brain, pituitary, brown adipose tissue	Brain, skin, placenta
Subcellular location	Endoplasmic reticulum (liver); basolateral plasma membrane (kidney)	Microsomal membranes	Microsomal membranes
Effect of thiouracils	Inhibition	Almost none	None
Effect of thyrotoxicosis	Increase	Decrease	Increase
Effect of hypothyroidism	Decrease	Increase	Decrease

control of thyroid hormone, which is partly explained by substrate-induced inactivation of the enzyme.

The *Type III deiodinase* catalyzes only inner ring deiodination with intermediate K_m and V_{max} values. It is likely involved in the clearance of plasma T_3 and the production of plasma rT_3. It may protectagainst exposure to high levels of active thyroid hormone, particularly in fetal tissues and the placenta. Its regulation is less well understood.

Nondeiodinative pathways of thyroid hormones are quantitatively less important, accounting for ~19% of T_4 degradation. Conjugation of the phenolic hydroxyl group of iodothyronines with sulfate or glucuronic acid leads to the formation of T_4 sulfate and T_3 sulfate (T_4S and T_3S), or T_4 glucuronide and T_3 glucuronide (T_4G and T_3G). Conjugation increases the water solubility of the substrates, thus facilitating their urinary and biliary clearance. Only small amounts of iodothyronine sulfates are, however, present in serum, urine, and bile. This has been explained by strong enhancement of inner ring deiodination of iodothyronines upon sulfation: inner ring deiodination of T_4S into rT_3S and of T_3S into $3,3'-T_2S$ is enhanced 200-fold and 40-fold, respectively, compared to that of T_4 and T_3. This suggests that sulfate conjugation results in irreversible inactivation of thyroid hormone. The effect of sulfation appears to be specific for type I deiodinase, as deiodination of sulfated substrates are not catalyzed by type II and III deiodinases. The physiological relevance of sulfate conjugation (catalyzed by sulfotransferases present in liver but also in other organs like brain and kidney) is further appreciated in conditions like nonthyroidal illness, fasting, and fetal life characterized by a low activity of type I deiodinase. Under these circumstances, T_3S accumulates in serum, and T_3 may be recovered by hydrolysis of T_3S by tissue sulfatases and bacterial sulfatases in the intestine. Glucuronidation of iodothyronines is catalyzed by liver uridine 5'-diphosphate-glucuronyltransferases. T_4G and T_3G are excreted in the bile. Bacterial β-glucuronidases in the intestine may hydrolyze the glucuronides to some extent with reabsorption of the liberated iodothyronines, thus constituting an enterohepatic cycle of thyroid hormones. Still other but relatively minor metabolic pathways are ether bond cleavage providing diiodotyrosine, and oxidative deamination of the alanine side chain converting T_4 into tetraiodothyroacetic acid (T_4A, or Tetrac) and T_3 into triiodothyroacetic acid (T_3A, or Triac). Although T_3A has a higher affinity for the β_1-T_3 receptor than T_3, its bioactivity in vivo is low due to a short half-life.

Clinical relevance

The extrathyroidal outer ring deiodination of T_4 generates 80% of the daily production of the active hormone T_3. It is thus feasible to treat thyroid hormone deficiency with a single daily dose of the prohormone T_4 (if T_3 is chosen, several daily dosages would be required in view of its shorter half-life): the activity of type I deiodinase provides a continuous production of T_3 with a rather constant serum T_3 concentration over the day. The deiodinases further allow fine-tuning of T_3 production in several tissues according to local need: this is especially true in the brain where modulation of the activity of type II and type III deiodinases protects to a certain extent against both local thyroid hormone excess and thyroid hormone deficiency.

Conditions like fasting and systemic illness, as well as a number of drugs (e.g., amiodarone), inhibit the uptake of thyroid hormones into target cells and the activity of type I deiodinase, generally resulting in low T_3 and high rT_3 serum concentrations. Other drugs (e.g., the anticonvulsive agents phenytoin and carbamazepine and the antituberculosis drug rifampicin) and xenobiotics (such as polychorobiphenyls) induce hepatic thyroid hormone glucuronidation. Still others (e.g., cholestyramine and colestipol) interfere with the enterohepatic cycle of thyroid hormones. The increased T_4 disposal requires a slight increase in T_4 secretion, which sometimes cannot be met in subjects with (subclinical) thyroid failure.

THYROID HORMONE RECEPTORS AND BIOLOGICAL EFFECTS

The major mechanism of action of thyroid hormones is through binding to specific, high-affinity low-capacity nuclear T_3 binding sites in target tissues. These nuclear thyroid hormone receptors (TR) associate with specific nucleotide sequences of the promoter region of T_3-responsive genes called thyroid hormone response elements (TRE), which result in modulation of gene transcription. The biological effects of thyroid hormone are thus predominantly *genomic effects*.

The K_a of T_3 binding to TR is in the order of 10^{10} to 10^{11} M/l, 10 times higher than that of T_4 binding; it strengthens the notion that T_4 mainly serves as a prohormone of T_3. The total nuclear T_3 binding capacity in various tissues is generally in good agreement with thyroid hormone responsiveness of these tissues, being, for example, high in liver and anterior pituitary and low in spleen and testis. The hepatocyte contains about 5000 nuclear T_3 binding sites, of which 50% are occupied with T_3 under normal circumstances; bound T_3 is largely derived from plasma T_3 and to a lesser extent from T_3 locally generated out of T_4. In contrast, the anterior pituitary has 8000 to 10 000 receptor molecules per nucleus with a receptor occupancy of 80%. Bound T_3 is derived equally from plasma T_3 and from T_4 locally converted into T_3 through type II deiodinase. In cerebral cortex the receptor occupancy is even higher (90%), with most T_3 coming from locally converted T_4.

Differences between tissues also exist in the distribution of the various TR subtypes (Tab. 10.5). TR belong to a superfamily of nuclear receptors, together with receptors for steroids, vitamin D, vitamin A, and its metabolite 9-cis retinoic acid (RXR). These receptors all consist of an amino-terminal A/B domain involved in transactivation, a DNA-binding domain C, and the carboxy-terminal D/E/F domains involved in ligand binding, dimerization, and transactivation. TR are encoded for by two genes. The TRα gene is located on chromosome 17. Alternative splicing gives rise to several isoforms. $TR\alpha_1$ binds T_3 with high affinity, but $TR\alpha_2$ does not bind T_3, as the distal part of the ligand-binding domain at the carboxy-terminus has been replaced by larger amino acid sequences coded by a separate exon. $TR\alpha_2$ apparently acts as a constitutive repressor, possibly by competing with other TR for DNA binding sites. The $TR\beta$ gene is located on chromosome 3. The two isoforms $TR\beta_1$ and $TR\beta_2$ arise from the use of different promoter regions of the $TR\beta$ gene, which alter the choice of upstream exons encoding for the amino terminus of the protein. Whereas $TR\beta_1$ and $TR\beta_2$ both bind T_3 with high affinity, the expression of $TR\beta_1$ is observed in many tissues, but that of $TR\beta_2$ is restricted to brain and anterior pituitary.

There exists a high degree of homology between $TR\alpha$ and $TR\beta$ proteins: the amino acid sequence is similar for 86% of domain C, 72% of domain D, and 82% of domain E. Domain C consists of 68 amino acids; it includes two groups of four cysteine residues tetrahedrally coordinated with a zinc atom to form two "fingers," constituting the DNA-binding motif. A region called the P box at the base of the first zinc finger preferentially recognizes the hexameric nucleotide sequence AGGTCA, allowing interaction with the major groove of DNA. Some thyroid hormone response elements (TREs) use other nucleotides in the core sequence. The zinc finger motifs and a region in domain E contain residues mediating protein-protein interaction, allowing dimerization of receptor proteins. Thyroid hormone response elements in many promotors consist of two closely spaced repeats of the core sequence; both the receptor protein and its dimerization partner can thus bind to a separate core sequence (hence called "half-site"). The spacing and orientation of the core half-sites dictate which receptors bind to a particular response element. TR homodimers are prevalent on everted repeat (TGACCTnnnnnnAGGTCA) and palindromic (AGGTCATGACCT) configurations of TRE. The favored dimerization partner of TR is the retinoid X receptor (RXR); the TR-RXR heterodimer binds preferentially at direct repeats separated by four nucleotides (DR4; AGGTCAnnnnAGGTCA), the TR component being bound to the downstream (or 3') half-site. RXR, however, also forms heterodimers with the vitamin D receptor (VDR), and the retinoic acid receptor (RAR) that bind to the same direct repeats. The specificity of response elements is determined by the number of spacings between the half-sites (DR3 for VDR dimers, DR4 for TR dimers, and DR5 for RAR dimers). TR, uniquely, can also bind as a monomer to a slightly extended half-site (TAAGGTCA). The DNA binding of the TR-RXR heterodimer is much more stable than of TR homodimers or monomers.

Thyroid hormone receptors function as transcription factors activated by the binding of T_3 to a hydrophobic pocket consisting of 11 α-helices in the hormone-binding domain E. Unliganded TR bound to TREs may silence transcription. This silencing effect is presumably mediated by proteins called co-repressors, which do not bind to DNA but interact with the carboxy-terminal domain of TR and components of the basal transcription machinery like TF-IIB or TATA binding protein. Identified co-repressors are nuclear receptor co-repressor (N-CoR) and silencing mediator for retinoid and thyroid hormone receptors (SMRT). Binding of T_3 induces conformational changes of the receptor protein; it disrupts the TR homodimer whereas the heterodimer remains stable, and dissociates co-repressors that result in de-repression. Transcription activation may be enhanced by association with co-activators binding to TR at a C-terminal amphipathic α-helix. Putative co-activators include steroid receptor co-activator-1 (SRC-1), receptor-interacting protein 140 (RIP 140) and CREB-binding protein (CBP; CREB = CAMP response element - binding protein).

The biological effects of thyroid hormone can be summarized as stimulation of growth and differentiation, and of metabolism in general. The enhancement of numerous pathways by thyroid hormone manifests itself as an increased oxygen consumption and heat production. This is not due to uncoupling of mitochondrial oxidative phos-

Table 10.5 Characteristics of thyroid hormone receptor (TR) subtypes

TR Subtype	$TR\alpha_1$	$TR\alpha_2$	$TR\beta_1$	$TR\beta_2$
Size (kD)	47	55	53	58
No. of amino acids	410	492	461	514
T_3 binding	Yes	No	Yes	Yes
DNA binding	Yes	Yes	Yes	Yes
Heterodimer formation	Yes	No	Yes	Yes
Tissue distribution +++	Brain	Brain		
++	Heart, kidney, pituitary	Heart, kidney, pituitary	Liver, heart, kidney, brain, pituitary	Brain, pituitary
+	Liver	Liver		

phorylation (this early hypothesis on the mechanism of action of thyroid hormone has proven to be false). Many if not most effects of thyroid hormone can now be explained from the binding of thyroid hormone receptors to thyroid hormone response elements, which result in transcription activation, induction of specific mRNAs, and modulation of protein synthesis. A number of T_3-responsive genes have been identified, which contain a (not always classical) TRE in the promoter region and respond to T_3 with an increased gene expression both at the mRNA and at the protein level. Important examples are growth hormone (resulting in growth and differentiation, and lipogenesis); lipogenic enzymes such as malate dehydrogenase (resulting in FFA production and ATP consumption); phosphoenolpyruvate carboxykinase (resulting in gluconeogenesis and ATP consumption); $Na^+K^+ATPase$ (resulting in faster repolarization of the membrane action potential, and ATP consumption); actomyosin-ATPase (resulting in a higher velocity of muscle contraction and ATP consumption); sarcoplasmic reticulum -$Ca^{++}ATPase$ (resulting in a higher velocity of muscle relaxation and ATP consumption); mitochondrial enzymes such as α-glycerophosphatedehydrogenase, succinate dehydrogenase and cytochrome C-oxidase (resulting in ATP production and O_2 consumption); and several Purkinje cell-expressed genes such as myelin basic protein and Pcp-2 (involved in brain development). T_3 thus, in general, stimulates protein synthesis (it also increases ribosomal RNA), but in some instances inhibition is observed, such as the T_3-induced suppression of TSHα and TSHβ gene expression in the pituitary. Thus far no evidence has been obtained for a specific "negative" TRE mediating inhibitory effects on protein synthesis, although the negative TREs often contain only a single binding site for TR not allowing dimerization. A few examples are known of an effect of T_3 on translation. The expression of TR isoforms may change under certain physiological and pathophysiological conditions: $TR\alpha_1$ seems to be preferentially expressed during fetal life, and the number of TR in liver decreases during fasting and critical illness. The unanticipated complexity of TR and transcription regulation raise many unanswered questions. Nevertheless, the available data suggest that the biologic effects of thyroid hormones can largely be explained by regulation of gene expression.

This is not to say that *nongenomic effects* do not exist. Proposed non-nuclear pathways for thyroid hormone action are direct effects of T_3 upon plasma membrane transport of amino acids and glucose, on K^+-channels in the plasma membrane of the sinoatrial pacemaker cells and of smooth muscle cells in blood vessels, and on mitochondrial respiratory activity via adenine nucleotide (ADP/ATP) translocase. Specific mitochondrial T_3 receptors have indeed been demonstrated, but the issue remains controversial. Recent studies surprisingly indicate that $3,5-T_2$ and $3,3'-T_2$ stimulates resting metabolism in hypothyroid rats, apparently not mediated via TR but via mitochondrial respiration. Consensus exists that the regulation of brain T_4 5'-deiodinase activity (type II) by thyroid hormone involves a unique, non-nuclear site of hormone action.

Clinical relevance

Elucidation of the molecular mechanism of the action of thyroid hormone has made it clear that probably no single gene is exclusively regulated by T_3, as numerous other transcription factors besides TR will bind to the promoter region and influence gene expression. It follows that though many of the symptoms and signs of thyroid hormone deficiency or excess are understood in molecular terms, no single peripheral tissue function test of thyroid hormone action will be very specific for thyroid hormone, restricting their usefulness in the diagnosis of hypothyroidism or hyperthyroidism. The biologic effects of thyroid hormone in target tissues are highly modulated in a tissue- and cell-specific manner, possibly contributing to the variation in clinical presentation among patients with hypothyroidism or hyperthyroidism.

Whereas mutations in the TRα gene are unknown, genomic mutations in the TRβ gene are inherited in an autosomal dominant manner, resulting in thyroid hormone resistance syndromes. The mutations occur in the hormone binding domain of $TR\beta_1$, resulting in a lower affinity for T_3 binding. Mutated TRβ receptors are still capable to form dimers and to bind to TREs, but transcription is tampered, leading to hypothyroid effects in tissues with predominant expression of TRβ. The TSH-mediated increase of plasma T_4 and T_3 concentrations may, however, cause hyperthyroid effects in tissues with abundant expression of nonmutated $TR\alpha_1$.

Suggested readings

BARTALENA L. Recent achievements in studies of thyroid hormone binding proteins. Endocr Rev 1990;11:47-64.

BRAVERMAN LE, UTIGER RD (eds). Werner and Ingbar's The thyroid, a fundamental and clinical text, 7th ed. Philadelphia-New York: Lippincott-Raven, 1996.

BRENT GA. The molecular basis of thyroid hormone action. N Engl J Med 1994;331:847-53.

FRANKLYN JA, CHATTERJEE VKK. Molecular biology of thyroid hormone action. In: Weetman AP, Grossman A (eds). Pharmacotherapeutics of the thyroid gland. Berlin-Heidelberg-New York: Springer-Verlag, 1997;151-70.

GROSSMANN M, WEINTRAUB BD, SZKUDLINKSI MW. Novel insights into the molecular mechanisms of human thyrotropin action: structural, physiological, and therapeutic implications for the glycoprotein family. Endocr Rev 1997;18:476-501.

HENNEMANN G, VISSER TJ. Thyroid hormone synthesis, plasma membrane transport and metabolism. In: Weetman AP, Grossman A (eds). Pharmacotherapeutics of the thyroid gland, Berlin-Heidelberg-New York: Springer-Verlag, 1997;75-118.

KIMURA S. Thyroid-specific enhancer-binding protein. Role in thyroid function and organogenesis. Trends Endocrinol Metab 1996;7:247-52.

McLACHLAN SM, RAPOPORT B. The molecular biology of thyroid peroxidase: cloning, expression and role as autoantigen in autoimmune thyroid disease. Endocr Rev 1992;13:192-206.

MENDEL CM. The free hormone hypothesis: a physiologically based mathematical model. Endocr Rev 1989;10:232-74.

OPPENHEIMER JH, SCHWARTZ HL. Molecular basis of thyroid hormone-dependent brain development. Endocr Rev 1997;18:462-75.

STOCKIGT JR, LIM CF, BARLOW JW, TOPLISS DJ. Thyroid hormone transport. In: Weetman AP, Grossman A (eds). Pharmacotherapeutics of the thyroid gland. Berlin-Heidelberg-New York: Springer-Verlag, 1997;119-50.

VASSART G, DUMONT JE. The thyrotropin receptor and the regulation of thyrocyte function and growth. Endocr Rev 1992;13:596-611.

Diagnostic procedures

Albert G. Burger

The thyroid holds important stores of hormones. The blood also represents a large reservoir of circulating thyroxine (T_4), which is mainly bound to the interalpha glycoprotein thyroxine-binding globulin (TBG). Other T_4-binding proteins are transthyretin (prealbumin) and albumin. Of these three proteins, TBG has the highest affinity for T_4: its Ka is 1×10^{10} M^{-1} compared to 7×10^7 and 7×10^5 M^{-1} for transthyretin and albumin. The maximal binding capacity of TBG is about 250 nmol/l serum (20 µg/100 ml). Under most physiopathological conditions, TBG is the limiting buffering system that determines the ratio of protein bound to free T_4 (fT_4). This ratio is highly in favor of protein binding since the free fraction represents only 0.02% of the total serum T_4. There are 3 mechanisms that account for altered effective TBG concentrations. (1) *The inherited altered trait of X-linked absence (1:5000 births) or X-linked increased TBG (1:25 000) concentrations.* In addition, many point mutations have been described that result in many genetic variants (TBG Chicago, etc.); perhaps the most striking one is found in Australia, where close to 30% of the Aborigines present with a genetic variant. In most instances the affinity of TBG for T_4 is decreased, which can be explained by direct effects of the amino acid substitution and/or as a secondary altered glycosylation of the protein. (2) *The serum TBG concentrations may vary as a function of its glycosylation.* A highly glycosylated TBG will have a longer half-life. Estrogens are known to have this effect. In pregnancy, TBG concentrations are very high. Androgens and glucocorticoids have the opposite effect. TBG concentrations can also increase because of increased synthesis stimulated by thyroid hormones and estrogens, among others. (3) *Competition for the T_4 binding site of TBG by substances such as phenytoin, high doses of salicylate, and free fatty acids (FFA).* Phenytoin, rifampicin, and carbamazepine also alter T_4 metabolism by accelerating its hepatic metabolism. Of particular clinical importance is the displacing of T_4 from TBG by high free fatty acid levels. This may occur in vivo, particularly under heparin treatment, which activates serum lipase activity. More importantly, FFA can also be generated in vitro either in the presence of heparin or by repeated freezing and thawing of serum. This can result in increases of FFA levels to 3

mmols/l or more, and such values artifactually increase the free T_4 levels.

Normal thyroid function is dependent on an adequate intranuclear concentration of 3,5,3'-triiodothyronine (T_3), which is again a function of the transfer of T_3 and of T_4 from plasma to the cell. For both hormones only the free fraction can enter the peripheral cell. If the free concentration falls, a normally functioning thyroid will be stimulated by thyroid-stimulating hormone (TSH) to secrete more hormones in order to restore an adequate free concentration in the periphery and, particularly, in the pituitary, being the sensor. This will occur when fT_4 concentrations change due to altered TBG levels. Yet the kinetics of the protein changes are slow (half-life: 6 hours for transthyretin, 4 days for TBG), and the changes in TSH secretion are rapid. Therefore, changes in the binding capacity of serum proteins in general, and specifically in TBG, do not induce measurable changes in fT_4 and TSH.

TBG binds T_3 with a lower affinity than T_4 (affinity constant for T_3, 5×10 M^{-8}), and its serum levels are less affected by changes in serum proteins. Despite this, and the fact that T_3 is the active thyroid hormone, other factors markedly reduce the diagnostic value of T_3: (1) T_3 is primarily an intracellular hormone; serum represents no more than 15 to 20% of its whole body pool; (2) its production is mainly non-thyroidal and markedly influenced by the metabolic state of the organism; (3) its production and degradation are controlled by monodeiodination.

Regarding the last point, the production of T_3 reflects 5'-monodeiodination, while its degradation is also controlled by conjugation. Even though each of these pathways may vary, the degradation rate of T_3 is reasonably constant even when there are major changes in T_3 production. Therefore, T_3 levels are a reflection of its production and not of its degradation.

Three different ways of production can be distinguished: (1) the peripheral deiodination from T_4 (liver, kidney, muscle), (2) its local production in brain and pituitary, and (3) its thyroidal origin. The peripheral production is quantitatively the most important factor and is controlled by a key enzyme, the 5'-monodeiodinase type 1. However, in most catabolic states (fever, infection, terminal cancer, and major cardiac events), as well as in hypothyroidism, T_3 production and the activity of 5'-monodeiodinase type 1 are markedly reduced, which results in a fall of serum T_3 levels. This is most clearly documented during fasting, and it is quite certain that the switch from carbohydrate to fatty acid fuel plays a crucial role. Recently severe selenium deficiency has also been recognized to reduce the 5'-monodeiodinase type 1 activity and possibly also of the two other enzymes involved in monodeiodination: 5'-monodeiodinase type 2 (T_4 to T_3) and 5'-monodeiodinase type 3 (T_4 to reverse T_3 [rT_3]). All three are selenoproteins.

In contrast to the periphery, pituitary T_3 production is not decreased in severe illness; it is, however, inhibited with increasing T_4 concentrations. Inversely, decreasing T_4 levels will favor the generation of T_3. As a consequence in hypothyroidism, the decrease of intrapituitary T_3 will be retarded in comparison to serum T_3. In the euthyroid or hyperthyroid state, however, 5'monodeiodinase type 2 activity will be completely inhibited. The intrapituitary T_3 will be similarly regulated in other peripheral tissues. The regulation of T_3 production in the brain is even more complex, the description of which is beyond the scope of this chapter.

The thyroidal control of T_3 production also requires further description. The proportion of T_3 versus T_4 on thyroglobulin will depend on thyroidal stimulation and on the iodine balance. Strong stimulation by TSH or TSH receptor antibodies and a relative or absolute deficiency in intrathyroidal iodide will favor thyroidal T_3 production. In addition, in a very active gland stimulated by TSH or TSH receptor antibodies, thyroidal 5'-monodeiodinase type 1 activity will be strongly stimulated. This results in an increased intrathyroidal T_3 production in primary hypothyroidism, in hyperthyroidism, and in iodine deficiency. For clinical practice this is important, since the end result is that serum T_3 levels are a poor indicator of thyroid dysfunction. Free T_3 levels may correlate better, although one exception should be mentioned: subclinical hyperthyroidism results from an increase of serum T_3, so-called "T_3 toxicosis". However, even here, T_3 has lost its diagnostic value, since serum TSH levels will be an even more sensitive indicator of subclinical hyperthyroidism. In hypothyroidism, serum T_3 levels tend to remain within the normal range despite increased serum TSH levels. Reverse T_3 is the inactive counterpart of T_3 and has been advocated as a diagnostic tool in the past, but it is currently not considered valid. Nevertheless, it is an interesting parameter that gives a good mirror image of T_4 to T_3 conversion, even though its production may also depend on a specific enzyme converting T_4 to rT_3.

Methods of serum free T_4 and T_3 measures

As mentioned above, the biologically active free T_4 (fT_4) represents an extremely small fraction of the total, including inactive T_4. No fully satisfactory fT_4 measure is currently available. The best methods of measurement are those in which free T_4 is measured directly as a fraction of added ^{125}I T_4, or by radioimmunoassay (RIA) in the absence of serum proteins. Two techniques fulfill this criteria, which are the ultrafiltration and equilibrium dialysis methods. The latter method was the first reliable one; it can, however, yield falsely elevated values if free fatty acids are artificially increased by the presence of in vitro heparin or by repeated freezing and thawing. Both methods are cumbersome and cannot be used in routine work.

Two different approaches for measuring free T_4 indirectly are available. One is still widely used in the United States, which is the free T_4 or T_3 index test and based on the fact that the product of total serum T_4 times the result of the T_3 resin uptake gives an arbitrary index that roughly correlates with free T_4 values. The T_3 resin uptake methods are based on the following principle: since the serum protein binding of T_4 is mainly dependent on TBG, an increase of it will shift the equilibrium between TBG and free T_4 in favor of TBG. If ^{125}I T_3 or T_4 is added, a higher percentage will be bound to TBG, yet in any case the binding to TBG would be so strong, and the free fraction of T_3 or T_4 so small, that one could not measure it. A competitor is then added, such as resins or antibodies, which bind 15 to 30% of the ^{125}I T_3 in normal serum. Artifactual results with T_3 resin uptake methods are frequent and similar to the ones found using free commercial fT_4 methods (see below).

The free T_4 concentrations are far too low to be measured directly. Commercial companies have developed easily measurable T_4 analogs which do not bind to TBG and are distributed only within the free hormone fraction. In addition, this fraction is artificially increased by competitors of T_4 for TBG. These methods have the advantage over the free T_4 index in that they yield absolute concentrations of free T_4, and their interpretation is clear. However, due to their technical features, they are also prone to artifactual values, particularly in systemic illness where unknown competitors for T_4 binding to TBG have been described. In summary, the newer commercial methods will have a tendency toward inappropriately low values in severe illnesses and with decreased serum protein concentrations. Some of these problems can be overcome by more cumbersome techniques (two-step methods), but even these methods are not free of artifactual results. The latter tend to give values that are too high during severe illness. Nevertheless, in ambulatory medicine, these commercial methods are very satisfactory and render total T_4 and T_3 methods unnecessary. The clinician should rely first on serum TSH; serum free T_4 and T_3 levels are useful adjuncts for the refinement of diagnosis and treatment and for excluding some extremely rare thyroidal conditions (see below).

In conclusion, among thyroid hormones, only fT_4 measurements are necessary, despite some technical limitations. Total T_4 and total or free T_3 have only a confirmative value and are therefore mostly unnecessary for establishing a diagnosis. Among thyroid function tests, serum TSH is the first choice (see below).

Measuring serum TSH values is the first line diagnostic test. Its sensitivity is very high, and its specificity slightly lower (90%) since drugs and severe illness can decrease serum TSH levels in euthyroid subjects. The extraordinary role of serum TSH as a diagnostic parameter is based on the fact that it is the most sensitive parameter of peripheral thyroid hormone action. It increases exponentially when serum fT_4 decreases. Yet this peripheral action has at least three particularities that differentiate it from the clinically more relevant effects of T_3 on heart, liver, brain, and other tissues. These are: (1) the intrapituitary production of T_3 from T_4: the complex regulation of intrapituitary T_3 production, particularly important in the hypothyroid state, has already been mentioned. With the exception of the brown adipose tissue of small rodents, the complex intracellular regulation of thyroid hormone metabolism in the pituitary and brain is not found in other peripheral tissues; (2) the action of thyroid hormones in the pituitary is inhibitory: in contrast to peripheral effects that are stimulatory. Even with the most modern measurements of serum TSH, the severity of thyroid hormone excess cannot be measured. Nevertheless, one can distinguish between subclinical and clinical hyperthyroidism (see below); (3) the role of the hypothalamus for TSH secretion: TRH, somatostatin, dopamine, and others each have independent functions in the control of the TSH-producing cell. This makes the control of serum TSH secretion particularly complex, and it seems unlikely that it represents the mirror image of the peripheral control of thyroid hormone action.

Clinical use of serum TSH measures At present, serum TSH is measured with immunometric assays. As signals, ^{125}I has recently been replaced with chemiluminescent probes. Progress has been constant in this field; the lower detection limit of the newest assays is 0.002 mU/l or lower (third generation immunometric assays). However, the clinical relevance of such a low limit of detection is not yet established. For practical purposes, it is more important that the day-to-day variation be evaluated by each laboratory. Many of the new immunometric assays will have a coefficient of variation (SD/mean) of less than 5%, with serum TSH values of 0.5 mU/l or more, and 15 to 50% with values of 0.002 to 0.1 mU/ml. It is not clear how reproducible these assays are if different laboratories and commercial products are used. Furthermore, the clinician should be aware that these assays measure only the immunological and not the biological properties of TSH, and that there is strong evidence of discordance between these two parameters in primary and hypothalamic hypothyroidism and, possibly, in severely ill patients.

As in all pituitary hormones, TSH is secreted in a pulsatile manner and has a circadian rhythm. The TSH spikes do not exceed 0.5 mU/ml. Serum TSH levels are highest in the evening at 23 hours, during the first hours of sleep. The peak is displaced in night workers. In young subjects, the mean serum TSH levels are in the morning 0.9 ± 0.3 (standard error of the mean) and at 23 hours 1.9 ± 0.6 mU/l. In the elderly, serum TSH levels tend to be slightly lower (0.7

± 0.6 and 1.3 ± 0.9 mU/l, respectively). These fluctuations are rarely critical for the clinical evaluation of thyroid function. The normal range extends from 0.4 to 4 mU/l. In subjects with no thyroid hormone treatment, serum TSH levels can be grouped into three classes (Fig. 11.1). (1) *Serum TSH 0.1 to 0.4 mU/l (for some authors up to 0.6 mU/l)*. If repeatedly found at intervals of 3 months, this slight decrease of serum TSH is compatible but not diagnostic of partial thyroid autonomy. The cause of such autonomy might be a hot nodule, a multinodular goiter, or euthyroid Graves' disease. In these cases recent iodine contamination may play an important role. In the sick patient with non-thyroidal illness, such values can also represent the expression of blunted thyroid function, particularly if the patient receives drugs such as glucocorticoids, dopamine, or dopamine agonists. The clinical evaluation and follow-up of the patient will be the most important steps to clarify the diagnosis. In these situations, the determination of serum T_3 may be able to confirm T_3-toxicosis. Reverse T_3 values are useless and serum free T_4 will mostly be within the normal range, though in systemic illness it may be decreased. Such serum TSH levels are rarely found in pituitary or hypothalamic insufficiency, but when these conditions occur, the changes in thyroid function are mostly of secondary importance. Other pituitary insufficiencies

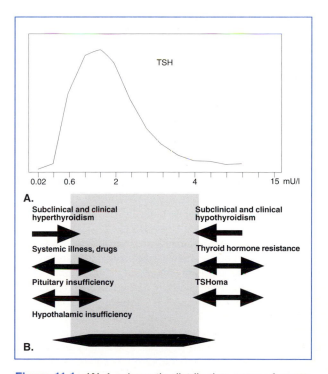

Figure 11.1 **(A)** A schematic distribution curve of serum TSH concentrations in the general population. **(B)** Shaded areas indicate the distribution of serum TSH concentrations in different disease conditions affecting thyroid function. The wider or thinner parts of each area represent the more or less dense distribution of serum TSH concentrations. Vertical lines indicate the upper and lower limits of the normal range.

are more pronounced. In the case of a clinical suspicion of thyroid autonomy, a thyroid scintiscan and measuring thyroid autoantibodies will be the most helpful. (2) *Serum TSH 0.05 to 0.1 mU/l (for some authors 0.02 to 0.1 or 0.2 mU/l).* The differential diagnosis is similar to that stated above. In addition, serum free T_4 levels and/or free T_3 levels tend to be at the upper limit or slightly increased and may confirm subclinical hyperthyroidism. Low serum TSH levels are the goal of T_4 treatment in patients with differentiated thyroid cancer. Serum fT_4 levels will be at the upper limit of normal, and in one-third of these patients fT_4 levels will be slightly increased. Serum T_3 levels will be in the normal range. This can be explained by the absent thyroidal component of T_3 production. Low serum TSH levels are frequent in panhypopituitarism but not in hypothalamic disease. It is rather rare to find such low serum TSH levels in systemically ill patients unless they have been treated with large doses of dopamine and/or glucocorticoids. (3) *Serum TSH below 0.02 mU/l.* Such values are only encountered in endogenous hyperthyroidism and possibly in severe panhypopituitarism. Some assays are able to measure levels as low as 0.002 mU/l. So far there are no data correlating the very low serum TSH levels with the clinical severity of hyperthyroidism.

It is now well-established that the reactivation of TSH secretion during treatment for hyperthyroidism may lag behind the normalization of peripheral thyroid hormones, and that clinical manifestations may last for several weeks and even months. There is so far no clear explanation for this, but it is important to realize that in these situations serum TSH is not a valid parameter of euthyroidism.

Use of TSH measurements in case of abnormal fT_4 values

Two diagnostic pitfalls can occur when serum TSH measurement is the only thyroid hormone parameter measured. Serum levels of TSH may be normal, slightly decreased, or increased in the case of thyroid hormone resistance, with frankly increased serum fT_4 and fT_3 levels. In the case of a pituitary TSH-secreting adenoma, called TSHoma, serum TSH levels are normal or moderately increased (up to 20 mU/l, rarely higher) despite clinical hyperthyroidism, with increased serum fT_4 and fT_3 levels.

Serum TSH measurements are essential for excluding thyroid dysfunction in two situations with apparently increased fT_4 levels. One abnormality consists of T_4 binding to serum transport proteins. There can be a congenitally high affinity and capacity binding of albumin or transthyretin for T_4. T_3 is much less affected. In addition, some neuroendocrine tumors secrete very large amounts of normal transthyretin (familial dysalbuminemic hyperthyroxinemia, FDH, and familial or acquired hyperthyroxinemia due to transthyretin excess). The affected subjects are euthyroid, as their free T_4 values, measured by ultrafiltration or equilibrium dialysis, and T_4 production rates are normal. Yet commercial kits for fT_4 measurements can yield artifactually greatly increased fT_4 values, even though newer versions of these kits avoid such errors. Few laboratories are equipped to identify these

proteins with ^{125}I T_4 electrophoresis of serum proteins. If this methodology is not available, differential diagnosis with pituitary tumors or thyroid hormone resistance should include serum T_3, serum alpha subunit, a TRH test, and possibly magnetic resonance imaging of the pituitary. Serum T_3 and the alpha subunit are increased in TSHomas; in thyroid hormone resistance the alpha subunit is not increased and in dysalbumenic hyperthyroxinemia T_3 and alpha subunit are normal. Basal serum TSH and the TRH test are normal in case of abnormalities in serum transport proteins, while in thyroid hormone resistance the response to TRH tends to be exaggerated. In most but not all cases of TSHomas there will be no response to TRH stimulation. The value of this test is therefore only indicative.

Another artifactual increase of fT_4 values is encountered in the presence of autoantibodies to T_4 or T_3, even though most modern kits are no longer affected by such antibodies. In this case, a normal serum TSH and TRH test will exclude any thyroid dysfunction.

Artifacts of TSH measures

There is only one condition where serum TSH values can be artifactually increased, namely in the presence of antibodies against mouse IgG in the patient's serum. Monoclonal mouse IgGs are part of all immunometric assays and will therefore be trapped by these antibodies. The most recently developed immunometric assays have overcome this problem. If necessary, the artifactual increase in serum TSH can be diagnosed by omitting anti-TSH antibodies in the assay and/or by a TRH test. It will show a complete non-response to TRH, which may hint to this artifact or to a TSHoma.

The well-established, overwhelming diagnostic power of serum TSH measurements can raise two questions. (1) Should one restrict the first line diagnostic parameters of thyroid dysfunction to TSH only and omit fT_4 measures? This might be justified for systematic screening, yet fT_4 measurements are inexpensive and will primarily be ordered during further work-up of the patient's thyroid disease. (2) Should serum TSH be used systematically as a screening test of the adult population above 50 years of age and repeated at regular intervals (every 5 years, for instance)? There is already a precedent, as neonatal screening with TSH exists. The cost of this test has markedly decreased since its inception and will probably decrease even further, making such a proposal become a realistic prospect.

TRH test

The main indications for this test (200 μg iv, blood sampling at 0, 15, 30, 60, and 120 minutes) are pituitary diseases. For primary thyroid dysfunction it has lost all of its indications except those mentioned above.

Measuring the alpha subunit of TSH, the common subunit of all pituitary glycoproteins, is important in case of TSHomas and, obviously, in gonadotropinomas.

THYROGLOBULIN

Thyroglobulin (TG) is released from normal thyroid glands. Disruption of the normal thyroid structure results in leakage of TG and high serum levels. Serum TG levels can be detected in subjects with a normal thyroid, with the levels higher in goitrous patients than in patients without thyroid disease. In multinodular goiter, TG levels can reach very high levels that overlap with those found in metastatic cancer patients. Marked and transient increases can be seen after ^{131}I treatment and after thyroid surgery. High levels are also found in stimulated thyroids, for instance, in Graves' disease and in functioning (and occasionally even non-functioning) thyroid adenomas.

Diagnostic procedures

Measurement of serum TG levels has improved due to the advances of immunometric assays. At the present time an assay should have a functional sensitivity (with a coefficient of variance of 10%) of less than 1 µg/l, and interference of TG antibodies in its measurement should be rare. This point is particularly important, since such an interference results in false low TG levels, which in the follow-up of thyroid cancers is a serious drawback. Therefore, two additional controls are obligatory: (1) TG antibodies should be measured, although their interference in TG measurement is not strictly a reflection of their titer; and (2) pure TG should be added to a separate sample of the patient serum. A recovery of 80% or more of the added TG excludes any major interference. Nevertheless, technical improvements of immunometric assays circumvent most of these problems since antibody interference is only seen in 1% of cases.

TG measurements are useful in neonatology, where low levels are found in thyroid agenesis or dysgenesis, and high levels are found in thyroid hormone resistance and in some rare inborn errors of thyroid hormone synthesis. They are a valuable adjunct to scintigraphy and thyroid ultrasound.

Low TG values are an excellent means to differentiate between thyrotoxicosis factitia and endogenous hyperthyroidism. In the presence of a normal-sized or even moderately-increased thyroid, the ingested L-thyroxine will suppress TG levels to values below 10 µg/l. In the presence of very large goiters, TG levels will often not be suppressible.

TG values can be of value during treatment of hyperthyroidism and during remission. In addition, in subacute thyroiditis an increase of TG levels has been documented. The measurement of TG values in these clinical situations is not frequently used.

TG measures are not useful in the differential diagnosis between benign nodular goiter and thyroid carcinoma, since in both conditions TG levels tend to be increased and overlap. In an occasional patient with an unidentified pulmonary or bone metastasis, a very high TG level may help to establish the origin of the tumor.

The greatest merit of TG measurements comes from the surveillance of differentiated follicular or papillary thyroid cancer since it allows for an easy detection of recurrences (Tab. 11.1). TG levels are a function of the tumor mass and tumor differentiation. TG levels tend to be lower in more aggressive tumors and are absent in undifferentiated cancers. Since even in cancers TG production is dependent on TSH stimulation, it is essential to measure its level not only under L-thyroxin treatment but also during withdrawal of treatment. This is because TG levels tend to increase by a factor of 4 to 5 in hypothyroidism. An absent increase of TG levels in hypothyroidism should be suspicious for artifactual TG levels due to some protein and/or antibody interference. Artifactually low levels due to TG autoantibodies should be thought of as well.

Thyroglobulin is only part of necessary controls in the follow-up of thyroid cancers. There is a complementarity between TG levels, ^{131}I whole body scans, neck ultrasound, and occasionally magnetic resonance. The following examples illustrate the importance of complementarity: occasionally scintiscans can be positive with TG levels of 5 and less µg/l. It is more frequent to find moderately increased TG levels and negative scintiscans. This usually indicates the presence of tumor tissue but, as an alternative, artifactual TG levels must also be considered possible. In this context, a TG level that does not increase after withdrawal of thyroid hormones and the increase of serum TSH should be regarded as highly suspicious and potentially an artifact.

AUTOANTIBODIES

For clinical use, three types of antibodies are of interest: the anti-thyroperoxidase (anti-TPO), the antithyroglobulin antibodies, and the anti-TSH receptor antibodies. Among the anti-TSH receptor antibodies, one can distinguish blocking and stimulating antibodies. It is possible that the recently discovered anti-sodium-iodide symporter antibodies may also play a clinical role in the near future.

The thyroid antibodies belong to the IgG class. Only for anti-TPO antibodies have there been described some rare cases of complement fixing and cytotoxic activity. The antigenic sites of TPO have been well-characterized; there are six of them. For anti-TG and anti-TSH receptor antibodies, this is less well-known since the antigenic sites are mainly conformational and not linear. Indications to measure thyroid antibodies can serve diagnostic, follow-up, and screening purposes.

TPO antibodies are the most sensitive antibodies for the diagnosis of any thyroid autoimmune process, and they are widely used in combination with the thyroid hormone tests for diagnosing the etiology of a thyroid disease. Their presence confers an increased risk in developing hypothyroidism and is an indication for clinical follow-up. They are also useful in the follow-up of Graves' disease since their titer may reflect the activity of the disease. In Hashimoto's thyroiditis, the follow-up of these patients with measurements of antibodies may be confusing and is not generally recommended. There is no specific indication for TG antibodies since they are identical with the ones enumerated above. On a rare occasion, however, the TPO antibodies may be negative while TG antibodies will reveal thyroid disease.

The TSH receptor antibodies are mostly not useful for the diagnosis of Graves' disease but, similar to the action of TPO antibodies, their titer may follow the activity of the disease. They can also be present in primary hypothyroidism and in postpartum thyroiditis and are therefore not absolutely diagnostic for Graves' disease.

There is one uncommon but clear indication for measuring these antibodies, namely in pregnant patients with Graves' disease in whom the thyroid has been removed. In this case, one has no clinical indication about the severity of the autoimmune process and, on rare occasions, placental transfer of a high titer of TSH receptor antibodies may cause neonatal hyperthyroidism. Screening with anti-TPO antibodies is advocated during pregnancy since their presence indicates increased risk for a postpartum thyroiditis.

Diagnostic procedures

In vivo isotope imaging

Diagnostic in vivo isotopic imaging will yield information on thyroidal uptake of the isotope and functional morphology of the thyroid. Two isotopes, the ^{123}I (iodine-123) and the ^{99n}Tc (technetium-99n), are nearly exclusively used. There is still some indication for ^{131}I (iodine-131) for whole body scintigraphy of patients with thyroid cancers. The place for other isotopes, such as thallium and gallium, has not been established. Thallium has been used for identifying thyroid metastases and ^{67}GA (gallium-67) is taken up by inflammatory cells, particularly mast cells, and can therefore be used in some cases of destructive thyroiditis such as subacute thyroiditis (Tab. 11.2).

Iodine-123   The physical characteristics of the iodine isotope ^{123}I are given in Table 11.2. It is close to an ideal isotope in that the irradiation of the thyroid is minimal. In an empty stomach with intact acidity, the iodide is specifically taken up by the gastric mucosa. Thyroidal uptake occurs very rapidly. If food has been ingested, the uptake may be delayed and occur by intestinal absorption.

^{123}I uptake is dependent on the activity of the sodium-iodide symporter, formally called "iodide trapping" of the thyroid. Once transported into the cell, the free intrathyroidal iodide is immediately incorporated into thyroglobulin. Thus, the free iodide pool of the thyroid is only increased under pathological conditions. This can be tested by the perchlorate discharge test (see below). Once stored in the colloid as thyroglobulin, the labeled thyroxin will remain for a long time in the thyroid, depending on the total amount of stored colloid. In most conditions, the reserve of thyroglobulin is enormous and, therefore, the turnover of this iodide is slow, even though the most recently formed colloid will be preferentially resorbed and secreted. As a rule of thumb, only 1 to 2% of the accumulated dose will be secreted per day. The disappearance of the isotope will therefore be mainly a function of its physical half-life (for ^{123}I, 13 hours). During secretion, most of the ^{123}I will be secreted as T_4, and to a lesser extent as T_3, and only a minor part of iodide will be lost.

Iodine contamination is one of the major technical problems resulting in invalid thyroid imaging. In subjects with a normal thyroid and a daily iodide intake of 200 to 400 µg/day, a single dose of 30 mg of iodide together with the tracer will reduce the uptake to background levels. A similar effect can be obtained with half the dose of iodide given over several days. However, it should be noted that this applies for a completely normal thyroid. In areas of moderate iodine deficiency where small multinodular goiters are frequent, the suppression of ^{123}I uptake by iodine needs higher and longer treatment with similar or higher doses. Accidental iodine contamination is a frequent event since during axial tomography large amounts of iodine-containing contrast media are injected. These substances are highly water-soluble and are eliminated within 4 to 6 weeks. Iodide is rapidly eliminated by the renal route (clearance 50 ml per minute) and in renal insufficiency correspondingly decreased.

At the present time the major culprit of long-term iodine contamination is amiodarone. This drug and its biologically active metabolite desethylamiodarone have an approximate half-life of 4 to 6 weeks. However, iodine

Table 11.1 Diagnostic use of serum thyroglobulin levels in differentiated thyroid cancer

TSH <0.1 mU/l	TSH >30 mU/l	^{131}I scintigraphy	Loco-regional tumor	Distant metastasis
<5 µg/l	<5 µg/l	Negative (exceptionally positive)	No	No
< 5 µg/l	4 to 5 x increase	Positive or negative	Yes	Unlikely
5 to 20	No change	Negative	Artifactual TG(?)	—
5 to 20	4 to 5 x increase	Positive or negative	Yes	Likely
> 20	4 to 5 x increase	Positive (exceptionally negative)	Yes	Yes

(TSH = thyroid-stimulating hormone.)

contamination from its degradation products can last for months and up to 1 to 2 years.

Historically, other organic iodine compounds can be responsible for even longer-lasting contaminations. For instance, dyes used for myelography have given rise to life-long contamination and can even pass the placenta with consequent low thyroidal uptake in the children.

Among the non-iodinated substances interfering in thyroidal uptake, methimazole, propylthiouracil, and perchlorate should be mentioned; the latter being a specific inhibitor of the iodide symporter. In severe non-thyroidal illness, thyroid function and thyroid uptake may be depressed. Drugs such as glucocorticoids (30-60 mg of prednisone) and dopamine and its analogues have multiple impacts, but the most significant one is a reduction of TSH secretion with a following reduction of thyroid function. Older literature mentions sulfonamides as well, but the more modern drugs of this class have not been reported to interfere.

^{99m}Tc pertechnetate (^{99m}Tc)

^{99m}Tc is close to ideal for studying the trapping of iodide by the thyroid. It is easily available and of low cost. Since it can only give information on anion trapping, the measurements are performed within an hour after intravenous injection. The thyroidal uptake of ^{99m}Tc is approximately 10 times lower than for ^{123}I (0.4 to 4%). The precise normal range will also be dependent on iodine intake and must therefore be validated for each laboratory. Compared to ^{123}I, ^{99m}Tc may occasionally show uptake of cold nodules, which may be taken erroneously for functioning nodules.

It should be noted that on many occasions thyroid imaging with isotopes can be favorably replaced by ultrasonography. The indications for scintigraphy could be summarized as follows: in hyperthyroidism ^{99m}Tc is as effective as ^{123}I for the differential diagnosis of nodular or diffuse goiter. If the thyroid is diffusely enlarged without concomitant exophthalmos or pretibial myxedema, the positive uptake will allow for the exclusion of silent and/or subacute thyroiditis, and it will help in establishing a diagnosis of thyrotoxicosis factitia and/or iodine contamination.

In the case of multinodular goiter with a moderate decrease of serum TSH (<0.6 mU/l), the scintigraphy may confirm autonomous regions.

In the case of very painful thyroid and inflammatory symptoms, an absent thyroid uptake may confirm the diagnosis of subacute thyroiditis.

In the case of an isolated thyroid nodule, no uptake will identify a cold nodule. However, ^{99m}Tc may be taken up by cold nodules, giving the erroneous impression of a functional nodule. This investigation has been superseded by cytology.

In conclusion, in most cases ultrasound evaluation of the thyroid gland is as useful as or better than scintigraphy. Nevertheless, the two examinations can be complementary. Scintigraphy will allow for the identification of an inactive nodule of the thyroid, which the ultrasound may reveal to be cystic, mixed, or solid. In multinodular goiter, the scintigraphy will clearly give the patchy appearance of the functioning and, possibly also, autonomous tissue. However, its value to describe inactive or cold nodules in this situation is limited.

Iodine-131

The disadvantage of the ^{131}I isotope is its rather large delivered dose of irradiation to the patient. In thyroid cancer patients, ^{131}I has kept its place for diagnostic procedures. During the follow-up of these patients, whole body scintigraphies are obtained with ^{131}I during intense TSH stimulation, which is classically obtained by stopping T_4 or T_3 substitution, or more recently by injecting recombinant human TSH.

Hypothyroidism is obtained by switching 7 weeks before ^{131}I treatment to T_3 substitution, which must be

Table 11.2 Isotopes used for thyroid imaging

	^{123}I	^{131}I	^{125}I	^{99m}Tc	Thallium-201	F-18-Thioglucose
Half-life	13 h	8 d	60 d	6 h	73 h	110 m
Emission	Gamma	Beta, gamma	Gamma	Gamma	Gamma	Beta +, gamma
Radiation exposure (rad)/mCi	13	1300	790	0.13	—	—
Diagnostic dose uCi	300	50	—	2000	—	—
Route	Oral	Oral	—	iv	iv	iv
Absorption	Gastric	Gastric	Gastric	—	Taken up by inflammatory cells	Taken up by tumor cells
Maximal uptake	4 to 8 h	4 to 8 h	4 to 8 h	20 to 40 min	—	—
Artifacts						

stopped 12 to 14 days before giving the dose. Serum TSH levels should increase to more than 30 mU/l. The efficiency of the whole body scan or treatment can be increased by concomitant regimen recommendations such as avoidance of iodized salt and iodide-rich bread, eggs, and fish. A small dose of diuretics (thiazides) can also be recommended to decrease the circulating iodide pool. Large diagnostic doses of ^{131}I are used (5 to 10 mCi), since the uptake of the cancerous cell is much lower than normal and is mostly markedly below 0.5% of the administrated dose. The whole body scintigraphy is performed 3 to 4 days after administration of the radioactive iodide. A ^{131}I scintigraphy or therapy should not be repeated before 8 to 12 weeks since it induces a stunting effect (transiently abolished uptake).

This technique is very sensitive for detecting small metastases and in most cases correlates very well with the presence of serum thyroglobulin (TG) levels. However, it has been reported that there can be some dissociation and that serum TG levels can be increased even in the absence of residual ^{131}I iodide uptake. If one can exclude an artifactual increase of thyroglobulin (presence of autoantibodies due to thyroglobulin, etc.), it is thought that these patients have metastases and should benefit from a more complete work-up with subsequent surgery and/or ^{131}I treatment (see above).

Rare and/or experimental methods for thyroid imaging

Perchlorate discharge tests can only be performed with ^{123}I or [131]I. It is a rarely-used test that was initially utilized for detecting inherited defects of intrathyroidal iodine metabolism (absence of sodium-iodide symporter, absence of thyroglobulin, and dehalogenase defect). Its diagnostic value was for acquired small iodine organification defects that can be seen in autoimmune thyroiditis and Graves' disease treated with [131]I. This test currently has no place in routine diagnostic procedures.

Methodology: 3 hours after giving ^{123}I, give 1g perchlorate orally and measure the uptake of the gland at 3 hours and 1 hour after perchlorate. A decrease of more than 15% of the 3-hour uptake is significant. The test can be made more sensitive by giving 500 µg KI together with the [123]I.

Positron emission tomography with fluoro-deoxyglucose is a very promising technique for detecting highly metabolically active tissue. The active principle, deoxyglucose, can be taken up by cells but cannot be metabolized. Malignant cancer cells have a high glucose metabolism, and therefore metastasis of poorly differentiated thyroid cancers that may no longer retain ^{131}I may concentrate fluoro-deoxyglucose and become visible with this technique. Normal thyroid tissue will not concentrate fluoro-deoxyglucose.

Ultrasonography

This technique is unsurpassable for evaluating the anatomy and size of the thyroid. It should, however, be clear that this technique will not enable diagnosis of benign or malignant lesions nor permit the evaluation of thyroid function. Though this last point may appear trivial, recent improvements using the Doppler-ultrasonography have made deductions from thyroidal blood flow on thyroid activity. At the present time, such statements have not been confirmed and it is generally accepted that echography Doppler techniques do not add anything to regular ultrasonography.

An echographic report should at least describe the longitudinal and horizontal maximal length of both glands and report on additional structures such as a pyramidal lobe and adjacent lymph nodes. The size of nodules is also necessary information, but the size measures should not be overevaluated since they will depend on the experience of the examiner, the pressure that is applied by the ultrasound probe, and the quality of the equipment. This should be kept in mind when one gives much importance to size changes over time of thyroid nodules and goiters.

The report should also describe the structure of the gland, the homogeneity of the tissue, and intensity of the signal. The gland may appear hypodense in inflammatory processes (subacute and autoimmune thyroiditis) and in Graves' disease, but also in thyroid lymphomas. Cysts and calcifications are also well-demonstrated.

The great value of ultrasonography for the detection of malignant lesions comes from the identification of nodules and their better localization for fine needle biopsy. In many centers ultrasonography has to a large extent replaced isotopic scintigraphy of the thyroid.

FINE NEEDLE BIOPSY

Fine needle biopsy is an essential part of investigation for thyroid nodules with a diameter of 15 mm or more. Its use is widely accepted for the differential diagnosis between benign thyroid nodules, multinodular goiter, and thyroid cancer. Its use in inflammatory disease such as subacute thyroiditis and autoimmune thyroiditis has not been widely accepted. Hot or toxic nodules do not need to be biopsied since the reports of well-documented malignant, hyperactive nodules are extremely rare, and surgery will mostly be the choice for these diseases. Such lesions can be suspected in the presence of a moderately decreased or suppressed serum TSH value and are an indication for isotopic thyroid imaging.

The success of fine needle biopsy depends on some imperative rules. (1) The biopsy should be performed by an experienced expert in the field who can easily locate the lesion by palpation and/or ultrasound. (2) In order to achieve a 96 to 98% accuracy, at least 6 to 8 clusters of cells must be seen. This means in most cases that an equal number of punctures have to be performed. (3) The cytologist must show a continued interest in this field, and there should be a close collaboration between the clinician and the pathologist. Reviewing in common of the slides is certainly of educational practice.

If these premises are respected, fine needle biopsy has a remarkable success rate and has reduced surgical intervention substantially. Before the introduction of this technique, approximately half of the patients with a thyroid nodule were operated on, and now in most centers approximately one-fifth of all patients are operated on.

If the technical conditions are fulfilled, the cytological diagnosis can be classified as benign, malignant, or suspect cells. *Benign cells* refer to benign follicular cells and have a macrofollicular aspect. In the case of cystic material, follicular cells in sufficient amounts must be present. When suspect cells are present, many endocrinologists will choose surgery, but depending upon the clinical picture, repeated cytology and close follow-up is an alternative. *Malignant cells* are in differentiated thyroid cancers and are mainly seen with papillary cancers. Poorly differentiated, anaplastic cancers and lymphomas are for the most part easily diagnosed.

Suggested readings

Beck-Peccoz P, Brucker-Davis F, Persani L, Smallridge RC, Weintraub BD. Thyrotropin-secreting pituitary tumors. Endocr Rev 1996;17:610-38.

Danforth E, Burger AG. The impact of nutrition on thyroid hormone physiology and action. Ann Rev Nutr 1989;9:201-27.

Ekins R. Measurement of free hormones in blood. Endocr Rev 1990;11:5-46.

Faber J, Waetjen I, Siersbaek-Nielsen K. Free thyroxine measured in undiluted serum by dialysis and ultrafiltration: effects of non-thyroidal illness, and an acute load of salicylate or heparin. Clin Chim Acta 1993;223:159-67.

Guadaño-Ferraz A, Obregon MJ, St Germain DL, Bernal J. The type 2 iodothyronine deiodinase is expressed primarily in glial cells in the neonatal rat brain. Proc Natl Acad Sci USA 1997;94:10391-6.

Hamburger JI. Diagnosis of thyroid nodules by fine needle biopsy: use and abuse. J Clin Endocrinol Metab 1994;79:335-9.

McKenzie JM, Zakarija M. Clinical review 3. The clinical use of thyrotropin receptor antibody measurements. J Clin Endocrinol Metab 1989;69:1093-6.

Meier C, Burger AG. Effects of pharmacological agents on thyroid hormone synthesis. In: Braverman LE, Utiger RD (eds). The thyroid. 7th ed. Philadelphia: Lippincott-Raven, 1997; 276-85.

Rago T, Vitti P, Chiovato L, et al. Role of conventional ultrasonography and color flow-Doppler sonography in predicting malignancy in cold thyroid nodules. Eur J Endocrinol 1998;138:40-6.

Refetoff S, Murata Y, Mori Y, Janssen OE, Takeda K, Hayashi Y. Thyroxine-binding globulin: organization of the gene and variants. Horm Res 1996;45:128-38.

Spencer CA, Takeuchi M, Kazarosyan M. Current status and performance goals for serum thyrotropin (TSH) assays. Clin Chem 1996;42:140-8.

Spencer CA, Takeuchi M, Kazarosyan M. Current status and performance goals for serum thyroglobulin assays. Clin Chem 1996;42:164-73.

Stockigt JR. Serum thyrotropin and thyroid hormone measurements and assessment of thyroid hormone transport. In: Braverman LE, Utiger RD (eds). The thyroid. 7th ed. Philadelphia: Lippincott-Raven, 1997; 377-96.

Weetman AP, McGregor AM. Autoimmune thyroid disease: further developments in our understanding. Endocr Rev 1994;15:788-830.

Hyperthyroidism and thyrotoxicosis

Luigi Bartalena, Paolo Vitti

KEY POINTS

- *Thyrotoxicosis* defines the hypermetabolic state caused by thyroid hormone excess at the tissue level, while *hyperthyroidism* indicates the increased thyroid hormone synthesis and secretion. All patients with hyperthyroidism have thyrotoxicosis, whereas not all patients with thyrotoxicosis (e.g., those with destructive thyroiditis or thyrotoxicosis factitia) are hyperthyroid.
- Graves' disease is the most common form of hyperthyroidism, accounting for 60 to 90% of cases in iodine-sufficient areas.
- Laboratory diagnosis of hyperthyroidism relies on the finding of increased serum concentrations of free thyroid hormones and suppressed serum concentration of thyrotropin. Graves' disease is an autoimmune disease characterized by the presence of serum anti-thyroglobulin, anti-thyroid peroxidase, and TSH receptor antibodies, which may be helpful in the differential diagnosis of hyperthyroidism.
- Treatment of hyperthyroidism due to Graves' disease can be carried out by antithyroid drugs (thionamides), radioiodine, or thyroidectomy. The choice of treatment depends on several factors, including the age of the patient, goiter size, concomitant ophthalmopathy, and other special situations, including pregnancy.
- Severe forms of Graves' ophthalmopathy can be treated by high-dose glucocorticoids, orbital radiotherapy, and orbital decompression.
- Treatment of toxic adenoma and toxic multinodular goiter is carried out by radioiodine or thyroidectomy. Antithyroid drugs are used only in preparation to the above treatments.

The hypermetabolic state caused by thyroid hormone excess at the tissue level is defined as *thyrotoxicosis*. Under most circumstances, this is due to increased thyroid hormone synthesis and secretion, i.e., due to *hyperthyroidism*. However, the two terms are not synonymous, because thyrotoxicosis may not be related to thyroid hyperfunction, but to thyroidal-destructive processes or to exogenous thyroid hormone intake. While hyperthyroidism is associated with high thyroidal radioactive iodine uptake (RAIU), thyrotoxicosis not due to hyperthyroidism is characterized by low/suppressed RAIU values (Tab. 12.1).

Clinical manifestations of thyrotoxicosis (Tab. 12.2) range from scanty and subtle manifestations to overt and severe signs and symptoms. Most signs and symptoms are common to all types of thyrotoxicosis; whereas ophthalmopathy, localized (pretibial) myxedema, and thyroid acropachy are specific to Graves' disease; and thyroid pain and tenderness are typical of subacute thyroiditis.

Some types of thyrotoxicosis are uncommon or remarkably rare. The most common cause is Graves' disease, which accounts for 60 to 90% of the cases of thyrotoxicosis in iodine-sufficient areas.

Table 12.1 Causes of thyrotoxicosis

With high thyroidal radioactive iodine uptake

Common types
  Graves' disease
  Toxic adenoma
  Toxic multinodular goiter
  Iodine-induced thyrotoxicosis[1]

Uncommon types
  Congenital hyperthyroidism
  Hashimoto's thyroiditis
  TSH-induced hyperthyroidism
  TSH-secreting pituitary adenoma
    selective pituitary resistance to thyroid hormone
  Trophoblastic tumors

With low thyroidal radioactive iodine uptake

Common types
  Thyroiditis
    subacute (de Quervain's) thyroiditis
    silent (painless) thyroiditis
    post-partum thyroiditis
  Iodine-induced thyrotoxicosis[1]

Uncommon types
  Thyrotoxicosis factitia
  Metastatic thyroid carcinoma
  Struma ovarii

[1] It may be associated both with low/suppressed or with normal/elevated thyroidal radioactive iodine uptake.

Table 12.2 Symptoms and signs of thyrotoxicosis

	Frequency (%)
Symptoms	
Nervousness	99
Palpitations	90
Increased sweating	90
Heat intolerance	89
Fatigue	88
Weight loss	85
Dyspnea	80
Increased appetite	65
Eye symptoms[1]	55
Friable hair and nails	40
Increased bowel movements	33
Diarrhea	23
Menstrual disturbances	18
Signs	
Tachycardia	100
Goiter[2]	97
Tremors	97
Skin changes	97
Hyperkinesis	80
Thyroid bruit[1]	77
Lid lag and retraction	60
Ophthalmopathy[1]	30
Atrial fibrillation	10
Onycholysis	10
Localized (pretibial) myxedema[1]	5
Vitiligo[1]	5
Acropachy[1]	<1

[1] In Graves' disease.
[2] Diffuse in most Graves' disease, nodular in toxic adenoma and multinodular goiter, absent in some forms of iodine-induced thyrotoxicosis, thyrotoxicosis factitia, struma ovarii.

GRAVES' DISEASE

Graves' disease is an autoimmune thyroid disease, characterized by goiter, hyperthyroidism, ophthalmopathy, and, less frequently, dermopathy (localized or pretibial myxedema) and acropachy. Hyperthyroidism may be present in the absence of eye disease and vice versa. In endemic goiter regions, Graves' disease may develop in a pre-existing nodular goiter (so-called Marine-Lenhart syndrome).

Epidemiology

Graves' disease is the most common form of hyperthyroidism in iodine-sufficient areas. The annual incidence in Minnesota has been reported to be 0.3 cases/1000 individuals. In the Wickham survey in England, its prevalence was 2.7% in women and 0.23% in men. The female/male ratio is about 7:1, and the peak age of distribution is in the 3rd and 4th decades of life. Eye disease is severe only in 3 to 5% of cases. The onset of hyperthyroidism and ophthalmopathy usually show a close temporal relationship, generally occurring within 18 months from each other. Localized myxedema occurs in 12 to 15% of patients with concomitant severe eye disease.

Etiopathogenesis

Graves' disease is of autoimmune origin, related to the generation of thyroid antigen-specific T lymphocytes, the development of humoral and cell-mediated immune reactions, and the infiltration of the thyroid gland by immune effector cells. The ultimate cause of hyperthyroidism is from autoantibodies interacting with the TSH receptor on thyrocyte cell membrane and stimulating thyroid cell growth and function (TSH receptor antibody, TRAb). TSH receptor antibody is detectable in 80 to 90% of untreated Graves' patients. Circulating antibodies directed against thyroid peroxidase (anti-thyroid peroxidase) or thyroglobulin (anti-thyroglobulin) are demonstrable in most Graves' patients. A genetic susceptibility to thyroid autoimmunity is suggested by the familial predisposition found in more than half of Graves' patients, the frequent finding of circulating autoantibodies in relatives of Graves' patients, the high concordance rate in monozygotic twins, and the positive association with human leukocyte antigen (HLA) haplotypes (HLA-B8 and DR3 in Caucasians, HLA-B35 in Japanese, and HLA-Bw46 in Chinese populations). These HLA haplotypes are not necessarily disease genes, but they carry a greater risk for the development of Graves' disease. Other candidate genes, such as immunoglobulin G heavy chain or T cell receptor genes, are under investigation. Environmental factors (bacterial or viral infections) may cause the expression of HLA class II antigens and induce thyroid autoimmune disease in genetically predisposed individuals. Stress may also constitute a precipitating factor for Graves' disease.

The pathogenesis of Graves' ophthalmopathy is less clear. Autoreactive T cells directed against antigens shared by the thyroid and orbit might be recruited by adhesion molecules and infiltrate the retro-orbital tissue and the perimysium of extra-ocular muscles. There, together with macrophages, they produce cytokines; these in turn stimulate fibroblasts to secrete glycosaminoglycans, which are ultimately responsible for most clinical manifestations of ophthalmopathy. The nature of shared antigen(s) is uncertain; TSH receptor or its variants might be involved. The pathogenesis of dermopathy might be similar to that of ophthalmopathy.

Pathophysiology

The thyroid gland is usually hypertrophic and hyperplastic, and lymphocytic and plasma cell infiltration may be so marked to form lymphoid germinal centers. The vascularity of the gland is increased. The extra-ocular muscles of patients with ophthalmopathy are swollen, due to the proliferation of perimysial fibroblasts, lymphocytic infiltration, and edema, but myocytes are normal. Expansion of retro-ocular tissue volume occurs as a consequence of fibroblast proliferation and orbital edema due to increased glycosaminoglycan secretion. Similar changes are present in localized myxedema.

Clinical findings

Symptoms and signs include manifestations common to all forms of thyrotoxicosis, and specific features of Graves' disease (Tab. 12.2).

Symptoms and signs

Thyroid The thyroid gland is usually symmetrically enlarged, its consistency is generally firm, and thrills and bruits may be present on the gland. Goiter is absent in 3% of cases.

Skin and appendages Skin is warm, thin, and moist, and patchy vitiligo may be present. Hair is fine and friable, nails are soft and friable, and onycholysis is frequent. Localized myxedema is usually in the pretibial region, but other areas – including feet, toes, and upper extremities – may be involved. It presents as raised, light-colored or yellow-reddish lesions with an orange peel appearance, and is sometimes pruritic. Thyroid acropachy is characterized by swelling of the soft tissues of hands and feet, with clubbing of fingers and toes.

Cardiovascular system Tachycardia and palpitations are frequent. Systolic blood pressure is often increased, while diastolic blood pressure is decreased. A systolic murmur may be heard, which is often related to mitral valve prolapse. Premature heart beats and atrial fibrillation may occur. Cardiomegaly and heart failure (often resistant to digoxin) may develop even in the absence of underlying heart disease. Angina and myocardial infarction may occur.

Alimentary system Despite an increased appetite, weight loss is very common. Nausea and vomiting are occasionally present. Increased frequency of bowel movements and diarrhea may occur. Atrophic gastritis of autoimmune origin may be encountered in Graves' disease. Liver dysfunction is not infrequent in untreated patients, but liver function tests usually normalize upon restoration of euthyroidism.

Nervous system Nervousness, anxiety, emotional instability, hyperactivity, insomnia, and fine tremors are frequently observed in thyrotoxicosis. Frank psychosis and seizures are rare.

Muscles Muscular weakness is a frequent complaint, and muscular atrophy is encountered in most severe cases. Myasthenia gravis may be associated with Graves' disease. Hypokalemic periodic paralysis may be exacerbated or triggered by thyrotoxicosis.

Skeletal system Thyroid hormone excess causes a loss of bone mass, and osteoporosis is severe and premature in patients previously thyrotoxic. Linear bone growth may be accelerated in thyrotoxic children. Hypercalcemia may occur due to thyroid hormone action on bone metabolism.

Hematopoietic system Pernicious anemia occurs in 3% of Graves' patients, and circulating autoantibodies to gastric parietal cells are found in 30% of cases. Normocytic anemia or iron-deficient anemia related to malnutrition may be present. Graves' disease is occasionally associated with autoimmune thrombocytopenic purpura.

Reproductive system Menstrual function is often disturbed, and amenorrhea may develop. Fertility is often reduced, and the frequency of miscarriages is increased in untreated women. In men, gynecomastia, impotence, and reduced sperm count can occur.

Intermediate metabolism Oxygen consumption is increased. Diabetes mellitus may be exacerbated by thyrotoxicosis. Serum cholesterol is decreased due to its increased degradation, and plasma triglycerides may be decreased as well.

Eyes Eyelid retraction is frequent in all types of thyrotoxicosis, causing a bright-eyed stare. True ophthalmopathy is specific of Graves' disease and includes: soft tissue involvement that is responsible for lacrimation, redness, a burning sensation, photophobia, and a gritty sensation in the eyes; proptosis (exophthalmos); extra-ocular muscle dysfunction causing diplopia; exposure keratitis due to proptosis and lagophthalmos; and optic neuropathy that may cause blindness (Tab. 12.3). Eye signs may be present in the apparent absence of thyroid dysfunction (so-called Euthyroid Graves' Disease).

Diagnostic procedures

Laboratory findings Laboratory investigation is especially important in doubtful cases, particularly in the absence of goiter and eye disease. The combination of increased serum free thyroid hormone and suppressed TSH establishes the diagnosis of thyrotoxicosis. Serum free thyroxine (fT_4) (and TSH) measurement is usually sufficient to diagnose hyperthyroidism, but serum free 3,5,3'-triiodothyronine (fT_3) determination is also useful because of the occurrence of 3,5,3'-triiodothyronine (T_3)-toxicosis with normal or high-normal serum fT_3. Determination of anti-thyroid peroxidase and anti-thyroglobulin antibodies, positive in more than 90% and 50% of cases, respectively, helps to distinguish autoimmune from non-autoimmune thyrotoxicosis. TSH receptor antibody is present in most untreated Graves' patients and is helpful in doubtful cases.

Imaging studies The 24-hour thyroidal radioactive iodine uptake value is increased, but it may be lower than the 3-hour value in cases with rapid iodine turnover; it is useful, in doubtful cases, to rule out low-RAIU thyrotoxicosis (Tab. 12.1). A thyroid scan will show typical diffuse and homogeneous goiter, and it will also help to detect possible hypofunctioning ("cold") areas. Thyroid ultrasound usually shows an enlarged gland with a hypoechoic pattern associated (at echo-color-Doppler sonography) with increased blood flow. Computed tomography (CT) scan and magnetic resonance imaging (MRI) are important diagnostic tools in Graves' ophthalmopathy, especially in the absence of hyperthyroidism, or when ocular involvement is unilateral or asymmetrical. CT scan and MRI reveal swelling of extra-ocular muscles, increased volume of retro-ocular tissue, proptosis, and provide important information on compression of the optic nerve at the orbital apex. CT scan and MRI are useful to rule out other causes of proptosis (Tab. 12.4).

Treatment

The ideal treatment of Graves' disease and associated ophthalmopathy would be the elimination of its cause. Since this goal cannot be achieved, current treatment is aimed at reducing excess thyroid hormones by inhibiting their synthesis pharmacologically, or by ablating thyroid tissue with radioiodine or thyroidectomy. Management of ophthalmopathy is directed at controlling inflammatory manifestations, essentially by steroids and/or orbital radiotherapy, or directed at expanding the available space for the increased orbital content by orbital decompression.

Hyperthyroidism

The choice of treatment (Tab. 12.5) depends on several factors, including age, goiter size, presence of ophthalmopathy, availability of an expert surgeon, undue concern with radioiodine therapy, and compliance with a strict medical regimen.

Thionamides Thionamides (methimazole, carbimazole, propylthiouracil) inhibit thyroid peroxidase, blocking organification of iodide, coupling of iodotyrosines, and synthesis of thyroid hormones. Whether thionamides may also affect the immune mechanisms of Graves' disease is still a matter of argument. Propylthiouracil also inhibits peripheral monodeiodination of thyroxine (T_4) to T_3. Carbimazole is promptly converted to its active form, methimazole. Methimazole has greater intrinsic activity and longer duration of action than propylthiouracil (Tab. 12.6). The prevalence of adverse effects of thionamides is less than 5% (Tab. 12.7). *Agranulocytosis* (granulocyte count $<0.5 \times 10^9/l$) occurs in 0.1 to 0.5% of patients, may develop suddenly, usually within the first few months of treatment, and is very uncommon when using low doses of methimazole. It is a potentially lethal complication, manifests with signs of infection (fever, sore throat), and must be promptly treated with thionamide withdrawal, antibiotics, and granulocyte colony-stimulating factor. Recovery usually takes place in about two weeks. While other major side effects – such as severe liver dysfunction, vasculitis, and lupus-like syndrome – require prompt discontinuation of the drug, minor side effects are often transient and do not necessarily call for interruption of treatment. Substitution of one thionamide for the other

---

Table 12.3 Symptoms and signs of Graves' ophthalmopathy

Symptoms

Excessive lacrimation
Burning sensation
Gritty ("sandy") sensation
Ocular pain, either spontaneous or with eye movements
Photophobia
Diplopia
Blurred vision
Sight loss

Signs

Palpebral edema and hyperemia
Increased palpebral width with lid retraction
Edema of caruncle
Conjunctival hyperemia and chemosis
Lagophthalmos
Exophthalmos
Increased intra-ocular pressure
Restriction of eye movements
Corneal lesions (keratitis, ulcer)
Optic neuropathy

Table 12.4 Causes of proptosis

Graves' ophthalmopathy
Orbital tumors
  Lymphoma
  Hemangioma
  Optic nerve glioma
  Meningioma
  Rhabdomyosarcoma
  Metastases
Orbital inflammatory processes
  Pseudotumor
  Myositis
Orbital granulomatous processes
  Sarcoidosis
  Wegener's granulomatosis
Vascular disorders
  Carotid-cavernous fistula
Miscellanea
  Cushing's syndrome
  Liver cirrhosis
  Amyloidosis

may be advised, but cross-sensitivity is common. Treatment is usually started with 20 to 40 mg methimazole (200-400 mg propylthiouracil) per day, the lowest dose ensuring euthyroidism is maintained for 18 to 24 months. Hyperthyroidism recurs in about 60% of patients, more commonly within 3 to 6 months after treatment discontinuation. Factors increasing the likelihood of relapse of hyperthyroidism include large goiter, younger age, higher TSH receptor antibody at diagnosis, persistence of detectable TSH receptor antibody at the end of treatment,

persistence of high T_3/T_4 ratio during treatment, and the need for relatively high doses of thionamides to maintain euthyroidism.

Radioiodine This is an effective form of treatment and particularly indicated when the goiter is not large, in older patients, when cardiac complications are present, and in recurrent hyperthyroidism after thionamide treatment (Tab. 12.5). It is frequently followed by hypothyroidism, which should be considered an expected outcome rather than a complication. Since the resolution of hyperthyroidism after radioiodine requires several weeks, pretreatment with thionamides may be advised to deplete intrathyroidal hormone stores. If hyperthyroidism is not cured, a second dose of radioiodine is administered 6 to 12 months after the first one. When hypothyroidism develops, L-thyroxine replacement therapy is instituted, taking into account that replacement doses in these patients are often lower than that in athyreotic patients. Radioiodine therapy is safe, with no evidence of a higher risk for future carcinogenesis, congenital malformations, or other abnormalities in the offspring. It can be used in women of childbearing age, but pregnancy should be avoided for 6 to 12 months after treatment. It is contraindicated *during* pregnancy. Radioiodine therapy may be followed by the progression of ophthalmopathy, which can be prevented by a short course of glucocorticoids (prednisone 0.4-0.5 mg/kg body weight per day for 2 to 3 weeks, followed by gradual tapering of the dose, and drug withdrawal after 3 months).

Table 12.5 Main therapeutic options for hyperthyroidism due to Graves' disease

Thionamides

Mechanism of action	Inhibition of thyroid hormone synthesis and secretion, inhibition of peripheral conversion of T_4 to T_3 (propylthiouracil)
Goal	Permanent remission of hyperthyroidism, i.e., euthyroidism
Indications	Young age, small goiter, absence of ophthalmopathy, preparation to surgery, preparation to radioiodine (especially in the elderly), pregnancy, neonatal period
Limitations	High recurrence rate of hyperthyroidism, possible side effects

Radioiodine

Mechanism of action	Destruction of thyrocytes by β-radiation
Goal	Thyroid ablation, i.e., hypothyroidism
Indications	Age >18 yr, small/moderate goiter, ophthalmopathy, refusal of or contraindications to surgery, recurrence after or intolerance to thionamide treatment, elderly
Contraindications	Pregnancy
Complications	Possible exacerbation of ophthalmopathy (preventable by glucocorticoids)

Thyroidectomy

Mechanism of action	Removal of tissue responsible for excessive thyroid hormone synthesis
Goal	Thyroid ablation, i.e., hypothyroidism
Indications	Young age, large goiter (especially in the presence of tracheal or esophageal compression), ophthalmopathy, refusal of or contraindications to radioiodine therapy, pregnancy (in exceptional cases), recurrence after or intolerance to thionamide treatment, suspicion of associated malignancy
Contraindications	Systemic contraindications to surgery
Complications	Laryngeal nerve paralysis, hypoparathyroidism

Thyroidectomy Surgery (near-total or total thyroidectomy) is indicated in patients with large goiters. Surgery is indicated in patients with symptoms of tracheal compression (especially in younger patients below 18 years of age), when there is suspicion of associated malignancy, and also when the patient is reluctant to receive radioiodine therapy (Tab. 12.5). Thyroidectomy is indicated in pregnant women who are allergic to thionamides, or when patients are not complying with antithyroid drug treatment. Thyroidectomy seems to affect the course of ophthalmopathy less than radioiodine. In the case of persistent hyperthyroidism after thyroidectomy, radioiodine should be administered, because the risks of a second operation are higher. Complications of thyroidectomy include laryngeal nerve paralysis and hypoparathyroidism. In the hands of expert surgeons, these complications occur in 3% or less of cases.

Other drugs Beta-adrenergic antagonists ameliorate tremors, palpitations, and anxiety and are used in association with thionamides. Inorganic *iodide* (Lugol's solution, saturated solution of potassium iodide) rapidly blocks thyroid hormone release, though this effect is transient and followed by the recurrence of thyrotoxicosis. Its use is therefore limited to preparation for surgery (usually 5 drops of Lugol's solution 2 to 3 times per day for 7 to 10 days) and to thyroid storm (see below). Similar considerations can be drawn for *radiologic contrast agents* (iopanoic acid, sodium ipodate). The use of *potassium perchlorate* is limited by its toxicity, and this drug is currently employed almost exclusively in amiodarone-induced thyrotoxicosis (see below). *Lithium carbonate* is a weak antithyroid drug with little application in the management of hyperthyroidism. *Glucocorticoids* are used in association with thionamides in severe thyrotoxicosis, in view of their inhibitory action on peripheral monodeiodination of T_4 to T_3.

Ophthalmopathy

Mild ocular manifestations require only local supportive measures, including the following: guanethidine or β-adrenergic blocking eye drops to reduce lid retraction; methylcellulose eye drops to control the gritty, foreign body sensation; sunglasses to ameliorate photophobia; tapering of the eyelids at night if lagophthalmos is present; and prisms for mild diplopia (Tab. 12.8). For severe ophthalmopathy, the three main forms of treatment are by high-dose glucocorticoids, orbital radiotherapy, and orbital decompression. Other treatments, such as immunosuppressive drugs, iv immunoglobulins, somatostatin analogues, and plasmapheresis have either provided unsatisfactory results or need to be validated by properly performed clinical trials. *Glucocorticoids*, employed for their antiinflammatory and immunosuppressive actions, can be administered either orally, intravenously, or locally (retrobulbar or subconjunctival route). The rationale for the use of *orbital radiotherapy* resides in the antiinflammatory action of radiotherapy and in the radiosensitivity of lymphocytes infiltrating the retro-orbital tissue. The association of glucocorticoids and radiotherapy appears to

Table 12.7 Adverse effects of thionamides

	Frequency
Mild leukopenia	12-25%
Agranulocytosis	0.1-0.5%
Aplastic anemia	Very rare
Thrombocytopenia	Very rare
Skin rash	Relatively frequent
Urticaria	Relatively frequent
Itching	Relatively frequent
Aplasia cutis congenita (methimazole)[1]	Very rare
Hepatocellular necrosis (methimazole)	Very rare
Cholestasis (propylthiouracil)	Very rare
Arthralgias, fever	Uncommon
Lupus-like syndrome	Very rare
Vasculitis	Very rare
Nephrotic syndrome	Very rare
Loss of taste	Very rare
Overall frequency of thionamide adverse effects	<5%

1 Only a few cases have been described, not definitely linked to methimazole.

Table 12.6 Pharmacological features of methimazole and propythiouracil

	Methimazole	Propylthiouracil
Relative potency	10	1
Absorption after oral administration	Complete	Complete
Half-life in the circulation (h)	4-6	1-2
Binding to serum proteins	Very low	75%
Duration of action (h)	24	12-24
Placental transfer	Low	Lower
Milk transfer	Low	Lower

provide better results, exploiting the rapidity of glucocorticoid action, and the slower, but persistent effect of irradiation. The efficacy of glucocorticoids and orbital radiotherapy is greater when ophthalmopathy is of recent onset and active; thus, identification of patients who have active disease and are likely to respond to treatment is indicated (Tab. 12.9). While high-dose glucocorticoids carry the risk of major side effects, orbital radiotherapy is substantially devoid of risks. *Orbital decompression* is aimed at removing part of one or more walls of the orbit; its major indications are longstanding and severe proptosis, especially if unresponsive to glucocorticoids and/or orbital radiotherapy, and optic neuropathy. Its major drawback, especially with the transantral approach, is the development of post-surgical diplopia. Infrequent complications include sinusitis, numb lip, and cerebrospinal fluid leak. *Extra-ocular muscle surgery* for residual diplopia or eyelid surgery for lid retraction must be postponed until any eye disease is stable and inactive for at least 4 to 6 months. Cigarette smoking may negatively influence the course of ophthalmopathy and should be stopped.

Localized myxedema

In asymptomatic cases, no treatment is required. In all other cases, topic glucocorticoids are used, e.g., nighttime application of a glucocorticoid cream under occlusive plastic film dressing.

Table 12.8 Treatment of Graves' ophthalmopathy

Mild ophthalmopathy

Treatments	Effective on
Guanethidine or β-adrenergic eye drops	Lid retraction
Methylcellulose eye drops	Lacrimation, burning sensation
Sunglasses	Photophobia
Nighttime tapering of eyes	Lagophthalmos
Prisms	Mild diplopia

Severe ophthalmopathy

Effective treatments	
High-dose glucocorticoids	Active ophthalmopathy
Orbital radiotherapy	Active ophthalmopathy
Orbital decompression	Active or inactive ophthalmopathy, not responsive to steroids or radiotherapy, predominant and marked proptosis
Rehabilitative surgery (eye muscles, eyelids)	To be performed at least 6 months after rendering ophthalmopathy stable and inactive with other treatments

Treatments ineffective or to be validated
Immunosuppressive drugs
Somatostatin analogues
Intravenous Immunoglobulins
Plasmapheresis

Table 12.9 Method to assess activity of Graves' ophthalmopathy

Ocular manifestations

Spontaneous retrobulbar pain
Pain with eye movements
Eyelid erythema
Eyelid edema
Conjunctival injection
Chemosis
Swelling of caruncle

Scoring

Give one point for any manifestation
Activity score = sum of the points (from 0, no activity; to 7, very high activity)

(From Mourits MP, Koornneef L, Wiersinga WM, et al. Clinical criteria fur the assessment of disease activity in Graves' disease ophthalmopathy: a novel approach. British Journal of Ophthalmology 1989;73:639-44.)

Special situations

Concomitant hyperthyroidism and ophthalmopathy Correction of hyperthyroidism by antithyroid drugs is usually associated with amelioration of eye disease, though this treatment is often followed by the recurrence of thyroid hyperfunction, which may have detrimental effects on ophthalmopathy. Radioiodine therapy – and to a much lesser extent, thyroidectomy – may be soon followed by an exacerbation of ocular manifestations. However, the definitive control of hyperthyroidism is likely to have long-term beneficial effects on ophthalmopathy due to removal of the thyroidal source of antigens shared by the thyroid and the orbit. In addition, worsening of ophthalmopathy after radioiodine can be prevented by the concomitant administration of steroids (see above). Thus in patients with relevant ophthalmopathy, a definitive treatment of hyperthyroidism by radioiodine or thyroidectomy is indicated; it should be undertaken under the protection of middle-dose glucocorticoids if eye disease is mild or moderate, or followed by combined high-dose glucocorticoids and orbital radiotherapy if ophthalmopathy is severe.

Pregnancy Hyperthyroidism in pregnancy carries the risk of abortion, preterm delivery, lower birthweight, and neonatal mortality. It therefore requires prompt control. *Thionamides* represent the first choice treatment, radioiodine is contraindicated, and thyroidectomy should be restricted to exceptional cases performed in the third trimester. Both methimazole and propylthiouracil cross the placenta (Tab. 12.6) and can cause fetal hypothyroidism and goiter if their dose is excessive. Aplasia cutis has very rarely been reported in the offspring of mothers treated with methimazole during pregnancy. Thionamides should be given at the lowest dose maintaining maternal free thyroid hormones in the high-normal range. Low doses of thionamides are usually required. Combining high-dose thionamides with L-thyroxine is contraindicated, because L-thyroxine (which barely crosses the placenta) will maintain the mother euthyroid, but the high doses of thionamides will render the fetus hypothyroid. Although thionamides are transferred to the milk (Tab. 12.6), low doses of the drug do not affect thyroid function of the neonate; accordingly, breast-feeding can be allowed. Beta-adrenergic antagonists should be avoided, because they may be associated with a small placenta, intrauterine growth retardation, impaired response to anoxic stress, postnatal bradycardia, and fetal hypoglycemia.

Neonatal and fetal hyperthyroidism Neonatal thyrotoxicosis may develop due to transplacental TSH receptor antibody transfer from the mother. It is not common, but it is more likely in Graves' women with hyperthyroidism in remission after radioiodine or thyroidectomy and persistently elevated TSH receptor antibody levels. It is transient, with spontaneous remission taking place in 3 to 12 weeks, but it requires prompt treatment with thionamides (methimazole, 0.5-1 mg/kg body weight per day or propylthiouracil, 5-10 mg/kg body weight per day) and β-adrenergic antagonists. Iodide (1 drop of Lugol's solution every 8 hours) may be added to thionamides. Fetal thyrotoxicosis may also occur, as suggested by a heart rate >160 bpm; the mother is treated with thionamides in order to maintain fetal heart rate at about 140 bpm.

Hyperthyroidism in children and adolescents Thionamides are the first choice of treatment for children and adolescents below 18 years of age. Treatment may be continued for long periods (3 to 4 years or more). Ablation therapy should be carried out if hyperthyroidism recurs thereafter. Thyroidectomy is indicated when goiter is large or compliance with medical therapy is poor. Radioiodine is also effective and probably safe in this category of patients; however, since studies on potential long-term effects in patients treated so precociously are lacking, its use should possibly be avoided before attainment of adulthood.

Hyperthyroidism in the elderly The goals of treatment are rapid control of hyperthyroidism, avoidance of recurrences, and prevention of cardiac complications. To this end, after restoration of euthyroidism by antithyroid drugs, definitive treatment (usually by radioiodine) should be carried out. This could possibly be followed by the resumption of thionamide therapy after 2 weeks while waiting for the complete effect of radioiodine.

Thyrotoxic storm Thyrotoxic storm is a serious but rare complication of hyperthyroidism, characterized by severe manifestations of hypermetabolism (fever, profound sweating, dehydration, restlessness, insomnia, tremulousness). It occurs in patients whose hyperthyroidism is not diagnosed or is inadequately treated. It may be precipitated by surgery, infections, and traumas. It should be promptly treated with: (1) high doses of thionamides; (2) iodide or iodinated contrast agents, to be started 12 to 24 hours after thionamides; (3) glucocorticoids, to reduce peripheral conversion of T_4 to T_3; (4) β-adrenergic antagonists, even in the presence of heart failure, to reduce peripheral effects of thyroid hormones; (5) the treatment of underlying non-thyroidal illness by antibiotics, digoxin, or diuretics; (6) correction of dehydration by intravenous fluids; and (7) normalization of body temperature by cooling blankets and pharmacological agents (acetaminophen, chlorpromazine, meperidine). Plasmapheresis or peritoneal dialysis may be indicated to remove excess thyroid hormones from the circulation.

TOXIC ADENOMA

Toxic adenoma is an autonomously functioning, benign thyroid nodule causing thyrotoxicosis.

Epidemiology

The frequency of toxic adenoma ranges from 1.5 to 44% of cases of thyrotoxicosis. In most iodine-sufficient areas the frequency is about 10% or lower, though it may be higher in iodine-deficient areas. It is more frequent in women (the female/male ratio is 5:1 in Europe) and more common in middle-aged subjects. The onset of thyrotoxicosis may occur several years after the development of the nodule and is more frequent in nodules larger than 3 cm. Loss of function may rarely occur.

Etiopathogenesis

Toxic adenoma may be a solitary nodule in an otherwise normal thyroid gland or within a goiter. Recent evidence suggests that most toxic adenomas are due to somatic mutations in the gene encoding the TSH receptor, leading to its constitutive activation. These mutations have been detected in the adenomatous tissue, but not in the surrounding normal tissue. Another mutation causing constitutive activation of adenylate cyclase and the cAMP cascade less frequently described in toxic adenoma involves the α-subunit of the stimulatory guanine nucleotide-binding (G) protein.

Pathophysiology

Toxic adenoma may present as a benign encapsulated tumor, or as a hyperplastic lesion well-circumscribed from the surrounding tissue, but not encapsulated.

Clinical findings

Symptoms and signs of thyrotoxicosis are similar to, although usually milder than, those described for Graves' disease, but ophthalmopathy, localized myxedema, and acropachy are absent. If the nodule is large enough, it may cause symptoms related to tracheal and/or esophageal compression.

In addition to common laboratory tests for the diagnosis of thyrotoxicosis (see paragraph on Graves' disease), a thyroid scan provides a clue to the diagnosis. It will show prevalent tracer uptake in the nodule ("hot nodule"), with little or no uptake in the surrounding tissue. Ultrasound shows the presence of extranodular tissue. Echo-color-Doppler-sonography shows increased peripheral vascularity of the nodule.

Treatment

The use of antithyroid drugs is indicated only for the preparation of definitive treatment with radioiodine or surgery, and it is invariably followed by the recurrence of thyrotoxicosis after drug withdrawal. If radioiodine therapy is selected, relatively higher doses than in Graves' disease are employed. If patients are pre-treated with thionamides, they should be discontinued 3 weeks before radioiodine administration to be sure that extranodular tissue is functionally suppressed. Surgery is indicated when the nodule is large (>4 cm), especially in the presence of tracheal and/or esophageal compression, or when the patient is young and refuses radioiodine therapy (Tab. 12.10). Nodulectomy or lobectomy is indicated in true toxic adenoma, whereas subtotal thyroidectomy is advisable when a hot nodule develops in a multinodular goiter. Recently percutaneous 95% ethanol intranodular injections (1.5 ml/g of tissue) have been utilized, though persistence of hyperthyroidism occurs in about 30% of cases. This treatment represents an alternative when patients have contraindications to surgery, however, it is not indicated when multiple hyperfunctioning nodules are present or of a size larger than 3 cm.

Table 12.10 Therapeutic options for toxic adenoma

	Indications

Thyroidectomy	Young-adult age
	Large adenoma (>4 cm)
	Refusal of radioiodine
	  therapy
	Tracheal/esophageal
	  compression

Radioiodine	Older age Small adenomas (<4 cm) Contraindications to surgery

**Percutaneous
  intranodular
  ethanol injections**
	Single adenoma (<3 cm)
	Refusal of radioiodine
	  therapy
	Contraindications to
	  surgery

TOXIC MULTINODULAR GOITER

Toxic multinodular goiter is due to the presence, within a multinodular goiter, of multiple hyperfunctioning nodules or areas of autonomously functioning thyroid follicles scattered throughout the gland. It develops very slowly and insidiously, being commonly found in older patients with long-standing multinodular goiter. It is more frequent in iodine-deficient areas, where its onset may be related to an increased iodine supply. Ophthalmopathy, localized myxedema, and acropachy are absent. Due to the age of the patients, cardiovascular manifestations (tachyarrhythmias, heart failure) may be prominent. A thyroid scan will show a non-homogeneous distribution of tracer, with hyperfunctioning and hypofunctioning areas. Treatment is either radioiodine therapy or near-total/total thyroidectomy, the choice being based on the same considerations discussed in the paragraph on toxic adenoma. Antithyroid drugs are used only in preparation to ablative therapy.

THYROIDITIS

Transient thyrotoxicosis occurs in approximately 50% of patients with *subacute (De Quervain's) thyroiditis*. It follows the release of preformed thyroid hormones and is due to the destructive process. Thyrotoxicosis may last 4 to 10 weeks, is typically followed by a euthyroid phase, a hypothyroid phase and, eventually, by a recovery phase. The course of the disease may be accelerated by glucocorticoid administration. Signs and symptoms of thyrotoxicosis are associated with a painful, tender, and enlarged thyroid; an increased erythrocyte sedimentation rate; and mild leukocytosis. Serum free thyroid hormones are increased, serum TSH is suppressed, and serum thyroglobulin is increased. Thyroidal radioactive iodine uptake is very low or suppressed (Tab. 12.1). Salicylates or glucocorticoids are indicated to abate the inflammatory process (see Chap. 15). Thionamides are not indicated due to the destructive nature of thyrotoxicosis, while β-adrenergic antagonists control tachycardia.

Thyrotoxicosis may occur in *silent or painless thyroiditis*, which is an autoimmune disease, as suggested by its association with other autoimmune disorders, and by the predominant lymphocytic and plasma cell infiltration. Symptoms and signs of thyrotoxicosis are typical; the thyroid gland is usually enlarged and firm, but non-tender. The clinical course of the disease is similar to that of subacute thyroiditis, and hypothyroidism is permanent in about 10% of cases. Thyroidal radioactive iodine uptake is low/suppressed (Tab. 12.1), and serum thyroglobulin is increased, which is at variance with thyrotoxicosis factitia (see below). Anti-thyroid antibodies are generally present in the circulation, but TSH receptor antibody is absent. Erythrocyte sedimentation rate is normal. Treatment during the thyrotoxic phase is limited to β-adrenergic antago-

Table 12.11 Iodine-containing substances
Drugs
Amiodarone
Benziodarone
Expectorants
Iodochlorohydroxyquinoline
Povidone-iodine
Iodoform gauze
Iodine tincture
Solutions
Lugol's solution
Saturated potassium iodide solution
Iodinated glycerol
Radiologic contrast agents
Sodium ipodate
Iopanoic acid
Diatrizoate
Metrizamide
Diatrizoate

nists. *Post-partum thyroiditis* occurs within one year after delivery in women with circulating anti-thyroid antibodies and is otherwise similar to silent thyroiditis. Thyrotoxicosis is of short duration, lasting 2 to 6 weeks, and in most cases requires treatment only with β-adrenergic antagonists.

Hashimoto's thyroiditis may rarely be associated in its early phase with thyrotoxicosis, so-called Hashitoxicosis, probably related to the transient predominance of TSH receptor antibody with thyroid-stimulating activity on TSH receptor antibody with thyroid-blocking activity (see chapter on Thyroiditis).

IODINE-INDUCED THYROTOXICOSIS

Iodine-induced thyrotoxicosis (IIT) is reported with increased frequency due to widespread use of iodine-containing substances and drugs (Tab. 12.11). Iodine-induced thyrotoxicosis accounts for 0.2 to 10% of thyrotoxicosis, may develop both in patients with underlying thyroid abnormalities (goiter, latent Graves' disease, autonomously functioning nodules), and in subjects with apparently normal thyroid glands. It is more frequent in iodine-deficient than in iodine-sufficient areas, probably because the iodine load may unmask underlying thyroid autonomy. Among the different forms of iodine-induced thyrotoxicosis, *Amiodarone-induced thyrotoxicosis* (AIT) is a difficult therapeutic challenge, because it occurs in patients who often have serious heart problems for which this iodine-rich drug is very effective. In addition, the long half-life of amiodarone results in iodine release for several months after drug withdrawal. Thus, discontinuation of amiodarone treatment does not per se guarantee remission of thyrotoxicosis. Essentially, two forms of amiodarone-induced thyrotoxicosis are recognized: *Type I*, occurring in an abnormal thyroid gland, in which iodine load leads to increased thyroid hormone synthesis and secretion; and *Type II*, occurring in an apparently normal thyroid gland, in which thyrotoxicosis is the consequence of an amiodarone- (or iodine-) induced thyroid destructive process. Despite the iodine load, thyroidal radioactive iodine uptake is maintained or high in Type I AIT, while it is very low/suppressed in Type II AIT. Evidence of thyroid destruction in Type II AIT is provided, in addition to increased serum thyroglobulin levels, by the finding of very high circulating levels of interleukin 6. Urinary iodine excretion is greatly increased. Mixed forms of AIT may occur not infrequently.

Treatment of iodine-induced thyrotoxicosis, including amiodarone-induced thyrotoxicosis, with radioiodine is not feasible due to the normally low radioactive iodine uptake values and the high iodine content of the thyroid. Thyroidectomy during uncontrolled thyrotoxicosis and in the presence of large intrathyroidal stores of thyroid hormones is hazardous. In severe cases plasmapheresis can be performed, but its effectiveness is transient. Treatment of Type I amiodarone-induced thyrotoxicosis is usually carried out by a combination of thionamides (methimazole 30-40 mg/day) and potassium perchlorate (0.5 g twice a day). The latter drug inhibits iodide uptake and favors release of excess intrathyroidal iodide, which still is not organified. Administration of potassium perchlorate for more than 6 weeks should be avoided. In Type II AIT, thionamides and potassium perchlorate have low efficacy due to the destructive nature of the process. Glucocorticoids, however, are usually effective. Methylprednisolone is administered in daily doses of 40 mg for 2 to 3 weeks, the dose is gradually tapered, and then withdrawn after 3 months. Mixed forms are usually treated with a combination therapeutic regimen including thionamides, potassium perchlorate, and glucocorticoids. Once euthyroidism is restored, further therapeutic measures depend on the underlying thyroid disease.

UNUSUAL FORMS OF THYROTOXICOSIS

TSH-INDUCED HYPERTHYROIDISM

TSH-induced hyperthyroidism may be caused either by a TSH-secreting pituitary adenoma or by selective pituitary resistance to thyroid hormones.

TSH-secreting pituitary adenoma

TSH-secreting pituitary adenoma is a rare condition (280 cases so far described) in which free thyroid hormones are increased, TSH is normal or increased, TSH α-subunit is increased, and the ratio TSH α-subunit/TSH is usually >1. Goiter is present, ophthalmopathy, localized myxedema, and acropachy are absent. Magnetic resonance imaging (MRI) usually detects a pituitary tumor that may be either a micro- or a macroadenoma (0.5% of pituitary adenomas). Familial cases have not been described. The disease is treated by adenomectomy with or without external radiotherapy. Recurrences are common. Dopamine agonists and somatostatin analogues have proven effective in controlling hyperthyroidism. Thionamides, radioiodine, and thyroidectomy are not a correct therapeutic approach to the disease.

Selective pituitary resistance to thyroid hormone

Selective pituitary resistance to thyroid hormone is part of a spectrum of thyroid hormone resistance syndromes, which is due to mutations in the thyroid hormone β-receptor gene. In generalized resistance to thyroid hormones, both pituitary and peripheral tissues have, to a different extent, reduced sensitivity to hormone action. These patients are euthyroid or even hypothyroid. In selective pituitary resistance to thyroid hormone, some or all thyroid hormone-target tissues are normally sensitive to thyroid hormone action. The pituitary is resistant at the same time, and thus thyrotoxicosis develops. The biochemical picture is similar to that produced by TSH-secreting pituitary adenomas, with the exception that the TSH α-subunit is normal and the ratio of TSH α-subunit/TSH is <1. No pituitary tumor is detectable by MRI. The disease is familial, though the phenotype of the disease may vary in different members of the family. Treatment is carried out by β-adrenergic antagonists and thionamides. Some evidence suggests that triiodothyroacetic acid reduces TSH secretion with minimal thyromimetic effects and should probably be preferred to triiodothyronine. However, the long-term efficacy of triiodothyroacetic acid has to be established.

THYROTOXICOSIS FACTITIA

Thyrotoxicosis factitia is due to the surreptitious ingestion of excess thyroid hormones, and it should be distinguished from iatrogenic thyrotoxicosis caused by excessive doses of thyroid hormones administered by the physician or inadvertently taken by the patient. To the latter category belongs the so-called "hamburger thyrotoxicosis", two epidemics of which occurred in the United States after ingestion of trimmed bovine meat that contained thyroid tissue. Thyrotoxicosis factitia should be considered primarily a psychiatric disorder. Patients are almost invariably women, often overweight, who have a difficult relationship with their partner and try to call his

attention through their "sickness", or are driven by the idea that thyroid hormone makes them look younger and lose weight. They strenuously deny deliberate thyroid hormone intake. The clinical and biochemical picture is typical of thyrotoxicosis, goiter is absent, and thyroidal radioactive iodine uptake is very low/suppressed. Serum thyroglobulin determination is a clue to diagnosis, being very low or undetectable in thyrotoxicosis factitia, and at variance with other forms of low-RAIU thyrotoxicosis (subacute thyroiditis, amiodarone-induced thyrotoxicosis) (Tab. 12.12). Treatment of thyrotoxicosis requires only thyroid hormone withdrawal, possibly associated for a short time with β-adrenergic antagonist administration. Psychiatric aid is essential.

CONGENITAL HYPERTHYROIDISM

Congenital hyperthyroidism is a very rare type of thyrotoxicosis due to germline mutations of the TSH receptor, leading to its constitutional activation in all thyroid follicular cells. This situation is similar to that observed in many toxic adenomas, except that in the latter mutations are somatic. Described in few families, its inheritance appears to be autosomal dominant. It is characterized by diffuse goiter with high thyroidal RAIU. Thyroid autoantibodies, and in particular TSH receptor antibody, are absent, as well as ophthalmopathy, localized myxedema, and acropachy. Treatment resides in thyroid ablation by either radioiodine or thyroidectomy.

METASTATIC THYROID CARCINOMA

Follicular thyroid carcinoma that metastasize mainly to lung and bone rarely causes thyrotoxicosis if the bulk of metastatic tissue is large. Treatment is radioiodine therapy, which has occasionally been reported to cause thyrotoxic storm.

STRUMA OVARII

Struma ovarii is a very rare type of thyrotoxicosis due to functioning thyroid tissue within an ovarian teratoma or dermoid. Goiter is absent, and RAIU is suppressed over

---

Table 12.12 Differential diagnosis of main forms of low-radioactive iodine uptake thyrotoxicosis

	Thyroid pain	Serum thyroglobulin	Urinary iodine excretion
Subacute thyroiditis	Present	Elevated	Normal
Iodine-induced thyrotoxicosis	Absent	Elevated	Elevated
Thyrotoxicosis factitia	Absent	Low/undetect	Normal

the thyroid, though it is present over the ovarian tumor. Surgery is the elective treatment of this neoplastic and potentially malignant disorder.

TROPHOBLASTIC TUMORS

Trophoblastic tumors, either hydatidiform moles or chorioocarcinomas, can cause thyrotoxicosis, but the precise

prevalence of the latter is not known. The thyroid gland is normal or slightly enlarged, ophthalmopathy and thyroid autoantibodies are absent, and thyroidal RAIU is increased. Features of the trophoblast tumor are present, often with metastatic diffusion in the case of choriocarcinoma, and very high serum and urine concentrations of β-subunit of chorionic gonadotropin are found. Uterine ultrasonography confirms the presence of the tumor. Treatment requires surgery and, in the case of choriocarcinoma, chemotherapy. Pre-surgery treatment of thyrotoxicosis due to trophoblastic tumors is carried out by potassium iodide per os or sodium iodide intravenously.

Suggested readings

BARTALENA L, BOGAZZI F, MARTINO E. Adverse effects of thyroid hormone preparations and antithyroid drugs. Drug Saf 1996;15:53-63.

BARTALENA L, MARCOCCI C, PINCHERA A. Treating severe Graves' ophthalmopathy. In: Davies TF (ed). Newer aspects of clinical Graves' disease. London: Baillière's Clinical Endocrinology and Metabolism 1997;11:521-36.

BECK PECCOZ P, BRUCKER-DAVIS F, PERSANI L, SMALLRIDGE RC, WEINTRAUB BD. Thyrotropin-secreting pituitary tumors. Endocr Rev 1996;17:610-38.

BURCH HB, WARTOFSKY L. Graves' ophthalmopathy: current concepts regarding pathogenesis and management. Endocr Rev 1993;14:747-84.

BURROW GN. Thyroid function and hyperfunction during gestation. Endocr Rev 1993;14:194-202.

CHIOVATO L, SANTINI F, PINCHERA A. Treatment of hyperthyroidism. Thyroid International 1995;2:1-12.

DREMIER S, COPPÉE F, DELANGE F, VASSART G, DUMONT JE, VAN SANDE J. Clinical review 84. Thyroid autonomy: mechanism and clinical effects. J Clin Endocr Metab 1996;81:4187-93.

MARIOTTI S, FRANCESCHI C, COSSARIZZA A, PINCHERA A. The aging thyroid. Endocr Rev 1995;16:686-715.

MARTINO E, AGHINI-LOMBARDI F, MARIOTTI S, BARTALENA L,

BRAVERMAN LE, PINCHERA A. Amiodarone: a common source of iodine-induced thyrotoxicosis. Horm Res 1987;26:158-71.

PERRILD H, JACOBSEN BB. Thyrotoxicosis in childhood. Eur J Endocrinol 1996;134:678-85.

ROSS DS. Current therapeutic approaches to hyperthyroidism. Trends Endocrinol Metab 1993;4:281-7.

ROTI E, MINELLI R, SALVI M. Clinical review 80. Management of hyperthyroidism and hypothyroidism in the pregnant women. J Clin Endocrinol Metab 1996;81:1679-82.

TORRING O, TALLSTEDT L, WALLIN G, et al. Graves' hyperthyroidism; treatment with antithyroid drugs, surgery, or radioiodine – A prospective, randomized study. J Clin Endocrinol Metab 1996;81:2986-93.

VITTI P, RAGO T, CHIOVATO L, et al. Clinical features of patients with Graves' disease undergoing remission after antithyroid drug treatment. Thyroid 1997;7:369-75.

WEETMAN AP, McGREGOR AM. Autoimmune thyroid disease: further developments in our understanding. Endocr Rev 1994;15:788.

WIERSINGA WM. Amiodarone and the Thyroid. In: Weetman AP, Grossman A (eds). Pharmacotherapeutics of the thyroid gland, handbook of experimental pharmacology, vol. 128. Berlin-Heidelberg: Springer-Verlag, 1997;225-87.

WIERSINGA WM. Graves' ophthalmopathy. Thyroid International 1997;3:1-9.

COLOR ATLAS

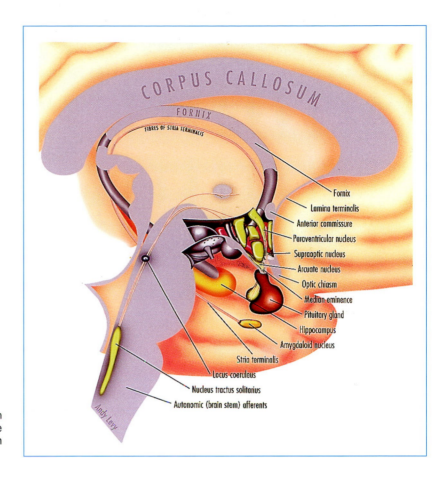

CORPUS CALLOSUM

FORNIX

FIBRES OF STRIA TERMINALIS

Fornix
Lamina terminalis
Anterior commissure
Paraventricular nucleus
Supraoptic nucleus
Arcuate nucleus
Optic chiasm
Median eminence
Pituitary gland
Hippocampus
Amygdaloid nucleus
Stria terminalis
Locus coeruleus
Nucleus tractus solitarius
Autonomic (brain stem) afferents

Andy Levy

Figure 4.1 The brain and brain stem in cross section, showing detail of the hypothalamus and pituitary with brain stem and limbic afferents.

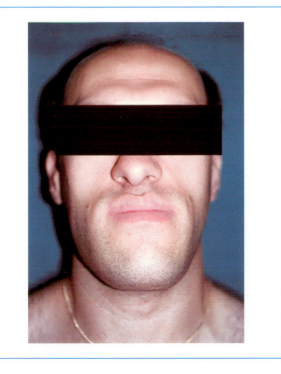

Figure 6.5 Facial features of acromegaly in a 42-year-old man. Note the frontal and mandibular prominence and the enlargement of nose and lips.

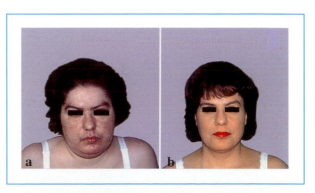

a   b

Figure 6.10 Regression of Cushing's features after successful transsphenoidal selective adenomectomy in a 38-year-old woman with Cushing's disease.

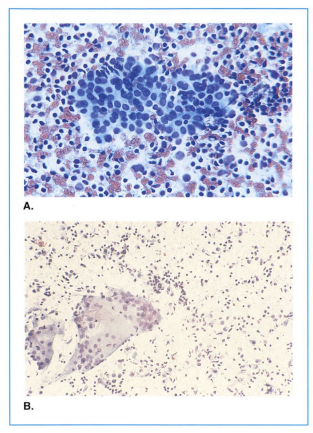

A.

B.

Figure 15.2 Fine-needle aspiration cytology. (**A**) Hashimoto's thyroiditis: oxyphil cells (Hürthle or Askanazy cells) and lymphocytes in different stages of maturation (Papanicolaou stain; x 200). (**B**) Subacute thyroiditis: leukocytes and giant multinucleated cells (Papanicolaou stain; x 200). (Courtesy of Dr. G. Di Coscio, Section of Pathology, Department of Oncology, University of Pisa).

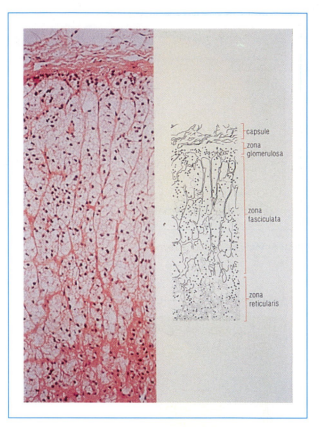

capsule

zona glomerulosa

zona fasciculata

zona reticularis

Figure 26.2 Histology of the different zones of the adrenal gland. (Reproduced with permission from James VHT. Adrenal cortex physiology. In: Besser GM, Cudworth AG, [eds.] Clinical endocrinology. London: Chapman and Hall, 1987, Chap. 6, 6.2.)

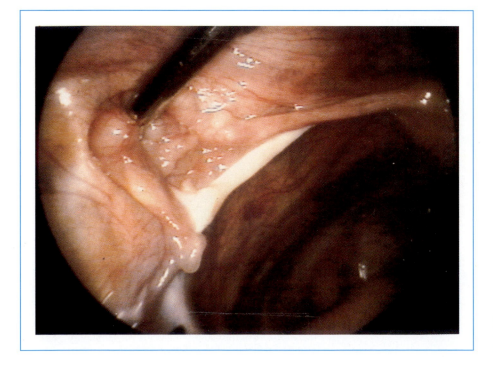

Figure 45.2 Streak ovary in a 20 year patient with pure gonadal dysgenesis (46, XX.)

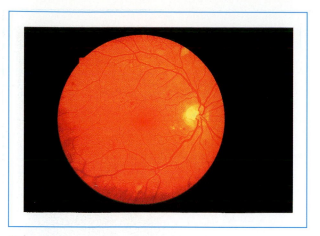

Figure 59.4 Background retinopathy.

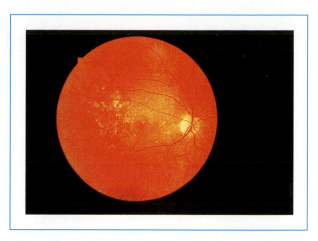

Figure 59.8 Clinically significant macular edema after photocoagulation.

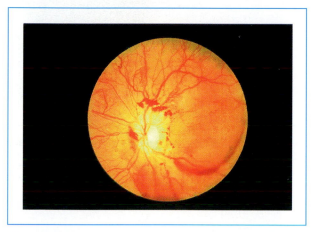

Figure 59.5 Proliferative retinopathy with preretinal hemorrhages above the optic disc, and a vitreous hemorrhage below.

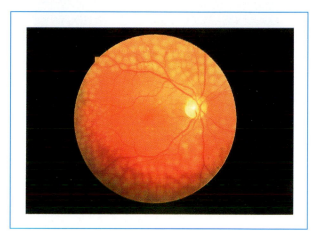

Figure 59.9 Panretinal photocoagulation.

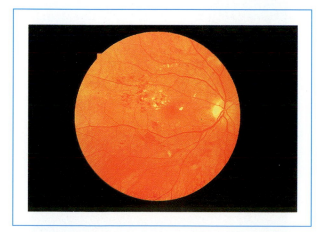

Figure 59.6 Clinically significant macular edema before photocoagulation.

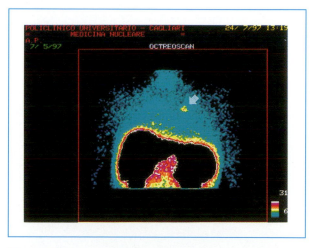

Figure 70.2 (^{111}In-DTPA-D-Phe)-Octreotide scintigraphy (Octreoscan®) in a case of ectopic ACTH syndrome due to malignant thymoma in a 32-year-old man. An area of clear uptake is seen in the mediastinum (arrow), corresponding to the primary tumor. (By courtesy of Dr. M. Piga, Nuclear Medicine, University of Cagliari.)

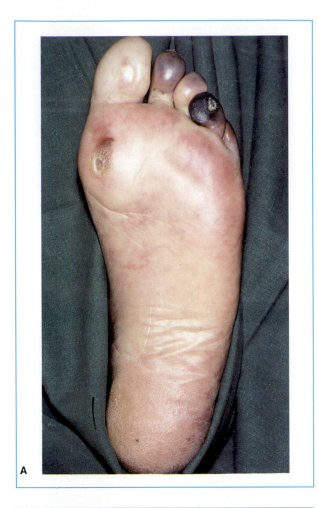

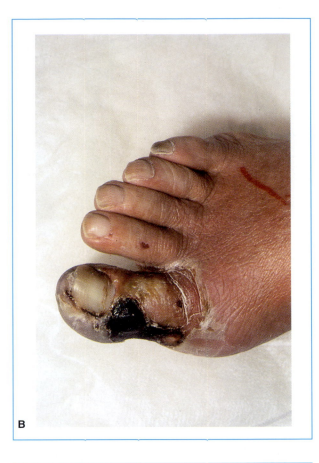

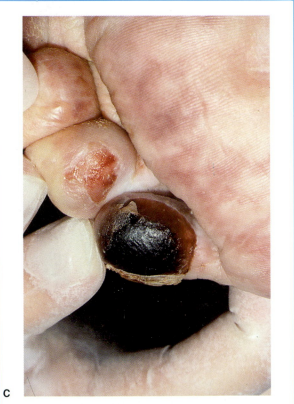

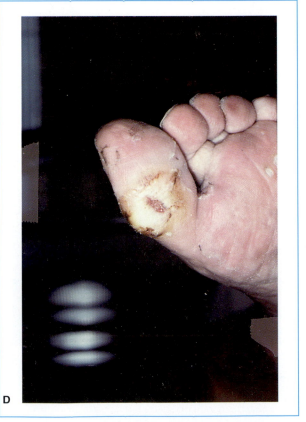

Figure 59.15 Typical localization and aspect of foot ulcers (A-D).

Hypothyroidism

John H. Lazarus

▰ KEY POINTS ▰

- Hypothyroidism may be primary (thyroid failure), secondary (pituitary failure), or tertiary (hypothalamic failure). The most common cause of hypothyroidism is autoimmune Hashimoto's thyroiditis.
- The clinical presentation of hypothyroidism is variable and may involve many systems, particularly the cardiovascular and neurological systems. Myxedema coma is rare but is a medical emergency for which specific and supportive treatment is available.
- Drug-induced hypothyroidism (e.g., lithium or amiodarone) must be recognized. It is not necessary to discontinue the drug in most cases.
- Postpartum thyroiditis is associated with transient hypothyroidism in 40 to 50% of anti-thyroid-peroxidase-positive women. Twenty percent develop permanent hypothyroidism.
- Severe iodine deficiency leads to hypothyroxinemia, which is particularly important in pregnant women because of the critical requirement of thyroxine for fetal brain maturation.
- Congenital hypothyroidism occurs at a frequency of 1 in 4000 live births.

Primary hypothyroidism is caused by a thyroid disorder that results in the failure of thyroid hormone production by the gland. Secondary hypothyroidism results from a defect in the production of thyroid-stimulating hormone (TSH) from the pituitary or from the defective action of TSH on the thyroid. Tertiary hypothyroidism occurs when a pathological process (e.g., tumor or infiltration) reduces the secretion of hypothalamic thyrotropin-releasing hormone (TRH). Hypothyroidism is common. The prevalence in the Whickham Survey was 1.5% in women and less than 1% in men. Recent follow-up data indicate a continuing risk of developing thyroid failure, particularly if positive thyroid auto-antibodies are present. There is a female/male ratio of about 5 to 1.

The most common cause of primary thyroid failure is Hashimoto's thyroiditis; other frequent causes of primary hypothyroidism include post-radioiodine hypothyroidism, post-thyroidectomy, and drugs (e.g., lithium, amiodarone). Destruction of pituitary thyrotropes by tumor or infiltrative disease results in secondary hypothyroidism.

Hypothalamic pressure or destruction due to tumor-causing reduction or loss of TRH produces tertiary hypothyroidism. Other causes are shown in Table 13.1.

HASHIMOTO'S AUTOIMMUNE THYROIDITIS

Hashimoto's autoimmune thyroiditis is an autoimmune disease characterized by the presence of goiter and circulating antithyroid antibodies, and it presents clinically in the euthyroid or hypothyroid state.

Epidemiology

Chronic autoimmune thyroiditis, as seen by necropsy evidence, is present in 27% of adult women and 7% of adult men. The prevalence of hypothyroidism that is not due to iatrogenic causes is about 10 per 1000 women and less than 1 per 1000 men. Approximately 50% of patients pre-

Table 13.1 Etiology of hypothyroidism

Primary hypothyroidism
  Congenital hypothyroidism
  Iodine deficiency
  Thyroid destruction
  Autoimmune thyroiditis
  Post-thyroidectomy
  Post-radioiodine therapy
  Post-external radiotherapy
  Thyroid infiltration
  Drugs (e.g., iodine, lithium, amiodarone, interferon
    alpha, interleukin 2)

Secondary hypothyroidism
  Pituitary disease

Tertiary hypothyroidism
  Hypothalamic disease

Transient hypothyroidism
  Subacute thyroiditis
  Silent thyroiditis
  Post partum thyroiditis
  Drug-induced
  Thyroiditis due to TSH receptor-blocking antibodies

senting with a small- or moderately-sized goiter have a variable degree of thyroid failure, which ranges from the elevation of TSH with normal thyroxine (T_4) and 3,5,3'-triiodothyronine (T_3) levels to severe hypothyroidism. Titers of thyroid antibodies are high, and the disease occurs in all age groups. Like other thyroid autoimmune diseases, it is 4 to 6 times more frequent in women. It is less common in children, and titers of antibodies are lower than in adults. Hashimoto's autoimmune thyroiditis is more commonly seen at presentation in the elderly, although the progression to the hypothyroid state in elderly euthyroid patients with thyroid antibodies is less than that observed in middle aged subjects.

Etiopathogenesis

Hashimoto's autoimmune thyroiditis is of autoimmune origin and characterized by the aberrant expression of HLA-DR (class II) molecules on thyrocytes, which permits autoantigen presentation to T helper lymphocytes. T helper lymphocytes then induce B lymphocytes to generate antibody. However, this scenario may not represent the initiating factor in thyroidal autoimmune destruction but act more as an amplification mechanism to perpetuate the immune attack. An inherited defect in antigen specific T suppressor cell function may be present, which leads to an augmentation of the immune response due to stimulation of T helper cells by interleukin 2. However, there is not complete agreement with this concept. More than 90% of patients with Hashimoto's disease have circulating antibodies against thyroid peroxidase (previously known as the microsomal antigen). Anti-thyroglobulin antibodies occur in a lesser number and are not thought to contribute to cytotoxicity as do anti-thyroid peroxidase antibodies. The latter are complement-dependent and may interact with cytokines such as interferon gamma and interleukin 2 to produce cell damage. The genetic predisposition to develop autoimmune hypothyroidism should not be overlooked, but the precise factors that trigger the autoimmune response are not known.

The discovery of hypothyroidism in Hashimoto's disease due to blocking of the TSH receptor by TSH receptor-blocking antibodies has increased our understanding of the pathophysiology of this condition. It is now speculated that these antibodies may cross the placenta to cause transient neonatal hypothyroidism.

Pathology

The thyroid gland may vary in size from a large nodular goiter to an atrophic gland in Hashimoto's disease. The range of severity can be from scattered clusters of infiltrating lymphocytes up to extensive chronic inflammation and scarring with almost complete loss of follicular epithelium. There is in situ immune complex deposition and basement membrane changes in the gland, with expression of major histocompatibility complex antigens on the thyroid cells. Focal lymphocytic thyroiditis is common and represents early autoimmune disease. Lymphoid follicles containing polyclonal B cells occur frequently. In hypothyroid patients the gland is small and fibrotic with scattered groups of lymphocytes and plasma cells.

Clinical findings

The clinical hallmark of Hashimoto's disease is an irregular firm goiter of any size, though typically 2 to 3 times normal, and seen in a woman who may be euthyroid or manifest symptoms and signs of hypothyroidism (Tab. 13.2). Adult hypothyroidism may be very insidious in its onset. A high index of clinical suspicion is important.

Symptoms and signs

Skin and appendages The skin is dry, cold, and thick. The patient may experience hair loss. The facies are coarse, and there is swelling of the face that occludes the malar angle. The tongue is thickened.

Cardiovascular system Angina may occur. Bradycardia is present with a low-voltage electrocardiogram accompanied by pericardial effusion (anterior and posterior).

Nervous system Apathy and sleepiness are common. Memory impairment, difficulty in concentrating, and depression are often found. Carpal tunnel syndrome may occur due to compressive paresthesiae of the median nerve. The myotonic ankle reflex may be used as a sensi-

Table 13.2 Clinical features of hypothyroidism

Symptoms	Signs
Cold intolerance	Coarse facies
Weight increase	Edema
Dry skin	Bradycardia
Hair loss	Myotonic ankle reflex
Aches and pains	Dry skin
Paresthesiae	Joint effusions
Memory impairment	Cognitive impairment
Poor concentration	Psychosis
Depression	Hypothermia
Constipation	Hair loss
Sleepiness	Anemia
Apathy	Hoarse voice
Tiredness	Thick skin
Slow speech	Titubation
Menstrual irregularities	Thick tongue
Dyspnea	Pericardial effusion
Galactorrhea	

tive clinical discriminator. Cognitive impairment and head titubation may occur. Frank psychosis is seen in severe hypothyroidism (myxedema madness).

Musculoskeletal system Muscular aches and pains in the arms and legs may be accompanied by joint pain and effusion.

Alimentary system Appetite is poor, but there is weight increase due to fluid accumulation. Constipation is common. Atrophic gastritis may be present.

Urogenital system The bladder is atonic, resulting in urinary retention. Menstrual irregularities are frequent. Miscarriage is more common than normal.

Symptoms such as lethargy, mild depression, variation in menstruation, and weight increase are common and non-specific, but they may point to the diagnosis of the hypothyroid state. The plethora of symptoms means that patients may be referred to a variety of clinics, such as gynecology, psychiatry, neurology, and cardiology. The duration of illness should be ascertained, as this often relates to the time taken to achieve full recovery. A family history of autoimmune endocrinopathy should be obtained. Recent pregnancy may suggest post partum hypothyroidism. Patients with subclinical hypothyroidism are common. The diagnosis is often made by chance in a patient who has presented with non-specific complaints and had thyroid tests performed as part of a screening process.

Diagnostic procedures

Laboratory findings A subnormal total or free thyroxine, together with an elevated TSH, confirms the primary hypothyroid state. The sensitivity of the modern assays has made the TRH test redundant. Investigation of pituitary hypothyroidism will be prompted by the initial finding of a low T_4 and low TSH. Appropriate pituitary function tests and radiology must be arranged and the same procedures followed for suspected tertiary hypothyroidism. Care must be taken not to confuse apparently subnormal hormone values with a low T_3 or euthyroid sick syndrome. Serum T_3 concentrations are a poor indicator of the hypothyroid state and should not be used.

Cardiac evaluation is important in primary hypothyroidism, especially in middle-aged to elderly patients, and if angina has been noted or there is evidence of pre-existing heart disease. Usually this will be apparent in the history, and an electrocardiogram will show classic low-voltage changes with bradycardia. Echocardiographic assessment may be necessary in more severe cases to show anterior and posterior pericardial effusion.

Other end organ effects of thyroid hormone that may be abnormal in thyroid failure are the ankle reflex time (measured as the half time of relaxation), and the elevation of serum cholesterol. Hypothyroidism is associated with an elevation in plasma total cholesterol, low-density lipoprotein cholesterol, and plasma triglycerides. Interestingly, high-density lipoprotein cholesterol has also been found to be elevated in hypothyroidism, as well as the lipoproteins apolipoprotein A-1 and apolipoprotein E. These changes are reversed with thyroxine therapy. A normochromic normocytic anemia and mild hyperprolactinemia may also be seen.

In compensated (subclinical hypothyroidism), the decreasing thyroidal production of T_4 causes the serum free-T_4 concentration to decrease, which produces an increased TSH output from the pituitary. The increased TSH output will maintain free-T_4 concentration at the bottom end of the normal reference range. Peripheral tests of thyroid function are not helpful in diagnosis because their specificity is too low.

A hallmark of autoimmune thyroid disease is the presence of circulating thyroid autoantibodies. These are produced against three well-characterized autoantigens, thyroglobulin (Tg), thyroid peroxidase (TPO), and the TSH receptor. Routine measurement of anti-thyroglobulin and anti-TPO antibodies should be performed in the evaluation of almost all hypothyroid patients. In Japan there appears to be a significant incidence of hypothyroidism due to TSH receptor blocking antibodies; the titer of these may decrease over time, resulting in a return to euthyroidism in some patients. This phenomenon is rare in Europe and the Americas, perhaps related to different ambient iodine concentrations. Anti-thyroglobulin and anti-TPO antibodies are measured by hemagglutination inhibition, enzyme-linked immunosorbent assay, or radioimmunoassay.

Imaging studies Assessment of the hypothyroid patient with Hashimoto's disease should include evaluation of the goiter by appropriate imaging and fine needle aspiration biopsy if indicated. Cardiac function should be assessed before treatment is started. The presence of other associated autoimmune endocrinopathies (e.g., Addison's disease, pernicious anemia, premature ovarian failure) must be ascertained. The presence of a rapidly growing large goiter in an elderly hypothyroid patient is suggestive of a thyroid lymphoma, and fine needle aspiration biopsy is indicated. As a general rule, this biopsy is not performed in patients with hypothyroidism. However, if there is a goiter with a dominant nodule, fine needle aspiration biopsy will be necessary to exclude malignancy.

Treatment

Levo-thyroxine substitution therapy should be started once the diagnosis of hypothyroidism is established. Levo-T_4 is preferred to T_3 because of its longer half-life and greater chance of compliance with once-a-day therapy. In the absence of severe cardiac manifestations, 0.1 mg is a reasonable starting dose in an adult. The patient should be reviewed in 6 to 8 weeks and the dose increased to 0.15 mg per day. Underlying this straight-forward approach are two questions: How much reliance can be placed on the patient's perceived response to T_4, and what level of thyroid hormones (assuming they are measured) is reasonable while the patient is on therapy? It should be noted that there is considerable variation in patient response to T_4 because of differential thyroid hormone receptor isoform tissue concentration. The patient's account of improvement, or lack of it, with T_4 therapy should be assessed carefully; serum T_3 concentration during T_4 therapy must be in the normal range, as should that of TSH. Serum T_4 may exceed the upper limit of normal on T_4 therapy without ill-effect. Often, a high T_4 and normal T_3 is accompanied by a suppressed TSH (second or third generation assay), but this is not an indication that the dose of T_4 should be reduced if the patient has responded satisfactorily. Clinically, such a response as this implies a normal pulse rate and complete resolution of presenting symptoms and signs. Occasionally cardiac symptoms such as palpitations will occur with a normal replacement T_4 dose; in this case a β-adrenergic blocker drug is indicated. Apparent lack of response to T_4 is not uncommon and should raise the possibility of (1) poor compliance with therapy, (2) presence of anemia, particularly pernicious anemia, (3) persisting underlying psychiatric abnormality, (4) other autoimmune disease such as Addison's disease (this should have been recognized at presentation), and (5) other non-thyroid-related disease. Note that hypothyroid myopathy can take up to one year to resolve completely.

Subclinical hypothyroidism

The decision to treat subclinical hypothyroidism has been difficult because of its non-specific symptomatology. However, there are new data showing a definite association of subclinical hypothyroidism with depressive symptomatology. Furthermore, carefully performed controlled trials of thyroxine therapy have demonstrated significant improvement in symptomatology when assessed in a double-blind fashion. There is no doubt that the most effec-

tive method of monitoring thyroxine replacement therapy is by the measurement of serum TSH. Studies have shown that the normal replacement dose of T_4 is about 150 to 165 µg per day. Excess T_4 therapy is associated with symptoms of hyperthyroidism such as tachycardia and weight loss. There has been concern as to the deleterious effects of excess T_4 on bone density, particularly in postmenopausal patients on long-term treatment in whom the TSH level is subnormal. However, no evidence of an increased fracture rate in these groups has been found, and even in thyroid cancer patients receiving TSH-suppressive doses of T_4 bone density is within normal limits.

Pregnancy and thyroxine therapy

There is no contra-indication to pregnancy in a woman already on T_4 treatment. There is now evidence from carefully observed clinical studies that the dose of T_4 should be increased by at least 50 µg and possibly double that in early gestation (as soon as pregnancy is confirmed). Serum T_4 and TSH levels must be monitored throughout the duration of pregnancy.

HYPOTHYROIDISM FOLLOWING DESTRUCTIVE THERAPY FOR HYPERTHYROIDISM

Treatment

Surgical treatment

Hypothyroidism occurs in about 25% of patients during the first year following thyroid surgery (range 5 to 80%) and in 2 to 5% per year thereafter. Predictive factors for the development of hypothyroidism in this setting include postoperative remnant size, anti-TPO, and anti-thyroglobulin antibody titers, and the degree of thyroidal lymphocytic infiltration. It should be remembered that the natural history of Graves' disease is known to result in hypothyroidism in a significant minority of patients, even in untreated subjects. Thus, surgery may merely hasten this process. With the availability of current accurate laboratory evaluation of thyroid function, the condition is readily diagnosed and easily treated with thyroxine.

Radioiodine therapy

Hypothyroidism following radioiodine therapy is thought to be inevitable by some groups. Indeed, some clinicians intentionally render patients hypothyroid with large ablative doses of radioactivity and commence the patient immediately on thyroxine replacement therapy. Clearly, the amount of activity of ^{131}I administered is an important predictor of the development of hypothyroidism, but it is not the only predictor. Goiter size, ambient iodine concentration, the presence of thyroid anti-TPO antibodies, and the method of dosage calculation are also of relevance. A recent series of patients treated with radioiodine have shown that hypothyroidism occurred in 10% of patients at 1 year and 50% at 10 years. A continuing cumulative hypothyroid rate of 3% per annum is on-going after that period. Thus, the hypothyroid rate will vary depending on the philosophy of dosimetry. All patients receiving radioiodine should have life-long regular follow-up to aid detection of hypothyroidism. In some centers this is performed by a method of computerized registry.

HYPOTHYROIDISM DUE TO ENDEMIC GOITER

The classic picture of endemic cretinism has been described for at least three centuries.

Etiopathogenesis

Iodine

Severe iodine deficiency is the principal cause of cretinism. There is a correlation between the degree of iodine deficiency and the incidence of cretinism. Correction of the iodine deficiency reduces the incidence of the disorder. More recently the concept of iodine deficiency disease has been recognized to spread over a wide spectrum of disorders, ranging from mild psychomotor retardation to severe hypothyroid cretinism. Studies in iodine-deficient areas have indicated that iodine deficiency during gestation results in hypothyroidism in the offspring. This is due to the lack of sufficient thyroid hormones in the fetus to ensure adequate brain development. Maternal thyroid hormones are known to cross the placental barrier to supply the fetus during the first trimester before fetal thyroid function is established. In iodine-deficient regions, maternal hypothyroxinemia reduces the availability of thyroxine to the fetus, resulting in the impairment of neural maturation. The prevalence of neonatal hypothyroidism is a very sensitive indicator of iodine deficiency in a geographical region.

Other goitrogens

Other factors also contribute to the incidence of hypothyroidism in iodine-deficient areas. Naturally occurring goitrogens such as the thiocyanate ion found in Cassava act as co-goitrogens in the presence of iodine deficiency. Other staple foods, such as millet and various vegetables, are also known to contain goitrogens. Selenium, a trace metal, is a vital constituent of the type I deiodinase enzyme that converts thyroxine to triiodothyronine. Selenium deficiency has been shown to contribute to the hypothyroidism seen in iodine-deficient areas. The presence of thyroid growth blocking antibodies in neonatal hypothyroidism has been found by some but by no means all workers.

Treatment

Iodine deficiency affects around one billion people worldwide and is readily correctable, usually by the provision of iodized salt. Hypothyroid persons should be treated in the standard way with thyroxine. A trial of thyroid hormone administration should always be tried, even in cretins in the older age groups, as some modest improvement in mentation may still be observed.

DRUG-INDUCED HYPOTHYROIDISM

Iodide

Excess iodide ingestion results in an acute transient inhibitory effect on iodide organification. In some susceptible people the thyroid cannot escape from this effect on the organification mechanism, and hypothyroidism results after prolonged administration of iodine. Goiter also occurs following excess iodide with or without accompanying hypothyroidism. Iodine is found in various drugs such as amiodarone, topical antiseptics, radiology contrast agents, and vitamins, as well as many proprietary preparations. Withdrawal of the iodine-containing substance nearly always relieves the hypothyroidism.

Lithium

Lithium (usually administered as lithium carbonate) is effective in the treatment and prophylaxis of bipolar manic depressive psychosis. The cation inhibits the release of thyroid hormones from the thyroid and, in patients with thyroid antibodies, increases the titer of both anti-TPO and anti-thyroglobulin antibodies. Hypothyroidism occurs in about 5% of patients receiving the drug. The drug should not be stopped if this happens: treatment with thyroxine will restore euthyroidism.

Amiodarone

Amiodarone, which is often used for life-threatening cardiac arrhythmias, contains 37% iodine and also has a structural similarity to thyroxine. In iodine-sufficient areas, the iodine overload may result in hypothyroidism. The reduced thyroid function is also due to the inhibition of the conversion of T_4 to T_3 by the drug. As with lithium, this drug should not be discontinued, and the patient should be given thyroxine therapy. The diagnosis of hypothyroidism must be established, as amiodarone administration also causes abnormalities in thyroid function tests even in the euthyroid state.

Cytokines

Treatment of malignant disease or chronic hepatitis B or C with interferon alpha may induce the appearance of thyroid antibodies (anti-TPO and anti-thyroglobulin), leading to hypothyroidism. Similar events occur following therapy with interleukin 2 in patients with cancer.

POST PARTUM HYPOTHYROIDISM

Post partum thyroiditis is an autoimmune condition with

many immunological similarities to Hashimoto's thyroiditis, except that in some 70% of cases the condition is transient. It is a destructive thyroiditis occurring after pregnancy and is associated with the so-called "immune rebound" seen at that time. It occurs in 50% of women who have been observed to be thyroid-antibody positive (usually anti-TPO) during early pregnancy. Of these, approximately two-thirds will develop hypothyroidism at around 19 weeks post partum. Twenty to 30% of these women will go on to develop permanent hypothyroidism requiring life-long thyroxine therapy. Transient hypothyroidism is often accompanied by definite hypothyroid symptoms and should be treated with thyroxine. Thyroxine may be stopped after one year to establish whether the condition is transient or not.

SUBACUTE THYROIDITIS

Patients with subacute thyroiditis usually have neck pain, thyroid tenderness, and symptoms of inflammatory illness. The disease is characterized by thyroid follicular destruction attributed to viral infection with resulting transient hyperthyroidism due to thyroid hormone release from the damaged follicles. In severe cases patients also develop hypothyroidism, which lasts 4 to 8 weeks. Recovery to the euthyroid state is seen in 90% of patients, who eventually have normal thyroid ultrasound morphology. During the recovery or the hypothyroid phase, the thyroid test results may be confusing, particularly if the patient is seen for the first time at this stage. Specific treatment for the hypothyroidism is rarely required.

SILENT THYROIDITIS

The pathology and course of silent thyroiditis are similar to post partum thyroiditis. About 40% of patients develop a hypothyroid phase that follows the hyperthyroid phase; the hypothyroidism usually lasts between 4 to 16 weeks and occasionally persists indefinitely (in less than 5%). If the hypothyroid symptoms persist, sufficient thyroxine should be given to relieve the symptoms but not to suppress the TSH level to normal, as a raised TSH level is thought to speed the recovery process. If hypothyroidism lasts more than 6 months, it is most likely permanent, and further trials of withdrawal of T_4 are unnecessary.

CONGENITAL HYPOTHYROIDISM

Epidemiology

In countries where this condition is routinely screened for incidence, congenital hypothyroidism occurs in 1/4000 live births. This relates to the occurrence of permanent hypothyroidism due to conditions listed in Table 13.3, but it is important to note that the condition also may be tran-

Table 13.3 Etiology of congenital hypothyroidism

Permanent
Thyroid dysgenesis
Thyroid agenesis
TSH
  defective synthesis (central hypothyroidism)
  hyporesponsiveness
  hyperresponsiveness
Stimulating G-protein deficiency
Iodide transport defect
Iodide organification defect
Thyroglobulin synthesis defect
Iodotyrosine deiodinase deficiency

Transient
Maternal antithyroid drug ingestion
Excess maternal iodide ingestion
  (e.g., amniofetography)
TSH receptor-blocking antibodies
Extreme prematurity
Transient hyperthyrotrophinemia

sient. Screening for congenital hypothyroidism is usually performed by estimating TSH in neonatal blood samples obtained by heel prick at around 5 days postnatal. The sample is presented for analysis as a dried blood spot on filter paper. This method will miss central hypothyroidism, which occurs in 1/100 000 births.

Clinical findings

The cause of congenital hypothyroidism should be determined. A thyroid scan using ^{123}I or ^{99m}Tc pertechnetate will indicate the presence or absence of thyroid tissue or any evidence of ectopia. Thyroid ultrasonography may also yield information on the size and location of the thyroid gland. Further diagnostic tests include the urinary iodine excretion, the thyroidal radioiodine uptake if thyroid tissue is present, and the perchlorate discharge test. Measurement of serum thyroglobulin should also be performed; this will indicate the presence of functioning thyroid tissue. Specific information can also be obtained by estimation of the saliva/blood ratio of radioiodine and the measurement of low molecular peptides in the urine. Recently, molecular biological techniques have become available to determine specific mutations or deletions in the transmembrane or extracellular domain of the TSH receptor. This type of analysis is yielding important information about the role of the receptor in congenital hypothyroidism.

Treatment

Following the discovery of raised TSH in a blood spot, confirmation should be obtained in a serum sample and a full clinical examination should be performed. Although neonatal hypothyroidism is not apparent in 50% of infants with this disorder, there is a higher incidence of other congenital abnormalities. Further evaluation of the cause of the hypothyroidism should then be done (see investigations above). Thyroxine therapy must be started as soon as possible, because any delay will adversely affect the subsequent IQ of the child. Careful titration of the thyroxine dose must be maintained; an initial dose of 10 to 15 µg/kg per day should be given and increased as necessary in order to reduce the TSH level to <20 mU/l in the majority of infants. If necessary, thyroxine may be stopped at around 2 years of age to reassess thyroid function in suspected cases of transient hypothyroidism. Treatment of central hypothyroidism must include careful assessment of other pituitary hormone deficiencies in addition to T_4.

MYXEDEMA COMA

This is a rare but recoverable cause of coma. It is essentially very severe hypothyroidism and is characterized by hypothermia and impaired consciousness. It may be precipitated by infection, congestive heart failure, cerebrovascular accidents, hypothermia, and some drugs. There is accompanying respiratory depression and typical external features of thyroid failure (dry skin, loss of hair, and coarse facies). The clinical picture is often complicated by neuropsychiatric features such as confusion, paranoia, and hallucinations. Cardiac findings may include bradycardia, low-voltage ECG, and pericardial effusion on echocardiography. Therapy must be cautious (see below).

Clinical findings

The classic features of hypothyroidism, coarse facies, bradycardia, dry skin, and hair loss should be assessed. A myotonic ankle jerk is easily the most discriminatory clinical feature. The thyroid gland should be palpated. The typical Hashimoto gland is firm and lobulated. Features of associated organ-specific diseases such as vitiligo, pernicious anemia, and type 1 diabetes mellitus should be looked for. In secondary or tertiary hypothyroidism, the sallow waxy appearance of pituitary hypothyroidism may be apparent.

Treatment

Treatment must be immediate. Correction of hypothermia and appropriate ventilatory support should be given. Thyroxine should be given intravenously, as nasogastric tube administration is uncertain due to aspiration and malabsorption. 3,5,3'-Triiodothyronine should also be given intravenously in a dose of T_3 20 µg twice per day to start. Hypotension, hyponatremia, and possible adrenocortical insufficiency should be corrected.

OTHER CAUSES OF HYPOTHYROIDISM

Radiotherapy

External radiotherapy to the neck for treatment of Hodgkin's and non-Hodgkin's lymphoma results in hypothyroidism in 25 to 50% of patients. Hypothyroidism also occurs in patients receiving external radiotherapy for tumors of the head and neck, and in those having total body irradiation prior to bone marrow transplantation. The hypothyroidism in all of these cases usually presents within 1 year of treatment; a significant incidence of subclinical hypothyroidism is seen following external radiotherapy.

Chemotherapy

Chemotherapy also results in hypothyroidism, though much less so than after radiotherapy.

Infiltration

Infiltration of the thyroid due to a variety of disease processes causes hypothyroidism; some of these conditions are associated with autoimmune thyroiditis as well (Tab. 13.4). In general, the incidence of thyroid failure in these diseases is low, but it is of obvious importance in view of the long duration of the primary condition.

Central hypothyroidism

Central hypothyroidism is due to an abnormality of the pituitary and/or hypothalamus. The most common cause in an adult is a pituitary tumor (functioning or non-functioning adenoma or craniopharyngioma). Infections such as tuberculosis, toxoplasmosis, and abscess, as well as infiltrations (Tab. 13.4), must also be considered. Occasionally other tumors (e.g., glioma, metastatic tumors, and meningiomas) may cause hypothyroidism by pressure effects on the hypothalamus or pituitary.

Resistance to the effect of thyroid hormone

This comprises a syndrome of reduced responsiveness of target tissues to the action of thyroid hormone and is associated with mutations in the T_3 binding domain of the thyroid hormone receptor β-gene. This results in the variable reduction in the affinity of the receptor for T_3 and in interference with the function of the normal thyroid hormone receptors. Biochemically, there are elevated levels of serum thyroid hormones with measurable TSH. Although the majority of patients are metabolically euthyroid, some show clinical and laboratory features of thyroid hormone deficiency, such as mild to moderate growth retardation and delayed bone maturation.

Table 13.4 Infiltrations of the thyroid
Riedel's thyroiditis Cystinosis Hemochromatosis Scleroderma (systemic sclerosis) Sarcoidosis Amyloidosis

Suggested readings

AMINO N. Hypothyroidism: etiology and management. In: Wheeler MH, Lazarus JH (eds). Diseases of the thyroid. London: Chapman & Hall, 1994;245-68.

NYSTRÖM E, CAIDAHL K, FAGER G, WIKKELSÖ C, LUNDBERG P-A, LINDSTEDT G. A double-blind cross-over 12 month study of L-Thyroxine treatment of women with "subclinical" hypothyroidism. Clin Endocrinol 1988;29:63-75.

OPPENHEIMER JH, SCHWARTZ HL, STRAIT KA. An integrated view of thyroid hormone actions in vivo. In: Weintraub BD (ed). Molecular endocrinology: basic concepts and clinical correlation. New York: Raven Press, 1995; 249-68.

TOFT AD. Thyroxine therapy. New Eng J Med 1994;331:174-80.

TUNBRIDGE WM, EVERED DC, HALL R, et al. The spectrum of thyroid disease in the community: the Whickam survey. Clin Endocrinol 1977;7:481-93.

Nontoxic goiter

Gianfranco Fenzi, Paolo E. Macchia

▇ KEY POINTS ▇

- Goiter is a chronic enlargement of the thyroid gland not due to neoplasm or inflammatory process, the volume of each lobe resulting larger than the terminal phalanx of the thumb of the person examined with normal thyroid function tests.
- Goiter is termed endemic when it is present in more than 5% of the total population, or in more than 10% of schoolchildren in a definite geographic area. Goiter is termed sporadic if it is present in less then 5% of the general population in a definite geographic area.
- Endemic goiter is an adaptive disease that develops in response to inadequate iodine intake from the diet.
- Nodules may be a consequence of long-standing goiter, and they may become hyperfunctioning.
- Suppressive therapy with levothyroxine may reduce recently developed diffuse goiter. Nodular goiters are generally unaffected by the treatment, although further volume increases may be stopped.
- Levothyroxine therapy should be individually adjusted in order to obtain thyrotropin suppression with the least necessary dose. In elderly patients or in those with cardiac problems therapy may be started with extreme caution, if at all.
- Iodine supplementation in food (salt, etc.) may completely prevent endemic goiter.

Goiter is a chronic enlargement of the thyroid gland not due to neoplasm or inflammatory process, the volume of each lobe resulting larger than the terminal phalanx of the thumb of the person examined. Thyroid enlargement can be of variable size, with or without nodules, presenting with various pathological aspects. Nontoxic goiter can be subdivided into endemic, sporadic, and familial goiter.

ENDEMIC GOITER

Goiter is defined as endemic when it is present in more than 5% of the total population, or in more than 10% of schoolchildren in a definite geographic area. Nutritional iodine deficiency is the main cause of endemic goiter. Table 14.1 shows the grading of goiter according to the criteria recently proposed by the World Health Organization.

Table 14.1 Classification of goiter size

Grade	Thyroid inspection and/or palpation
0	No palpable or visible goiter
1	Enlarged thyroid palpable but not visible when the neck is in neutral position
2	Enlarged thyroid visible in neutral position

(According to the WHO/UNICEF/ICCIDD consultation on IDD indicators.)
(WHO = World Health Organization; UNICEF = United Nations International Children's Emergency Found; ICCIDD = International Council for Control of Iodine Deficiency Disorders; IDD = Iodine Deficiency Disorders.)

Goiter endemia should be characterized not only by the prevalence of the goiter, but also by the severity of iodine deficiency (Tab. 14.2). In severe endemias the disease appears early in the life, increasing to a peak during puberty and young adult life. The prevalence is generally higher in females, but this difference is reduced in severe iodine deficient areas.

In addition to endemic goiter, iodine deficiency (if severe) is also responsible for endemic cretinism, hypothyroidism with or without stunted growth, and for an increased incidence of prenatal and/or neonatal death (Tab. 14.3). A higher prevalence of endemic goiter has been reported in mountainous regions, such as the Himalayas, Andes, and previously Alps, but it can also be elevated in lowlands far from the sea as in continental Europe, Asia, and Central Africa (Fig. 14.1). In the large majority of affected areas, a reduced iodine content was observed in drinking water and in food. In fact, approximately 150 µg/day of iodide are necessary, but higher amounts are required in special situations such as pregnancy, nursing, and puberty (Tab. 14.4).

Pathophysiology

Endemic goiter is an adaptive disease that develops in response to inadequate iodine intake from the diet. When dietary iodide intake is insufficient, compensatory mechanisms will intervene to maintain normal secretion of thyroid hormones: an increase in iodide trapping, increased thyroglobulin production, and preferential secretion of tri-iodothyronine (T_3). These effects are mainly due to an increased pituitary secretion of thyrotropin (thyroid-stimulating hormone [TSH]), which is also responsible for the stimulation of thyroid cell replication and growth, ending in an increase of the volume of thyroid gland (Fig. 14.2).

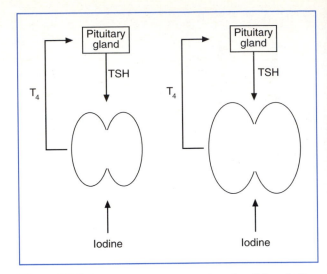

Figure 14.2 Pathogenesis of endemic goiter. When iodine intake is insufficient, T_4 secretion decreases and TSH secretion from the pituitary increases. The increased TSH produces a slow, progressive growth of the thyroid, resulting in the formation of goiter.

If iodide supplementation decreases to less than 50 µg/day, the adaptive mechanisms are not sufficient and clinical hypothyroidism may develop. The prolonged stimulation of the thyroid gland by TSH is thus responsible for the development of goiter. However, goitrogenic factors in the diet or environment other than iodine deficiency could play a role in goiter formation (Tab. 14.5).

SPORADIC GOITER

Sporadic goiter is defined as the presence of goiter in <5% of the general population in a geographic area. Sporadic goiter is present all over the world, and more frequently in females.

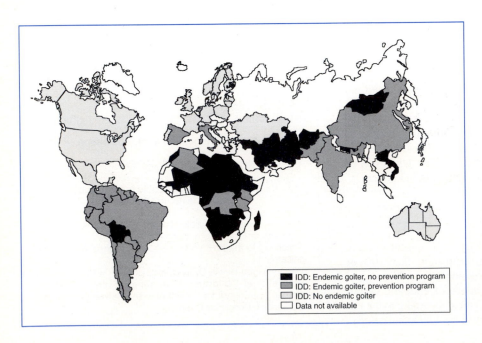

IDD: Endemic goiter, no prevention program
IDD: Endemic goiter, prevention program
IDD: No endemic goiter
Data not available

Figure 14.1 Geographical distribution of iodine deficiency and endemic goiter. Severe iodine deficient areas are illustrated as black, grey are areas where prevention programs are in progress, and light-grey depicts the areas where the iodine deficiency and the endemic goiter disappeared due to effective iodine prophylaxis programs.

Table 14.2 Classification of degrees of iodine deficiency

Grade	Urinary iodine excretion	Clinical manifestations
I (mild)	50-99 µg/l	Euthyroidism
II (moderate)	25-49 µg/l	Subclinical hypothyroidism
III (severe)	<20 µg /l	Hypothyroidism, cretinism

Table 14.4 Recommended daily dietary iodine intake

Adult	150 µg
Pregnancy	220 µg
Lactation	290 µg
Infants	
0 - 6 months	110 µg
6 - 12 months	130 µg
> 1 - 8 years	90 µg
9 - 13 years	120 µg
≥ 14 years	150 µg

Pathophysiology

The etiology of the sporadic goiter is still not well-defined. It is possible that the a cause is a reduced intrathyroidal concentration of iodine not due to dietary deficiency, but rather to metabolic disorders of iodine metabolism. Estrogens could play a critical role, as demonstrated by the higher incidence in females, especially during puberty and pregnancy. This is possibly due to an increase in urinary iodine excretion. Very high levels of human chorionic gonadotropin (hCG) during pregnancy may induce thyroid stimulation and growth similar to TSH, due to the interaction of hCG with the TSH receptor (specificity spillover). Finally other environmental factors may play a role, such as the introduction of natural goitrogens from vegetables and chemicals.

Diffuse goiter should be considered an initial manifestation of thyroid growth derived from low or moderate goitrogenic stimuli. If these stimuli continue over time, some cells and follicles will be selectively chosen for growth irrespective from the surrounding non-predisposed cells; thus, part of the thyroid gland will undergo nodular transformation, being the nodules the final expression of the growth of the selected follicles.

As observed in clinical practice, when thyroid scintiscan is performed, nodular goiters present irregular radioisotope uptake. Some nodules concentrate the tracer with higher avidity, other less intensely or even not at all ("hot, warm, cold" nodules), suggesting that some cells and follicles are also favored in their function. It is conceivable that these cells, which undergo autonomous proliferation and/or function, present alterations in the control of cell proliferation.

Specific gain-of-function mutations of the TSH receptor have been reported in solitary toxic "autonomous" and in hyperfunctioning "hot" nodules in multinodular goiters, particularly in patients from iodine-deficient areas. Rarely, somatic mutations of the Gs protein were also found. It is possible that various endogenous and/or environmental factors can induce such somatic gain-of-function, gain-of-growth mutations.

Table 14.3 Iodine deficiency disorders

Fetus

Abortions
Stillbirths
Increased prenatal and infant mortality
Endemic cretinism
  Neurologic
    Mental deficiency
    Deaf-mutism
    Spastic diplegia
    Squint
  Myxedematous
    Mental deficiency
    Hypothyroidism
    Dwarfism

Neonate

Goiter
Overt or subclinical hypothyroidism

Infant-child

Goiter

Adolescent

Juvenile hypothyroidism
Impaired mental and physical development

Adult

Goiter and its complications
Hypothyroidism
Endemic mental retardation
Decreased fertility rate

(Adapted from Delange FM, Ermans AM. Iodine deficiency. In: Breverman LE, Utiger RD [eds]. The thyroid. 7th ed. Philadelphia: Lippincott-Raven, 1996.)

Table 14.5 Goitrogenic factors in endemic goiter

Iodine deficiency

Natural goitrogens (thioglucosides)
Excess iodine
Excess calcium, fluoride, or lithium
Bacterial pollution of the water
Genetic factors
Autoimmunity

The pathological picture in goiter varies depending upon the duration of the disease. In the beginning, diffuse hypertrophy, hyperplasia, and an increased vascularization of the gland are observed; later, the architecture of the thyroid gland is lost, and some areas containing colloid appear. More often these areas alternate with localized areas of focal hyperplasia. Some well-defined nodules have characteristics of neoplasia, areas of hemorrhage, and calcifications.

Clinical findings

Unless there has been a recent rapid enlargement, a longstanding goiter suggests benign disease. A detailed list of drugs the patient is taking should be recorded, with particular reference to those with known goitrogenic action or those containing iodine. Severe tenderness suggests subacute thyroiditis. Sudden pain in a nodule or in an apparently normal gland is most likely the result of hemorrhage. Local symptoms of goiter are uncommon, and large goiters are usually well-tolerated, unless partly or wholly retrosternal, when difficulty in swallowing and shortness of breath are common. Recurrent laryngeal nerve stretching and/or compression associated with hoarseness are rare.

A familial goiter developing in adult life is likely due either to iodine deficiency or to autoimmune thyroiditis, while in childhood it suggests iodine deficiency or dyshormonogenesis.

The majority of patients with goiter are euthyroid. Symptoms of hypothyroidism are often mild and so slow in developing that the patient may feel they are merely due to natural aging. On the other hand, goitrous patients may often present with symptoms suggesting hyperthyroidism, such as anxiety, weight loss, palpitations, and sweating. These symptoms may reflect a concomitant emotional disorder, but they can also be due to the toxic evolution of a long-standing nontoxic goiter, especially in aging patients. Finally, as the patient becomes aware of his/her goiter, it is common for him or her to attribute a variety of local and general complaints to the thyroid condition, although careful evaluation will reveal that they are not dependent on the thyroid enlargement.

For local examination of the neck, the patient should be seated in a well-lit place, ideally facing a window. The physician should pay attention to any neck enlargement and/or lumps, and to its (their) mobility on swallowing. The normal thyroid is infrequently visible, even with the neck fully extended. Therefore, a visible thyroid is enough to establish the presence of a goiter. Mobility during swallowing distinguishes thyroidal from other masses arising in the neck. However, when the goiter is so large as to occupy all the space available in the neck, or in cases of Riedel's thyroiditis or invasive carcinoma, movement on swallowing is lost.

In palpation of the neck, the examiner should outline the thyroid gland and determine the limits of the borders of the lateral lobes. The normal gland can usually be appreciated on palpation, and it feels rubbery. The gland is considered enlarged when the lateral lobes are larger than the terminal phalanx of the thumb of the subject. When a nodule is found, the physician should evaluate its size and establish whether it is solitary or associated with other nodules. Tenderness is typical of acute or sub-acute thyroiditis or recent hemorrhage. In Hashimoto's thyroiditis the gland is firm and nodular, whereas a stony hard consistency is more suggestive of thyroid carcinoma or Riedel's thyroiditis. The presence of the pyramidal lobe is typical of diseases characterized by diffuse thyroid enlargement, and it should be distinguished from the delphian (pre-tracheal) lymph node. A vascular thrill may be felt and is suggestive of hyperthyroidism. In this case, a continuous systolic bruit is commonly heard.

In patients with a large retrosternal or nodular goiter, raising the arms produces congestion of the face and respiratory distress. This is a result of further narrowing of the thoracic inlet, already occupied by the retrosternal goiter, which increase compression of the veins and trachea (Pemberton's sign).

Palpation often reveals nodules that require further evaluation. Palpation cannot distinguish solid from cystic thyroid nodules, but a very hard and firm nodule and the concomitant presence of cervical lymphadenopathy may increase the suspicion of thyroid malignancy.

Deviation and/or compression of the trachea may cause dyspnea, cough, and inspiratory stridor. Hoarseness may indicate involvement of the recurrent laryngeal nerve, which should be confirmed by laryngoscopy. Hoarseness may also be observed when thyroid inflammation spreads beyond the capsule, or when a rapidly enlarging thyroid nodule stretches the nerve.

When a nodule is present, it must be ascertained as to whether it is benign or malignant. An increased serum concentration of calcitonin in a patient with a thyroid nodule is always indicative of medullary thyroid cancer. The cytological examination of material obtained by fine needle aspiration allows for the recognition of papillary and undifferentiated thyroid malignancies, although follicular cancer cannot easily be identified by this technique (see Chap. 16).

To assess whether thyroid enlargement, particularly nodular, is producing any significant compression and/or displacement of neighboring structures, an X-ray of the neck and the chest on both orthogonal positions should be performed. At the level of the neck, displacement and/or narrowing of the trachea can be observed (Fig. 14.3), and examination with barium may occasionally demonstrate displacement of the cervical esophagus in patients with large goiters. Less penetrating pictures may show intrathyroidal calcification and will also indicate the size of the goiter and its retrosternal extension.

Diagnostic procedures

Although nontoxic goiter is characterized by euthyroidism, it may evolve into hyperthyroidism or hypothyroidism. For this reason TSH and free thyroid hormone assays should be performed when goiter is observed.

The development of ultrasensitive TSH assays has made it possible to measure serum TSH very precisely

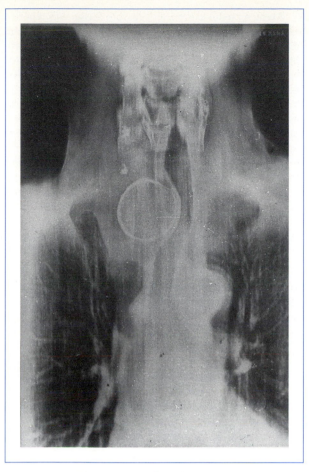

Figure 14.3 X-ray tomography of a large nodular goiter with calcification and retrosternal extension. Note the displacement and narrowing of the trachea.

and to differentiate between normal and low values of preclinical hyperthyroidism.

These sensitive TSH assays also permit a more precise definition of the upper limit of normal values, which is useful in the diagnosis of preclinical hypothyroidism. Serum free thyroid hormone measurement is also useful to assess the thyroid state.

Although measurement of urinary iodine excretion is the only way to confirm and quantitate iodine deficiency in a particular area, individual determinations are of limited value since the excretion of iodine varies considerably from day to day, depending on the variation of iodine intake. Thus, when a patient resides in an area previously not evaluated for iodine deficiency, a large number of urinary samples from that area are required to establish the role of iodine deficiency in goiter development.

Imaging studies High resolution ultrasonography confirms the presence of a nodule felt by palpation and precisely assesses the volume of the gland. Furthermore, ultrasonography often shows that a nodule that was apparently solitary on palpation is actually associated with other smaller nodules. This technique also allows for the distinction between solid and cystic lesions and for the confirmation of the thyroidal origin of a neck lump. Finally,

sonography can be used to perform a more precise fine needle aspiration of a thyroid nodule, confirming the presence of the needle within the nodular lesion to be sampled. Recently, color flow Doppler sonography, by providing a noninvasive, real-time display of thyroid vascularity, has provided useful information on thyroid hyperfunction as well as on the vascular pattern of the nodules.

Scintigraphy is useful in evaluation if one or more nodules are evolving to functional autonomy. The association of scintigraphy with a perchlorate discharge test can establish if an organification defect is present.

Treatment

Medical treatment

Since TSH is a growth factor for thyroid cells, therapy should be aimed at suppressing TSH secretion. This is obtained by giving thyroid hormones in a dose appropriate to inhibit pituitary TSH secretion, while maintaining serum free T_3 (fT_3) and free T_4 (fT_4) in the normal range.

The thyroid hormone of choice is levothyroxine (L-T_4) administered in an individually adjusted dose from 1.5 to 2.2 µg/kg daily. It is a good procedure to reach this dose progressively during several weeks. The treatment should continue indefinitely. Desiccated thyroid preparations are obsolete since the amounts of T_4 and T_3 in the tablet are not well-titered and the preparations contain variable amounts of T_3. Levotriiodothyronine (L-T_3) is not recommended because of its short half-life and fluctuating levels following administration that require trice a day dosing. Moreover, with the L-T_4 therapy, the patient will regulate the amount of T_3 available to the target tissues through peripheral deiodination of exogenous T_4.

L-T_4 treatment often results in a slow regression of goiter. This effect is mainly observed when the goiter is diffuse, small- to medium-sized, and recently developed. Nodular goiters are far less frequently influenced by L-T_4 therapy, and the aim of treatment is to prevent further enlargement of the nodule(s). Before starting L-T_4 treatment, the patient should be monitored for cardiovascular disease. Therefore, in patients with underlying cardiovascular diseases, the risks of L-T_4 therapy would be greater than the beneficial effects. The finding in patients with clinically euthyroid goiter of serum TSH values below the normal range should call for caution, since underlying hyperfunctioning "autonomous" tissue or nodule(s) are almost certainly present. L-T_4 therapy in such cases is useless and potentially dangerous because toxic symptoms can rapidly occur.

In patients older than sixty years, suppressive L-T_4 treatment should be started very cautiously, if at all, and only if the advantages are clearly evident (such as in subclinical hypothyroidism). In any case, it is worth noting that the amounts of L-T_4 required for suppression of TSH secretion in such patients is lower than in younger patients.

Several reports have indicated that long-term treatment with L-T_4 may impair cardiac function and reduce bone mass. The most recent studies, however, have clearly stated that the accurate monitoring of L-T$_4$ doses in each individual (keeping serum fT$_3$ and possibly fT$_4$ values in the normal range) may avoid these unwanted effects on the heart and/or bone. However, a completely suppressed serum TSH for a long period of time should be avoided, except in patients with treated thyroid cancer.

Radioiodine may be considered in patients in whom hyperthyroidism has developed as a consequence of autonomous hyperfunctioning nodules. Some authors have reported successful treatment with radioiodine in reducing goiter mass in patients with large substernal and multinodular nontoxic goiters, and it is especially useful in patients in whom surgery is at high-risk and compressive symptoms require therapy.

Surgical treatment

Surgery is indicated in large nodular goiters that produce compression and/or dislocation of the neck structures (particularly the trachea), and in goiters extending substernally in the mediastinum. The extent of thyroid resection may vary from lobectomy, to subtotal thyroidectomy, to near-total thyroidectomy. The latter should be considered in large multinodular goiters involving both lobes and in patients who cannot afford to be treated with L-T$_4$ "suppressive" therapy after surgery. In fact, nodular recurrence in the remaining thyroid tissue is frequently observed after surgery when L-T$_4$ suppressive therapy is not started within 2 to 3 months. This can be due to the growing potentiality of the remaining thyroid cells under the continuous stimulation of TSH.

Prophylaxis

Iodine prophylaxis is the best approach to eradicate iodine deficiency and consequent disorders. Iodination methods include iodination of water, iodination of salt or bread, and the use of iodized oil. The use of iodized salt has been demonstrated to be the best way to provide iodine to the population. However, in particular areas where supplementation of salt is difficult or even impossible, iodized oil given intramuscularly or orally is also effective. Consumption of iodized salt is the simplest and most effective system to provide the appropriate amount of iodine to the diet. Addition of potassium iodide or, even better, iodate (for its stability), provides a consumer with 20 to 50 µg of iodine per g of salt. From the very first campaigns in the United States in 1917, the effectiveness of this method was confirmed in various countries (Switzerland, India, Mexico, Greece, and so on). The efficacy of iodine prophylaxis was demonstrated not only in the rapid reduction of goiter prevalence from above 20-30% to <5% of the population, but also in the disappearance of the other conditions and disorders due to iodine deficiency (Tab. 14.3).

An increased occurrence of thyrotoxicosis was reported as the main complication of iodine prophylaxis. This condition was observed soon after the beginning of iodine prophylaxis, especially in older subjects with nodular goiter, and was transient. It was likely due to an underlying toxic nodular goiter or Graves' disease that was fueled with iodine to increase secretion of T$_4$. The thyrotoxicosis was usually mild and easily managed. Continued iodine prophylaxis resulted in a prevalence of Graves' disease similar to that observed in the iodine sufficient areas, while the thyrotoxicosis from nodular goiters drastically diminished. This indicates that iodine prophylaxis was also able to prevent the "autonomous" nodular evolution of the goiter.

FAMILIAL GOITER

Goiter is defined as being familial when it is observed in different members of the family; it is generally transmitted as an autosomal recessive disorder due to errors in the hormonogenesis pathway. Goiter may be present at birth or seen later during childhood or adult life.

Hypothyroidism and goiter are now prevented in nations where effective congenital hypothyroidism screening programs are performed in the general population. Patients with familial goiter present at birth with elevated serum TSH values associated with low-normal T$_4$ and normal T$_3$. The early treatment of these patients will prevent the goiter formation.

Iodine pump defects

Recently, mutations in the sodium/iodine symporter have been reported, that impair the iodine uptake not only by the thyroid gland, but by the salivary gland and gastric mucosa. The diagnosis is based on low radioiodine thyroid uptake and also on reduced concentration of the isotope in saliva after oral administration of tracer radioiodine. Diagnosis is confirmed by the response to treatment with high doses of iodine, which enter the thyroid gland by passive diffusion.

Organification defects

Alterations of the iodine incorporation into the thyroglobulin molecule have been reported in animals and in patients with thyroperoxidase abnormalities. The diagnosis is made by the perchlorate discharge test: oral administration of perchlorate produces a rapid discharge of more than 15% of the radioiodine previously concentrated by the gland as assessed by measuring thyroid uptake for additional 1-2 hours.

Pendred's syndrome

This disease is characterized by goiter, mild hypothyroidism, and a neurological hearing defect. The syndrome is considered to be among the organification defects, and the gene involved in this disease was very recently characterized. Mutations in this gene, which encodes a protein called Pendrin, have been found in several families with this syndrome.

Defects in diiodotyrosine deiodination

Familial goiter is characterized by a deficiency in thyroid iodotyrosine dehalogenase and clinically presents with goiter, mild hypothyroidism, and high to very high radioiodine uptake, followed by a relatively rapid decline of the radioiodine in the gland. Administration of perchlorate does not result in radioiodine discharge since much of the radioiodine is in the form of radiolabeled monoiodotyrosine and diiodotyrosine. The enzyme is also deficient in peripheral tissues, especially in the liver and kidney. High values of labeled monoiodotyrosine and diiodotyrosine found in blood and excreted in urine after the administration of tracer doses of radioiodine confirm the diagnosis.

Treatment

In general, treatment of patients with hereditary defects in thyroid hormone synthesis is the same as for any other hypothyroid patient of the same age. Early treatment is mandatory in order to prevent cerebral damage.

Suggested readings

BIKKER H, WULSMA T, BAAS F, DE VIJLDER JJ. Identification of five novel inactivating mutations in the human thyroid peroxidase gene by denaturating gradient gel electrophoresis. Hum Mutat 1995;6:9-16.

DELANGE FM. The disorders induced by iodine deficiency. Thyroid 1994;4:107-28.

DELANGE FM, ERMANS AM. Iodine deficiency. In: Breverman LE, Utiger RD (eds). The thyroid. 7th ed. Philadelphia: Lippincott-Raven, 1996;296-316.

EVERETT LA, GLASER B, BECK JC, et al. Pendred syndrome is caused by mutations in a putative sulphate transporter gene (PDS). Nature Genet 1997;17:411.

FENZI GF, MARCOCCI C, AGHINI-LOMBARDI F, PINCHERA A. Clinical approach to goitre. Baillières Clin Endocrinol Metabol 1988;2:671-82.

HUYSMANS DA, HERMUS AR, CORSTENS FH, et al. Large, compressive goiters treated with radioiodine. Ann Intern Med 1994;121:757-62.

MEDEIROS-NETO G, STANBURY JB. Inherited disorders of the thyroid system. Boca Raton: CRC Press, 1994.

MATSUDA A, KOSUGI S. A homozygous missense mutation of the sodium/iodide symporter gene causing iodide transport defect. J Clin Endocrinol Metab 1997;82:3966-71.

MICRONUTRIENT DEFICIENCY INFORMATION SYSTEM. Global prevalence of iodine deficiency disorders. MDIS working paper no.1. Geneva: WHO-Nutrition Unit Publishers, 1993.

PETER HJ, BÜRGI U, GERBER H. Pathogenesis of non toxic diffuise and nodular goiter. In: Breverman LE, Utiger RD (eds). The thyroid. 7th ed. Philadelphia: Lippincott-Raven, 1996; 890-5.

POHLENZ J, MEDEIROS-NETO G, GROSS JL, SILVEIRO SP, KNOBEL M, REFETOFF. Hypothyroidism in a Brazilian kindred due to iodide trapping defect caused by a homozygous mutation in the sodium/iodide symporter gene. Biochem Biophys Res Commun 1997;240:488-91.

STUDER H, GERBER H, PETER HJ. Natural heterogeneity of thyroid cells: the basis for understanding thyroid function and nodular goiter growth. Endocrin Rev 1989;10:125-35.

TOFT A. Thyroxine therapy. N Engl J Med 1994;331:174-80.

Thyroiditis

Luca Chiovato, Enio Martino

KEY POINTS

- Thyroiditis encompasses a heterogeneous group of acute, subacute, and chronic inflammatory disorders of the thyroid, of which etiologies range from autoimmune to infectious origins. Patients can be euthyroid, may experience transient phases of thyrotoxicosis and/or hypothyroidism, or may progress to permanent hypothyroidism.
- Chronic autoimmune thyroiditis presents with two clinical entities: a goitrous form (Hashimoto's thyroiditis) and an atrophic form (atrophic thyroiditis or primary myxedema).
- Treatment with immunosuppressive agents (corticosteroids) is not recommended in autoimmune thyroiditis. Lifelong substitution therapy with L-thyroxine is indicated in hypothyroid patients.
- Among children living in areas of iodine sufficiency, juvenile lymphocytic thyroiditis is the cause of euthyroid goiter in about one-half to two-thirds of patients.
- Silent thyroiditis is characterized by transient thyrotoxicosis with low thyroid radioiodine uptake and a small, painless, nontender goiter.
- The postpartum rebound of immunity may be accompanied by destructive thyroiditis (postpartum thyroiditis), resulting in transient thyrotoxicosis evolving to hypothyroidism, or hypothyroidism alone, followed by gradual recovery.
- Subacute thyroiditis is a spontaneously remitting, painful, inflammatory disease of the thyroid, probably of viral origin. Treatment involves the administration of salicylates, other non steroidal anti-inflammatory drugs, or corticosteroids.
- The differential diagnosis of anterior neck pain includes subacute thyroiditis, hemorrhage into a thyroid nodule, Hashimoto's thyroiditis of acute onset (rare), acute suppurative thyroiditis, pharyngitis, globus hystericus, and rapidly growing malignancies (anaplastic carcinoma or lymphoma).
- Acute suppurative thyroiditis is a rare, serious, bacterial inflammatory disease of the thyroid. Infection to the thyroid occurs by hematogenous seeding, via the lymphatics, by extension from adjacent infected structures, by direct trauma, or through persistent thyroglossal duct or left pyriform sinus fistula.
- Riedel's thyroiditis is a rare chronic inflammatory disorder of unknown etiology, characterized by dense fibrosis of the thyroid and adjacent tissues. A generalized fibrosing disease (fibrous mediastinitis, retroperitoneal fibrosis, retro-orbital fibrosis, sclerosing cholangitis, and pancreatitis) occurs in one-third of patients.

The term *thyroiditis* encompasses a heterogeneous group of inflammatory disorders involving the thyroid gland, of which the etiologies range from autoimmune to infectious origins. The clinical course may be acute, subacute, or chronic. A classification of thyroiditis is depicted in Table 15.1.

Table 15.1 A classification of thyroiditis

I. Autoimmune thyroiditis
  Chronic autoimmune thyroiditis
    Hashimoto's thyroiditis
    Atrophic thyroiditis
    Focal thyroiditis
    Juvenile thyroiditis
  Silent thyroiditis
  Postpartum thyroiditis
 	
II. Subacute thyroiditis
 	
III. Acute suppurative thyroiditis
 	
IV. Rare forms of infectious thyroiditis
 	
V. Riedel's thyroiditis

AUTOIMMUNE THYROIDITIS

Chronic autoimmune or lymphocytic *thyroiditis* presents with two clinical entities: a goitrous form (*Hashimoto's thyroiditis*), and an atrophic form (*atrophic thyroiditis* or primary myxedema). Clinical variants include *juvenile thyroiditis* (lymphocytic thyroiditis of childhood and adolescence) and focal or *minimal thyroiditis*. *Silent* (painless) *thyroiditis* and *postpartum thyroiditis* also recognize an autoimmune origin, but in most cases their clinical courses are transient.

Organ-specific autoimmunity is the cause of Hashimoto's thyroiditis and atrophic thyroiditis. In both diseases the thyroid is infiltrated by lymphocytes, thyroid antibodies are present in serum, and there is a clinical or immunological overlap with other autoimmune diseases. Chronic autoimmune thyroiditis occurs frequently in certain families, particularly among the female members. Susceptibility genes include major histocompatibility complex (MHC) class I, class II, and class III genes, T-cell receptor and immunoglobulin genes, and cytokine regulatory genes. In Caucasian patients, a weak association of HLA-DR5 with Hashimoto's thyroiditis and of HLA-DR3 with atrophic thyroiditis was reported. Autoimmune thyroiditis is more common in patients with Down's syndrome or Turner's syndrome than in the general population. Endogenous susceptibility factors include sex hormones, which determine the marked prevalence of thyroid autoimmunity in women, and glucocorticoids. Environmental factors such as infectious agents, therapeutically administered interferon (IFN) alpha and interleukin (IL) 2, physical and emotional stress, and increased iodine intake may be important for the development of autoimmune thyroiditis. The mechanisms leading to the activation of thyroid-reactive T cells in autoimmune thyroiditis are discussed in Chapter 72. Once activated, autoreactive T-helper cells recruit cytotoxic T cells and B cells into the thyroid. The direct killing of thyroid cells by cytotoxic T

cells expressing perforin is probably the main destructive mechanism. T cells also cause tissue injury by release of cytokines. Interleukin (IL) 1, tumor necrosis factor alpha, and interferon gamma variably impair thyroid function. Thyrocyte apoptosis may contribute to follicular destruction. Thyroglobulin (Tg) antibodies (TgAb) may form Tg-TgAb immune complexes along the basal membrane of thyroid follicles. Thyroid peroxidase (TPO) antibodies (TPOAb) fix complement, but they probably exert a secondary destructive mechanism, requiring a primary disruptive event to allow antibody access to the intrafollicular site of TPO expression. Tissue injury itself causes complement activation and accounts for the presence of membrane attack complexes of complement on thyroid cells. Antibody-dependent, cell-mediated cytotoxicity involving natural killer cells is an additional mechanism of tissue destruction. Thyroid-stimulating hormone (TSH)-receptor antibodies (TRAb) blocking the action of TSH (TSH-blocking Ab, TSHBAb) occur in up to 20% of patients with atrophic thyroiditis and contribute to the development of hypothyroidism and thyroid atrophy. Antibodies to the Na+/I-symporter may also be involved in the pathogenesis of thyroid dysfunction. Antibodies to thyroxine (T4) and 3,5,3'-triiodothyronine (T3) are occasionally found in patients with autoimmune thyroiditis, but, with rare exceptions, do not affect thyroid function.

Goitrous *Hashimoto's thyroiditis* is characterized by lymphocytic infiltration with plasma cells and germinal centers, follicular destruction, colloid depletion, and fibrosis. Thyroid cells may show an oxyphilic cytoplasm (Hürthle or Askanazy cells). In *atrophic thyroiditis*, the gland is reduced in size, with lymphocytic infiltration and fibrosis replacing the thyroid parenchyma. Thyroid follicle destruction is mild and lymphocytic infiltration is minimal in focal thyroiditis. In *juvenile thyroiditis* oxyphil cells, fibrosis, and germinal centers are less prominent or absent. In *silent* and *postpartum thyroiditis* the thyroid is infiltrated with lymphocytes and thyroid follicles are collapsed, but germinal centers and Hürthle cells are absent.

CHRONIC AUTOIMMUNE THYROIDITIS

Epidemiology

Chronic autoimmune thyroiditis is the most common cause of spontaneously acquired hypothyroidism in populations with sufficient iodine intake. Severe forms of autoimmune thyroiditis are detected at autopsy in 5 to 15% of women and in 1 to 5% of men. The disease is most often diagnosed between the ages of 50 and 60 years, and it is 5 to 7 times more frequent in women than in men. The prevalence of thyroid antibodies, which correlates with at least some degree of autoimmune thyroiditis, increases from 6 to 15% in the second to third decades of life to more than 21 to 27% in women 60 years old or older. In communities with sufficient iodine intake, elevated serum TSH concentrations mainly result from chronic autoimmune thyroiditis. In these populations, subclinical hypothyroidism is found in 8 to 17% of subjects older than 55 to 60 years, and overt hypothyroidism is found in 1.7 to 3% of elderly women. The rate of hypothyroidism is higher in women than in men, and higher in whites than in blacks. In recent years, chronic autoimmune thyroiditis has been diagnosed more frequently than in the past due to both improved diagnostic procedures and to an increased number of affected cases. The increased iodine consumption that occurred in Western countries in the past few generations may explain this phenomenon.

Clinical findings

Patients may present with a goiter, with hypothyroidism, or both. In many patients the diagnosis is made because tests done for unrelated complaints reveal thyroid dysfunction or thyroid antibodies. On physical examination most Hashimoto's glands are diffusely enlarged, but one lobe may be larger than the other, and the pyramidal lobe may be palpable. The goiter is generally moderate in size, though massive enlargements may occur. The gland is nontender, firm or rubbery in consistency, with a bosselated surface. If left untreated, the goiter either remains unchanged or enlarges gradually over many years. A feeling of tightness in the neck may occur, but compression of the trachea is uncommon. Rapid growth of the goiter and compressive symptoms should raise the suspicion of thyroid lymphoma.

Patients may present with complaints of hypothyroidism, but for each patient with overt thyroid failure, several have subclinical hypothyroidism. Patients with atrophic thyroiditis exclusively present with hypothyroidism. The incidence rate for the development of hypothyroidism in women increases with age, with 51% of cases diagnosed between 45 and 64 years of age. Thyrotoxicosis (*Hashitoxicosis*) rarely occurs, due to a combination of Hashimoto's thyroiditis with Graves' disease in the same patient or to the transient discharge of preformed thyroid hormones as a result of the inflammatory process. Hyperthyroidism in patients with a combination of Graves' and Hashimoto's disorders is produced by TSH-receptor antibodies with thyroid stimulating (TSAb) activity and is indistinguishable from that of only Graves' disease. The only differences with Graves' disease are that the goiter is firmer, the titers of TPOAb and TgAb are higher, and the chance of spontaneous remission of hyperthyroidism is higher.

Diagnostic procedures

Laboratory evaluation includes tests for thyroid autoimmunity, thyroid echography, and assays for TSH and free T_4 (fT_4). Serum *TPOAb* are detectable in up to 95% of patients with Hashimoto's thyroiditis and 90% of those with atrophic thyroiditis. *TgAb* are less frequently positive in patients with both types of autoimmune thyroiditis. High titers ($\geq 1/1000$) of TPOAb and/or TgAb are almost exclusively observed in clinically overt thyroid autoimmune diseases, but low or undetectable titers are encountered in a few patients with chronic autoimmune thyroiditis (seronegative Hashimoto's thyroiditis). Conversely, low to medium titers of TPOAb and/or TgAb are found in a minority of normal subjects, and in patients with nontoxic goiter, subacute thyroiditis, or thyroid carcinoma. Thus, the diagnostic specificity of thyroid antibody tests is not absolute. Antibodies to thyroid hormones may interfere with the measurement of serum T_4 or T_3 and result in falsely high or low thyroid hormone levels, depending on the assay used.

Thyroid radionuclide scan is not crucial to the diagnosis, and shows either a diffuse, patchy uptake or a pattern that may mimic hypofunctioning or hyperfunctioning nodules (pseudo toxic adenoma). Values of thyroid radioactive iodine uptake (RAIU) may be normal, low, or high in Hashimoto's thyroiditis. An ultrasound pattern of the thyroid, characterized by a diffusely reduced echogenicity, is found in chronic autoimmune thyroiditis (Fig. 15.1). In the assessment of most patients fine needle aspiration biopsy (FNAB) is not necessary, but it is advisable in those with suspicious nodules or a rapidly enlarging goiter in order to rule out malignancy. Cytological smears of Hashimoto's thyroiditis are rich in lymphocytes and oxyphil cells (Fig. 15.2, see Color Atlas).

An increase in serum TSH concentration, either at the basal level or after TRH stimulation, may occur long before any decline in serum fT_4 levels (subclinical hypothyroidism). Decreased serum concentrations of fT_4, and less frequently of free T_3 (fT_3), are observed in overt hypothyroidism; but low serum fT_3, and less frequently fT_4 levels, may be found in patients with non-thyroidal illnesses. An increased serum TSH concentration is the single best diagnostic test for primary hypothyroidism. Because rare cases of peripheral resistance to thyroid hormones are an exception to this rule, fT_4 assays are needed as a second key test.

The diagnosis of chronic autoimmune thyroiditis is based on the detection of a typical Hashimoto's goiter and/or hypothyroidism (either overt or subclinical). Positive tests for thyroid antibodies support the diagnosis, but they are not completely specific. Thyroid echography, by showing a hypoechogenic pattern of the goiter in Hashimoto's thyroiditis or a gland reduced in size in atrophic thyroiditis, provides confirmatory evidence. In euthyroid patients with seronegative Hashimoto's thyroiditis, the ultimate diagnosis may require FNAB. In iodine-deficient areas, differentiation of Hashimoto's thyroiditis from nontoxic multinodular goiter with focal thyroiditis may be difficult, and intermediate conditions are encountered. Differentiation between Hashimoto's thyroiditis with a prominent "nodule" and thyroid carcinoma requires FNAB. A rapidly enlarging nodule with regional lymphadenopathy suggests thyroid malignancy.

Complications

Up to 5% of patients with thyroid-associated ophthalmopathy have chronic autoimmune thyroiditis with hypothyroidism. A peculiar encephalopathy with stroke-

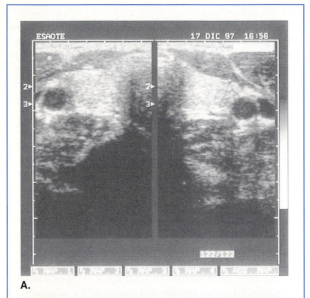

A.

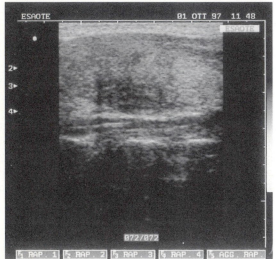

B.

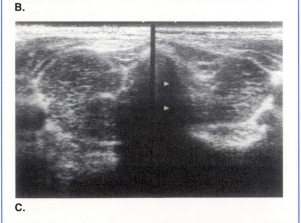

C.

Figure 15.1 Thyroid ultrasound. (**A**) Normal thyroid. (**B**) Subacute thyroiditis: multiple ill-defined hypoechogenic areas in the parenchyma. (**C**) Hashimoto's thyroiditis: diffuse hypoechogenic pattern of the parenchyma. (Courtesy of Dr. T. Rago, Department of Endocrinology, University of Pisa.)

like episodes, seizures, or altered consciousness has been observed in euthyroid patients with Hashimoto's thyroiditis, though rarely. Patients with chronic autoimmune thyroiditis are prone to develop other autoimmune conditions, as suggested by the presence in their serum of autoantibodies to adrenal cortex (1-2%), pancreatic islet cells (1-3%), gastric parietal cells (10-30%), intrinsic factor (1%), DNA, mitochondria, phospholipids, or IgG. Chronic autoimmune thyroiditis is a component of type 2 autoimmune polyglandular syndrome, a condition characterized by the coexistence of two or more of the following disorders: Addison's disease, autoimmune thyroiditis, insulin dependent diabetes mellitus, atrophic gastritis with or without pernicious anemia, vitiligo, alopecia, myasthenia gravis, and hypophysitis. Other disorders that may also occur in association with chronic autoimmune thyroiditis are premature ovarian failure, celiac disease, psoriasis, rheumatoid arthritis, systemic lupus erythematosus, Sjögren's syndrome, polymyalgia rheumatica, temporal arteritis, chronic active hepatitis, biliary cirrhosis, and systemic sclerosis. Focal thyroiditis is seen in many patients with papillary thyroid carcinoma, and it may represent a secondary immune response to the cancer. In patients with Hashimoto's thyroiditis, the prevalence of primary lymphomas of the thyroid is 80 times greater than expected, and most patients with this malignancy have pre-existent Hashimoto's thyroiditis. Despite this increased incidence, lymphomas of the thyroid remain rare tumors.

Treatment

Immunosuppressive agents such as corticosteroids are not recommended in a benign disease that can be safely and economically treated with L-thyroxine (L-T_4). Corticosteroids cause some regression of Hashimoto's goiter and decrease thyroid antibody titers, but the activity of the disease returns after treatment is withdrawn.

Patients with overt hypothyroidism require substitution therapy with L-T_4 at a dose that normalizes serum TSH levels. The average daily replacement dose of L-T_4 in adults is 1.6 µg/kg body weight. Full replacement doses are 75-100 µg per day in most women and 100-150 µg per day in most men. Elderly hypothyroid patients require a dose 20 to 30% lower. In hypothyroid patients with coexistent cardiac disease, L-T_4 therapy should be initiated with 12.5-25 µg per day, followed by careful increments of 12.5-25 µg per day every 4 to 8 weeks. L-T_4 substitution may precipitate angina or myocardial infarction in the elderly with coronary artery disease, but it ameliorates reversible coronary dysfunction inherent with hypothyroidism and produces beneficial effects on hypothyroid hyperlipidemia. Coronary by-pass or angioplasty can be safely performed before starting L-T_4 administration. Long-term L-T_4 substitution was not found to reduce bone mineral density, provided that serum TSH concentrations are kept in the normal range. Successful L-T_4 therapy is often accompanied by a decrease in thyroid antibody titers in patients with elevated serum TSH levels before treatment. Indications for L-

T_4 substitution therapy in subclinical hypothyroidism are not univocal, but an improvement in some hypothyroid features was observed in two placebo-controlled trials of L-T_4 therapy. Restoration of normal TSH levels with L-T_4 also produces a slight reduction in the elevated serum cholesterol levels sometimes observed in patients with subclinical hypothyroidism. We advise replacement therapy when serum TSH concentration is higher than 10 mU/l, and in those patients with borderline high serum TSH (5-10 mU/l) and positive thyroid antibody who are at high risk for progression to overt hypothyroidism. The presence of goiter and symptoms consistent with thyroid hormone deficiency favor treatment. Substitution treatment should be lifelong because hypothyroidism tends to recur when therapy is discontinued. A spontaneous recovery of thyroid function that persists when L-T_4 treatment is withdrawn occasionally occurs when hypothyroidism has been precipitated by dietary or pharmacological iodine overload, by administration of lithium or cytokines, or when TSHBAb present in serum before starting L-T_4 treatment disappear in the subsequent follow-up. The permanence of such remissions is uncertain, but most of these patients might not remain euthyroid during the follow-up. Untreated euthyroid patients with autoimmune thyroiditis require periodic thyroid function tests: once a year in patients with Hashimoto's thyroiditis and every 6 months in those with a gland reduced in size.

The proper treatment of euthyroid Hashimoto's goiter is controversial. The use of L-T_4 may be considered for two main reasons. The first is that an average of 30% reduction in goiter size was observed in several trials, although in our and other's experience shrinkage of goiter is mainly observed in patients with elevated serum TSH levels before L-T_4 treatment. The second reason pertains to the possible evolution to hypothyroidism and to the fact that L-T_4 therapy may limit a further growth of goiter. The decision to treat with L-T_4 is optional. Surgery is indicated, though this happens rarely, in cases of extremely large Hashimoto's goiters with obstructive symptoms, or when associated thyroid malignancy is suspected. L-T_4 therapy is mandatory after surgery, as hypothyroidism invariably results.

Prognosis

Overt hypothyroidism can develop in patients who are euthyroid or have subclinical hypothyroidism when first seen, but the progression is slow and takes several years. Temporary remissions of subclinical hypothyroidism may also occur. In the follow-up study performed in Whickham, the annual rate of developing overt hypothyroidism was 4.3% in women with both raised serum TSH (>6 mU/l) and positive thyroid antibodies, 2.6% if only TSH was raised, and 2.1% if only thyroid antibodies were positive. Even a serum TSH level at the upper limit of the normal range (>2-4 mU/l) was associated with an increased probability of hypothyroidism. Graves' hyperthyroidism occasionally develops in patients with hypothyroidism caused by chronic autoimmune thyroiditis and is believed to result from a change in the nature of TSH-receptor anti-

bodies from blocking to stimulating. The opposite evolution from hyperthyroidism to hypothyroidism may also occur due to changes in the biological activity of TRAb or to the progressive destruction of thyroid parenchyma produced by autoimmune thyroiditis. Hypothyroidism due to chronic autoimmune thyroiditis ultimately supervenes in 10 to 20% of patients with Graves' hyperthyroidism who remain in remission after anti-thyroid drugs. Euthyroid patients with chronic autoimmune thyroiditis are more susceptible to the antithyroid effects of excess iodine, and amiodarone is a common cause of iodine-induced hypothyroidism in these patients. Hypothyroidism may develop in up to one-third of patients treated with lithium and is more common in those with thyroid antibodies. Therapy with IFN-α, IL-2 or granulocyte-macrophage colony-stimulating factor may be associated with the development of thyroid antibodies, transient thyrotoxicosis, hypothyroidism or both, primarily in patients who have thyroid antibodies before therapy. Smoking increases the risk of hypothyroidism in patients with autoimmune thyroiditis.

JUVENILE THYROIDITIS

Among children and adolescents living in areas of iodine sufficiency, *juvenile (lymphocytic) thyroiditis* is the cause of euthyroid goiter in one-half to two-thirds of patients. Atrophic thyroiditis may also occur and is associated with hypothyroidism. Thyroid antibodies are less frequently positive than in adults. FNAB may be needed to establish the diagnosis. In a 20-year follow-up study of goitrous juvenile thyroiditis, spontaneous resolutions occurred in about 25%, but hypothyroidism developed in 33% of patients. Elevated serum TSH indicates the need for L-T_4 therapy. If serum TSH is normal, L-T_4 may not diminish thyromegaly, but the effects of hypothyroidism will be prevented in those patients progressing to thyroid failure.

SILENT THYROIDITIS

Silent (painless) thyroiditis is characterized by transient thyrotoxicosis with low RAIU, and a small, painless, nontender goiter. Silent thyroiditis occurs either sporadically or in the postpartum period (postpartum thyroiditis). The overall prevalence of silent thyroiditis as a cause of thyrotoxicosis ranges from 4 to 15%, but the latter figure appears high. A seasonal and geographic variation in the prevalence has been reported, with those areas previously iodine-deficient, but recently exposed to sufficient iodine, having a greater prevalence. The female/male ratio is approximately 2/1. Thyrotoxicosis results from damage of the follicular cells by the inflammatory process, with leakage of preformed thyroid hormones in the bloodstream. The inflammatory process impairs the capacity of the thyroid to make thyroid hormone. As a consequence, patients undergo a euthyroid phase and then, when thyroidal hormone stores are depleted, become hypothyroid. Most cases of silent thyroiditis recognize an autoimmune pathogenesis. Silent thyroiditis has been reported in patients with other autoimmune disorders, with a personal or family history of thyroid autoimmunity, and in those experiencing a rebound of immunity after treatment of Cushing's syndrome. An infectious etiology has been hypothesized in some patients, but no infective agent has been identified. Excess iodide intake, amiodarone, IFN-α and IL-2, simple palpation, or parathyroid surgery have been reported as initiating events of silent thyroiditis.

Silent thyroiditis presents with a relatively abrupt onset of symptoms of mild thyrotoxicosis (tachycardia, heat intolerance, sweating, nervousness, and weight loss). The thyroid may be normal in size (50% of cases), or a small, modestly firm, nontender goiter may be palpable. After 2 to 9 weeks thyrotoxicosis subsides, and patients progress to euthyroid and hypothyroid phases before recovering normal thyroid function. About 40% have a hypothyroid phase, which usually lasts between 4 and 10 weeks. Euthyroidism is ultimately restored in most cases, but persistent hypothyroidism may also develop (5%). Recurrences may develop in up to 11% of cases. Impaired thyroid reserve or goiter may occur after a bout of silent thyroiditis.

Free T_4 and free T_3 are elevated in the thyrotoxic phase, but the increase of T_4 relative to T_3 is disproportionate owing to the release of preformed thyroid hormones into the circulation. Serum Tg and urinary iodide concentrations are also increased. Radioactive iodine uptake is suppressed (often 1-2% at 24 hours). The erythrocyte sedimentation rate is normal or only slightly elevated. The white blood cell count is usually normal. TPOAb and TgAb are present in sera of 60% and 25% of patients, respectively. Serum TSH levels are low in the thyrotoxic phase, but they may increase to hypothyroid levels before recovery. Silent thyroiditis should be considered in all cases of thyrotoxicosis with low RAIU and a nontender gland. Other causes of thyrotoxicosis with low RAIU should be excluded, such as thyrotoxicosis factitia (serum Tg is low), iodine-induced hyperthyroidism (uri-

nary iodine excretion >1000 μg/24 h), or ectopic thyroid hormone production (*struma ovarii*). Differentiation from Graves' hyperthyroidism is important (Tab. 15.2). FNAB reveals lymphocytic thyroiditis, but it is usually not necessary to make the diagnosis. Thyroid ultrasound shows decreased echogenicity.

Anti-thyroid drugs or radioiodine are inappropriate for the treatment of silent thyroiditis, because thyrotoxicosis is due to the release of preformed thyroid hormones. Thyrotoxic symptoms are managed with β-adrenergic blocking agents, such as propranolol (20 to 40 mg orally 3 to 4 times daily). Prednisone, started at 40 to 60 mg per day orally and then tapered over 4 weeks, causes a decline of T_4 and T_3 serum concentrations within 7 to 10 days. L-T_4 replacement therapy is usually not needed because symptoms of hypothyroidism are often mild and transient. When hypothyroidism is symptomatic, a suboptimal replacement dose of L-T_4 should be given, and then it should be tapered after 6 months and the patient should be checked to determine whether recovery has occurred.

AUTOIMMUNE THYROIDITIS DURING PREGNANCY AND POSTPARTUM

Chronic autoimmune thyroiditis, mainly asymptomatic, is relatively common in women of childbearing age. During pregnancy all autoimmune reactions are inhibited by a number of physiologic factors, and following delivery there is a reversal of these alterations with a rebound of autoimmune phenomena. Thus, TPOAb, TgAb, and TRAb decrease or may even disappear during the third trimester of pregnancy, but a rebound increase is observed after delivery. Most patients with asymptomatic chronic autoimmune thyroiditis remain euthyroid during pregnancy, but a few show a mild deterioration of thyroid function with a slight increase in serum TSH (up to 5-10 mU/l) at the end of pregnancy. It is therefore recommended that in these women serum TSH and fT$_4$ levels are checked between 28 and 32 weeks of gestation. Hypothyroid patients with autoimmune thyroiditis on replacement therapy frequently require an increase in the dose of L-T_4 during pregnancy, which mainly occurs in the first trimester of gestation and is highlighted by an

---

Table 15.2 Differentiation between silent thyroiditis and Graves' disease

	Silent thyroiditis	Graves' disease
Onset	Abrupt	Gradual
Severity of thyrotoxicosis	Mild-moderate	Moderate-marked
Duration of symptoms	<3 months	>3 months
Thyroid bruit	Absent	May be present
Ophthalmopathy, dermopathy	Absent	May be present
T_3 (ng/ml)/T_4 (μg/dl) ratio	<20/1	Mostly >20/1
RAIU	Low	High
TSH-R antibodies	Usually negative	Usually positive
Thyrotoxicosis	Transient	Persistent

(T_3 = triiodothyronine; T_4 = thyroxine; TSH-R = thyroid-stimulating hormone receptor; RAIU = radioactive iodine uptake.)

elevation in serum TSH level. The dose of L-T$_4$ should be adjusted to keep serum TSH within normal limits. TPOAb and TgAb cross the placenta, but they do not directly damage the fetal thyroid. Because of this, the incidence of congenital hypothyroidism is not increased in neonates of mothers with autoimmune thyroiditis. The rare neonates born to mothers with atrophic thyroiditis and serum TSHBAb may develop transient neonatal hypothyroidism, hence the determination of TSH-receptor antibodies in pregnant women with atrophic thyroiditis is indicated.

The rebound of immunity that follows delivery may be accompanied by destruction thyroiditis resulting in transient thyrotoxicosis evolving to hypothyroidism, or by hypothyroidism occurring de novo, followed by gradual recovery (*postpartum thyroiditis, PPT*). The incidence of PPT ranges from 1.1 to 16.7% in different studies. Risk factors for the development of PPT include: positive TPOAb in the first trimester of pregnancy, type I diabetes mellitus, a history of chronic autoimmune thyroiditis or Graves' disease, or a previous episode of PPT during a preceding pregnancy. Circulating TPOAb are found in the majority of women with PPT. Thyroid biopsies show diffuse lymphocytic infiltration.

The classical clinical course (Fig. 15.3) is observed in about 26% of patients. The first phase, within 2 to 3 months after delivery, is characterized by mild symptoms of thyrotoxicosis and lasts from 1 to 6 weeks. Mild hypothyroidism of 2 to 6 weeks' duration may then occur between 3 and 8 months after delivery. Lack of energy, poor memory, dry skin and cold intolerance predominate. Postpartum depression is more common in women with positive thyroid antibodies irrespective of their thyroid status. A small, diffuse, firm, nontender, usually painless

goiter is palpable. Spontaneous recovery of thyroid function occurs in most patients. Transient thyrotoxicosis alone or transient hypothyroidism alone occurs in 38% and 36% of patients, respectively. Persistent hypothyroidism develops in 20 to 30% of patients.

Postpartum thyroiditis is suspected in women who have fatigue, palpitation, emotional lability or goiter during the first year after delivery. Thyroid hormone and TSH changes are similar to those found in silent thyroiditis. High titers of TPOAb are found in most patients. Serum Tg is elevated. Diffuse or multifocal reduction of thyroid echogenicity is found at ultrasound. The differential diagnosis with Graves' hyperthyroidism, which may actually appear or relapse in the postpartum period, is based on the same criteria suggested for silent thyroiditis (Tab. 15.2). RAIU evaluation using ^{123}I may be ordered, but breast feeding should be interrupted for at least 3 days. Long-term follow-up of thyroid function is mandatory in patients with PPT.

Administration of β-adrenergic blocking drugs ameliorates symptoms of thyrotoxicosis. In patients with marked hypothyroid symptoms, L-T$_4$ treatment at medium-low dose (50-75 µg/day) is required, and it should be maintained for the first year after parturition. Thereafter an attempt to withdraw therapy should be done to check whether hypothyroidism is transient or permanent.

SUBACUTE THYROIDITIS

Subacute (granulomatous) thyroiditis is a spontaneously remitting, painful, inflammatory disease of the thyroid, probably of viral origin. It is the most frequent cause of anterior neck pain. The disease is most prevalent in the temperate zone, has a seasonal distribution (summer and fall), and afflicts more frequently women between the third and sixth decades of life. Subacute thyroiditis is often preceded by an upper respiratory tract infection and occurs in coincidence with outbreaks of viral diseases (mumps, measles, influenza). Elevated titers of viral antibodies (coxsackievirus, adenovirus, mumps) have been found in convalescent sera of patients with subacute thyroiditis, but a specific viral agent has not been identified. While subacute thyroiditis is not an autoimmune disease, serum thyroid antibodies may appear transiently during the course of the disorder. Following recovery, all elements of the immune response disappear, except in rare patients who progress to persistent hypothyroidism. Histopathological changes include infiltration with neutrophils and mononuclear cells, disruption of follicles, and a typical lesion characterized by a central core of colloid surrounded by a large number of individual histiocytes (giant multinucleated cells) (Fig. 15.2, see Color Atlas). With recovery inflammation recedes and follicular regeneration appears. The release of preformed thyroid hormones from disrupted follicles is responsible for the initial thyrotoxicosis. Later in the disease, when thyroid hormone stores are depleted, hypothyroidism ensues

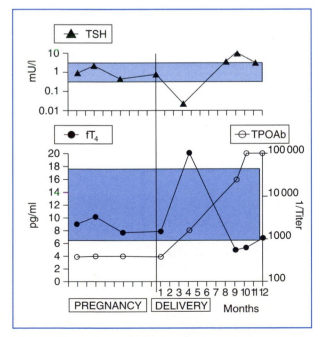

Figure 15.3 A case of postpartum thyroiditis. The shaded area indicates the normal range. (TSH = thyroid-stimulating hormone; fT$_4$ = free thyroxine; TPOAb = thyroid peroxidase antibodies.)

and serum TSH concentration rises. With recovery, the thyroid rebuilds its hormone stores, serum T_4 rises, and serum TSH normalizes.

There is usually a viral prodrome with myalgias, low-grade fever, sore-throat and dysphagia, or an upper respiratory tract infection. Anterior neck pain occurs abruptly, is sometimes unilateral, and may radiate to the ear, mandible or occiput. With progression of the disease, pain may shift to the contralateral lobe (creeping thyroiditis). Moving the head, swallowing, or coughing aggravate the pain. In a few patients, however, pain is entirely lacking. Systemic symptoms (malaise, fatigue, myalgia, and fever) may occur together with symptoms of thyrotoxicosis. On palpation the thyroid is slightly to moderately enlarged, sometimes asymmetrical or even nodular, firm, and exquisitely tender and painful. Pain causes the patient to withdraw from the fingers of the examiner. The course of the disease may last 2 to 6 months without treatment. Thyrotoxicosis occurs during the initial inflammatory phase in half of the patients, and persists for 3 to 8 weeks. An interval of euthyroidism may then occur, followed in one- to two-thirds of patients by transient hypothyroidism. Most patients enter a recovery stage in 4 to 8 weeks and regain normal thyroid function. Some patients with subacute thyroiditis go directly from the painful to the recovery phase. Recurrences are reported in about one-fifth of the patients. While permanent hypothyroidism is rare (1-5%), the disease may evolve into chronic autoimmune thyroiditis. A few patients have been reported to progress to Graves' disease.

Patients with subacute thyroiditis have an elevated erythrocyte sedimentation rate (>55 mm/h), normal or slightly elevated leukocyte counts, and increased serum IL-6 and Tg concentrations during the thyrotoxic phase. Thyroid antibodies (mainly TgAb) are transiently detectable at low titer in a minority of patients. Serum T_4 and T_3 concentrations may be high, normal or low depending on the phase of the disease (Tab. 15.3). The serum TSH level is low but not completely suppressed during the thyrotoxic phase, it is usually high in the hypothyroid phase, and it normalizes during recovery. During the thyrotoxic phase RAIU is less than 2 to 5% at 24 hours. Isotope thyroid scans show a cold area in the involved section of the gland, a patchy and irregular pattern, or no uptake at all. Thyroid ultrasound shows multi-

ple ill-defined hypoechogenic areas in the parenchyma (Fig. 15.1).

Table 15.4 summarizes the differential diagnosis of a painful anterior neck. With hemorrhage into a pre-existing thyroid nodule, pain is localized, erythrocyte sedimentation rate is not markedly elevated, and fever and bacterial toxicity are absent. Hashimoto's thyroiditis of acute onset may be associated with pain, but RAIU is rarely completely suppressed. Acute suppurative thyroiditis is differentiated by a much greater inflammatory reaction, high leukocytic counts, and febrile responses. Thyroid palpation excludes pharyngitis. In globus hystericus, patients complain of pressure or feeling a ball in the throat, but there is no specific thyroid enlargement or tenderness. During thyrotoxicosis, Graves' disease can be differentiated by the lack of accompanying neck pain and by the elevated RAIU. In patients with sudden painful enlargement of the thyroid gland, FNAB is indicated to exclude malignancies with extensive infiltration of the gland (anaplastic carcinoma or lymphoma).

Treatment

In milder cases, salicylates or non steroidal anti-inflammatory drugs provide some relief of pain and tenderness. In more severe subacute thyroiditis, corticosteroids (prednisone: 40 to 60 mg/day, or analogues at equivalent anti-inflammatory dosage) have a more dramatic and rapid effect. Relief of local and constitutional symptoms often occur within 24 hours. The corticosteroid is slowly tapered over the next 6 to 8 weeks and then discontinued.

Table 15.4 Differential diagnosis of anterior neck pain

Subacute thyroiditis
Acute hemorrhage into a thyroid nodule or cyst
Acute suppurative thyroiditis
Painful Hashimoto's thyroiditis
Infected thyroglossal duct cyst
Infected branchial cleft cyst, or cystic hygromas
Rapidly enlarging thyroid carcinoma
Cellulitis of anterior neck
Radiation thyroiditis
Musculoskeletal disorders
Pharyngeal inflammatory disease
Globus hystericus

Table 15.3 Laboratory findings during different phases of subacute thyroiditis

Phase	T_4 and/or T_3 level	TSH level	RAIU value
Thyrotoxic	High	Low	<5%
Hypothyroid	Low	Low, normal or high	Normal to high
Recovery	Normal	High to normal	High to normal

(T_4 = thyroxine; T_3 = triiodothyronine; TSH = thyroid-stimulating hormone; RAIU = radioactive iodine uptake.)

In 10 to 20% of patients recurrences occur as the dosage is reduced, which necessitates the restoration of a higher dose once again. Antibiotics are of no value. Thyroidectomy is rarely if ever indicated, but it should be considered in rare patients with a prolonged and recurrent course and with pain unresponsive to anti-inflammatory therapy. Symptoms of thyrotoxicosis should be managed with β-adrenergic blocking agents (propranolol: 20-40 mg, 3 to 4 times daily). Anti-thyroid drugs and radioiodine are ineffective. The hypothyroid phase is usually mild, thus L-T_4 replacement is needed only in a few patients. It is prudent to periodically check thyroid status after recovery from subacute thyroiditis.

ACUTE SUPPURATIVE THYROIDITIS AND RARE FORMS OF INFECTIOUS THYROIDITIS

Acute suppurative thyroiditis is a rare, serious, bacterial inflammatory disease of the thyroid. Etiologic agents include *Staphylococcus aureus, Streptococcus pyogenes, Streptococcus pneumoniae*, Enterobacteriaceae (*Escherichia coli, Pseudomonas aeruginosa, Salmonella typhi*), and anaerobes of the oropharyngeal cavity. Infection to the thyroid occurs by hematogenous seeding from distant foci, by extension from adjacent infected structures, by direct trauma, through a persistent thyroglossal duct or left pyriform sinus fistula. Patients present with severe anterior neck pain of abrupt onset, dysphagia, dysphonia, fever, rigor, and diaphoresis. Palpation shows a unilateral or less-frequently bilateral tender swelling of the thyroid that may be fluctuant and is associated with cervical lymphadenopathy. The skin over the infected nodule is erythematous and warm. The white cell count and erythrocyte sedimentation rate are elevated. Thyroid antibodies are absent. Serum T_4 and T_3 levels are usually normal as well as thyroid RAIU. Isotope scans reveal a "cold" defect in the involved lobe. Ultrasonography shows an enlarged irregular mass of mixed echogenicity with sonolucent areas. The presence at fine-needle aspiration of purulent material is confirmatory of suppurative thyroiditis and allows for the identification of the causative agent. The thyroid is rarely the seat of tuberculosis, syphilis, fungal infections (*Aspergillus* species), or parasites. *Pneumocystis carinii* infection of the thyroid has been reported in patients with AIDS.

Treatment

Therapy of acute suppurative thyroiditis requires the administration of appropriate antibiotics based on the findings of the culture from a fine-needle aspirate, and surgical drainage (or excision) of any area of fluctuance or abscess. While awaiting the results of the culture, a combined regimen of nafcillin (due to the high frequency of infection with *S. aureus*) and gentamicin or a third generation cephalosporin would be appropriate in adults. In children, first line antimicrobial therapy should be directed to the oropharyngeal flora using cefoxitin or clindamicin. If a pyriform sinus fistula is identified, fistulectomy is warranted. Permanent sequelae are uncommon.

RIEDEL'S THYROIDITIS

Riedel's thyroiditis (sclerosing thyroiditis, invasive fibrous thyroiditis) is a rare, chronic inflammatory disorder of unknown etiology, characterized by dense fibrosis involving the thyroid and adjacent tissues. It occurs mainly in middle-age or elderly women. A generalized fibrosing disease is suggested by the association in one-third of patients with extracervical fibrosclerosis, which include fibrous mediastinitis, retroperitoneal fibrosis, retro-orbital fibrosis, sclerosing cholangitis, and pancreatitis. Pathology consists of an exuberant fibrosis with marked eosinophil infiltration involving the thyroid gland and extending beyond the capsule. A patient will present with a long history of a painless, progressively increasing anterior neck mass. Pressure symptoms (dysphagia, cough, hoarseness, stridor, attacks of suffocation) may appear. Examination reveals a stony-hard or woody thyroid mass that varies in size from small to very large, may involve one or both lobes, and is fixed to surrounding structures. Most patients are euthyroid. Thyroid antibodies are present in up to 45% of patients. Serum calcium may be low due to parathyroid invasion. Ultrasound and computerized tomography are useful to show the extent of the lesion. White cell count and erythrocyte sedimentation rate may be slightly elevated. Differentiation from thyroid carcinoma or lymphoma of the thyroid requires open biopsy, since FNAB may be difficult to interpret. Surgical treatment is necessary to relieve pressure on the trachea and to establish diagnosis. Subtotal thyroidectomy is hazardous, and wedge resection of the isthmus is the procedure of choice. While corticosteroids are of little or no value, Tamoxifen was recently suggested to have some effect. The course of the lesion may be slowly progressive, may stabilize, or remit. Mortality rate due to asphyxia ranges from 6 to 10%. Extrathyroidal fibrotic lesions may complicate the prognosis.

Suggested readings

BASGOZ N, SWARTZ MN. Infections of the thyroid gland. In: Braverman LE, Utiger RD (eds). Werner and Ingbar's the thyroid. 7th ed. Philadelphia: Lippincott-Raven Publishers, 1996;1049-56.

BOTTAZZO GF, MIRAKIAN R, DREXHAGE HA. Adrenalitis, oophoritis and autoimmune polyglandular disease. In: Rich RR, Fleischer TA, Schwartz DB, Shearer WT, Strober W (eds). Clinical immunology, principles and practice. St. Louis: Mosby, 1996;1523-36.

CHIOVATO L, FILETTI S, PINCHERA A. Clinical aspects of autoimmune thyroiditis. In: Andreoli M, Shields M (eds). Frontiers in endocrinology: Highlights in molecular and clinical endocrinology. Rome: Ares-Serono Symposia Publications. 1994;123-32.

CHIOVATO L, MARIOTTI S, PINCHERA A. Thyroid disease in the elderly. Baillière's Clin Endocrinol Metab 1997;11:251-70.

DAYAN C M, DANIELS GH. Chronic autoimmune thyroiditis. N Engl J Med 1996;335:99-107.

LAZARUS JH. Silent thyroiditis and subacute thyroiditis. In: Braverman LE, Utiger RD (eds). Werner and Ingbar's the thyroid. 7th Ed. Philadelphia: Lippincott-Raven Publishers, 1996;577-91.

LAZARUS JH. Postpartum thyroiditis. Thyroid International 1996;5:1-12.

MARTINO E, AGHINI-LOMBARDI F, BARTALENA L. Enhanced susceptibility to amiodarone-induced hypothyroidism in patients with thyroid autoimmune disease. Arch Int Med 1994;154:2722-6.

MESTMAN JH, GOODWIN M, MONTORO MM. Thyroid disorders of pregnancy. Endocrinol Metab Clin North Am 1995;24:41-71.

PINCHERA A, FENZI GF, BARTALENA L, CHIOVATO L, MARCOCCI C. Thyroiditis. In: De Visscher M (ed). The thyroid gland. New York: Raven Press, 1980;413-41.

VOLPE R. Autoimmune thyroiditis. In: Braverman LE, Utiger RD, (eds). Werner and Ingbar's the thyroid. 6th ed. Philadelphia: JB Lippincott, 1991;921-41.

VOLPE R. Subacute and sclerosing thyroiditis. In: DeGroot LJ (ed.). Endocrinology. Philadelphia: WB Saunders, 1995;742-51.

VOLPE R. Autoimmune thyroid diseases. In: Braverman LE (ed). Diseases of the thyroid. Totowa: Humana Press, 1997;125-54.

WANG C, CRAPO LM. The epidemiology of thyroid disease and implications for screening. Endocrinol Metab Clin North Am 1997;26:189-218.

WEETMAN AP. Chronic autoimmune thyroiditis. In: Braverman LE, Utiger RD (eds). Werner and Ingbar's the thyroid. 7th Ed. Philadelphia: Lippincott-Raven Publishers, 1996;738-48.

Thyroid cancer

Furio Pacini, Martin J. Schlumberger

■ KEY POINTS ■

- Thyroid carcinoma is the most common malignancy of the endocrine glands, though it only represents 1% or less of all human cancers.
- The great majority (60 to 80%) of cancers of the follicular thyroid epithelium are well-differentiated, papillary and follicular carcinomas that have a good prognosis, particularly in young patients.
- Thyroid cancer is one of the most curable cancers, with very high long-term survival rates for the well-differentiated histotypes.
- Some patients are at high-risk for recurrent disease or even death. Most of these patients can be identified at the time of diagnosis by using well-defined prognostic indicators.
- The incidence of thyroid nodules is about 1 per 1000 persons per year. Incidence of thyroid carcinoma ranges from 0.5 to 10 cases per 100 000 persons per year. Thus, 0.5 to 10% of thyroid nodules harbor a cancer.

Thyroid carcinoma is the most common malignancy of the endocrine glands, although it makes up only 1% or less of all human cancers. Cancers of the follicular thyroid epithelium include papillary and follicular histotypes, usually referred to as "differentiated thyroid carcinomas", and undifferentiated (or anaplastic) carcinoma. Those of the parafollicular epithelium (the C cells) are represented by medullary thyroid carcinoma.

The great majority (60-80%) are well-differentiated, papillary and follicular carcinomas that have a good prognosis, particularly in young patients. Undifferentiated thyroid carcinoma accounts for less than 10% of cases, is found in older age groups, and carries a very poor prognosis. Medullary thyroid carcinomas account for 5 to 10% of all thyroid carcinomas; they are differentiated carcinomas that retain the ability to secrete large amounts of calcitonin, and they are genetically determined in one-fourth of the cases. Much less frequent malignancies of the thyroid are lymphomas, sarcomas, and metastases from other cancers.

CANCERS OF THE FOLLICULAR THYROID EPITHELIUM

Epidemiology

The incidence of thyroid nodules is about 1 per 1000 persons per year. Incidence of thyroid carcinoma ranges from 0.5 to 10 cases per 100 000 persons per year. Thus, 0.5 to 10% of thyroid nodules harbor a cancer. This figure reflects well the incidence of clinically important thyroid carcinomas, but the diagnostic improvement, primarily by ultrasound and fine needle aspiration cytology (FNAC), increases the detection of minimal thyroid carcinomas that likely have no clinical relevance. Likewise, an accurate pathological examination of resected multinodular goiters may detect many occult tumors. Thus, the precise incidence of thyroid carcinoma is difficult to define.

Differentiated thyroid cancers are two to four times more frequent in women than in men. However, the female predominance decreases in prepubertal and post-menopausal ages, suggesting that sex hormones could have a pathogenetic role.

Thyroid cancer is one of the most curable cancers, with very high long-term survival rates, at least for the well-differentiated histotypes. However, some patients are at high-risk for recurrent disease or even death. Most of these patients can be identified at the time of diagnosis by using well-defined prognostic indicators.

Etiopathogenesis

Oncogenes

Gene rearrangements involving the RET and TRK proto-oncogenes have been demonstrated to be causative events specific to a subset of the papillary histotypes. The oncogenic activation of these genes is accomplished by the fusion of their tyrosine kinase domain with unlinked amino-terminal sequences of other genes in the same or other chromosomes of RET and TRK. TRK oncogenes are created by rearrangement of the NTK1 gene, which encodes a receptor for nerve growth factor; this links it to at least three different activating genes. In the case of RET rearrangements, the resulting chimeric oncogenes were called PTC as an acronym for papillary thyroid cancer. Three chimeric forms have been identified so far (RET/PTC 1, 2, and 3). Although strictly associated with papillary thyroid carcinoma, RET/PTC is found in only 3 to 33% of the cases not associated with radiation. In papillary thyroid carcinomas occurring after irradiation, the frequency of RET/PTC activation is between 60 and 80%, as in children of Belarus, who were heavily exposed to radiation after the Chernobyl nuclear disaster, and in patients who received external radiation treatment during childhood. The oncogene involved in these radiation-induced tumors is mainly RET/PTC 3, while in spontaneous tumors the RET/PTC 1 is predominant. This suggests that RET/PTC 3 could be specifically linked to radiation as a mutagenic event. Alternatively, RET/PTC activation, particularly type 3, might be a distinctive feature of papillary tumors arising in young patients (most Belarus cancers were diagnosed in children) independent of irradiation. The latter hypothesis is supported by a significant correlation between high rates of RET/PTC activation and lower age at diagnosis in Italian patients not exposed to radiation.

Mutated forms of the H-*ras* , K-*ras* , and N-*ras* oncogenes were found in differentiated thyroid cancer, but mutations are not specifically restricted to malignant lesions. Thus, mutations of the *ras* gene family might represent an early event in thyroid tumorigenesis. Activating mutations of genes encoding the thyroid-stimulating hormone (TSH) receptor and the subunit of the Gs protein, similar to those found in toxic adenomas, have been reported in few follicular carcinomas. Inactivating mutations of the p53 tumor-suppressor gene are rare in patients with differentiated thyroid carcinomas but common in those with undifferentiated thyroid carcinomas.

Ionizing radiation

External irradiation to the neck during childhood increases the risk of papillary thyroid carcinoma. The latency period between exposure and diagnosis is at least 5 years, the incidence is maximal after about 20 years, remains high for about 20 years, and then decreases gradually. There is a linear relationship between radiation doses from 10 to 1500 cGy and the number of thyroid cancers. Beyond this point the risk of thyroid cancer decreases, probably due to thyroid cell death. A major risk factor is a young age at the time of irradiation; after the age of 15 or 20 years, the risk is not increased. In children exposed to a dose of 1 Gy to the thyroid, the excess risk of thyroid cancer is 7.7.

Diagnostic or therapeutic administration of radioactive iodine (^{131}I) does not seem to be associated with an increased risk for thyroid cancer. However, the increased incidence of papillary thyroid cancer in children in the Marshall Islands after atomic bomb testing and, more recently, in Belarus and Ukraine after the Chernobyl nuclear reactor accident suggest a direct carcinogenic effect of radioactive isotopes of iodine. In contrast to the cancers observed after external irradiation, the post-Chernobyl cancers developed in children and young adults after a very short mean latency period (6.5 years in average) between exposure and diagnosis. Whether these discrepancies are due to different radiation doses to the thyroid, or to the very young age of the patients when the growing thyroid is particularly sensitive to radiation, or to a combination of these and other environmental (iodine deficiency) factors is still a matter of discussion.

Other factors

In countries where iodine intake is adequate, differentiated thyroid cancers account for more than 80% of all thyroid carcinomas, with the papillary histotype being the most frequent form (70-80%). In iodine-deficient areas, a relative increase of follicular and anaplastic cancers is the rule, although there is no definite demonstration of an increased number of thyroid cancers.

Cases of familial papillary thyroid cancer have been reported in about 3% of patients. A high incidence of thyroid carcinomas have been reported in association with adenomatous polyposis coli and Cowden's disease (the multiple hamartoma syndrome).

Pathology

Papillary carcinoma

The typical appearance of papillary thyroid carcinoma is that of an unencapsulated neoplasm with papillary and follicular structures and characteristic nuclear changes. The papillae have a fibrovascular core covered by a single layer of neoplastic cells. The typical nuclear features include large-size clear nuclei and nuclear grooves. Cytoplasmic invaginations into the nuclei, termed pseudoinclusions, are also typical. Psammoma bodies, present in 40 to 50% of the cases, consist of degenerative calcified changes within papillae, and they are almost pathognomonic of papillary thyroid carcinoma. The tumor spreads through lymphatics to the regional lymph nodes and less frequently to the lung. The histological features described above account for the classical form of papillary carcinoma (nearly 70% of the total). The remaining cases are composed of several variants, including the encapsulated variant, the follicular variant, the tall-cell variant, the diffuse sclerosing variant, and the clear-cell variant (Tab. 16.1).

Follicular carcinoma

Follicular carcinoma is characterized by follicular differentiation, without the nuclear features typical of papillary carcinomas. Capsular and vascular invasion are key features that distinguish between benign and malignant follicular proliferation, and they must be carefully searched for. The pattern of invasion may vary from a minimally invasive to a widely invasive form. The growth pattern may also vary, ranging from diffuse solid growth with a high degree of atypias to a macrofollicular structure resembling that of the normal thyroid. Lymph node involvement and multicentricity are rare, while distant metastases, mainly to the lung and bone, are relatively frequent due to hematogenous spread.

Hürthle cell carcinoma

In 1988 the World Health Organization formally classified these tumors as an oxyphilic variant of follicular carcinoma, but some authors believe that they should be classified separately as Hürthle cell carcinomas because of their peculiar behavior, which is different from both follicular and papillary well-differentiated thyroid carcinomas. Hürthle cell carcinomas represent 3 to 10% of all thyroid tumors and account for 15 to 20% and 2 to 8% of follicular and papillary carcinomas, respectively. Hürthle cells are large, polygonal, eosinophilic cells with hyperchromatic nuclei and fine granular acidophilic cytoplasm. True Hürthle cell tumors are well-encapsulated lesions, while nonencapsulated Hürthle cells cannot be considered as a neoplastic process, but rather an association with other benign (Hashimoto's thyroiditis, Graves' disease, nodular goiter) and malignant (well-differentiated thyroid cancer) thyroid diseases.

Although preferentially classified among follicular tumors, Hürthle cell carcinomas are usually more aggressive and metastasizing, and they are less prone to take up radioiodine and produce thyroglobulin than well-differentiated thyroid carcinomas. This is also true for the Hürthle cell variant of papillary thyroid carcinoma. The peak incidence is in the 5th and 6th decades of life. Women are more frequently affected than men. Previous neck irradiation was reported in 39% of patients.

Diagnosis of a Hürthle cell tumor is usually made by FNAC. However, as in the case of follicular tumors, no differentiation is possible between adenoma and carcinoma by cytology or in most cases even by frozen section. Capsular and vascular invasion at final histology is the diagnostic clue. Initial therapy, as in other high-risk thyroid cancers, is total thyroidectomy and careful lymph node dissection if regional node metastases are present. Radicality of the initial surgical treatment is particularly important in Hürthle cell carcinomas, because they often fail to concentrate radioiodine.

Undifferentiated (anaplastic) carcinoma

Undifferentiated thyroid cancer (large-cell type) represents about 10% of all thyroid carcinomas. It is prevalent in the elderly, frequently with longstanding simple or multinodular goiters. Tumors may represent the transition from a benign or well-differentiated lesion to an undifferentiated one, possibly due to the loss of function of the p53 tumor-suppressor gene by somatic point mutations. It presents as a large mass with necrotic areas, and it is extremely aggressive both locally and at a distance. When spreading locally, it invades soft tissues of the neck, trachea, and esophagus, frequently making radical surgery impossible. Metastases to the lung are common, and early death usually occurs within 12 months.

The rare small-cell histotype, previously considered a variant of undifferentiated thyroid carcinoma, was shown by immunohistochemical studies to be either medullary and follicular carcinomas or a small-cell lymphoma.

Diagnosis

Clinically evident thyroid nodules are found in about 4 to 5% of the general population. Since most thyroid nodules are benign, the differential diagnosis between benign and malignant nodules is crucial for the selection of patients to be treated by surgery. Recently, fine needle aspiration cytology allowed for an improvement in the diagnosis of the nature of thyroid nodules, which has lead to a significant reduction in the number of benign nodules treated by surgery.

Differentiated (papillary and follicular) thyroid carcinomas usually present as asymptomatic thyroid nodules, but sometimes metastatic lymph nodes may be the first manifestation. More rarely, distant metastases to the lung or bone from follicular carcinoma may be the presenting

Table 16.1 Histological variants and their relative proportions in papillary thyroid carcinoma

Variant	Relative %
Classical type	70
Encapsulated	10
Follicular	10
Tall-cell	4
Diffuse sclerosing	3
Clear-cell	2
Others	1

symptom. Hoarseness, dysphagia, and/or dyspnea may seldom be the hallmark of the tumor, which is indicative of an advanced stage of disease. The nodule is usually single, firm, and freely moveable during swelling, and it is scarcely distinguishable from a benign lesion. Carcinoma should be suspected when the nodule is single in an otherwise normal thyroid, when it is found in children or adolescents, in men, and in association with ipsilaterally enlarged lymph nodes. Previous history of irradiation to the neck and/or head during childhood is an important risk factor for the development of papillary thyroid carcinoma. The final diagnosis must rely upon the results of FNAC, which should be performed in any palpable nodule. Three cytologic results are possible: benign, malignant, or indeterminate (or suspicious). False negative and false positive results are rare. Thyroid ultrasonography is useful for guiding aspiration of poorly palpable nodules.

Undifferentiated carcinoma presents as a rapidly enlarging thyroid mass. The tumor is hard and fixed to neck structures. Local symptoms such as dysphagia and dysphonia are frequent due to infiltration of the esophagus and the recurrent laryngeal nerves, respectively. Involvement of the skin, with ulceration, is also possible.

Measurement of serum TSH and thyroid hormones is not helpful in the differential diagnosis of benign and malignant nodules, but only in the assessment of the functional thyroid status. Measurement of serum thyroglobulin, essential for the follow-up of differentiated thyroid cancer after total thyroidectomy, gives no clue toward the pre-surgical diagnosis, and it should not be performed. In contrast, four recent, independent prospective studies showed that routine measurement of circulating calcitonin in thyroid nodules made the preoperative diagnosis of medullary thyroid carcinoma more accurate than fine needle aspiration cytology. Accordingly, serum calcitonin measurement should be included in the diagnostic evaluation of thyroid nodules. In addition, a familial history of medullary thyroid carcinoma should raise the suspicion of hereditary medullary carcinoma.

Clinical and laboratory features associated with a high risk of cancer are summarized in Table 16.2, and a practical diagnostic approach to patients with thyroid nodules is schematically represented in Figure 16.1.

Prognosis

The overall survival rate of differentiated thyroid carcinoma at 10 years is between 80 and 95%. Five to 20% of patients have local or regional recurrences, and 10 to 15% have distant metastases. Prognostic indicators for recurrent disease and death are the patient's age at diagnosis, the histotype, and the extension of disease. Several staging systems have been proposed and aimed at identifying high-risk patients who would require the most aggressive forms of therapy. The most widely used system is the tumor-node-metastases (TNM) classification: few patients

Table 16.2 Clinical and laboratory features suggesting the malignant nature of a thyroid nodule

History
External radiation during childhood
Familial history of medullary cancer
Age < 20 or > 60 yr
Male sex

Thyroid nodule
Rapidly growing (especially during L-thyroxine)
Firm or hard or pain
Fixed to soft tissue

Others
Lymphadenopathy
Dysphagia, hoarseness
Elevated serum calcitonin

have a high risk of death from thyroid carcinoma, more than 80% are at low risk, and some have an elevated risk of recurrence but a low risk of death. The latter includes younger (<16 years) and older patients (>45 years), patients with certain histotypes (tall-cell, columnar-cell and diffuse sclerosing variants among papillary carcinomas; the widely invasive variant of follicular carcinoma; the Hürthle cell and the insular carcinomas), those with large tumors, with tumors extending beyond the thyroid capsule, or with lymph node metastases. The assessment of these prognostic indicators should dictate the initial treatment and the subsequent follow-up.

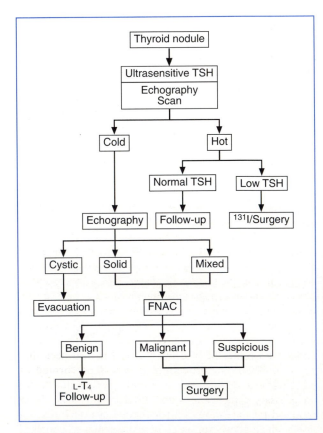

Figure 16.1 Thyroid nodule: diagnostic approach.

Surgery of the primary tumor and lymph node metastases

The initial treatment for differentiated thyroid cancer is surgery. Although some controversy exists regarding the extent of thyroid surgery, total thyroidectomy or "near-total" thyroidectomy – a procedure intended to leave no more than 2 to 3 g of thyroid tissue – should be preferred. At least three main arguments justify this approach. First, papillary carcinomas are multicentric in 30 to 80% of the cases, according to different series. Second, removal of most of the thyroid tissue will facilitate post-surgical ablation of any thyroid residue by radioiodine therapy. Third, total ablation of the thyroid gland is the prerequisite for the subsequent detection (and subsequent treatment) of local or distant metastases by whole body scanning and serum thyroglobulin measurement. The argument against a radical surgical procedure is essentially the increased risk of surgical complications such as recurrent laryngeal nerve injuries and hypoparathyroidism. These complications are almost absent in the hands of an experienced surgeon, and they should not be promoted as reasons against total or near-total thyroidectomy. Some authors guide their surgical decision on the basis of prognostic factors. "Low-risk" patients, who might be treated with limited surgery (lobectomy plus isthmectomy), are those with papillary tumors, aged less than 40 years, with a single nodule less than 1 to 2 cm in size, no clinical evidence of local or distant metastases, and no history of previous exposure to external radiation. Follicular carcinomas should always be treated with total thyroidectomy, and a completion thyroidectomy should be performed in patients who have undergone a lobectomy for a presumed benign tumor that proved to be follicular carcinoma at definitive histology.

There is considerable evidence that recurrence rates and death rates are higher when less radical thyroidectomies are performed. In a series of the Mayo Clinic, the extent of surgery significantly affected the risk of local recurrence in papillary carcinomas. In a series from Ohio State University, both the 30-year cancer recurrence rate and the 30-year cancer-specific mortality were higher after subtotal than after total or near-total thyroidectomy. Likewise, at the University of Chicago, performance of less extensive initial surgery in papillary carcinomas (lobectomy or bilateral subtotal thyroidectomy) was associated with a nonsignificant trend to increased risk of death and a significantly increased risk of recurrence. Both risks were significantly higher when tumors larger than 1 cm in size were treated with less extensive surgery.

Surgical treatment of cervical lymph node metastases varies from removal of only macroscopically affected nodes ("node picking") to the classical radical neck dissection. The latter procedure is rarely performed in patients with differentiated thyroid cancer due to its unnecessary complications and disfiguration. It has been replaced by the "modified (or functional) neck dissection", which allows for an *en bloc* dissection of lymphatics of the neck while preserving other functionally important neck structures. A prophylactic modified neck dissection is not recommended in most cases of differentiated thyroid cancer. Most authors advocate a disease-related strategy, based on routine removal of lymph nodes of the central neck compartment (paratracheal and tracheoesophageal chains), including the superior mediastinum and the region around the thymus gland, while reserving a modified neck dissection for patients with clinically evident lymph node metastases in the lateral neck. This strategy seems the most appropriate, especially given that in patients who are apparently free of lymph node metastases, a lateral modified neck dissection, if needed, can be easily and safely performed later. In patients with no evidence of lymph node involvement, other authors advocate intra-operative node sampling to decide whether a modified neck dissection is needed.

Radioiodine (^{131}I) ablation of post-surgical thyroid remnants

Post-surgical thyroid remnants should be ablated by therapeutic doses of radioiodine because destruction of residual thyroid cells facilitates subsequent follow-up. This is based on serum thyroglobulin measurement, diagnostic radioiodine whole body scanning, and ^{131}I therapy. Furthermore, ^{131}I may destroy microscopic foci of multicentric papillary carcinoma and decrease subsequent tumor recurrence.

Postoperative ^{131}I therapy is performed 4 to 6 weeks after surgery, without thyroid hormone administration in the interim. Some centers measure thyroid bed uptake using a tracer dose of ^{131}I and then give a standard therapeutic dose of [131]I (between 30 and 100 mCi), followed by the institution of L-thyroxine suppressive therapy. Whole body scanning is performed 7 to 15 days after treatment, depending on ^{131}I uptake. In patients who have undergone a total or near-total thyroidectomy, total ablation is achieved in 60 to 80% of the patients either after 30 or 100 mCi doses. Thus, the use of lower (30 mCi) doses is probably to be preferred. Other centers prefer to start with a diagnostic ^{131}I whole body scan with a 1 to 2 mCi tracer dose and then treat the patients with therapeutic doses according to the results of the diagnostic scan. A post-therapy scan is also performed.

Diagnostic and therapeutic follow-up

It is well-known that the great majority of local recurrences and/or distant metastases develop or are detected in the first 2 to 3 years after the diagnosis. However, in a minority of cases, distant metastases may develop even 20 years after initial treatment, suggesting that follow-up of differentiated thyroid cancer should go on throughout the patient's life.

Five to 20% of patients with differentiated thyroid cancer have local or regional recurrences. These are usually due to persistent or recurrent disease in thyroid remnants or lymph nodes after incomplete initial treatment, or to aggressive tumors. Local or regional disease may be detected by palpation, ultrasonography, CT scan, or whole body scan performed either after a diagnostic or a therapeutic dose of [131]I.

The frequency of distant metastases in differentiated thyroid carcinoma ranges between 10 and 18% of cases. Although distant metastases may be the presenting symptom, they are usually discovered at the time of the primary diagnosis or soon after thyroidectomy; or they may develop later, even 20 years after the initial treatment. Metastases to the lung is the most common site of distant metastases, followed by bone metastases. The combination of lung and bone disease is found in about one-third of the patients with distant metastases. Other less common localizations are brain, liver, and skin, which usually occur in the presence of lung and/or bone metastases. The pattern of metastatic lung involvement may vary from one or more macronodules (>1 cm in diameter) to a diffuse micronodular spread; this is usually not detectable by chest X-ray, and sometimes not even by CT scan, but it is easily diagnosed with ^{131}I whole body scanning. Mediastinal lymph node metastases are also frequently present, particularly in papillary tumors. Bone metastases are associated primarily with the follicular histotype and tend to occur in older patients. Vertebrae, pelvis, and ribs are the sites more frequently affected, but any skeletal segment may be affected. Single lesions are present in one-third of patients. Most metastases are detectable both by whole body scanning and X-ray film, but 25% are evidenced only by whole body scanning. The latter group is likely to respond to ^{131}I therapy.

The diagnostic and therapeutic strategies for monitoring patients with differentiated thyroid carcinoma are well-established and are very effective in identifying and treating most patients who are not cured after initial treatment. Essentially, after total thyroidectomy and radioiodine ablation of thyroid residues, two powerful tools are available to raise the suspicion for local or distant metastases and to localize them: serum thyroglobulin (Tg) measurement and ^{131}I whole body scanning, respectively. Radioiodine therapy and reoperation are very effective treatments for patients with metastases from well-differentiated carcinomas.

Clinical findings

Diagnostic procedures

Clinical, ultrasonographic, and radiographic examination Clinical examination with accurate palpation of the thyroid bed and lymph node chains of the neck is performed every 6 to 12 months in thyroid cancer patients. Ultrasonography of the neck may integrate the clinical examination. Tiny, oval lymph nodes detected either by palpation or by ultrasound may be a normal finding in the neck and should not create unnecessary concern. If there is a suspicion of lymph node metastases, an ultrasono-

graphic-guided fine needle aspiration for cytology and Tg measurement should be performed. Routine chest and bone X-ray is of little diagnostic value in the early diagnosis of distant metastases to the lungs or bones, particularly in patients with undetectable serum Tg levels. However, they are useful for monitoring the evolution of known metastatic disease; they are also useful in patients with negative ^{131}I whole body scanning but elevated serum Tg levels indicative of metastases that do not take up radioiodine.

Serum Tg measurement Tg is produced and secreted by normal and neoplastic follicular cells but not by other cell systems in the body. Thus, serum Tg measurement is a specific and sensitive tumor marker of differentiated thyroid cancer: after total thyroid ablation, serum Tg levels are undetectable in patients free of disease, while detectable and often elevated serum Tg concentrations are found in patients with persistent or recurrent disease. Two important factors must be considered when interpreting serum Tg values: the level of serum TSH and the presence of circulating anti-Tg autoantibodies. Tg production by neoplastic cells is, at least partially, under TSH control. As a consequence, serum Tg concentrations are lowered, even to undetectable levels, during TSH suppression by thyroid hormone administration and are increased after drug withdrawal. Serum Tg results are artifactually affected by circulating anti-Tg antibodies, which are present in about 15% of patients and interfere in the Tg assay, producing false positive or negative results depending on the assay used.

As a rule, patients with undetectable serum Tg levels off L-thyroxine therapy may be considered free of disease, while in patients with distant metastases serum Tg concentrations are elevated after withdrawal of L-thyroxine (L-T$_4$) therapy and are reduced but still detectable during L-T$_4$ treatment. In cases of lymph node metastases, serum Tg may be low or undetectable during L-T$_4$ therapy but becomes elevated after L-T$_4$ withdrawal (Tab. 16.3). Comparison of serum Tg measurements and ^{131}I whole body scanning has demonstrated solid agreement between the two techniques. Detectable serum Tg levels are usually associated with positive whole body scanning, indicating the presence of residual or metastatic disease. Undetectable serum Tg levels are found in patients with negative scans, which indicates that the patient is in remission. However, serum Tg predicts better than whole body scanning the presence of metastases in about 13% of patients who have increased serum Tg levels but negative basal whole body scanning. In these patients, abnormal foci of ^{131}I uptake can be demonstrated only after the administration of therapeutic doses of [131]I.

[131]I whole body scan Metastatic well-differentiated thyroid cancer retains the ability of normal follicular cells to concentrate iodine, which represents the basis for the diagnostic and therapeutic use of ^{131}I in metastatic thyroid cancer. Radioiodine uptake by metastatic tissue is dependent on TSH stimulation, which requires a state of hypothyroidism. For this reason, total thyroidectomy and ablation of post-surgical thyroid residues are the funda-

mental prerequisites for radioactive imaging. The other important practice is the withdrawal of L-T$_4$ therapy for a period of time long enough to induce high serum levels of endogenous TSH. The lowest serum TSH value for an adequate incorporation of ^{131}I in neoplastic tissues is around 30 µU/ml, usually reached after 30 to 45 days off L-T$_4$, and 2 weeks off L-triiodothyronine. Unfortunately, this period of hypothyroidism is very unpleasant for many patients. Intramuscular injection of recombinant human TSH is a promising alternative for the execution of ^{131}I whole body scanning, because thyroxine treatment does not need to be discontinued. Pilot trials comparing the results of whole body scanning performed after recombinant TSH and after L-T$_4$ withdrawal have shown very good concordance between the two techniques. Another requirement for effective ^{131}I uptake is the lack of recent assumption of stable iodine that would prevent the uptake of radioactive iodine by the metastases. Since insufficiently high serum TSH levels and contamination by iodine are the most frequent causes of false negative ^{131}I whole body scanning, serum TSH concentration and urinary iodine excretion must be checked before performing ^{131}I whole body scanning and ^{131}I therapy.

Whole body scanning is performed 48 to 72 hours after the administration of 2 to 5 mCi of ^{131}I. Higher doses are not indicated because they could produce a sublethal (stunning) radiation effect in the metastatic cells that would prevent the subsequent uptake of the therapeutic dose of ^{131}I. If no abnormal ^{131}I uptake is found, despite elevation of serum Tg, a therapeutic dose of ^{131}I (100 mCi) should be administered and a post-therapy scan obtained 5 to 7 days later. This procedure will allow for the identification of small foci of ^{131}I in more than 80% of the patients with negative basal scan and elevated serum Tg concentrations. If no localization is found, the search for metastases should include chest X-ray, CT scan, bone scintigraphy, and liver ultrasound. Whenever a metastasis has been localized by whole body scanning, a complete radiological assessment should also be obtained. In bone metastases, the aim is to assess whether the localization is accessible to radical surgical therapy. With lung metastases, it is crucial to establish whether there are one or more macronodular lesions or multiple micronodules that are not visible with plain chest X-ray but only by CT scan. This is of relevant prognostic utility, since diffuse lung metastases, undetectable by X-ray but able to take up radioiodine (such as those frequently encountered in children) are highly responsive to treatment with ^{131}I.

Clinical, biochemical, scintigraphic evaluation and radioiodine therapy, if needed, should be performed every 6 to 12 months in patients with persistent disease. Patients considered disease-free (i.e., negative scan and undetectable serum Tg off L-T$_4$) may be followed annually with clinical examination and serum Tg measurement. Any other test is unnecessary as long as serum Tg remains undetectable. If serum Tg becomes detectable on L-thyroxine, ^{131}I whole body scanning should be immediately planned.

Treatment

Local and regional recurrences

Recurrences in the neck after primary surgery may develop in the thyroid bed and the surrounding soft tissues or in the regional lymph nodes. They both carry an unfavorable prognosis, and most of the patients dying from differentiated thyroid cancer are in this group. The prognosis is better when the recurrent cancer is diagnosed by ^{131}I scintigraphy rather than clinically, and when it is able to concentrate iodine.

Any clinically detectable local recurrence should be treated by surgery, although radical reoperations involving central dissections are difficult and expose the risk of complications of the parathyroid glands and recurrent laryngeal nerve. Recurrent disease in the lateral cervical nodes is easier to treat surgically, as the operative field has usually not been previously operated on. The surgical procedure to be preferred is a modified radical neck dissection. When lymph node recurrences concentrate iodine, treatment with ^{131}I is an effective alternative to reoperation. Two to three therapeutic courses of ^{131}I are usually effective in treating over 60% of the patients. If the disease persists after two to three ^{131}I doses, reoperation may be considered, preferably with the use of an intraoperative probe. Local recurrences that cannot be completely excised and do not take up ^{131}I can benefit from external radiotherapy.

Distant metastases

Effective treatment depends largely on the size, location, number of metastatic lesions, and their ability to take up

---

Table 16.3 Percent of patients with detectable serum Tg after total thyroidectomy, during L-thyroxine (L-T$_4$) suppressive therapy, and after withdrawal, in the series of Villejuif and Pisa

	On L-T$_4$		Off L-T$_4$	
	Villejuif	**Pisa**	**Villejuif**	**Pisa**
Total remission	5/349 (1.4%)	36/517 (6.9%)	11/95 (11.5%)	126/136 (92.6%)
Lymph node metastases	19/24 (79.1%)	52/66 (78.7%)	26/27 (96.3%)	126/136 (92.6%)
Distant metastases	162/165 (98.1%)	138/153 (90.2%)	181/181 (100%)	290/292 (99.3%)

radioiodine. Micronodular diffuse lung metastases and, to a lesser extent, small metastatic bone foci revealed by whole body scanning in the absence of radiographic changes, have the greatest chance of cure. This is particularly true in children, who often have a diffuse pattern of metastatic pulmonary spread and do exceptionally well with radioiodine therapy. Macronodules in the lung and large bone metastases have a poor prognosis. Loss of radioiodine uptake is also a negative prognostic indicator. All together, these findings emphasize the concept that early recognition and early treatment of distant metastases is of paramount importance upon the final outcome.

Surgical treatment Lung metastases are frequently cured by radioiodine therapy, leaving the choice of surgical therapy to the treatment of a minority of selected cases. Patients eligible for surgery are those with a single macronodular lesion, or more than one in the same lobe; with or without mediastinal lymph node involvement, particularly when they are devoid of radioiodine uptake. The rationale is that some of them may achieve long-term remission, and, in less-advanced cases (one single pulmonary nodule), even definitive cure.

Bone metastases are relatively insensitive to radioiodine therapy. Bone surgery may be palliative in cases of pathological fractures or to ameliorate neurological symptoms due to spinal cord compression by vertebral metastases, or curative in the case of single, localized metastases. With large metastases that are not radically resectable, surgery may help to reduce tumor mass, which allows for a more effective action of radioiodine therapy.

Brain metastases are extremely rare and have a very poor prognosis. Although they can usually take up ^{131}I, the therapy of choice is surgery whenever feasible because of severe neurological symptoms.

Radioiodine treatment ^{131}I therapy in the management of distant metastases achieve complete responses in 35 to 45% of cases. Lung metastases, particularly micronodular, are more responsive than bone metastases. In adult patients, the treatment dose is usually 100 to 150 mCi, repeated every 6 to 8 months. Lower doses (empirically 1 mCi/kg body weight) should be employed in children with lung metastases, particularly of the diffuse type, to avoid the risk of radiation-induced pulmonary fibrosis.

There is a group of patients (15 to 20%) with elevated serum Tg levels and no uptake in diagnostic whole body scanning. The site of metastatic involvement in such patients, usually the lung or mediastinal lymph nodes, may be detected by whole body scanning performed 5 to 7 days after the administration of high doses of ^{131}I (100 mCi). This procedure is also of therapeutic value, as indicated by the finding that a few days after the administration of ^{131}I therapy there is a transient increase in serum Tg concentrations. This can be explained as massive release into the circulation of stored Tg by radiation-damaged tumoral cells. Furthermore, a progressive normaliza-

tion of whole body scanning and serum Tg levels over the years and the normalization of chest CT scans in patients with radiographic evidence of micronodular lung metastases were observed in patients periodically treated with this modality of treatment.

Side effects after the administration of therapeutic ^{131}I doses are frequent, but they are mild and transient. They consist mainly of gastrointestinal symptoms, nausea, occasionally vomiting, and acute sialoadenitis. An overall increase in the risk of leukemia (5 cases per 1000 treated patients) was found from a review of several published series. The risk increases by increasing cumulative doses, reducing the intervals between each treatment, and giving total blood doses per treatment greater than 2 Gy. Pancytopenia was reported in 4.4%, anemia in approximately 25%, and thrombocytopenia in one-third of patients treated with mean ^{131}I doses of 536 mCi. Another rare complication of radioiodine therapy is radiation-induced pulmonary fibrosis, which may develop in patients repeatedly treated for lung metastases, particularly of the diffuse type. Children seem to be particularly prone to this complication. Finally, it was reported that in men both transient and permanent testicular damage, limited to the germinal epithelium, and in women transient ovarian failure, occurred in those who were treated with high doses of ^{131}I. ^{131}Iodine-induced genetic damage in offspring of patients treated with ^{131}I has not been documented. The only reported anomaly was an increased frequency of miscarriage in women treated with ^{131}I during the years prior to conception.

The importance of L-thyroxine suppressive therapy

Both function and growth of metastatic thyroid cells are under TSH control. It is a common observation that bone or lung metastases increase in size and take up radioiodine after L-T$_4$ withdrawal, while a reduction in size and no uptake is observed on L-T$_4$. Serum Tg, a marker of cell function, increases dramatically during hypothyroidism, while it returns to low levels during hormone therapy. Thyroid hormone therapy significantly influences both recurrence rate and survival as an independent variable. In this regard, suppression of endogenous TSH to undetectable levels is to be regarded as a true anti-neoplastic therapy and should never be omitted in patients with active disease.

The drug of choice is L-thyroxine and the effective dosage is between 2.2 to 2.8 µg/kg body weight. Higher dosages are usually required in children. In any patient, an attempt should be made to use the smallest dose necessary to suppress TSH secretion. The adequacy of therapy is monitored by serum TSH measurements. Serum TSH should be undetectable, but levels less than 0.1 µU/ml may be accepted. Serum fT$_3$ and fT$_4$ should be in the normal range to avoid iatrogenic thyrotoxicosis. When these guidelines are followed, L-T$_4$ suppressive therapy is safe and is devoid of long-term side effects on the heart or bone.

The shift from suppressive therapy to replacement therapy may be considered in patients who have well-documented stable and complete remission, as assessed by negative ^{131}I whole body scan and undetectable serum Tg off L-T$_4$ therapy.

UNDIFFERENTIATED THYROID CARCINOMA

Undifferentiated thyroid carcinoma is among the most aggressive malignant tumors in man and represents approximately 5 to 15% of thyroid carcinomas. Its peak incidence is in the seventh decade, with almost no sex predilection. Bad prognosis is not ameliorated by surgery, chemotherapy, or radiotherapy. Total thyroidectomy should be attempted, but the infiltration of soft tissues of the neck almost invariably makes radical surgery impossible. External radiotherapy is used after surgery, but it is usually unsatisfactory. Several chemotherapeutic protocols, including single (doxorubicin) and combination (doxorubicin plus cisplatin) drugs, have been totally disappointing. The combination of radiotherapy and chemotherapy has been employed with little advantage. With any form of treatment, mean survival ranges between 3 and 6 months from the diagnosis, although individual survival exceeding 2 to 3 years have been reported.

Since radical surgery is rarely feasible, a novel approach is to use hyperfractionated radiotherapy in combination with chemotherapy as initial treatment, leaving surgery as a second step. The aim is to control and reduce the primary tumor with medical therapy, thus giving the surgeon more chances to perform a radical thyroidectomy. Further radiotherapy and chemotherapy may be added after surgery to stabilize the results of treatment. Using this integrated therapeutic approach, complete local control was obtained in 5 of 16 patients and 3 patients survived more than 20 months in one study.

MEDULLARY THYROID CARCINOMA

Medullary thyroid carcinoma (MTC) is a tumor of the parafollicular thyroid cells (C cells), which synthesize and release calcitonin (CT). The embryologic origin of C cells is from the neural crest, from which they migrate during fetal life to reach their final destination. Within the thyroid, C cells are preferentially located at the junction between the upper one-third and lower two-thirds of both thyroid lobes. This is the region where most MTCs will develop. Despite close contact between parafollicular and follicular cells, no paracrine interaction exists between these two types of cells.

The product of the C cells is a 32-amino acid hormone, calcitonin, the gene of which acts with an alternative RNA splicing, coding for calcitonin in the normal C cells and for another peptide, calcitonin gene-related peptide, in several cells of the central nervous system. At variance with the normal C cells, neoplastic C cells are able to produce both calcitonin and calcitonin gene-related peptide. The action of calcitonin after it is released into the bloodstream is to bind to specific receptors on osteoclasts, thus inhibiting bone resorption. Calcitonin release is regulated by the extracellular concentration of calcium. Other substances, primarily pentagastrin, may stimulate calcitonin

secretion. On this basis, both calcium infusion and pentagastrin injection are commonly used as stimulating agents in the diagnosis and follow-up of MTC.

Pathophysiology

Medullary thyroid carcinoma is a rare tumor, accounting for about 10% of all thyroid carcinomas. Most MTCs (nearly 80%) occur as sporadic tumors with a peak of incidence in the fourth and fifth decades, the rest (20%) occurs as inherited tumors, usually earlier in life, associated with other endocrine neoplasms as part of familial syndromes known as multiple endocrine neoplasias type 2 (MEN 2, see Chapter 71). Germline point mutations of the RET proto-oncogene, a gene coding for a tyrosine kinase membrane receptor, were demonstrated as causative of MEN 2 with a very high specificity. Somatic point mutations and also deletions of the same gene were found in nearly 50% of the sporadic MTC.

Sporadic medullary thyroid carcinoma presents as a white-red, hard lesion. At microscopy, it presents as sheets of spindle or rounded cells, typical of endocrine tumors. Nuclei are usually uniform with rare mitosis. Secretory granules are found in the cytoplasm. Deposits of amyloid, a product of the CT gene, are frequently found and are a distinctive feature of MTC. Sometimes MTC can mimic other thyroid tumors, mainly Hürthle cell, anaplastic, and even papillary carcinomas. In these cases, immunohistochemistry with anti-calcitonin antibodies will help in establishing the diagnosis. Accompanying C cell hyperplasia, a distinctive feature of familial MTC, is seldom also found in sporadic cases.

The metastatic spread of MTC to regional lymph nodes is very frequent, even in the earliest phase of the disease. Metastatic nodes that are not clinically evident are frequently found by the surgeon when careful exploration of the central neck compartment and lateral chains is performed. Distant metastases, usually slowly growing, are also frequent, both at diagnosis or during follow-up. The sites most frequently affected are the liver, lungs, and skeleton.

Clinical findings

Medullary thyroid carcinoma usually presents as a thyroid nodule, cold at thyroid scan, and not distinguishable from thyroid nodules of any other nature. Cervical lymph node involvement is very frequent. Diagnosis can be suspected only if there is a familial history of MTC, or in the presence of secretory diarrhea, typically, but not frequently, associated with MTC. Most of the time the diagnosis is made at histology. Cytology is an excellent diagnostic procedure for thyroid carcinoma in general, however, the specific diagnosis of MTC may be underscored with routine staining, especially if the pathologist is not alerted by suspicion of MTC. In several recent prospective series of unselected thyroid nodules undergoing diagnostic evaluation, routine measurement of serum calcitonin allowed the pre-operative diagnosis of unsuspected MTC in a surprisingly high number of patients, with a diagnostic accuracy superior to FNAC (Tab. 16.4). Thus, serum calcitonin measurement should be considered in the diagnostic evaluation of thyroid nodules.

Treatment

The outcome of sporadic MTC is largely dependent upon the effectiveness of the first surgical procedure. Minimal therapy for MTC is total thyroidectomy with dissection of

Table 16.4 Medullary thyroid cancer (MTC) diagnosed by routine measurement of serum calcitonin (CT) and by FNAC in nodular thyroid diseases

Authors	Patients	MTC detected by CT	MTC detected by FNAC
Pacini, 1994	1385	8 (0.57%)	2 (0.14%)
Rieu, 1995	469	4 (0.84%)	1 (0.21%)
Vierhapper, 1997	1062	13 (1.22%)	–
Niccoli, 1977	1167	12 (1.02%)	3 (0.25%)

the central node compartment, which is the first site of lymphatic spread. Dissection of other lymph node chains depends on the clinical presentation. After surgery, one should allow for the clearance of calcitonin from the circulation before measuring serum calcitonin concentration. If after 30 to 40 days basal and pentagastrin-stimulated serum calcitonin concentrations are undetectable, the patient has many chances to achieve definitive cure. Unfortunately, even after careful surgery, no more than 40 to 50% of the patients are cured. Many have sustained increased serum calcitonin, which is evidence of persistent disease. The localization of suspected metastases is based on diagnostic imaging techniques, including neck and liver ultrasound, CT scan of the mediastinum and lung, and bone scintigraphy. Several other scanning techniques, such as MIBG, ^{99m}TcDMSA, and radiolabeled somatostatin analog scanning can detect macroscopic lesions, but their usefulness in detecting microscopic disease is usually poor. In selected cases, venous catheterization for the measurement of serum calcitonin has been successfully employed.

From a practical point of view, once local disease is detected in the neck, a second operation is indicated. If no disease is found, despite elevation of serum calcitonin, it is probably better to wait and to re-evaluate the patients every 6 to 12 months; particularly in light of other treatment modalities, such as external radiotherapy and chemotherapy, being entirely disappointing in the treatment of MTC. Considering all of the stages of MTC, the usual 10-year survival in several series is around 50 to 60%. Survival may be prolonged and the quality of life acceptable even in the presence of diffuse metastatic involvement.

Suggested readings

AIN KB. Papillary thyroid carcinoma. Endocrinol Metab Clin North Am 1995;24:711-60.

CARUSO D, MAZZAFERRI EL. Fine-needle aspiration in the management of thyroid nodules. Endocrinologist 1991;1:194-202.

FAGIN JA. Molecular genetics of human thyroid neoplasms. Annu Rev Med 1994;45:45-52.

HAY ID. Papillary thyroid carcinoma. Endocrinol Metab Clin North Am 1990;19:545-76.

HESHMATI HM, GHARIB H, VAN HEERDEN JA, SIZEMORE GW. Advances and controversies in the diagnosis and management of medullary thyroid carcinoma. Am J Med 1997;103:60-9.

MAXON HR III, SMITH HS. Radioiodine-131 in the diagnosis and treatment of metastatic well differentiated thyroid cancer. Endocrinol Metab Clin North Am 1990;19:685-718.

MAZZAFERRI EL. Management of a solitary thyroid nodule. N Engl J Med 1993;328:553-9.

NIKIFOROV YE, ROWLAND LM, BOVE KE, MONFORTE-MUNOZ H, FAGIN JA. Distinct pattern of ret oncogene rearrangements in morphological variants of radiation-induced and sporadic thyroid papillary carcinomas in children. Cancer Res 1997;57:1690-4.

PACINI F, FONTANELLI M, FUGAZZOLA L, et al. Routine measurement of serum calcitonin in nodular thyroid diseases allows the preoperative diagnosis of unsuspected sporadic medullary thyroid carcinoma. J Clin Endocrinol Metab 1994;78:826-29.

PACINI F, FUGAZZOLA L, LIPPI F, et al. Detection of thyroglobulin in fine needle aspirates of nonthyroidal neck masses: a clue to the diagnosis of metastatic differentiated thyroid cancer. J Clin Endocrinol Metab 1992;74:1401-4.

PACINI F, LIPPI F, FORMICA N, et al. Therapeutic doses of iodine-131 reveal undiagnosed metastases in thyroid cancer patients with detectable serum thyroglobulin levels. J Nucl Med 1987;28:1888-91.

PACINI F, VORONTSOVA T, DEMIDCHIK EP, et al. Post-Chernobyl thyroid carcinoma in Belarus children and adolescents: comparison with naturally occurring thyroid carcinoma in Italy and France. J Clin Endocrinol Metab 1997;82:3563-9.

SCHLUMBERGER MJ. Papillary and follicular thyroid carcinoma. N Engl J Med 1998;338:297-306.

SCHLUMBERGER M, DE VATHAIRE F, CECCARELLI C, et al. Exposure to radioactive iodine-131 for scintigraphy or therapy does not preclude pregnancy in thyroid cancer patients. J Nucl Med 1996;37:606-12.

Thyroid function in nonthyroidal illness

Elio Roti, Roberta Minelli, Mario Salvi

KEY POINTS

- In nonthyroidal illness, low serum 3,5,3'-triiodothyronine (T_3) and free T_3 concentrations; normal or decreased serum thyroxine (T_4) and free T_4 concentrations; and increased serum reverse T_3 (rT_3) concentrations; and normal, decreased, or increased serum thyroid-stimulating hormone concentrations have been observed. Decreased serum T_3 and increased rT_3 concentrations are due to decreased T_4 and rT_3 5'-monodeiodination, respectively.
- The mechanisms of decreased 5'-monodeiodination activity are related to reduced caloric intake, decreased selenium tissue concentrations, and decreased T_4 tissue uptake. The changes of serum thyroid hormone concentrations are not related to specific diseases but rather to the severity of disease.
- Patients with nonthyroidal illness and abnormal thyroid function results are in general considered euthyroid.
- Thyroid function testing in patients with nonthyroidal illness is not necessary except in patients with suspected hyperthyroidism or hypothyroidism. Final diagnosis of thyroid function can be postponed except when the altered thyroid state is responsible for severe complications, mainly cardiovascular complications.
- In patients with nonthyroidal illness, normal serum thyroid-stimulating hormone and fT_4 concentrations unequivocally define a condition of euthyroidism. Free T_4 results may be falsely altered depending upon the assay methods employed.
- Thyroid hormone administration to patients with nonthyroidal illness with low serum thyroid hormone concentration does not have any consistent benefit, and it is not recommended by the majority of specialists.

The terms nonthyroidal illness (NTI) or euthyroid sick syndrome describe various clinical conditions not due to thyroid diseases. These illnesses are characterized by abnormal results of thyroid function tests, primarily decreased serum triiodothyronine (T_3) and free T_3 (fT_3), increased reverse T_3 (rT_3), normal thyrotropin (thyroid-stimulating hormone [TSH]) and, in more severe conditions, decreased thyroxine (T_4) and free T_4 (fT_4) concentrations.

In some circumstances, other changes in thyroid function tests can be observed, such as decreased or increased serum TSH, increased total T_4, and normal T_3 and rT_3 concentrations. Recently it has been reported

that T_3 sulfate (T_3S), a product of the peripheral catabolism of thyroid hormones, is increased in the serum of patients with NTI. Despite the presence of abnormal thyroid function tests, patients with NTI are considered euthyroid.

The abnormal thyroid function tests in nonthyroidal illness, however, are not due to thyroid or hypothalamic-pituitary diseases but are due to different pathologically or pharmacologically induced conditions. In Table 17.1 we report the illnesses more frequently associated with changes in thyroid function tests. In general, different diseases cause similar changes in thyroid function tests and

Table 17.1 Conditions of nonthyroidal illness

Metabolic diseases	Fasting Diabetic ketoacidosis Protein-calorie-malnutrition
Infective diseases	Malaria Tubercolosis HIV infection Sepsis
Surgical procedures	Coronary bypass Transplant Caesarean section Other surgical procedures
Renal diseases	Chronic renal failure Nephrosic syndrome
Liver diseases	Hepatitis Cirrhosis
Cardiac diseases	Miocardial infarction
Pulmonary diseases	Pneumonitis
Psychiatric diseases	Primary depression
Tumors	
Burns	

their derangement from normal range limits is related to the severity of the disease.

Many drugs may cause changes in thyroid function tests as well (Tab. 17.2). The mechanisms responsible for the occurrence of abnormal thyroid function tests involve changes in thyroid hormone production, transport, distribution, and metabolism, occasionally accompanied by altered pituitary TSH secretion.

Epidemiology

Low T_3 syndrome, which is characterized by decreased serum T_3, increased rT_3, normal T_4, and normal TSH concentrations, has been reported in as high as 70% of hospitalized patients. The mean value of serum T_3 concentrations in patients with NTI is approximately 40% of the normal level. Serum fT_3 values decline as well but less markedly, reaching values of approximately 60% of normal values. Low serum T_4 and T_3 concentrations are seen in patients with more severe conditions of nonthyroidal illness and in general in those with poor prognoses. This condition has been observed in 2.9 to 4.4% of patients in intensive care units. In intensive care patients, abnormal serum TSH values have been observed in 22% of the cases. Low serum TSH concentrations were observed in 13% of the patients. Finally, in euthyroid patients with nonthyroidal illness, increased concentrations of T_4 have been reported in 4 to 33% of cases. The severity of the dis-

eases and the pharmacological treatments are important variables determining the different prevalence of abnormal thyroid function profiles; patients in intensive care units most likely have the highest prevalence of abnormal thyroid function tests due to nonthyroidal illness.

SPECIAL NONTHYROIDAL ILLNESS CONDITIONS

In general, low T_3 and increased rT_3 are the most frequently abnormal tests observed in nonthyroidal illness. As the severity of the disease proceeds, low T_4 and low TSH values occur as well. However, in some conditions this pattern is not observed. In renal diseases low T_3 concentrations are accompanied by normal serum rT_3 concentrations because tissue uptake of rT_3 is increased. In acute viral hepatitis, serum total T_4 concentrations are increased because hepatic stores of thyroxine-binding globulin (TBG) are released into the circulation, and therefore the binding capacity of TBG for T_4 is increased. In acute psychiatric disorders serum T_4 concentrations are also increased, due to an activation of the pituitary-thyroid axis. In patients affected with the human immunodeficiency virus (HIV), during the asymptomatic period of the disease, serum T_4 and T_3 are within the normal range limits; as the disease proceeds, serum T_4 and T_3 concentrations decline as in patients with other nonthyroidal illness conditions.

Etiopathogenesis

The most frequently investigated condition of nonthyroidal illness is fasting, and this condition may be paradigmatic of all other conditions of nonthyroidal illness. A few hours after the onset of fasting, serum total and free T_3 concentrations markedly decrease. In this condition the production rate of T_3 from T_4 is decreased due to reduced 5'-monodeiodination activity. The decreased peripheral T_3 production of patients with nonthyroidal illness has been related to many possible mechanisms, such as decreased tissue T_4 uptake; decreased selenium tissue concentrations, which as selenocysteine has a relevant role in the activity of 5'-deiodinase; increased serum rT_3 concentrations, which have an inhibitory action on 5'-monodeiodination activity; and decreased serum T_3 binding. High serum rT_3 concentrations are mainly due to decreased peripheral clearance as a consequence of the decreased tissue uptake and 5'-monodeiodination. The decrement of serum T_4 concentrations, which is observed in severe conditions of nonthyroidal illness, is mainly due to decreased binding of the hormone to the serum carrier proteins related to the presence of an abnormal thyroxine-binding globulin; to the presence of serum inhibitors of the binding of T_4 to thyroxine-binding globulin; to decreased serum albumin concentrations; in the most severe cases of nonthyroidal illness, to decreased TSH stimulation of the thyroid gland. Cytokines have a central role in the activation of these mechanisms. Administration of cytokines to experimental animals and healthy volunteers resulted not only in changes of thyroid function tests, but also in changes of other endocrine glands, particularly in the activation of pituitary-adrenal axis with increased cortisol secretion, which reduces peripheral production of T_3. Furthermore, cytokines per se, and endogenous and also exogenous glicoactive steroids, inhibit TSH release. In rare conditions serum T_4 concentrations may be increased. This occurs primarily in relation to increased serum thyroxine-binding globulin concentrations, such as during acute viral hepatitis, and to a transiently increased T_4 production in response to TSH stimulation, such as during acute psychiatric disorders.

In some conditions serum TSH concentrations are also modified: they can be decreased as in patients treated with glucocorticoids and dopamine; and increased, such as in the recovery phase of very severe nonthyroidal illness conditions, which is possibly related to markedly decreased serum T_4 and T_3 concentrations that activate the negative feedback mechanism of TSH secretion.

The metabolic conditions of patients with nonthyroidal illness

Except for a few conditions, such as patients with anorexia nervosa, patients affected by nonthyroidal illness are judged clinically euthyroid. The reduction in serum T_3 and T_4 concentrations may suggest the presence of hypothyroidism, however, normal serum TSH concentrations indicate that, at least at the pituitary level, thyroid hormones exert complete biological activity. It may be argued that in severe nonthyroidal illness, low serum T_4 and T_3, and normal or low TSH concentrations correspond to a situation of central hypothyroidism. This possibility is supported by the observation that in patients recovering from severe nonthyroidal illness, the increase of serum TSH concen-

trations precedes the normalization of serum thyroid hormone concentrations. Low tissue T_3 concentrations at autopsy in patients who died of nonthyroidal illness suggests that patients affected by nonthyroidal illness may be hypothyroid. Decreased liver concentrations of malic-dehydrogenase and glycerophosphate dehydrogenase, decreased cardiac Ca^{2+}-activated myosin ATPase, and decreased serum concentrations of angiotensin-converting enzyme suggest decreased thyroid hormone action in target tissues. In contrast, normal metabolic rate, normal systolic time interval, normal Achilles' tendon reflex, normal serum sex hormone-binding globulin (SHBG), and osteocalcin concentrations suggest normal thyroid function. In the past it has been suggested that the decrement of serum thyroid hormone concentrations was compensated by an increased post-receptor response to thyroid hormones. More recently, it has been observed that in diseased human liver, gene expression of thyroid hormone receptor α and β variants was normal, as well as the expression of sex hormone-binding globulin, thyroxine-binding globulin, cortisol-binding globulin, and transthyretin RNAs, thus suggesting that at least in patients with chronic liver diseases, the condition of euthyroidism is maintained.

Clinical findings

Demonstrating that patients with nonthyroidal illness have abnormal thyroid function tests is not necessary. Thyroid function evaluation in patients with nonthyroidal illness is appropriate when history and signs of thyroid

Table 17.2 Drugs and X-ray contrast dyes affecting thyroid function tests

	T_4	fT_4	T_3	fT_3	rT_3	T_3S	Basal TSH	TSH response to TRH
Dopamine	↓	↓	↓	↓			↓	↓
Glucocorticoids	↓	=	▼		▲		↓	↓
Radiopaque dyes	=↑	=	▼	↓	▲	▲	=↑	↑=
Propranolol		=	=	↓		–	=	=
Amiodarone		↑	↑	▼	↓	▲	↑	↑
Heparin	=	↓	=	↓			=	=
IL-1β	↓	↓	↓				↓	↓
IFN-α	=	=	↓		↑		↓	↓
Endotoxin	↓	↓	↓		↑		↓	
Fenclofenac		↓	↓					↓

(= no change; ↑ increased; ↓ decreased; ▼ markedly decreased; ▲ markedly increased.)

dysfunction are present, particularly atrial fibrillation and cardiac failure nonresponsive to treatment. Patients treated with amiodarone and interferon and those administered with X-ray contrast dyes are also candidates for thyroid function testing. Considering the variable changes in thyroid function tests occurring during nonthyroidal illness, we believe that in most of the cases TSH and fT_4 measurements will permit an accurate evaluation of thyroid function. When both tests result within the normal range limits, patients will be unequivocally euthyroid. Suppressed serum TSH concentrations (< 0.1 mU/l) by second generation assay do not define the existence of thyrotoxicosis with absolute certainty. In fact, it has been reported that only 24% of patients with nonthyroidal illness with suppressed serum TSH concentration were hyperthyroid, whereas 41% of the patients had suppressed serum TSH concentrations as a consequence of nonthyroidal illness per se, and 35% of the patients had steroid treatment. When thyroid function evaluation is conducted by third generation TSH assay, suppressed serum TSH concentrations are due to thyroid disease in 73% of the cases, whereas in the remaining cases suppressed concentrations are due to nonthyroidal illness and steroid treatment. Thus, TSH measurement by third generation assay will define thyroid function in most of the patients. Elevated serum fT_4 concentrations in nonthyroidal illness patients with suppressed serum TSH concentrations apparently may confirm a diagnosis of hyperthyroidism, however, it should be pointed out that falsely elevated serum fT_4 concentrations may occur when a two-step fT_4 assay is employed. This phenomenon, due to factors inhibiting the binding of T_4 to carrier protein, is particularly evident in heparinized patients. It has been reported that elevated serum fT_4 concentrations are more frequently due to an assay artifact than to true hyperthyroidism. If the condition of the patient is not critical, deferring thyroid function testing after the resolution of the nonthyroidal illness will permit a definitive diagnosis. In addition, increased serum TSH concentrations, in a range of 6 to 20 mU/l, does not conclusively diagnose primary hypothyroidism; it has been reported that in 72% of the cases, the increment of serum TSH concentrations was due to nonthyroidal illness, particularly in patients recovering from a severe nonthyroidal illness process. It is important to realize that the measurement of serum fT_4 concentrations by one-step or analog methods may give falsely low results. Thus, these methods are not valid to confirm a diagnosis of primary hypothyroidism. In cases of elevated serum TSH concentrations, a definitive diagnosis of primary hypothyroidism can be suspected when patients have a history of thyroid diseases and when they consume drugs containing iodine or lithium. Positive serum antithyroid peroxidase antibodies (AbTPO) will support the diagnosis of primary autoimmune hypothyroidism.

In the presence of low serum fT_4, fT_3, normal, or low TSH concentrations, one can suspect the presence of central hypothyroidism. Signs of failure of other pituitary target glands such as adrenal glands and gonads may alert the physician. A definitive diagnosis, and therefore treatment of central hypothyroidism during nonthyroidal illness, is required if signs of adrenal failure are suspected. If adrenal failure is not suspected, the diagnosis can be postponed until after the resolution of the nonthyroidal illness process.

TRUE HYPOTHYROIDISM AND HYPERTHYROIDISM IN NONTHYROIDAL ILLNESS PATIENTS

Untreated hypothyroid patients affected by nonthyroidal illness processes, such as fasting, do not show any significant change of serum TSH concentrations. Therefore it is unlikely that nonthyroidal illness will mask a diagnosis of primary hypothyroidism. More difficult is to solve the question of whether nonthyroidal illness will mask a thyrotoxic condition. In patients with unequivocal clinical signs of hyperthyroidism affected by nonthyroidal illness, elevated serum fT_4 and fT_3 and suppressed TSH concentrations, by third generation assay, confirm the diagnosis of thyrotoxicosis. The diagnosis of subclinical hyperthyroidism in patients with a concomitant nonthyroidal illness process is extremely difficult. In this condition, suppressed serum TSH concentrations are expected to be accompanied by normal fT_4 and fT_3 values. The presence of clinical signs of Graves' disease or toxic nodular goiter may address the diagnosis. In these conditions radioactive iodine thyroid uptake, thyroid scintigraphy, determination of antithyroid peroxidase antibodies and thyrotropin receptor antibodies may allow for the diagnosis of true hyperthyroidism.

Treatment

The administration of thyroid hormones to patients with nonthyroidal illness has been suggested in view of some indices of reduced thyroid function. Since T_3 is the hormone more frequently reduced, and because T_4 to T_3 5'-monodeiodination is impaired in patients with nonthyroidal illness, treatment with T_3 rather than T_4 has been suggested. In patients who underwent cardiac bypass, the administration of T_3 at the doses of 0.03 to 0.2 μg/kg body weight has been followed by an amelioration of cardiac output and a decrement of peripheral vascular resistance. However, T_3 treatment did not change the prevalence of cardiac arrhythmias, the need for inotropic drugs and, in general, the morbidity and mortality of the patients. Even in patients with severe burns, T_3 treatment was not accompanied by a significant amelioration of the clinical condition. Finally, the administration of T_4 at the dose af 1.5 μg/kg body weight for 14 days to patients with nonthyroidal illness did not change the mortality rate of T_4-treated patients, which was 73% versus 75% of control patients, despite a significant increase observed in serum T_4 and T_3 concentrations. It has been reported that the administration of T_3 to patients with renal failure and to fasting subjects increased protein catabolism. This result suggests a detrimental effect of thyroid hormone replacement in patients with nonthyroidal illness. In view of these results, we and many other authors do not advocate thyroid hormone treatment in patients with nonthyroidal illness.

BARTALENA L, BROGIONI S, GRASSO L, MARTINO E. Interleukin-6 and the thyroid. Eur J Endocrinol 1995;132:386-93.

CHOPRA I J. Euthyroid sick syndrome: is it a misnomer? Endocr Rev 1997;82:329-334.

DOCTER R, KRENNING EP, DE JONG M, HENNEMANN G. The sick euthyroid syndrome: changes in thyroid hormone serum parameters and hormone metabolism. Clin Endocrinol (Oxf) 1993;39:449-518.

HEUFELDER AE, HOFBAUER LC. Human immunodeficiency virus infection and the thyroid gland. Eur J Endocrinol 1996;134:669-74.

KAPTEIN EM. Thyroid hormone metabolism and thyroid diseases in chronic renal failure. Endocr Rev 1996;17:45-63.

KAPLAN MM, LARSEN PR, CRANTS FR, DZAU VJ, ROSSING TH, HADDOW JE. Prevalence of abnormal thyroid function test results in patients with acute medical illnesses. Am J Med 1982;72:9-16.

KLEMPERER JD, KLEIN I, GOMEZ M, et al. Thyroid hormone treatment after coronary-artery bypass surgery. N Engl J Med 1995;333:1522-27.

NICOLOFF JT, LOPRESTI JS. Nonthyroidal illness. In: Braverman LE, Utiger RD (eds). The thyroid. 7 th ed. Philadelphia: Lippincott-Raven, 1996; 286-96.

ROTI E, MINELLI R, GARDINI E, BRAVERMAN LE. The use and misuse of thyroid hormone. Endocr Rev 1993;14:401-423.

SLAG MF, MORLEY JE, ELSON MK, CROWSON TW, NUTTALL FQ, SHAFER RB. Hypothyroxinemia in critically ill patients as a predictor of high mortality. JAMA 1981;245:43-45.

STOCKIGT JR. Guidelines for diagnosis and monitoring of thyroid disease: nonthyroidal illness. Clin Chem 1996;42:188-192.

STOCKIGT JR. Update on the sick euthyroid syndrome. In: Braverman LE (ed). Contemporary endocrinology: diseases of the thyroid. Totowa: Humana Press, 1997; 49-68.

UTIGER RD. Altered thyroid function in nonthyroidal illness and surgery. To treat or not to treat. N Engl J Med 1995;7:1562-63.

WARTOFSKY L, BURMAN KD. Alterations in thyroid function in patients with systemic illness: the "euthyroid sick syndrome". Endocr Rev 1994;3:210-247.

WARTOFSKY L. The low T_3 or "sick euthyroid syndrome": Updated 1994. Endocr Rev 1994;3:248-251.

WEHMANN RE, GREGERMAN R, BURNS WH, SARAL R, SANTOS GW. Suppression of thyrotropin in the low-thyroxine state of severe nonthyroidal illness. N Engl J Med 1985;312:546-52.

Calcium and bone metabolism

18

Calcium and bone metabolism: basic concepts

Jan A. Fischer

This is an overview of the present knowledge regarding mineral and bone metabolism. Different related diseases are summarized with reference to genetic, physiological, and pathophysiological mechanisms. The reader is referred to chapters with sections on calcium and bone metabolism that include a detailed analysis of the etiology, prevalence, pathology, clinical manifestations, diagnosis, and treatment of the various diseases.

Calcium and phosphate are the predominant constituents of bone mineral, or apatite. Over 99% of total body calcium is found in the skeleton, the remainder being distributed in intra- and extracellular fluids. Serum levels of total calcium have a generally reported normal range of 2.1-2.6 mmol/l or 8.4-10.4 mg/100 ml (this range can vary depending on the laboratory and has been reported to be smaller in research-oriented laboratories). Forty-five percent of the serum calcium is protein-bound, mainly to albumins, and complexed to bicarbonate, phosphate, and citrate; 55% is in free ionized form. For practical purposes, total serum calcium alone is measured. During bone formation, the protein matrix, consisting primarily of collagen type 1, is synthesized, and calcium phosphate is subsequently deposited.

Raised and decreased serum levels of calcium define hyper- and hypocalcemia (Tab. 18.1). Diseases associated with hypercalcemia are treated in Chapters 19 and 20 such as familial primary hyperparathyroidism, which occurs alone and in multiple endocrine neoplasia (MEN), frequently in MEN type 1 and rarely in MEN type 2 (Tab. 18.2). Hypocalcemia is reviewed in Chapter 21.

The extracellular concentration of free ionized calcium is maintained at around 10^{-3} mol/l. The regulation of electric transmission in the nervous system, muscular contraction, hormone secretion, and renal tubular concentrating ability crucially depends upon the serum levels of free calcium. Calcium imbalance can thus cause significant deleterious effects. Hypercalcemia is revealed by dehydration as a result of polyuria, anorexia, vomiting, nephrolithiasis, and ectopic calcifications, which are best

Table 18.1 Regulation of serum calcium

Factors increasing serum calcium concentration

Parathyroid hormone (PTH)
Parathyroid hormone-related protein (PTHrP)
Vitamin D
Calcium
Thyroxine
Estrogen (in breast carcinoma and metastases)
Thiazide diuretics
Lithium

Factors lowering the serum calcium concentration

Calcitonin and related peptides (Fig. 18.1)
Cortisone
Phosphate
Bisphosphonates
Low magnesium
Loop diuretics (e.g., furosemide)

visualized in the cornea. Acute severe hypercalcemia may lead to stupor and coma. Subtle signs include constipation, muscle weakness, fatigability, and depression. These characteristic symptoms occur irrespective of the etiology of hypercalcemia (Tab. 18.1). Hypocalcemia results in tetany, and in severe cases epileptic seizures. After hyperventilation, prolonged vomiting, and administration of alkali, the ionized fraction of the serum calcium is lowered while total calcium remains normal.

The concentration of intracellular free cytosolic calcium is about 10^{-7} mol/l and therefore 10 000 times lower than extracellular calcium levels. The extraordinary gradient between the outside and inside of the cell is regulated through several mechanisms. Among these mechanisms are calcium uptake via voltage-dependent and second messenger-operated calcium channels, facilitated and passive diffusion, sodium/calcium exchange, and a calcium/magnesium ATPase expelling calcium from cells.

A novel calcium receptor recognizing extracellular calcium has recently been cloned (Tab. 18.2). Mutations that inactivate this calcium sensor result in familial hypocalciuric hypercalcemia in heterozygotes, and result in severe neonatal hyperparathyroidism in homozygotes (see Chap. 19). Activating mutations are responsible for a rare form of hypoparathyroidism with hypocalcemia, accompanied by low to normal serum levels of parathyroid hormone (PTH) (see Chap. 21).

In addition to cyclic 3',5'-adenosine monophosphate (cyclic AMP), increased cytosolic calcium is an important intracellular signaling pathway. Raised calcium leads to increased cell division and, when uncontrolled, to malignant transformation and tumor formation. Cyclic AMP is the predominant mediator of the actions of parathyroid hormone, parathyroid hormone-related protein (PTHrP), calcitonin, calcitonin gene-related peptide (CGRP), amylin, and adrenomedullin. Cell division is lowered in the majority of cells when cyclic AMP production is increased. Differentiation occurs during the development and renewal of tissues.

A PTH/PTHrP receptor is linked through guanine nucleotide binding protein (G)-coupled mechanisms to the activation of the cyclic AMP and calcium signaling pathways (Tab. 18.2). An inactivating mutation of the PTH/PTHrP receptor occurs in Blomstrand chondrodysplasia. Downstream inactivating mutations of the stimulating G protein subunit ($G_{s\alpha}$) are associated with pseudohypoparathyroidism type Ia, pseudopseudohypoparathyroidism, and Albright's osteodystrophy (see Chap. 21). In pseudohypoparathyroidism type Ib with absent signs of Albright's osteodystrophy, $G_{s\alpha}$ activity is normal. Yet, the diagnosis of pseudohypoparathyroidism types Ia and Ib is established on the basis of absent or low urinary cyclic AMP responses to the administration of exogenous

parathyroid hormone. In pseudopseudohypoparathyroidism, the urinary cyclic AMP excretion is stimulated by parathyroid hormone as in normal subjects. While the test is crucial for the diagnosis of pseudohypoparathyroidism, the molecular mechanism remains to be elucidated. Therefore, the hypothesis that target organ resistance to parathyroid hormone and clinical hypoparathyroidism are caused by an inactivating mutation of one $G_{s\alpha}$ allele alone is questionable, however the genetic defect of hormone resistance in target organs such as of PTH and thyroid-stimulating hormone may be caused by transcription from only one paternal allele. Activating mutations of the PTH/PTHrP receptor are, on the other hand, the cause of Jansen's metaphyseal chondrodysplasia. Those of $G_{s\alpha}$ are associated with fibrous dysplasia (McCune-Albright osteodystrophy) (Tab. 18.2) (see Chap. 23).

Major regulators of calcium metabolism are PTH, PTHrP, and the D vitamin (Tab. 18.3). The secretion of parathyroid hormone is inversely related to the serum calcium concentration. As a result, the secretion of parathyroid hormone is raised in calcium and vitamin D deficiencies. It is also raised in target organ resistance to parathyroid hormone, such as in pseudohypoparathyroidism. In these conditions, secondary hyperparathyroidism occurs without exception. Patients are hypocalcemic or normocalcemic. Raised serum levels of parathyroid hormone are the most sensitive index of a calcium deficiency, followed by lowered concentrations of 25(OH)vitamin D. The causes are insufficient synthesis in the skin because of limited exposure to sunlight, and inadequate intake of the parent vitamin D. This results in infantile rickets in children not subjected to prophylaxis with vitamin D and in an increased incidence of fractures of the hip, particularly in elderly women with osteoporosis (see Chaps. 22 and 25). Rickets and osteomalacia have in common insufficient mineralization of the skeleton and wide osteoid seams. In the cases of calcium and vitamin D deficiencies, patients also have secondary hyperparathyroidism. Major

Table 18.2 Molecular defects in disorders of calcium and bone metabolism

	Mutation	
	Activating	**Inhibiting**
Calcium-sensing receptor	Hypoparathyroidism	Hypocalciuric hypercalcemia (heterozygotes)
		Neonatal hyperparathyroidism (homozygotes)
PTH/PTHrP receptor	Jansen's metaphyseal chondrodysplasia	Blomstrand chondrodysplasia
$G_{s\alpha}$ protein	Fibrous dysplasia (McCune-Albright syndrome)	Pseudohypoparathyroidism type Ia and Pseudopseudohypoparathyroidism
1α-vitamin D hydroxylase	–	Vitamin D-resistant rickets type I
Vitamin D receptor	–	Vitamin D-resistant rickets type II
PHEX[1]	–	X-linked hypophosphatemia
Menin[2] (tumor suppressor gene)	–	Multiple endocrine neoplasia type 1
RET protooncogene	–	Multiple endocrine neoplasia type 2
Collagen type I	–	Osteogenesis imperfecta
Tissue non-specific alkaline phosphatase	–	Hypophosphatasemia

[1] PHEX (endopeptidase) (The Hyp Consortium, Nature Genetics 1995;11:130.)
[2] Menin (Chandrasekharappa SC et al., Science 1997;276:404-7.)

Table 18.3 Regulation of the serum calcium concentration and the skeleton

	Serum calcium	Serum PTH	Bone density	Bone formation	Bone resorption
PTH	↑	↑	↑ to ↓	↑	↑
PTHrP	↑	↓	↑ to ↓	↑	↑
Vitamin D	↑	↓	↑	↑	↑
Thyroxine	↑	↓	↓	(↑)	↑
Cortisone	↓	↑	↓	↓	(↓) to ↑
Estrogens	↓	↓	→	→	↓
Growth hormone	→	→	↑	↑	↑
Calcium	↑	↓	→	→	↓
Calcitonin	↓	↑	→	→	↓
Phosphate	↓	↑	→ to ↑	→	↓
Bisphosphonates	↓	↑	↑	→	↓

causes of secundary hyperparathyroidism are deficient biosynthesis of vitamin D due to inadequate ultraviolet irradiation, deficient biosynthesis of vitamin D due to insufficient nutritional intake associated with intestinal malabsorption, and steatorrhea in patients with celiac gluten-sensitive disease, chronic pancreatic insufficiency, and primary biliary cirrhosis. The most frequent cause of osteomalacia is chronic renal failure with an inadequate conversion of 25(OH)- into the biologically most active $1,25(OH)_2$ vitamin D, which occurs almost exclusively in the kidneys. Exceptions are granulomatous tissues such as in sarcoidosis and tuberculosis, where raised synthesis occasionally leads to hypercalcemia.

Target organs of PTH and PTHrP are the skeleton and the kidneys. Bone formation is stimulated following pulsatile administration of parathyroid hormone. A sustained increase of parathyroid hormone, such as presumably seen in some patients with primary hyperparathyroidism and hypercalcemia, enhances bone resorption. Serum levels of calcium are also raised through stimulation of the renal tubular reabsorption of calcium. They are raised indirectly through the activation of renal 1α-vitamin D hydroxylase, resulting in increased biosynthesis of $1,25(OH)_2$ vitamin D, which stimulates intestinal calcium absorption. In addition to parathyroid hormone, low nutritional calcium and phosphate activate the 1α-vitamin D hydroxylase. A rare cause of severe osteomalacia is vitamin D-dependent rickets type I with the inadequate formation of $1,25(OH)_2$ vitamin D due to mutations of the renal 1α-vitamin D hydroxylase (see Chap. 22). In type II vitamin D-resistant rickets, inactivating mutations of the vitamin D receptor lead to elevated but functionally inadequate serum levels of $1,25(OH)_2$ vitamin D.

Since skeletal apatite consists of calcium and phosphate, decreased mineralization of the skeleton is not only associated with an inadequate supply of calcium, but also with an inadequate supply of phosphate. This occurs with excessive use of laxatives, such as aluminum hydroxide administered in chronic renal failure patients on dialysis, and in patients with renal tubular dysfunctions with the suppressed reabsorption of phosphate. The latter patients are hypophosphatemic. The hereditary condition is termed X-linked hypophosphatemia with mutations in the PHEX (phosphate-regulating gene with homologies to endopeptidases on the X-chromosome) (Tab. 18.2). Serum levels of parathyroid hormone are normal and therefore not the cause of renal phosphate wastage in this condition. Most likely a novel hypothetical hormone, "phosphatonin," possibly activated by PHEX, causes the inhibition of renal phosphate reabsorption. This etiology is supported in patients with tumor-induced hypophosphatemic osteomalacia, which resolves following surgical removal.

Parathyroid hormone-related protein (PTHrP) is the most frequent cause of malignancy-associated hypercalcemia (see Chap. 20). Unlike PTH, which is only formed in the parathyroid glands, PTHrP is synthesized in many tissues. It may act in an autocrine or paracrine fashion to stimulate bone resorption; it may also stimulate chondrogenesis, and the relaxation of the smooth musculature of blood vessels and the uterus. These actions are the same as those of parathyroid hormone and mediated through the same PTH/PTHrP receptor. A specific action of PTHrP not shared by parathyroid hormone is the stimulation of placental calcium transport.

Hypocalcemia occurs in patients with hypoparathyroidism and undetectable or low serum levels of parathyroid hormone. It is a result of agenesis or dysgenesis of the parathyroid glands, surgical removal, autoimmune destruction, or hypomagnesemia (see Chap. 21). In pseudohypoparathyroidism with target organ resistance and secondary hyperparathyroidism, serum levels of calcium are normal or decreased, and they are usually higher than those in hypoparathyroid patients. Other causes of hypocalcemia are vitamin D-deficiency and the inadequate biosynthesis of $1,25(OH)_2$ vitamin D (see above). For unknown reasons, hypocalcemia also occurs in acute pancreatitis. Calcitonin – together with the structurally related peptides calcitonin gene-related peptide (CGRP), adrenomedullin, and amylin – lower raised serum levels of calcium in hyper- but not normocalcemic patients via the inhibition of osteoclastic bone resorption (Fig. 18.1). CGRP released from afferent nerve fibers is effective in the skeleton in paracrine fashion. Unlike calcitonin, CGRP stimulates bone formation. CGRP and adrenomedullin are potent vasodilators. Calcitonin is used therapeutically in part due to its analgesic properties in patients with osteoporosis to inhibit postmenopausal bone loss; like calcitonin phosphate lowers serum levels of calcium by inhibiting osteoclastic bone resorption, such as in hyperphosphatemic chronic renal failure patients. A similar mechanism of action is involved with bisphosphonates used in the prevention and treatment of osteoporosis. Estrogen suppresses bone breakdown and is also used for the prophylaxis and treatment of postmenopausal osteoporosis (Tab. 18.3) (see Chap. 25).

As a result of bone formation, parathyroid hormone stimulates the synthesis of insulin-like growth factor (IGF) in osteoblasts. The actions of insulin-like growth

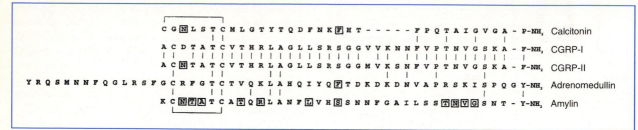

Figure 18.1 Amino acid sequences of human calcitonin, calcitonin gene-related peptides (CGRP) types I and II, adrenomedullin, and amylin.

factor are modulated by the presence of several ill-defined binding proteins and proteases, with some activating and some inhibiting its effects. Insulin-like growth factor and bone morphogenetic factors related to transforming growth factor-β are abundant in the skeleton. They stimulate bone formation primarily by autocrine and paracrine mechanisms, however, the therapeutic importance of bone morphogenetic factors is so far limited to its local administration to stimulate the implantation of bone explants in the filling of bone defects. Insulin-like growth factor and transforming growth factor-β cannot be used systemically in osteoporotic patients for the stimulation of bone formation because of the accompanying side effects.

Thyroxine and cortisone stimulate bone resorption, which leads to osteoporosis and skeletal fractures.

With calcitonin, estrogen, and bisphosphonates, bone resorption is suppressed while bone formation remains unaffected. Bone loss can therefore be prevented or suppressed, though the bone that was already lost is not replaced in old age. Stimulation of bone formation is therefore an important therapeutic goal. At this point in time this can be achieved in humans with fluoride and with parathyroid hormone. As sodium fluoride is not extensively used because of its narrow dose window, this leaves parathyroid hormone as an important agent to stimulate the synthesis of insulin-like growth factor among the growth factors of osteoblasts and bone formation. Therapeutic use is hampered, however, because a non-injectable form of administration or a peroral mimic still needs to be developed.

Suggested readings _____

BILEZIKIAN JP, MARCUS R, LEVINE MA (eds). The parathyroids: basic and clinical concepts. New York: Raven Press, 1994;859.

BILEZIKIAN JP, RAISZ LG, RODAN GA (eds). Principles of bone biology. San Diego: Academic Press, 1996;1398.

MUFF R, BORN W, FISCHER JA. Calcitonin, calcitonin gene-related peptide, adrenomedullin and amylin: homologous peptides, separate receptors and overlapping biological actions. Europ J Endocrinol 1995;133:17-20.

STREWLER GJ, ROSENBLATT M. Mineral metabolism. In: Felig F, Baxter JD, Frohman LA (eds). Endocrinology and mineral metabolism. 3rd ed. New York: McGraw-Hill, 1995;1407-516.

Primary hyperparathyroidism

Jeffrey O'Riordan

KEY POINTS

- Primary hyperparathyroidism is a common condition. It can be asymptomatic but can also cause serious disability due, for example, to renal calculi or bone disease.
- The cornerstone of diagnosis is the demonstration that hypercalcemia exists and that other causes of hypercalcemia can be excluded. Finding raised immunoassayable parathyroid hormone supports the diagnosis if renal function is normal.
- Particular care is needed if there is a family history of hypercalcemia. Isolated familial hyperparathyroidism occurs. However, more commonly in a familial context, hyperparathyroidism is part of a multiple endocrine neoplasia syndrome (particularly type 1, but also type 2). The multiple endocrine neoplasia type 1 syndrome is due to mutation of the MEN1 gene, encoding a putative protein, while MEN2 is due to a mutation in the RET oncogene. If there is a family history of failed neck surgery for presumed primary hyperparathyroidism, then benign familial hypercalcemia should be suspected. This is accompanied by hypocalciuria, hence the alternative name familial hypercalcemia with hypocalciuria. This is due to a mutation in the calcium receptor, which in homozygote children is a serious condition, but it is usually asymptomatic in heterozygotes.
- The preferred treatment for primary hyperparathyroidism is surgical. Only a specialized parathyroid surgeon should be asked to do this operation. Surgery of the neck for a second time is particularly difficult and should be preceded by using all possible preoperative localization techniques. The results of surgery are good, but if postoperative hypoparathyroidism develops, this will require long-term therapy, usually with a 1-hydroxylate form of vitamin D, such as calcitriol or alphacalcidol. This requires careful, life-long monitoring.
- If a patient is asymptomatic and it is decided that surgery should not be undertaken, it is advisable to measure serum calcium annually.

Hyperparathyroidism results from excessive secretion of parathyroid hormone. In "primary hyperparathyroidism" the underlying disorder is in the parathyroid glands themselves. This may be due to an adenoma in one or more glands or, alternatively, there may be hyperplasia of all parathyroid tissue. In "secondary hyperparathyroidism" the excessive secretion is in response to hypo- or normocalcemic stimuli, such as occurs in renal failure or malabsorption, or in vitamin D deficiency. The response is generally only partially effective, and the patient retains raised concentrations of parathyroid hormone. The term "tertiary hyperparathyroidism" is used in situations in which there is hypercalcemia with parathyroid overactivity in the presence of a condition that would be expected to cause secondary parathyroid overactivity. However, progression from secondary to tertiary hyperparathyroidism has only rarely been recorded, with the exception of renal transplantation, so the etiological connection is generally uncertain.

Epidemiology

The overall incidence of hyperparathyroidism is about 1 in 2000. Two-thirds of patients with primary hyperparathyroidism are female. The condition can occur at any age, including the neonatal period. However, it is uncommon under the age of 10 in either sex, with the exception of neonatal hyperparathyroidism in the familial homozygous form of hypocalciuric hypercalcemia (see below). In males over the age of 20 the incidence remains quite steady throughout life, but in females there is a considerable increase with age, reaching a peak between 50 and 70 years.

Etiology

Etiology is generally unknown, though the condition can follow 30 or 40 years after irradiation of the neck in childhood. Both monoclonal and polyclonal origins of parathyroid tumors are possible. Parathyroid hyperplasia may be due to a circulating mitogenic factor, however a single parathyroid tumor is more likely to be monogenic in origin, resulting from a point mutation. In primary hyperparathyroidism and in multiple endocrine neoplasia types 1 and 2 (MEN), there may be a single adenoma or hyperplasia affecting some or all the parathyroid glands. Allelic loss of parts of chromosome 11 can occur in the abnormal parathyroid tissue in primary hyperparathyroidism. A gene abnormality has been mapped to the region 11q13, and clonal rearrangement of this area has been found in a few patients with parathyroid tumors; within that region is the oncogene PRAD-I, which may be important in the genesis of parathyroid tumors in some patients.

Recently the gene causing multiple endocrine neoplasia type 1 was cloned: it encodes a protein called "menin" of unknown function, presumably it is a tumor suppressor gene, since mutations of it cause multiple endocrine tumors. In multiple endocrine neoplasia type 2, mutations of the RET proto-oncogene are associated with medullary carcinoma of the thyroid, and presumably also with primary hyperparathyroidism when the parathyroid gland is affected in that syndrome.

Pathophysiology

In 80% of patients with primary hyperparathyroidism there is a single adenoma. In the majority of the remainder there is hyperplasia of one or more glands. The distinction between an adenoma and a hyperplastic gland depends in essence in seeing a rim of normal tissue in the adenoma. Unless the histological section goes through that region, the correct diagnosis will be missed, particularly if only a single gland is affected. Microscopic recognition of overactive parathyroid tissue is itself difficult, since the appearance of normal glandular tissue is similar to that of overactive tissue. Thus, the best differentiation is on the basis of the size of the tissue and its weight. In normal subjects a total weight of 4 glands is about 120 mg, with a volume of about 0.12 ml. In hyperparathyroidism the abnormal gland may weigh between 0.2 and 50 g.

Clinical findings

The clinical presentation of primary hyperparathyroidism is quite variable: some patients present with renal calculi, others with the symptoms of hyperparathyroid bone disease, and in many the condition may appear to be asymptomatic. It is a matter for concern that there is often a considerable delay in making the diagnosis even when the clinical features are clear cut. It is not uncommon for symptoms to be present for as long as 7 years even when the patient has renal calculi or severe hyperparathyroid bone disease, and in 10% of patients symptoms of either of these may have been present for longer than 8 years.

Symptoms and signs

Renal stones are present in about one-third of patients and can produce the same features as stones due to any other cause. The symptoms are commonly renal colic, hematuria, or urinary tract infections. Anuria can be produced if both ureters are blocked at the same time, or if there is only one ureter containing an obstructing stone in a patient with a single-functioning kidney. The stones are usually formed in the renal papillae and may be single or multiple, small or large (and they may be staghorn). Bladder calculi occasionally form, especially if there is underlying disease of the bladder such as a tumor or a diverticulum. Nephrocalcinosis (calcification within the renal substance) can also develop; which is usually asymptomatic, but renal failure and its accompanying symptoms can occur.

Currently hyperparathyroid bone disease is present in only 5 to 10% of primary hyperparathyroid patients; the incidence has relatively declined over the past 50 years since the condition was first recognized and as other forms of presentation have been recognized. There has also most likely been a decrease in the absolute incidence as well. In many patients the changes in bone are asymptomatic (being recognized by a reduction of bone density and/or the presence of minor changes on X-rays, particularly of the fingers), but serious symptoms can occur such as bone pain and weakness, causing great difficulty in walking. The pain can be diffuse, affecting the spine, chest, and limbs. Weakness is usually associated with the presence of radiologically-extensive bone disease, and it is in the form of a proximal myopathy, causing difficulty in walking upstairs or getting up from lying flat. It is often difficult to distinguish between a true myopathy and the weakness due to severe bone pain.

Weight loss and lethargy can be the presenting features of hyperparathyroidism, and anemia can also be attributable to the condition. There may also be symptoms due to hypercalcemia per se, including thirst and polyuria, constipation, and depression, which can result from a serum calcium above 3.5 mmol/l (14 mg/100 ml).

With the advent of biochemical screening, which includes measurement of serum calcium, a large proportion (perhaps even more than 50%) of patients with hyperparathyroidism are now found "by accident". Many, but not all, of these cases will actually be asymptomatic, and if there are any symptoms that have led to the blood test being done, they are not necessarily attributable to the elevation of serum calcium. That elevation itself is usually relatively small (up to 2.75 mmol/l; 11.0 mg/100 ml).

In general, hyperparathyroidism does not cause physical signs, but hypertension may be present, as may be anemia and weight loss. The absence of some physical signs, such as those of thyrotoxicosis or lymphadenopathy, hepatomegaly (with or without jaundice), and splenomegaly, are important in excluding other causes of hypercalcemia (see below and Tab. 19.1). Severe hyperparathyroid bone disease is accompanied by serious signs, with difficulty in walking up or down stairs, sitting up from the prostrate position, weakness of abduction of the shoulders, elevation of the leg off a couch, or getting up from squatting. These active movements may be accompanied by severe pain, which can also be caused when the ribs are sprung by compression with sudden release. Pseudo-clubbing may be present (resulting from shortening of the distal phalanges). Subconjunctival calcification is occasionally seen but is not diagnostic. Bone tumors due to underlying osteitis fibrosa cystica, may, rarely, cause a palpable swelling, such as of the tibia.

Diagnostic procedures

There are two important facets of investigating patients suspected of having primary hyperparathyroidism. The first is to obtain positive support for the diagnosis, and the second is to exclude other causes of hypercalcemia or show that there is a cause other than parathyroid overactivity for the elevation of serum calcium. It has to also be appreciated that a patient may have more than one cause for hypercalcemia, such as coexistent hyperparathyroidism (due to a parathyroid adenoma) and sarcoidosis; the etiological significance of such coexistence is not clear. Hyperparathyroidism can also coexist with a

benign gammopathy or with multiple myeloma. In addition, patients with Paget's disease can have hyperparathyroidism independent of that bone disease.

Serum calcium

Detection of hypercalcemia is mandatory in making the diagnosis of primary hyperparathyroidism. Measurement of serum calcium in a laboratory that uses reliable techniques with a tight normal range (e.g., 2.20-2.60 mmol/l; 8.8-10.4 mg/100 ml) is essential. If the quoted normal range is greater, it is likely that unreliable methods are being used. It is wise to have multiple samples measured to avoid laboratory errors, so three or four measurements in the course of a week are advisable. Some of these should be taken after overnight fasting since the effect of dietary calcium intake, albeit small, is then avoided. Whenever possible stasis should be avoided; venous stasis leads to hemoconcentration and a rise in serum albumin, and hence a rise in total serum calcium because approximately half of the total serum calcium is bound to proteins (mostly albumin). There are a number of ways of to correct for changes in albumin. One method is correcting to a serum albumin of 41 g/l and assuming that 6 g of albumin bind 0.1 mmol of calcium per liter. Allowance can then be made for deviation in serum albumin from 41 g/l. On this basis, an observed serum calcium of 2.60 mmol/l (10.4 mg/100 ml) with an albumin of 35 corrects to 2.70 mmol/l (10.8 mg/100 mmol) and is clearly raised, while with an albumin of 47 g/l it is corrected to 2.50 mmol/l (10.0 mg/100 ml) and so is normal. Measurement of ionized calcium does not give any practical advantage and is not necessary, even though the techniques of measuring it have improved. It is important to note that the total serum calcium in a patient can fluctuate so that readings slightly above and strictly within the normal range may be observed on successive days, giving rise to the entity sometimes referred to as "normocalcemic hyperparathyroidism".

Serum phosphate

Parathyroid hormone causes phosphaturia and hypophosphatemia, but in practice the measurement of serum phosphate is not of great diagnostic value. The result is dependent on diet and fasting and is modified by changes in renal function.

Serum alkaline phosphatase

If serum alkaline phosphatase is raised and liver function is normal, and there is hypercalcemia, it is likely that the patient has hyperparathyroid bone disease. Apart from measuring standard liver function tests (such as bilirubin and transaminases), it can be useful to measure serum γ-glutamyltransferase since if that is raised, an elevated alkaline phosphatase is likely due to liver disease. Measurement of isoenzymes of alkaline phosphatase are not reliable in general and have no practical advantage. In

---

Table 19.1 Causes of hypercalcemia

Hyperparathyroidism
  Malignant diseases (with or without metastases to
    bone), including lymphoma
  Sarcoidosis
  Multiple myeloma
  Thyrotoxicosis
  Drug-induced
    Vitamin D intoxication
    Thiazide diuretics
    Milk alkali syndrome
  Familial hypercalcemia with hypocalciuria

interpreting a value for alkaline phosphatase, it is important to know the normal adult range for alkaline phosphatase in the laboratory used, since quoted values vary considerably from place to place. In investigating growing children, it also has to be remembered that the upper limit of the normal alkaline phosphatase is two to three times greater than it is in adults.

Plasma protein

At the same time as measuring serum albumin, total plasma proteins should be measured as a way of detecting a dysproteinemia. Fractionation of plasma proteins and electrophoresis are useful in demonstrating the existence of a paraprotein, which is suggestive of multiple myeloma.

Serum parathyroid hormone

Current techniques for measuring circulating parathyroid hormone can be extremely useful in the diagnosis of parathyroid overactivity. The values given by different methods vary considerably, however, since they measure fragments of the intact hormone to varying degrees; this has to be taken into account in interpreting the numbers generated. With currently used techniques, it is unusual for people with hyperparathyroidism to have normal values of circulating parathyroid hormone.

Measurement of vitamin D metabolites

Circulating 25-hydroxyvitamin D, either derived from vitamin D_3 (also called cholecalciferol) or vitamin D_2 (also called ergocalciferol), is a good reflection of vitamin D status. As such, it is useful in demonstrating the presence of vitamin D intoxication due to excessive ingestion of vitamin D. To produce hypercalcemia, it is necessary to take between 50 000 and 100 000 units of vitamin D daily (1.25-2.5 mg daily). Preparations containing this much vitamin D are not readily available. Hence, vitamin D intoxication is more likely in professions allied to medicine and nursing, in those manufacturing vitamin D on an industrial scale, or in those using large amounts of it for food supplementation.

Parathyroid hormone stimulates the activity of the 1α-hydroxylase that converts 25-hydroxyvitamin D to 1,25-dihydroxyvitamin D, so it might be expected that in hyperparathyroidism the circulating concentration of 1,25-dihydroxyvitamin D would be raised. This is sometimes true, however the concentration can also be normal, and in patients with impaired renal function it can be below normal. The assay is particularly valuable in establishing that hypercalcemia is due to excess 1,25-dihydroxyvitamin D, such as in sarcoidosis when extrarenal 1α-hydroxylase activity is increased.

Urine calcium and creatinine clearance

Parathyroid hormone causes hypercalciuria. However, in about one-third of patients with hyperparathyroidism, urinary excretion of calcium over a 24-hour period is normal; thus, it is unwise to use the demonstration of hypercalciuria for the diagnosis of parathyroid overactivity. Further, measurement of urinary calcium excretion in the fasting state does not add greatly to the diagnostic usefulness unless familial hypercalcemia with hypocalciuria is suspected.

The measurement of serum creatinine (besides creatinine clearance) as a measurement of renal function is important in the assessment of the effects of hypercalcemia and any coexistent renal calculi. Moreover, the contribution of immunoreactive parathyroid hormone fragments in serum due to decreased metabolism in renal failure can be indicated.

Hematological tests

A routine blood count is useful for the detection of anemia or the presence of abnormal white cells, suggestive of, for example, lymphoma. The sedimentation rate may be elevated and raise suspicion of the existence of multiple myeloma in a patient with hypercalcemia. Examination of bone marrow is important if myeloma is suspected. It can also be useful in demonstrating the presence of malignancy of other types, sarcoid granulomata.

X-rays

A chest X-ray may demonstrate the presence of a primary tumor or secondary deposits (e.g., from a silent hypernephroma). Skeletal X-rays are critical to the demonstration of the existence of hyperparathyroid bone disease. An X-ray of the hands may show subperiosteal erosions, usually best seen on the radial side of the middle phalanges. In more gross cases, there may be the so-called "brown tumors" of osteitis fibrosa cystica. These cystic lesions, which on section may be brown because of previous hemorrhage, are most easily seen in the long bones, the pelvis, the skull, and in the ribs and clavicles. In the skull there also may be a so-called "salt and pepper" appearance, and in the clavicles there may be erosion of the medial ends.

Bone density

A reduction in bone density is an important indication, in patients who are otherwise asymptomatic, that surgical removal of parathyroid tumors is advisable (see below).

Ultrasound

Ultrasound is important in two ways in patients with hypercalcemia: firstly, in identifying the location of abnormal parathyroid glands in the neck, and secondly, in examining the abdomen. These are discussed below.

Localizing parathyroid tumors Ultrasound is probably the best way of localizing overactive parathyroid glands in the neck. The technique, however, is "observer-dependent". Hence, its significance declines unless the observer is experienced – not just in ultrasound, but specifically in the use of ultrasound for localizing parathyroid tissue.

There is a risk of erroneously thinking that a parathyroid has been found (false positives).

PRIMARY HYPERPARATHYROIDISM • 225

Ultrasound of the abdomen Ultrasound of the abdomen is valuable since a number of relevant abnormalities can be identified with this scanning modality. The presence of renal calculi can obviously be detected ultrasonically, even if they were not clinically suspected and have not been shown on X-ray of the abdomen. Any obstruction, either to a single renal calyx or to the ureter, can also be demonstrated. This technique can also be used to detect important, non-parathyroid causes of hypercalcemia, such as a hypernephroma or ovarian tumor; the presence of metastases in the liver can also be revealed. In patients with multiple endocrine neoplasia type 1, the presence of associated pancreatic tumors can also be demonstrated. In sarcoidosis, the finding of an enlargement of the liver and/or the spleen may be valuable, and enlargement of retroperitoneal glands may make it possible to establish the diagnosis with a biopsy when other techniques have failed.

Differential diagnosis

The important causes of hypercalcemia are listed in Table 19.1. It may be useful to consider some of the problems of diagnosis that arise. A useful clue to the correctness of the diagnosis of hyperparathyroidism is if it is established that the hypercalcemia has been of long-standing. Generally the serum calcium of a patient with this condition remains elevated and unchanged over many years. If it is known that in relatively recent times the patient had a normal serum calcium, then another cause should be strongly suspected. On the other hand, having a history of renal calculi over many years is a lesser indication, since renal calculi are quite commonly due to causes other than hyperparathyroidism; hypercalcemia associated with the presence of renal calculi may therefore have an origin outside the parathyroid. Serum levels of parathyroid hormone are normal or low as a result of the suppression of parathyroid hormone secretion. This is due to hypercalcemia other than that caused by primary hyperparathyroidism.

Malignant disease

Hypercalcemia can occur in malignant disease with or without metastases to the bone. In the latter case there is generally production of parathyroid hormone-related peptide (considered in greater detail in Chapter 20, Malignancy-associated hypercalcemia). In practice, if there are metastases to bone, the diagnosis is generally clear cut. Difficulties occasionally arise when there is no obvious primary tumor, such as a neoplasm of kidney or ovary, in which case ultrasound of the abdomen can be valuable.

Sarcoidosis

Occult sarcoidosis is probably the most common cause of diagnostic difficulties, with symptoms such as malaise and lethargy being wrongly attributed to hyperparathyroidism causing hypercalcemia. The diagnosis of sarcoidosis can be difficult to establish if, for example, there is no lymphadenopathy, pulmonary infiltration, or splenomegaly. A steroid suppression test using 40 mg hydrocortisone, three times per day for 10 days, is valuable in this context, although it must be said that the elevated serum calcium (corrected for albumin) may not have fallen to normal within the usual 10-day period of the test. If there is a suspicion that the calcium is falling, the steroid administration should be continued for a total of 3 weeks and extra measurements of serum calcium should be made in that period. Conversely, normocalcemia is occasionally produced with steroids in patients with hyperparathyroidism (although this is of no diagnostic or therapeutic value). Sometimes that fall in serum calcium is only apparent, and it is actually due to hemodilution produced by water retention with steroid administration. Correction for this is possible by taking into account the fall in serum albumin that accompanies it. At times, however, even corrected calcium falls in hyperparathyroid patients with steroids, so caution is needed in interpreting the results of a suppression test. This should be used to increase the level of suspicion rather than to make a firm diagnosis.

A positive Kweim test may support the diagnosis of sarcoidosis. This skin test should probably not be performed until at least 2 months after any administration of steroids, even in the doses used in the steroid suppression test. It is necessary to use an antigen in the Kweim test, one that has been adequately validated or the value of the test is limited. Ultimately the diagnosis of sarcoidosis depends on the results of a biopsy. If there is lymphadenopathy, then the choice of the site to be biopsied is simple. In some cases liver biopsy, scalene node biopsy, or renal biopsy have established the diagnosis; occasionally cervical gland biopsy during exploration of the neck for presumed hyperparathyroidism has established the correct diagnosis. In some cases it is not possible to get histological proof of the diagnosis and it has to be assumed that steroid-suppressible hypercalcemia is due to occult sarcoidosis. In that situation finding an elevated concentration of circulating 1,25-dihydroxyvitamin D in the presence of a normal concentration of 25-hydroxyvitamin D (which itself excludes the diagnosis of excessive ingestion of vitamin D) may also support the diagnosis of sarcoidosis. The elevated 1,25-dihydroxyvitamin D concentration falls to normal in a steroid suppression test if it is due to sarcoid.

Multiple myeloma

Hypercalcemia found during investigation of an illness and suspected of being due to hyperparathyroidism is sometimes due in fact to multiple myeloma. There may be symptoms compatible with both diagnoses, including bone pain. Myeloma may cause radiological changes, including the presence of lytic lesions or vertebral collapse. The finding of a paraproteinemia or the presence of Bence Jones protein in the urine may indicate myeloma.

It is important, however, to distinguish the protein abnormalities in myeloma from those of a benign gammopathy. Bone marrow biopsy may be necessary in which an excess of plasma cells in the marrow is sought.

Thyrotoxicosis

Hypercalcemia in this condition is well-recognized. The diagnosis may not be clinically obvious, with the usual manifestations of thyrotoxicosis being missed or absent, so the measurement of serum thyroxine and thyroid stimulating hormone in the investigation of hypercalcemia is important.

Milk alkali syndrome

Excess ingestion of milk and alkali can increase serum calcium. This is often accompanied by impairment of renal function. The biochemical abnormalities revert to normal when the oral intake is corrected for approximately 6 weeks, during which time any indigestion can be controlled with histamine$_2$ antagonists. It is often difficult to obtain the appropriate history – the difficulty can be as great as getting a true indication of excessive alcohol intake. Careful questioning is necessary in a hypercalcemic patient who complains of indigestion. Having said that, it is remarkable how many of the population, at least in the United Kingdom, take proprietary antacids. Because peptic ulceration is probably exacerbated by hypercalcemia, the antacid intake is not necessarily the cause of the hypercalcemia.

Familial hypercalcemia with hypocalciuria

Familial hypercalcemia with hypocalciuria (FHH) is due to mutations in the gene for the calcium receptor (see Chap. 18). The condition can cause major diagnostic problems unless the family history is already known. The difficulties are compounded by the fact that hyperparathyroidism can occur as a familial entity without there being any other features of multiple endocrine adenomatosis, hence the presence of a family history of hypercalcemia does not exclude hyperparathyroidism. However, if there is a family history of failed parathyroid surgery, FHH should be seriously considered, as it is possible that a mutation in the gene for the calcium receptor is the prime problem. In general this is a completely benign condition, although there are occasional reports of its association with renal calculi and pancreatitis. Recognition of familial hypercalcemia with hypocalciuria is important because parathyroid surgery will not help the condition.

Treatment

Medical treatment

Medical treatment has a small part to play in the management of hyperparathyroidism unless the serum calcium is symptomatic and itself a cause for concern, and this is usually only if the serum calcium is greater than 3.5 mmol/l (14 mg/100 ml). At that point rehydration and promotion of a diuresis (with a loop diuretic such as furosemide) is appropriate. Thiazide causing hypercalcemia is contraindicated in this situation. It may be necessary to give intravenous pamidronate (a bisphosphonate), since that can restore serum calcium to normal. This can be useful if there are reasons for delaying surgery, or if time is needed to make a firm diagnosis and to exclude other causes of hypercalcemia such as sarcoidosis. Recently calcium receptor antagonists have been described, but their effectiveness is limited as they only have a transient effect (for perhaps a few hours), and they only reduce serum calcium by less than 1 mmol/l (2.5 mg/100 ml), which is a trivial difference. A more potent compound with prolonged action would be valuable.

Surgical treatment

Surgery should be considered as the definitive treatment, of which there are two questions to consider: "Who should do it?" and "What are the indications?". The answers to the first of these questions is easy. The operation should be done by an experienced parathyroid surgeon. Such surgeons are not common. Somebody who has done two or three parathyroid explorations a year for 10 years should not be considered "experienced" in this context. It is probably reasonable to say that the first hundred such operations done by a single surgeon are relatively difficult and thereafter become much easier. Such statements are of course difficult to prove. However, it is well-recognized that a parathyroid tumor can have a variable location, including behind the esophagus, high in the neck, low in the upper mediastinum, or completely enclosed within the thyroid; and even though these facts are well known, such locations still defeat an inexperienced operator. It is not uncommon on reexploration of the neck to find that either the top has been removed from a dumb-bell shaped tumor, or that the abnormal gland is found in a previously unexplored tissue plane. It should be noted that even if the tumor is in the superior mediastinum, it is usually accessible to an experienced parathyroid surgeon through a standard incision low in the neck without the need to split the sternum.

If the patient is symptomatic, perhaps with renal calculi or parathyroid bone disease, or the bone density is low compared to a reference group of the same age, there is of course a significant problem and surgery is necessary. If, however, the patient appears to be asymptomatic or the hypercalcemia is found on "routine blood tests", the situation is more difficult (Tab. 19.2). A number of such cases have shown that there can be little change over a period of say 5 to 10 years. Rarely a change has been documented with relatively mild hypercalcemia (say 2.7 mmol/l; 10.8 mg/100 ml), progressing over a year or more to a much more serious situation (say 3.5 mmol/l; 14.0 mg/100 ml), with the onset of symptoms. It is not possible to predict which patients will change in this way. Another problem is posed by the fact that, rarely, a parathyroid carcinoma is found in the asymptomatic group. Its early removal is advantageous. If an experienced surgeon is available and the patient is fit, a strong case for surgery can be made on the basis that the operation is safe. In those circumstances, the risk of hypoparathyroidism post-operatively and the development of a recurrent laryngeal nerve palsy caused by the operation are both small. Moreover, it is surprisingly common for patients who have appeared to be asymptomatic beforehand to spontaneously say that they feel better when the adenoma has been removed. If a decision has been made not to operate, it is important to avoid excessive anxiety, either in the patient or the medical attendants. There is no point in measuring the serum calcium every few months, as that merely engenders anxiety about changes in successive readings that are probably not significant. If no operation is planned, it is probably reasonable simply to check the calcium annually.

A description of the surgical technique to be used is beyond the scope of this chapter, but a few points should be noted. Frozen sections should be available at the time of surgery to verify findings. A statement that the gland has been identified by looking at it is of little value if it has not been confirmed histologically. A drawing of the operative findings to show the relationship between the thyroid and the abnormal parathyroid is valuable even if it is not feasible to say whether the gland removed is an upper or lower one. Documentation of the size of the gland removed is also important. Unless there is a clearly enlarged gland, it is unlikely to be significant. Another requirement is the availability of an anesthetist experienced in the specific needs for successful surgery, including the use of hypotension to reduce bleeding. This must be balanced against the risk of hypotension affecting renal function, which may already be impaired by stones or hypercalcemia.

From the medical standpoint, the essential thing is to document that serum calcium falls after surgery to normal and remains normal. For this purpose, serum calcium should be measured daily for one week and then 3 to 4 times per year for 2 years. After a successful parathyroidectomy, calcium will fall to normal within 2 to 3 days and remain normal. Rarely, it takes 6 or 7 days for this to happen. Having come down to normal, if all abnormal parathyroid tissue has been removed, it will remain normal. If the operation has failed, hypercalcemia is usually demonstrable again within one week. Careful monitoring is therefore needed in that period, since if further surgery is necessary, it is best done within 10 days of the first operation before scar tissue has formed. The surgical approaches to be used, if such a rapid reexploration is needed, will depend on the original findings. Total thyroidectomy is one possibility at the second operation, since even if the thyroid appeared to be normal, an adenoma could be invisible within it. If the exploration of the neck is not feasible within 10 days, then it is best deferred for 3 months, by which time the increased vascularity of the scar tissue will have subsided. In patients with parathyroid carcinoma, initial surgery will usually produce normocalcemia, though hypercalcemia usually returns within two years, providing the basis for normal follow-up.

Failed surgery

Reexploration of the neck is far more difficult for the surgeon and more hazardous for the patient. It is therefore appropriate to review the diagnosis before it is undertaken and to consider whether the original indications justify the added risk. For example, if the original symptoms were minor and if the hypercalcemia was marginal, it would be reasonable to not do more apart from observation. The risk of recurrent laryngeal nerve palsy is greater after a second operation, and the risk of postoperative hypoparathyroidism is also increased especially if normal glands have previously been removed at the first operation.

As well as reviewing the diagnosis, it is appropriate in this situation to consider using all possible preoperative localization techniques in patients who have had failed

Table 19.2 Indications for surgical removal of parathyroid tumors

	High priority	Intermediate priority	Advisable
Serum calcium	>3 mmol/l (>12 mg/100 ml)	>2.75 mmol/l (>11 mg/100 ml)	<2.75 mmol/l (<11 mg/100 ml) but above normal
Skeleton	Osteitis fibrosa, fast bone mineral loss	Postmenopausal status, decreased bone mineral density	
Renal	Deteriorating glomerular filtration rate (GFR), nephrocalcinosis, nephrolithiasis	Age-related reduced GFR	
Other	Recurrent pancreatitis	Ulcer disease	Asymptomatic, hypertension, psychiatric symptoms

(From Fischer JA. Asymptomatic and symptomatic primary hyperparathyroidism. Clin Invest 1993;71:505-18.)

neck explorations. Those techniques can be used in sequence to focus attention on suspicious areas. The ultrasound examination can be repeated, and radioisotope scans done using two isotopes, so that uptake by the thyroid can be subtracted. Over the years a variety of isotope techniques have been advocated; initial reports have always been encouraging, but none has become "indispensable". Parathyroid venous sampling can be useful. In this technique blood is taken from the major veins of the neck and from as many small thyroid veins as can be entered, using a catheter passed up the inferior vena cava up to the neck. A skilled, practiced radiologist is needed, and the procedure is time consuming. Samples can then be assayed for parathyroid hormone and "a hot spot" sought when the results are charted on a drawing showing the sites of sampling. Any of these techniques may produce suggested evidence for focusing analysis of high-resolution computer technology scanning (which is better than magnetic resonance imaging because of the problems of movement artifact in the latter). Computer technology scans should extend from the angle of the jaw down to the aortic arch. The key to localization may depend on detecting areas of asymmetry in regions where symmetry would be expected. In practice it is unlikely that an adenoma smaller than 1 cm in diameter would be identified by computer technology scanning.

The most successful technique for localizing parathyroid tumors is probably parathyroid angiography. Again, this needs a radiologist who is experienced in the particular technique. This is often a neuroradiologist who does spinal angiography. It is essential to use contrast media that do not carry a risk of spinal artery thrombosis, which can cause Brown Séquard syndrome. With angiography it is possible to demonstrate tumors that have not been detected preoperatively by any other method, either in the neck or in the mediastinum. Because of the difficulty of the method however, it can only be used in relatively few cases, in those in whom previous neck surgery has been unsuccessful.

SPECIAL SITUATIONS

It is appropriate to consider the problems of hyperparathyroidism and of parathyroid surgery that arise in some specific circumstances.

Pregnancy

Sometimes hyperparathyroidism is diagnosed during pregnancy – usually because of a renal calculus causing abdominal pain. Hyperparathyroidism is typically a benign condition in pregnancy. Surgery during pregnancy is best avoided. It is quite clear that moderate hypercalcemia is generally well-tolerated by the fetus. The existence of maternal hypercalcemia may only be recognized post partum when an otherwise healthy child has a hypocalcemic attack in the neonatal period as a result of

suppression of the parathyroid glands by the fetal hypercalcemia produced by an elevated maternal calcium. Generally the infant's parathyroid recovers spontaneously, although treatment may be needed for some time. Occasionally, however, hyperparathyroidism causes serious problems to the mother during pregnancy and spontaneous abortion can occur. If parathyroid surgery is thought to be necessary, then it is best done in the middle trimester.

Multiple endocrine neoplasia

The indications for surgery in this condition are the same as for uncomplicated primary hyperparathyroidism. The only question is the type of surgery to be done. The problem is that after surgery in this condition there is tendency for the hyperparathyroidism to recur after an interval that may extend over many years, even if at first it has seemed successful. Generally in multiple endocrine neoplasia there is parathyroid hyperplasia rather than a single adenoma, though glands that seem normal during initial surgery may subsequently become overactive. For this reason it had been suggested that there should be an attempt to remove all parathyroid tissue and to reimplant a small piece in the muscle of the forearm. It was thought that if this tissue became overactive, it could be easily subsequently removed. However, removal of the glandular tissue from the forearm is not at all easy, and there is a tendency for it to spread microscopically within the muscle. Moreover, there is always the dilemma as to whether the overactive tissue is really to be found in the forearm or whether it is to be developed in the neck, where originally it had not been found. It seems more reasonable therefore, in multiple endocrine neoplasia, to perform a radical operation with the intention of causing hypoparathyroidism, and accepting the need for long-term medical treatment for that. The efficacy of such a policy, however, remains to be established by long-term follow-up.

Hyperparathyroidism in children

Hyperparathyroidism in children is fortunately rare. No pediatric surgeon is experienced in parathyroid surgery, few parathyroid surgeons are experienced in pediatric surgery, and so the problems are considerable. Exploration of the neck of children is not at all easy, and the criteria for identifying an abnormal gland in the neck of an adult do not apply in the child. The life-threatening form of neonatal hyperparathyroidism in homozygous patients with a calcium receptor defect require total removal of the parathyroid glands. Otherwise, it is better to avoid surgery in children. If there is failure-to-thrive, however, this would be a strong indication, as would be the presence of hyperparathyroid bone disease seen on X-ray of the wrists or knees.

Parathyroid carcinoma

As in the case of malignancy of other endocrine glands, the diagnosis of parathyroid carcinoma can be quite difficult unless there is metastasis outside the capsule.

Sometimes the histological appearance of malignancy is found in patients with a relatively small gland and relatively minor elevation of serum calcium. Generally, however, patients with parathyroid carcinoma have very large tumors (often weighing more than 10 g) and usually the serum calcium is quite high (greater than 3 mmol/l; 12 mg/100 ml). There is often marked hyperparathyroid bone disease and/or large renal calculi. The metabolic disturbance is generally corrected with removal of all visible parathyroid tissue, upon which treatment for hypoparathyroidism may then be necessary. Any hyperparathyroid bone disease will heal with this regime. Generally, however, the condition recurs within 2 years, replacement therapy becomes unnecessary, and serum calcium rises. Nevertheless, the outlook can be remarkably good. Even if the original presentation has been dramatic, the patient may, with recurrence of the tumor, remain physically well despite a calcium of say 3.5 mmol/l (14.0 mg/100 ml), as high as that which caused major symptoms initially. Generally, when hyperparathyroidism recurs, it is due to diffuse local infiltration, though sometimes there may be a recurrence of a local mass instead. Surgically it is difficult to deal with the situation if there is local infiltration, but removal of a recurrent mass, despite the presence of surrounding scar tissue, is often feasible. Distant metastases, in the lung or the pleura, for example, may not develop for as long as 10 years. If they are present, removal of those metastases is justifiable since "debulking" of the tumor load can be very effective, restoring serum calcium to normal for perhaps a year or more. Chemotherapy in this situation has remarkably little to offer.

Malignant hypercalcemia

Occasionally patients present with life-threatening hypercalcemia, such as 5 mmol/l (20 mg/100 ml) or greater with only a short history. This situation must be approached as an emergency and plans made to deal with it swiftly. It should be possible to reach a diagnosis of hyperparathyroidism within two days and then to undertake emergency surgery. In that time relatively little investigation is feasible. The ones to be done should be those that will either produce positive support for the diagnosis

of hyperparathyroidism or those that will exclude the presence of another cause. The investigations to be done will include examination of plasma proteins and a blood count, looking for multiple myeloma, a chest X-ray, looking for malignant disease (either primary or secondary) and X-ray of the hands looking for evidence of parathyroid bone disease. A skeletal survey looking for malignant deposits, an ultrasound examination of the neck and abdomen (looking for a parathyroid tumor or other disease) will all be useful. While these tests are being done, the patient should be rehydrated and attempts made to reduce the serum calcium with intravenous pamidronate.

Treatment of postoperative hypocalcemia

Hypoparathyroidism probably occurs postoperatively in a few percent of the cases after parathyroid surgery. The more parathyroid glands are removed, the greater the risk. If within a week of surgery, hypocalcemia develops, it is probably useful to give calcium supplement and, if possible, definitive treatment should be deferred for a couple of weeks to see if spontaneous recovery occurs. Should definitive treatment be needed, it is best done with 0.5 to 2.0 µg 1-hydroxylate forms of vitamin D, that is, 1,25-dihydroxycholecalciferol or α-calcidol. The maintenance dose of calcitriol is usually about 0.25 to 1.0 µg per day and that of α-calcidol about 1-2 µg per day. If the patient had severe hyperparathyroid bone disease preoperatively, then postoperative hypocalcemia is to be expected due to the "hungry bone" syndrome. The requirement for treatment is then likely to be great and the dose of calcitriol, for example, may need to be as high as 10 µg per day with large calcium supplements. The doses should be reduced as the bone disease heals, as reflected by a fall in alkaline phosphatase towards normal. When the bone disease is healed and alkaline phosphatase approaches normal (which may take 4 to 6 months) a decision has to be made as to whether long-term treatment is needed. If life-long medication is needed, serum calcium will need to be measured 3 to 4 times a year to avoid vitamin D intoxication.

Suggested readings

BRESLAU NA, PAK CYC. Asymptomatic primary hyperparathyroidism. In: Coe FC, Favus MF (eds). Disorders of bone and mineral metabolism. New York: Raven Press, 1992;523-38.

FISCHER JA. "Asymptomatic" and symptomatic primary hyperparathyroidism. Clin Investig 1993;71:505-18.

HEATH H, HODGSON SF, KENNEDY MA. Primary hyperparathyroidism. Incidence, morbidity, and potential economic impact in a community. N Engl J Med 1980;302:189-93.

POTTS JT JR. Management of asymptomatic hyperparathyroidism: a report on the NIH consensus development conference. Trends Endocrinol Metab 1992;10:376-9.

SILVERBERG SJ, BILEZIKIAN JP. Primary hyperparathyroidism: still evolving? J Bone Miner Res 1997;12:856-62.

Malignancy-associated hypercalcemia

Horacio Plotkin, Andrew F. Stewart

KEY POINTS

- Malignancy-associated hypercalcemia can be divided into four subcategories, which are, in descending order of frequency: humoral hypercalcemia of malignancy, local osteolytic hypercalcemia, overproduction of 1,25 vitamin D by malignant lymphomas, and authentic ectopic hyperparathyroidism.
- Malignancy-associated hypercalcemia is by far the most common form of hypercalcemia among hospitalized patients, and it is second in frequency to hyperparathyroidism among outpatients.
- The onset of malignancy-associated hypercalcemia indicates a very poor prognosis: 50% survival is approximately 30 days.
- It is critical to specifically seek and exclude other treatable forms of hypercalcemia in patients with cancer.
- Immediate therapy for malignancy-associated hypercalcemia should be directed at increasing renal calcium excretion and inhibiting osteoclastic bone resorption.
- The only effective long-term therapy of malignancy-associated hypercalcemia is successful treatment of the underlying malignancy. Therefore, anti-tumor therapy should be selected and implemented at an early stage in patients with malignancy-associated hypercalcemia.

There are four major categories of malignancy-associated hypercalcemia: (1) humoral hypercalcemia of malignancy, (2) local osteolytic hypercalcemia, (3) ectopic hyperparathyroidism, and (4) secretion of the active form of vitamin D by lymphomas. In this chapter, the causes, pathophysiology, differential diagnosis, and treatment of hypercalcemia resulting from cancer will be discussed.

The development of hypercalcemia in a patient with cancer predicts a very poor prognosis: 50% of patients die within 30 days of the onset of hypercalcemia. Death frequently occurs as a result of the development of hypercalcemia-induced renal failure and/or coma.

Malignancy-associated hypercalcemia is common, occurring in up to 25% of patients with squamous carcinoma of the oropharynx, up to 30% of patients with mul-

tiple myeloma, and up to 20% of patients with breast cancer. As is described in Table 20.1, while hypercalcemia has been reported to occur in association with almost every type of malignancy, it is particularly likely to occur in patients with squamous carcinomas arising at any site, with renal and gynecological carcinomas, with hematologic malignancies and lymphomas, and with carcinoma of the breast. Conversely, hypercalcemia rarely occurs in association with certain common neoplasms such as carcinoma of the colon, gastric carcinoma, small cell carcinoma of the lung, or prostate carcinoma. The failure of the latter two tumor types to lead to the development of hypercalcemia on a regular basis is particularly surprising, given the predilection for these tumors to involve the skeleton, and for small cell carcinoma to cause other endocrine paraneoplastic syndromes such as the syndrome of inappropriate secretion of antidiuretic hormone (SIADH) and syndromes of ectopic adrenocorticotropic hormone production. These observations make the point that skeletal involvement and ectopic hormone production alone are not sufficient to lead to hypercalcemia: a tumor must produce the right "hormone" or cytokine, and it must produce this hypercalcemic factor in a location and quantity that gives it access to the skeleton.

The malignancy-associated hypercalcemia field has received much attention over the past two decades for two reasons. First, there have been dramatic discoveries regarding the pathogenesis and diagnosis of the syndrome. Second, there have been equally dramatic advances in the therapy of the syndrome.

Local osteolytic hypercalcemia

The first subtype of malignancy-associated hypercalcemia to be described in pathophysiological terms was the hypercalcemia observed in patients with breast cancer and multiple myeloma. In a large series of such patients reported in 1936, Gutman et al. observed that virtually all patients with malignancy-associated hypercalcemia due to these two malignancies also had extensive skeletal metastatic disease. More modern series have confirmed these observations, and it is now clear that one mechanism responsible for hypercalcemia is direct skeletal involvement with tumors. The tumor types commonly associated with this type of hypercalcemia in modern series are shown in Table 20.1. Local osteolytic hypercalcemia accounts for approximately 20% of patients with malignancy-associated hypercalcemia. The trabecular and cortical bone surfaces in patients with myeloma and breast cancer are covered with osteoclasts actively resorbing bone in response to cytokines or paracrine factors produced by the malignant cells. Skeletal tumor metastasis

alone, however, is not adequate to cause hypercalcemia, as underscored by the observations noted above that tumors such as small cell carcinoma of the lung and prostate carcinoma, both of which regularly involve the skeleton, rarely cause hypercalcemia. Thus, hypercalcemia that occurs in tumors that involve the skeleton must result from the secretion of specific cytokines and paracrine factors that activate osteoclasts. The list of such cytokines includes interleukin 1, interleukin 6, tumor necrosis factor-beta (also called lymphotoxin), parathyroid hormone-related protein, and prostaglandins of the E series. This list has grown in recent years, and it will certainly continue to grow as new cytokines are discovered.

From a clinical biochemical standpoint, since the hypercalcemia results from excessive release of calcium from the skeleton, one finds reductions in parathyroid hormone, and resultant normal to high-normal serum phosphorus values, a low-normal fractional excretion of phosphorus, a high-normal tubular maximum for phosphorus excretion, hypercalciuria, and reductions in plasma $1,25(OH)_2$ vitamin D. Hypercalcemia in these patients is the result of osteoclastic bone resorption occurring at an accelerated rate, such that the rate of calcium entry into the extracellular fluid exceeds the ability of the kidney to clear calcium. Intestinal calcium absorption does not contribute to the syndrome, as would be predicted by the reductions in $1,25(OH)_2$ vitamin D. As one would also expect, extensive skeletal tumor involvement is typically observed by skeletal radiographs, bone biopsy, and/or autopsy. Interestingly, while the bone scintigraphic scan is extensively positive in patients with solid tumor metastasis (e.g., breast carcinoma) in malignancy-associated hypercalcemia, it may be negative in multiple myeloma despite extensive marrow involvement, reflecting the requirement for osteoblast activation for detection using scintigraphic methods. The diagnosis of local osteolytic hypercalcemia is one of exclusion: the diagnosis is established by excluding other causes of hypercalcemia (Tab. 20.2) and by demonstrating that the patient in question fulfills the criteria outlined above.

Humoral hypercalcemia of malignancy

Humoral hypercalcemia of malignancy was first described in 1941. It is the most common of the subtypes of malignancy-associated hypercalcemia, accounting for approximately 80% of unselected patients in most recent series. The types of tumors that most often cause this syndrome are listed in Table 20.1. It is important to note, with two important exceptions, that these tumors are distinct from those that most often cause local osteolytic hypercalcemia. Humoral hypercalcemia malignancy most often (and some would say, by definition) occurs as a result of secretion by the offending neoplasm of parathyroid hormone-related protein (PTHrP). This peptide is produced in small amounts under normal circumstances by most normal cell types, where it serves paracrine or autocrine functions and does not enter the systemic circulation in significant quantities. However, when it is overproduced by malignant cells and enters the circulation in sufficient quantities, it is

---

Table 20.1 Subtypes of malignancy-associated hypercalcemia

Humoral hypercalcemia of malignancy

  Squamous carcinoma (lung, oropharynx, cervix, esophagus, etc.)
  Renal carcinoma
  Ovarian carcinoma
  Bladder carcinoma
  HTLV-1 lymphoma
  Breast carcinoma

Local osteolytic hypercalcemia

  Breast carcinoma
  Multiple myeloma
  Lymphoma

$1,25(OH)_2$ vitamin D-producing lymphomas

Ectopic hyperparathyroidism

Table 20.2 Differential diagnosis of hypercalcemia

Hyperparathyroidism

Malignancy-associated hypercalcemia

Granulomatous disorders
  Sarcoidosis, tuberculosis, etc.

Endocrine disorders
  Hyperthyroidism
  Pheochromocytoma
  VIPoma
  Addisonian crisis

Medications
  Vitamin D or A intoxication
  Lithium
  Hydrochlorothiazide
  Theophylline
  Estrogen or anti-estrogen (in the setting of breast
    cancer and skeletal metastases)

Milk-alkali syndrome

Parenteral nutrition containing calcium

Immobilization

Acute or chronic renal failure

Familial hypocalciuric hypercalcemia

Neonatal hypercalcemia

Hyperalbuminemia

---

able to interact with the shared parathyroid hormone (PTH)/PTHrP receptor and mimic the actions of PTH on the kidney and skeleton. Thus, PTHrP secretion in humoral hypercalcemia of malignancy is not really "ectopic", since PTHrP is normally produced by the same cells that gave rise to the malignancy. Given the above, the clinical biochemical abnormalities in humoral hypercalcemia of malignancy are predictable: circulating PTHrP concentrations are elevated, serum calcium is elevated as a result of osteoclastic bone resorption, and parathyroid hormone is suppressed. Since PTHrP mimics the action of PTH, phosphaturia and hypophosphatemia occur as long as renal function is preserved. Hypercalciuria occurs since the filtered load of calcium is elevated. Some investigators have suggested that PTHrP stimulates renal calcium reabsorption with a potency analogous to that of PTH, while others have suggested that PTHrP has weak calcium reabsorptive actions on the renal tubule. Unlike patients with hyperparathyroidism in whom $1,25(OH)_2$ vitamin D concentrations are elevated as a result of PTH action on the proximal renal tubule, the concentrations of this active vitamin D metabolite are reduced in patients with humoral hypercalcemia of malignancy. The pathophysiological basis for this observation is unknown. Given the clinical biochemical phenomenology described above, one can construct a pathophysiologic scenario in patients with humoral hypercalcemia of malignancy: hypercalcemia occurs, as in local osteolytic hypercalcemia, as a result of excessive osteoclastic bone resorption with skeletal calcium delivery into the extracellular fluid at a rate that exceeds the ability of the kidney to clear it. Excessive PTHrP-mediated renal calcium reabsorption may contribute to the syndrome, although, as noted above, this is a matter of some debate.

Intestinal calcium absorption does not occur since $1,25(OH)_2$ vitamin D concentrations are low.

As might be expected, skeletal metastases are not a prominent feature of this syndrome. Most patients have no skeletal metastases; some patients do have skeletal metastases, but in general, the number of metastases is fewer than five, and they do not contribute to the development of hypercalcemia in an important way.

The diagnosis of humoral hypercalcemia of malignancy is suspected in patients who fulfill the above criteria and in whom no other cause of hypercalcemia can be found. The diagnosis can be confirmed, if necessary, by finding an elevated concentration of PTHrP in the circulation.

Authentic ectopic hyperparathyroidism

Prior to the discovery of PTHrP as the cause of humoral hypercalcemia of malignancy, it was widely believed that the condition was due to the secretion of PTH by tumors, and the syndrome bore names such as "ectopic hyperparathyroidism" or "pseudohyperparathyroidism". By the mid- to late 1980's, most investigators in this area felt that all cases of humoral hypercalcemia of malignancy were due to PTHrP and that ectopic secretion of PTH did not occur. This perception has changed over the last several years, with the publication of five well-documented cases of what can only be described as authentic ectopic PTH secretion. The typical clinical presentation of ectopic parathyroid hormone secretion in these reports has been as follows: a patient presents with an elevated serum calcium concentration in the setting of elevated PTH concentrations, as determined using a sensitive and specific two-site PTH immunoradiometric assay. The combination of an elevated PTH and hypercalcemia leads to a surgical exploration of the neck, which reveals four normal parathyroid glands. Attention is then focused on identifying a non-parathyroid source of PTH, and a tumor is discovered. Four out of five patients described to date were 69 years old or older, the one exception being a 25-year-old man with a PTH-producing thymoma. The histological type of the tumor differed in each of the cases and has included a small cell carcinoma of the lung, an ovarian adenocarcinoma, a primitive neuroectodermal malignancy, a thymoma, and a squamous cell carcinoma of the lung. In all cases, circulating PTH was found to be 10 to 70 times the upper limits of normal. PTHrP values were normal when measured. In the case of the ovarian adenocarcinoma, ectopic expression of the PTH gene was found to result from a gene rearrangement that placed the PTH gene under the control of an ovarian promoter. The mechanisms responsible for the ectopic expression of PTH in the other tumors are not clear.

These patients present a particularly difficult diagnostic challenge since they present with the classical biochemical findings of primary hyperparathyroidism, and because the syndrome is rare and not widely recognized.

The syndrome should be considered in all patients with hypercalcemia and particularly those in whom parathyroid exploration for a putative parathyroid adenoma is unsuccessful.

Hypercalcemia due to 1,25 vitamin D-producing lymphomas

In 1984, two groups described unusual patients with lymphomas who were hypercalcemic and in whom the hypercalcemia appeared to be due to the production of the active form of vitamin D [1,25(OH)$_2$ vitamin D (calcitriol)] by the lymphomas. Since then, approximately 30 additional patients have been described. Thus, these patients account for well under 1% of patients with malignancy-associated hypercalcemia. In these patients, a lymphoma that may or may not involve the skeleton produces excessive quantities of this active vitamin D metabolite, and this in turn causes hypercalcemia by stimulating osteoclastic bone resorption in the skeleton and by stimulating intestinal calcium absorption. Hypercalcemia occurs when the combined rates of bone resorption and intestinal calcium absorption exceed the ability of the kidneys to clear calcium. The hypercalcemia leads to a reduction in PTH secretion, and therefore phosphorus concentrations are normal or high-normal. PTHrP concentrations are undetectable. In cases where the lymphoma is localized to a single site, such as the spleen, surgical resection of the lymphoma will correct the hypercalcemia, underscoring the point that this type of hypercalcemia, as in humoral hypercalcemia of malignancy and ectopic HPT, is also "humoral".

No single type of lymphoma is associated with this syndrome. Both non-Hodgkin's and Hodgkin's lymphomas may be responsible, and they may be well- or poorly-differentiated, nodular, or diffuse.

From a pathogenic standpoint, one must wonder why malignant lymphoid tissue would produce 1,25(OH)$_2$ vitamin D. As it turns out, 1,25(OH)$_2$ vitamin D is a normal product of lymphoid tissues, and it appears to play a local paracrine role under normal circumstances in lymphocyte and macrophage differentiation, proliferation, immune recognition, and, in macrophages, in phagocytosis. In certain lymphomas, 1,25(OH)$_2$ vitamin D is overproduced, enters the systemic circulation, and has effects on systemic calcium homeostasis. In this way, the syndrome is very much like the hypercalcemia that accompanies sarcoidosis and other granulomatous diseases, in which the same pathophysiology pertains.

The treatment of patients with malignancy-associated hypercalcemia is discussed below in more detail. It is important to note, however, that these patients represent a special subgroup of patients with malignancy-associated hypercalcemia, for, like hypercalcemic patients with sarcoidosis, they do require a reduction in calcium and vitamin D intake, and glucocorticoids represent an attractive treatment modality.

Other types of malignancy-associated hypercalcemia

The four patient groups described above account for more than 99% of the patients with malignancy-associated hypercalcemia. Nonetheless, there are rare patients encountered with malignancy-associated hypercalcemia in whom other mechanisms appear to apply. For example, we have reported a patient with an ovarian carcinoma, with suppressed PTH and 1,25(OH)$_2$ vitamin D and no evidence for PTHrP production, but with no skeletal involvement and in whom hypercalcemia reversed following oophorectomy. Clearly this was a case of "humoral hypercalcemia" in a patient with cancer, but none of the usual "humors" could be implicated.

Similarly, occasional patients with renal carcinoma and hypercalcemia have been reported in whom prostaglandins of the E series have been implicated pathogenically.

Clinical findings

Patients with malignancy-associated hypercalcemia virtually always have advanced disease at the time of onset of hypercalcemia, and, with very few exceptions, the tumor burden is large when hypercalcemia occurs. One way to interpret this observation is that tumors are inefficient at producing and/or processing the cytokines and "humors" that cause malignancy-associated hypercalcemia, so that a large tumor burden must be present before hypercalcemia can occur. In practical terms, this means that tumors in patients with malignancy-associated hypercalcemia are not occult or difficult to localize: rather, they are large and obvious at presentation and do not typically require an extensive search before they are found. If a tumor is not discovered after a careful physical exam, mammography, a complete blood count, a urinalysis, and a chest radiograph, one should begin to look hard for other explanations for the hypercalcemia (see Differential Diagnosis below and Tab. 20.2).

Hypercalcemia leads to reductions in the level of consciousness, ranging from mild confusion to deep coma. The degree of neurologic alteration is a result not only of the degree of hypercalcemia, but also of the rate of change in the serum calcium: a patient with chronic hypercalcemia may tolerate a serum calcium in the 16 mg/dl (4 mM) range with little neurologic deficit, while an acute rise to 12 mg/dl (3 mM) may be sufficient to induce stupor or coma in other patients. The effect of serum calcium on neurologic function is also influenced by the underlying level of function of, and interacting medications in, the patient in question. For example, an elderly person with mild Alzheimer's disease who is using narcotics for pain control is likely to display more profound degrees of neurologic dysfunction for a given degree of hypercalcemia than a 20-year-old patient taking no medications.

Hypercalcemia also induces polyuria and polydipsia. The mechanisms responsible for his phenomenon are not completely clear, but the recent discovery of the parathyroid gland calcium receptor and the presence of this receptor in the concentrating portions of the distal nephron suggests that this receptor may interfere with urinary concentrating ability.

Hypercalcemia regularly leads to reductions in renal function, which may be mild or may be severe. Mechanisms for renal failure include: (1) dehydration from the nephrogenic diabetes insipidus described in the preceding paragraph, (2) the acute vasoconstrictive effect of hypercalcemia on the renal afferent arteriole, (3) nephrocalcinosis from calcium phosphate salt precipitation in the interstitium, or (4) ureteral obstruction from renal calculi. In general, if hypercalcemia is corrected rapidly, renal function returns to normal. If chronic hypercalcemia is allowed to continue for weeks or months, particularly if it is accompanied by elevations in the serum phosphorus, permanent renal damage occurs.

Hypercalcemia may also cause shortening of the Q-T interval on the electrocardiogram. It is often assumed that hypercalcemia may predispose a patient to serious ventricular arrhythmias, but reports of this are rare.

Differential diagnosis

The disorders that must be considered in the differential diagnosis in a patient being evaluated for a diagnosis of malignancy-associated hypercalcemia are summarized in Table 20.2. Two important points should be made here. First, in most instances, the diagnosis of malignancy-associated hypercalcemia is one of exclusion: the diagnosis can only be made when other causes of hypercalcemia have been eliminated. Second, while the above is intuitive, it is critically important to individually consider and exclude the diagnoses in Table 20.2 in every case, for while malignancy-associated hypercalcemia is in general poorly responsive to treatment, all of the other disorders listed in Table 20.2 are amenable to treatment. Thus, to assign a diagnosis of malignancy-associated hypercalcemia is to assign a very poor prognosis. This is not a trivial point, for the authors have repeatedly observed hypercalcemia occurring in patients with cancer in whom the hypercalcemia resulted from a "benign" cause. Examples include hyperthyroidism in a woman with breast cancer, tuberculosis in a man with squamous carcinoma of the lung, and immobilization hypercalcemia in a young man with leukemia. In each of these instances, hypercalcemia reversed with treatment of the underlying disorder and in each case, the status of the patient in question was viewed in a very different light when a "benign" cause for the hypercalcemia was discovered.

Treatment

A critical decision that must be made when confronted with a patient with malignancy-associated hypercalcemia is whether treatment is appropriate. As noted earlier, patients with malignancy-associated hypercalcemia have a very poor prognosis: the 50% survival from the time of diagnosis of hypercalcemia is approximately 30 days.

Thus, in many instances, if a patient has been treated previously with aggressive chemotherapy, surgery, and radiation, the most appropriate therapy would be no therapy at all. In addition, one might be less inclined to treat an elderly person with another underlying disease such as Alzheimer's disease. On the other hand, patients with malignancy-associated hypercalcemia may commonly present with hypercalcemia as their initial abnormality, before having received anti-neoplastic therapy. An example might be a 45-year-old woman with estrogen receptor-positive breast cancer or a 55-year-old previously healthy man with multiple myeloma. In such patients, aggressive therapy would most often be warranted.

A second important point is that the only effective long-term therapy of malignancy-associated hypercalcemia is effective treatment of the underlying neoplasm. Anti-hypercalcemic therapy with the agents listed below is not effective over the long-term. Thus, if treatment is to be effective, anti-tumor therapy (surgery, radiation, chemotherapy) should be initiated immediately, using the anti-hypercalcemic agents listed in Table 20.3 as temporizing measures while awaiting a response to anti-tumor therapy.

Saline infusion at a rate of 200 to 400 ml per hour is given in an effort to (1) increase the glomerular filtration rate and therefore the filtered load of calcium, and (2) inhibit calcium reabsorption in the proximal tubule. The rate of infusion is guided by the cardiovascular status.

A loop diuretic such as furosemide, 20 to 40 mg, is given intravenously every 4 to 12 hours once the patient is well-hydrated with saline, in an effort to block calcium reabsorption in the thick ascending limb of Henle's loop. It is critical to withhold this therapy until the patient is well-hydrated, because further reductions in the glomeru-

---

Table 20.3 Treatment of malignancy-associated hypercalcemia

Tumor therapy
   Surgery
   Radiotherapy
   Chemotherapy

Anti-hypercalcemic therapy
   Saline infusion
   Loop diuretics (no chlorothiazides)
   Oral phosphorus replacement
   Reduction in oral calcium intake
   Discontinue calcium in TPN
   Mobilization
   Glucocorticoids
   Mithramycin (plicamycin)
   Gallium nitrate
   Calcitonin
   Bisphosphonates
      Pamidronate
      Clodronate
   Dialysis

(TPN = total parenteral nutrition.)

lar filtration rate will further reduce the filtered load of calcium and prevent the diuretic-induced fall in serum calcium. Careful attention must be given to the monitoring and replacing of potassium and magnesium. Diuretics of the chlorothiazide family should not be given, because they stimulate calcium reabsorption in the distal tubule and may worsen hypercalcemia.

Patients with malignancy-associated hypercalcemia regularly become hypophosphatemic regardless of the underlying cause of the hypercalcemia. Saline, furosemide, PTHrP, calcitonin therapy, anorexia, and antacids – all of which are given regularly to, or are produced in, patients with malignancy-associated hypercalcemia – all lead to hypophosphatemia. Since hyperphosphatemia can worsen hypercalcemia and make hypercalcemia more difficult to treat, it is important to judiciously replace phosphorus deficits with oral phosphorus supplements. These supplements can be given as oral neutral phosphate in doses of 250 mg four times per day in patients who have phosphorus concentrations below 3.0 mg/dl (1.0 mM). Strict attention must be given to the serum phosphorus and creatinine, since hyperphosphatemia in the setting of hypercalcemia will abruptly precipitate nephrocalcinosis and renal failure.

Patients with malignancy-associated hypercalcemia have reductions in plasma $1,25(OH)_2$ vitamin D. For this reason, they cannot effectively absorb calcium from the diet. For this reason, and since calcium-containing foods such as ice cream and milkshakes may be an important part of the diet of a patient with malignancy-associated hypercalcemia, it is not necessary, and may actually be counterproductive from a nutritional standpoint, to restrict calcium intake. The exception to this rule is the patient with a $1,25(OH)_2$ vitamin D-producing lymphoma who will hyperabsorb calcium from his or her diet. These patients, like those with sarcoidosis, should have their calcium intake restricted.

Peripheral hyperalimentation solutions may contain significant amounts of calcium. This may be important pathophysiologically, particularly in patients with reductions in renal function. This source of calcium entry into the extracellular fluid is frequently overlooked. Parenteral alimentation solutions that do not contain calcium can be obtained and should be substituted in this circumstance.

Immobilization may lead to hypercalcemia in patients with multiple myeloma, breast cancer, and other malignancies. For this reason, when possible, hypercalcemic patients should be encouraged to ambulate regularly. Weight-bearing exercise can effectively correct hypercalcemia in some patients. Clearly, this is not always possible, but in many instances it is possible.

Glucocorticoids can be very effective in reversing the hypercalcemia associated with breast and hematologic malignancies. Unfortunately, they may also interfere with certain chemotherapeutic regimens. Further, the time required for a response to glucocorticoids may be as long as 1 to 2 weeks. For these reasons, and because of the recent arrival of more effective therapies in the form of the bisphosphonates, glucocorticoids are not commonly used in the management of malignancy-associated hypercalcemia. In unusual cases, however, they may be very useful.

Mithramycin (also called plicamycin), gallium nitrate, and calcitonin have all been used as anti-resorptive (i.e., anti-osteoclastic) therapies in patients with malignancy-associated hypercalcemia. Mithramycin is effective but is limited by its toxicity over the long-term. It may still prove useful in the occasional patient who does not respond to other therapies. Gallium nitrate has been reported to be very effective, but its use is limited by the requirement for continuous intravenous administration. Calcitonin is also useful in the occasional patient with malignancy-associated hypercalcemia, but its use is limited by the temporary nature if its hypocalcemic response, the small magnitude of the fall in serum calcium it produces, and the recent introduction of more effective therapies.

A major advance in the therapy of malignancy-associated hypercalcemia has been the development and application of bisphosphonates. These agents are clearly the drugs of choice for malignancy-associated hypercalcemia. They are potent inhibitors of osteoclast-mediated bone resorption and are very effective in treating malignancy-associated hypercalcemia of all types. Further, they produce very few side effects. They must be given parenterally, but generally the responses they induce last for 1 to 4 weeks. The specific bisphosphonates that are available vary by country, but dichloromethylene bisphosphonate (clodronate) and aminopropylidine bisphosphonate (APD, pamidronate) are widely available for the treatment of malignancy-associated hypercalcemia. The dose of pamidronate is 60 to 90 mg infused in saline over several hours, ideally 12 to 24 hours. Other new agents will become available, and in some countries they already are. These include tiludronate, ibandronate, risedronate, alendronate, and others.

Finally, hypercalcemia may occur in patients with renal failure. If this occurs, many of the therapies shown in Table 20.3 cannot be given or will not be effective. In such patients, it should be remembered that dialysis against a low calcium dialysate is a very effective means of reducing the serum calcium. While this is not appropriate in most patients, it may be reasonable in a new, previously untreated patient with myeloma with renal failure due to light chain nephropathy, or in a young woman with breast cancer with transient renal failure due to aminoglycoside antibiotics.

Acknowledgement

This chapter was prepared thanks to the support of the Department of Veterans Affairs, and NIH Grant DK 51081.

BRESLAU NA, MCGUIRE JL, ZERWEKH JE, FRENKEL ED, PAK CYC. Hypercalcemia associated with increased serum calcitriol levels in three patients with lymphoma. Ann Int Med 1984;100:1-7.

BURTIS WJ, BRADY TG, ORLOFF JJ. Immunochemical characterization of circulating parathyroid hormone-related protein in patients with humoral hypercalcemia of malignancy. Engl J Med 1990;322:1106-12.

GARRETT RI, DURIE BGM, NEDWIN GE, et al. Production of the bone-resorbing cytokine lymphotoxin by cultured human myeloma cells. N Engl J Med 1987;317:526-32.

GUISE TA, YIN JJ, TAYLOR SD, et al. Evidence for a causal role of parathyroid hormone-related protein in the pathogenesis of human breast cancer-mediated osteolysis. J Clin Invest 1996;98:1544-9.

MUNDY GR. Hypercalcemia in hematologic malignancies and in solid tumors associated with extensive localized bone destruction. In: Favus M (ed). Primer on the metabolic bone disease and disorders of mineral metabolism. 3rd ed. Philadelphia: Lippincott-Raven, 1996;203-6.

NAKAYAMA K, FUKUMOTO S, TAKEDA S, et al. Differences in bone and vitamin D metabolism between primary hyperparathyroidism and malignancy-associated hypercalcemia. J Clin Endocrinol Metab 1996;81:607-11.

NIELSEN PK, RASMUSSEN AK, FELDT-RASMUSSEN U, BRANDT M, CHRISTENSEN L, OLGAARD K. Ectopic production of intact parathyroid hormone by a squamous cell lung carcinoma in vivo and in vitro. J Clin Endocrinol Metab 1996;81:3793-6.

NUSSBAUM SR, GAZ RD, ARNOLD A. Hypercalcemia and ectopic secretion of parathyroid hormone by an ovarian carcinoma with rearrangement of the gene for PTH. N Engl J Med 1990;323:1324-8.

ROSENTHAL NR, INSOGNA KL, GODSALL JW, SMALDONE L, WALDRON JW, STEWART AF. 1,25 dihydroxyvitamin D-mediated humoral hypercalcemia in malignant lymphoma. J Clin Endocrinol Metab 1985;60:29-33.

SEYMOUR JF, GAGEL RF, HAGEMEISTER FB, DIMOPOULOS MA, CABANILLAS F. Calcitriol production in hypercalcemia and normocalcemia patients with non-Hodgkin lymphoma. Ann Int Med 1994;121:33-40.

SHANE E. Hypercalcemia: pathogenesis, clinical manifestations, differential diagnosis, and management. In: Favus M (ed). Primer on the metabolic bone disease and disorders of mineral metabolism. 3rd ed. Philadelphia: Lippincott-Raven, 1996;177-81.

STEWART AF. Humoral hypercalcemia of malignancy. In: Favus M (ed). The American Society for Bone and Mineral Research Primer on metabolic bone diseases and disorders of mineral metabolism. 3rd ed. New York: Raven Press, 1996; 198-203.

STEWART AF, INSOGNA KL, BROADUS AE. Malignancy-associated hypercalcemia. In: DeGroot L (ed). Endocrinology. 3rd ed. Philadelphia: W.B. Saunders, 1995;1061-74.

YANG KH, STEWART AF. Therapy of hypercalcemia. In: Mazzaferri EL, Bar RS, Kreisberg RA (eds). Advances in endocrinology and metabolism. Vol. 4. St. Louis: Mosby, 1993;305-34.

YANG KH, STEWART AF. The PTH-related protein gene and protein products. In: Bilezikian JP, Raisz L, Rodan G (eds). Principles of bone biology. San Diego: Academic Press, 1996;347-76.

Hypoparathyroidism and pseudohypo-parathyroidism

Geoffrey N. Hendy, David Goltzman

■ KEY POINTS ■

- Hypoparathyroidism is a disorder in which hypocalcemia and hyperphosphatemia occur as a result of deficient parathyroid hormone secretion. The hypoparathyroidism may be transient or permanent.
- Hypoparathyroidism most commonly occurs as a result of surgical excision of, or damage to, the parathyroid glands.
- Developmental defects of the parathyroid gland and defects in parathyroid hormone biosynthesis or secretion occur rarely.
- Congenital resistance to parathyroid hormone occurs in the syndromes referred to as pseudohypoparathyroidism.
- Acute or severe symptomatic hypocalcemia is treated with intravenous calcium infusion. Intravenous vitamin D therapy is not needed.
- The mainstay of chronic treatment is oral calcium and vitamin D. A thiazide diuretic may be added to reduce hypercalciuria and raise the serum calcium.

Maintenance of the concentration of calcium in extracellular fluid within a narrow normal range of 8.5 to 10.0 mg/dl (2.1 to 2.5 mM) is critical for many physiological processes. The parathyroid gland plays a key role in calcium homeostasis by sensing a decrease in ambient calcium concentration and responding appropriately by synthesizing and secreting more parathyroid hormone (PTH). Parathyroid hormone acts on the kidney to enhance renal calcium reabsorption and promote the conversion of 25-hydroxyvitamin D to 1,25-dihydroxyvitamin D. This active metabolite of vitamin D increases gastrointestinal absorption of calcium and, with PTH, induces skeletal resorption, which causes increases in the extracellular fluid calcium concentration. The parathyroid gland senses the normalization of the ambient calcium concentration and reduces PTH release. PTH also modulates the extracellular concentration of other ions, the most important of which is phosphate. PTH-induced skeletal lysis increases extracellular phosphate as well as calcium levels. A compensatory decrease in extracellular fluid phosphate is brought about by the action of PTH to inhibit renal phosphate reabsorption, thereby producing phosphaturia.

In target issues, PTH binds to a plasma membrane G-protein-coupled receptor (PTHR), which also binds the related ligand PTH-related peptide (PTHrP). A second receptor, PTHR2, which binds PTH but not PTHrP, is expressed in the brain but not bone and kidney, and its involvement in any disease process is unknown. The results of interaction of PTH with its receptor in bone and kidney have classically been interpreted to be the stimulation of the enzyme adenylate cyclase on the inner surface of the plasma membrane, although the same receptor can couple to phosphatidylinositol turnover as well. The product of the adenylate cyclase activity, cyclic AMP, activates protein kinase A, while the products of phospholipase C activity – inositol-(1,4,5)-trisphosphate (IP_3) and diacylglycerol – mobilize intracellular Ca^{2+} stores and activate protein kinase C activity, respectively. Thus, a cascade of events is initiated leading to the final cellular response to the hormone.

Hypoparathyroidism is a disorder in which hypocalcemia and hyperphosphatemia occur as a result of deficient parathyroid hormone (PTH) secretion. The hypoparathyroidism may be transient or permanent, and there are a considerable number of etiologies of each type. Functional or biochemical hypoparathyroidism, as in the various forms of pseudohypoparathyroidism, occurs when adequate circulating concentrations of PTH are unable to function optimally in target tissues and maintain blood calcium levels within the normal range.

The clinical forms and causes of hypoparathyroidism due to decreased secretion of PTH are presented in Table 21.1.

PARATHYROID GLAND ABLATION OR DESTRUCTION

Surgical excision

Hypoparathyroidism most commonly occurs as a result of surgical excision of, or damage to, the parathyroid glands. This can take place during total thyroidectomy for thyroid cancer, radical neck dissection for laryngeal or esophageal

---

Table 21.1 Pathophysiologic classification of hypoparathyroid states

Parathyroid gland ablation or destruction

Surgical excision
Autoimmune
Irradiation
Neoplastic infiltration
Granulomatous disease
Metal overload (Wilson's disease; hemochromatosis)

Developmental defects of the parathyroid gland

Idiopathic hypoparathyroidism
DiGeorge syndrome
Kearns-Sayer syndrome
MELAS syndrome
X-linked recessive hypoparathyroidism
Kenny-Caffey syndrome
Barakat syndrome

Defects in parathyroid hormone (PTH) biosynthesis or secretion

Impaired production of PreProPTH mRNA (autosomal recessive)
Impaired translocation of PreProPTH (autosomal dominant)
Overactive calcium-sensing receptor (autosomal dominant)
Neonatal hypocalcemia
Hypomagnesemia

Resistance to parathyroid hormone action

Hypomagnesemia
Pseudohypoparathyroidism

---

carcinoma, or repeated surgery for hyperparathyroidism. The resulting hypoparathyroidism may be transient; or it may be permanent as manifested by prolonged hypocalcemia that may develop either immediately, weeks, or years after neck surgery. Transient hypocalcemia commonly occurs immediately after removal of a parathyroid adenoma because of inadequate secretion of PTH by the previously suppressed remaining parathyroid tissue. However, these parathyroid glands generally resume normal function within a short time even after long-term suppression. In those patients having significant preoperative hyperparathyroid bone disease, the postoperative hypocalcemia may be exaggerated because of increased movement of plasma calcium into the remineralizing skeleton: the so-called "hungry bone syndrome". The incidence of permanent hypoparathyroidism after initial neck exploration for primary hyperparathyroidism is about 1% of patients. In those patients with parathyroid hyperplasia or undergoing repeated neck exploration to identify an adenoma, the incidence of hypoparathyroidism may be greatly increased. In those cases, parathyroid tissue can be autotransplanted into the brachioradialis in the forearm or sternocleidomastoid muscle at the time of parathyroidectomy, or it can be cryopreserved for later transplantation if required.

Autoimmune disorders

Isolated or idiopathic hypoparathyroidism can be found as one of a heterogeneous group of rare disorders. Although most cases are sporadic, familial occurrence is also known. The disorder may occur as an autoimmune disorder either alone or with other endocrine deficiencies, as in a pluriglandular autoimmune syndrome, or it may be associated with diverse developmental abnormalities such as lymphedema, nephropathy, nerve deafness, or Fallot's tetralogy. The diversity of the various syndromes suggests that PTH deficiency is not due to an intrinsic defect of the parathyroid gland itself.

In type 1 autoimmune polyglandular disease, the most commonly associated manifestations are hypoparathyroidism with mucocutaneous candidiasis and Addison's disease. Additional features of the syndrome include pernicious anemia, chronic active hepatitis, alopecia, gonadal failure, and thyroid disease. Patients may not express all elements of the basic triad. The disease, which is also known as the autoimmune polyendocrinopathy-candidiasis-ectodermal dystrophy syndrome, presents in infants or young children. It may be apparently sporadic or inherited in an autosomal-recessive manner, and the gene, which maps to chromosome 21q22, encodes a putative transcriptional regulator.

Antibodies directed against parathyroid tissue have been detected in over 30% of patients with isolated disease, and in over 40% of patients having hypoparathyroidism combined with other endocrine deficiencies. Recently, antibodies against the extracellular domain of the parathyroid calcium-sensing receptor have been reported in more than 50% of a group of patients with either type 1 autoimmune polyglandular syndrome or acquired hypoparathyroidism associated with autoimmune hypothyroidism. It remains uncertain as to whether the autoantibodies are of primary or secondary importance in the pathogenesis of the disease.

Irradiation and other causes of parathyroid gland destruction

Hypoparathyroidism can occur in those patients receiving extensive radiation to the neck and mediastinum. Metastatic neoplasia or granulomatous infiltration of the parathyroid glands are rare causes of clinical hypoparathyroidism. In addition, hypoparathyroidism can occur in metal overload diseases such as hemochromatosis or Wilson's disease, or it can be associated with transfusion therapy for thalassemia in which the metal ions deposit in the parathyroid glands.

DEVELOPMENTAL DEFECTS OF THE PARATHYROID GLAND

Idiopathic hypoparathyroidism

Familial isolated hypoparathyroidism has been described in which the PTH deficiency is inherited in an autosomal-dominant, autosomal-recessive, or X-linked manner. In most families, the affected status is not linked to the PTH gene, which is located on chromosome 11p15.

DiGeorge syndrome

Hypoparathyroidism can occur as part of a complex congenital defect. An example is the DiGeorge syndrome, in which patients suffer from neonatal hypocalcemic seizures and severe infections. The syndrome arises from a failure to develop the derivatives of the third and fourth pharyngeal pouches leading to agenesis or hypoplasia of the parathyroid glands and thymus. Additional deformities of the ear, nose, mouth, and aortic arch and congenital heart defects may occur. Although many cases of DiGeorge syndrome occur de novo, autosomal dominant inheritance is common. An association between several overlapping syndromes – including DiGeorge syndrome, velocardiofacial (Shprintzen) syndrome, conotruncal facial abnormality, and sporadic or familial cardiac defects – and microdeletions on chromosomes 22q11 or 10p has been noted. The major features of the 22q microdeletion disorders have been referred to by the acronym CATCH 22, for cardiac defect, abnormal facies, thymic hypoplasia, cleft palate, hypocalcemia, and 22q11 deletions. The role of several genes in the deleted portion of chromosome 22q11 in the etiology of DiGeorge syndrome and the embryological development of the parathyroid is presently being investigated.

Kearns-Sayer syndrome and MELAS

Hypoparathyroidism can occur in two disorders associated with mitochondrial dysfunction. These are the Kearns-Sayer syndrome, in which progressive external opthalmoplegia and pigmented retinopathy occur before 20 years of age, and the "MELAS" syndrome, comprised of mitochondrial encephalopathy, lactic acidosis, and stroke-like episodes. Both of these syndromes can occur with insulin-dependent diabetes mellitus and hypoparathyroidism. Kearns-Sayer syndrome can be associated with short stature, primary gonadal failure, and nerve deafness. In a single patient with MELAS, hypoparathyroidism, and diabetes mellitus, a point mutation in the mitochondrial leucine tRNA gene was identified. A patient with Kearns-Sayer syndrome, hypoparathyroidism, and sensory neural deafness had a deletion of 40% of the mitochondrial genome. The role of these mitochondrial mutations in the etiology of hypoparathyroidism remains to be clarified.

X-linked recessive hypoparathyroidism

In two multigeneration families with X-linked recessive hypoparathyroidism, the mutant gene was localized to the distal end of the X chromosome on band Xq26-27. A role of the gene in parathyroid gland development was suggested by the neonatal onset of hypocalcemia, and by the finding of parathyroid agenesis at autopsy of a patient from one of the families.

Kenny-Caffey and Barakat syndromes

In another congenital disorder, the Kenny-Caffey syndrome, hypoparathyroidism (again probably due to an embryological defect in parathyroid development) can be associated with growth retardation, osteosclerosis, cortical thickening of the long bones, and delayed closure of the anterior fontanel. No gross abnormalities were identified in the PTH gene. Hypoparathyroidism is also a part of several single familial syndromes that include the Barakat syndrome, which is associated with nerve deafness and steroid-resistant nephrosis resulting in renal failure.

DEFECTS IN PARATHYROID HORMONE (PTH) BIOSYNTHESIS OR SECRETION

In a few cases of familial isolated hypoparathyroidism a mutation in the PTH gene has been identified. For example, in one family with autosomal-recessive hypoparathyroidism, a donor splice site mutation at the exon 2-intron 2 junction of the PTH gene was identified. This led to exon skipping that resulted in the loss of exon 2, which encodes the initiation codon and signal peptide responsible for appropriate translation of the preproPTH mRNA and translocation of the precursor polypeptide, respectively. A missense mutation in the signal sequence of the precursor, preproPTH, was found in one patient with autosomal dominant hypoparathyroidism. The resultant defective processing of preproPTH to proPTH is thought to lead to reduced production of the hormone, although it is not entirely clear why hormone synthesis from the patient's remaining normal gene copy did not increase to compensate for this.

Gain of function mutations in the calcium-sensing receptor gene (CASR) located on chromosome 3q13.3-21 have now been identified in several families previously diagnosed with autosomal dominant hypocalcemia, autosomal dominant hypoparathyroidism, or hypocalcemic hypercalciuria. In the parathyroid, the activated CASR chronically suppresses PTH secretion, and in the kidney it induces hypercalciuria, which contributes to the hypocalcemia.

Neonatal hypocalcemia

After birth, there is a natural fall in serum calcium concentrations such that many normal infants have levels <8 mg/dL (<2.0 mM) during the first 3 weeks of life. In some infants, within the first days of life there is an exaggeration of the normal fall in serum calcium that is probably due to a deficient release of PTH by immature parathyroid glands. The course is self-limited, although symptoms such as muscular twitching or convulsive seizures should be treated with oral or intravenous calcium. Infants born to mothers with hyperparathyroidism or hypercalcemia may be more severely affected, as their parathyroid activity will have been more markedly suppressed in utero by the maternal hypercalcemia.

RESISTANCE TO PARATHYROID HORMONE ACTION

Hypomagnesemia

Whereas modest magnesium deficiency either due to defective intestinal absorption or renal tubular reabsorption leads to increased PTH secretion; more severe deficits cause impaired PTH secretion with ensuing hypocalcemia and tetany. Additionally, resistance to the action of PTH may occur, but all of the defects are reversible with restoration of the normal serum magnesium concentration.

Pseudohypoparathyroidism

Several clinical disorders characterized by end-organ resistance to PTH have been described that are associated with hypocalcemia and hyperphosphatemia. However, the increased secretion of PTH and target tissue are unresponsive to the hormone, as exemplified by the absence of a normal increase in urinary cAMP excretion after the administration of biologically active exogenous PTH. These disorders have been collectively termed pseudohypoparathyroidism (PHP) (Fig. 21.1). The biochemical characteristics of these disorders as compared to hypoparathyroidism are outlined in Table 21.2. Pseudohypoparathyroidism type Ia (PHPIa) is sometimes associated phenotypically with resistance to the action of several hormones in addition to PTH that act via adenylate cyclase. These include thyroid-stimulating hormone

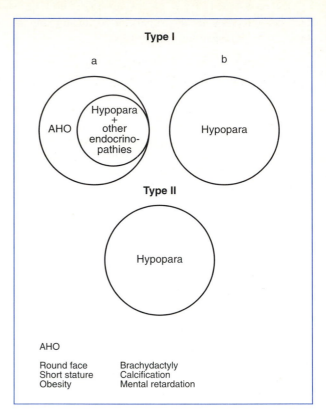

Figure 21.1 Classification of pseudohypoparathyroid states. Both type I and II syndromes are characterized by resistance to exogenous PTH; however, in the former, the resistance is at the level of the receptor-G-protein-adenylate cyclase complex; whereas in the latter, resistance is distal to cyclic AMP generation. Type Ia is distinguished from type Ib by the presence of AHO (Albright's hereditary osteodystrophy), and other endocrinopathies, in addition to hypoparathyroidism. Note that the "calcifications" of AHO are also described as "ectopic ossifications". Type Ic (not shown in figure) is distinguished from type Ia by the presence of normal levels of $G_{s\alpha}$ protein.

and gonadotropins, resulting in hypothyroidism and gonadal failure, respectively.

Pseudohypoparathyroidism type Ia patients exhibit a distinctive physical appearance, referred to as Albright's hereditary osteodystrophy (AHO), with characteristic skeletal and developmental defects. The stigmata of AHO include short stature, round facies, brachydactyly, obesity, metastatic subcutaneous calcifications (also described as ectopic ossifications), and a tendency towards mental retardation. In some PHPIa patients, AHO may be subtle or, rarely, absent. The relationship between the biochemical abnormalities – hypocalcemia and hyperphosphatemia – and AHO remain unclarified some 55 years after the initial description of the disease. In certain families, only some affected members demonstrate both AHO and PTH resistance, and other affected members have AHO only with no endocrine dysfunction, a disorder termed pseudo-pseudohypoparathyroidism (PPHP) by Fuller Albright.

Pseudohypoparathyroidism type Ia is inherited in an autosomal dominant fashion. The molecular defect has

Table 21.2 Biochemical characteristics of hypoparathyroidism and pseudohypoparathyroidism

Condition	Biochemical characteristics						
	Serum PO_4	PTH	25(OH)D	1,25(OH)$_2$D	PTH infusion U_{cAMP}	U_{PO_4}	Multiple endocrine defects
Hypoparathyroidism	↑	↓	→	↓	→	→	Yes/No *
Pseudohypoparathyroidism							
Type Ia	↑	↑	→	↓	↓	↓	Yes
Type Ib	↑	↑	→	↓	↓	↓	No
Type Ic	↑	↑	→	↓	↓	↓	Yes
Type II	↑	↑	→	↓	→	↓	No

(↑ = increased; ↓ = decreased; → = normal; * = depends upon the etiology.)
(Adapted from Streeten EA, Levine MA. Hypoparathyroidism and other causes of hypocalcemia. In: Becker KL [ed]. Principles and practice of endocrinology and metabolism, 2nd ed. Philadelphia: J.B. Lippincott, 1995;532-46.)

been identified as a reduction in the activity of the $G_{s\alpha}$ subunit, which transduces signals between G-protein coupled hormone receptors and adenylate cyclase. Several different deactivating mutations in the $G_{s\alpha}$ gene (GNAS1) on chromosome 20q13.11 have been reported in PHPIa patients.

There is a marked excess of maternal transmission in AHO, implicating genomic imprinting in the disease. Full expression of GNAS1, which occurs in maternally transmitted cases, leads to PHPIa (AHO plus hormone resistance). However, partial expression (AHO alone), as in pseudo-pseudohypoparathyroidism, is generally observed with paternal expression. Despite the strong clinical evidence supporting the disease being under imprinted control, it has been difficult to demonstrate this experimentally in human tissues. This points to the possibility of cell-type specific or subtle quantitative imprinting effects. Ablation of the $G_{s\alpha}$ gene in mice has confirmed that maternal transmission of the deleted allele results in PTH resistance but paternal transmission does not.

Apparent cases of PHP1a have been characterized in which no mutations of the $G_{s\alpha}$ gene have been found, suggesting that PHPIa can arise from more than one type of defect in PTH signaling. Alternatively, some evidence exists that antagonists to circulating PTH may be present in some of these patients. Additionally, patients with brachydactyly and mental retardation, resembling AHO but with normal $G_{s\alpha}$ levels, have microdeletions of chromosome 2q27, which indicates that genes important for skeletal and neurodevelopment lie within this region.

Pseudohypoparathyroidism type Ib is not associated with a reduction in $G_{s\alpha}$ expression or AHO. Patients show a defect in renal PTH signaling but an apparently normal response to PTH in bone, which suggests a defect in either renal PTHR function or expression. Ablation of the PTHR in mice shows that severe skeletal malformations are a consequence of disruption of receptor signaling, indicating that mutations in the PTHR coding sequence are an unlikely site for the defect in PHPIb. This

has been confirmed by direct studies of genomic DNA from patients with PHPIb, which failed to identify any mutations either within protein-coding exons or the gene promoter regions. Additionally, preliminary linkage analyses using polymorphic markers at or near the PTHR on chromosome 3p21.1-22 have indicated that mutations in multigeneration families giving rise to PHPIb phenotypes may reside outside the PTHR locus. The existence of multiple promoters in the PTHR gene, one of which may be kidney-specific, does, however, open the possibility to the defect lying in an essential renal transcriptional regulator or RNA splicing factor. Alternatively, the defect may lie in a factor required for PTH-stimulated generation of cAMP, but acting downstream of the receptor. Tissue-specific factors that regulate G protein signaling – the so-called RGS proteins – have been identified. However, to be implicated in PHPIb, such a factor would be required to be not only specific to the kidney, but also to the PTH signaling pathway. Disruption of its expression would not perturb the expression of other genes essential for normal kidney function.

In patients with pseudohypoparathyroidism type Ic, multiple hormone resistance and AHO is found in the presence of normal $G_{s\alpha}$ activity. The defect may be in other components of the receptor-adenylate cyclase system, such as the catalytic unit. Finally, patients with pseudohypoparathyroidism type II have a normal urinary cAMP response to PTH but an impaired phosphaturic response. The defect could be in protein kinase A, one of its substrates or targets, or in a component of the PTH-protein kinase C signaling pathway.

Clinical findings

The signs and symptoms of hypoparathyroidism of any etiology include evidence of latent or overt enhanced neuromuscular excitability (Tab. 21.3) because of the decreased extracellular fluid ionized calcium concentration. The effect is potentiated by hyperkalemia and hypomagnesemia. There is variation among patients in the severity of symptoms. Patients may have circumoral numbness, paresthesias of the distal extremities. or muscle cramping progressing to carpopedal spasm or tetany. Laryngospasm or bronchospasm and seizures of all types may also occur. Other manifestations include fatigue, irritability, and personality disturbances. Severe hypocalcemia may be associated with prolongation of the Q-T interval on the electrocardiogram. This is reversible with correction of the hypocalcemia. Patients having idiopathic hypoparathyroidism or pseudohypoparathyroidism with chronic hypocalcemia may also have calcification of the basal ganglia or more widespread intracranial calcification that may be detected by skull X-ray or CT scan, extrapyramidal neurological symptoms, subscapsular cataracts, and abnormal dentition.

Increased neuromuscular irritability may be demonstrated by eliciting Chvostek's sign or Trousseau's sign. Chvostek's sign is spasm of the facial muscles in response to tapping just anterior to the ear. It should be noted that 20% of normal individuals will demonstrate a slight positive reaction to this. Trousseau's sign is carpopedal spasm induced by inflation of a blood pressure cuff to 20 mmHg above systolic blood pressure for 3 minutes. A positive response reflects the heightened irritability of nerves undergoing pressure ischemia.

In hypoparathyroidism serum calcium concentrations are decreased (typically 6 to 7 mg/dl [1.50-1.75 mM]), and serum phosphate levels are increased (6 to 9 mg/dl [1.93 - 2.90 mM]). Serum immunoreactive PTH levels are low or undetectable, except in cases of PTH resistance (e.g., pseudohypoparathyroidism) when they are elevated or at the upper limit of normal. Usually serum concentrations of $1,25(OH)_2D$ are low. In hypoparathyroidism, serum alkaline phosphatase is normal. Despite an increase in the fractional urinary excretion of calcium due to the absence of PTH, intestinal calcium absorption and bone resorption are both low. Therefore the filtered load of calcium and the 24-hour urinary excretion of calcium are also reduced.

Table 21.3 Clinical features of hypocalcemia

Neuromuscular irritability
  Paresthesias
  Laryngospasm
  Bronchospasm
  Tetany
  Seizures
  Chvostek's sign
  Trousseau's sign
  Prolonged Q-T interval on ECG

(ECG = electrocardiogram.)
(Adapted from Shane E. Hypocalcemia: pathogenesis, differential diagnosis and management. In: Favus MJ [ed]. Primer on the metabolic bone diseases and disorders of mineral metabolism. 3rd ed. Philadelphia: Lippincott-Raven, 1996;217-9.)

Nephrogenous cyclic AMP excretion is low and renal tubular reabsorption of phosphate is elevated. After administration of exogenous biologically-active PTH (the Ellsworth-Howard test), the urinary cyclic AMP and phosphate excretion increase markedly except in pseudohypoparathyroid patients. Decreased parathyroid gland reserve can be detected by an ethylene-diaminetetraacetate infusion study, however, this test is generally not required and should be done with caution.

Treatment

The goal of treatment of hypoparathyroid states is to raise the serum calcium to sufficiently high concentrations such that acute symptoms can be alleviated and complications of chronic hypocalcemia can be prevented. The calcium concentration required for this purpose is generally in the low-normal to mid-normal range.

Acute or severe symptomatic hypocalcemia is best treated with intravenous calcium infusion. Intravenous vitamin D therapy is unnecessary. Generally 1 to 3 g of calcium gluconate (10 to 30 ml of 10% calcium gluconate containing 93 to 279 mg elemental calcium) can be infused over a 10 to 20 minute period followed by continuous infusion of about 100 mg/h of elemental calcium (e.g., 100 ml of 10% calcium gluconate in a liter of 5% dextrose in water). Serum calcium concentrations should be measured at frequent intervals. Calcium chloride (10%) can also be used for infusion purposes but is more likely to cause phlebitis. Hyperphosphatemia, alkalosis, and hypomagnesemia should be corrected concomitantly if present. If a patient is receiving a digitalis-like drug, electrocardiographic monitoring should be performed to prevent digitalis toxicity, which can occur as the serum calcium is raised.

Oral calcium and vitamin D should be started as soon as possible to allow reduction and discontinuation of the intravenous calcium.

The mainstay of chronic treatment is oral calcium and vitamin D. Generally 1 to 3 g of elemental calcium per day is required. This can be administered in several forms; thus, 1 g of elemental calcium is present in 2.5 g calcium carbonate, 5 g calcium citrate, 8 g calcium lactate, or 10 g calcium gluconate. Calcium carbonate is generally the least expensive form. Vitamin D is preferentially administered as calcitriol [$1,25(OH)_2D$] (0.25 µg to 1 µg daily). Nevertheless, if cost is a factor, pharmacologic doses of cholecalciferol or ergocalciferol (25 000-100 000 U or 0.63-2.5 mg per day) or calcidiol (25-200 µg per day) may be used. Cholecalciferol and ergocalciferol have the longest duration of action and can result in prolonged toxicity. Serum calcium and 24-hour urinary calcium excretion should be monitored closely when therapy is started and until the patient is stabilized. Because of the absence of the renal calcium reabsorptive effect of parathyroid hormone in hypoparathyroid states, hypercalciuria may occur as treatment is initiated and may occur even prior to the normalization of the serum calcium. Consequently, only a low-normal serum calcium may be attainable in order to prevent chronic hypercalciuria and nephrocalcinosis. If the serum calcium attainable with oral calcium and calcitriol is below the normal range (e.g., below 8 mg/dl or 2mM) and the patient remains symptomatic, then a thiazide diuretic may be added to reduce hypercalciuria and raise the serum calcium.

As the serum calcium is normalized, elevated serum phosphate concentrations generally decline, but phosphate binding gels such as aluminum hydroxide are occasionally helpful in reducing phosphate during the start of therapy.

Suggested readings

ALBRIGHT F, BURNETT CH, SMITH PH. Pseudohypoparathyroidism: an example of "Seabright-Bantam syndrome". Endocrinology 1942;30:922-32.

BARAKAT AY, D'ALBORA JB, MARTIN MM, JOSE PA. Familial nephrosis, nerve deafness, and hypoparathyroidism. J Pediatr 1977;191: 61-4.

BERGADA I, SCHIFFREN A, ABU SRAIR H-A, et al. Kenny Syndrome: description of additional abnormalities and molecular studies. Human Genet 1988;80:39-42.

HARVEY JN, BARNETT D. Endocrine dysfunction in Kearns-Sayre syndrome. Clin Endocrinol 1992;37:97-103.

HERRERA M, GRANT C, VAN HEERDEN JA, FITZPATRICK LA. Parathyroid autotransplantation. Arch Surg 1992;127:825-9.

HONG R. The DiGeorge anomaly. Immunodefic Rev 1991;3:1-14.

ILLUM F, DUPONT E. Prevalence of CT-detected calcification in the basal ganglia in idiopathic hypoparathyroidism and pseudohypoparathyroidism. Neuroradiology 1985;27:32-7.

LEVINE MA. Pseudohypoparathyroidism. In: Bilezikian JP, Raisz LG, Rodan GA (eds). Principles of bone biology. San Diego: Academic Press 1996;853-76.

LI X, SONG Y-H, RAIS N, et al. Autoantibodies to the extracellular domain of the calcium sensing receptor in patients with acquired hypoparathyroidism. J Clin Invest 1996;97:910-4.

MCKUSICK VA. Mendelian inheritance in man: catalogues of autosomal dominant, autosomal recessive, and X-linked phenotypes. 14th ed. Baltimore: The Johns Hopkins University Press, 1994.

OKANO O, FURUKAWA Y, MORII H, FUJITA T. Comparative efficacy of various vitamin D metabolites in the treatment of various types of hypoparathyroidism. J Clin Endocrinol Metab 1982;55:238-43.

O'RIORDAN JLH. Treatment of hypoparathyroidism. In: Bilezikian JP, Levine MA, Marcus R (eds). The parathyroids. New York: Raven Press, 1994;801-4.

SHANE E. Hypocalcemia: pathogenesis, differential diagnosis, and management. In: Favus MJ (ed). Primer on the metabolic bone diseases and disorders of mineral metabolism, 3rd ed. Philadelphia: Lippincott-Raven, 1996;217-9.

STREETEN EA, LEVINE MA. Hypoparathyroidism and other causes of hypocalcemia. In: Becker KL (ed). Principles and practice of endocrinology and metabolism, 2nd ed. Philadephia: J.B. Lippincott, 1995;532-46.

THAKKER RV. Molecular basis of PTH underexpression. In: Bilezikian JP, Raisz LG, Rodan GA (eds). Principles of bone biology. San Diego, Academic Press, 1996;837-51.

Rickets and osteomalacia

Francis H. Glorieux

In the strict sense of the term, rickets is caused by any interference with the process of endochondral bone formation, which is comprised of the sequence of events that takes place in the epiphyseal growth plates and results in the lengthening of the long bones. The other processes that involve rapid matrix mineralization during growth include remodeling of cancellous bone (to accommodate for the development of the marrow cavity) and apposition of periosteal bone (to increase bone width and cortical thickness). Remodeling (to ensure bone tissue renewal and maintain mineral homeostasis) remains active throughout life. Defective mineralization of newly formed matrix (osteoid tissue) throughout the skeleton results in its excessive accumulation, or osteomalacia. Thus, rickets occurs during growth in children, while osteomalacia occurs in both children and adults.

Pathophysiology

Bone formation and skeletal growth require the controlled production of a matrix (cartilage in the epiphyseal plate, and osteoid in metaphyseal areas and at sites of intramembranous bone formation) that will rapidly calcify when adequate concentrations of extracellular calcium and phosphate are available. The mineral phase will first be amorphous and then becomes crystalline in the form of hydroxyapatite, with the basic formula $Ca_{10}(PO4)_6(OH)_2$. Failure to mineralize because of an inadequate supply of mineral will result in an excessive accumulation of unmineralized matrix. This will cause the characteristic swelling around the growth plates, which is particularly evident at the wrists and ankles, and at the costochondral junction of the ribs where they form the classic rosary. The alteration of the natural sequence of endochondral bone formation will also slow down the growth in length of the various pieces of the axial and appendicular skeleton, resulting in an overall decrease of the linear growth rate that, in the extreme cases, may be completely arrested.

Poorly mineralized bone is weakened and will bend or twist under the weight of the body and the pull of muscles. Fractures may occur, though more frequently skeletal deformities will appear, such as genu varum, genu valgum, coxa vara, tibial and femoral torsion, pelvic deformities, chest deformations, scoliosis, and kyphosis. In the infant, delayed mineralization of the skull may result in craniotabes. Thoracic deformities include pigeon breast deformity and lower rib cage flaring due to softening of the ribs and depression at the sites of insertion of the diaphragm (Harrison's groove).

In reaction to the hypocalcemia characteristic of the calcipenic forms of rickets, secondary hyperparathyroidism develops and leads to increased bone resorption. This will in turn lead to a progressive decrease in bone mass and severe osteopenia, further compromising bone integrity. By contrast, osteopenia never occurs in the phosphopenic forms of rickets, and osteomalacia as normocalcemia does not trigger excessive parathyroid reaction.

A number of schemes have been proposed to classify the various forms of rickets. As bone mineral is mostly made of calcium and phosphate, rickets and osteomalacia may arise from either primary calcipenia or primary phosphopenia. In each of the two categories, there are acquired and inherited forms (Tab. 22.1). The intent here is not to discuss in detail all of the reported forms but, rather, to concentrate on those that most frequently present clinically, as well as to discuss the most recent insights into the genetics and the molecular mechanisms underlying some of the heritable forms of rickets.

Clinical findings

Symptoms and signs

In calcipenic rickets, the initial reaction to inadequate intestinal calcium absorption is hypocalcemia, which may cause tetany or convulsions. In a second stage, secondary hyperparathyroidism corrects the calcemia at the expense of bone mass. Increased resorption will translate into progressive osteopenia and restore normal serum calcium levels. It is at this stage that the radiologic changes become evident. The renal response to increased parathyroid hormone secretion includes increased reabsorption of calcium. A further response is the reduced reabsorption of phosphate, which leads to increased phosphaturia; if sustained,

Table 22.1 Classification of rickets and osteomalacia

Calcipenic forms

Dietary calcium deficiency
Simple vitamin D deficiency
Vitamin D deficiency secondary to
    fat malabsorption
    liver disease (?)
    renal insufficiency
Heritable forms
    pseudo-vitamin D deficiency (PDDR)
    25 OHD-1α-hydroxylase defect
    hypocalcemic vitamin D-resistant rickets (HVDRR)
    alterations of the vitamin D receptor (VDR)

Phosphopenic forms

Insufficient intake
    prematurity
    total parenteral nutrition
    use of phosphate binders
Increased renal loss
    Fanconi syndrome by tubular damage
    tumor-induced rickets and osteomalacia (TIO)
Heritable
    increased renal loss
    familial hypophosphatemia
    sex-linked dominant (XLH)
    sporadic form (new mutations)
    autosomal dominant
    hypercalciuric form (HHRH)

this results in hypophosphatemia, thus further compromising the mineralization process. In a third stage, with further bone demineralization, the calcemic response to parathyroid hormone decreases and hypocalcemia reappears.

In phosphopenic rickets, since serum calcium remains normal, there are no clinical signs of nerve irritability, nor secondary hyperparathyroidism. Hence, osteopenia is absent. The hallmark of this form of rickets, except in the rare cases where there is insufficient phosphate intake, is increased renal loss, which may have different mechanisms (see below). It is usually more severe in the acquired forms (e.g., tumor-induced rickets) than in the familial forms of hypophosphatemia.

Serum alkaline phosphatase activity is uniformly elevated in all forms of rickets, and the levels reflect the severity of the bone disease. Normal values are up to 300 IU/l in growing individuals and up to 100 IU/l in adults. Although alkaline phosphatase is not specific to bone, the bone isozyme represents over 80% of the total activity in growing individuals who have no liver dysfunction. There is thus no need to assess the bone-specific isozyme activity in children, as the simple testing of total alkaline phosphatase activity is adequate in evaluating the severity and monitoring the treatment of rickets. In adults, bone-specific alkaline phosphatase evaluation has been recommended instead.

Serum 25 hydroxy-vitamin D [25-(OH)D] concentrations are depressed in vitamin D-deficiency rickets, usually to below 14 ng/ml (34 nmol/l). In all other forms of rickets, concentrations are either normal (14-45 ng/ml or 34-91 nmol/l), or they are very much elevated in cases of prior treatment with large amounts of vitamin D at the time of referral of a vitamin D refractory form.

Serum concentrations of 1,25-dihydroxy vitamin D [$1,25(OH)_2D$] vary widely. Normal values are 27-56 pg/ml (65-134 pmol/l). The concentrations are elevated in cases of calcium deficiency, target organ resistance by alterations of the vitamin D receptor (HVDRR), and the hypercalciuric form of familial hypophosphatemia (HHRH). In simple vitamin D deficiency they may be either low, normal, or elevated. The reason for the normal or elevated levels is uncertain, but it may be related to a maximal upregulation of the 1α-hydroxylase enzyme (due to the substrate deficiency) when the blood sample is obtained after brief exposure to sunlight or the ingestion of a small amount of vitamin D.

In vitamin D pseudo-deficiency (PDDR), serum $1,25(OH)_2D$ is markedly decreased and is sometimes undetectable. It does not increase significantly after administration of large amounts of vitamin D, reflecting the defect in 1α-hydroxylase activity. Interestingly, the serum concentration is similarly decreased in tumor-induced rickets (TIO). The ability of TIO patients to maintain normocalcemia despite depressed levels of $1,25(OH)_2D$ has yet to be explained.

Diagnostic procedures

The most marked changes occur at the cartilage-metaphysis junction just under the growth plates. The space is widened by the accumulation of uncalcified cartilage, which in turn causes fraying, cupping, widening, and fuzziness of the zone of provisional calcification. These changes are better and earlier detected in the most active growth plates, which are in the distal ulna and femur and the proximal and distal tibia. Changes in the diaphyses may not be evident when metaphyseal changes are first detected; they will appear later as coarse trabeculation and, in cases of increased resorption, as cortical thinning and subperiosteal erosion. A sign of hyperparathyroidism is the disappearance of the lamina dura that normally surrounds tooth sockets. In adults, diaphyseal cortical defects appear as Looser's zones or pseudo-fractures.

Treatment

Vitamin D_2 or D_3 is used in the treatment of vitamin D-deficiency rickets. Initial doses may vary from 2-5000 IU per day. Such low dosages decrease the probability of toxic effects and do not mask non-nutrient forms of rickets. Healing requires 6 to 12 weeks of therapy. The most sensitive biochemical index of healing is a return to normal of serum alkaline phosphatase activity. When achieved, vitamin D supplementation may be reduced to the recommended daily allowance of 400 IU.

An adequate calcium intake is necessary to avoid severe hypocalcemia following the inception of vitamin D therapy and to ensure the healing of bone. Dietary intake or supplementation should provide about 50 mg/kg per day of elemental calcium in the growing child, and 800 to 1000 mg per day in the adult patient.

The vitamin D metabolites or their analogs should never be used in the treatment of vitamin D deficiency. These therapies should be restricted to the treatment of the various heritable forms of rickets (see below).

HERITABLE CALCIPENIC RICKETS

Patients whose rickets are similar to vitamin D-resistant (hypophosphatemic) rickets in terms of requiring large therapeutic doses of vitamin D and yet differ markedly in clinical and biochemical features have been recognized as suffering from a separate disorder. The clinical course of this disorder is similar to that of rickets due to simple vitamin D deficiency, despite adequate availability of vitamin D. The disorder was therefore named "pseudo-vitamin D-deficiency rickets". It was noted that therapy with very large doses of vitamin D resulted in remission of the disease, and hence the disease was also called vitamin D-dependent rickets. Gaining an understanding of the abnormalities in vitamin D metabolism led to the recognition that this condition was likely due to a defect in the renal 1α-hydroxylase enzyme. It is characterized by a low serum 1,25(OH)$_2$D concentration and a rapid and complete therapeutic response to small doses of calcitriol [1,25(OH)$_2$D$_3$]. Subsequently another condition HVDRR was recognized that develops despite high circulating concentrations of calcitriol. It is due to end organ resistance to 1,25(OH)$_2$D, consecutive to a spectrum of mutations affecting the vitamin D receptor (VDR) in target tissues.

PSEUDO-VITAMIN D DEFICIENCY

Almost all of the clinical and biochemical features of pseudo-vitamin D deficiency (PDDR) are similar to those of vitamin D-deficiency rickets. Clinically, the child is well at birth, and then within the first year of life he or she develops hypotonia, muscle weakness, an inability to stand or walk, growth retardation, convulsions, frontal bossing, and the signs of severe rickets, which are rachitic rosary, thickened wrists and ankles, bowed legs, and fractures. A history of adequate intake of vitamin D is usually obtained. Laboratory investigations (Tab. 22.2) reveal hypocalcemia with secondary hyperparathyroidism and associated increased urinary cAMP and amino-acid excretion, elevated serum alkaline phosphatase activity, either hypo- or normophosphatemia, hyperphosphaturia, and low urinary calcium excretion and decreased intestinal absorption of calcium. Because the condition is inherited as an autosomal recessive trait, the incidence of parenteral consanguinity is high. It is particularly frequent in French-Canadians from the Saguenay region of Québec, where the estimated gene frequency is 0.02.

The pathogenesis of this disorder was elucidated by studying vitamin D metabolism in affected patients. It was observed that massive doses of vitamin D$_3$ and high doses of 25-(OH)D$_3$, but only small doses of 1,25(OH)$_2$D$_3$, were required to correct the clinical and biochemical abnormalities found in PDDR patients. This observation provided indirect evidence that the condition was due to an inborn error of vitamin D metabolism affecting the renal 1α-hydroxylase enzyme that converts 25-(OH)D to 1,25(OH)$_2$D. Studies of circulating vitamin D metabolites in patients further supported this hypothesis. The serum 25-(OH)D concentration is normal in untreated patients and is high in patients treated with vitamin D, whereas the serum concentration of 1,25(OH)$_2$D is low in untreated patients (Tab. 22.2), and it remains low in patients treated with vitamin D$_3$. The absence of 1α-hydroxylase activity has been documented in decidual cells of human placenta, which thus represents another target for the PDDR mutation.

Table 22.2 Biochemical and genetic details of the various forms of rickets

Type	Serum				Urine		Chromosomal location	Gene
	Ca^{2+}	PO$_4^{3-}$	1,25(OH)$_2$D$_3$	PTH	PO$_4^{3-}$	Ca^{2+}		
Vitamin D deficiency	↓/N	↓/N	↓	↑	↑	↓		
Renal tubular defect								
XLH	N	↓	↓/N	N	↑	↓/N	Xp22.1	PHEX
HHRH	N	↓	↑↑	N	↑	↑↑	?	?
TIO	N	↓	↓↓	N	↑	↑/N	?	?
Vitamin D metabolism defect								
PDDR	↓	↓/N	↓	↑	↑	↓	12q14	1α-OHase
HVDRR	↓	↓/N	↑↑	↑	↑	↓	12q12-q14	VDR

N = normal; ↓ = decreased; ↑ = increased. In all disorders, the serum 25-hydroxyvitamin D$_3$ concentrations are normal (except vitamin D deficiency) and serum alkaline phosphatase activity is usually elevated.
(PHEX = phosphate regulating gene with homologies to endopeptidases on the X chromosome; 1α-OHase = renal 1α-hydroxylase gene; PTH = parathyroid hormone; XLH = X-linked hypophosphatemic rickets; HHRH = hypophosphatemic rickets with hypercalciuria; TIO = tumor induced rickets; PDDR = pseudo-vitamin D deficient rickets; HVDRR = hypocalcemic vitamin D resistant rickets; VDR = vitamin D receptor gene.)

The recommended treatment for PDDR is replacement therapy with calcitriol. An initial dose of 1 to 3 μg per day will induce the resolution of rickets within 7 to 9 weeks. The maintenance dose is about half the initial dose and will probably need to be continued throughout life. The required dose is remarkably stable, with only temporary interruption during prolonged immobilization and increasing dosage during pregnancy (unpublished data).

Linkage studies in affected French-Canadian families have mapped the PDDR gene to chromosome 12q14. The gene encoding the 1α-hydroxylase enzyme has recently been cloned and mapped to an identical location, demonstrating that it is the target of the PDDR mutation. Studies are under way to precisely characterize the mutations in the affected families.

HEREDITARY 1,25(OH)$_2$D-RESISTANT RICKETS

Hereditary 1,25(OH)$_2$D-resistant rickets (HVDDR) is an autosomal recessive disorder in which there is end organ resistance to 1,25(OH)$_2$D. The clinical features are similar to those found in PDDR, with two major exceptions: (1) in HVDRR, the circulating concentrations of 1,25(OH)$_2$D are markedly elevated (as high as 1000 pg/ml [2400 pmol/l]), and (2) alopecia totalis may occur in some patients. It is an early onset disease, with variable severity in its clinical and biochemical manifestations, suggesting heterogeneity in the underlying defects.

The resistance to 1,25(OH)$_2$D$_3$ therapy is also variable. Some patients have improved following therapy with very large doses of vitamin D or calcitriol. In patients who are refractory to vitamin D therapy, alternative treatment with oral calcium supplements has been tried with limited success. However, long-term nocturnal intravenous calcium infusions have successfully resolved rickets and promoted mineralization in HVDRR patients, though there are considerable practical difficulties with this therapy.

The elevated serum concentrations of 1,25(OH)$_2$D in patients with HVDRR suggested an abnormality in the mode of action of the metabolite within the target tissues. Its functions are mediated by an intracellular receptor that binds DNA and concentrates the hormone in the nucleus in a fashion analogous to the classical steroid hormones. The interactions between 1,25(OH)$_2$D and its intracellular receptor have been studied using cultured skin fibroblasts from control subjects and HVDRR patients. Several defects have been identified and include a complete absence of receptors, a decreased number of receptors with normal affinity, a normal receptor-hormone binding but a subsequent failure to translocate the complex to the nucleus, and a post-receptor defect in which normal receptors are present but there is a deficiency in the induction of the 25-(OH)D-24-hydroxylase enzyme in response to 1,25(OH)$_2$D. Thus, the heterogeneity suggested from clinical observations is demonstrated at the molecular level with various combinations of defective recep-

tor-hormone bindings and expressions. The 1,25(OH)$_2$D receptor (VDR) is closely related to the thyroid hormone receptors and represents another member of the trans-acting transcriptional factors, which includes the steroid and thyroid hormone receptors.

Genetic abnormalities of the human VDR gene have been identified in HVDRR patients. The human VDR gene consists of 9 exons; exons 2 and 3 encode the DNA binding domain, while exons 5 to 9 encode the vitamin D binding domain. The gene has been mapped to chromosome 12q12-q14 in man, which is in close vicinity to the locus for the gene causing renal 1α-hydroxylase deficiency (PDDR). Mutational analysis of the VDR gene in HVDRR patients has demonstrated an array of nonsense and missense mutations affecting different parts of the receptor. Recently, null mutant (that is, "knockout") mice for VDR have been produced by targeted gene disruption. They exhibit all of the features consistent with the HVDRR phenotype. This mouse model will help to further elucidate the physiologic role of VDR in the vitamin D signaling pathway.

HERITABLE PHOSPHOPENIC RICKETS

X-LINKED HYPOPHOSPHATEMIC RICKETS (XLH)

Pathophysiology

The first familial occurrence of vitamin D-resistant rickets was described in a mother, her son, and her daughter. Skeletal deformities were used as the discriminant for the affected phenotype and an autosomal dominant mode of inheritance was proposed. However, it was observed that the severity of skeletal deformities varied and that some hypophosphatemic females had no evidence of bone disease. When hypophosphatemia was used as the discriminant, an X-linked dominant mode of inheritance was established. The males are uniformly more severely affected than the females, who sometimes have no evidence of rickets. This variability in female patients, which is expected in an X-linked disease, can be explained by the Lyon hypothesis of X-chromosome inactivation, which states that one of the X chromosomes in a pair is randomly inactivated in each cell of the early female embryo. The subsequent daughter cells have the same X chromosome inactivated as their mother cell. Thus a female hypophosphatemic patient is a mixture of cells, some of which have an active normal X chromosome and some of which have an active "hypophosphatemic" X chromosome. The relative proportions of each cell type vary from female to female due to the randomness of the inactivation process, and this would in turn determine the variable expression of the X-linked hypophosphatemic rickets gene in females. Further support for this comes from phosphate infusion studies in hypophosphatemic patients and normals. These studies demonstrated that hypophosphatemic males (hemizygotes) had decreased maximum tubular capacity for reabsorbing phosphate (TmP), while hypophosphatemic females (heterozygotes) had a TmP that was intermediate between that of normals and hypophosphatemic males. About one-third of the patients present with a negative family history but cannot otherwise be differentiated from the XLH form. Some such "sporadic" female subjects have given birth to affected babies, implying that they in fact carry new XLH mutations. It also indicates that the mutation rate for the trait is rather high.

Family segregation studies have led to the mapping of the HYP gene to the short arm of the X chromosome (Xp22.1). Using the powerful technique of positional cloning, a consortium of researchers was able to identify the gene. Sequence analysis revealed that it encoded a protein that had similarities with the family of endopeptidase genes – such as neutral endopeptidase, endothelin-converting enzyme-1, and the Kell-antigen – hence the gene was called PHEX (phosphate-regulating gene with homologies to endopeptidases on the X chromosome).

Mutational analysis of the PHEX gene in XLH patients has identified a number of different genetic abnormalities, including nonsense mutations that result from frameshifts due to base pair deletions and insertions, missense mutations, splice site mutations, and genomic deletions. These mutations indicate that a loss of function of PHEX is involved in the etiology of this form of hypophosphatemic rickets. However, the mechanisms whereby PHEX mutations lead to the XLH phenotype remain to be elucidated; first the tissues in which PHEX is expressed must be determined, and second its physiologic role in these organs must be defined. The putative substrate that PHEX cleaves has yet to be identified as well, and it is postulated that it may possibly be a phosphate-regulating hormone, referred to as "phosphatonin". Phosphatonin may also be secreted by some tumors associated with hypophosphatemic osteomalacia (see below).

Clinical findings

Symptoms and signs

X-linked hypophosphatemic rickets is the first recognized and most frequent form of familial rickets. Albright coined the term "vitamin D-resistant rickets", as the patients he described presented with changes in mineral metabolism that could only be overcome by very large daily doses of vitamin D.

The classic triad consists of hypophosphatemia, rickets, and osteomalacia, causing limb deformities and growth retardation. Although low serum phosphate is evident early after birth, it is only at the time of weight bearing that progressive leg deformities (more often in varum than in valgum) and departure from normal growth rate become obvious. It is striking that, despite these symptoms, affected children are not sick. They never present with tetany or convulsion. They are normally active and never experience myopathy. Tooth eruption is often delayed, but teeth have normal enamel, in opposition with the enamel hypoplasia evident in the calcipenic forms of rickets.

The major abnormalities are hypophosphatemia and hyperphosphaturia resulting from a low reabsorption threshold for renal phosphate. Renal function is otherwise normal and glycosuria, aminoaciduria, and acidification defects are notably absent. Normal serum calcium and an absence of secondary hyperparathyroidism in untreated patients are also important diagnostic features (Tab. 22.2). Urinary calcium excretion is low as well, and intestinal absorption of calcium and phosphate is slightly impaired. Serum alkaline phosphatase activity, which varies with age and correlates with the rate of bone formation, is elevated in affected individuals with rickets, but it is normal in hypophosphatemic individuals without active bone disease. The circulating concentration of 25(OH)D is normal in hypophosphatemic patients, and 1,25(OH)$_2$D is either normal or slightly decreased. It has been argued that 1,25(OH)$_2$D levels are inappropriately low in the face of chronic hypophosphatemia. Whatever the cause, this relative decrease in 1,25(OH)$_2$D synthesis is not severe enough to significantly impair intestinal calcium absorption. Normocalcemia is the rule, and there is no secondary hyperparathyroidism.

Diagnostic procedures

On X-rays, active rickets is present, which reflects the mineralization defect. There are no signs of subperiosteal erosion or excessive bone resorption. Bone density (by dual-energy X-ray absorptiometry) is normal to high normal. Thus, on histologic sections, there is no osteopenia, which is in sharp contrast with what is observed in calcipenic rickets (with secondary hyperparathyroidism). However, there is severe osteomalacia, which is characterized by excessive accumulation of unmineralized osteoid tissue and very little resorption activity. In keeping with a sex-linked dominant mode of inheritance, the disease manifestations are more severe in males than in females, some of whom may be asymptomatic, have no skeletal involvement, and exhibit only hypophosphatemia. They represent the "carriers" for the trait and provide evidence that hypophosphatemia cannot solely explain the bone changes.

Treatment

In the past, XLH was traditionally treated with large doses of vitamin D. Infants received 10 000 to 25 000 IU per day of vitamin D, and older children up to 300 000 IU per day. This resulted in significant improvement of the rickets and reduced the need for corrective osteotomies of the tibia and femora. However, hypophosphatemia persisted, growth rate was not markedly improved, and vitamin D intoxication with hypercalcemia and renal damage sometimes occurred. To offset the phosphate loss, oral phosphate supplements (1 to 4 g per day) were administered at frequent intervals (4 to 5 times a day) and were effective in producing normophosphatemia. However, the hypocalcemic effect of phosphate therapy often induced secondary hyperparathyroidism. Large doses of vitamin D were added to prevent that, which in turn increased the risk of vitamin D intoxication and renal damage. A combination of calcitriol (0.5-1.0 μg day) plus phosphate seems to be the most effective treatment for this disease. This combined therapy results in improved phosphatemia and growth velocity. It also resolves rickets and osteomalacia as assessed by a fall in serum alkaline phosphatase activity, and it normalizes radiographs and bone histology. However, complications of treatment do still occur, with nephrocalcinosis developing in some patients. This side-effect, detected by systematic ultrasonic imaging of the kidneys, had first been attributed to the heavy prolonged phosphate load administered to XLH patients. The similar incidence of nephrocalcinosis in XLH and PDDR patients, however, demonstrates that it is the daily administration of calcitriol and not phosphate that is the triggering factor. Except in cases of repeated intoxication (overdosage) with vitamin D and calcitriol, nephrocalcinosis has not been linked to alteration of kidney function. Phosphate-induced secondary hyperparathyroidism is a constant concern, and in some patients it may become autonomous and require surgery. The growth-promoting effects of therapy are not always striking, particularly in boys. For that reason, the adjunct of recombinant growth hormone as a third therapeutic component has recently been advocated. Definite positive effects have been observed in young XLH patients. Larger scale studies will be necessary to definitively establish the balance between the long-term benefits and the potential negative side-effects of this therapeutic regimen.

TUMOR-INDUCED OSTEOMALACIA

Tumor-induced (or oncogenic) rickets and osteomalacia (TIO) is a rare, acquired disorder characterized by hypophosphatemia, hyperphosphaturia, and low circulating $1,25(OH)_2D$ levels in addition to rickets and osteomalacia. It occurs in previously unaffected individuals. There are striking similarities between this tumor-induced form of hypophosphatemia and XLH. There are also important differences. TIO patients may have undetectable serum concentrations of $1,25(OH)_2D$ despite hypophosphatemia. The mechanisms by which TIO patients are able to maintain normocalcemia despite an evident defect in $1,25(OH)_2D$ synthesis have not been elucidated. Unlike XLH patients, TIO patients often suffer from a severe, crippling, proximal myopathy. Aminoaciduria, most frequently glycinuria, and glycosuria are occasionally present. Typical rachitic changes are present on radiographs of bone metaphyses. Osteopenia, pseudo-fractures, and coarse trabeculation also occur. On histologic sections, almost all surfaces are covered by thick osteoid seams with no evidence of increased resorption.

The tumors associated with TIO are usually of mesenchymal origin and include hemangiomas, angiosarcomas, giant cell tumors of bone, sclerosing angiomas, hemangiopericytomas, and non-ossifying sarcomas.

These tumors are often small, difficult to locate, and they may involve any organ. Frequently reported locations are the soft palate and the plant of the foot. Tumors of epithelial origin, for example breast and prostatic carcinomas, have also been observed to be associated with this disorder. It has been postulated that the tumors may secrete phosphatonin, which would inhibit the renal tubular reabsorption of phosphate. The role of this possible humoral factor, which may represent a substrate for PHEX (see above) in the control of phosphate homeostasis, remains to be elucidated.

A complete surgical removal of the tumor rapidly corrects all of the abnormalities. When the tumor is not clearly identified or cannot be fully removed, medical therapeutic intervention is warranted. As in XLH, it is based on the association of $1,25(OH)_2D_3$ (1-2 μg/day) and phosphate salts (2-4 g day). Little information is available regarding the long-term effects of such treatment. It is likely that the same secondary effects observed in treated XLH patients (nephrocalcinosis and secondary hyperparathyroidism) may also develop in treated TIO subjects. Thus, careful monitoring of urinary calcium and parathyroid and renal function is mandatory.

HEREDITARY HYPOPHOSPHATEMIC RICKETS WITH HYPERCALCIURIA

Tieder et al. reported nine children who presented with hypophosphatemic rickets and hypercalciuria who were all part of a single large pedigree. There were a number of individuals in the pedigree with "idiopathic hypercalciuria" in whom no bone disease has been identified.

The hereditary hypophosphatemic rickets with hypercalciuria (HHRH) clinical syndrome resembles that of XLH patients: they have lower limb deformities and stunted growth. Muscle weakness, which is not part of XLH, has been reported in some patients. On X-rays, active rickets and osteopenia are evident. The mode of inheritance is most likely autosomal recessive.

Biochemically, normocalcemia, increased alkaline phosphatase activity, and hypophosphatemia due to increased renal phosphate loss are found. Hypercalciuria is most evident after a meal or an oral calcium load; it disappears after a 15-hour fast. The salient abnormality is an elevated serum concentration of $1,25(OH)_2D$, which is the probable cause of increased intestinal calcium absorption. It has been suggested that these high concentrations of $1,25(OH)_2D$ are the expected response to hypophosphatemia, in contrast to the "inappropriately low" levels of the metabolite in XLH serum. This hypothesis remains untested.

The genetic defect in HHRH is unknown. There has been no report of attempts to locate the HHRH locus on the genome in order to establish possible linkage with genes involved in the control of phosphate transport.

Treatment is based on supplementation with high doses of phosphate salts (1-3 g per day in 4 to 5 divided doses). Within a few weeks of treatment, muscle strength and bone pain improve substantially, and the patient's growth rate increases with the healing resolution of the rachitic lesions. Unlike XLH, there is no need for calcitriol as an adjunct to phosphate therapy, as basal circulating levels are very high. There is no report on long-term effects of the treatment. Noticeably, the common complications found in XLH patients (nephrocalcinosis and hyperparathyroidism) are not encountered in HHRH patients.

FANCONI SYNDROME

The Fanconi syndrome is characterized by multiple defects of the proximal renal tubule. There is renal wastage of amino acids; glucose; bicarbonate, leading to metabolic acidosis; phosphate, leading to hypophosphatemia; sodium; uric acid; proteins; and potassium, leading to hypokalemia. The clinical manifestations include rickets, lower limb deformities, and impaired linear growth.

Serum calcium is normal, and calciuria varies. Clearly, hypophosphatemia is the major factor underlying rickets and osteomalacia. It is possible, however, that acidosis plays a contributing role, since bone serves as a buffer for hydrogen ion excess. The excess acid is buffered by calcium carbonate, which leads to the dissolution of bone mineral and may cause hypercalciuria. Circulating levels of $1,25(OH)_2D$ are normal in Fanconi syndrome, a finding that is similar to what is observed in XLH patients.

Rickets is treated, as in XLH, with a combination of phosphate and $1,25(OH)_2D_3$. Dosage and monitoring follow the same guidelines as in XLH. Alkali therapy may be used to correct the metabolic acidosis and potassium supplements used to control hypokalemia.

The Fanconi syndrome is often idiopathic. It may also be caused by toxic agents, including mercury, lead, cadmium, streptozotocin, and outdated tetracycline. It may also be found in association with inborn errors of metabolism that affect proximal renal tubule function, which include glycogen storage disease, galactosemia, cystinosis, tyrosinemia, and hereditary fructose intolerance.

Suggested readings

ALBRIGHT F, BUTLER AM, BLOOMBERG E. Rickets resistant to vitamin D therapy. Am J Dis Child 1937;54:529-47.

DREZNER MK. Clinical disorders of phosphate homeostasis. In: Feldman D, Glorieux FH, Pike JW (eds). Vitamin D. San Diego: Academic Press, 1997;733-54.

ECONS MJ, DREZNER MK. Tumor-induced osteomalacia - unveiling a new hormone. N Engl J Med 1994;330:1679-81.

GLISSON F. De rachitide sive morbo puerili qui vulgo, the ricket dictur. London, 1650.

GLORIEUX FH. Rickets, the continuing challenge. N Engl J Med 1991;325:1875-7.

GLORIEUX FH, CHABOT G AND TAU C. Familial hypophosphatemic rickets: pathophysiology and medical management. In: Glorieux FH (ed). Rickets. Vol. 21. New York: Nestlé Nutrition Workshop Series, Raven Press, 1991;185-202.

GLORIEUX FH, MARIE PJ, PETTIFOR JM, et al. Bone response to phosphate salts, ergocalciferol and calcitriol in hypophosphatemic vitamin D resistant rickets. N Engl J Med 1980;303:1023-31.

GLORIEUX FH, ST-ARNAUD R. Vitamin D pseudo-deficiency. In: Feldman D, Glorieux FH, Pike JW (eds). Vitamin D. San Diego: Academic Press, 1997;755-64.

MALLOY PJ, PIKE JW, FELDMAN D. Hereditary 1,25-dihydroxyvitamin D resistant rickets. In: Feldman D, Glorieux FH, Pike JW (eds). Vitamin D. San Diego: Academic Press, 1997;765-87.

SAGGESSE G, BARONCELLI G, BERTELLONI S, et al. Long-term growth hormone treatment in children with hypophosphatemic rickets: effects on growth, mineral metabolism and bone density. J Pediatr 1995;127:395-402.

THE HYP CONSORTIUM. A gene (PEX) with homologies to endopeptidases is mutated in patients with X-linked hypophosphatemic rickets. Nat Genet 1995;11:130-6.

TIEDER M, MODAI D, SAMUEL R, et al. Hereditary hypophosphatemic rickets with hypercalcuria. N Engl J Med 1985;312:611-7.

TIEDER M, MODAI D, SHAKED U, et al. "Idiopathic" hypercalciuria and hereditary hypophosphatemic rickets; two phenotypical expressions of a common genetic defect. N Engl J Med 1987;316:125-9.

Miscellaneous bone diseases

Socrates E. Papapoulos

KEY POINTS

- The precise cause of Paget's disease of bone has not yet been determined, but available evidence favors a paramyxovirus infection of genetically predisposed individuals. Bone scintigraphy is the most sensitive method of detecting Pagetic lesions, but it is not specific. It should always be included in the investigation of affected patients, and radiographs should be subsequently made of areas with increased uptake of the radioisotope. In Paget's disease bone resorption is coupled to bone formation, which is reflected in measurements of biochemical indices of bone turnover. Bisphosphonates are the treatment of choice for Paget's disease. Newer, nitrogen-containing bisphosphonates bring about long-lasting remission with relatively short exposure to the drug in the majority of patients. Asymptomatic patients with localization in skeletal areas, with a risk of complications, should be considered for treatment with available bisphosphonates.
- Fibrous dysplasia can be monostotic or polyostotic and can be associated with pigmented skin lesions and various hyperfunctioning endocrinopathies. Biochemically and radiologically it mimics Paget's disease.
- Skeletal involvement is very common in patients with Gaucher's disease and is a major cause of morbidity. Enzyme replacement therapy arrests the progression and reverses hematological and visceral complications of Gaucher's disease but its effect on skeletal complications remains to e established.
- Osteopetrosis is very rare and in humans mainly due to impaired function of the osteoclasts.
- Osteogenesis imperfecta is characterized by low bone mass and increased bone fragility. The severity of the disease varies widely and depends largely on the clinical type. No clear genotype-phenotype relations have been established. Osteogenesis imperfecta type I may run a very mild course presenting later in life as osteoporosis. Bisphosphonate (mainly pamidronate) therapy of a small number of patients has been very successful.

PAGET'S DISEASE OF BONE

Paget's disease is a focal disorder of bone remodeling caused by abnormally increased bone resorption. The primary abnormality occurs in the osteoclasts, which increase in number and size in affected skeletal sites while the rest of the skeleton is spared. The result is increased bone resorption followed by a secondary increase in the rate of bone formation due to the coupling of these two processes and, thus, a high rate of bone turnover. Because of the accelerated rate of bone turnover, bone packets lose their lamellar structure, resulting in the appearance of woven bone with a characteristic mosaic pattern, which is of poor quality and susceptible to fractures.

Pathophysiology

Paget's disease affects slightly more men than women and seldom presents before the age of 35 years. Its prevalence increases with age and it affects 2 to 5% of those above 50 years, making it the most common bone disorder after osteoporosis. There is a geographical variation, the disease being common in central, western, and parts of southern Europe, the United States, Australia, New Zealand, and some countries of South America; Paget's disease is uncommon in Scandinavia, China, and Japan. A familial aggregation of the disease has also been noted, and current studies investigate a possible linkage to chromosome 18. There is considerable evidence supporting a viral etiology of Paget's disease with a member of the paramyxovirus family (measles virus, respiratory syncytial virus, canine distemper virus). However, not all studies have confirmed that, and the nature of the virus is still debated. Additional studies with bone marrow of patients with Paget's disease provided evidence of an abnormal bone marrow microenvironment in Pagetic lesions. This led to the hypothesis that locally produced factors, such as the cytokine interleukin-6, may play an autocrine/paracrine role and determine the preferential differentiation of early osteoclast precursors to abnormal osteoclasts and thus contribute to the pathogenesis of the disease. Therefore, although the precise cause of the disease has not been determined, the evidence favors a paramyxovirus infection in genetically predisposed individuals.

The most commonly affected bones are the pelvis (in about two-thirds of patients), the spine, the femora, and the skull, but practically all bones of the skeleton can be affected. About one third of the patients have only one lesion; the frequency of single lesions varies among the different series, which probably reflects referral patterns, and is higher in asymptomatic patients. The anatomical distribution of Pagetic lesions in an individual patient remains largely unchanged throughout life. This knowledge is important for reassuring patients with limited bone involvement who fear that they may develop extensive disease with time.

Clinical findings

Symptoms and signs

The majority of patients are asymptomatic. The disease is diagnosed incidentally during radiological examination because of another reason or an otherwise unexplained increase in serum alkaline phosphatase activity. Precise data about the proportion of symptomatic patients are not available and quoted figures vary widely. The prevalence of symptomatic disease in a large population of patients was estimated to be between 4 and 5% in Sheffield, United Kingdom. In symptomatic patients in our Department, the median duration of symptoms before referral was 5 years (range 0 to 25 years), and the median age

at referral was 63 years for men and 67 years for women. In Paget's disease, morbidity is determined by the damage caused and the progression of the disease at affected sites, as well as by the number and localization of the lesions. It should be noted, however, that extensive disease as originally described by Sir James Paget is nowadays rare, occurring in less than 5% of symptomatic patients. This may be not only due to the limited chances of an individual developing extensive disease, but also to actual changes in disease patterns.

Pain is the presenting symptom in over 80% of patients with Paget's disease. It is related to the extent and site of the disease but is not specific. It can be the result of the disease process or of complications at the site of the lesion or adjacent structures. Pain due to secondary osteoarthritis is common, occurs mainly in the hips, the knees, and the vertebrae, and it may make the assessment of the relative contribution of bone and joint pains to the patient's disability difficult. In such cases the origin of pain can be assessed retrospectively after treatment that primarily reduces the disease-related pain. *Deformity* is present in about 15% of patients at the time of diagnosis and affects weight-bearing bones, mainly the tibia and the femur; the most common deformity is bowing of the limb. In addition, characteristic deformities and enlargement of affected bones may occur at the jaw or the skull. *Fractures* are the presenting symptom in about 9% of patients; they occur more commonly in long bones and may be fissures or complete fractures. A very serious but uncommon (<1%) complication is the development of *osteosarcoma* in Pagetic lesions. *Neurological* complications include irreversible hearing loss in about one third of the patients with skull disease, spinal or brain stem compression, and, very rarely, hydrocephalus. Hypervascularity of affected bones may cause ischemia of adjacent structures as a result of the *steal syndrome*. When localized in the lower limbs, it can present as difficulty in walking (mimicking intermittent claudication); in the skull it may be responsible for headaches and, rarely, for mental dysfunction; it may also contribute to hearing loss. The *skin* above affected bones may be warm due to increased blood flow and bone turnover locally; it is usually seen in long bones and the skull. High output *cardiac failure*, commonly described in earlier publications, is rarely seen today. Reported associations with other conditions include urolithiasis, gout, and hyperparathyroidism.

Diagnostic procedures

In Paget's disease, a high rate of bone turnover is reflected in a directly proportional increase in biochemical indices of bone resorption and formation; urinary hydroxyproline and serum alkaline phosphatase, respectively, are the most frequently studied. The levels can be found within the reference range in about 10% of patients with limited skeletal involvement, while patients with skull disease tend to have higher values. Assays for the determination of biochemical indices of bone turnover more specific than hydroxyproline and alkaline phosphatase have been developed. For bone resorption these include pyridinium cross links, in particular deoxypyridinoline, and peptides of the cross-linking domains of type I collagen (N-telopeptides or C-telopeptides).These collagen degradation products, which are not affected by the diet of the patient, have been found to be elevated in urine and more recently in blood of patients with Paget's disease. For bone formation, serum assays for bone-specific alkaline phosphatase are available, as well as for other secretory products of the osteoblasts such as osteocalcin and procollagen carboxy- and amino-terminal propeptides. Serum osteocalcin levels are found within the normal range in about 50% of patients and are not useful in the management of the disease.

Despite the large changes in the rate of bone turnover, extracellular calcium homeostasis is generally maintained, but disturbances may occur. Serum calcium concentrations are normal but hypercalcemia may develop in immobilized, untreated patients with extensive skeletal involvement or may be due to concurrent primary hyperparathyroidism. The incidence of the latter is thought to be increased in Paget's disease. Serum calcitriol concentrations are usually within the reference range, but raised circulating parathyroid hormone with normal serum calcium concentrations (secondary hyperparathyroidism) have been reported in up to 20% of patients with Paget's disease, and there is also an increased incidence of hypercalciuria.

Abnormally increased bone resorption may be detected radiologically as a decrease in the density of affected bones; a wedge- or flame-shaped segment of bone resorption may be seen in long bones and extensive osteolytic areas in the skull (osteoporosis circumscripta). Older lesions usually have a mixed sclerotic and lytic appearance. The involved parts are enlarged and deformed, and the cortex can be thickened and dense (Fig. 23.1). Cyst-like lytic lesions interrupting the continuity of the cortex and fissure fractures in the cortex of long bones can increase the risk of complete fractures. The radiological changes are characteristic of the disease. Differential diagnosis includes bone metastases, particularly from prostate cancer and fibrous dysplasia. Bone scintigraphy is not specific, but it is more sensitive than plain radiographs, with about 15% of the lesions detected by scintigraphy having normal radiographic appearance. In addition, scintigraphy is the best method for assessing the extent of the disease. A bone scan should always be included in the investigation of a patient with Paget's disease, and radiographs of the areas with increased uptake of the radioisotope should be subsequently made.

Treatment

During the past 25 years, the management of patients with Paget's disease has changed dramatically with the discovery of the therapeutic potential of the calcitonins and the bisphosphonates. Other less-frequently used treatments include plicamycin (mithramycin) and gallium nitrate. When given parenterally, all calcitonins suppress the rate of bone turnover by about 50% and bring about clinical and radiological improvement. Calcitonin also has analgesic effects. Intranasal calcitonin, which is the most common form used, is less effective. In most patients, however, incomplete responses are obtained, and bone

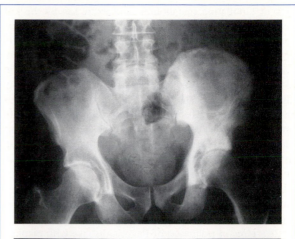

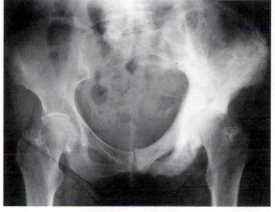

Figure 23.1 Radiographs of the pelvis from two patients with Paget's disease, demonstrating the typical changes of the disease and different degrees of secondary osteoarthritis of the hip joint, and also illustrating the progressive course of complications.

turnover reverses quickly to pretreatment values after stopping treatment. Moreover, resistance to treatment may develop. The well-described but poorly understood "escape" phenomenon is in part due to the generation of neutralizing antibodies to salmon calcitonin; this, together with the need for frequent injections, make long-term management of the disease with calcitonin difficult. Side effects of parenteral calcitonin treatment include nausea, vomiting, hot flashes, and diarrhea, while intranasal calcitonin has fewer side effects. The long-term safety profile of the calcitonins is excellent.

Bisphosphonates are currently the treatment of choice for Paget's disease because they suppress disease activity more completely than the calcitonins, and their effect persists after the discontinuation of treatment. Bisphosphonates are synthetic, bone-seeking compounds that are used in the management of skeletal disorders. Their specific pharmacological properties include poor intestinal absorption, selective uptake at active bone sites, suppression of osteoclast-mediated bone resorption, long skeletal retention, lack of circulating metabolites, and excretion by the kidneys. The structure of the bisphosphonate molecule allows for numerous substitutions, which have resulted in the development of various clinically useful compounds with considerable differences in antiresorptive potency, activity to toxicity ratio, and mechanism of action. Thus, although all bisphosphonates share a number of common properties, there are also differences among them, and results obtained with one compound should not be readily extrapolated to the whole class. Their mechanism of action includes inhibition of the activity of mature osteoclasts and/or the formation of new osteoclasts from their precursors. Bone selectivity, the lack of circulating metabolites, and specific antiresorptive action make bisphosphonates ideal agents for the management of Paget's disease.

The aims of treatment of Paget's disease with bisphosphonates are: (1) normalizing the activity of the disease with the shortest possible exposure to the drug; (2) reducing skeletal morbidity and improving the quality of life; (3) preventing complications; (4) making it convenient for the patient; and (5) producing no significant side effects. For understanding the action of bisphosphonates in Paget's disease and for the design of optimal treatment strategies, knowledge of certain pharmacodynamic principles of bisphosphonate treatment is essential. When a potent bisphosphonate is given to a patient with Paget's disease, the initial effect is the suppression of bone resorption. This occurs within a few days, during which the rate of bone formation is not affected (Fig. 23.2). The latter decreases secondarily at a slower rate because of the coupling between bone resorption and formation, so that a new equilibrium is reached within 3 to 6 months. Thus, a potent bisphosphonate given at the right dose eventually decreases the rate of bone turnover, even if administered for a short period of time. In Paget's disease with increased bone turnover, the dose that reaches the bone surface at any particular time is more important for the optimal suppression of disease activity rather than the total dose of the bisphosphonate. Therefore, higher doses given over short periods of time should be used, which contrasts with the approach in osteoporosis in which lower doses are given over longer periods. Practically all bisphosphonates, either approved or still in clinical development, have been used in the treatment of patients with Paget's disease. These are registered in various countries, and the recommended regimens are shown in Table 23.1.

Etidronate was the first bisphosphonate given to patients with Paget's disease. Its overall effectiveness is similar to that of parenteral calcitonin, but it has the advantage that it can be given orally, and its effect on bone turnover persists after stopping treatment. This effect is incomplete, however, and the therapeutic window of etidronate is narrow; doses that effectively suppress bone resorption are close to those that induce abnormal mineralization of newly formed bone (osteomalacia). Because of these and the availability of newer potent bisphosphonates, etidronate should not be used anymore in the treatment of Paget's disease.

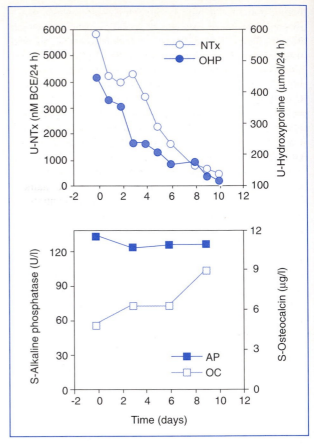

Figure 23.2 Biochemical indices of bone turnover in serum (S) and urine (U) in a patient treated with a nitrogen-containing bisphosphonate for 10 days. (OHP=hydroxyproline; NTx=N-telopeptide of collagen type I; AP=alkaline phosphatase; OC=osteocalcin.)

Bisphosphonate therapy is associated with clinical, radiological, and histological improvement. The response depends largely on the compound used, newer bisphosphonates containing a nitrogen atom in their molecule such as alendronate, ibandronate, olpadronate, pamidronate, and risedronate are especially effective and bring about the most consistent responses. Clinical responses

Table 23.1 Recommended doses and routes of administration of bisphosphonates registered for the treatment of Paget's disease of bone

Generic name	Dose
Alendronate	Oral, 40 mg/d for 6 months
Clodronate	Oral, 1600 mg/d for 3 or 6 months
	iv, 300 mg/d for 5 days
Etidronate	Oral, 400 mg/d for 6 months
Pamidronate*	iv, 30 to 60 mg/d for 3 days
Risedronate	Oral, 30 mg/d for 2 months
Tiludronate	Oral, 400 mg/d for 3 months

* Lower dose recommended by the company, higher dose recommended by investigators.

include the disappearance or significant reduction in pain due to the disease in over 80% of patients. However, in about 75% of patients with associated osteoarthritis, pain does not respond to treatment and analgesics or non-steroidal anti-inflammatory drugs can then be used. If the hip joint is affected, this may require corrective surgery (hip replacement). About half of the patients with pain associated with deformity of the femur or the tibia respond favorably to treatment, but persistent pain following effective treatment may require osteotomy. These complications emphasize the need for early intervention. There have been reports of improvement of spinal cord compression with bisphosphonate treatment, however hearing loss is not affected, though its progression is arrested. Fracture frequency appears to decrease after treatment with clodronate or pamidronate but not after etidronate. Radiological improvement can be impressive if the lesions are lytic and are localized in the long bones or the skull (Fig. 23.3). In other areas improvement occurs slowly. Changes are sometimes difficult to demonstrate outside specialized units, which follow standard X-ray protocols.

The first measurable effect of bisphosphonate treatment is the decrease in the rate of bone resorption. This is followed by a secondary decrease in the rate of bone formation, which results in a new steady state at a lower rate of bone turnover 3 to 6 months after the start of treatment. The antiresorptive efficacy of treatment is evaluated by measuring collagen type I degradation products. The overall efficacy of treatment is measured with serum alkaline phosphatase activity. Because the changes in bone remodeling following bisphosphonate therapy are predictable, it is not necessary to prolong treatment until the lowest level of serum alkaline phosphatase is reached. Short treatment courses with potent bisphosphonates are sufficient to achieve remissions in the majority of patients. With some of the newer bisphosphonates, remissions can be achieved in over 80% of patients. It should be noted that while in the past, the effectiveness of treatment was assessed by the degree of suppression of the initial values of indices of bone turnover, today this should only be assessed by the ability of the bisphosphonate to reduce these biochemical indices into the normal range.

The duration of remissions depends on the lowest level of serum alkaline phosphatase achieved with treatment. Suppression to well within the reference range should, therefore, be a main aim of treatment. Once remission is achieved, recurrences occur slowly, and follow-up of patients once or twice a year with measurement of their serum alkaline phosphatase activity is usually sufficient.

In the past, treatment was given only to symptomatic patients and to those requiring orthopedic surgery to reduce the excessive bleeding from Pagetic bone during the operation. Available treatments are safe and effective, hence they should also be offered to asymptomatic patients if they are young or have localizations of the disease that bear a risk for complications. Examples of this are the disease being localized around large joints and causing osteoarthritis, at the skull with potential hearing loss, in weight bearing long-bones causing a risk of deformities and fractures, and in the spine causing osteoarthritis and spinal compression with neurological consequences.

Bisphosphonate therapy has relatively few side effects. Mild gastrointestinal complaints have been reported with low frequency with all bisphosphonates. Amino-bisphosphonates, such as oral alendronate and pamidronate, can induce more severe gastrointestinal side effects, including heartburn, nausea, and vomiting in a few patients associated with esophagitis or gastritis. Oral bisphosphonates should always be given in the fasting state, in an upright position with a full glass of water, and never with food or calcium supplements, which reduce their already low intestinal absorption. Rapid intravenous injection of bisphosphonates may chelate calcium in the circulation and form complexes that can be nephrotoxic. Biphosphonates should, therefore, be given parenterally by slow intravenous infusion. Some novel potent bisphosphonates, such as ibandronate, may eventually be administered by intravenous injection, while clodronate can be given intramuscularly. Aminobisphosphonates should never be administered intramuscularly because they can cause severe local irritation. The first treatment with a nitrogen-containing bisphosphonate may increase body

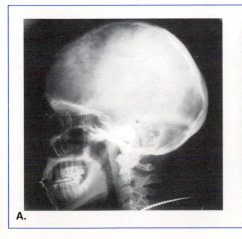
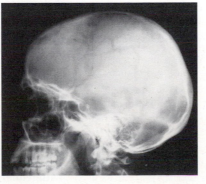

A.   B.

Figure 23.3 Radiographs of the skull of a patient with Paget's disease with osteoporosis circumscripta before (**A**) and after (**B**) treatment with pamidronate. Note the recalcification of the large lytic area.

temperature and induce flu-like symptoms (acute phase reaction). This has been reported with alendronate, ibandronate, neridronate, olpadronate, and pamidronate, but not with clodronate, etidronate, or tiludronate, which do not contain a nitrogen atom in their structures. This reaction is transient, subsides without any specific treatment, does not occur upon continuation of treatment or in patients previously treated with a nitrogen-containing bisphosphonate, and is probably caused by the release of inflammatory cytokines such as interleukin-6 and tumor necrosis factor-α.

FIBROUS DYSPLASIA

Fibrous dysplasia is a sporadic skeletal disorder characterized by the progressive replacement of normal bone architecture by abnormal fibrous tissue, which can cause pain, fractures, deformities, and nerve compression. The disease is divided into monostotic and polyostotic forms. Polyostotic fibrous dysplasia may be associated with pigmented skin lesions and various hyperfunctioning endocrinopathies. McCune, Bruch, Albright and colleagues described polyostotic fibrous dysplasia, café-au-lait spots, and precocious puberty in girls for the first time in 1937. This association has been termed the McCune-Albright syndrome and was subsequently shown to include multiple endocrinopathies such as gonadotropin-independent precocious puberty in girls and boys, autonomous thyroid nodules, acromegaly, hypercortisolism, and hypophosphatemic rickets and osteomalacia. There is no familial aggregation of the disease.

Fibrous dysplasia is a developmental disorder associated with mutations of the gene encoding the α subunit of the stimulating G protein $G_{s\alpha}$, which leads to the constitutive activation of adenylyl cyclase. Mutations have been identified in different endocrine and nonendocrine tissues, including bone. The mechanisms by which these activating mutations of $G_{s\alpha}$ lead to the characteristic bone lesions of fibrous dysplasia are not known.

Clinical findings

Symptoms and signs

Polyostotic fibrous dysplasia typically begins in infancy and childhood, before the age of 10 years, but the age of diagnosis is variable. Isolated lesions of the monostotic form develop in the second to third decade of life, and if small they remain asymptomatic and may be discovered accidentally on radiographs performed for an unrelated reason. Bone lesions can cause *pain, deformities,* and pathological *fractures.* When facial bones are affected, deformities and *visual* and *hearing* loss may occur as a result of cranial nerve compression. Any bone may be involved but long bones; particularly the femur, the tibia,

and also facial bones and the ribs are frequently affected in the monostotic form of the disease. The polyostotic form also involves the pelvis, the humerus, the radius, the scapula, and the clavicle. Vertebral lesions are rather uncommon. The lesions may be segmented and found only on one side of the body or distributed throughout the skeleton. They are usually progressive. Development of new lesions is, however, uncommon. Malignant transformation is rare and has been estimated to occur in about 0.5% of cases, particularly if a bone lesion has been previously irradiated. Patients with the McCune-Albright syndrome may have café-au-lait pigmented *skin lesions* with irregular borders (coast of Maine), which distinguishes them from those of neurofibromatosis, which have a smooth border (coast of California). The skin lesions have a characteristic distribution and tend to localize on the side of the bone lesions. *Endocrine dysfunction* depends on the gland involved and includes precocious puberty, hyperthyroidism, acromegaly with associated hyperprolactinemia and Cushing's syndrome. In some patients with the McCune-Albright syndrome, generalized bone disease characterized by proximal myopathy, renal phosphate wasting and rickets or osteomalacia has been described.

Diagnostic procedures

Biochemical parameters of calcium metabolism are normal unless the disease is accompanied by hypophosphatemic osteomalacia. In this case, serum phosphate and tubular maximum reabsorption of phosphate over the glomerular filtration rate (TmP/GFR) are low, serum alkaline phosphatase activity is increased, and serum calcitriol is low. Depending on the extent of the disease, biochemical indices of bone turnover can be increased to levels similar to those of patients with Paget's disease. In patients with the McCune-Albright syndrome, endocrine function tests can be abnormal depending on the endocrine gland involved. Bone histology shows a vascular stroma with an excess of fibroblasts, woven bone with increased osteoid, and in some cases with raised numbers of osteoclasts.

On plain radiographs, the lesions are radiolucent and have a ground-glass appearance. In the long bones they are usually localized in the diaphyses or the metaphyses and only rarely in the epiphyses, and they are associated with thinning and scalloping of the cortex and expansion of the affected bone area (Fig. 23.4). Periosteal new bone formation is usually absent. Deformities may be marked; the so-called "sheperd's crook" appearance of the femur is characteristic. Skull lesions are lytic or sclerotic and the latter are more frequently seen in the skull than in other skeletal sites. Vertebral fractures are rare. Bone scintigraphy shows increased uptake of the radioisotope in affected areas and is more sensitive than plain radiographs in detecting the extent of the lesions.

Differential diagnosis

Differential diagnosis includes Paget's disease of bone, enchondromatosis, and brown tumors of osteitis fibrosa cystica of hyperparathyroidism. Monostotic fibrous dys-

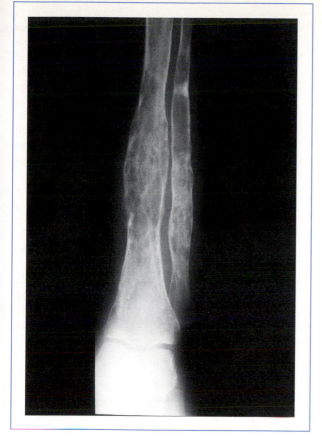

Figure 23.4 Radiograph of the lower leg of a patient with polyostotic fibrous dysplasia with characteristic changes.

plasia should be further differentiated from solitary bone cysts such as aneurysmal bone cysts and tumors e.g., when the disease is localized in the jaw.

Treatment

Orthopedic management consists of stabilizing fractures and correcting and preventing deformities. Large lytic lesions may be treated with bone grafts, which may stabilize the bone and reduce the pain. Decompression operations may be required for sclerotic progressive lesions of the skull that lead to nerve compression. Amino-bisphosphonates, in particular intravenous pamidronate, suppress bone turnover, decrease bone pain, arrest the progress of the disease, and in some cases induce recalcification of the bone lesions. The optimal frequency of administration as well as the dose of the bisphosphonates still need to be defined. Fibrous dysplasia with increased bone turnover can be treated with bisphosphonates as in Paget's disease. However, while the short-term response may be the same as in Paget's disease, the long-term response is different. For example, in Paget's disease, a short course of a potent bisphosphonate can be followed by a long-term remission. This is not the case in fibrous dysplasia, which requires more frequent therapy. In girls with the McCune-Albright syndrome testolactone, an aro-

matase inhibitor that blocks the conversion of androgen to estrogen, decreased serum estradiol levels and reduced the frequency of menses. Some patients, however, escape from the effect of this treatment after 1 to 3 years.

GAUCHER'S DISEASE

Gaucher's disease is an autosomal recessive lipid storage disorder due to deficiency (or deficient activity) of the lysosomal enzyme glucocerebrosidase (acid β-glucosidase) that results in the accumulation of glucocerebroside (glucoceramide), primarily in cells of the monocyte-macrophage lineage. These cells are known as Gaucher's cells. The gene of the enzyme has been located to chromosome 1, and numerous mutations have been identified.

Clinical findings

Three clinical types of the disease are recognized based on the presence and progression of neurological manifestations. The most common type is the non-neuropathic variant of the disease and occurs in nearly 99% of patients. The prevalence of Gaucher's disease varies between 1 in 40 000 to 1 in 200 000 being much more common in Ashkenazi Jews of Eastern European origin.

Symptoms and signs

Gaucher's disease is a multisystemic disorder involving the liver, spleen, lymph nodes, bone marrow and, less frequently, the lungs, skin, and gastrointestinal tract. Because of this, clinical presentation and severity vary widely.

Skeletal involvement is common in patients with type 1 Gaucher's disease, affecting more than 80% of patients and is a major cause of morbidity. There is, however, a large variation in the age of onset, the extent, and the progression of skeletal disease. Because of the variability of bone lesions, their origin at the bone marrow-bone interface, and the general effect of the disease on bone mass, the skeletal complications of Gaucher's disease are considered as metabolic bone disease in a broader context. The pathogenesis of the bone disease is unclear, but it is related to the presence of Gaucher cells in the bone marrow. These cells presumably stimulate the formation and/or activity of osteoclasts through the production of bone-resorbing cytokines or of other bone cells through the production of growth factors.

Clinical manifestations of skeletal complications of Gaucher's disease are not related to the distribution of the disease to various organs or to any particular genotype, but correlate with the extent of skeletal involvement. Bone disease is progressive; complications are arbitrarily divided into those complications that give rise to symptoms, and those that are only detected by specific investigations. Of the former, *pain* is the most common and serious symptom. It can be nonspecific, presenting as a dull pain that is usually not associated with other signs or symptoms and resolves without specific treatment. Severe, excruciating pain may occur in up to 40% of patients as a result of the so-called "*bone crisis*" due to a bone infarction. This is usually localized and is accompanied by pyrexia and leucocytosis; it usually does not respond to common analgesics, and clinically resembles an attack of sickle cell anemia. It is one of the most distressing complications of the disease and resolves after 1 to 3 weeks. Pathological *fractures* either of long bones or the vertebrae is another cause of pain. *Avascular necrosis,* with its characteristic clinical picture and its disabling consequences, can occur in nearly half of the patients with involvement of the femoral head. Finally, secondary *osteoarthritis* of a severity requiring hip replacement may develop. Of the complications that do not directly give rise to symptoms, osteopenia is common. In a recent cross-sectional study of 61 adults with type 1 disease, the bone mineral density of both the axial and the appendicular skeleton was below reference values of the same age and sex. This suggests that the whole skeleton is affected in Gaucher's disease. The degree of osteopenia is an independent predictor of the severity of bone involvement, assessed radiologically, and bone mineral density measurements have been proposed as sensitive indicators of skeletal involvement in Gaucher's disease.

Diagnostic procedures

The diagnosis can be made on bone marrow aspirates by the demonstration of the presence of typical Gaucher's cells. However, pseudo-Gaucher's cells may also be found in the bone marrow of patients with some hematological malignancies or congenital anemias. For this reason, sensitive assays for measuring enzyme activity in leukocytes or skin fibroblasts are required for diagnosis. Tartrate-resistant acid phosphatase and angiotensin-converting enzyme activities are elevated or normal in the blood of patients with Gaucher's disease and are not specific. Recently the activity of the enzyme chitotriosidase was found to be elevated in the plasma of patients with Gaucher's disease and is used as a marker to follow the effectiveness of therapy.

Radiographic appearances are characteristic of the disease. Erlenmeyer flask deformities of the distal femur and the proximal tibia are distinctive but not pathognomonic (Fig. 23.5). Thinning of the cortex and areas of osteolysis, as well as, of osteosclerosis most likely resulting from local infiltration of the marrow by Gaucher cells and subsequent repair of the lesions also occur. Plain radiographs are insufficiently sensitive to detect the extent of bone disease and its response to treatment. The best imaging method for the assessment of bone involvement in Gaucher's disease is through magnetic resonance, and the recently developed quantitative magnetic resonance methodology in which the fat content of the marrow of vertebral bodies can be measured. Bone scintigraphy with

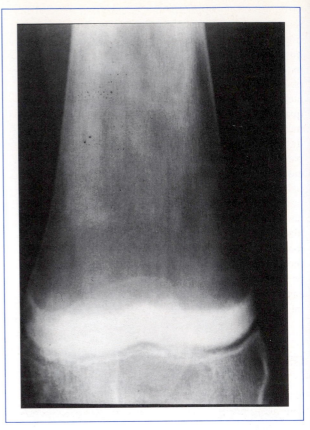

Figure 23.5 Radiograph of the distal femur of a young patient with Gaucher's disease with the characteristic Erlenmeyer flask appearance and an area of metaphyseal sclerosis due to inhibition of bone resorption by bisphosphonate (pamidronate) treatment.

Tc-labeled bisphosphonate is not specific, but it may help in the differential diagnosis of a bone crisis. Biochemical indices of bone turnover show wide variation, and can be increased or normal, but in bone biopsies low bone turnover has generally been detected. The mechanisms underlying these differences are not well understood and may be related to the wide spectrum of the disease, as well as to the timing of the investigations.

Treatment

Management of the disease consists of nonspecific and disease- and bone-specific interventions. Nonspecific measures include bed rest; sufficient fluid intake; potent analgesics; prevention of secondary osteomyelitis during bone crises; orthopedic operations for fractures, avascular necrosis, and joint disease; and early mobilization and physiotherapy in the case of vertebral fractures.

In recent years, the standard treatment for Gaucher's disease has been revolutionized by the development of replacement therapy with the enzyme glucocerebrosidase, which is prepared from natural sources (alglucerase) or by recombinant technology (imiglucerase). This was shown to arrest the progression and to reverse hematological and visceral complications of the disease. An optimal dose remains to be defined. With regard to skeletal complications, some reports show improvement, while others show no effect, which may be related to the different doses used. Moreover, hematological improvements are more obvious than bone responses, which are much slower and lack reliable objective endpoints for their assessment. The quantitative magnetic resonance and bone mineral density measurements may be helpful in this respect, but definite data are not yet available. The bisphosphonate pamidronate has been used in patients with Gaucher's disease with skeletal complications and reduced the bone pain and frequency of bone crises; in a few cases this treatment normalized abnormally increased biochemical parameters of bone resorption. In view of the well-recognized effects of bisphosphonates in patients with low bone mass from other causes, the combination of enzyme replacement therapy with bisphosphonate treatment may be envisaged for the future management of the bone disease in Gaucher's patients. Reliable data in support of this therapeutic concept remain to be established.

OSTEOPETROSIS

Osteopetrosis (marble bone disease) is the prototype of sclerosing bone dysplasias. It is the result of impaired function of the osteoclasts that fail to resorb calcified cartilage or bone. It is a rare disorder, but because its fundamental defect lies in the osteoclasts, it has been very informative to biologists studying the process of osteoclastogenesis and bone resorption. The disease is heterogeneous and two main clinical forms are recognized: (1) An infantile, malignant form with autosomal recessive transmission, which, if not treated, leads to death in infancy or early childhood, and (2) An autosomal dominant adult, benign form that is often asymptomatic. A number of variants with clinical expressions of different severity between the two main forms have also been described. Of these, the best-characterized is a syndrome presenting with osteopetrosis, cerebral calcifications, and renal tubular acidosis due to deficiency of the enzyme carbonic anhydrase type II. This enzyme is responsible for the production of protons in the osteoclasts, which are necessary for normal bone resorption. This heterogeneity implies that multiple genes are involved in the pathogenesis of the disease. Extensive studies have been performed in murine models of osteopetrosis. For example, there is a naturally occurring mouse model, the op/op mouse, in which osteopetrosis is due to the deficient production of colony stimulating factor-1 (CSF-1 or M-CSF), a cytokine essential for osteoclastogenesis. In this model, osteoclasts are absent, while in the human disease osteoclasts are present but are not functional. Treatment of the mice with exogenous CSF-1 results in osteoclast formation and resolution of the osteopetrosis. Other animal models include mice with disruptions of the *src-* or the *c-fos* proto-oncogenes. Further studies in these models may be relevant to the pathogenesis of human osteopetrosis.

Clinical findings

Symptoms and signs

Malignant osteopetrosis presents in infancy with failure to thrive, hepatosplenomegaly, anemia, multiple cranial nerve palsies, deafness, blindness, recurrent infections, and bleeding disorders. Eruption of dentition is usually delayed. Bones, although very dense, are of poor quality and fracture easily. The hematological consequences of the osteopetrosis are due to the occupancy of the marrow spaces by calcified cartilage, which cannot be resorbed to enlarge the marrow cavity. If untreated, the condition is fatal. Adult osteopetrosis may run a benign course and remain undiagnosed. Sometimes facial palsy, anemia, or deafness from cranial nerve compression may occur, or pathological fractures may draw attention to the condition.

Diagnostic procedures

There are generally no abnormalities in the biochemical parameters of calcium and bone metabolism, but hypocalcemia and secondary hyperparathyroidism may occur. Acid phosphatase and creatine kinase (the brain isoenzyme) activities may be increased in serum. Bone histology in infantile osteopetrosis usually reveals numerous osteoclasts lacking ruffled borders. In other forms of osteopetrosis, the number of osteoclasts can be increased, normal, or decreased. Areas of calcified cartilage persist in mature bone, which is pathognomonic. The bone has a woven appearance, and there may also be an excess of osteoid.

The principal radiographic feature of osteopetrosis is generalized symmetrical osteosclerosis with modelling abnormalities. In younger patients, the osteosclerosis is more prominent in the skull, while a bone-within-bone appearance is commonly seen in the vertebrae. Osteomyelitis can occur in all forms of osteopetrosis. Fractures are typically transverse and may be complicated by delayed union. Radiographic features of rickets have been described in some patients, as well as alternate bands of increased and normal density in long bones of adult patients, suggesting periods of exacerbations and remissions of the disease.

Treatment

The treatment of choice of infantile osteopetrosis is bone marrow transplantation, which has been successful in many patients. However, not all patients benefit from this procedure because of the heterogeneity of the molecular basis of the disease. Due to the activation of osteoclasts and the subsequent massive resorption of the calcified cartilage, successful bone marrow transplantation may be complicated by hypercalcemia. This is also a sign that the transplantation of bone marrow has been successful. The hypercalcemia is transient and usually mild or moderate and can be treated with intravenous saline alone. Severe, hypercalcemia may, however, develop in some patients requiring treatment with antiresorptive agents, which can be very effective and do not interfere with normal osteoclastic resorption in the long-term. Other therapeutic measures include a low-calcium diet alone or in combination with high doses of calcitriol and treatment with recombinant human interferon γ. In patients with osteopetrosis due to deficiency of carbonic anhydrase type II, bicarbonate supplements are given, but the long-term results of this intervention are not known.

OSTEOGENESIS IMPERFECTA

Osteogenesis imperfecta is an autosomal dominant genetic disorder of the connective tissue due to quantitative or qualitative abnormalities of the principal protein of the bone matrix collagen type I resulting in low bone mass and increased bone fragility. Osteogenesis imperfecta is also called brittle bone disease. Collagen type I is present in additional tissues such as dentine, the sclerae, skin, joints, tendons and heart valves with signs and symptoms observed in affected patients. Osteogenesis imperfecta is thought to occur in 1 in 20 000 births but this is not a reliable estimate, since many cases are diagnosed later in life and some lethal perinatal cases may be misdiagnosed. The severity of the disease varies widely from lethal cases in the perinatal period to undiagnosed or accidentally discovered cases in adulthood. Patients have normal intelligence. All forms of the disease result from mutations of type I collagen. Many such mutations have been identified, but so far no clear phenotype-genotype correlations have been established. To account for the clinical heterogeneity the disease is commonly classified into four types, originally proposed by Silence (Tab. 23.2). This useful classification does not, however, completely separate the various clinical expressions of the disease.

Table 23.2 Clinical classification of osteogenesis imperfecta

Type I	Mild bone fragility, little or no deformity, normal or slightly reduced stature, blue sclerae, hearing loss, normal teeth or dentinogenesis imperfecta; the most frequent type occurring in about 60% of patients with osteogenesis imperfecta
Type II	Lethal in perinatal period, severe bone disease, multiple fractures, marked long bone deformities, platyspondyly
Type III	Progressive deformities, scoliosis, very short stature, sclerae variable, hearing loss, and dentinogenesis imperfecta common
Type IV	Moderate bone disease and deformities, normal sclerae, short stature, dentinogenesis imperfecta common, hearing loss may develop

---

Clinical findings

The clinical presentation of the disease is dominated by bone fragility and deformities that depend largely on the clinical type of the disease. The main feature is *fractures*, mainly of the appendicular, but also of the axial skeleton. In osteogenesis imperfecta type I, fractures are relatively infrequent when compared to the other types, but osteopenia is prominent. The frequency of fractures decreases dramatically after puberty and increases again later in life, especially in women after the menopause. Osteogenesis imperfecta type I may run a very mild course and remain undiagnosed until later in life and then presents as "osteoporosis". Fractures are much more frequent in osteogenesis imperfecta type IV, and *bone deformities* are also common. The most severe of the non-fatal forms of the disease is osteogenesis imperfecta type III, in which there are progressive skeletal deformities and multiple fractures. Because of the fractures and the corrective surgery associated with them, patients with osteogenesis imperfecta type III are confined to wheel chairs. Fracture complications include severe angulation, which limits the function, non-union, and in a few cases hyperplastic callus formation. Apart from deformities resulting from the fractures, scoliosis is common, especially in severe disease. Other deformities include bowing of the tibia, skull deformities, protrusio acetabuli, coxa vara, genu valgum, and deformities of the chest wall. *Stature* is normal or a little shorter in patients with osteogenesis imperfecta type I, while it is severely decreased in the other types, with most of the patients falling under the 5th percentile for height. Characteristic *blue sclerae* are described in patients with osteogenesis imperfecta type I but not with type IV. In type III, the color of the sclerae is variable. The color of the sclerae cannot always be assessed with confidence and may change with increasing age. *Hearing loss* is very common. It usually appears in adulthood and is sensorineural rather than conductive. *Dentinogenesis imperfecta* occurs in about 25% of patients of each clinical type, but it is relatively uncommon in patients with mild disease and very common in those with severe disease. The presence or absence of dentinogenesis imperfecta has led some authors to distinguish osteogenesis imperfecta type I into types IA and IB. *Joint hypermobility* is common and occurs in 70% of patients. It is attributed to underdevelopment of the ligaments. Interestingly, joint pains are a prominent clinical feature in adult patients with mild disease. The *skin* is usually thin and bruises easily, and cardiac abnormalities, such as mitral valve prolapse, are uncommon. Pulmonary insufficiency is usually the cause of death in the lethal type, but pulmonary function in other clinical types is variable.

Diagnostic procedures

Biochemical findings pertinent to calcium and mineral metabolism are usually normal, as are the levels of the calciotropic hormones parathyroid hormone and calcitriol. In children external calcium balances are usually positive, which is in contrast to idiopathic juvenile osteoporosis. Some patients may have hypercalciuria; it is not clear whether this is related to the disease process or is the result of immobilization. Biochemical indices of bone turnover are usually found within the reference range, but increases in both serum alkaline phosphatase activity and in urinary hydroxyproline excretion have been reported. Bone biopsies from patients with osteogenesis imperfecta show thin osteoid seams and decreased calcification rates, but bone turnover may also be increased. Hypercellularity is usually found reflecting compensatory efforts of the osteoblasts. There appears to be an imbalance between bone formation and bone resorption, which is supported by recent reports of measurements of new biochemical indices of bone turnover. The diagnosis can be established by the clinical presentation. In doubtful cases, skin fibroblast cultures reveal abnormalities of collagen synthesis. In children, the disease should be differentiated from idiopathic juvenile osteoporosis and from child abuse.

Characteristic of all types of osteogenesis imperfecta is the generalized osteopenia confirmed by bone mineral measurements at various ages. Radiographic appearances are variable and depend on the severity of the disease. Generally there are modelling defects with thinning of the cortices. The metaphyseal-epiphyseal architecture in the lower extremities is normal in patients with mild disease. In severe cases, the diaphysis of long bones is narrow with an enlarged dysplastic metaphyseal-epiphyseal area. Deformities can occur as a result of fractures. Irregular calcified radiolucencies at the end of long bones can be seen in children, particularly children with osteogenesis imperfecta type III, giving the so-called "popcorn" appearance. Vertebral deformities, in some cases with total vertebral collapse can be recognized at any age (Fig. 23.6).

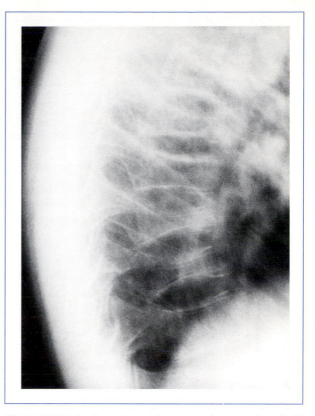

Figure 23.6 Radiographs of the spine of a prepubertal girl with osteogenesis imperfecta type I and multiple vertebral deformities.

Treatment

Various bone-acting drugs have been tried in the treatment of children and adults with osteogenesis imperfecta with limited success. Efforts have been focused on surgical corrections, rehabilitation of patients, and management of non-skeletal features of the disease. Recently there have been new approaches to the management of patients with osteogenesis imperfecta. Growth hormone has been administered to children with various clinical types of the disease. Overall, this treatment increased growth velocity as well as the rate of bone turnover, but there are no concrete data about a possible reduction of the incidence of fractures. In a series of open, long-term studies involving a small number of patients, treatment with the bisphosphonates pamidronate (orally or intravenously) and olpadronate (orally) led to clinical improvements and reversal of vertebral deformities. It also increased calcium balance and bone mineral density in some prepubertal children. These findings were considered sufficient to justify the planning of controlled studies with nitrogen-containing bisphosphonates, which are currently underway. A recently developed animal model of osteogenesis imperfecta, together with in vitro attempts for potential gene therapy, provide new dimensions in the future management of patients with the disease.

Suggested readings

BRUMSEN C, HAMDY NA, PAPAPOULOS SE. Long-term effects of bisphosphonates on the growing skeleton; studies of young patients with severe osteoporosis. Medicine (Baltimore) 1997;76:266-83.

DELMAS PD, MEUNIER PJ. The management of Paget's disease of bone. N Engl J Med 1997;336:558-66.

FLEISCH H. Bisphosphonates in bone disease: from the laboratory to the patient. 3rd ed. New York: Parthenon Publishing Group, 1997.

GRABOWSKI GA, BARTON NW, PASTORES G, et al. Enzyme therapy in Type 1 Gaucher disease: comparative efficacy of mannose-terminated glucocerebrosidase from natural and recombinant sources. Ann Intern Med 1995;122:33-9.

INCERTI C. Gaucher's disease: an overview. Sem Hematol 1995; 32 (Suppl 1):3-9.

KANIS JA. Pathophysiology and treatment of Paget's disease of bone. London: Dunitz, 1997.

LIENS D, DELMAS PD, MEUNIER PJ. Long-term effects of intravenous pamidronate in fibrous dysplasia of bone. Lancet 1994;343:953-4.

Loria-Cortez R, Quesada-Calvo E, Corder-Chaverri E. Osteopetrosis in children: a report of 26 cases. J Pediatr 1977;91:43-7.

Mankin HJ, Doppelt SH, Rosenberg AE, Barranger JA. Metabolic bone disease in patients with Gaucher's disease. In: Avioli LV, Krane SM, eds. Metabolic bone disease and clinically related disorders. 2nd ed. Philadelphia: WB Saunders, 1990;730-52.

Papapoulos SE. Paget's disease of bone: clinical, pathogenetic and therapeutic aspects. Baillières Clin Endocrinol Metab 1997;11:117-43.

Schwindinger WF, Levine MA. McCune-Albright syndrome. Trends Endocrinol Metab 1993;4:238-42.

Smith R. Osteogenesis imperfecta. Clin Rheum Dis 1986;12: 655-87.

Siris ES. Seeking the elusive etiology of Paget's disease: a progress report. J Bone Miner Res 1996;11:1599-601.

Whyte MP. Osteogenesis imperfecta. In: Favus MJ, ed. Primer on the metabolic disease and disorders of mineral metabolism. 3rd ed. Philadelphia: Lippincott-Raven 1996;382-5.

Whyte MP. Sclerosing bone dysplasias. In: Favus MJ, ed. Primer on the metabolic bone diseases and disorders of mineral metabolism. 3rd ed. Philadelphia: Lippincott-Raven 1996;363-7.

Ectopic calcification and ossification

Socrates E. Papapoulos

▰ KEY POINTS ▰

- Three general mechanisms are responsible for ectopic (heterotopic) mineralization: metastatic calcification, dystrophic calcification, and heterotopic ossification.
- Metastatic calcification occurs in conditions associated with hypercalcemia and/or hyperphosphatemia.
- Tumoral calcinosis is a heritable form of metastatic calcification that can be successfully managed by restriction of dietary phosphate and the use of phosphate binders.
- Dystrophic calcification occurring in patients with connective tissue disorders is termed "calcinosis" and can be particularly severe in patients with dermatomyositis. Diltiazem and probenecid have been very effective in the management of a few patients with calcinosis associated with juvenile dermatomyositis.
- Fibrodysplasia (myositis) ossificans progressiva, a rare but dramatic form of ectopic ossification, can be suspected at birth by the presence of short, malformed great toes.
- The etiology of heterotopic ossification following total hip replacement is unknown. Various agents have been used to treat or prevent this complication, but results have been equivocal.

Ectopic (or heterotopic) mineralization is characterized by extraskeletal deposition of calcium salts, most commonly phosphate as amorphous salt or as hydroxyapatite crystals. When this involves formation of true bone, it is termed ectopic (heterotopic) ossification as opposed to calcification, which is used in the literature to describe all other forms of ectopic mineralization. The pathogenesis of the disorder is incompletely understood, and three general mechanisms have been proposed to account for it. First, metastatic calcification due to an abnormal calcium-phosphate solubility product in extracellular fluid, as occurs, for example, in hypercalcemia and/or hyperphosphatemia independently of their cause. Second, dystrophic calcification, which occurs in the presence of normal extracellular concentrations of calcium and phosphate and is attributed to changes of the soft tissue. Third, hetero-topic ossification, which can be either congenital or acquired, and its pathogenesis is largely unknown. Ectopic mineralization can occur according to these three mechanisms in a variety of disorders, which are listed in Table 24.1.

METASTATIC CALCIFICATION

Metastatic calcification occurs in conditions associated with hypercalcemia and/or hyperphosphatemia. In hypercalcemia, calcium deposits can be found in the conjunctiva and the cornea of the eye, the kidneys, the lungs, and the stomach. The reason for the preferential deposition of calcium phosphate in these organs may be associated with the higher local pH, which facilitates the formation of cal-

Table 24.1 Disorders associated with ectopic mineralization

Metastatic calcification

Hypercalcemia
　　Milk alkali syndrome, vitamin D intoxication,
　　　sarcoidosis, hyperparathyroidism (autonomous)
Hyperphosphatemia
　　Hypoparathyroidism, renal failure, vitamin D
　　　intoxication, tumoral calcinosis, cell lysis following
　　　chemotherapy for leukemia

Dystrophic calcification

Calcinosis (circumscripta or universalis)
　　Dermatomyositis, scleroderma, lupus erythematosus
Post-traumatic
Tuberculous lesions
Monkeberg's medial calcinosis

Ectopic ossification

Congenital
　　Fibrodysplasia (myositis) ossificans progressiva
　　Pseudohypoparathyroidism and pseudopseudohy-
　　　poparathyroidism
Acquired
　　Myositis ossificans; post-traumatic (spinal cord
　　　injury, hip surgery, burns)
　　Hematomas
　　Ankylosing spondylitis, diffuse idiopathic skeletal
　　　hyperostosis
Other types
　　Chondrocalcinosis, urinary stones

(Adapted from Fawthrop FW, Russell RGG. Ectopic calcification and ossification. In: Nordin BEC, Need AG, Morris HA,
(eds). Metabolic bone and stone disease. 3rd ed. Edinburgh:
Churchill Livingstone, 1993;325-38; and from Whyte MP.
Extraskeletal (ectopic) calcification and ossification. In: Favus
MJ [ed]. Primer on the metabolic bone diseases and disorders
of mineral metabolism. 3rd ed. Philadelphia: Lippincott-Raven,
1996;422-30.)

cium phosphate crystals at a lower solubility product. Any hypercalcemic disorder may be associated with metastatic calcifications if the elevation of plasma calcium is sufficiently high and prolonged. This is, however, more likely to occur in conditions where hypercalcemia is accompanied by higher plasma levels of phosphate, such as vitamin D intoxication and the milk alkali syndrome. Chronic hyperphosphatemia can cause the same effect if this is of sufficient severity, even if plasma calcium concentration is low, as for example in hypoparathyroidism. In this condition extraskeletal deposition of calcium phosphate is frequently seen, with calcification of the basal ganglia in the brain being characteristic. Metastatic calcification occurs more commonly in patients with chronic renal failure, especially in those in whom hyperphosphatemia is inadequately controlled. In some cases this may be severe and can give rise to clinical manifestations such as pruritus, band keratopathy, and persistent and irritating conjunctivitis, in addition to arterial and visceral calcifications. Nephrocalcinosis is a special form of metastatic calcification in the kidney, distinct from the deposition of calcium salts within the renal tubular lumen associated with renal stone disease. It can occur in hypercalcemic conditions such as primary hyperparathyroidism, vitamin D intoxication, and the milk alkali syndrome, but also in the absence of hypercalcemia as in renal tubular acidosis. A heritable form of metastatic calcification is tumoral calcinosis, which is characterized by large periarticular calcifications involving the large joints. Patients have increased plasma phosphate and renal tubular reabsorption of phosphate and, paradoxically, some of them also have increased circulating concentrations of calcitriol. This further increases the intestinal absorption of calcium and phosphate. The pathogenesis of these changes is unknown. Restriction of dietary phosphate and the use of phosphate binders have been very effective in the management of patients with tumoral calcinosis, and even dissolution of calcified masses has been reported.

DYSTROPHIC CALCIFICATION

Soft tissue calcification is a non-specific response to tissue damage, which occurs despite normal calcium-phosphate solubility products. The etiology is unknown, but it is thought that during injury substances with nucleating properties, normally present only in bone collagen, are exposed to tissue fluids initiating the calcification. The nature of these substances is unknown, but in some studies bone matrix glycoproteins have been identified at sites of ectopic calcification. Whether these have been absorbed at these sites from the circulation or whether a population of stem cells that is normally present in these sites was stimulated by the tissue damage to develop further and to produce them is not known. Moreover, the significance of these matrix glycoproteins in the pathogenesis of dystrophic calcification remains to be determined.

Examples of dystrophic calcification include heart valve calcification after rheumatic fever, and a rare form of inherited arterial calcification called Monckeberg's medial calcinosis. These are distinct from the calcification of blood vessels (and cartilage) that occurs with normal aging in the absence of injury. Other examples of dystrophic calcification are healed tuberculous lesions and calcifications of certain tendons after injury.

Dystrophic cutaneous or subcutaneous calcification occurring in patients with connective tissue disorders such as scleroderma, dermatomyositis and lupus erythematosus is termed calcinosis. It can be limited to the skin or to extensor aspects of joints (circumscripta), or it can also involve the deep fascia (universalis). These forms of calcinosis are distinct from tumoral calcinosis, which is a form of metastatic calcification (see section on metastatic calcification). An example of calcinosis circumscripta are the calcifications around the fingertips that can be seen in patients with scleroderma and other connective tissue diseases. These deposits may induce an inflammatory reaction, pain, or tenderness and may ulcerate through the surface. Calcinosis universalis occurs mainly in dermatomyositis, but an idiopathic form affecting children and infants without dermatomyositis also exists. In dermatomyositis, calcinosis usually develops 2 to 3 years after the onset of the disease and often follows episodes of inflammation. The calcification may be progressive, leading to considerable disability, especially in children. Adequate control of the disease with prednisone or other immunosuppressive drugs reduces the risk of calcinosis. Limited studies with warfarin, colchicine, biphosphonates, and phosphate binders have not produced consistent results. Recently, the calcium channel blocker diltiazem has been successfully used in the treatment of calcinosis associated with juvenile dermatomyositis and scleroderma. Probenecid, which promotes phosphate excretion, has been reported in the past to be effective; a recent study showed dramatic improvement and resolution of calcinosis in a patient with juvenile dermatomyositis. These approaches should be seriously considered in the management of patients with dermatomyositis, particularly for those who are young and have progressive calcinosis.

ECTOPIC OSSIFICATION

Fibrodysplasia (myositis) ossificans progressiva is the most dramatic form of ectopic bone formation. It is a rare, autosomal dominant disorder with an estimated incidence of one per two million live births in Great Britain. It is characterized by congenital malformations of the great toes and progressive disabling heterotopic osteogenesis in predictable anatomic and temporal patterns. The presence of short, malformed great toes at birth can raise suspicion of the disease before the formation of heterotopic bone. Spontaneous, painful soft tissue swellings that are red and tender appear during the first decade of life and are associated with low-grade fever and elevated erythrocyte sedimentation rate. These lesions develop rapidly (within days) and can be induced by minor trauma or intramuscular injections, for example during immunization in childhood. Areas mainly affected include the paraspinal muscles of the back and the limb and shoulder girdles. Severe scoliosis and immobilization of the neck, shoulders, and joints gradually develop. The disease runs a variable course with periods of remissions and exacerbations, but most affected individuals become wheelchair-bound by the age of 30 years. Starvation may result from ankylosis of the jaw, and pneumonia may occur as a complication of fixation of the chest wall, which might, in addition, lead to respiratory failure and death. Radiographic appearance is that of soft tissue calcification. Biochemical parameters of mineral metabolism are usually normal. The etiology of the disease is unknown, but recent studies revealed increased levels of bone morphogenetic protein 4 and its encoding mRNA in lymphocytes of affected patients. Bone morphogenetic proteins belong to the transforming

growth factor beta (TGFβ) superfamily of peptides and are potent inducers of endochondral bone formation and fracture healing. It should be recognized, however, that further progress in elucidating the etiology of the disease will not be easy due to its rarity and due to the inability to obtain tissue for examination, other than blood, from affected individuals. There is no effective treatment for the disease. Attempts with various agents, including the bisphosphonate etidronate, have generally not been successful. Anecdotal experience suggests, however, that if etidronate is given at high doses (preferably intravenously), which are known to inhibit the mineralization of newly formed bone, very soon after the onset of the acute symptoms, it may alleviate the symptoms and restrict the development of the calcification. Surgical removal of ectopic bone is followed by recurrence, and intramuscular injections should be avoided.

Debilitating ossifications, particularly around joints, are a characteristic feature of certain patients with pseudo- and pseudo-pseudohypoparathyroidism (see Chap. 21).

"Myositis ossificans" is the term used to describe acquired heterotopic ossification associated with hip surgery, neurological disorders, burns, or trauma. Patients with spinal cord injuries and paraplegia frequently develop ectopic bone formation, most commonly adjacent to the hip joints outside the joint capsule. In susceptible individuals it occurs within months of the injury, and its etiology is unknown. It appears that its incidence is decreasing in recent years, possibly as a result of better overall management of these patients. Heterotopic ossification is also a well-recognized complication of total hip replacement. It starts within a few weeks after surgery and is completed after about 6 months. Although common, it causes symptoms such as pain and limitations in joint movements in a minority of patients. The cause is unknown. Over the years there have been several attempts to treat or prevent this complication, but results have been equivocal. Some studies have reported favorable results with the use of nonsteroid anti-inflammatory drugs (NSAIDs) such as indomethacin, and with warfarin or etidronate. The latter has also been given to patients with ectopic ossification resulting from spinal cord injury. In cases of repeat hip surgery following ectopic ossification, etidronate is recommended at a dose of 20 mg/kg orally 1 month before and 3 months after the operation. Results are not, however, predictable.

Heterotopic ossification in the spine also occurs in the absence of trauma as in diffuse idiopathic skeletal hyperostosis or Forestier's disease and in ankylosing spondylitis where it can be readily recognized radiologically.

Suggested readings

COHEN RB, HAHN GV, TABAS JA, et al. The natural history of heterotopic calcification in patients who have fibrodysplasia ossificans progressiva: a study of forty four patients. J Bone Joint Surg Am 1993;75:215-9.

EDDY MC, LEELAWATTANA R, MCALISTER WH, WHYTE MP. Calcinosis universalis complicating juvenile dermatomyositis: resolution during probenecid therapy. J Clin Endocrinol Metab 1997;82:3536-42.

FAWTHROP FW, RUSSELL RGG. Ectopic calcification and ossification. In: Nordin BEC, Need AG, Morris HA (eds). Metabolic bone and stone disease. 3rd ed. Edinburgh: Churchill Livingstone, 1993;325-38.

PACHMAN LM. Juvenile dermatomyositis: pathophysiology and disease expression. Pediatr Clin North Am 1995;42:1071-98.

SHAFRITZ AB, SHORE EM, GANNON FH, et al. Overexpression of an osteogenic morphogen in fibrodysplasia ossificans progressiva. New Engl J Med 1996;335:555-61.

THOMAS BJ. Heterotopic bone formation after total hip arthroplasty. Orthop Clin North Am 1992;23:347-58.

WHYTE MP. Extraskeletal (ectopic) calcification and ossification. In: Favus MJ, (ed). Primer on the metabolic bone diseases and disorders of mineral metabolism. 3rd ed. Philadelphia: Lippincott-Raven, 1996;422-30.

Osteoporosis

Elaine Dennison, Cyrus Cooper

███ **KEY POINTS** ██████████████████████

- Osteoporosis is a skeletal disorder characterized by low bone mass and micro-architectural deterioration of bone tissue, with consequent increases in bone fragility and fracture risk. Osteoporosis is now firmly established as one of the major disorders associated with aging.
- These fractures, usually of the hip, spine, and wrist, now constitute a growing public health problem.
- Guidelines for defining osteoporosis, which incorporate both low bone mineral density and fracture risk, have been provided by the World Health Organization.
- Measurement of bone mineral density is most commonly made by dual energy X-ray absorptiometry, although other techniques, including computed X-ray tomography and ultrasound, are currently being evaluated.
- Treatment strategies include a population-based or high-risk approach. Mass screening cannot be justified at this time.
- A number of effective drugs are now available, which act by either decreasing bone resorption or stimulating bone formation.

Osteoporosis is a skeletal disorder characterized by low bone mass and micro-architectural deterioration of bone tissue, with a consequent increase in bone fragility and susceptibility to fracture. It is a widespread condition and is often unrecognized in clinical practice, which may have devastating health consequences through its association with fragility fractures. An expert panel convened by the World Health Organization (WHO) has suggested that osteoporosis be defined as when bone mineral density measurements in women fall below more than 2.5 standard deviations (SD) below the young normal mean. This definition also incorporates fracture risk by classifying the subset of women with low bone density and a previous fracture as sufferers of severe or established osteoporosis. Population-based data from the United States suggests that while the majority of white women under 50 years of age have normal bone density, osteoporosis becomes increasingly prevalent with advancing age (Fig. 25.1). Because life expectancy is increasing, it is ensured that this is a health problem clinicians will increasingly encounter in their practice. By age 80 years, for example,

70% of women will have bone mass values below the 2.5 SD threshold. Sixty percent of this group will have experienced one or more fractures at the hip, spine, distal forearm, proximal humerus, or pelvis.

Epidemiology

Fractures of the hip, spine, and forearm are the clinical consequences of reduced bone density. Epidemiological studies from North America have estimated the lifetime risk of common fragility fractures to be 17.5% for hip fracture, 15.6% for clinically diagnosed vertebral fracture, and 16% for distal forearm fracture among white women aged 50 years. Corresponding risks among men are 6%, 5%, and 2.5%. Figures for a British population are given in Table 25.1. Although all three fractures are more common among women than men, the ratio describing incidence in the two sexes is not the same for all fracture types, and it varies considerably with age. Figure 25.2 shows age-specific incidence rates for hip, vertebral, and distal forearm

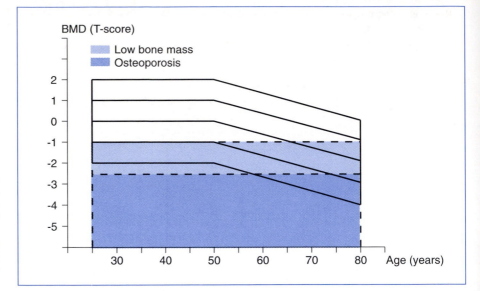

Figure 25.1 WHO classification of osteoporosis. Assessment of fracture risk and its application to screening for postmenopausal osteoporosis. (From Kanis JA, and the World Health Organisation Study Group. Osteoporosis International 1994;4:368-81.)

fractures in men and women, using data derived from the population of Rochester, Minnesota, USA. The sex difference in fracture rate is more pronounced in white populations, with Asian and black populations tending toward similar rates in men and women. This is commonly attributed to the differing relative contribution of bone strength and trauma to fracture risk at each site.

As the elderly proportion of the population increases, the fracture rate is predicted to rise, with projections in Europe of an 80% increase in fracture rate by the year 2025. Reported medical costs for initial stabilization of a hip fracture range from US$ 1900 in Portugal to US$ 9000 in Greece. Added to this must be the cost of institutional care for a large number of patients. Although it is primarily hip fracture that is associated with hospitalization and failure to return home, there are considerable costs associated with outpatient visits, nursing care, and days off work for all fracture types. In the United Kingdom (population 60 million), the annual cost to the healthcare system from osteoporotic fractures has been estimated at US$ 1200 million.

Fracture incidence is bimodal, with peaks in youth and in the very elderly. In young people, fractures of the long bones predominate, often following substantial trauma, and the incidence is greater in young men than in young women. Most fractures in the elderly, in contrast, are due to minor or moderate trauma. They usually occur in falls from the standing position, but they have been known to occur spontaneously, and they occur more frequently in the winter months in temperate countries. In addition, the majority occur during falls indoors rather than as a result of slipping on icy surfaces. One explanation that has been suggested to account for this observation is that neuromuscular function may be impaired at lower temperatures. Alternatively, bone density may suffer adversely from reduced vitamin D production in winter as a result of reduced sunlight exposure.

Vertebral fractures show a more linear pattern of increasing incidence with age among women than men,

Table 25.1 Lifetime risk of the common age-related fractures in British men and women aged 50 years

Lifetime risk of fracture	Men (%)	Women (%)
Hip	3	14
Vertebral (spine)[1]	2	11
Distal forearm (wrist)	2	13

[1] Data for clinically diagnosed vertebral deformities.

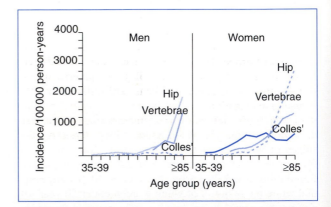

Figure 25.2 Incidence rates of hip, forearm (Colles') and clinically diagnosed spine fractures. Data derived from Rochester, USA. (From Cooper C, Melton LJ. Epidemiology of osteoporosis. Trends in Endocrinology and Metabolism 1992;3:224-9.)

and they are associated with excess mortality, possibly through coexisting frailty. It has been noted that among patients with clinically diagnosed vertebral deformity in Rochester, Minnesota, USA, observed mortality was greater than predicted over a 5-year period among both men and women. This contrasts with a finding of no excess mortality among women with vertebral deformity in whom no clinical intervention was required. More information is required to interpret these observations.

Accurate epidemiological data on vertebral fractures have been difficult to collect to date for two reasons. Firstly, efforts have been hampered by the lack of a universally recognized definition of vertebral deformity from lateral thoracolumbar X-rays, and secondly, by the fact that the majority of vertebral fractures are asymptomatic. The application of recently developed definitions to various population samples in the United States has permitted estimation of the incidence of new vertebral fractures in the general population. The incidence of all vertebral deformity has been estimated to be about three times that of hip fracture for post-menopausal white women. The age-adjusted female:male ratio for these deformities is 1.9, with only about one-third recognized clinically (Tab. 25.2). The most frequently affected levels are thoracic 8 to 12 and lumbar 1, the weakest regions in the spine. Trauma plays a far larger role in the etiology of male vertebral collapse, especially in younger patients.

To address this issue further, a multinational, cross-sectional population-based study (the European Vertebral Osteoporosis Study, or EVOS) was commenced in Europe in 1989; this aimed to evaluate the true prevalence of vertebral deformity in individuals 50 and older in different regions of Europe. While investigators found men to have higher deformity prevalence rates in the younger age groups, this pattern was reversed at about the age of 70 when an exponential increase in vertebral deformity was noted in women. It seems likely that vertebral deformity in middle-aged individuals is a consequence of high trauma or osteoarthritic change, while deformities occurring later in life are more clearly attributable to osteoporosis. Prevalence of vertebral deformity as described in the EVOS study is shown in Figure 25.3. Pronounced geographic differences also became apparent. The prevalence of vertebral deformities was higher in Scandinavian countries, where 20% of women and 16% of men had vertebral deformities, compared with 11% women and men in Eastern Europe. The reason for such dramatic differences are not apparent, but methodological factors, including sampling error and recall bias, are unlikely to be the whole explanation.

The epidemiology of wrist fracture seems distinct from its counterparts described above. Distal forearm fracture

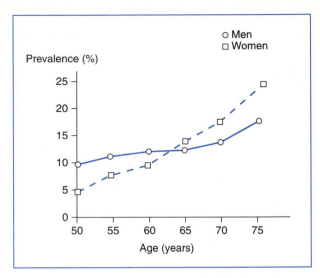

Figure 25.3 Prevalence of vertebral deformity with age. (From O'Neill TW, Felsenberg D, Varlow J, Cooper C, Kanis JA, Silman AJ. The prevalence of vertebral deformity in European men and women: the European Vertebral Osteoporosis Study. Journal of Bone and Mineral Research 1996;11:1010-28.)

almost always results as a consequence of a fall onto an outstretched hand. These fractures show a steep rise in incidence during the perimenopausal period among women, but a plateau thereafter. In men there is no apparent increase in incidence of wrist fracture with age. In white women, the incidence increases linearly between the ages of 40 and 65 and then stabilizes, while in men the incidence remains constant between 20 and 80 years. A much stronger sex ratio exists for this fracture than for most others, which has been estimated to be 4:1 in favor of women. A winter peak is again demonstrated, but this is probably due to falls outside on icy surfaces. The plateau with age in women may be due to the mode of falls; later in life a woman is more likely to fall onto a hip than an outstretched hand as her neuromuscular coordination deteriorates.

Hip fracture increases exponentially with age in both men and women. Although hip fractures occur 15 years later, on average, than spine and wrist fractures, they are associated not only with a greater risk of functional impairment and institutionalization, but also with a 20% mortality rate within the first year. Most deaths observed with hip fracture occur soon after the fracture. Excess mortality is particularly marked in men over 75, which may reflect co-morbidity, dementia and a range of attributes related to secondary osteoporosis. Overall, 90% of hip fractures occur among people aged 50 years and older, with 80% occurring in women. Quality of life in survivors may also be severely impaired; one year post-fracture, 40% of patients are unable to walk independently, 60% are unable to do at least one activity of daily living, and at least 80% are unable to do at least one independent activity of daily living, such as shopping or driving.

Table 25.2 Outcome of vertebral fracture	
Hospitalization	2-10%
Clinical attention	40%
Incident vertebral fractures	100%

Secular changes in hip fracture incidence are known to occur; in England and the Netherlands the age-adjusted incidence of hip fracture has increased 30% in the last 15 years. Possible explanations for this trend include decreasing bone quality through this century, an increasing tendency to fall through ill health as the elderly population becomes more frail, and increased height in recent generations. In the United Kingdom, hip axis length and femoral neck length increased significantly between the late 1950s and 1990, and studies have suggested that geometry at the hip may be an important fracture determinant. While bone mineral density consistently emerges as the most valuable predictor of osteoporotic fracture, tendency to fall is another important mechanism, which will be addressed later.

Pathophysiology of fracture

Bone mass

The two determinants of bone fracture rate are bone strength and trauma (Fig. 25.4). Bone density is an important determinant of bone strength, but many other qualities, including its micro-architecture and the relative proportion of non-mineralized osteoid, are also important. The extent to which these other factors may be measured noninvasively remains less clear.

At the cellular level, bone is a structure in a constantly dynamic state, capable of remodeling in response to stress or to repair a fracture. This is normally achieved through a coupled process of bone resorption and formation,

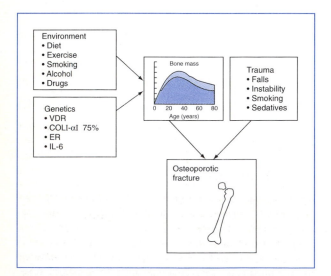

Figure 25.4 Pathogenesis of osteoporotic fracture: genes and environment. (COLI = collagen type I; ER = estrogen receptor; IL = interleukin; VDR - vitamin D receptor. (From Ralston SH. Pathophysiology of osteoporosis. In: Compston JE [ed]. Osteoporosis - New perspectives on causes, prevention and treatment. Royal College of Physicians of London, 1996.)

achieved by osteoclast and osteoblast lines, respectively; in a healthy adult the rate of bone resorption roughly approximates the rate of bone formation. Bone loss results from the disturbance in the equilibrium of bone remodeling. The bone matrix is normally replaced at an annual turnover rate of approximately 25% in cancellous bone and 2 to 3% in cortical bone. The remodeling process occurs in discrete pockets of bone separated both geographically and chronologically from each other. Activation of resorption depends on the retraction of lining cells, derived from osteoblasts, that normally cover all bone surfaces. Osteoclast precursors then settle on the revealed surface, where they fuse to form differentiated osteoclasts. It is not clear what initiates activation at any site, but one possibility is that changes in stress-generated potentials or local factors released from aging bone may be important. The resorptive phase of the cycle lasts about 10 to 14 days, and it is probably followed by apoptosis of the osteoclast. Once activation has occurred and the osteoclasts have resorbed a predetermined volume of bone, they are replaced by mononuclear cells. This is followed by osteoblast replication and differentiation in the resorption cavity, where osteoid is produced, and mineralization occurs after 25 to 35 days. A complete remodeling cycle takes several months. The entire group of cells involved in removing and replacing a packet of bone is called a bone remodeling unit. Disruption of this cycle, either reflecting accelerated bone breakdown or diminished bone formation, will lead to bone loss, the former of which is probably more important in osteoporosis. Alterations in bone remodeling determine the changes in cancellous microstructure associated with bone loss. High turnover states predispose to trabecular perforation and erosion, with consequent reduction in connectivity. This will have an adverse effect on bone strength and is probably irreversible. Conversely, the trabecular thinning associated with low turnover states is accompanied by better preservation of bone architecture and bone strength and is potentially reversible.

Peak bone mass

Bone mass in later life depends upon the peak attained at skeletal maturity and subsequent age-related bone loss. Both males and females increase bone mass in the prepubertal and pubertal years. Although the peak bone mass of men is greater than that of women, bone density is similar in both sexes for hip and spine. There appears to be some increase in bone density once linear growth is complete, but the determinants of this remain unclear. Twin studies suggest a strong genetic contribution to bone density, but environmental factors such as hormonal status, physical activity, and calcium intake are also important.

Much genetic research in recent years has concentrated on the identification of genes thought to regulate bone mineral density, either directly or indirectly through other factors, such as body build. The discovery of the vitamin D receptor gene was initially hailed as a breakthrough in the genetic field and has been extensively studied. What seems likely is that the vitamin D receptor genotype is modified by environmental factors. Geneticists have studied other candidate genes, in particular the collagen I-αI gene and the estrogen receptor gene. However, it is important to remember that other factors controlling the tendency to fall, including balance and vision, may be under partial genetic control and may also predict fracture risk.

It is currently unclear whether post-menopausal and age-related bone loss are under genetic control. Family history of fracture remains a risk factor after adjusting for bone mineral density, suggesting that genetic factors may be acting on other aspects of bone quality or structure. This concept is supported by ultrasound studies of twin pairs that suggest that broadband ultrasound attenuation and velocity of sound are both influenced by genetic factors, irrespective of bone mineral density.

The early environment is also a determinant of peak bone mass. Recent studies have demonstrated that growth in infancy is a determinant of adult bone mass. The mechanism underlying this association is believed to be the programming of a range of metabolic and endocrine systems. Programming is the term used for persisting changes in structure and function caused by environmental stimuli during critical periods of early development. In general, the earlier in life that undernutrition occurs, the more likely it is to have permanent effects on body build. There are several mechanisms whereby such adversity could compromise the skeleton. These include interactions of an adverse environment with gene expression, the programming of endocrine systems such as the growth hormone/insulin-like growth factor I axis, the hypothalamic-pituitary-adrenal axis or the parathyroid hormone/vitamin D axis, and finally the coupling between osteoblast and osteoclast activities.

Determinants of bone loss

In both sexes bone loss begins at the age of 35, but it varies in timing and magnitude at different skeletal sites. Superimposed on this age-related decline is an accelerated phase of loss during the estrogen-deficient years following menopause. Bone loss continues through later life and may be accelerated by a number of factors. The role of calcium in the retardation of bone loss has been the subject of much debate. Calcium absorption decreases with age in both sexes as a result of lower vitamin D intake and synthesis. Dietary intake of calcium may also be lower in older age groups, and these factors together may lead to secondary hyperparathyroidism. Calcium in elderly post-menopausal women retards loss, but it has not been shown to have the same beneficial effect in younger women. An inverse relationship between smoking and bone density is well-established and is due to multiple factors including an earlier menopause, reduced body weight, and enhanced metabolic breakdown of exogenous estrogens. Heavy alcohol consumption is associated with decreased bone density, but moderate consumption may be beneficial. Its deleterious effects are multifactorial, which include adverse effects on protein and calcium metabolism, mobility, gonadal function, and a direct toxic effect on osteoblasts. Weightbearing exercise has an important effect on bone density, and immobilized indi-

viduals lose bone rapidly. Mechanical loading and high body mass index appear to exert their effects through mediators such as nitric oxide and prostaglandins; high frequency, high impact exercise cycles appear to be most beneficial. Secondary causes of increased bone loss include hyperthyroidism, steroid therapy, and hypogonadism in men.

Biomechanical factors

A number of risk factors for hip fracture besides low bone mass have been identified, which are completely or partially modifiable. Sedative use, including short-acting sedatives, is a common risk factor; it has been estimated that approximately 10% of all hip fractures in the Netherlands could be attributed to the use of such drugs. Many elderly people have substantial impairments of visual function, which may also be important. Impaired depth perception (due to unilateral visual function) and declines in the ability to recognize contrast may be more important than impaired acuity. Another fracture determinant, muscle weakness, is also treatable; one study found that the ability to stand up from a chair without using one's hands was the best neuromuscular function predictor of hip fracture risk after adjusting for body mass and other risk factors. Exercise programs have been shown to improve physical strength and function in the elderly.

The pronounced differences in the incidence patterns of hip, spine, and forearm fractures are also most likely largely determined by the types of falls in the elderly. Epidemiological and biomechanical studies have suggested that subjects who directly injure their hip during a fall are at considerably increased risk of sustaining a hip fracture, while those who fall backward and land on an outstretched hand tend to sustain wrist fractures. The age-related decline in neuromuscular function, which reduces the ability to stretch out an arm while falling, thus explains the plateau in forearm fractures and accompanying rise in hip fractures among women aged 75 years and over. The geometry of the proximal femur has also been discussed as a further independent risk factor for fracture.

Clinical findings

Bone measurement

Measurements of bone mineral density are central to the diagnosis of osteoporosis, since the disorder is defined in terms of bone mass as described at the beginning of this chapter. Bone mineral is normally evenly distributed throughout the bones in the body. The aim of measurement is to predict individuals at the highest risk of fracture by virtue of their low bone density.

Currently available techniques for measuring bone mass include single and dual energy X-ray absorptiometry (DXA), computed X-ray tomography, and ultrasound. Some of the properties of these methods are summarized in Table 25.3.

Dual energy X-ray absorptiometry (DXA) Estimates of the accuracy error of dual energy X-ray absorptiometry range from 2 to 10% and are greatest at the lumbar spine, particularly from scanning at the lateral position. The precision of measurement is 1 to 2%; for this reason, repeat scans cannot be usefully performed to assess treatment response at intervals of less than 6 months. In addition, osteoarthritis, vascular calcification, and fractures confound anteroposterior measurements at the lumbar spine, making the interpretation of scans particularly difficult in the elderly, among whom these conditions are prevalent. Due to calibration differences, the development of commercial DXA systems by several manufacturers has highlighted difficulties in the direct comparison of measurements obtained on different instruments. The problem of discordance between ultrasound and DXA measurements is even greater. Dual energy X-ray absorptiometry has become established as the assessment method of choice in clinical practice for many reasons. It can measure bone mineral at clinically relevant sites (primarily the hip and spine), giving values that have been shown in numerous studies to be clinically relevant for fracture prediction. It is a precise technique, involving only a small amount of radiation exposure. It tends, however, to be relatively expensive and based in hospitals.

A number of approaches have been used to convey the information obtained from a DXA scan to a clinician and patient. The actual value obtained is g/cm^2 and cannot be interpreted in isolation. The results can be expressed as a Z score, representing a comparison of the subject's bone density to another of the same age, or alternatively as a T score, representing a comparison of bone density of others of the same age to that of 25 year old women. There are strengths and weaknesses to each of these approaches. However, the WHO classification relates to the T score,

that is, their definition of osteoporosis is a bone mineral measurement of more than 2.5 SD below the young normal mean. At the present time, this is the most widely used classification system.

Ultrasound Quantitative ultrasound measurement, which remains a research tool at the present time, provides two indices of skeletal status: broad-band ultrasound attenuation, and speed-of-sound or ultrasound velocity. These measurements are thought to give information on bone stiffness and micro-architecture in addition to bone mineral density. Ultrasound systems are portable, relatively inexpensive, involve no radiation dose, and are acceptable to the patient. Their main limitation, however, is the paucity of accuracy and clinical data available to support their use. Two prospective studies suggest that quantitative ultrasound may be as good as DXA in predicting hip fracture among very elderly (75+ years) subjects. However, precision error is high, results from different machines cannot be compared, and clinically relevant sites cannot yet be measured.

Quantitative computed tomography Quantitative computed tomography enables differential measurement of cortical and cancellous bone in the spine or peripheral skeleton, but the radiation dose is relatively high. In addition, this high precision technique is unfortunately not readily available in many centers. Unlike other techniques described, quantitative computed tomography measures volumetric bone density as g/cm^3. Dual energy X-ray absorptiometry, in contrast, makes a measurement of bone mineral content (g), which can be converted to an areal bone density by dividing bone mineral content by the area of bone in the forearm, spine, or hip. Areal bone density therefore reflects bone size as well as true bone density, and although this influence can be reduced by mathematical correction, it cannot be eliminated.

Table 25.3 Methods of bone mineral measurement

Technique	Site	Precision error (%)	Accuracy error (%)	Duration of examination (min)	Absorbed dose (Mrem)
Older techniques					
SPA	Proximal radius	2-3	5	15	10
DPA	Spine, hip, regional, total body	2-4	4-10	20-40	5
QCT	Spine	2-5	5-20	10-20	100-1000
Never developments					
SXA-R	Distal radius, calcaneus	1-2	5	10-20	5-10
DXA	Spine, hip, regional, total body	1-2	3-5	5	1-3
QCT-A	Spine, hip	1-2	5-10	10	100-300
Ultrasound	calcaneus	2-6	–	2-5	Nil

(SPA = single-photon absorptiometry; SQA-R = rectilinear SPA; DPA = dual-photon absorptiometry; DXA = DPA with a dual energy X-ray source; QCT = Quantitative computed tomography; QCT-A = QCT with advanced software and hardware capabilities.)

As more accurate technology has been developed and enabled us to measure bone density noninvasively, controversy has raged over who exactly should undergo measurement.

It has now been agreed that those individuals at high risk of osteoporosis, by virtue of fulfilling one or more of the criteria shown in Table 25.4, should be assessed, though the mass screening of post-menopausal women to target hormone replacement is not justifiable. In some groups, it may be appropriate to initiate osteoporosis treatment without bone mineral measurement, although the physician may find measurements useful for monitoring the efficacy of treatment. The clinical indications include women who have experienced premature menopause (where scanning may be useful in ensuring compliance with medication), women with multiple vertebral fractures (spine bone mineral density measurements may be inaccurate due to interference by osteoarthritis), and individuals on high-dose glucocorticoid therapy.

For clinicians treating men, diagnostic dilemmas exist: definitions of osteoporosis have been established for women only, forcing the use of the criteria originally defined for females. In general, a diagnosis of male osteoporosis is made if bone mineral density measurement gives a value of greater than 2.5 SD below the female age-matched mean.

The relationship between bone mineral density and fracture risk is similar to the relationship between hypertension and stroke; strong graded relationships exist between the risk factor and its clinical outcome, but the former is not an essential prerequisite for the latter. A recent meta-analysis yielded a relative risk of 2.6 for hip fracture, with each SD decrease in bone density at the hip below the age-adjusted mean. At the spine the relative risk for vertebral fracture was 2.3 for each SD decrease in

bone density at that site. Measurement of bone density at any site, however, gave a significantly increased relative risk of fracture for low bone mineral density. Although we are able to predict fracture risk with these tools, we are still unable to identify those individuals who will sustain a fracture.

Biochemical markers

Although biochemical markers may be used to monitor bone turnover, currently they are predominantly used as a research tool. Potential uses for the future include:
- prediction of bone loss/fracture/response to therapy;
- monitoring of therapy;
- monitoring of the effect of the disease/drug on bone;
- study of the pathogenesis of osteoporosis.

Markers may be divided principally into two groups: resorption markers and formation markers. Some of the principal biochemical markers are displayed in Table 25.5. While breakdown markers may change in approximately 20 days, formation markers require a 50-day interval before any significant change becomes apparent. Circulating levels of each of these markers can be influenced by factors other than bone turnover, including excretion from other tissues of origin, their metabolic clearance, and analytical aspects of the assay. Several studies using these markers have shown a sustained increase in bone turnover in late post-menopausal and elderly women, triggered by their menopause. In addition, prospective studies have shown an association of osteoporotic fractures with bone turnover, independent of bone mass. These studies suggest that a combined approach encompassing clinical risk factors, bone mass, and bone turnover may be useful, although the optimal combination according to age has not yet been defined. Treatment with antiresorptive drugs induces a rapid decrease of bone turnover markers, correlated with the long-term effect of such treatments on bone mass. This may be of particular clinical relevance, as bone marker measurement might be reasonably expected to produce the same information within 3 to 6 months that would otherwise be provided by a DXA scan over a year after initiating therapy. The precision of bone mass measurements, and the change in bone

---

Table 25.4 Clinical indications for bone densitometry

Presence of strong risk factors:

Premature menopause (<45 yr)
Prolonged secondary amenorrhea
Primary hypogonadism
Corticosteroid therapy (>7.5 mg/d for 1 year or more)
Anorexia nervosa
Malabsorption
Primary hyperparathyroidism
Organ transplantation
Chronic renal failure
Myelomatosis
Hyperthyroidism
Prolonged immobilization
Radiological evidence of osteopenia or vertebral
  deformity, or both
Previous fragility; fracture of the hip, spine, or wrist

Monitoring of therapy:

Hormone replacement therapy in patients with
  secondary osteoporosis
Newer drugs, e.g., bisphosphonates, calcitonin, vitamin
  D metabolites, sodium fluoride

Table 25.5 Biochemical markers

Markers of bone formation

Osteocalcin
Bone isoenzyme of alkaline phosphatase
Procollagen propeptides of type I collagen

Markers of bone resorption

Pyridinium cross-links (pyridinoline/deoxypyridinoline)
Hydroxyproline
Hydroxylysine glycosides
Tartrate-resistant acid phosphatase

density that might reasonably be expected, would preclude confidence in earlier bone density measurements. In the same way, repeated bone marker measurements are likely to improve the management of osteoporotic patients by detecting noncompliant patients and nonresponders. Of note, however, markers are of unequal specificity and sensitivity, suggesting that to attempt to draw some meaningful conclusion by deriving a value from the comparison of the increase of a formation and resorption marker may be unhelpful.

Treatment

Drugs used to treat osteoporosis may be grouped into those that decrease bone resorption and those that increase bone formation, as described in Table 25.6. The effect of each form of treatment on bone mineral density over time is illustrated in Figure 25.5.

Antiresorptive treatment

Antiresorptive drugs are most effective when bone turnover is increased, and their effect is greater on cancellous bone than cortical bone. The most commonly used drugs in this category are estrogen, calcium, the bisphosphonates, calcitonin and calcitriol.

Estrogen and related compounds Although menopause is a physiological event, the resulting estrogen deficiency is a significant factor in the pathophysiology of many diseases, notably cardiovascular disease and osteoporosis. Currently, hormone replacement therapy is the treatment of choice for preventing bone loss in post-menopausal women. It has been shown in case control and cohort studies to be associated with reduced fracture risk. There is no evidence that adding progesterone to the regimen reduces this protection. However, some issues remain unresolved. Firstly, there is evidence that if hormone replacement therapy is used only for the first 10 post-

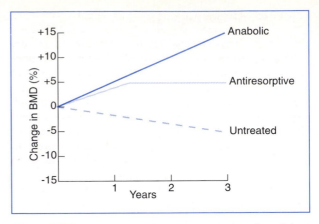

Figure 25.5 Characteristics changes in bone mineral density associated with anabolic and antiresorptive agents. (From Compston JE. Mechanisms of drug-induced effects on bone. In: Compston JE [ed]. Osteoporosis - New perspectives on causes, prevention and treatment. Royal College of Physicians of London, 1996.)

menopausal years, that its effects may not persist over the age of 75, and therefore would not protect against hip fracture. Efficacy of treatment appears to vary by site, providing more benefit at the spine than at the hip, and may decrease with time. Diminished compliance with age may also be an issue. Any decision on whether to prescribe hormone replacement therapy is unlikely to be made solely for the prevention of osteoporosis. Instead, it represents a balance of protection against coronary heart disease and osteoporosis, but with a possible excessive risk of breast cancer. Risk of endometrial cancer associated with estrogen use can be eliminated by the prescription of a combined estrogen/progesterone preparation, which will produce regular withdrawal bleeds. It has been estimated that about 20% of British women currently take hormone replacement therapy, possibly reflecting women's dislike of the recurrence of menses, and fears surrounding reports of increased cancer risk. Preparations marketed as rare/no bleed have recently become available, which may improve uptake, particularly in the elderly, and preparations are available in a variety of forms, including patches. There are few absolute contraindications to estrogen therapy, but they include active endometrial or breast cancer, pregnancy, undiagnosed abnormal vaginal bleeding, severe active liver disease, acute deepvein thrombosis and thromboembolic disease, and recent hormone-dependent cancers. Relative contraindications might include uncontrolled hypertension, previous pulmonary embolus, systemic lupus erythematosus, endometriosis, fibroids, previous breast cancer or a strong family history of the disorder. The debate on breast cancer risk remains controversial, with some studies suggesting a relative risk of up to 2 in users. It has been difficult to accurately estimate risk, as those women who use hormone replacement therapy may have their condition detected, and therefore treated earlier, with a consequent reduction in mortality.

There has been much recent interest in the use of other hormonal agents. Tibolone is a synthetic compound with

---

Table 25.6 Drugs used in the prevention and treatment of osteoporosis

Antiresorptive agents

Hormone replacement therapy
Selective estrogen receptor modulators
Bisphosphonates
Calcitonin
Calcium
Vitamin D
Anabolic steroids

Anabolic agents

Sodium fluoride
Parathyroid hormone peptides
?High-dose estrogens

combined estrogenic, prostagenic, and androgenic properties. It prevents post-menopausal bone loss and increases bone mineral density, but its long-term effects on bone loss and cardiovascular disease are unknown. Attention has also focused on the estrogen agonist/antagonists such as tamoxifen and raloxifene. The latter has been shown to prevent bone loss at axial and appendicular sites, while inhibiting the progression of estrogen-dependent breast tumors in animals and human studies. It has no action on uterine tissue, and as such makes it a potential candidate for treatment of osteoporosis. Such agonists/antagonists are now classified as selective estrogen receptor modulators (SERM), and they may be developed into alternatives to hormone replacement therapy in the future.

Bisphosphonates Bisphosphonate treatment acts as a potent antiresorptive agent by binding selectively to the hydroxyapatite crystals of bone and preventing the osteoclast from breaking it down. The drug is retained in the skeleton under osteoid for up to 10 years, although biologically inactive, which has lead to fears about its long-term safety. There have also been concerns that the drugs may lead to a decline in bone turnover, with consequent inability to repair microfractures. Over the past few years, a number of new bisphosphonates have become available for clinical testing, several of which have been used in treating osteoporosis. By preventing remodeling cycles, these drugs act to increase bone mass. The activity of these drugs on bone resorption varies greatly from one drug to another.

Etidronate was the first bisphosphonate to be used for the treatment of post-menopausal osteoporosis. In two important studies, etidronate was given in a dose of 400 mg daily for 2 weeks to women with established osteoporosis, followed by calcium with or without vitamin D for a further 3 months, upon which the cycle was repeated. These studies showed a gain in lumbar spine bone mineral density, which was maximal in the first year of treatment. Results for a double-blind, randomized, placebo-controlled trial of continuous bisphosphonate as pamidronate have also been shown, and display statistically significant increases in spine and femoral neck bone mass versus placebo, with reduced vertebral fracture rates in the treatment group.

Subsequent studies using continuous treatment with alendronate at a dose of 10 mg per day showed a similar pattern of response, with significant increases in both spine and femoral neck bone mineral density in the treated group, with the greatest increase seen in the first 6 months of treatment. The alendronate study showed a 48% reduction in the incidence of new fractures after 3 years of treatment, although to achieve sufficient statistical power, all of the treatment groups in the alendronate study (including the 5 mg daily dose group) were pooled. More recently, a large study randomizing 2,027 women with low femoral neck bone density and vertebral deformity to placebo or alendronate showed that alendronate reduced the risk of clinical vertebral fractures by 55%, and of hip fractures by 51%. This well-conducted study demonstrates for the first time efficacy of the bisphosphonates against hip fracture among women with vertebral fracture.

All bisphosphonates are poorly-absorbed from the gastrointestinal system, and wide variations in how much drug each individual patient absorbs may exist. Studies are therefore underway to see if intermittent intravenous pulses of bisphosphonate may have a role.

Side effects of these drugs include reports of esophageal ulceration in those individuals taking alendronate. Correct schooling of patients in how to take their medication is therefore very important.

Calcium Calcium is required for bone mineralization and also functions as an antiresorptive agent by raising circulating ionized calcium concentration and suppressing the parathyroid hormone level. Calcium is an important determinant of peak bone mass. Dietary requirements increase during puberty, when up to 400 mg of calcium enters the skeleton each day. It has been suggested that up to 1600 mg calcium daily may be required by adolescents to achieve an optimal peak bone mass: considerably higher than current intakes for British and American teenagers. Different guidelines exist for calcium intake around the world, reaching a 1000 mg per day recommendation for American perimenopausal women on estrogen, to 1500 mg per day for their postmenopausal counterparts not taking estrogen. Ecological studies have proved to be confusing on this subject, with the highest fracture rates observed in countries with the highest calcium intake, although this cannot be translated into recommendations for an individual.

The role of calcium intake in the pathogenesis of age-related bone loss remains controversial. Four randomized, placebo-controlled studies in recent years have supported the proposal that supplemental calcium reduces bone loss in adult women. These studies have used varying calcium supplements from 800 mg to 1700 mg per day in women who were late postmenopausal or elderly. Although these studies have suggested that this diminished bone loss may be translated into reduced fracture rate, they have not been large enough to confirm this convincingly for calcium alone. Previous studies have shown an apparent reduction in vertebral fractures in women with osteoporosis treated with calcium, but these studies were not randomized. Studies to date have focused on women, and limited data are available in men.

Vitamin D Vitamin D treatment has also been used in trials in combination with calcium. Vitamin D insufficiency is increasingly recognized as a cause of secondary hyperparathyroidism, increased bone turnover, and bone loss in the elderly. The elderly are particularly vulnerable to vitamin D deficiency because skin production of the vitamin declines with aging, they spend less time outside in sunlight, and they may have reduced vitamin D absorption efficiency. Vitamin D supplements have been shown to reduce femoral neck bone loss in both free-living and institutionalized elderly individuals. However, studies that have attempted to translate this into fracture risk have proved to be more confusing. A Dutch study showed no reduction in fracture incidence with vitamin D supplementation when the intervention group included free-living men and women, while a French study demonstrated lower fracture rates in elderly nursing home residents who received a higher dose of vitamin D supplementation in combination with calcium. Raised serum levels of parathyroid hormone highlight reduced serum 25(OH)D in free-living women in comparison to the others. Therefore, while caution needs to be exercised in extrapolating these results to the more mobile elderly, in whom winter vitamin D levels may be expected to be higher, there may be a place for vitamin D/calcium supplementation in the institutionalized elderly. Further debate has focused on the best way to administer this treatment, with the suggestion that only annual injection of vitamin D may be cost-effective. Intestinal absorption of calcium is known to decline with age, as does renal function, reducing the capacity to hydroxylate 25-hydroxyvitamin D to $1,25(OH)_2D$.

Active metabolites of vitamin D Calcitriol, as the active metabolite of vitamin D, diminishes with aging. These reduced levels relate to decreased intestinal calcium absorption. It has been shown that in postmenopausal osteoporosis, malabsorption of calcium occurs, and it can be normalized by calcitriol administration. A number of small studies have suggested that treatment with this agent can improve bone mineral density, but there has been only one large study that suggested that calcitriol was able to reduce the incidence of vertebral fractures, and possibly, but not conclusively, peripheral fractures. Its main use at the present time appears to be in the treatment of glucocorticoid-related osteoporosis. Its main side-effect is the risk of hypercalcemia, for which monitoring is required.

Calcitonin Calcitonin is a peptide hormone synthesized and secreted by the C cells of the thyroid. Calcitonin suppresses bone resorption by inhibiting the recruitment and activity of osteoclasts. Studies attempting to elucidate this drug's contribution to management of osteoporosis have given varying results, possibly because of the uncertainty about the optimum dosage for treatment. However, intranasal calcitonin has been shown to preserve bone density in postmenopausal women with osteoporosis and to reduce the incidence of osteoporotic fractures. Use of this drug has been hampered in clinical practice by practical difficulties of administration, usually as salmon calcitonin by injection or intranasal spray, and by its expense. It has, however, found a role in controlling the acute pain of vertebral fractures by virtue of its analgesic properties.

Formation-stimulating drugs

In contrast to the large number of antiresorptive agents that induce a small increase in bone mass (typically less than 10%), bone-forming agents are fewer and their role in clinical practice less fully evaluated. The main agents that have been used or tested so far are fluoride salts, parathyroid hormone, peptide growth factors, and strontium.

Fluoride Fluoride salts are the only agents clinically available. These drugs act to either increase the activation of new bone remodeling units or to increase the activity of individual osteoblasts. Recent controlled trials have not settled uncertainties about the effectiveness of fluoride therapy in decreasing vertebral fracture rate in established osteoporosis. While it is uncontested that fluoride treatment has a potent anabolic effect on bone, concerns persist about the quality of the newly synthesized bone. Fluoride has anabolic effects on the skeleton by causing osteoblast proliferation and stimulating new bone formation. Excessive exposure leads to a condition called fluorosis characterized by abnormal, poorly mineralized bone. Treatment may increase bone mass without reducing the fracture rate. Two large randomized trials of fluoride using a dose of 75 mg per day in the United States showed an increase of 8% annually in lumbar spine bone density in women with established osteoporosis, but radial bone was lost at a rate of 2% per year. The treatment did not reduce fracture risk. A European study evaluating the effect of a lower dose of fluoride in combination with calcium and vitamin D found that the addition of fluoride to the regimen was no more effective for the reduction of vertebral fractures. However, other studies have suggested a reduction in fracture rate takes place for women with established vertebral osteoporosis taking fluoride at a dose of 50 mg per day or less. No controlled trials have shown a decrease in the incidence of non-vertebral fractures in the treated group.

Other agents Currently there are other bone-forming agents used in research only. There has been interest in parathyroid hormone and parathyroid peptides, while strontium has provoked interest due to its ability to increase bone mass and markers of bone turnover in postmenopausal osteoporotic women. Anabolic steroids, used occasionally in the elderly to improve muscle mass as well as bone mass, act primarily to decrease bone turnover rather than to increase bone formation. The therapeutically most promising agents is probably parathyroid hormone.

Prevention

As a considerable amount of bone may have been lost by the time a fracture occurs, the prevention of bone loss is likely to be a more effective strategy for reducing fracture incidence than treating established disease. There are two general strategies that may be employed to achieve this: the population approach and the high-risk approach. A population-based strategy is aimed at increasing the peak bone mass of the entire population in a positive direction. Such measures would involve alterations in lifestyle such as improving nutrition (possibly including calcium supplementation), reducing cigarette and alcohol consumption, and participating in high-impact weight bearing exercise; beneficial not only for the small increase in bone mineral density it affords, but also for the improvement in coordination it produces. Substantial differences exist in the fracture rates between populations, which are not fully explained by variation in bone density. Environmental factors related to bone strength and the risk of falling have therefore been implicated to partially explain this, and it is hoped that addressing these issues may provide another public health measure to reduce the scale of the problem in the future.

In the elderly, avoidance of falls is a particularly important issue. It has been demonstrated that in this group, the more risk factors that exist for falling, the greater the risk of hip fractures, regardless of bone mass. Simple measures in the home to reduce the risk of falling should include removing loosefitting rugs and ensuring adequate lighting, and medication should be reviewed where appropriate. In individuals who still remain at risk of falling, physiotherapy to improve balance and demonstrate "safe" ways to fall have a role. In addition, studies of hip protectors in the elderly (which cover the greater trochanter and disperse the energy of a fall) have shown a reduction in fracture risk. Unfortunately, while extremely effective, poor compliance due to the discomfort and inconvenience of wearing these appears to preclude widespread use at present.

In contrast to a population-based approach, a high-risk strategy would target those individuals found to be at high fracture risk during a screening measure, most commonly by DXA. It is, however, now commonly accepted that a mass screening program would not be an effective means of reducing fracture incidence in the general population. The clinical indications for bone densitometry delineated above remain the guidelines for clinical use of this technology. Although we are currently able to predict the fracture risk from bone mineral density measurements, there have been no studies to prove that this information is translated into reduced fracture risk as a result of enhanced compliance with efficacious treatments such as hormone replacement therapy.

SPECIAL FORMS

Glucocorticoid-induced osteoporosis

Osteoporotic fracture is now well-recognized as a complication of long-term steroid therapy. Fractures are commonly seen at sites of high trabecular bone content, and it has been suggested that the threshold for fracture is higher in steroid-treated individuals, with therapeutic implications. Glucocorticoid-induced bone loss affects both cortical and trabecular bone, with the most rapid bone loss in the first 6 months of therapy. This represents a period of increased bone loss and rapid turnover, followed by a slower phase representing reduced bone formation with relatively normal bone turnover. The relationship between dose and duration of glucocorticoid therapy and bone loss

is uncertain. Some studies have demonstrated a correlation between cumulative dose and bone loss, but the confounding effects of disease activity and other drugs have made many studies difficult to interpret.

Glucocorticoids exert their effects on bone at a number of levels. In vivo, they promote negative calcium balance by reducing intestinal calcium absorption and also by reducing renal tubular reabsorption. This may provoke hyperparathyroidism and increased bone loss. In vitro, glucocorticoids have a direct effect on osteoblast function that results in decreased bone formation, and they also have an indirect effect on osteoclasts that results in increased resorption.

Guidelines for the management of patients on maintenance steroid therapy differ in different countries, but in the United Kingdom, lifestyle advice would be given to everyone, and bone mineral density would be measured if treatment continued for longer than 6 months. Hormone replacement therapy would be recommended if this revealed a result more than 1 SD below the age-matched mean, or if prednisolone was given at a dosage greater than 15 mg per day. Alternatively, deflazocort could be substituted for prednisolone. Bisphosphonates, calcitriol, and testosterone replacement in men are also commonly used therapies.

Male osteoporosis

Men have greater bone mass than women, due primarily to their larger bones rather than to an increased bone density. They also experience less age-related endocortical bone resorption and more periosteal bone formation than women, all contributing to greater bone mass in later life. Testosterone, probably through the peripheral conversion to estrogen, is an important determinant of the attainment of adult bone mass and the prevention of bone resorption, and falling hormone levels with age may partially explain the reduction in bone mass in later life. There has also been some evidence that men who suffer osteoporotic fractures have smaller bones than their gender-matched controls.

In contrast to women, in whom a cause for osteoporosis can only rarely be found, up to 50% of male osteoporotics have a readily identifiable etiological factor. Well-known causes include hypogonadism and hypercortisolism, either endogenous such as Cushing's disease, or due to glucocorticoid therapy. There appears to be an important contribution from alcoholism, often in combination with excess tobacco use and lack of exercise.

Currently, however, decisions to treat men are still largely determined by trial results in women, both in terms of the cut-off criteria for osteoporosis definition, and in the evaluation of therapeutic options. One additional treatment often used in clinical practice, however, is anabolic steroid therapy, including Deca-Durabolin and testosterone, along with the monitoring of prostate function and serum lipids.

Suggested readings

BLACK DM, CUMMINGS SR, KARPF DB, et al. Randomised trial of effect of alendronate on risk of fracture in women with existing vertebral fractures. Fracture Intervention Trial Research Group. Lancet 1996;348:1535-41.

COOPER C, FALL C, EGGER P, HOBBS R, EASTELL R, BARKER D. Growth in infancy and bone mass in later life. Annals Rheum Diseases 1997; 56:17-21.

DAWSON-HUGHES B. Calcium, vitamin D and vitamin D metabolites. In: Papapoulos SE, Lips P, Pols HAP, Johnston CC, Delmas PD (eds.). Osteoporosis. Amsterdam: Elsevier Science B.V., 1996.

HARRIS ST, WATTS NB, JACKSON RD, et al. Four-year study of intermittent cyclic etidronate treatment of postmenopausal osteoporosis: three years of blinded therapy followed by one year of open therapy. Am J Med 1993;95:557-67.

KANIS J.A. Assessment of fracture risk and its application to screening for postmenopausal osteoporosis: synopsis of a WHO Report. Osteoporosis Int 1994;4:368-81.

LIBERMAN UA, WEISS SR, BROLL J, et al. Effect of oral alendronate on bone mineral density and the incidence of fractures in postmenopausal osteoporosis. The Alendronate Phase III Osteoporosis Treatment Study Group. N Engl J Med 1995;333:1437-43.

MARSHALL D, JOHNELL O, WEDEL H. Metaanalysis of how well measures of bone mineral density predict occurrence of osteoporotic fractures. BMJ 1996;312:1254-9.

REID IR, WATTIE DJ, EVANS MC, GAMBLE GD, STAPLETON JP, CORNISH J. Continuous therapy with pamidronate, a potent bisphosphonate, in postmenopausal osteoporosis. J Clin Endocrinol Metab 1994;79:1595-9.

RIGGS BL, HODGSON SF, O'FALLON WM, et al. Effect of fluoride treatment on the fracture rate in postmenopausal women with osteoporosis. N Engl J Med 1990;322:802-9.

TERMINE JD. Selective estrogen receptor modulators (SERMS) as an alternative to estrogen replacement therapy. Bone 1997; 20:122S.

TILYARD MW, SPEARS GFS, THOMPSON J, DOVEY S. Treatment of postmenopausal osteoporosis with calcitriol or calcium. N Engl J Med 1992;326:357-62.

The adrenal glands

26

The adrenal cortex: basic concepts and diagnostic procedures

André Lacroix, Annie Clavier

Embryology

The adrenal cortex originates from mesenchymal cells attached to the coelomic cavity, which is adjacent to the urogenital ridge. The cortex is invaded during the second month of its development by neuroectodermal cells, which will form the distinct inner adrenal catecholamine-producing medulla. The adrenal becomes larger than the kidney by midgestation, primarily because of the inner cortical fetal zone that occupies most of the adrenal mass. The outer "definitive" zone occupies only one-fourth of the cortex at birth, and it includes the zonae glomerulosa and fasciculata; the fetal zone disappears by one year of age and is replaced by the zona reticularis.

Adrenal anatomy

Each adrenal gland is roughly pyramidal in structure, 2 to 3 cm wide, 4 to 6 cm long, and 1 cm thick, weighing 4 to 6 g (Fig. 26.1). The adrenal medulla, which is mostly concentrated at the upper caudal pole, represents approximately 10% of the adrenal weight. Each gland is surrounded by loose connective tissue, by a fibrous capsule, and by perirenal fat. Both glands lie in the upper retroperitoneum on either side of the spine and consist of medial and lateral limbs that diverge inferiorly. The right gland is located below the liver at the upper pole of the right kidney, where its medial and lateral limbs form a configuration of an inverted V. The medial limb is lateral and parallel to the right crus of the diaphragm, which can serve as a reference to assess the normal width of the gland. The lateral limb is lower, more horizontal, and lies parallel to the posterior aspect of the inferior vena cava. The right adrenal vein is, thus, very short, as it drains directly into the closely located inferior vena cava. The left adrenal gland is lower than the right one, and it lies medial to the upper pole of the left kidney. The shorter medial and lateral limbs form a thicker confluence creating an arrowhead configuration. The left adrenal vein is longer than the right and drains into the left renal vein. The arterial supply to both glands is symmetrical with numerous (10-12) small

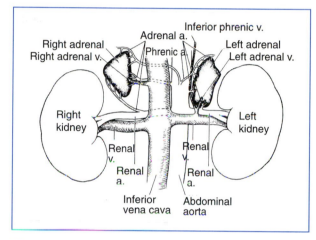

Figure 26.1 Anatomy of the adrenal glands. (From Miller WL, Tyrrell JB. The adrenal cortex. In: Felig P, Baxter JD, Frohman LA [eds.]. Endocrinology and metabolism. 3rd ed. New York: McGraw-Hill, 1995;557.)

arteries identified as the inferior group arising from the renal arteries, the medial group arising from the aorta, and the upper pole group arising from the inferior phrenic arteries. The small arteries branch out to form a dense subcapsular plexus, draining into the rich radial capillaries and sinusoidal plexus of the cortex. The venous drainage traverses the medulla to drain into the central vein. Some arterial medullary branches penetrate directly through the cortex to provide the arterial supply to the medullary sinusoids, bathing the chromaffin cells prior to draining into the same central adrenal vein. Efferent sympathetic and parasympathetic axons penetrate the cortex to reach the adrenal medulla; however, sympathetic axons also contribute to regulate cortical arteriolar blood flow. In addition, axons containing catecholamines and other neurotransmitters such as neuropeptide Y and others innervate glomerulosa cells, and they modulate cell growth and function. Similarly, axons originating from the adrenal medulla and containing neuromediators such as vasoactive intestinal polypeptide, atrial natriuretic peptides are also present in close proximity to glomerulosa cells.

Adrenocortical histology

The adrenal cortex is composed of three concentric zones (Fig. 26.2, see Color Atlas) with distinct steroid biosynthetic capacities. The outer zona glomerulosa lies just under the adrenal capsule and constitutes approximately 15% of the width of the cortex; its poorly demarcated nests of cells are responsible for the biosynthesis of mineralocorticoids and aldosterone. The fasciculata zone constitutes approximately 75% of the cortex, composed of radial cords of clear cells due to their rich lipid droplet content. The innermost zona reticularis is dense and composed of irregular, lipid-poor cords of cells, making up 10% of the cortex. The latter two zones are responsible for the synthesis of cortisol and adrenal androgens. Dehydroepiandrosterone (DHEA) is sulfated mostly in the zona reticularis. Recent studies indicate the presence of numerous prolongations of adrenal medullary cells into the adrenal cortex, suggesting a role of modulation of adrenal cortical function by neurotransmitters and peptides synthesized by the adrenal medullary neurons.

Steroid biosynthesis

Sources of cholesterol for adrenal steroidogenesis

Steroidogenesis results from specific sequential enzymatic conversions of cholesterol substrate into steroid hormones, which exert a wide variety of biological activities (Tab. 26.1). Approximately 80% of adrenal cholesterol sources are provided by circulating low density lipoprotein (LDL). The adrenal cells can also synthesize cholesterol de novo from acetyl coenzyme A.

Cholesterol side chain cleavage by CYP11A1

A series of steroidogenic enzymes are compartmentalized either in the mitochondria or in the endoplasmic reticulum. Several of these enzymes belong to the superfamily of mixed function oxidase genes known as cytochrome P450. Free cholesterol must be transported to the inner mitochondrial membrane by interacting with several proteins, including a sterol carrier protein and a steroidogenesis activator protein (SGAR). The first rate-limiting step in steroidogenesis involves the removal of six carbons from the lateral chain of cholesterol by the integral inner mitochondrial membrane P450 side chain cleavage (CYP11A1) enzyme to generate pregnenolone (Fig 26.3).

The activities of 3β-HSD II: progesterone and 17-hydroxyprogesterone synthesis

The newly synthesized pregnenolone is returned to the cytosol, where a series of microsomal enzymes convert it sequentially to 11-deoxycortisol and deoxycorticosterone.

Table 26.1 Nomenclature for steroidogenic enzymes now utilized

Trivial name	Past	Current
Cholesterol side-chain cleavage enzyme; desmolase	P450scc	CYP11A1
3β-Hydroxysteroid dehydrogenase	3β-HSD	3β-HSD II
17α-Hydroxylase/17,20-lyase	P450c17	CYP17
21-Hydroxylase	P450c21	CYP21A2
11β-Hydroxylase	P450c11	CYP11B1
Aldosterone synthase; corticosterone 18-methylcorticosterone oxidase/lyase	P450C11AS	CYP11B2

The adrenal and gonadal type II 3β-hydroxysteroid dehydrogenase (3β-HSD II) (a non-P450 enzyme bound to the endoplasmic reticulum) catalyzes the conversion of Δ^5-3β-hydroxysteroids such as pregnenolone or 17-hydroxypregnenolone to their Δ^4-3-ketosteroids such as progesterone and 17-hydroxyprogesterone. The low activity of 3β-HSD II in the fetal gland explains the high production of adrenal androgens such as DHEA, a Δ^5-3β-hydroxysteroid, compared to the low production of cortisol, a Δ^4-3-ketosteroid in the fetal adrenal.

The activities of CYP17: 17α-hydroxylase and 17,20-lyase activities

The hydroxylation of pregnenolone or of progesterone at their carbon-17 is essential for the glucocorticoid pathway. This enzyme is absent in the zona glomerulosa cells where pregnenolone and progesterone are precursors to the formation of mineralocorticoids, which lack a hydroxyl group in position C-17. The CYP17 can also remove the two-carbon side chain at the C-17 to generate dehydroepiandrosterone from 17-hydroxypregnenolone, or androstenedione from 17-hydroxyprogesterone.

The activities of CYP21A2: synthesis of 11-deoxycortisol and deoxycorticosterone

This single enzyme (CYP21A2) is responsible for the conversion of progesterone to deoxycorticosterone in the zona glomerulosa, and of 17-hydroxyprogesterone to 11-deoxycortisol (compound S) in the zona fasciculata. Its deficiency results in the most common of the congenital adrenal hyperplasias, with deficiencies of glucocorticoid and mineralocorticoid synthesis leading to increased adrenocorticotropic hormone (ACTH) and adrenal androgen production, and to salt-wasting.

The conversion of 11-deoxycortisol to cortisol by CY11B1

CY11B1 is located in the inner mitochondrial membrane. It is responsible for the last step in cortisol biosynthesis in which 11-deoxycortisol is hydroxylated in position C-11 to form cortisol in fasciculata cells.

Aldosterone biosynthesis

The CYP11B2 (also known as aldosyntase) is expressed only in glomerulosa cells and is located in the inner mitochondrial membrane. It is capable of catalyzing the last three steps of aldosterone synthesis, namely the 11β-hydroxylation of deoxycorticosterone to corticosterone, the 18-hydroxylation of corticosterone, and the 18-methyl oxidation of 18-hydroxycorticosterone to aldosterone.

Adrenal androgen synthesis

Androgens secreted by the adrenal cortex are mainly DHEA and its sulfate, dehydroepiandrosterone sulfate (DHEAS); in fact, they constitute the most abundant steroids secreted by the adrenals. They are produced from 17-hydroxypregnenolone via the 17,20-lyase activity of CYP17. Most of the DHEA and DHEAS serve as precursors for more potent androgens and estrogens, to which they are converted in peripheral tissues. However, a small proportion is converted in the adrenal to androstenedione by the action of 3β-hydroxysteroid dehydrogenase.

Regulation of aldosterone secretion

See Chapter 34.

Regulation of glucocorticoid secretion

The secretion of cortisol is regulated by several levels of signals and interactions between the brain, the hypothalamus, the pituitary, and the adrenal glands (Fig. 26.4).

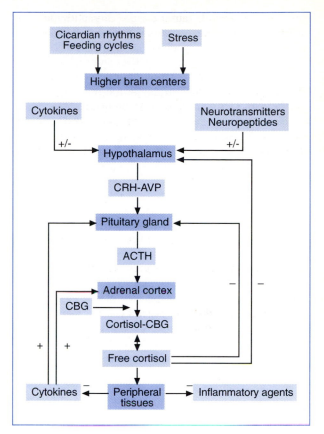

Figure 26.4 Regulation of the hypothalamic-pituitary-adrenal axis. (CRH = corticotropin-releasing hormone; ACTH = adrenocorticotropic hormone; CBG = corticosteroid-binding globulin.)

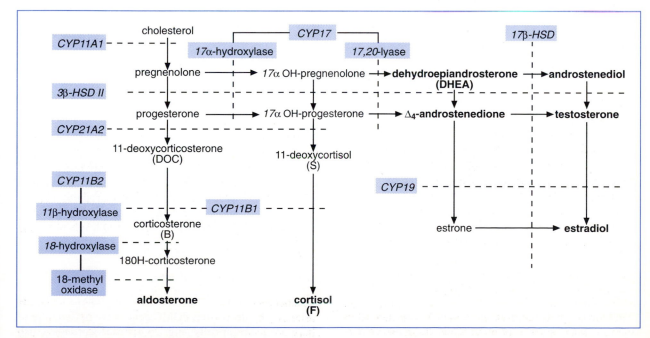

Figure 26.3 Main steroid biosynthetic pathways.

Under various stimuli such as stress, diurnal rhythms, or feeding cycles, brain neurotransmitters and neuropeptides induce the release of hypothalamic hormones, mainly corticotropin-releasing hormone (CRH) and arginine vasopressin. CRH and AVP reach the pituitary via the portal blood flow, where they stimulate the release of corticotropin (ACTH) into the general circulation. A negative feedback loop is exerted by the inhibitory effect of cortisol on the synthesis and secretion of CRH, and arginine vasopressin at the hypothalamic level, and of ACTH at the pituitary level.

Pulsatile secretion and diurnal rhythm

ACTH is secreted in brief pulsatile episodes followed by rapid, concomitant rises in plasma cortisol levels. A slower decline of cortisol results from its longer plasma half-life of approximately 80 minutes. The diurnal rhythm results from an increased amplitude (but not frequency) of ACTH pulses that start in the second half of the night around 2 to 4 a.m. Plasma cortisol concentration reaches its maximum a few hours before and lasts 1 hour after awakening. Plasma cortisol then declines progressively during the day to reach its nadir in late evening. However, additional peaks of ACTH and cortisol follow meals at lunch and sometimes at dinner, and they are dependent on the stimulation of the axis primarily by the protein content of the meal.

Regulation of cortisol secretion by stress

Acute physical or psychological stress stimulates the hypothalamic release of ACTH secretagogues such as CRH and arginine vasopressin. Surgery is one of the most potent stimuli of the hypothalamic-pituitary-adrenal axis, which is also stimulated by severe trauma, burns, illnesses, fever, hypotension, exercise, hypoglycemia, cold exposure, and smoking. Hypoglycemia stimulates the medial-basal hypothalamus, releasing CRH and arginine vasopressin, but it exerts no direct effect at the pituitary corticotrope cell level. In surgical stress, the afferent nerve impulses from the surgical incision are necessary to activate the axis. Pretreatment with glucocorticoids can inhibit the response of the axis in minor stress, but not totally in severe stress. Cytokines such as interleukins 1 and 6, and tumor necrosis factor, which are all released during infection, also stimulate the axis at the hypothalamic or pituitary levels.

Corticotropin-releasing hormone

Corticotropin-releasing hormone (CRH) is a 41-aminoacid peptide synthesized by neurons in the paraventricular hypothalamic nucleus, which project their axons to the median eminence to secrete their products in the portal blood flow. These neurons may also synthesize other ACTH secretagogues, such as arginine vasopressin. CRH binds to its specific cell surface receptor, which is coupled

to adenylate cyclase to generate cAMP, which activates protein kinase A. This results in the stimulation of transcription, increased mRNA levels of pro-opiomelanocortin (POMC), the polypeptide precursor of ACTH, and increased maturation and secretion of ACTH. Chronic CRH stimulation will induce corticotrope cell hyperplasia.

POMC and ACTH

Pro-opiomelanocortin is a 241-amino acid polypeptide precursor protein capable of being matured into several hormones and peptides, including lipotropins, melanocyte-stimulating hormones, β-endorphins, in addition to ACTH. POMC is processed by specific prohormone convertases in the different tissues where it is expressed, such that the cleavage products are tissue-specific.

The main product of POMC processing in anterior pituitary corticotrope cells is ACTH. ACTH is a 39-amino acid peptide capable of stimulating secretion of glucocorticoids, androgenic steroids, and to a lesser extent of mineralocorticoids from the adrenal cortex. In addition, in humans, where very little maturation of melanocyte-stimulating hormones is present, ACTH itself stimulates melanin synthesis in skin melanocytes. The first 18 amino-terminal amino acids maintain all of its biological activity. Synthetic ACTH (1-24) is the form most commonly used for clinical purposes. Intermediate lobe-type peptides such as α-melanocyte-stimulating hormone, β-endorphin, and γ-lipotropin can be produced in ACTH-producing nonpituitary tumors.

ACTH acts by binding to its specific cell surface receptor (Fig. 26.5), which is coupled to $G_{s\alpha}$ and to adenylate cyclase. ACTH binding increases cAMP levels intracellularly, which activates a cAMP-dependent protein kinase (protein kinase A) and phosphorylation of several proteins implicated in its biological activities. The acute effects of ACTH are exerted within minutes, mainly by activating existing CYP11A1 to convert cholesterol to pregnenolone. The still incompletely understood mechanisms appear to necessitate the function of the recently characterized steroidogenic acute regulatory protein (StAR) and its transcription factors, including steroidogenic factor 1 (SF-1).

The chronic effects of ACTH involve increases in gene transcription of most of the steroidogenic enzymes, which include CYP11A1, CYP17, CYP21A2, and CY11B1. ACTH also increases the synthesis of other key proteins for steroidogenesis such as LDL receptors, adrenodoxin, and many other growth factors and their receptors to maintain adrenal size and function. In the chronic absence of ACTH, the adrenal cortex becomes atrophic; this can be reverted to normal function and size by administering exogenous ACTH or by restoring normal levels of ACTH over a prolonged period.

Glucocorticoid negative feedback

Glucocorticoids inhibit the release and synthesis of ACTH primarily by decreasing POMC gene transcription in pituitary corticotroph cells (Fig. 26.4). Glucocorticoids also block the stimulatory effect of CRH on ACTH synthesis

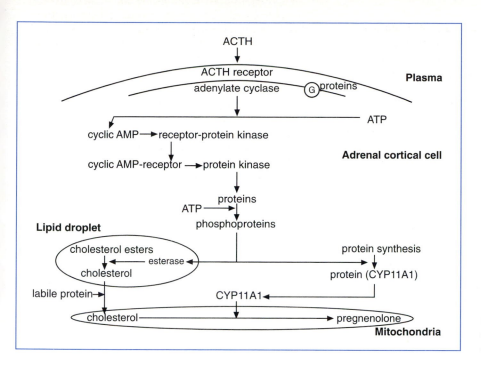

Figure 26.5 Simplified mode of action of ACTH on the adrenal cortical cell.

and release by the pituitary. In addition, glucocorticoids inhibit the production and secretion of CRH and vasopressin in the hypothalamic paraventricular nuclei. This regulation of ACTH by glucocorticoids is responsible for the decreased or undetectable levels of ACTH in individuals receiving supraphysiological doses of glucocorticoids or in those with excess cortisol production from an adrenocortical tumor (Cushing's syndrome). The importance of the suppression of the CRH-ACTH-adrenal axis depends upon the intensity and duration of steroid overexposure. After withdrawal of excess glucocorticoid exposure, a progressive recuperation of the CRH, followed by ACTH, and then of the adrenal cortex size and function will require several weeks or up to 12 to 18 months, depending on the intensity of the previous suppression. Conversely, ACTH levels will be elevated in patients where cortisol production is decreased, such as in Addison's disease.

Steroids in circulation and cortisol metabolism

In physiological conditions, only 3 to 10% of circulating cortisol is free. Approximately 85% of cortisol is bound to corticosteroid-binding globulin (CBG, or transcortin). DHEA, DHEAS and androstenedione, the adrenal androgens, are 90% bound to albumin and 3% to testosterone-binding globulin (TeBG).

CBG is a 383-amino acid (59 kd) glycosylated alpha-2-globulin that is produced mainly by the liver, and it has one binding site for cortisol per molecule. CBG increases two- to threefold with exposure to estrogens or during pregnancy. This effect is dose-dependent, achieving a maximal effect in 3 to 5 days, and returns to normal in 2 to 3 weeks after cessation of exposure.

The steroids fixed on proteins are biologically inactive, which is why ACTH and cortisol production are influenced only by the free cortisol levels. Bound cortisol is protected from degradation and thus constitutes a reservoir to limit rapid fluctuations of free cortisol. Bound cortisol ensures a uniform delivery and distribution to individual target cells.

Cortisol is metabolized by several enzyme systems. These include liver 5α- and 5β-reductases and 3α-hydroxysteroid dehydrogenases to generate tetrahydrocortisol (THF) from cortisol, or tetrahydrocortisone (THE) from cortisone. The sum of these metabolites form the urinary 17-hydroxycorticosteroids. Cortisol can also be oxidized to form ketones in carbons 17 and 11; it can be hydroxylated in position 6 to form 6β-hydroxycortisol. Cortisol is inactivated into cortisone by 11β-hydroxysteroid dehydrogenase in kidney and other extrahepatic tissues. Cortisol metabolites are rendered more water soluble by conjugation with glucuronic acid or sulfate. DHEA, DHEAS, and androstenedione are metabolized to primarily form androsterone and etiocholanolone, the main components of 17-ketosteroids.

Mechanisms of action of glucocorticoids

Glucocorticoid receptors

Free cortisol most likely enters the target cell membrane by passive cell diffusion, but this is not fully elucidated as yet. Intracellularly, cortisol binds to its specific glucocorticoid type II receptor (GR), which is a well-characterized member of the steroid, thyroid, vitamin D, and retinoid nuclear receptor superfamily. The GR is a single chain polypeptide of 94 kd and forms a complex with other proteins, such as heat shock protein (hsp90). It has a high affinity for glucocorticoids. Upon the binding of cortisol to the carboxy-terminal ligand binding domain of GR, hsp90 dissociates from the complex, and the mid-portion of the GR (the zinc-finger DNA-binding domain) acquires a high affinity to bind to specific regions of DNA, the so-called glucocorticoid response elements (GRE). Dimers of the GR are usually necessary to initiate the binding to GRE. The GRE are usually located in proximity to the promoter regions of target genes. Interaction of the GR with GRE and with other transcription factors increase or decrease the transcriptional activity of the various target genes of glucocorticoids, resulting in modifications of the amount of the regulated protein and of the biological responses of the target cells.

Mineralocorticoid receptors

Aldosterone binds to a glucocorticoid type I or mineralocorticoid receptor (MR), which is structurally very similar (107 kd) to other steroid hormone receptors. The MR binds mineralocorticoids and glucocorticoids equally well. However, in mineralocorticoid target tissues, cortisol is converted to the inactive cortisone by 11β-hydroxysteroid dehydrogenase type II, thus preventing a continuous MR activation by high circulating concentrations of cortisol.

Biological effects of glucocorticoids

The biological activities of glucocorticoids are summarized in Table 26.2.

Carbohydrate metabolism

Glucocorticoid deficiency results in fasting hypoglycemia, whereas hypercortisolism induces insulin resistance and hyperglycemia. Overall, glucocorticoids increase plasma levels of glucose via multiple actions on carbohydrate metabolism. Glucocorticoids activate glycogen synthetase and inactivate glycogen phosphorylase, which results in increased stores of glycogen in the liver. By increasing the availability of glucogenic amino acids from muscles, glucocorticoids stimulate liver gluconeogenesis and glucose production. Key enzymes of gluconeogenesis such as glucose-6-phosphatase and phosphoenol-pyruvate carboxykinase (PEPCK) are regulated through specific GRE located in the 5'-flanking regions of their genes. Glucocorticoids also have a permissive effect on the gluconeogenic function of other hormones such as glucagon and epinephrine. Glucocorticoids inhibit glucose uptake in peripheral tissues in part by inhibiting glucose transporters in cells.

Lipid metabolism

Glucocorticoids activate lipolysis in adipose cells, providing more glycerol for gluconeogenesis and increasing free fatty acids for energy utilization. Chronic exposure to excess cortisol leads to a striking redistribution of fat, which accumulates in dorsocervical, supraclavicular, trunk, mediastinum, and mesenteric-abdominal regions by mechanisms that are not well understood.

Protein metabolism

Glucocorticoids exert a catabolic effect on muscle proteins, causing breakdowns that liberate gluconeogenic amino acids. Glucocorticoid excess results in proximal muscle wasting and profound myopathy. Suppression of synthesis of several proteins of connective tissues, such as collagen, and inhibition of fibroblast growth and function results in thinning of skin, poor wound healing, friable connective tissue, easy bruising, and characteristic purple striae of skin on the abdomen, thighs, and/or arms.

Bone and calcium homeostasis

Glucocorticoid excess causes osteopenia by a variety of effects on bone and calcium regulation. Trabecular bone in the spine is depleted more than cortical bone in the hip. Glucocorticoids inhibit osteoblast function, collagen synthesis, and new bone formation, which is prominently reflected by a decrease in serum alkaline phosphatase and osteocalcin levels. Glucocorticoids exert direct effects on osteoblasts, but they also modulate the production of several bone growth factors and their receptors. Osteoclast numbers and bone resorptive activity are also increased. Glucocorticoids enhance the bone resorptive activity of parathyroid hormone (PTH) by increasing PTH receptors in osteoblasts. A decrease in calcium absorption in the gut results from opposing effects of glucocorticoid and vitamin D on intestinal calcium transport. An important increase in urinary calcium loss results from decreasing renal calcium reabsorption, which is coupled to the increase in calcium filtering from the increased bone resorption. In children, excess glucocorticoids result in the inhibition of linear skeletal growth and short stature. This probably results from the catabolic effects of glucocorticoids on bone formation, connective and muscle tissues, and protein metabolism in general.

Hematopoietic and immune systems: the anti-inflammatory activity

Glucocorticoids induce a marked decrease in circulating T lymphocytes and to a lesser extent of B lymphocytes, eosinophils and monocytes; CD4 or helper T cells are more sensitive than B cells, whereas CD8 or cytotoxic T cells are relatively insensitive. In opposition, they increase the mobilization and demargination of granulocytes from the bone marrow into the circulation where neutrophil counts are increased. T-cell functions are inhibited in part by the inhibitory effects of glucocorticoids on interleukin 2, a potent T-cell growth factor. Early B-cell activation and proliferation are also inhibited. Glucocorticoids inhibit the differentiation of monocytes into macrophages and inhibit their phagocytic and cytotoxic functions. Glucocorticoids also enhance lymphocyte-programmed cell death or apoptosis.

Effects of glucocorticoids on immune and inflammatory activities result largely from their effects on various cytokines. The production of IL-1, TNF, IL-2, IL-6, interferon-γ, IL-3, and GM-CSF can be inhibited by physiological levels of glucocorticoids. In addition, they block the activities of other important mediators of inflammation such as prostaglandins, bradykinin, serotonin, histamine, collagenase, and elastase. Glucocorticoids protect from endotoxic shock by blocking the exaggerated response of TNF and the immune system to infections (Fig 26.4).

Glucocorticoids have thus become widely utilized in the systemic or local treatment of a large spectrum of inflammatory conditions. In addition, they play a significant role in the treatment of cancers of the lymphoid system. However, immunosuppression and an increased susceptibility to acquire new infections or to reactivate latent infections can result from supraphysiological levels of glucocorticoids.

Table 26.2 Biological activities of glucocorticoids

	Actions	Glucocorticoid excess	Glucocorticoid deficiency
Carbohydrates	↑ Glycogen synthetase Inactivate glycogen phosphorylase ↑Liver glucogenesis, glucose production ↓ Glucose uptake in peripheral tissues Permissive role (catecholamine-glucagon)	Insulin resistance Hyperglycemia	Fasting hypoglycemia
Lipids	↑ Lipolysis in adipose cells ↑ Free fatty acid	Striking redistribution of fat	
Proteins	Catabolic effect on muscle ↓ Fibroblast and epithelial growth and function	Proximal muscle wasting Poor wound healing Friable connective tissues	
Caloric intake	Regulate appetite	Increased appetite Weight gain	Anorexia Weight loss
Bone and calcium	↓ Osteoblast function, collagen synthesis ↓ New bone formation ↑ Osteoclast number, bone resorptive activity ↑ PTH activity Regulate gut calcium absorption, renal calcium reabsorption	Osteoporosis Hypercalciuria Kidney stones	Mild hypercalcemia
Hematopoietic and immune systems	↓ Circulating T lymphocytes and B lymphocytes ↓ Eosinophils, monocytes ↓ T-cell function (IL-2, IL-1, TNF, etc.) ↓ Early B-cell activation and proliferation ↑ Mobilization, demargination of granuclocytes ↑ Apoptosis ↓ Differentiation of monocytes into macrophages ↓ Phagocytic functions	↑ Susceptibility to infections Mild polycytemia	Normochromic normocytic anemia
Central nervous system	Regulate neuronal and glial function	Psychological disturbances Memory loss Sleep disturbances Psychosis	Depression Apathy, lethargy Psychosis
Cardiovascular system	Actions on vascular smooth muscle and endothelial cells Regulate synthesis of vasoactive substances and their receptors Modulate renin-angiotensin system	Hypertension ↑ Vascular reactivity	Hypotension
Electrolytes	Modulate vasopressin synthesis ↑ Glomerular filtration rate ↑ Expression of atrial natriuretic peptides ↑ Renal K$^+$ secretion	Hypokalemia Kaliuresis Alkalosis	Hyponatremia with normal potassium ↓ Free water clearance

(IL-1 = interleukin 1; IL-2 = interleukin 2; TNF = tumor necrosis factor.)

Glucocorticoids and the central nervous system

Glucocorticoids exert numerous effects on human behavior, including alterations of mood, cognition, sleep patterns, and reception of sensory input. Close to 50% of patients with exogenous or endogenous hypercortisolism present with psychological disturbances, mostly depression. Euphoria can also be present, particularly with exogenous glucocorticoids. Manic behaviors and occasional frank psychosis can be induced by high amounts of steroids. Adrenal insufficiency can also be manifested by depression, apathy, lethargy, or psychosis. Memory loss and difficulties in retaining new acquisitions is noted in individuals exposed to excessive glucocorticoids. Atrophy of hippocampal structures implicated in memory have been described in patients with hypercortisolism; more diffuse patterns of cerebral atrophy have also been reported in patients with pituitary or adrenal causes of endogenous hypercortisolism.

Cardiovascular effects

Glucocorticoids exert important permissive effects on the vascular reactivity of several vasoactive agents such as angiotensin II, norepinephrine, vasopressin, and endothelin. Thus, independent of the blood volume effects of mineralocorticoids, glucocorticoids play a role in the maintenance of normal blood pressure. In hypocortisolism, patients exhibit hypotension that responds poorly to vasoconstrictors. High blood pressure in hypercortisolism is not clearly explained by the mineralocorticoid effects, nor by the stimulation of the production of angiotensinogen. Plasma renin activity is usually normal or slightly decreased. Glucocorticoids appear to increase the expression of the receptors for several of the vasoconstrictive agents, including β-adrenergic receptors. In addition, increased vascular reactivity may result from their effects in increasing voltage-dependent Ca^{2+} channels in vascular smooth muscle cells. An increased amount of glucocorticoids presenting to mineralocorticoid target tissues, such as the kidney, may also overflow the inactivating capacity of 11β-hydroxysteroid dehydrogenase (inactivation of cortisol to cortisone) and induce some mineralocorticoid effects of cortisol. The inhibition of vasodilator factors such as kallikrein and prostaglandin E_2 may also contribute to the hypertension.

Electrolyte metabolism

Glucocorticoid deficiency results in a decrease in free water clearance and dilutional hyponatremia with normal potassium levels; this is different from the hyponatremia, hyperkalemia, and depletion in plasma volume that results from mineralocorticoid deficiency. Decreased cortisol levels are associated with a reduction in the inhibitory feedback of glucocorticoids in the synthesis of vasopressin in hypothalamic paraventricular nuclei; an inappropriate secretion of vasopressin occurs, which then induces the water retention and hyponatremia. Glucocorticoids increase epithelial Na^+ absorption and K^+ secretion directly in renal collecting ducts and in colon cells. Glucocorticoids increase the expression of atrial natriuretic peptides (ANP) in the heart and in the circulation, and they increase the number of their receptors in endothelial cells. Cortisol is thus important in allowing the normal excretion of sodium loads.

Synthetic glucocorticoids and their relative potency

See Chapter 31.

DIAGNOSTIC PROCEDURES

A summary of the procedures available for the diagnosis of adrenocortical dysfunctions is given in Table 26.3.

Cortisol assays in blood, saliva, and urine

Serum or plasma levels of cortisol are now most often measured using direct radioimmunoassay kits or automated immunofluorometric assays. These assays all measure total plasma cortisol, that is, primarily the CBG-bound fraction and the small, free fraction.

Normal plasma concentrations vary according to diurnal rhythms. They vary from 170 to 800 nmol/l (6-28 µg/dl) within an hour of the usual awakening time, decrease to ranges of 85 to 400 nmol/l (3-14 µg/dl) in late afternoon, and reach nadirs of less than 140 nmol/l (5 µg/dl) during the early hours of sleep. If one wishes to screen for hypocortisolism, a fasting morning plasma cortisol should be determined. In patients with hypercortisolism, plasma cortisol levels may be in the normal range or elevated in the morning, but they remain more or less at the same levels during the whole day and thus lose the diurnal rhythm. In suspected hypercortisolism, it is therefore useful to determine the plasma cortisol level in the evening as well as in the morning. Several factors must be considered in the interpretation of plasma cortisol levels. Alterations in CBG levels will modify total plasma cortisol levels. Estrogen administration or birth control pills will elevate total plasma cortisol up to 1400 nmol/l or more; diurnal rhythm will be maintained with afternoon levels, which would be approximately 50% of morning levels. However, the free plasma cortisol level and urinary 24-hour free cortisol excretion remain normal.

Plasma free cortisol diffuses well into the saliva independently of saliva flow rate, which allows for an immediate estimation of plasma free cortisol. A sample of 2.5 ml of saliva is collected after rinsing the mouth and is stored frozen until it is assayed by competitive binding assay or radioimmunoassay for cortisol. Morning values range between 6 to 32 nmol/l (0.2-1.1 µg/dl) in men and 5 to 18 nmol/l (0.2-0.6 µg/dl) in women; levels decrease to 2 to 4 nmol/l at 8 p.m. in both sexes. Salivary cortisol determinations are particularly useful in ambulatory patients, who are required to collect serial samples, such as in the investigation and medical follow-up of hypercortisolism.

Urinary free cortisol excretion is the result of the glomerular filtration of plasma free cortisol, hence it can reflect an index of integrated 24-hour plasma free cortisol levels. It is usually measured by radioimmunoassay (after extraction), by immunofluorometric assays, or with spectrophotometric detection during high-pressure liquid chromatography. Normal levels range between 50 to 330 nmol per 24 hours and must be interpreted with urinary creatinine levels to assess the validity of the collection method. It is imperative that the technique of urine collection is explained well to the patient and that the completeness of the collection is respected. This is not a valid test to diagnose hypocortisolism as it is not very sensitive to discriminate between normal and decreased levels. However, it is the measurement of choice for the screening of hypercortisolism, as it reflects the rapidly increasing free cortisol fraction when CBG becomes saturated.

Measurement of plasma ACTH

This peptide can now be measured in unextracted plasma with sensitive two-site immunoradiometric assay or by radioimmunoassay. Plasma ACTH levels vary normally between 2 to 11 pmol/l (10-55 pg/ml) in the morning and decrease during the day often becoming less than 1.1 pmol/l by bedtime. A plasma ACTH assay must be interpreted simultaneously with a plasma cortisol determination. In primary adrenal insufficiency or in untreated congenital adrenal hyperplasia, morning ACTH levels will be elevated, while plasma cortisol will be low. In hypocortisolism secondary to hypothalamic or pituitary disease, morning ACTH will be relatively decreased when compared to the low plasma cortisol levels. In the presence of hypercortisolism (increased urinary free cortisol levels), the determination of plasma ACTH and cortisol levels will be most useful to distinguish between ACTH-dependent or ACTH-independent hypercortisolism. A primary adrenal source of excess cortisol excess or exposure to exogenous supraphysiological sources of glucocorticoids will result in low levels of ACTH. In hypercortisolism secondary to a pituitary corticotroph adenoma, ACTH levels will be either slightly elevated or will be inappropriately within the normal or upper-normal range despite elevated cortisol levels. If hypercortisolism results from the ectopic expression of ACTH and other POMC-derived peptides from an extrapituitary tumor, ACTH levels will usually be frankly elevated with high levels of plasma and urinary cortisol. Abnormal POMC products may be detected by specific assays.

Plasma renin and aldosterone measurements

In primary adrenal insufficiency or in salt-losing congenital adrenal hyperplasia, plasma aldosterone will be decreased and renin activity will be increased. In opposition, in adrenal insufficiency secondary to hypothalamic-pituitary disease or suppression by exogenous glucocorticoids, the renin-angiotensin-aldosterone axis will be normal. This is discussed in further details in the chapter on mineralocorticoids.

Table 26.3 Summary of initial diagnostic procedures to evaluate the hypothalamic-pituitary-adrenal axis

Appropriate tests	Suspected pathology hypocortisolism	Hypercortisolism
Plasma cortisol	Fasting, morning	Morning and evening Loss of diurnal rhythm
Urinary free cortisol	Not sensitive	Most sensitive Multiple determinations (cyclic diseases)
Dexamethasone suppression tests	No	Short overnight 1 mg test: cortisol 8 a.m. >140 nmol/l suspect between 70-140 nmol/l
Combined dexamethasone-CRH test	No	Cortisol >38 nmol/l, 15 min post-CRH
ACTH test	Cortisol <550 nmol/l (primary adrenal insufficiency or after a long ACTH deficiency)	For differential diagnosis
Metyrapone test	11-deoxycortisol <210 nmol/l (adrenal insufficiency)	For differential diagnosis
CRH test	ACTH <2 x basal values Cortisol <550 nmol/l (primary or secondary adrenal insufficiency)	For differential diagnosis
Insulin-induced hypoglycemia	Decreased response in all forms of hypocortisolism	Can be useful for differential diagnosis

Adrenal androgens and steroid precursors

DHEAS is produced almost exclusively by the adrenal, and hence it serves as a useful marker of the source (adrenal versus gonads) of excessive androgens in conditions of hyperandrogenism. DHEA and androstenedione, on the other hand, are not produced exclusively by the adrenal. Their levels are affected in part by the diurnal rhythm of ACTH, and their determinations are useful only in more limited situations of rare congenital adrenal hyperplasias or virilizing tumors. DHEAS has a longer half-life, and its plasma levels do not fluctuate as much with ACTH diurnal rhythm. Normal plasma DHEAS levels vary greatly for age and sex. The levels are very high during fetal life, are low during early childhood, increase to adult levels prior to puberty (adrenarche) (men: 2-10 μmol/l; women: 3-12.7 μmol/l), and begin a progressive decline of approximately 3% per year by age 25 to 30. DHEAS can be quite elevated in adrenal carcinoma, but it is usually normal or low in adrenal adenomas that secrete cortisol. DHEAS can be slightly increased in ACTH-dependent hypercortisolism, polycystic ovarian disease, and idiopathic hyperandrogenism.

Tests of adrenal reserve

ACTH stimulation tests

The ACTH stimulation test is performed most commonly as a short test using an IV bolus of 250 μg of ACTH 1-24 (cosyntropin), which is an analog with the full biological activity of ACTH. Blood samples for the determination of cortisol levels are collected before and 30 and 60 minutes after the administration of ACTH 1-24. In normal individuals, plasma levels of cortisol should increase above a value of 550 nmol/l (20 μg/dl) after 30 or 60 minutes. In complete primary adrenal insufficiency, no response of cortisol will be seen, while in partial primary disease a suboptimal response will be elicited. Under these circumstances, endogenous plasma ACTH levels should be elevated. If the adrenal insufficiency is secondary to a hypothalamic-pituitary deficiency of ACTH, the adrenal gland may have become atrophic depending on the duration of the ACTH deficiency. However, the adrenal gland should be capable of responding to exogenous ACTH with a short test with 250 μg of ACTH 1-24 (cosyntropin) if the atrophy is not long-standing. If the glands have become significantly atrophic, the response of the adrenal may require repeated stimulations with either 250 μg of ACTH 1-24 diluted in 500 ml of normal saline solution and infused over 8 hours daily up to 5 days, or intramuscular injections of ACTH in depot form every 12 hours for up to 4 days. Plasma and urinary free cortisol should be collected prior and daily during the test. A normal gland will increase plasma (above 550 nmol/l) and urinary values three- to fourfold, progressively. The short IV test is commonly used to assess whether the hypothalamic-pituitary-adrenal axis has recovered from its chronic suppression after withdrawal of exogenous glucocorticoid therapy, or removal of an endogenous source of excess cortisol. A normal response to 250 μg of ACTH 1-24 iv is a good indication that endogenous CRH and ACTH have recuperated sufficiently to restore adrenocortical size and function to normal. It must be cautioned, however, that in the case of a very recent suppression of ACTH (for example, a few days after the removal of a pituitary corticotroph adenoma, or shortly after the initiation of high doses of a potent glucocorticoid exogenously), the adrenal cortex may not have become atrophic yet and may respond to ACTH administration. This could erroneously lead to the conclusion of a normal response, while the capacity of the hypothalamic-pituitary response to an acute stress may actually be compromised. Under such circumstances, the response of the full axis to insulin-induced hypoglycemia or to metyrapone administration may be more reliable to evaluate the axis.

Metyrapone test

The metyrapone test is useful to assess both the adrenal and the pituitary reserve. Metyrapone inhibits adrenal CYP11B1 and thus blocks the conversion of 11-deoxycortisol (compound S) to cortisol. The resulting decrease in plasma cortisol levels stimulates CRH and ACTH release and steroidogenesis. An accumulation of the steroid precursors, and particularly of 11-deoxycortisol, can be detected as a result of the induced enzyme block.

Two procedures are used: (1) In the overnight test, a single dose of metyrapone (30 mg/kg) is administered orally, with a snack at midnight, and blood is drawn at 8 a.m. for 11-deoxycortisol and cortisol levels. The normal results are an 11-deoxycortisol level above 210 nmol/l (7 μg/dl) and a cortisol level <286 nmol/l (10 μg/dl); the low cortisol level indicates the adequate inhibition of CYP11B1. If the plasma ACTH level is determined, it should exceed 17 pmol/l (85 pg/ml). (2) The second, less often used procedure, is the 3-day test in which urines are collected during 24 hours for basal levels. The patient then takes 750 mg of metyrapone every 4 hours for 6 doses, and the urine specimens are collected during a second day and again during the next 24 hours for measurement of urinary 17-hydroxycorticosteroids and creatinine. The normal results are a two- to threefold increase above the baseline of the urinary 17-hydroxycorticosteroids, which include the metabolites of 11-deoxycortisol. The metyrapone test should be performed only as a second-line investigation: it is unnecessary and potentially dangerous - if baseline ACTH is elevated (primary adrenal failure), and/or if the short ACTH is abnormal. The metyrapone test becomes useful and safe in detecting a subtle secondary adrenal insufficiency when baseline ACTH and the short ACTH test are normal. This test is also useful in the etiological diagnosis of Cushing's syndrome (see Chap. 29).

Corticotropin-releasing hormone test

CRH directly stimulates the pituitary secretion of POMC, for example, ACTH, β-lipotropin, and β-endorphin. One μg/kg of human synthetic CRH or preferably ovine CRH, which has a longer half-life, is injected intravenously. ACTH and cortisol levels are determined 15 and 0 minutes before and 15, 30, 45, 60, 90, and 120 minutes after injection.

A normal response is an ACTH rise of two- to fourfold above the basal values with a peak 15 minutes after CRH, and an increase in plasma cortisol levels up to 550 to 690 nmol/l (20 to 25 µg/dl) in 30 to 60 minutes. Patients with primary adrenal insufficiency have high ACTH levels and low or subnormal cortisol levels. In pituitary deficiency, ACTH and cortisol responses are decreased. The ACTH response could be exaggerated and prolonged in hypothalamic diseases. The CRH test is not very useful in distinguishing primary from secondary adrenal insufficiency; an ACTH stimulation test is preferable. In hypercortisolism, however, the CRH test can be useful, since in Cushing's disease the response is normal or exaggerated (because there is a high density of CRH receptors on the pituitary tumor cells). In ectopic ACTH syndrome, there is usually no response (because there are generally no CRH receptors in nonpituitary tumor cells). In adrenal cortisol-secreting tumors, the ACTH levels are suppressed and do not respond to CRH.

Insulin-induced hypoglycemia test The insulin-induced hypoglycemia test is the most sensitive and accurate test of the hypothalamic-pituitary-adrenal reserve, but it is not simple to perform and can be dangerous. Hypoglycemia is a major stress, increasing CRH, ACTH, vasopressin, cortisol, GH, and prolactin release, and it activates the adrenergic system.

The test is performed after an overnight fast on a supine patient under the continued surveillance of a physician. Hypoglycemia is induced with the intravenous administration of 0.15 U/kg body weight (0.05 U/kg in children) of regular insulin. Plasma cortisol and glucose samples are drawn before and 30, 45, 60, and 90 minutes after insulin injection. The test is considered adequate if the glucose levels decrease below 2.2 mmole/l (40 mg/dl). The normal response is an increase of plasma cortisol above 550 nmol/l (>20 µg/dl). An adequate response excludes all hypothalamic-pituitary-adrenal anomalies. The test is abnormal in the case of hypopituitarism of any etiology, including acute or chronic treatment with synthetic glucocorticoids and primary adrenal insufficiency.

The dose of insulin must be adjusted according to the patient's conditions. It is increased to 0.2 to 0.3 U/kg in subjects with insulin resistance (acromegaly, diabetes, obesity or Cushing's syndrome). When an adrenal insufficiency is suspected, a lower dose (0.1 U/kg) is recommended. The test is contraindicated in patients with seizure disorders, cardiovascular and cerebrovascular ischemic diseases, and possibly in those older than 65 years.

Tests of hypothalamic-pituitary adrenal suppressibility: dexamethasone suppression tests

Dexamethasone is a potent synthetic glucocorticoid that inhibits pituitary ACTH release and consequently cortisol secretion. Dexamethasone is not detected by antibodies used for the measurements of cortisol in blood or urine and can thus be utilized without interfering with cortisol determinations. These tests are useful to eliminate diagnoses of endogenous cortisol hypersecretion (Cushing's syndrome).

The classic low-dose dexamethasone suppression test
Dexamethasone (2 mg/day) is administered orally for 2 days in eight divided doses. Normal individuals almost totally suppress cortisol production (24-hour urinary cortisol excretion <10 µg or 30 nmoles).

The short overnight 1 mg dexamethasone test The short overnight 1 mg dexamethasone test is often performed in first intention: 1 mg dexamethasone is administered orally at 11 p.m. and plasma cortisol is measured at 8 a.m. on the following morning. A plasma cortisol level below 140 nmol/l (5 µg/dl) excludes a diagnosis of Cushing's syndrome with rare exceptions. Most normal individuals suppress their plasma cortisol levels to less than 70 nmol/l (2.4 µg/dl). In addition, conditions that elevate blood CBG levels such as estrogens, drugs that increase dexamethasone catabolism such as phenytoin, or failure of the patient to take the dexamethasone will cause falsely elevated cortisol levels.

Combined dexamethasone-CRH test Recently a combined dexamethasone-CRH test was found to be the most reliable in distinguishing states of functional hypercortisolism (pseudo-Cushing's: affective disorders, alcoholism, exercise, or anorexia nervosa) from genuine Cushing's syndrome (see Chap. 29). Dexamethasone 0.5 mg is given orally every 6 hours for eight doses, ending 2 hours before the IV injection of 1 µg/kg ovine CRH. Plasma cortisol should be less than 38 nmol/l (1.4 µg/dl) 15 minutes following CRH injection in normal or pseudo-Cushing's states, whereas it is elevated in Cushing's syndrome. The differential etiology of hypercortisolism should then be assessed (as outlined further in Chapter 29).

Suggested readings

BERTAGNA X. Proopiomelanocortin-derived peptides. Endocrinology and Metabolism Clinics of North America. 1994;23:467-85.

CANALIS E. Mechanisms of glucocorticoid action in bone: implications to glucocorticoid-induced osteoporosis. J Clin Endocrinol Metab 1996;81:3441-7.

EHRHART-BORNSTEIN M, HINSON JP, BORNSTEIN SR, et al. Intraadrenal interactions in the regulation of adrenocortical steroidogenesis. Endocrine Review 1998;19:101-43.

GROSSMAN A. Corticotropin-releasing hormone: basic physiology and clinical applications. In: DeGroot LJ, Besser M, Burger HG, et al. (eds); Cahill GF Jr, Martini L, Nelson DH (cons. eds). Endocrinology, 3rd ed. Philadelphia: WB Saunders, 1995;341-54.

IMURA H. Adrenocorticotropic hormone. In: DeGroot LJ, Besser M, Burger HG, et al. (eds); Cahill GF Jr, Martini L, Nelson DH (cons. eds). Endocrinology, 3rd ed. Philadelphia: WB Saunders, 1995;355-67.

KAYE TB, CRAPO L. The Cushing syndrome: an update on diagnostic tests. Ann Intern Med 1990;112:434-44.

MIESFELD, RL. Biochemistry. In: DeGroot LJ, Besser M, Burger HG, et al. (eds); Cahill GF Jr, Martini L, Nelson DH (cons.

eds). Endocrinology, 3rd ed. Philadelphia: WB Saunders, 1995;1656-67.

MILLER WL, TYRRELL JB. The adrenal cortex. In: Felig P, Baxter JD, Frohman LA (eds). Endocrinology and metabolism, 3rd ed. New York: McGraw-Hill, 1995;555-711.

MUNCK A, NÁRAY-FEJES-TÓTH A. Glucocorticoid action. In: DeGroot LJ, Besser M, Burger HG, et al. (eds); Cahill GF Jr, Martini L, Nelson DH (cons. eds). Endocrinology, 3rd ed. Philadelphia: WB Saunders, 1995;1642-56.

ORTH DN, KOVACS WJ, DEBOLD CR. The adrenal cortex. In: Wilson JD, Foster DW, et al. (eds). Williams Textbook of endocrinology, 9th ed. Philadelphia: WB Saunders, 1998; 517-64.

SIMPSON ER, WATERMAN MR. Steroid hormone biosynthesis in the adrenal cortex and its regulation by adrenocorticotropin. In: DeGroot LJ, Besser M, Burger HG, (eds); Cahill GF Jr, Martini L, Nelson DH (cons. eds). Endocrinology, 3rd ed. Philadelphia: WB Saunders, 1995;1630-41.

TSIGOS C, CHROUSOS GP. Physiology of the hypothalamic-pituitary-adrenal axis in health and dysregulation in psychiatric and autoimmune disorders. Endocrinology and Metabolism Clinics of North America 1994;23:451-66.

YANOVSKI JA, CUTLER GB, CHROUSOS GP, et al. Corticotropin-releasing hormone stimulation following low-dose dexamethasone administration: a new test to distinguish Cushing's syndrome from pseudo-Cushing's states. J Am Med Soc 1993;269:2232-8.

Adrenocortical insufficiency

Pierre Thomopoulos

▮ KEY POINTS ▮

- Suspicion of chronic adrenocortical insufficiency should be confirmed by the rapid adrenocorticotropic hormone (ACTH) stimulation test. Isolated assays of plasma cortisol are frequently misleading.
- A normal result of the rapid ACTH test eliminates the diagnosis of primary adrenocortical insufficiency, but it does not exclude secondary insufficiency.
- Suspicion of secondary adrenocortical insufficiency with a normal result to the rapid ACTH stimulation test should be confirmed by a metyrapone test or the insulin hypoglycemia test.
- Acute adrenal insufficiency should be suspected in any case of circulatory failure of no obvious etiology. It is often preceded and accompanied by gastrointestinal symptoms. Treatment should be started immediately without waiting for the results of hormonal evaluation.
- Education of the patient and his or her family should include the instruction to make the appropriate increase in glucocorticoid dose at the onset of illness. A medical information card or bracelet should be supplied.

Impairment of the adrenal production of glucocorticoids (cortisol) and mineralocorticoids (aldosterone) leads to a life-threatening situation that is often misinterpreted and neglected. Yet, when the diagnosis is suspected, the confirmatory procedures and treatment are simple and rapidly efficacious.

Primary adrenal insufficiency (Addison's disease) is caused by damage of the adrenal glands. Secondary insufficiency results from inadequate adrenocorticotropic hormone (ACTH) and/or corticotropin-releasing hormone secretion. Both primary and secondary insufficiency are rare diseases. The prevalence of acquired primary insufficiency is estimated at 39 to 60 cases per 1 million people in Western countries, with most of the cases being diagnosed in the third to fifth decade of life. Adding to these patients the congenital and hereditary disorders of adrenal insufficiency, one could calculate a four-fold higher prevalence. In addition, iatrogenic adrenal insufficiency, secondary to exogenous glucocorticoid therapy, includes a large number of patients and implies similar risks of acute adrenal crisis.

Etiology

For most cases of adrenal insufficiency, impairment of hormonal production can take place over the course of many years, and the clinical picture is insidiously dominated by the features of the disorder. In such cases, second to making the correct diagnosis, it is important to investigate for the offending agent. This might lead to the discovery of extra-adrenal localizations of the disease requiring specific treatment, such as polyglandular disorders in cases of autoimmunity, or pulmonary and urogenital lesions in cases of tuberculosis. On the other hand, in some situations the signs of adrenal insufficiency may be buried under the manifestations of the causal disease, either during a chronic evolution (such as acquired immune deficiency syndrome [AIDS]) or in the course of an acute crisis (such as adrenal hemorrhage or necrosis of a pituitary adenoma).

PRIMARY ADRENOCORTICAL INSUFFICIENCY (ADDISON'S DISEASE)

Causes of primary adrenal insufficiency are reported in Table 27.1.

AUTOIMMUNE ADRENALITIS

Autoimmune adrenalitis is the most common cause of Addison's disease. It accounts for 75 to 80% of cases. Humoral and cellular immunity are both involved.

Antibodies to the adrenal cortex are detected in up to 70% of idiopathic insufficiencies. They inhibit adrenal steroidogenesis in vitro, and some of them are directed against enzymes of steroidogenesis ($P450_{17\alpha}$ or $P450_{C21}$). However, their titers progressively decrease and may completely disappear. In addition, the antibodies may exist in patients with other autoimmune diseases without adrenal insufficiency. Although their sensitivity and specificity are of limited value, their presence is the only direct marker of an autoimmune origin.

Lymphocytic infiltration of the adrenals is also observed early in the evolution of the disease. It is followed by gradual destruction of cortical cells and their replacement by fibrotic tissue. The gland becomes atrophic, although the adrenal medulla remains intact.

A special feature of autoimmune adrenal insufficiency is the frequent association to other autoimmune endocrine or nonendocrine disorders, which are observed in 50% of the cases. These associations are named polyglandular autoimmune syndromes and they present themselves into two different groupings, the type I and the type II. Polyglandular autoimmune syndrome type I is often familial, inherited in an autosomal recessive pattern. Its first manifestations are hypoparathyroidism and/or mucocutaneous candidiasis occurring during childhood. Addison's disease develops in 60% of the cases during adolescence.

Polyglandular autoimmune syndrome type II is by far the more frequent of the two syndromes. It is familial in half of the cases, and it occurs mostly between 20 and 40 years of age. It often develops in a sequence that starts with insulin-dependent diabetes, followed by Graves' disease, then Addison's disease, and finally hypothyroidism. Hypoparathyroidism and candidiasis are absent in polyglandular autoimmune syndrome type II.

Thus, the diagnosis of autoimmune adrenal insufficiency should lead to the detection of associated and possibly familial autoimmune diseases. A word of caution, however, should be stressed in regards to looking for hypothyroidism, since thyroid-stimulating hormone (TSH) levels may be increased, with normal total and free thyroxine, as a mere functional consequence of hypocortisolism. In this case TSH will normalize after steroid treatment is started.

The systematic search for adrenal insufficiency in cases of other, much more common, autoimmune endocrine diseases (that is, Hashimoto's thyroiditis, atrophic thyroiditis, Graves' disease, or insulin-dependent diabetes mellitus) is not productive since its prevalence in such patients is less than 2%.

INFECTIOUS ADRENALITIS

Adrenal tuberculosis is the second-most common cause of Addison's disease in most countries. It accounts for 20% of the cases. The adrenal glands are completely destroyed, including the medulla. They are taken over by caseous necrosis, which is progressively replaced by fibrosis. In patients during the early stage of the disease (less than 2 years duration) the computed tomography (CT) scan usually shows enlargement of the adrenals, with a central hypodense area of necrosis and peripheral contrast enhancement. Later on, the adrenals become atrophic, with calcification in half of the cases. However, a normal appearance of the glands does not exclude tuberculosis. Extra-adrenal tuberculosis usually accompanies the disease and should be investigated, especially in the lungs, gastrointestinal tract, and kidneys. In very uncommon cases, the recovery of adrenal function has been observed in response to antituberculous therapy.

Disseminated fungal infections can destroy the adrenal glands. This is especially true with histoplasmosis and paracoccidioidomycosis (South American blastomycosis). In contrast, North American blastomycosis, coccidioiodomycosis, and cryptococcosis are seldom involved. Syphilis has also become a rare cause.

INVASIVE DESTRUCTION OF ADRENALS

Metastatic involvement of the adrenals is common in lung, breast, stomach, colon cancer, and melanoma, as

---

Table 27.1 Causes of primary adrenal insufficiency

Autoimmune adrenalitis (80%)
Infectious adrenalitis
   Tuberculosis (20%)
   Histoplasmosis, paracoccidioidomycosis, blastomycosis,
     coccidioidomycosis, cryptococcosis
Invasive destruction
   Metastases
   Lymphoma
   Amyloidosis, sarcoidosis
AIDS (infectious or invasive destruction)
Adrenal hemorrhage
Iatrogenic (mitotane, ketoconazole, aminoglutethimide,
   metyrapone, etomidate, surgery)
Congenital and familial
   Adrenoleukodystrophy
   Adrenal hypoplasia
   Familial glucocorticoid deficiency

well as Hodgkin's and non-Hodgkin's lymphoma. Although overt Addison's disease is unusual, partial insufficiency may be detected in up to 20% of cases with bilateral adrenal metastases. Amyloidosis and sarcoidosis are rare invasive causes.

ACQUIRED IMMUNE DEFICIENCY SYNDROME

Patients with AIDS may have adrenal involvement through multiple mechanisms: infection by cytomegalovirus, tuberculosis, *mycobacterium avium-intracellulare*, toxoplasmosis, cryptococcosis, as well as invasion by Kaposi's sarcoma and lymphoma. Symptoms and signs of Addison's disease may be mistaken and imputed to AIDS itself. A systematic search for adrenal deficiency through the rapid ACTH test shows a decreased response in 8 to 14% of the patients, who are at risk of acute adrenal crisis and should receive benefit from hormonal replacement treatment. In addition, some drugs used in AIDS patients (ketoconazole, rifampin, phenytoin) may precipitate adrenal insufficiency.

IATROGENIC ADRENAL DEFICIENCY

Iatrogenic adrenal deficiency is a predicted situation in medically treated Cushing's syndrome. Mitotane blocks the synthesis of corticosteroids and, moreover, induces necrosis of the adrenal cortex, which may be permanent. Aminoglutethimide, metyrapone, and ketoconazole reversibly inhibit several steps of steroidogenesis.

Inhibition of cortisol synthesis may be an unexpected side effect in the treatment of fungal diseases by ketoconazole. This is also true for anesthesia induced by etomidate, which may persist for a few days after the end of the treatment.

Another class of drugs, including rifampin, phenytoin, and barbiturates, increases cortisol metabolism. These drugs have no adrenal side effects in normal people, but they may precipitate acute crisis in cases of undiagnosed insufficiency or in patients treated with a purely substitutive dose of steroids. A readjustment of the doses should be ordered when such medications are prescribed.

ADRENAL HEMORRHAGE

Adrenal hemorrhage is a cause of rapid and total destruction of adrenal glands, leading to acute adrenal insufficiency. In adults, it usually occurs after 50 years of age in patients on anticoagulant therapy. It can also complicate the antiphospholipid syndrome, which includes multiple venous and arterial thromboses and the presence of circulating anticoagulant.

Adrenal hemorrhage can also occur in patients with severe, often life-threatening illnesses, such as infection with sepsis, burns, major surgery, complicated pregnancy, trauma, severe cardiovascular disease, or acute renal failure. Its most common cause in children is meningococcal

or pseudomonas septicemia. In neonates, it may occur after a complicated delivery. A high mortality rate is linked to adrenal hemorrhage due to the acute onset of the adrenal insufficiency and to the association with severe illness.

Modern imaging technique by CT scan or magnetic resonance imaging (MRI) can establish the diagnosis by showing the adrenal enlargement. Density on unenhanced CT is increased, and intensity on T2 magnetic resonance images is high in acute hemorrhage. In patients successfully treated, the hematomas resolve and the glands become atrophic, and, in some cases, calcified.

CONGENITAL AND FAMILIAL ETIOLOGIES

Insufficiency due to disorders of adrenal steroid biosynthesis, with adrenal hyperplasia, is discussed further (see Chap. 28).

ADRENOLEUKODYSTROPHY

Adrenoleukodystrophy is a disease caused by the defective oxidation of very long chain fatty acids (VLCFA) in peroxisomes and their accumulation in central and peripheral nervous tissue, adrenals, gonads, and other organs. *Neonatal adrenoleukodystrophy* is a rare and distressing disease. Patients die before the age of five, with adrenal insufficiency always associated with (or preceded by) severe neurologic and mental deterioration. The number, size, and global function of peroxisomes are decreased. Inheritance is autosomal recessive.

Much more frequent is *X-linked adrenoleukodystrophy*. Its incidence is 1 in 20 000 males. It is due to the dysfunction of a peroxisomal protein, which leads to the impairment of the first step of VLCFA oxidation. Neurologic disorders appear mostly in childhood or adolescence, progressing within a few years to major cerebral deterioration. A milder form exists, beginning in late adolescence or early adulthood and characterized by demyelinization of spinal cord and peripheral nerves, with spasticity, sensory disturbances, and urinary and sexual dysfunction. Its progression is slow. In 80 to 90% of the cases these patients have adrenal atrophy and insufficiency, and in 30% of them testicular deficiency is also observed. Endocrine disorders precede neurologic symptoms in 30 to 40% of the cases. Moreover, 8% of the patients have isolated Addison's disease. Thus, in idiopathic adrenal deficiency of males with negative adrenal autoantibodies, it is important that adrenoleukodystrophy be considered. Diagnosis is based on the measurement of plasma VLCFA (C26, C25, C24 and the C26/C22 ratio) and is found in 30% of such patients. Diagnosis brings about neurological investigation and follow-up, to workups in other members of the family, and to potential benefit from specific diet counseling and other therapeutic interventions.

ADRENAL HYPOPLASIA

Adrenal hypoplasia prevalence is estimated at 1:12 500 live births. It presents as adrenal failure shortly after birth and is secondary to impaired development of the adult adrenal cortex. Inheritance is either autosomal recessive or X-linked. The latter is commonly associated with hypogonadotropic hypogonadism. In addition, it may coexist with glycerol kinase deficiency and/or Duchenne muscular dystrophy. The gene for X-linked adrenal hypoplasia has been identified and termed DAX1. It encodes for a protein belonging to the nuclear receptor superfamily and is expressed in the adrenal cortex, hypothalamus, and pituitary. The frequency of the combined loss of DAX1 with the contiguous loci for glycerol kinase and/or Duchenne dystrophy is responsible for the appearance of this complex syndrome. Diagnosis, which in the past was based on the measurement of plasma and urinary glycerol levels, may at present be established by direct study of the DAX1 gene.

FAMILIAL GLUCOCORTICOID DEFICIENCY

Familial glucocorticoid deficiency is a rare autosomal recessive disorder that usually presents in childhood as unresponsiveness to ACTH. Cortisol and adrenal androgen secretions are defective while, in most cases, the renin-angiotensin-aldosterone system is intact. The disease may be isolated, and mutations to the ACTH receptor have been reported in some families. Adrenal failure may also coexist with achalasia of the cardia and with alacrimia (absence of tears), featuring the so-called triple A syndrome, which is frequently associated with various and progressive neurologic disorders. ACTH receptors are normal in the latter.

Pathophysiology

Impairment of glucocorticoid secretion causes a decreased sense of well-being, gastrointestinal disturbances, hypoglycemia, water retention that aggravates the hyponatremia, and reduced vascular adrenergic tone. In addition, the decreased negative feedback by cortisol results in increased synthesis and secretion of corticotropin-releasing hormone by the hypothalamus, ACTH, and other pro-opiomelanocortin (POMC)-derived peptides by the pituitary. The melanocyte-stimulating action of these peptides is responsible for the hyperpigmentation of the skin and mucous membranes.

Mineralocorticoid deficiency leads to increased sodium renal loss with dehydration and hyponatremia, and increased renal retention of potassium and hydrogen ions with hyperkalemia and acidosis. The reduced intravascular volume is responsible for the hypotension, aggravated by the upright position, and the increased production of renin (and angiotensin II). Loss of adrenal epinephrine may also aggravate hypoglycemia and hypotension. Adrenal androgen deficiency may be manifest only in women as a decrease in axillary and pubic hair and libido.

In most cases the loss of adrenal function is progressive. Symptoms and signs appear when more than 90% of the glands are destroyed. Before that point, the increased ACTH and renin maximally stimulate the remaining cortical tissue, which may produce normal basal amounts of glucocorticoids and mineralocorticoids, but becomes unable to increase its secretion in response to stress. During this transient state of *partial deficiency* or *decreased adrenal reserve*, an acute crisis may be precipitated by surgery, trauma, or infection. In cases of adrenal hemorrhage, the abrupt loss of steroid production may result in adrenal crisis before skin hyperpigmentation has developed.

Clinical findings

The clinical features of Addison's disease (Tab. 27.2) are often misleading and may go unnoticed for months. In fact, most of the symptoms and signs taken separately are non-specific and follow a slow progression until their duration and association focus suspicion on the adrenal cortex. Weakness is a constant complaint, along with fatigue and malaise. Weakness occurs for usual, routine tasks and improves with rest, and it is frequently associated with myalgias and arthralgias. Postural dizziness or, less often, syncope are reported, and postural hypotension with tachycardia is observed. Thus, the existence of systolic hypertension is a strong indication to exclude the diagnosis of adrenal insufficiency. Moreover, spontaneous improvement of pre-existing hypertension is reported.

Gastrointestinal symptoms are common. Anorexia is almost constantly found among patients and associated with weight loss. Salt craving is reported by some patients, as well as an increased thirst for iced liquids.

Spontaneous hypoglycemia is infrequent in adults, while it is common in infants and children. It may be precipitated by infection, fever, or alcohol ingestion. In cases of previously existing diabetes, an unexpected improvement of the disease with increased sensitivity to the therapeutic agents is often observed. In women, amenorrhea with decreased axillary and pubic hair may occur. Loss of libido is reported frequently in both sexes.

Table 27.2 Clinical and laboratory features of chronic primary adrenal insufficiency

Weakness, malaise, depression
Dizziness, postural hypotension
Myalgias, arthralgias
Anorexia, salt craving
Weight loss
Hyperpigmentation
Hyponatremia
Hyperkalemia
Azotemia
Eosinophilia, lymphocytosis, normochronic anemia

In most patients, psychiatric symptoms are present, such as lack of initiative, impairment of memory, and depression. These manifestations may occasionally be misleading if they occur early in the disease and if they mimic classical psychiatric syndromes.

In contrast to the above symptoms and signs, hyperpigmentation is a highly specific sign of chronic adrenal insufficiency. It may be misdiagnosed as an effect of sun exposure. Indeed, it predominates in areas exposed to light. However, it also occurs in pressure or friction points (elbows, knees, knuckles, toes, waist), in palmar creases and nail beds, and in buccal mucosa and gums. Scars are also hyperpigmented if acquired after the onset of the disease. Vitiligo may coexist with hyperpigmentation in 10% of patients with autoimmune Addison's disease.

Diagnostic procedures

For patients with primary adrenal insufficiency, the routine laboratory findings frequently show hyponatremia, hyperkalemia, and mild acidosis. Fasting blood glucose is usually low to normal. A mild elevation of urea and creatinine is secondary to dehydration. Elevations of hepatic transaminases have been reported and, occasionally, a mild hypercalcemia may be observed. Moderate

eosinophilia, lymphocytocis and normocytic, normochromic anemia are common.

The diagnosis is confirmed by the rapid ACTH stimulation test (Fig. 27.1). This test can be done at any time of the day, since, in contrast to the circadian rhythm of basal cortisol, the stimulated cortisol concentration is independent of the time of day. It should be stressed that an isolated assay of plasma cortisol is frequently misleading, since it may be normal in partial chronic adrenal insufficiency and low in normal subjects. However, the observation of an absent or subnormal response of cortisol after ACTH stimulation is diagnostic of adrenal insufficiency. Basal plasma ACTH is clearly and constantly elevated, confirming the primary adrenal origin. In fact, during the transient phase of preclinical (incipient) adrenal insufficiency, isolated elevation of ACTH is observed before the cortisol response to ACTH becomes subnormal. Thus, ideally, basal plasma ACTH should be measured concomitantly to the ACTH stimulation test. In addition, aldosterone concentration is low, non-responsive to ACTH or to the upright position, and it is associated with high renin activity and concentration. It is not recommended to proceed to a more extensive hormonal exploration, which may show a mild elevation of TSH and prolactin. Their values return to normal after steroid treatment. Adrenal androgens (dehydroepiandrosterone, dehydroepiandrosterone sulfate, and androsterone) are low.

After the confirmation of Addison's disease, an adrenal CT scan should be performed. If bilateral adrenal enlargement is observed, further evaluation is indicated to determine the specific cause (tuberculosis, other granulomatous diseases, metastatic cancer, or hemorrhage). In the absence of glandular enlargement in males, screening for adrenoleukodystrophy by measurement of serum very long chain fatty acid should also be considered, unless association with other autoimmune diseases or positivity of adrenal autoantibodies makes the diagnosis of autoimmune adrenalitis obvious.

Treatment

Treatment for chronic primary adrenal insufficiency includes substitutions for both glucocorticoid and mineralocorticoid function. Cortisol (hydrocortisone) is a natural glucocorticoid and is usually prescribed at 20 to 30 mg per day. Two-thirds of the dose is given in the morning and one-third in the early afternoon, which reproduces roughly the circadian secretion of cortisol. Cortisol analogs may also be used in equivalent doses, which are 5 mg and 0.5 mg for prednisone and dexamethasone, respectively. Mineralocorticoid substitution is obtained by 9α-fluorocortisol at 0.05 to 0.2 mg per day given in the morning, with liberal salt intake.

The evaluation of glucocorticoid replacement is based on the clinical judgement of a patient's subjective feeling, and the aim of treatment should be to administrate the smallest dose that keeps the patient's well-being at a nor-

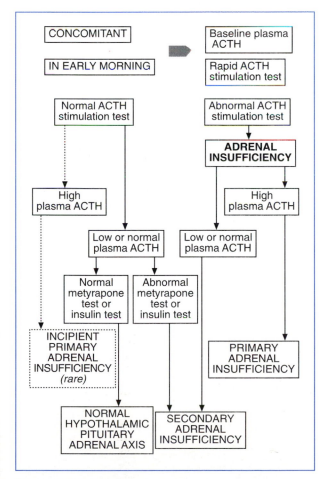

Figure 27.1 Diagnostic approach to primary and secondary adrenal insufficiency.

mal level. Mineralocorticoid adequacy is obtained when blood pressure, sodium, potassium, and plasma renin levels are normal without orthostatic hypotension and tachycardia. Increasing 9α-fluorocortisol doses in the summertime is required for some patients.

Educating the patient and his or her family members is crucial to avoid adrenal crises. They should be instructed to make the appropriate increase in glucocorticoid doses when needed, which must be doubled or tripled at the onset of minor illnesses for 24 or 48 hours. Similar increments are necessary, under medical supervision, for the administration of drugs that accelerate hepatic metabolism of cortisol, such as rifampin, phenytoin, phenobarbital, mitotane, and aminoglutethimide. Parenteral glucocorticoids should be prescribed (hydrocortisone phosphate or succinate, 100 mg, or dexamethasone sodium phosphate, 4 mg) and should be carried by the patient at all times. He or she should receive them immediately at times of vomiting or diarrhea, along with seeking medical attention. In addition, a medical information card or bracelet should be supplied that indicates the patient's diagnosis and treatment.

Moderately stressful situations, such as arteriography, CT scan, endoscopy, and barium enema should be covered by the administration of 100 mg iv hydrocortisone before the procedure. In cases of severe illness or trauma, patients should be treated as described below for acute adrenal insufficiency.

When major surgery is scheduled, the clinical and electrolyte status should be assessed and, eventually, corrected. In order to reproduce the normal increase of cortisol secretion during surgery, 100 mg hydrocortisone is given intravenously or intramuscularly before anesthesia, and another 50 mg iv or im in the recovery room. After that, iv or im are given every 6 hours for the first 24 hours. The dose is tapered by half per day, and maintenance doses are resumed in 3 to 5 days. Mineralocorticoid (9α-fluorocortisol) is re-introduced at the previously used dose as soon as that patient can take oral medications. However, in cases of complications, the high glucocorticoid dosage (200 to 400 mg per day) should be maintained.

During pregnancy the hormone replacement dosages are usually not modified. A slight increase in glucocorticoid or mineralocorticoid may be required in the second and third trimesters. During labor, hydration is provided by saline infusion, and 25 to 50 mg cortisol iv or im is administrated every 6 hours. At the time of delivery, the dosage is increased at 100 mg every 6 hours, then rapidly tapered to the usual oral dose within 3 days, while mineralocorticoid treatment is resumed.

SECONDARY ADRENAL INSUFFICIENCY

The etiology of secondary adrenal insufficiency (Tab. 27.3) includes the most common cause of adrenal insufficiency, namely, chronic administration of pharmacological

Table 27.3 Causes of secondary adrenal insufficiency

Long-term glucocorticoid administration
Selective cure of Cushing's syndrome
Pituitary adenomas
  non secreting
  secreting
Craniopharyngiomas
Metastatic tumors
Lymphocytic hypophysitis
Sarcoidosis, histiocytosis
Sheehan's syndrome
Pituitary surgery, radiotherapy
Isolated ACTH deficiency

dosages of glucocorticoids. This subject is discussed further in the chapter on glucocorticoid therapy (Chap. 31).

A similar situation occurs after the selective cure of *Cushing's syndrome* by removal of ACTH-secreting pituitary or non-pituitary or unilateral cortisol-secreting adrenal tumors. Progressive return to normal function is expected in such situations following an evolution that may take several months (or years).

Secondary adrenal deficiency is a component of *panhypopituitarism*, which may be caused by any process involving the pituitary or the hypothalamus. In this setting, growth hormone and gonadotropic insufficiencies are more frequently encountered than impairment of ACTH and TSH secretion. Hypothalamic lesions (craniopharyngioma, sarcoidosis, histiocytosis) and metastatic tumors are often associated with diabetes insipidus, while this is very rarely the case for adenomas of the pituitary. In patients with *secreting pituitary adenomas*, signs of adrenal deficiency may be obscured by the syndrome of oversecretion (e.g., acromegaly) and should be systematically evaluated. *Lymphocytic hypophysitis* is diagnosed more often, at present, through modern pituitary imaging techniques. It should be considered any time a pituitary mass is discovered during late pregnancy or after delivery. Progress in obstetrical care is responsible for the decreased incidence of pituitary infarction occurring after excessive blood loss at delivery (*Sheehan's syndrome*). Hemorrhage into a pituitary tumor (*pituitary apoplexy*) may lead to acute adrenal insufficiency. It has been possibly precipitated by stimulation tests (luteinizing hormone-releasing hormone, thyrotropin-releasing hormone, growth hormone-releasing hormone, corticotropin-releasing hormone alone or in combination) in some patients bearing macroadenomas.

Iatrogenic panhypopituitarism occurs after surgery to sellar or parasellar lesions. It is also a frequent, but often delayed, complication of radiotherapy. ACTH deficiency is observed in 30% of patients within 10 years after this treatment. This complication should be expected and evaluated not only after irradiation for hypothalamic and pituitary tumors, but also after such therapy for any cranial, facial, and otorhinolaryngeal process.

Isolated ACTH deficiency is an acquired rare disorder, probably due to an autoimmune process, and occurring mostly in middle-aged patients. It is a primary pituitary defect since ACTH fails to respond to stimulation by corticotropin-releasing hormone or vasopressin.

Pathophysiology

The main effect of ACTH deficiency is decreased secretion of cortisol and adrenal androgens. Initially, basal production is maintained, but the hormones cannot increase in times of stress. In time, basal secretion decreases and the adrenal glands become atrophic and unable to respond to acute stimulation by ACTH.

The renin-angiotensin-aldosterone system is initially preserved. Hyponatremia, when present, is due to glucocorticoid deficiency and water retention. However, in cases of profound and long-standing ACTH decrease, mineralocorticoid deficiency may develop, with hyporeninemia. Most often, the situation returns to normal after glucocorticoid treatment.

Clinical findings

The clinical presentation of secondary adrenal insufficiency is similar to those suffering from Addison's disease, with the exception of absent hyperpigmentation. In contrast, pallor of the skin is usually observed in hypopituitarism. Additionally, dehydration and hyperkalemia are usually absent. These patients have commonly-associated features of pituitary or hypothalamic tumor, such as headaches, visual defects, and hypo- or hypersecretion of other pituitary hormones.

Diagnostic procedures

Abnormal cortisol response to the rapid ACTH stimulation test, associated with normal or subnormal plasma ACTH levels, is diagnostic of secondary adrenal insufficiency (Fig. 27.1). The aldosterone increase after ACTH stimulation remains normal in these patients. However, in almost 30% of cases of ACTH deficiency, the cortisol response to rapid ACTH stimulation may be normal. In such situations, more specific information should be obtained by using the metyrapone test or insulin-induced hypoglycemia test. A subnormal response to either of these tests confirms secondary adrenal insufficiency in the presence of normal or low ACTH levels. These patients are further evaluated for deficiencies or oversecretions of the other pituitary hormones. In addition, the presence of mass lesions of the hypothalamus or pituitary is looked for by CT or MRI scan.

Treatment

Treatment for chronic secondary adrenal insufficiency is similar to that of primary deficiency, except that mineralocorticoids are seldom necessary. Glucocorticoids are used in addition to the substitution of the other pituitary hormones, as required.

ACUTE ADRENAL INSUFFICIENCY

Acute adrenal insufficiency is a medical emergency that is too often misdiagnosed. It may occur in a patient with known and treated adrenal insufficiency, in the presence of a stressful situation such as infection, trauma, or surgery, if the dose of glucocorticoid treatment has not been appropriately increased, or if the patient cannot retain medication because of vomiting. In such situations acute adrenal insufficiency develops rapidly – presenting with gastrointestinal symptoms, which include anorexia, nausea, vomiting and abdominal pain – and mimics an acute surgical abdomen. Fever is commonly associated and may be due to hypoadrenalism itself, as well as to an infection. Hypotension may develop into hypovolemic shock with apathy and confusion. In the previously undiagnosed patient, these clinical features are highly misleading, unless a history of symptoms of chronic insufficiency and the presence of hyperpigmentation (in the case of primary adrenal disease) suggests the diagnosis. In the case of adrenal hemorrhage causing acute destruction of the glands, the presenting features are abdominal or flank pain, in addition to rapidly developing signs of acute adrenal insufficiency.

Hyponatremia, hyperkalemia, lymphocytosis, and eosinophilia are frequently present. The confirmation of the diagnosis should not delay the institution of therapy. In the majority of cases, it is sufficient to obtain a plasma sample that will allow for the assay of cortisol (and ideally ACTH). If the plasma cortisol level is below 20 µg/dl (SI = 0.56 µmol/l) in the face of hypovolemia or shock, the diagnosis is confirmed. The measurement of ACTH in the same sample is not always possible in an emergency situation, since it requires that the blood sample is properly processed. A rapid (30-minute) ACTH stimulation test may be obtained, if desired, without delaying the appropriate therapy, by use of dexamethasone as a starting glucocorticoid, which does not interfere with cortisol assay.

Treatment. In the face of a strong clinical suspicion for acute adrenal insufficiency, blood is drawn for the measurement of electrolytes, glucose, cortisol and (if possible) ACTH, and treatment is instituted immediately, without waiting for the results. It includes vigorous intravenous rehydration by saline 0.9% or 5% glucose in 0.9% saline (e.g., 2 liters in 3 hours), which should be continued at a lower rate for the next 24 to 48 hours. Hydrocortisone iv 100 mg is injected as soon as possible, and given every 6 hours iv or im at the same dose for the first 24 hours. At this dosage cortisol has sufficient salt-retaining action so that mineralocorticoids are not necessary.

Any precipitating illness should be explored and appropriately treated. In the absence of complications, treatment can be tapered within 3 to 5 days and oral mineralocorticoids (9α-fluorocortisol 0.1 mg/day) are started when the patient is able to take food and when hydrocortisone has been decreased to less than 60 mg per day.

ISOLATED MINERALOCORTICOID DEFICIENCY

Isolated mineralocorticoid deficiency is a diagnosis considered in the presence of unexplained hyperkalemia when Addison's disease has been excluded. It is related either to *hyporeninism with secondary hypoaldosteronism*, or to *primary hypoaldosteronism with hyperreninism*. Resistance to aldosterone action is also an infrequent cause (*pseudohypoaldosteronism*).

Hyporeninemic hypoaldosteronism occurs mainly in 50- to 70-year-old persons with mild or moderate renal insufficiency, which does not explain the hyperkalemia. Half of the patients have diabetes, and the remainder suffer from interstitial nephritis, multiple myeloma, sickle cell anemia, AIDS, amyloidosis, or systemic lupus erythematosus. Diagnosis should eliminate spurious hyperkalemia (hemolysis, thrombocytosis, leukocytosis), as well as drugs that induce hyperkalemia (angiotensin-converting enzyme inhibitors, potassium-sparing diuretics, β-adrenergic antagonists, cyclooxygenase inhibitors, heparin). Hypochloremic acidosis is frequently associated and hyponatremia is only occasionally present. Plasma renin and aldosterone levels are low and they are not stimulated by upright posture or sodium depletion, while aldosterone increases after ACTH administration.

Treatment depends on the clinical findings. In the presence of hypertension or heart failure, diuretics (furo-semide) are the preferred therapy, which can ameliorate the hyperkalemia. Mineralocorticoid substitution (9α-fluorocortisol, starting at 0.1 mg/day) is reserved for the remainder.

Primary hypoaldosteronism with hyperreninism may be related to a rare congenital defect in aldosterone biosynthesis with salt wasting and hyperkalemia, which is transmitted as an autosomal recessive disease. Treatment provides the usual dosage of 9α-fluorocortisol. In addition, this may be an acquired condition. It may be observed during heparin therapy in predisposed patients (diabetics). It also occurs in over 50% of critically ill, hypotensive patients.

Pseudohypoaldosteronism. In rare cases, infants or children have salt wasting and hyperkalemia, despite elevated plasma renin and aldosterone levels. Pituitary-adrenal function is normal, and the patients do not respond to high doses of mineralocorticoids. An autosomal recessive transmission has been inconsistently reported. Treatment provides sodium and bicarbonate supplementation, which generally maintains the patients in good condition. Potassium-binding resins may be necessary to treat the hyperkalemia. This syndrome is related to inactivating mutations of the epithelial sodium channel. Partial unresponsiveness to mineralocorticoids occurs in pregnancy. It also occurs in a rare and peculiar familial syndrome called *pseudohypoaldosteronism type 2*, which has been described in children and young adults with hyperkalemia, hyperchloremia, metabolic acidosis, hypertension, and low plasma levels of renin and aldosterone. Large doses of mineralocorticoids are ineffective on hyperkalemia. This condition is successfully treated with thiazide diuretics.

Suggested readings

AUBOURG P, CHAUSSAIN J-L. Adrenoleukodystrophy presenting as Addison's disease in children and adults. Trends Endocrinol Metab 1991;2:49-52.

BLEVINS LS JR, SHANKROFF J, MOSER HW, LADENSON PW. Elevated plasma adrenocorticotropin concentration as evidence of limited adrenocortical reserve in patients with adrenomyeloneuropathy. J Clin Endocrinol Metab 1994;78:261-5.

BROSNAN CM, GOWING NFC. Addison's disease. B M J 1996;312:1085-7.

DE FRONZO R A. Hyperkalemia and hyporeninemic hypoaldosteronism. Kidney Int 1980;17:118-34.

KELJO DJ, SQUIRES RH JR. Clinical problem - solving. Just in time. N Engl J Med 1996;334:46-8.

KYRIAZOPOULOU V, PAPAROUSI O, VAGENAKIS A. Rifampicin-induced adrenal crisis in addisonian patients receiving corticosteroid replacement therapy. J Clin Endocrinol Metab 1984;59:1204-6.

LEIGH H, KRAMER SI. The psychiatric manifestations of endocrine disease. Adv Intern Med 1984;29:413-45.

LESHIN M. Polyglandular autoimmune syndromes. Am J Med Sci 1985;290:77-88.

MAJOR P, KUCHEL O, BOUCHER R, NOWACZYNSKI W, GENEST J. Selective hypopituitarism with severe hyponatremia and secondary hyporeninism. J Clin Endocrinol Metab 1978;46:15-9.

NERUP J. Addison's disease-clinical studies: a report of 108 cases. Acta Endocrinol (Copenh) 1974;76:127-41.

OELKERS W. Adrenal insufficiency. N Engl J Med 1996;335:1206-12.

RAO RH, VAGNUCCI AH, AMICO JA. Bilateral massive adrenal hemorrhage: a early recognition and treatment. Ann Intern Med 1989;110:227-35.

SELLMEYER DE, GRUNFELD C. Endocrine and metabolic disturbances in human immunodeficiency virus infection and the acquired immune deficiency syndrome. Endocr Rev 1996;17:518-32.

Biosynthetic disorders: congenital adrenal hyperplasia

Maria I. New

■ KEY POINTS

- Congenital adrenal hyperplasia is a family of inborn errors of steroidogenesis, primarily characterized by a specific enzyme deficiency that impairs cortisol production by the adrenal cortex, and can lead to sexual ambiguity in both genetic males and females.
- The enzymes most often affected are 21-hydroxylase and 11β-hdroxylase.
- Correct identification of the enzyme affected is achieved by the observation of clinical syndromes reflecting distinct hormonal patterns, and it is measured quantitatively as abnormally low or high glucocorticoid, mineralocorticoid, progestogen and/or sex steroid levels.
- In the classical forms of congenital adrenal hyperplasia, adrenal androgen *overproduction* causes virilization at birth in females and precocious development postnatally in both sexes, whereas *impairment* of androgen synthesis in adrenals and gonads causes insufficient virilization of males at birth and in both sexes failure of pubertal development.
- In the nonclassical form of 21-hydroxylase deficiency congenital adrenal hyperplasia, as with the classical form, both males and females may present with signs of androgen excess postnatally. Patients often present with short stature, hirsutism, premature development of pubic hair, severe cystic acne refractory to antibiotics, and oligomenorrhea, and may be infertile unless proper treatment is instituted.
- Hydrocortisone (cortisol) is the most often used compound for glucocorticoid replacement therapy for 21-hydroxylase deficiency and 11β-hydroxylase deficiency. Patients with nonclassical 21-hydroxylase deficiency are treated with low doses of dexamethasone.
- It has been shown that the prenatal treatment with dexamethasone of female fetuses affected with 21-hydroxylase (and recently with 11β-hydroxylase) deficiency can greatly reduce or prevent virilization of external genitalia, preventing the need for later genital surgery.

Congenital adrenal hyperplasia (CAH) is a family of inborn errors of steroidogenesis, primarily characterized by a specific enzyme deficiency that impairs cortisol production by the adrenal cortex, and can lead to sexual ambiguity in both genetic males and females. The enzymes most often affected are 21-hydroxylase, 11β-hydroxylase, and 3β-hydroxysteroid dehydrogenase, and less often, 17α-hydroxylase/17,20-lyase, and the steroidogenic acute regulatory protein (StAR) (Tab. 28.1).

Many of the corresponding genes for the described enzymes have been isolated and characterized, and specific mutations causing many cases of CAH have been identified. These advances have important implications for early prenatal diagnosis and prenatal treatment.

Adrenal steroidogenesis and fetal development The adrenal cortex produces cortisol and aldosterone by separate regulatory systems. The production of cortisol occurs in the zona fasciculata of the cortex, while aldosterone is produced in the zona glomerulosa (for a simplified scheme of adrenal steroidogenesis, see Fig. 26.1). Cortisol is synthesized under the trophic control of ACTH, forming a negative feedback loop in which high serum cortisol centrally inhibits and low serum cortisol stimulates release of ACTH. The adrenal enzyme deficiencies described above, causing impaired synthesis and decreased secretion of cortisol, thus lead to chronic elevations of ACTH, and overstimulation and consequent hyperplasia of the adrenal cortex.

Without these enzyme abnormalities, male genital differentiation in embryonic and fetal life is dependent on two functions of the testes: (1) the secretion of sufficient quantities of testosterone to direct the formation of the internal male genital structures from the wolffian ducts; and (2) the secretion of the anti-mullerian hormone glycoprotein to suppress development of the mullerian ducts, which would develop into the female internal structures (i.e., the fallopian tubes, uterus, cervix, and upper vagina). Testosterone, after peripheral conversion to dihydrotestosterone, is required for normal formation of the male external genitalia. Dihydrotestosterone is also responsible for the formation of the scrotum from the genital swellings, midline closure of the genital folds, elongation into the body of the phallus, and extension of the urogenital sinus by fusion along the ventral groove to form a penile urethra.

21-HYDROXYLASE DEFICIENCY

Clinical findings

Decreased cortisol synthesis owing to impaired steroid 21-hydroxylation is by far the most common biochemical cause of congenital adrenal hyperplasia, making up 90 to

Table 28.1 Clinical and laboratory features of various disorders of adrenal steroidogenesis

Deficiency (syndrome)	Genital ambiguity	Postnatal virilization	Salt metabolism	Diagnostic hormones	Treatment
21-Hydroxylase					
I. Classic					
Salt wasting	F	Yes	Salt wasting	17-OHP[a], Δ^4	HC, 15-20 mg/m²/d PO, and 9αFF, 0.05-0.2 mg/d PO
Simple virilizing	F	Yes	Normal (↑ renin)	17-OHP[a], Δ^4	HC (same); addition of 9αFF (same) if ↑ renin
II. Nonclassic	No	Yes	Normal		HC, 10-15 mg/m²/d or dexamethasone, 0.25-0.5 mg/d hs, or prednisone 5-10 mg/d
11β-Hydroxylase					
I. Classic (hypertensive CAH)	F	Yes	Salt retention	DOC[a], S	HC, 15-20 mg/m²/d
II. Nonclassic	No	Yes	Normal	S ± DOC	HC, dexamethasone, or prednisone as for NC 21-OHD
3β-Hydroxysteroid dehydrogenase					
I. Classic	M	Yes	Salt wasting	17-OHP[a], DHEA	HC and 9αFF as for SW 21-OHD[b]
II. Nonclassic	No	Yes	Normal	17-OHP, DHEA	HC as for NC 21-OHD
17α-Hydroxylase	M	No	Salt retention	DOC[a], B	HC, 15-20 mg/m²/d[b]
17,20-Lyase	M	No	Normal	None	HC, 15-20 mg/m²/d
StAR (lipoid hyperplasia)	M	No	Salt wasting	None	HC, 15-20 mg/m²/d 9αFF, 0.05-0.2 mg/d[b]

[a] Increased in serum of affected patients before or after ACTH stimulation.
[b] With addition of sex steroid replacement at puberty.
(17-OHP = 17-hydroxyprogesterone; Δ^4 = Δ^4-androstenedione; HC = hydrocortisone; 9αFF = fludrocortisone acetate; DHEA = dehydroepiandrosterone; StAR = steroidogenic acute regulatory protein; NC = nonclassic; SW = salt wasting.)

95% of cases. Complete and near-complete blocks of the 21-hydroxylase (21-OH) enzyme produce the classical form of CAH, which occurs in 1 in 15 000 live births worldwide and higher in certain ethnic groups. The degree of androgen excess causes external genital ambiguity in newborn females, and progressive postnatal virilization in males and females, including precocious pubic hair, advanced somatic and epiphyseal development and induced central precocious puberty in childhood. The allelically distinct, milder nonclassical form of 21-OH deficiency has a frequency of 1 in 100 in the heterogeneous population. The general timing of the appearance of symptoms is shown in Figure 28.1.

Classic 21-hydroxylase deficiency occurs in two forms: simple virilizing and salt wasting. In *simple virilizing* 21-hydroxylase deficiency, which occurs in approximately one-third to one-fourth of the cases, developmental genital anomalies are manifest in females in varying degrees of genital virilization. The extent of masculinization ranges from mild clitoral enlargement, through varying degrees of fusion of the labioscrotal folds (posterior to anterior), to the formation of a penile urethra. Since there is no anomalous production of anti-mullerian hormone in the gonadally normal female, females presenting with even extreme virilization from androgen excess will have normal development of their internal reproductive structures, allowing for childbearing if diagnosed and treated. In regards to the virilizing forms of CAH, progressive differentiation towards the male type in genetic females has been given a five-stage classification by Prader. Genital development in males is normal, which is why the syndrome often goes unrecognized until signs of androgen excess appear in later childhood.

In two-thirds to three-fourths of classical cases, *salt wasting* also occurs. Renal salt wasting results from inadequate secretion of salt-retaining steroids, especially aldosterone, and may be manifested soon after birth by a shock-like state with low serum concentrations of sodium, depleted fluid volume, and very high serum potassium

levels. While these crises are anticipated in females because of the genital ambiguity that promotes their immediate diagnosis, males may appear completely normal and are in jeopardy of entering a salt-wasting crisis at home. Salt losing in infancy from an aldosterone biosynthetic defect may improve with age, and possible adjustments in sodium intake and mineralocorticoid replacement in patients labelled neonatally as salt wasters can be made on the basis of careful monitoring of plasma renin activity.

Nonclassic 21-hydroxylase deficiency refers to the condition in which partial deficiencies of 21-hydroxylation produce late-onset less extreme hyperandrogenemia and milder symptoms (Fig. 28.1). Females do not demonstrate genital ambiguity at birth, though both males and females may manifest signs of androgen excess at any phase of postnatal development. In pubertal-age girls, menarche may be delayed, and in adolescent and young adult females, secondary amenorrhea is common. In women, hirsutism, oligomenorrhea or amenorrhea, and/or polycystic ovary disease may be seen. In males, oligospermia has been found in some cases. For men and women, adult stature below genetic potential, insulin resistance, and reduced fertility are also seen in untreated groups. See Table 28.2 for the diagnostic criteria for steroid 21-OH deficiency.

Diagnostic procedures

Hormonal diagnosis For classical 21-hydroxylase deficiency, progesterone, 17-hydroxyprogesterone, androstenedione, and testosterone are secreted in excess. The urinary excretion of the metabolites of these steroids is also increased. Hormonal diagnosis of 21-OH deficiency of any degree is best achieved by an ACTH stimulation test, which involves taking a blood sample to measure the serum 17-hydroxyprogesterone concentration before and 60 minutes after intravenous administration of 0.25 mg synthetic $ACTH_{1-24}$ (Cortrosyn). Testing should be done early in the morning since serum 17-hydroxyprogesterone concentrations are elevated at this time (morning salivary levels also correlate with serum concentration). Random basal serum concentrations may not differ from that of normal in non-classical patients. As seen in Figure 28.2, nomogram plots of baseline versus stimulated 17-hydroxyprogesterone concentrations result in three distinguishable groups: classical, nonclassical, and an overlap of heterozygotes and genetically unaffected. It should be noted that serum 17-hydroxyprogesterone may be elevated in premature infants and infants under stress, which can result in false-positives.

Molecular genetics The molecular genetic basis of 21-hydroxylase deficiency has been studied extensively. The gene encoding 21-hydroxylase (a microsomal cytochrome P450 termed P450C21) is located on the short arm of chromosome 6 in the HLA complex. The gene locus for the 21-OH enzyme is termed CYP21. Approximately 40

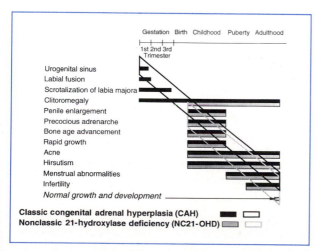

Figure 28.1 Clinical spectrum of steroid 21-OHD. There is a wide spectrum of clinical presentations ranging from prenatal virilization with labial fusion, to precocious adrenarche, to pubertal or postpubertal virilization.

> **Table 28.2** Diagnosis of the forms of steroid 21-hydroxylase deficiency

Indications for testing
The following clinical signs and symptoms should lead the physician to consider the diagnosis of steroid 21-hydroxylase deficiency:

In the neonate
Ambiguity of the genitalia in the genetic female, including clitoromegaly, fusion of the labia majora and minora, and urogenital sinus
History of a previously affected member of the family
Cryptorchid testes, not responsive to human chorionic gonadotropin (hCG)

In childhood
Advanced stature or advanced bone age
Precocious appearance of sexual hair
Seborrhea or acne; oily hair
Recession (frontal or temporal) of the hairline
Enlarged clitoris, fusion (posteroanterior) of the labia in genetic females
Enlarged penis relative to the size and volume of the testes in males
Early onset of puberty

At pubertal age and after puberty
Short stature with history of early growth
Excessive hair on the face, abdomen, inner thighs, or arms
Enlarged or enlarging clitoris in the female
Infertility in either sex

Testing
Give Cortrosyn (synthetic $ACTH_{1-24}$) 0.25 mg iv bolus at 8 a.m.
Obtain blood at the time of Cortrosyn administration (0 minutes) and again after 60 minutes
Separate serum samples (and freeze if necessary). Submit serum for 17α-hydroxyprogesterone measurement
Compare values with those shown on the nomogram (Fig. 28.2) and score for indicated 21-hydroxylase genotype

Interpretation of results
The coordinates of the baseline and ACTH-stimulated values form a regression line, and subjects aggregate into groups around the regression line. Patients with classic CAH have the most severe 21-hydroxylase deficiency. Patients with the symptomatic or asymptomatic nonclassic forms have a less sever deficiency, while heterozygotes for all three forms have an even milder deficiency that is unmasked only with ACTH stimulation. Those members of the general population who are in the heterozygote range may be carriers of a gene for 21-hydroxylase deficiency (Fig. 28.2)

CYP21 mutations causative of CAH have been identified and characterized, some of which have been linked to certain ethnic groups. It should be noted, however, that though the functional consequence of each DNA lesion generally corresponds to the clinical severity of the inherited disease, phenotype is not always as predicted by genotype. This remains to be explained.

11β-HYDROXYLASE DEFICIENCY

The second most common cause of CAH is 11β-hydroxylase deficiency, representing 5 to 8% of all cases in the general population, though it was found to be more common in an Israeli population of Moroccan Jewish origin. Like 21-OH deficiency, 11β-OH deficiency occurs late in cortisol synthesis, causing a shunting of accumulating precursor steroids into pathways of androgen biosynthesis, producing genital ambiguity in affected girls and postnatal hyperandrogenism in both sexes. In 11β-OH deficiency, an excess of the mineralocorticoid deoxycorticosterone (DOC) causes expanded fluid volume and

hypertension. As with 21-OH deficiency, cases of mild, late-onset forms of 11β-OH deficiency have also been reported.

The diagnosis of 11β-OH deficiency is established by means of an ACTH test similar to that for 21-OH deficiency, except that the important diagnostic hormones are deoxycorticosterone and 11-deoxycortisol, both of which are elevated, while plasma renin activity is markedly suppressed.

The human adrenal cortex expresses the 11β-hydroxylating enzyme responsible for completing cortisol biosynthesis (cytochrome P450c11) from CYP11B1, located on chromosome 8q. Numerous mutations in CYP11B1 have been identified in cases of 11β-OH deficiency.

3β-HYDROXYSTEROID DEHYDROGENASE

In 3β-hydroxysteroid dehydrogenase deficiency (3β-HSD), steroid synthesis in both the adrenal cortex and in the gonads is affected, and only largely inert steroid precursors are formed and secreted. Circulating androgen pre-

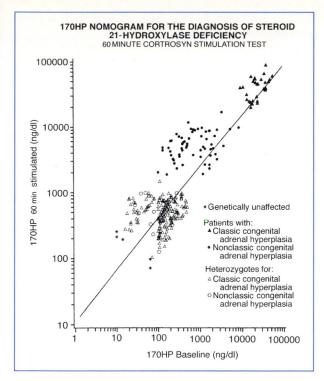

170HP NOMOGRAM FOR THE DIAGNOSIS OF STEROID 21-HYDROXYLASE DEFICIENCY
60 MINUTE CORTROSYN STIMULATION TEST

• Genetically unaffected

Patients with:
▲ Classic congenital adrenal hyperplasia
• Nonclassic congenital adrenal hyperplasia

Heterozygotes for:
△ Classic congenital adrenal hyperplasia
○ Nonclassic congenital adrenal hyperplasia

Figure 28.2 Nomogram relating baseline to corticotropin-stimulated serum concentrations of 17-hydroxyprogesterone. Scales are logarithmic. A regression line for all data points is shown.

cursors undergo conversion peripherally to potent androgens. In genetic females with the classical deficiency, virilization of the external genitalia occurs. In males, because of the testicular defect, prenatal differentiation of the external genitalia is incomplete. Thus, genital ambiguity results in both sexes. 3β-HSD deficiency may also exist in a milder, nonclassical form.

The severity of the enzyme defect may not be concluded on the basis of the appearance of the external genitalia at birth. A high ratio of $\Delta^5:\Delta^4$ steroids is diagnostic for 3β-HSD deficiency. An ACTH stimulation test highlights this abnormality. Serum pregnenolone, 17α-hydroxypregnenolone and DHEA concentrations are elevated, and the levels of the Δ^5 metabolites pregnenetriol and 16-pregnenetriol are elevated in the urine. A dexamethasone suppression test is indicated to rule out an adrenal or ovarian steroid-producing tumor.

Analysis of DNA from patients with classic 3β-HSD deficiency has confirmed a monogenic autosomal recessive mode of transmission for the HSD3B2 gene.

17α-HYDROXYLASE/17,20-LYASE DEFICIENCY

Steroid 17α-hydroxylase/17,20-lyase deficiency is an infrequent cause of CAH, accounting for about 1% of cases overall. Patients have a decreased ability to synthesize cortisol, leading to elevated ACTH, which increases serum levels of deoxycorticosterone and especially corti-

costerone, and resulting in low-renin hypertension, hypokalemia, and metabolic alkalosis. Both adrenal glucocorticoids and sex steroids are diminished. Isolated 17,20-lyase has also been observed, which results in deficient C19 sex steroids in the adrenals and gonads.

Affected females have normal genitalia at birth but at adolescence do not enter puberty. Affected males can be born with external female genitalia due to their deficient gonadal testosterone production, though a uterus and fallopian tubes do not develop since anti-mullerian hormone secretion by Sertoli cells inhibits mullerian duct development. The wolffian ducts are incompletely developed as well.

Hormonal diagnosis is made by the serum presence of very high corticosterone levels and high deoxycorticosterone levels, in addition to high levels of their metabolites. Because of the excess deoxycorticosterone, aldosterone levels may be low due to suppressed renin and hypokalemia, even though the aldosterone pathway is intact.

The CYP17 gene encodes the 17α-hydroxylase enzyme (also a cytochrome P450) and is located on chromosome 10, region q24-q25. To date about 17 mutations have been described.

LIPOID CONGENITAL ADRENAL HYPERPLASIA

Lipoid congenital adrenal hyperplasia is extremely rare. Cholesterol is not converted to pregnenolone, which profoundly impairs synthesis of all steroids and results in massive accumulations of cholesterol and cholesterol esters. Males are born with female-appearing external genitalia but have undescended testes, females have a normal genital phenotype at birth but remain sexually infantile without treatment, and all patients present with salt wasting. If not detected and treated, lipoid CAH is fatal in newborns.

Abnormalities of the steroidogenic acute regulatory protein (StAR) are responsible for this disorder. StAR is involved in the transfer of cholesterol from the outer to the inner mitochondrial membrane, where it is then converted to pregnenolone. The gene encoding StAR is on chromosome 8, region p11.2, where mutations were found that result in lipoid CAH.

Treatment

See Table 28.1 for a summary of treatment guidelines in CAH.

In CAH due to 21-hydroxylase deficiency, glucocorticoid replacement therapy not only replaces the deficient hormone but also reduces the overstimulation of the adrenal cortex by reducing the release of ACTH, thereby suppressing the overproduction of adrenal androgens. Hydrocortisone (cortisol) is the most often used compound for replacement therapy for 21-OH, 11β-OH, and 17α-hydroxylase deficiencies. Proper replacement therapy in 21-OH and 11β-OH deficiencies prevents further virilization, slowing accelerated growth and bone age advancement to a more normal rate, and allowing a normal onset of puberty. In 11β-OH and 17α-hydroxylase deficiencies, glucocorticoid treatment suppresses the oversecretion of deoxycorticosterone and leads to the remission of hypertension. Excessive glucocorticoid administration can cause cushingoid facies, growth retardation, and inhibition of epiphyseal maturation.

Hydrocortisone is a physiologic hormone and so minimizes complications. Oral administration is the usual mode of treatment, conventionally given daily in divided doses, as it is believed divided doses better suppress the production of adrenal androgens. Given in two doses of 10-20 mg/m^2 daily is adequate for the otherwise healthy child. The dosage may have to be increased for a few days to 2 to 3 times that of the normal daily dosage during times of nonlife-threatening illness or stress. Families should be given injection kits of hydrocortisone (50 mg for young children; 100 mg for older patients) for times of emergency. Up to 5 to 10 times the daily dosage may be required during surgical procedures. Patients who show a poor response to the standard dosage of hydrocortisone may have their dosage increased to 20-30 mg/m^2 per day, or their regimen may have to be changed to a synthetic hormone analog such as prednisone or dexamethasone. The use of these analogs require critical dosage adjustment since they are more potent and longer-acting.

Patients with salt-wasting CAH may also require mineralocorticoid replacement. A cortisol analogue, 21-acetyloxy-9α-fluorohydrocortisone (9α-FF), is used for its potent mineralocorticoid activity. A combination of hydrocortisone and 9α-FF has proven to be quite effective in the treatment of patients with salt-wasting 21-OH deficiency.

Patients with nonclassical 21-OH deficiency and nonclassical 3β-HSD deficiency are treated with glucocorticoids if they manifest symptoms of androgen excess. In cases of excess ovarian androgen production, women may have to be suppressed by the use of progestational and estrogenic agents by suppression of the release of gonadotropins. Other antiandrogen agents that may help include spironolactone and cyproterone acetate, and the androgen receptor blocker, flutamide. The aim of treatment in these patients is to minimize symptoms without giving rise to glucocorticoid side effects.

In lipoid congenital adrenal hyperplasia, as all steroidogenic enzymes are normal, a substrate for steroidogenesis can be used for the effective treatment of patients. Freely diffusable 20α-hydroxycholesterol is recommended, which must be implemented as a lifelong treatment plan.

Prenatal diagnosis and treatment

Prenatal treatment of female fetuses affected with 21-OH can greatly reduce or prevent virilization of external genitalia, preventing the need for later genital surgery. For this outcome, prenatal treatment in pregnancies at risk must be initiated before 10 weeks of gestation. Dexamethasone (20 µg/kg per day divided into 3 doses) given orally to mothers at-risk, blind to the status of the fetus, suppresses fetal adrenal androgen secretion. Depending on which procedure is available, either chorionic villus sampling (10 to 12 weeks of gestation) or amniocentesis (15 to 18 weeks of gestation) is performed. Fetal cells are cultured for karyotyping and DNA analysis for CAH mutations. If the fetus is male or unaffected, prenatal treatment is terminated. Prenatal treatment is continued to term for affected female fetuses.

Prenatal treatment for the fetus with low doses of dexamethasone does not appear to have any side effects even after in excess of 10 years' follow-up, despite some findings in rodents that high doses of dexamethasone resulted in cleft palate formation in utero and placental degeneration with fetal death. Maternal side effects, such as mood changes, weight gain, pedal and leg edema, and elevated blood pressure, all disappear upon discontinuation of treatment. Due to the positive genital outcome of their prenatally treated daughters, almost all women with complications report that they would undergo dexamethasone treatment again if they became pregnant.

Prenatal diagnosis of 11β-OH deficiency in at-risk pregnancies has been reported, and dexamethasone prenatal treatment for affected fetuses has been attempted and has been found to be as effective as prenatal treatment for 21-OH deficiency.

Acknowledgments

I wish to express my appreciation to Laurie Vandermolen for her editorial assistance.

Suggested readings

NEW MI, CRAWFORD C, WILSON RC. Genetic disorders of the adrenal steroidogenic enzymes. In: Emery AEH and Rimoin D (eds). Principles and practice of medical genetics. 3rd ed. New York: Churchill Livingstone, 1996:1441-76.

NEW MI, WHITE PC. Genetic disorders of steroid metabolism. In: R Thakker, Alberti KGMM, Burger HG, Cohen RD, et al. (eds). Genetic and molecular biological aspects of endocrine diseases. London: Baillière Tindall, 1995:525-54.

29

Cushing's syndrome

Xavier Bertagna, Jean-Pierre Luton

KEY POINTS

- Clinical suspicion of Cushing's syndrome is based on a combination of sensitive (central obesity) and specific (related to protein wasting) signs.
- Measuring cortisol in a 24-hour urinary collection is the easiest and best way to diagnose hypercortisolism.
- The final diagnosis requires sophisticated hormonal testing and imaging procedures best performed in specialized referral centers.
- Pituitary surgery by the transsphenoidal route offers a success rate and quality of cure that undoubtedly designates it as the best therapeutic option in Cushing's disease.

Epidemiology

Cushing's syndrome refers to the manifestations induced by chronic exposition to glucocorticoid excess and may result from various causes. It most commonly arises from iatrogenic causes, when glucocorticoids are given to treat inflammatory diseases; this is specifically dealt with in Chapter 31 "Glucocorticoid Therapy". The present chapter will be devoted to the sole spontaneous causes of chronic hypercortisolism (Tab. 29.1).

Cushing's disease is the most common cause of spontaneous Cushing's syndrome, occurring in 60 to 70% of Cushing's patients. It results from adrenocorticotropic hormone (ACTH) hypersecretion from pituitary corticotroph adenomas.

Ectopic ACTH syndrome is responsible for 5 to 10% of the cases of spontaneous Cushing's syndrome; it is caused by a variety of ACTH-secreting nonpituitary tumors.

About 20 to 30% of Cushing's syndromes are non-ACTH dependent and are caused by primary adrenocortical tumors.

Spontaneous Cushing's syndrome is rare; the estimated incidence is about 1 per 100 000 per year. There is a high female to male ratio (about 3-5:1), except in ectopic ACTH syndrome.

Table 29.1 Causes of spontaneous Cushing's syndrome

ACTH-dependent	
Pituitary ACTH oversecretion	
Cushing's disease	60-70%
CRH-secreting tumors	(rare)
Non pituitary ACTH oversecretion	
Ectopic ACTH syndrome	5-10%
ACTH-independent	
Unilateral adrenocortical tumor	
Adrenocortical adenoma	10-15%
Adrenocortical carcinoma	10-15%
Bilateral adrenocortical involvement	
Primary pigmented nodular	
adrenocortical dysplasia	(rare)
ACTH-independent bilateral	
macronodular adrenocortical hyperplasia	(rare)

Etiopathology

ACTH-DEPENDENT CUSHING'S SYNDROME

Cushing's disease

In Cushing's disease, pituitary ACTH oversecretion induces bilateral adrenocortical hyperplasia and an excess production of cortisol, adrenal androgens, and 11-deoxy-corticosterone.

A pituitary corticotroph adenoma is present – and can be detected at surgery – in the vast majority of patients with Cushing's disease. Most are microadenomas, arbitrarily defined as being less than 10 mm with a mean of approximately 5 mm.

The hallmark of ACTH oversecretion in Cushing's disease is its partial resistance to the normal suppressive effect of glucocorticoids. Because ACTH secretion by the pituitary tumor is not normally restrained, ACTH is over-produced and results in subsequent chronic hypercortisolism. Since peripheral tissues have retained their normal sensitivity to the action of cortisol, they appropriately develop the features of Cushing's disease.

The possibility that Cushing's disease may be caused by a primary hypothalamic defect, where corticotropin-releasing hormone (CRH) overactivity would induce corticotroph cell hyperplasia and ACTH oversecretion, is also advocated by some authors: it is based on the apparent lack of microadenomas in some patients, and on possible corticotroph cell hyperplasia.

The ectopic ACTH syndrome

Various tumors of nonpituitary origin ("nonpituitary tumors") can occasionally produce ACTH. The most frequent of them originate in the thorax; they are the highly aggressive small-cell carcinoma of the lungs, or the slow-growing bronchial or thymic carcinoid tumors. The other most frequent causes are other carcinoid tumors of gastric, pancreatic, and intestinal origin; and pheochromocytomas and medullary thyroid cancers.

The hallmark of the ectopic ACTH syndrome is that its production is completely unresponsive to glucocorticoid feedback, providing the basis of the hormonal investigation.

Corticotropin-releasing hormone-secreting tumors

Rare, hypothalamic tumors have been described, such as gangliocytomas, however more patients have presented with the ectopic CRH syndrome. The most frequent non-hypothalamic tumors responsible for CRH secretion have been the prostate, small cell lung cancers, colon carcinomas, nephroblastoma, thyroid medullary carcinomas, and bronchial carcinoids.

Effects of chronic ACTH oversecretion

In contrast with some other endocrine functions in man,

chronic adrenocortical stimulation by ACTH does not induce a desensitization state. Indeed, the opposite occurs: the adrenocortical response is amplified, and it is not unusual to observe a very high secretion of cortisol in face of "normal" (but constant and inappropriate) ACTH plasma levels.

In response to ACTH, various growth factors are secreted: IGF1, bFGF (basic fibroblast growth factor), and IGF2 participate in stimulating corticosteroid production, the growth of the adrenals, and the adrenal vascular system as well.

The mechanisms of adrenal androgen secretion are grossly parallel with that of cortisol. Thus DHEA, DHEA sulfate, and delta 4-androstenedione are elevated in ACTH-dependent Cushing's syndromes. Their peripheral transformation to testosterone and dihydrotestosterone may lead to a state of androgen excess in females.

Pathology of the adrenal

Whatever the cause of ACTH oversecretion, the most common adrenocortical lesion is bilateral simple diffuse hyperplasia. The two glands are symmetrically (and generally moderately) enlarged, weighing between 5 and 12 g each at operation. The glands are yellow or brown, and the cortex appears regularly widened on section.

A multinodular hyperplasia is present whenever one or several macroscopic yellow nodules are present. Such glands, in general, have a greater weight than in simple diffuse hyperplasia. The size of the nodules displays an extremely wide range of variation, from a few millimeters to several centimeters. Although as a rule they occur in both glands, marked asymmetry is occasionally seen, which may falsely indicate an autonomous adenoma-like lesion.

ACTH-INDEPENDENT SPONTANEOUS CUSHING'S SYNDROMES

Primary adrenocortical tumors: adenomas and carcinomas

Primary adrenocortical tumors cause approximately 20 to 30% of the cases of spontaneous Cushing's syndromes in adults. Benign adenomas and adrenocortical carcinomas distribute evenly. As for Cushing's disease, female preponderance is noted. Chronic glucocorticoid excess induces an appropriate suppression of pituitary ACTH. The contralateral and the non-tumorous ipsilateral adrenals are both atrophic. Cortisol secretion is autonomous and unresponsive to dexamethasone suppression tests.

Most benign adrenocortical adenomas respond to exogenously administered ACTH, and most adrenocortical carcinomas do not. Whereas benign tumors are usually small and exclusively secrete cortisol, malignant tumors are much larger, and they secrete a large array of steroid precursors and androgens.

Adenomas are encapsulated tumors, typically composed of a mixture of compact and clear cells with no nuclear abnormalities.

Carcinomas are larger tumors, often with features of

local invasiveness. They can contain areas of focal hemorrhage, necrosis, or broad fibrous connective tissue bands. Compact and clear cells are found: nuclear polymorphism, mitotic figures, and vascular invasion are indicative of malignancy.

Removal of a benign adrenal adenoma brings about an immediate and definitive cure with often transient, though sometimes long-lasting, hypocorticotropism. Malignant adrenocortical tumors are highly aggressive: in most series the survival rate is only 20% five years after diagnosis.

Primary pigmented nodular adrenocortical dysplasia

Primary pigmented nodular adrenocortical dysplasia is a rare condition that occurs primarily in childhood. Cortisol oversecretion is autonomous with hormone dynamics essentially similar to those encountered in cases of adrenocortical adenomas, yet this primary adrenal disorder is driven by bilateral adrenocortical lesions: the two glands harbor numerous nodular lesions, which typically appear brown or black. The size of the adrenals is classically not increased. Histologically, the nodules consist of typical compact adrenocortical cells with eosinophilic cytoplasm-containing brown pigment. The adrenocortical tissue that lies in between the nodules has been variously described as normal or more often atrophic. Other features add to the concept that adrenocortical nodular dysplasia is a separate entity. Indeed, it may be part of a more complex clinical spectrum called the Carney complex, which associates myxomas of the heart, skin, or breast; pigmented skin lesions; endocrine tumors; and peripheral nerve tumors (schwannomas). The Carney complex is often a hereditary condition transmitted as a Mendelian autosomal dominant trait, whose gene locus was recently situated on chromosome 2p16.

ACTH-independent bilateral macronodular adrenocortical hyperplasia

In ACTH-independent bilateral macronodular adrenocortical hyperplasia, bilaterally hyperplastic and nodular glands, often with large nodules, secrete excess cortisol, and pituitary ACTH is totally suppressed. This condition suggests that non-ACTH factors may induce cortisol hypersecretion by nodular and hyperplastic adrenocortical glands. A recent report convincingly demonstrated that such adrenocortical lesions had acquired an inappropriate sensitivity to gastric inhibitory polypeptide, which stimulated cortisol release in vivo and in vitro, also explaining why the patient had high plasma cortisol increases after meals.

Clinical findings

Symptoms and signs

Centripetal fat deposition is the most common manifestation of glucocorticoid excess and often the initial symptom of the patient. Although weight gain is classic, it may be minimal. The peculiar distribution of adipose tissue readily distinguishes it from simple obesity: fat accumulates in the face and the supraclavicular and dorsocervical fat pads, bringing about the typical moon facies and buffalo hump, which is most often accompanied by facial plethora. Fat also accumulates over the thorax and the abdomen, which becomes protrudent (Figs. 29.1 and 29.2, see Color Atlas). This acquired habitus change is best evidenced by comparison with anterior photographs.

Protein-wasting features

Not as frequent, but certainly crucial, are the clinical features that pertain to the protein-wasting effect of cortisol. Absent in simple obesity, they have a high diagnostic value and must be thoroughly investigated at examination.

Skin thinning due to the atrophy of the epidermis and the underlying connective tissue may be mild and is best appreciated by running the skin gently over the tibial crest; in some patients, the skin is so fragile that it can be scratched simply by removing a strip of adhesive tape. Skin thinning and tension over accumulated fat both account for the plethoric appearance of the face and the purple aspect of striae due to the streaks of capillaries that almost become visible. Striae are present in many patients and are most commonly located on the abdomen and the flanks, and also on the breasts, hips, and axillae. In contrast with the usually whitish and small striae often seen after pregnancy or rapid weight gain, the striae of Cushing's disease are typically purple to red, and more than 1 cm wide. Most patients complain of easy bruisability, whereas this is uncommon in simple obesity. In Cushing's disease, minimal trauma generates multiple ecchymotic lesions or purpura, especially on the forearm, and blood collection often results in large ecchymotics lesions. Minor wounds heal slowly and are the source of postoperative complications at the incision site. The most superficial wounds, particularly frequent on the lower extremities, may lead to indolent infection and ulceration that take months to disappear. Lower limb edema is frequent and does not always result from congestive heart failure but rather from increased capillary permeability. Protein wasting is responsible for a generalized tissue fragility. Surgeons usually find that the tissues tear easily. Spontaneous ruptures occur, mainly of tendons.

Muscle wasting is frequent and characteristically proximal, leading to fatigability and muscle atrophy, particularly in the lower limbs. The weakness may be so severe as to prevent the patient from getting up from a chair without help.

Bone wasting results in general osteoporosis. Particularly vulnerable is the vertebral body. Compression fractures of the spine are evident on plain X-rays in about 20% of the patients, and almost half of the patients complain of backache (Fig. 29.3, see Color Atlas). Kyphosis and loss of height, sometimes dramatic, are frequent. Pathological fractures can occur elsewhere, particularly in the ribs and pelvis.

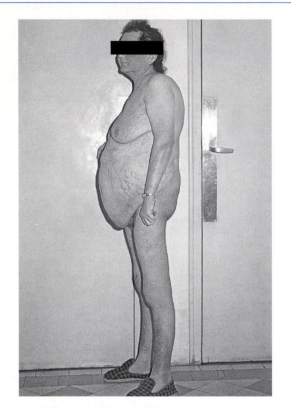

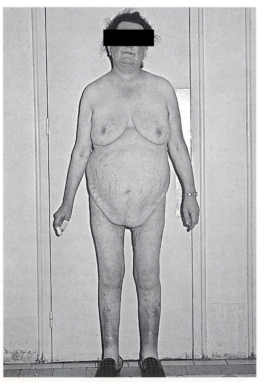

Figure 29.1 Typical aspect of a patient with Cushing's syndrome: centripetal fat depositing with truncal obesity contrasting with the muscular atrophy of the thighs and legs. (Personal collection, Pr. J-P. Luton.)

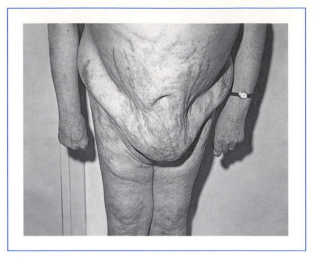

Figure 29.2 Typical aspect of large, purple striae. (Personal collection, Pr. J-P. Luton.)

There is an impaired defense mechanism against infections. Banal bronchopulmonary infections may take a most aggressive, life-threatening course. Superficial mucocutaneous infections are extremely frequent, such as tinea versicolor and ungual mycosis, which will only subside with the control of hypercortisolism.

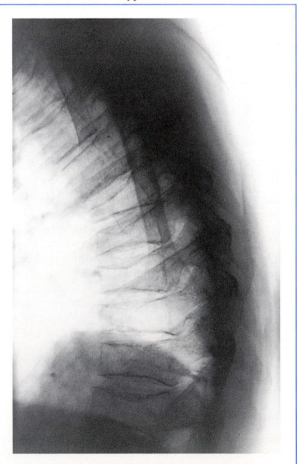

Figure 29.3 Spine osteoporosis. (Personal collection, Pr. J-P. Luton.)

Most patients have high blood pressure. It may occasionally be severe, inducing cardiac hypertrophy and eventually congestive heart failure. Increased susceptibility to both arterial and venous thrombosis is also present due to lipid and coagulation disturbances. Cardiovascular complications are the major threats of the disease and contribute greatly to its morbidity and mortality rate.

Hirsutism, due to a slight excess of adrenocortical androgens, is extremely frequent in women. Frank virilism (temporal hair loss, coarsening of the voice, clitoral hypertrophy) occasionally occurs and points to a specific cause of Cushing's syndrome, especially an adrenocortical carcinoma. Excess adrenal androgens and cortisol both suppress the gonadotroph function, which results in an array of gonadal dysfunctions: most female patients have oligomenorrhea or amenorrhea, and infertility is frequent. In male patients, the curtailed gonadotroph function induces a dramatic fall in testosterone, which is not compensated by the increased adrenocortical androgens. It results in a loss of libido and diminished sexual performance. Loss of sexual hair and reduced testis size are observed.

Psychic disturbances are extremely common. They are highly variable both in their expression and their severity, and they do not correlate with the intensity of the hypercortisolism. They are most often mild and limited to anxiety, increased emotional lability, and irritability or unwarranted euphoria. Sleep disorders are also frequent. Severe psychotic symptoms may occur, such as depression, maniac disorders, delusions and/or hallucinations, and may ultimately lead to suicide.

The clinical features of hypercortisolism cover a wide spectrum of symptoms and signs. Many of them – such as obesity, high blood pressure, and psychological disturbances – are extremely common, and yet Cushing's syndrome is rarely their cause. Abnormal fat distribution (central obesity) is the most sensitive sign, and evidence of protein wasting (osteoporosis, myopathy) is highly specific. In the absence of fat redistribution, the likelihood of Cushing's syndrome is slim; in the presence of protein waisting, weight gain is highly suggestive of Cushing's syndrome. This scheme provides a most useful guide that will prove highly beneficial for the clinical approach of many suspected cases.

Particular combinations of symptoms and signs

Though many patients with Cushing's syndrome present with a highly suggestive combination of symptoms and signs, as described above, in other cases the clinical picture is much less clear and even misleading, for reasons cited below.

Some patients exhibit the syndrome only partially, and one symptom can dominate the whole picture. It is not rare that an occasional patient has been misdirected for months or even years in rheumatologic or psychiatric wards before it is realized that he has a Cushing's syndrome.

Mild forms may be mistaken for all sorts of ill-defined conditions, such as polycystic ovary syndrome, essential hypertension, idiopathic cyclic edema, and idiopathic hirsutism. Some patients with Cushing's syndrome have a cyclical pattern in which episodes of active hypercortisolism are separated by periods of normal pituitary-adrenal activity of varying lengths. Some patients exhibit a fairly regular pattern of episodic hypercortisolism and complain of "swelling" from time to time. A slight delay in obtaining the necessary blood, salivary, or urine samples to establish the hypercortisolism explains how the diagnosis may be missed. The simplest way to make this diagnosis is to educate the patient to collect a 24-hour or overnight urine sample or bedtime saliva at the time when he feels symptoms have recurred.

In the mild forms of Cushing's syndrome, the diagnosis is often less apparent in men than in women. It is claimed that some persistent testicular androgens offer better protection against the protein-wasting effect of cortisol.

Cushing's disease usually presents as a slowly progressive pathologic condition with a mild degree of hyperandrogenism in females.

The ectopic ACTH syndrome is often diagnosed in patients who bear obvious and aggressive tumors. Classically, the clinical features are dominated by muscle wasting, weight loss, and hyperpigmentation. High levels of circulating cortisol and other mineralocorticoids (deoxycorticosterone) induce severe hypokalemia, and frank diabetes is often present. A rapid progression of the primary malignancy prevents the more classical features of Cushing's syndrome (central obesity) to appear. More recently, a completely different form of the ectopic ACTH syndrome with a mild clinical presentation has been described (see "Occult ectopic ACTH syndrome," below).

Adrenocortical adenoma usually presents with features of pure cortisol overproduction (absent or mild features of androgenism in females, lack of hyperpigmentation). Adrenocortical carcinomas typically secrete an array of steroids, particularly androgens; the rapid onset of frank virilism should be suspicious. Some tumors are large enough to be accessible at palpation.

In rare instances, the first presenting symptoms will be those of a tumor. The fine biological work-up of a pituitary macroadenoma may clearly indicate a state of ACTH hypersecretion in a patient who had no evident features of chronic hypercortisolism. These findings may even be secondarily encountered during the careful monitoring of what was primarily diagnosed as a nonfunctional pituitary adenoma, stressing the need for careful and prolonged follow-up of such patients. In other patients with large adrenocortical tumor and/or aggressive small cell carcinoma of the lungs, the clinical features of chronic hypercortisolism may be obscured by those of the primary malignancy.

Cushing's syndrome in children

In children, Cushing's syndrome almost invariably provokes growth retardation if not growth arrest. A decrease in growth rate may be the sole symptom in mild forms of the disease, where the final diagnosis is often delayed. Weight gain with centripetal obesity, as in adults, is present in most cases, however.

Cushing's syndrome in pregnant women

Pregnancy rarely occurs in a hypercortisolic woman because of the hypofertility associated with this condition. Among the few reported cases, there was an exaggerated prevalence of adrenocortical tumors.

In mild cases of Cushing's syndrome, the clinical diagnosis may be obscured by features frequently present in pregnancy, such as weight gain, high blood pressure, abdominal striae, and impaired glucose tolerance. However, the presence of exaggerated morphological changes, virilism, and especially catabolic features should raise suspicion.

Diagnostic procedures

Routine laboratory

Routine laboratory tests may provide some clue to the diagnosis, but their major function is to measure the severity of the disease. The test results are not only related to the rate of cortisol secretion, but also for each individual, to his or her personal sensitivity to glucocorti-

coids. They will be most useful for the follow-up of treated patients (Fig. 29.4).

Altered counts of circulating leukocytes are frequent, showing increased neutrophils and decreased lymphocytes and eosinophils.

Serum electrolytes are usually normal. In severe cases, hypokalemia, alkalosis, and hypernatremia develop in response to high levels of cortisol and deoxycorticosterone. Although some degree of glucose intolerance is observed in most patients, frank fasting hyperglycemia occurs in a minority of patients.

Chest X-ray and electrocardiogram results are normal except in cases of rib fractures, and cardiac enlargement due to high blood pressure. Kidney function and liver tests are normal. Serum IgG have been reported to be slightly depressed. Bone mass is reduced in most patients, as well as biochemical markers of bone formation such as osteocalcin.

Establishing the hypercortisolic state

Baseline measurements *Plasma cortisol* As a group, patients with Cushing's syndrome have higher morning plasma cortisol values, yet around 50% of patients fall within the normal range. Because patients with Cushing's syndrome typically lack a normal circadian rhythm, this overlap progressively disappears during the day. Late evening plasma cortisol has a good sensitivity.

Salivary cortisol Salivary cortisol is a perfect indicator of plasma free cortisol. It offers a convenient and non-

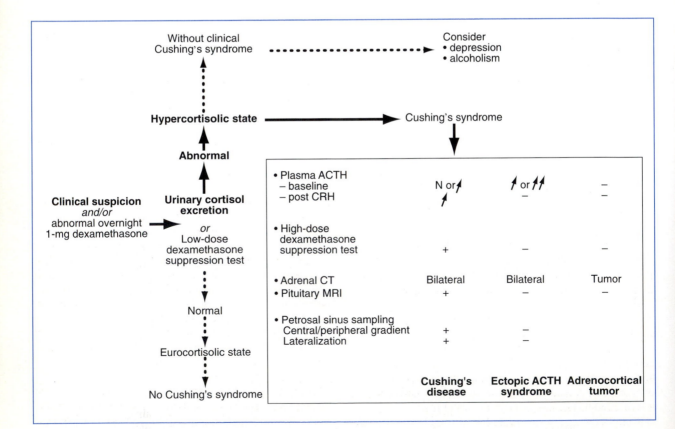

Figure 29.4 Diagnostic flow-chart in Cushing's syndrome.

stressful way of sample collection, even in outpatients. It can substitute for plasma cortisol with at least an equal performance.

24-hour urinary cortisol excretion (or urinary free cortisol) An almost perfect distinction is obtained between patients with Cushing's syndrome and normal subjects, provided that the urine collection is done accurately and that the laboratory has validated its normal values in a large population of normals (usually less than 90 µg/24h). This single basal measurement has a diagnostic accuracy comparable to the reference low-dose dexamethasone suppression tests.

Suppression tests

The classic low-dose dexamethasone suppression test In a normal individual, the administration of 0.5 mg dexamethasone, given every 6 hours for 8 doses (2 mg per day), induces almost complete suppression of ACTH and of cortisol secretion. Initially appreciated through measurement of the urinary 17-hydroxycorticosteroids, the suppressive effect of the low-dose dexamethasone test is now best evaluated by measuring urinary cortisol excretion on the second day (normal response: less than 10 µg by 24 hours). Since it was designed, the classic low-dose dexamethasone suppression test has been considered the most reliable means to achieve or eliminate the diagnosis of Cushing's syndrome. It remains the admitted reference test.

The overnight 1 mg-dexamethasone suppression test One mg of dexamethasone is administered orally between 11 and 12 p.m., and plasma cortisol is measured the next morning at 8 a.m. In normal subjects, plasma cortisol values will be suppressed below a definite limit (established by each laboratory, and depending on the assay method), which is usually less than 20 ng/ml for most immunoassays. Although it is convenient, this test has a low specificity, particularly in obese subjects.

Searching the cause of Cushing's syndrome

The assessment of the corticotroph function is the key to the hormonal evaluation.

Baseline plasma ACTH

The presence of detectable plasma ACTH (>5 pg/ml) coincident with hypercortisolism virtually excludes a primary autonomous adrenocortical tumor.

Patients with Cushing's disease have morning plasma ACTH levels that tend to be slightly elevated. ACTH is almost always measurable. Between one-half and two-thirds of the patients have values within the normal range, and the values of the others usually do not exceed 200 pg/ml.

Patients with the ectopic ACTH syndrome tend to have higher levels of ACTH than patients with Cushing's disease, yet the overlap between the two groups is wide.

Dynamics of the corticotroph function: the classic high-dose dexamethasone suppression test

Dexamethasone is given orally at the dose of 2 mg every 6 hours (8 mg per day) for 2 days. Urinary cortisol excretion is measured on the second day of dexamethasone administration and compared with its control value before dexamethasone administration. This test is positive in most patients with Cushing's disease: most suppress to less than 60% of their control values on the high-dose dexamethasone test.

The high-dose dexamethasone suppression test is negative in autonomous secreting adrenocortical tumors, and in the ectopic ACTH syndrome.

Direct assessment of the pituitary ACTH reserve: the CRH test

Synthetic ovine (or less often, human) CRH is administered iv, 100 µg or 1 µg/kg body weight, and plasma ACTH and cortisol are measured during the next 60 minutes. Patients with Cushing's disease are typically responsive (ACTH and/or cortisol plasma levels increase by more than 50% and/or 20%), and patients with the ectopic ACTH syndrome or adrenal tumor are typically unresponsive.

Tracking the ACTH source: bilateral inferior petrosal sinus sampling

Bilateral inferior petrosal sinus sampling allows for the collection of blood draining immediately from the pituitary gland. In difficult cases, this invasive procedure establishes whether ACTH oversecretion is of pituitary or nonpituitary origin. In patients with Cushing's disease and negative pituitary magnetic resonance imaging (MRI), it may help to lateralize the microadenoma before surgery.

Imaging studies

Pituitary magnetic resonance imaging

Performing MRI of the pituitary has significantly improved our ability to detect pituitary microadenomas in Cushing's disease (Fig. 29.5). T1-weighted MRI images should be obtained in the coronal plane with and without Gadolinium DPTA enhancement. A hypointense signal better delimited after enhancement is typical of a microadenoma, which can be seen in as many as 70% of the patients. In the rare cases with macroadenomas, MRI also helps to detect possible invasion of the cavernous sinus.

Adrenal computed tomography scan

As a result of chronic stimulation by excess ACTH, the two adrenal glands develop hyperplasia and exhibit computed tomography (CT) features that are essentially the same in Cushing's disease as they are in the ectopic ACTH syndrome. The two glands are usually moderately enlarged. There is no reliable measure of the adrenals, but a loss of normal concavity of their borders is considered pathological. Occasional nodules may be present, probably more frequently in Cushing's disease than in the ectopic ACTH syndrome. Macronodular hyperplasia develops in up to 15% of patients with Cushing's disease.

No adrenocortical tumor large enough to cause a Cushing's syndrome, that is, >1.5 cm, can escape the detection power of CT. A benign adrenocortical adenoma is readily visible in the fat-filled perirenal area of these patients; it is essential to appreciate the atrophic

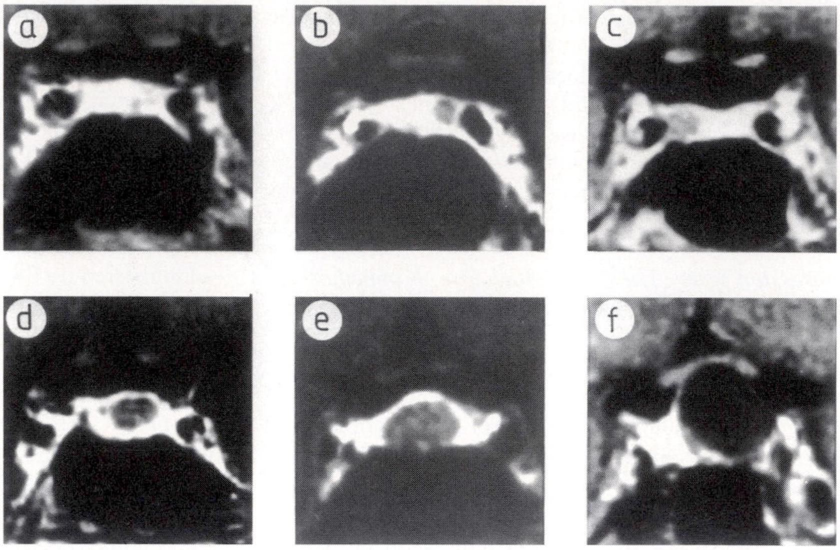

Figure 29.5 Pituitary corticotroph adenomas revealed by MRI in Cushing's disease. A typical hypointense signal is observed with T1-weighted images. (From Bertagna X, Raux-Demay MC, Guilhaume B, Girard F, Luton J-P. Cushing's disease. In: Melmed S [ed]. The pituitary. Cambridge MA: Blackwell Science, 1995;478-545.)

aspect of the contralateral gland by comparing its thickness with that of the diaphragma crus. Adrenocortical carcinomas, as a rule, are large and partly necrotic tumors. They may contain calcifications or hemorrhagic areas. At this stage MRI can be used as the most sensitive method in the preoperative assessment of vascular patency of the inferior vena cava and of locoregional invasion (liver, kidney, pancreas), using sagittal and coronal planes.

Searching a source of ectopic ACTH secretion In ectopic ACTH syndrome, most tumors are located in the thorax and readily detected by X-ray or CT scan. They are comprised of either the highly aggressive oat-cell carcinomas or the indolent bronchial carcinoids (Fig. 29.6). Bronchial carcinoid tumors may be small and undetectable for many years, resulting in "occult" ectopic ACTH syndrome. Recently, scintigraphy with labeled somatostatin analogues (Octreoscan) has provided a sensitive detecting tool. Ectopic ACTH secretion may also be caused by thymic or islet cell tumors, medullary thyroid carcinomas, pheochromocytomas, or other foregut carcinoid tumors, which can be searched by directed or specific imaging procedures.

Pitfalls in diagnosis

Drug interactions High estrogen states, as encountered in pregnancy or with oral contraceptive use, induce increased plasma corticosteroid-binding globulin levels. This modification is accompanied by a parallel increase in plasma cortisol. Persistence of a normal pituitary-adrenal axis is easily demonstrated by other indices: free plasma cortisol and salivary cortisol are normal and have normal circadian variations, and 24-hour urinary cortisol excre-

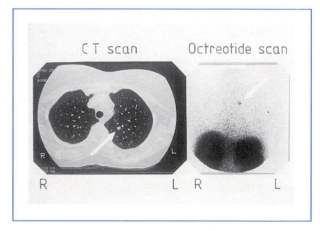

Figure 29.6 A questionable nodular lesion on the chest CT-scan (*left*) is confirmed by Octreoscan scintigraphy showing superimposable uptake (*right*) in a case of ACTH-secreting bronchial carcinoid. (With the permission of the Medicine Group Ltd-Publishing House, Abingdon Oxon.) (From Bertagna X. Cushing's syndrome. Medicine 1997;25:12-5.)

tion is normal. The classic low-dose dexamethasone test is normal. In late pregnancy the situation is more complex due to additional factors that profoundly modify the pituitary-adrenal homeostasis (see below).

Anticonvulsants such as phenytoin and barbiturates accelerate dexamethasone metabolism. Patients on these drugs have false-positive low-dose dexamethasone suppression tests.

Intercurrent pathological states Simple obesity was a major diagnostic problem when urinary 17-hydroxycorticosteroids were the standard markers of adrenocortical activity. It has now been amply demonstrated that the more appropriate parameters of baseline cortisol homeostasis (plasma and salivary cortisol, circadian rhythm, and urinary cortisol excretion), and the classic low-dose dexamethasone suppression test are all normal in simple obesity.

Chronic renal failure has been mistakenly associated with abnormal glucocorticoid regulation, including diminished suppressibility by dexamethasone. With the necessary precautions – plasma extraction or highly specific immunoassay – plasma cortisol is normal and normally suppressible by the classic low-dose dexamethasone test.

Hypercortisolic states without Cushing's syndrome

Various pathological or physiological conditions may be associated with biochemical, and sometimes clinical, evidence of endogenous glucocorticoid excess. In these situations, increased cortisol production is thought to be driven by pituitary ACTH oversecretion, secondary to a central nervous system disorder or to an appropriate adaptive reaction. This functional hypercortisolic state is usually mild and transient – regressing with its cause – and thus is not classically regarded as a cause of genuine Cushing's syndrome. It has long been recognized and is best studied in depressed patients.

Depression   Patients with severe endogenous depression often exhibit biochemical stigmata of hypercortisolism: plasma cortisol and urinary steroid excretion are increased, and they do not suppress normally on the classic low-dose dexamethasone test.

Whatever the exact pathophysiological mechanism, the hypercortisolic state that accompanies depression often creates a serious diagnostic problem. A depressed patient may present with obesity, mild hirsutism, slight hypertension, and moderate glucose intolerance. The question is, is he or she a depressed patient with transient functional hypercortisolism, or is he or she a true Cushing's syndrome with secondary depression? Although none of them is by itself absolutely conclusive, several features may more or less distinguish between the two conditions. Classically in depression: (1) the hypercortisolic state is clinically and biologically mild. Urinary cortisol excretion almost never exceeds three times the upper limit of normal; (2) the circadian pattern of plasma cortisol levels is less disrupted and sometimes a mere phase-shift phenomenon is observed; (3) cortisol response to insulin-induced hypoglycemia is present in depressed patients in contrast to patients with Cushing's syndrome of any cause, including Cushing's disease; (4) ACTH response to CRH is attenuated in contrast to the exaggerated response of Cushing's disease. Nevertheless, a wide overlap is observed; and finally (5) imaging investigations should find no evidence of adrenocortical or pituitary tumor.

Anorexia nervosa   Anorexia nervosa is associated with an array of neuroendocrine disorders among which sustained hypercortisolism is frequent. Increased urinary cortisol and lack of normal suppression by the classic low-dose dexamethasone test may be found. In contrast, with

depressed patients there is generally no clinical hesitation for the diagnosis.

Alcoholism   Patients with chronic alcoholism may present with clinical and biochemical features of glucocorticoid excess, creating a pseudo-Cushing's syndrome.

The simplest – and most effective – way to avoid a false diagnosis is to consider alcoholism and to observe the nice parallel decrease and normalization of cortisol indices and liver function tests during alcohol withdrawal in hospitalized patients.

Pregnancy   Normal pregnancy is associated with a profound hormonal turmoil that significantly alters glucocorticoid homeostasis.

In the first months of pregnancy, increased estrogens induce a two- to threefold rise in plasma corticosteroid-binding globulin, which culminates at about 3 months and plateaus thereafter. There is a parallel rise in plasma cortisol levels.

With time, more significant alterations develop that culminate in the last trimester when unequivocal features of a hypercortisolic state are found, at least from a biochemical point of view. The mean unbound and salivary cortisol and urinary cortisol excretion show a two- to threefold increase. Thirty percent of women have 24-hour urinary cortisol excretion above the upper limit of normal nonpregnant women, and most have an abnormal response to the classic low-dose dexamethasone suppression test. However, the biochemical abnormalities remain mild, and a normal circadian pattern for plasma and/or salivary cortisol is maintained.

Treatment

The morbidity and mortality of untreated chronic hypercortisolism demand that Cushing's syndrome be treated rapidly and actively in most patients.

The goals of treatment are to correct adrenocortical oversecretion, ablate or destroy the primary tumoral lesion, respect anterior pituitary functions and possibly restore a normal pituitary-adrenal axis, and eventually reverse the peripheral manifestations of steroid excess.

Cushing's disease

Transsphenoidal pituitary surgery   Prior to surgery, patients should be prepared so that severe hypertension and/or hyperglycemia be controlled, and infected areas eradicated. Under these strict conditions the transsphenoidal approach is considered a safe procedure. Mortality is occasionally reported as a consequence of meningitis.

A successful surgical outcome of selective adenomectomy characteristically induces a state of transient (although sometimes lasting up to several years) corticotroph deficiency during which steroid coverage is necessary. There is general agreement that this brings about a high immediate success rate of about 80%. These encouraging figures must be tempered by the fact that some patients who were immediate successes eventually relapse. It is recommended that all initially cured patients be regularly and indefinitely followed.

There are still patients who are unexpected failures either because the exploration cannot find the adenoma or because removal of an apparent adenoma does not control the hypercortisolism. The major causes of failure are anatomical due to the lateral extension, the small size, or the inaccessibility of the tumor.

Pituitary irradiation Conventional radiotherapy has long been used to directly suppress pituitary ACTH oversecretion. Its success rates vary between groups depending on the proposed criteria to define cure. Some groups have reported success rates in the 50% range. Most groups have delivered between 35 to 52 Gy with a daily fractional dose of approximately 200 cGy. Lower doses (20 Gy) have a high relapse rate. The response to radiotherapy is slow, taking months or years for a full effect.

Other modes of radiotherapy (heavy particles, stereotactic radiosurgery with the γ-knife) are very limited to specialized centers and require further evaluation.

Medical treatments towards the pituitary Various drugs have tentatively been used to try to suppress the oversecretion of pituitary ACTH. None of them (cyproheptadine, sodium valproate, bromocriptine, somatostatin) has convincingly shown a beneficial effect.

Anti-adrenocortical drugs. Op'DDD: an adrenolytic drug Among anti-adrenocortical drugs, Op'DDD [1-dichloro-2-(0-chlorophenyl)-2-(p-chlorophenyl)-ethane] has a unique adrenolytic action: it specifically destroys the adrenocortical cortex.

Patients with Cushing's syndrome almost invariably reduce their cortisol production on Op'DDD. Direct indicators of plasma free cortisol, such as salivary or urinary cortisol, are the best parameters. Decreased cortisol production is a slow phenomenon that manifests after 1 or 2 months of treatment.

Although Op'DDD is a highly effective adrenolytic drug with unique properties, its use as a sole therapeutic means in Cushing's syndrome has several limitations. Because of its numerous, rather than serious, side effects, its particular kinetics, and its highly variable bioavailability, it necessitates a close and repeated monitoring. Although its efficacy may last for years in a given patient, it is most often only transient. Its best indication is probably when a transient control of hypercortisolism is needed, such as when waiting for the full effect of pituitary irradiation to take place, or when preparing a severely ill patient for pituitary or adrenal surgery.

Inhibitors of cortisol synthesis In contrast with Op'DDD, all of those compounds exert an almost immediate effect on cortisol production. Yet, because they have no adrenolytic action, their long-term benefit in patients with Cushing's disease is countered by the inevitable increase in ACTH, which may overcome their partial blocking effect. This "escape" phenomenon is not observed in patients with Cushing's syndrome of non-pituitary origin.

Metyrapone inhibits 11β-hydroxylase, consequently blocking the last step of adrenal steroid biosynthesis in which the biologically inactive 11-deoxycortisol is converted to cortisol. Metyrapone often results in some general side effects such as nausea and dizziness. It increases the secretion of adrenocortical androgens and may result in intolerable worsening of hirsuties in female patients.

Aminoglutethimide blocks the first step in adrenal steroid biosynthesis. Its frequent side effects are somnolence, dizziness, and skin rash.

A new anticortisolic drug of the imidazole family, ketoconazole, has been found to inhibit various steps of adrenal and testicular steroidogenesis. Cortisol synthesis is inhibited at the levels of the 20- to 22-desmolase and 11β-hydroxylase. Several studies initiated in the late 1980's have shown the rapid cortisol-lowering action of ketoconazole in patients with Cushing's syndrome.

Total bilateral adrenalectomy The obvious and major advantage of total bilateral adrenalectomy is its unequaled efficiency to control the hypercortisolic state, the effect of which is constant and immediate. The important dogma is to operate on patients who have been prepared, that is, after a significant period of eucortisolic state, most often obtained by pharmacological means. Although it still remains a difficult surgical procedure, its mortality is now almost negligible, and its morbidity is greatly reduced with these precautions, provided that it is performed by a skilled and experienced surgical team. Laparoscopic surgery has recently offered a new approach that minimizes the postoperative discomfort to the patient.

Adrenalectomized patients will require life-long steroid treatment with glucocorticoids and mineralocorticoids with their unavoidable constraints, need for adaptation, education, and risk of acute adrenal insufficiency.

Unexpectedly, some patients resume endogenous cortisol secretion. This may even lead to a recurrence of their hypercortisolism years after a total bilateral adrenalectomy. This occurrence is not exceptional, being reported in as many as 10% of cases. It is due to the presence of some adrenal rests that have escaped the surgeon's knife, to accessory glands located in various sites that have regrown under the stimulatory action of chronically and highly elevated ACTH plasma levels.

Last but not least, in some patients, the drastic cortisol deprivation induced by adrenal surgery seems to trigger a definite boost in the growth and secretory activity of the pituitary tumor that was at the origin of the disease. Sellar deformations and clinical hyperpigmentation occur, with increased plasma ACTH levels, defining the Nelson's syndrome. These tumors often have a high aggressiveness, which may bear a significant morbidity and even mortality.

Thus, the high efficacy of adrenal surgery is counterbalanced by several disadvantages. It is reasonable to propose it only when pituitary directed treatments have failed or are contra-indicated.

The ectopic ACTH syndrome

Surgical removal of the responsible tumor immediately cures the hypercortisolism and is accompanied by a state of corticotroph insufficiency since the pituitary has been appropriately suppressed. This can be achieved only with the most indolent tumors such as bronchial carcinoids or the rare pheochromocytomas.

This ideal goal cannot be obtained in most cases, either because the tumor remains "occult," or, more frequently, because highly malignant tumors are not resectable. Specific chemotherapy may reduce ACTH secretion from an oat-cell carcinoma of the lung, and somatostatin analogs can lower ACTH secretion from most bronchial carcinoids.

In many patients, these therapeutic options cannot be utilized or do not prove inefficient. Adrenal-directed therapies must be proposed, either adrenal inhibition or, eventually, total bilateral adrenalectomy.

Adrenocortical tumors

Surgical removal of an adrenocortical adenoma permits a definitive cure. It is most often followed by a transient period of hypoadrenalism resulting from contralateral adrenocortical atrophy because pituitary ACTH has been chronically suppressed. Transient glucocorticoid coverage will be necessary.

Surgery is also the treatment of choice for adrenocortical carcinomas. In some cases an apparent total removal of the tumor is performed, though this does not eliminate the high risk of recurrence or metastases. Op'DDD is the drug of choice either as adjuvant therapy after apparent complete surgery, or in metastasized disease. In case of the failure of Op'DDD, other chemotherapeutic regimens have been proposed, such as VP-16 and cis-platin. In any

case, it remains a devastating disease with only about a 20% survival rate at 5 years after surgery.

Prognosis

Chronic hypercortisolism, per se, is a most severe condition with high morbidity and mortality rates. As reported in older series, it led to death in a majority of untreated patients. Cardiovascular complications were the predominant causes, followed by infections and suicide. Today, cardiovascular and psychiatric complications still remain the major life-threatening complications. The final prognostic of Cushing's syndrome lies on the severity of the hypercortisolic state and the aggressiveness of the responsible tumor.

The growth potential of the pituitary tumor may be another determinant of the final prognostic. Rare cases of spontaneous cure of Cushing's disease have been reported, which are thought to result from infarction and/or calcification of a pituitary tumor. In a minority of patients, tumor growth seems to be boosted by bilateral total adrenalectomy, eventually leading to the Nelson's syndrome. This rare occurrence is unpredictable. It is another argument that points to the pituitary as the more logical and first target when planning therapeutic strategies in Cushing's disease.

In ectopic ACTH syndrome the final prognosis relies, above all, on the primary tumor. The tumor may be highly malignant, such as is the small cell lung cancer, or, in contrast, quite indolent, as in the bronchial carcinoids.

A definitive cure is obtained after removal of an adrenocortical adenoma. In contrast, the adrenal cortical cancer bears a very poor risk, with only 20% survival rate at 5 years.

Suggested readings

ARON DC, TYRRELL JB (eds). Cushing's syndrome. Endocrinology and Metabolism Clinics of North America. Vol. 23. Philadelphia: W.B. Saunders Company, 1994.

ARON DC, TYRRELL JB, FITZGERALD PA, FINDLING JW, FORSHAM PH. Cushing's syndrome: problems in diagnosis. Medicine 1981;60:25-35.

BERTAGNA X, RAUX-DEMAY MC, GUILHAUME B, GIRARD F,

LUTON J-P. Cushing's disease. In: Melmed S (ed). The pituitary. Cambridge, MA: Blackwell Science, 1995;478-545.

MILLER JW, CRAPO L. The medical treatment of Cushing's syndrome. Endocr Rev 1993;4:443-58.

ORTH DN. Cushing's syndrome. N Engl J Med 1995;332:791-803.

WAJCHENBERG BL, MENDONCA BB, LIBERMAN B, et al. Ectopic adrenocorticotropic hormone syndrome. Endocr Rev 1994;15:752-87.

30

The incidentally discovered adrenal mass

Jean-Pierre Luton, Helen Mosnier-Pudar

KEY POINTS

- An expert clinical and biochemical work-up can detect a hypersecretory state, which requires a specific therapy (most often surgery). Pheochromocytoma should always be a concern in such cases.
- For nonhypersecretory incidentalomas, the possibility of a primary malignancy must be excluded, using principally imaging features. Early surgical management is the best likelihood of cure.
- Ultimately a metastatic malignancy, which would radically alter the staging of the primary neoplastic tumor, must be excluded.
- The management of an adrenal incidentaloma necessitates a multidisciplinary expertise: an endocrinologist, a radiologist, a surgeon, and a pathologist are all required.
- Excessive and/or aggressive explorations, including unwarranted surgery, must be avoided. The large majority of incidentally discovered adrenal masses are nonhypersecretory adrenocortical adenomas.

The term adrenal incidentaloma refers to an adrenal mass occasionally and unexpectedly discovered by an abdominal imaging procedure performed for reasons, *a priori*, unrelated to adrenal dysfunction. Widespread use of computed tomography (CT), magnetic resonance imaging (MRI), and ultrasonography makes it a common clinical problem and creates a potential dilemma for its management. The prevalence of adrenal incidentalomas by CT scan examination is estimated to be between 1 to 4%.

Finding an adrenal mass bears three threats to the subject:

- A hypersecretory, or potentially hypersecretory, lesion, which would require specific therapy (most often surgery). The possibility of a pheochromocytoma must always be kept in mind.
- A primary or metastatic malignancy. The diagnosis of

an adrenal carcinoma would lead to the proposal of early surgical management for the best likelihood of cure. However, the adrenals are a frequent site of remote metastasis. Most often adrenal metastases occur in the presence of obvious neoplastic dissemination, but occasionally they are the first site of tumor spread, and their recognition radically alters the staging of the primary neoplastic tumor.

- Excessive and/or aggressive explorations or even unwarranted surgery. The large majority of incidentally discovered adrenal masses are nonhypersecretory adrenocortical adenomas. These lesions occur equally in males and females, and they are uncommon under the age of 30 years. Higher prevalence is reported in black people, and in patients with diabetes mellitus, obesity, familial multiple endocrine neoplasia syndromes, and hypertension.

Etiology

The etiology of adrenal masses includes benign and malignant tumors from all zones of the adrenal cortex and medulla and metastases to the adrenals, as well as infiltrative diseases. Investigation of these masses may lead to the diagnosis of "pseudoadrenal" masses that correspond to tumors or artefacts arising from adjacent structures (such as the kidney, pancreas, spleen, lymph nodes, and vascular structures).

Because only a limited proportion of adrenal incidentalomas are eventually operated on, it is impossible to give the exact prevalence of each cause. Table 30.1 lists the various diagnoses that can be encountered. Different figures can be obtained from operated incidentalomas. The results of two recently published series show that the numbers are quite similar when obtained with 116 operated patients (out of 208) in a single center (Hôpital Cochin, Paris), or with 376 operated patients (out of 1004) in a large multicenter study in another country (National Italian Study Group on Adrenal Tumors) (Tab. 30.2). Approximately one-third of operated incidentalomas turned out to be potentially life-threatening lesions (secretory activity or a malignant nature). Considering that only about one-third of incidentalomas were operated on, and assuming that no "dangerous" lesions were missed, it appears that in approximately 10% of cases, the surgical approach is warranted and can be beneficial. The goal to strive for is to be able to safely and efficiently detect this small proportion of adrenal incidentalomas.

Clinical findings

Detection of hypersecretory – or potentially hypersecretory – adrenal masses

The detection of a hypersecretory or potentially hypersecretory adrenal mass relies heavily on both clinical and biological investigations. Indeed, conditions found initially for reasons unrelated to the adrenals ("incidentally") may retrospectively indicate strong clinical reasons to evoke an adrenal disease (high blood pressure, sudoral crisis, and so on).

Evidence of an excess secretion of cortisol, androgens, estrogens, mineralocorticoids, or catecholamines should be considered in the incidentaloma patient's personal and familial histories and upon physical examination. In the vast majority of cases these are not contributive, and CT and MRI are unable to distinguish hypersecretory from nonhypersecretory lesions. Thus an adequate biochemical screening of all adrenal masses is necessary.

Searching for pheochromocytoma Screening for pheochromocytoma is mandatory in all cases of incidentaloma, since this condition is a potentially lethal disorder with an unpredictable course. Urinary metanephrine in a 24-hour urine sample is the best biochemical screening test. We also advocate (^{131}I) metaiodobenzylguanidine (MIBG) scintigraphy for further evaluation of patients with suspicious biochemi-

Table 30.1 Etiological classification and relative frequency of various incidentally discovered masses of the adrenal gland

Adrenal cortex	
Adenoma	
Non-oncology and nonselected series	36-94%
Oncology patients	7-68%
Nodular hyperplasia	7-17%
Carcinoma	0-25%
Adrenal medulla	
Carcinoma	(*)
Ganglioneuroma	0-6 %
Pheochromocytoma	0-11 %
Other adrenal masses	
Angiomyolipoma	(*)
Abscess	(*)
Amyloidosis	(*)
Cysts	4-22 %
Fibroma	(*)
Granulomatosis (histoplasmosis, coccidiomycosis, blastomycosis, tuberculosis, sarcoidosis)	(*)
Hamartoma	(*)
Hematoma/hemorrhage	0-4 %
Hemangioma/lymphangiomas	(*)
Lipoma	0-11 %
Liposarcoma	(*)
Myelolipoma	7-15 %
Metastases	
Nononcology and nonselected series	0-21 %
Oncology patients	32-73 %
Pseudoadrenal masses (more common on the left side)	0-10 %
Diaphragmatic crura	(*)
Dilated inferior vena cava	(*)
Gallbladder	(*)
Kidney	(*)
Liver(*)	
Lymph nodes (para-aortic, pericaval, retropancreatic, retrocrural)	(*)
Omentum	(*)
Pancreas	(*)
Primary retroperitoneal neoplasms, hematomas, and cysts	(*)
Small and large bowel	(*)
Spleen/accessory spleen	(*)
Stomach/gastric diverticulum	(*)
Other vessels (especially aneurysms, varices, tortuousities, renal veins)	(*)
Technical artifacts (particularly in patients with prior abdominal surgery)	(*)

* Rare or not clearly defined in the literature.
(Adapted with permission from Kloos RT, et al. Incidentally discovered adrenal masses. Endocrine Rev 1995;16:460-84.)

cal results (elevated urinary metanephrine). Some authors propose to systematically perform it before operating (or biopsying) all apparently nonsecreting incidentalomas.

Searching for pre-toxic cortisol-secreting adenoma (pre-Cushing's syndrome) Clinically obvious manifestations of cortisol excess occur relatively late in the development

Table 30.2 Relevant etiology and their relative frequency in operated incidentalomas in two series

Masses etiology	Cochin Paris, France	NISGAT*
Pheochromocytoma	8,5%	11%
Pre-Cushing's syndrome	11,1%	13%
Conn's adenoma	2,5%	2,5%
Adrenal carcinoma	6,8%	11%
Metastases	7,7%	5%
Myelolipoma	1,7%	8%
Adrenal cyst	2,5%	5%
Neuronal tumor	5,1%	3%
Lymphangioma/angioma	9,4%	-
Liposarcoma	3,4%	-
Nonhypersecretory adrenal adenomas	24,1%	36,5%
Other tumors: renal carcinoma mesenchymoma bronchial cyst adrenal abcess	17,2%	5%

* National Italian Study Group on Adrenal Tumors.

an undiagnosed "pre-toxic" adrenocortical incidentaloma may precipitate an acute adrenal insufficiency crisis.

Searching for Conn's adenoma Elevated blood pressure and/or low serum potassium (≤ 3.5 mmol/l) are suggestive of mineralocorticoid excess and require further evaluation. Because asymptomatic aldosteronomas can occur, we advocate a systematic screening for mineralocorticoid excess. A simple and efficient method is used to measure the plasma aldosterone/renin ratio. Precaution should be taken that interfering medications have been discontinued for an appropriate interval.

Other secretory abnormalities High levels of dehydroepiandrosterone sulfate levels are occasionally found in adrenocortical carcinomas. Given the rarity of adrenocortical tumors secreting purely masculinizing or feminizing hormones, we do not routinely obtain testosterone or estradiol levels. High 17-hydroxyprogesterone baseline plasma levels may reveal rare cases of unknown congenital adrenal hyperplasia in men. The recommended minimal hormonal evaluation in clinically asymptomatic patients is shown in Table 30.2.

Detection of malignant adrenal tumors

When it is established that the incidentally discovered adrenal mass is nonhypersecretory, the possibility of primary or metastatic malignancy must be excluded.

Some benign lesions have typical morphologic features Some benign masses may have readily recognizable characteristics on CT scan and/or MRI. Those masses are myelolipomas, spontaneous adrenal hemorrhages, and adrenal cysts.

Several features suggest malignancy

Known extra-adrenal malignancy In patients with known malignancy, 8 to 38% have adrenal metastases at

of Cushing's syndrome. Thus it is not surprising to find some cases of incidentally discovered adrenal masses secreting cortisol at a rate not sufficient to cause overt Cushing's syndrome: hence the term, pre-Cushing's syndrome. By definition, the 24-hour urinary cortisol excretion is most often normal. The best diagnostic approach, therefore, is the overnight 1.0 mg dexamethasone suppression test. This test is mandatory since surgical removal of

Table 30.3 Recommended minimal hormonal screening tests for incidentally discovered adrenal masses in clinically asymptomatic patients

Hypersecretory state	Screening test
Pheochromocytoma	24-Hour urinary metanephrines
Pre-Cushing's syndrome	Overnight 1 mg dexamethasone suppression test[1]
Conn's adenoma	Plasma aldosterone/renin ratio[2]
Adrenocortical carcinoma	Serum dehydroepiandrosterone sulfate[3]
Congenital adrenal hyperplasia	Baseline 17-hydroxy-progesterone

[1] Some propose a higher dexamethasone dose (2 or 3 mg) for better specificity.
[2] Some propose to perform only on patients with hypertension and/or hypokalemia.
[3] Low sensitivity and specificity.

Table 30.4 Imaging characteristics and the nature of adrenal masses

Suggestive of benign masses	Suggestive of malignant masses
Small size	**Large size**
Round regular shape	Irregular shape, thick margins
Homogeneity	Necrosis
Low density on CT and low increase after contrast	High density on CT and high, non-homogeneous increase after contrast
Low T_2 weighted signal on MRI	High T_2 weighted signal on MRI
High lipid content	**Low lipid content**

autopsy; most commonly the primary malignancies originate from breast, lung, kidney, melanoma, or lymphoma. Conversely, in patients with no known primary malignancy, the overall rate for discovering a metastatic adrenal malignancy is low. It should be particularly looked for in case of bilateral tumors and/or when imaging characteristics are suspicious (Tab. 30.3): clinical examination, chest-X ray, abdominal and chest CT scan, and mammograms can be performed.

The large size of the tumor The probability of an adrenal mass being malignant has been shown to increase significantly with size (greatest diameter): a malignant/benign ratio of 8:1 has been reported for masses over 4 cm in diameter, thus prompting the suggestion for the systematic removal of masses above that size. However, management strategies based upon adrenal mass size alone are neither sensitive nor specific, and they cause one to miss smaller and perhaps more surgically amenable lesions. An alternative recommendation has been made that all lesions greater than 3 cm be removed. This approach would have as a consequence many more benign than malignant masses being subjected to surgical removal with the attendant costs and risks.

Demonstrable growth of the mass is suggestive of malignancy and necessitates surgery. For this reason nonoperated patients should be followed, though malignancy discovered by this method exposes patients to a delay in diagnosis and treatment.

Specific imaging features Besides the size, several other features, summarized in Table 30.4, may provide clues to the benign or malignant nature of the tumor.

Measuring the lipid content of a lesion appears to be a fairly good indicator, since adrenal adenomas typically have a high lipid content. This is easily measured by evaluating the spontaneous density of the adrenal mass on CT. An unenhanced CT attenuation under 10 Hounsfield units (HU) is suggestive of an adenoma. Above 10 HU, it is rarely an adenoma, and the diagnosis of pheochromocytoma, hematoma, and primary or secondary adrenal malignancy should be considered. Alternatively, MRI can provide another means to assess lipid content.

Lack of radiocholesterol uptake (NP59) Because nonhypersecretory adrenocortical adenomas typically concentrate iodocholesterol, whereas nonadrenocortical and/or malignant tissues do not, NP 59 scintigraphy has been proposed as a useful discriminating test. It has some serious limitations, however, which are primarily the size of the mass (which must be above 2 cm), its cost, the inevitable irradiation, and its restricted availability to only some specialized centers.

The indication for fine needle aspiration biopsy Fine needle aspiration biopsy is an invasive procedure that carries a well-documented, low but significant incidence of serious risks such as pneumothorax, bacteremia, and renal and hepatic hematoma, and a very low but identifiable risk of mortality. Furthermore, a histological distinction between benign and well-differentiated primary malignancy of the adrenal gland is often difficult. Fine needle aspiration biopsy is best able to distinguish between adrenal and nonadrenal tissue and may be useful in patients with known malignancies who are at risk for adrenal metastases.

Bilateral adrenal masses

Incidentally discovered bilateral adrenal masses represent 11 to 16% of adrenal masses.

They should be evaluated as already described, including searching for bilateral hypersecretory lesions.

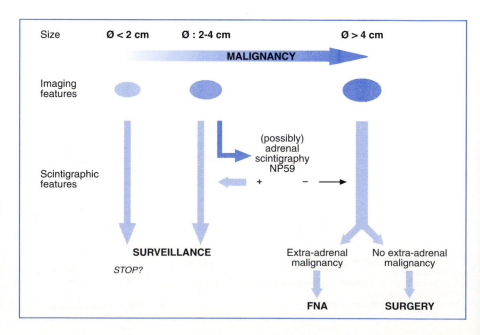

Figure 30.1 Recommendations for non hypersecretory adrenal incidentalomas. Size: best appreciated by CT scan; imaging features: see Table 30.4; scintigraphic features: + concordant uptake of iodocholesterol, – lack of iodocholesterol uptake; FNA: fine needle biopsy.

However, special attention should be given to some specific conditions: (1) primary adrenocortical insufficiency by adrenocortical destruction should be searched by plasma adrenocorticotropic hormone (ACTH) determination and the short ACTH-stimulation test; (2) congenital adrenal hyperplasia in men revealed by high 17-hydroxyprogesterone plasma levels; and (3) solid tumors, metastases, hematological malignancy, hemorrhage, infections (cytomegalovirus, mycobacterium, cryptococcosis), and granulomatous disease, which they most frequently represent.

Treatment

The combined expertise of endocrinologist and radiologist is required: (1) An expert clinical and biochemical work-up will detect a hypersecretory syndrome. (2) A *perfect imaging approach* (CT scan most often, or MRI) is crucial: it often reveals the incidentaloma; it immediately provides estimations of size, imaging characteristics, and so on; it should always identify the *lipid content* of the tumor; and it immediately diagnoses some specific lesions (such as myelolipoma and cysts).

After an adrenal incidentaloma has been deemed non-hypersecretory, the therapeutic strategy relies essentially on morphologic grounds (Fig. 30.1): (1) A "small size" (<2 cm) lesion that bears all of the imaging features in favor of a benign tumor should at the most be followed, or ignored. (2) All lesions that are "large" (>4 cm) and/or that bear suspicious imaging features must be submitted to further evaluation: fine needle aspiration in the rare cases of known malignancy, and surgery in other cases. (3) Lesions of "intermediary size" (2 to 4 cm) with benign imaging features may simply be followed; when a doubt remains concerning whether they are benign or not, further evaluations are necessary. Adrenal scintigraphy with NP 59 might prove useful. If necessary, surgery should be proposed. Those options rely on experience taken from various series and are inevitably somewhat empirical. The choice of cut-offs for the tumor size could be debated.

Suggested readings

BILBEY JH, MAC LOUGLIN RF, KURKJIAN PS, et al. MR imaging of adrenal masses: value of chemical shift imaging for distinguishing adenomas from other tumors. AJR, 1995;164:637-42.

KLOOS RT, GROSS MD, FRANCIS IR, KOROBIN M, SHAPIRO B. Incidentally discovered adrenal masses. Endocrine Rev 1995;16:460-84.

LEE MJ, HAHN PF, PAPANICOLAOU N, et al. Benign and malignant adrenal masses: CT distinction with attenuation coefficients, size, and observer analysis. Radiology 1991;179:415-8.

LEROY-WILLIG A, BITTOUN J, LUTON JP, et al. In vivo MR spectroscopic imaging of the adrenal glands: distinction between adenomas and carcinomas larger than 15 mm based on lipid content. Am J Roentgen 1989;153:771-3.

MANTERO F, MASINI AM, OPOCHER G, GIOVAGNETTI M, ARNALDI G. Adrenal incidentaloma: an overview of hormonal data from the National Italian Study Group. Horm Res 1997;47:284-9.

ROSS NS, ARON DC. Hormonal evaluation of the patient with an incidentally discovered adrenal mass. N Engl J Med 1990;323:1401-5.

Glucocorticoid therapy

T. Joseph McKenna

▰ KEY POINTS ▰

- Because of the high instances of side effects associated with the therapeutic use of glucocorticoids, the lowest effective dose should always be used. When using a pharmacological dose of glucocorticoids, it may be possible to achieve the required therapeutic effect using alternate-day treatment, which is associated with lower incidences of side effects. This strategy may be particularly successful in nephrotic syndrome, asthma, sarcoidosis, ulcerative colitis, and rheumatoid arthritis.
- Strategies that optimize glucocorticoid effect include the additional use of other immunosuppressive agents, and the employment of the optimum type of steroid and the optimum timing. For example, low-dose of long-acting glucocorticoid given at midnight may be more effective than higher doses of shorter-acting glucocorticoid given early in the day when used to suppress the hypothalamic-pituitary-adrenal axis, such as for patients with congenital adrenal hyperplasia.
- The "steroid withdrawal syndrome," characterized by the emergence of symptoms of adrenal insufficiency when reducing doses of glucocorticoid from pharmacological to physiological levels, may persist for months to years. Slowly tapering off glucocorticoid replacement – with symptoms eventually passing – and close clinical follow-up provide the most successful means of treating this condition, which presents a difficult management problem.
- Assessment of the recovery of the hypothalamic-pituitary-adrenal axis following exposure to pharmacological doses of glucocorticoids includes the measurement of morning plasma cortisol levels prior to glucocorticoid treatment on that day. Plasma cortisol levels greater than 400 nmol/l are usually indicative of adequate clinical recovery. The plasma cortisol response to the conventional dose of adrenocorticotropic hormone (ACTH), 250 μg iv, may be misleading. However, the cortical response to low-dose ACTH, 1 μg iv, has been reported to be more sensitive in the identification of secondary adrenal insufficiency.
- Activation of the entire hypothalamic-pituitary-adrenal axis in response to hypoglycemia is the gold standard for investigation. However, similar information can be obtained with lesser risk to the patient and demand on medical service by evaluating the 11-deoxycortisol and cortisol responses to the administration of a single dose of metyrapone given at night.

In this chapter, the types of steroid preparation available for therapeutic use and their duration of action and routes of administration will be considered. An emphasis will be placed on optimizing the therapeutic effect and minimizing the occurrence of adverse side effects. It is necessary to first have an appreciation of the mechanism by which steroids exert their physiological and pharmacological effects, and of the dissociation that occurs between the time during which the therapeutic steroid may be detected in systemic circulation and the duration of its biological effect.

The indications for treatment with glucocorticoids include steroid replacement, in which the essential aim is to achieve physiological equivalence under a variety of clinical situations. Non-replacement indications include the use of glucocorticoids where pharmacological effects are required, for example, to suppress an inflammatory or an immunological response. The pharmacological use of glucocorticoid treatment is effective in a large variety of conditions, including asthma, the inflammatory arthritides, autoimmune disorders, and to prevent or treat the process of transplant rejection. However, these beneficial effects may be offset considerably by the adverse effects of glucocorticoids, which may bring about marked compromise in the quality of life. For example, glucocorticoids may cause the development of crippling osteoporosis, and indeed may prove to be life-threatening due to a development such as fulminant infection in the immunocompromised host. In order to devise treatment strategies that obtain the optimum outcome, an understanding of the physiological and pharmacological principles involved is helpful.

MECHANISM OF STEROID HORMONE ACTION

Glucocorticoids are carried in the systemic circulation partially bound to carrier proteins such as corticosteroid binding-globulin and albumin. However, it is the unbound fraction that leaves the systemic circulation and gains access to the individual cells of tissue throughout the body. Within the cells the steroids bind to receptors. The glucocorticoid receptor is one of a family of related proteins which, through a mechanism of intracellular binding, facilitates physiological effects of thyroid hormones, vitamin D, retinoids, and adrenal steroids. When a glucocorticoid binds to a glucocorticoid receptor, it is associat-

ed with a number of intracellular proteins that are most likely necessary to ensure the complexing of glucocorticoid with its receptor, for example, heat shock proteins 70 and 90 and immunophilin. These proteins then dissociate from the complex, and the receptor undergoes conformational changes to facilitate translocation into the nucleus. In the nucleus, the glucocorticoid-receptor complex binds to specific glucocorticoid response elements that are associated with various genes. This association then triggers the characteristic glucocorticoid response of the cell. In many instances, this involves the activation of transcriptional processes that results in the generation of messenger RNA, which subsequently brings about the production of a new protein. This protein may be the end product necessary for the glucocorticoid effect in that tissue. Alternatively, in some tissues the binding of the steroid-glucocorticoid receptor complex to the glucocorticoid response elements in genes may result in the suppression of a characteristic tissue activity. For example, when supraphysiological doses of glucocorticoids are exhibited in cells responsible for the production of the ACTH parent molecule pro-opiomelanocortin, the production of pro-opiomelanocortin is inhibited. As a result, the secretion of ACTH falls, and the stimulus to further cortisol production is suppressed. It is probable that glucocorticoids bring about some of its anti-inflammatory/immunosuppressive effects in a similar manner, such as by suppressing cytokine production.

The time scale for the above sequence may be several hours to days. Thus, although circulating glucocorticoids are no longer detectable in systemic circulation, the intracellular processes involved in bringing about the characteristic steroid action may be on-going. Overall, there is relatively little difference in the half-life of various glucocorticoids in systemic circulation, but there is wide variation in the duration of biological actions stimulated by the steroids (Tab. 31.1).

INTERACTION BETWEEN ENDOGENOUS AND EXOGENOUS GLUCOCORTICOIDS

When considering the effects of glucocorticoids, the effect on endogenous glucocorticoid production should be

Table 31.1 Plasma half-life, duration of action, glucocorticoid and mineralocorticoid potencies and equivalent doses of some commonly used glucocorticoid preparations and of fludrocortisone

Steroid	Half-life (min)	Duration of action (h)	Relative potency Glucocorticoid	Mineralocorticoid	Replacement dose (mg)
Cortisol	80	8-12	1.0	1.0	20
Cortisone	30	8-12	0.8	0.8	25
Prednisone	60	12-36	3.5-4.0	0.8	5
Prednisolone	200	12-36	4.0	0.8	5
Methylprednisolone	200	12-36	5.0	0.5	4
Triamcinolone	200	12-36	5.0	0.0	4
Dexamethasone	300	36-72	30.0	0.0	0.5
Betamethasone	300	36-72	30.0	0.0	0.5
Fludrocortisone	240	12-24	10.0	125.0	2

particularly considered. Under physiological conditions, the hypothalamic-pituitary-adrenal (HPA) axis is activated just prior to a person's usual waking time. ACTH levels rise, and as a consequence, cortisol values increase and reach their highest levels soon after waking. Under non-stressed conditions, ACTH and glucocorticoid levels demonstrate a diurnal rhythm that falls over the following 4 to 6 hours, reaching low values that are then sustained until the next cycle occurs. Under conditions of stress, ACTH and cortisol levels will rise during the day, or the early morning rise might be sustained for a longer period than is normal, possibly throughout the whole day.

The administration of glucocorticoid that results in an excess of glucocorticoid prior to the time of the normal activation of the HPA axis will result in suppression of its activity. If glucocorticoid is administered over a short time period of 2 weeks or less, reactivation of the HPA axis occurs promptly. However, with longer and profound suppression, the time elapse before the reactivation of the HPA axis after steroid withdrawal is variably delayed and may be clinically significant.

GLUCOCORTICOIDS PREPARATIONS

Table 31.1 lists frequently used glucocorticoids and identifies their half-lives in plasma, approximate replacement dosage for each glucocorticoid, and their relative glucocorticoid and mineralocorticoid potencies. Figure 31.1 demonstrates the structures of these preparations. The activation of cortisone and prednisone requires reduction at the carbon atom 11 position in the steroid molecule. 11β-reduction occurs predominantly in the liver. Thus, cortisone and prednisone are only useful as glucocorticoids after they have gained access to the hepatic circulation and have been converted to hydrocortisone and prednisolone, respectively. Therefore, use of cortisone or prednisone topically or intra-articularly where local activity is required will be without effect. Furthermore, intramuscular injec-

tion of cortisone acetate is associated with much lower levels of plasma cortisol than when hydrocortisone is injected intramuscularly. For cortisol to appear in the circulation, hydrocortisone has merely to be absorbed from the injection site. In contrast, in the case of cortisone acetate, it must be absorbed and passed through the liver where conversion to cortisol takes place; slower absorption of cortisone acetate from the injection site may also contribute to the lower blood cortisol levels achieved than with intramuscular hydrocortisone. However, the disparity between cortisol levels resulting from oral administration of hydrocortisone or cortisone is less, since when cortisone is absorbed from the gastrointestinal tract it passes into the portal circulation, which perfuses the liver and provides the opportunity for the conversion of cortisone to cortisol.

A wide variety of steroid preparations are available, depending upon the route of administration. Most glucocorticoid preparations are absorbed well from the gastrointestinal tract, which is the preferred route for systemic delivery. Reference has already been made to the problems associated with the availability of cortisol arising from intramuscular administration of cortisone acetate. Triamcinolone acetonide given intramuscularly is absorbed very slowly and may have an effect that lasts for several days to weeks. When a rapid effect of glucocorticoid is required, such as for treatment of Addisonian crises or severe asthmatic attacks, highly soluble preparations should be used, e.g., such as hydrocortisone phosphate or hydrocortisone hemisuccinate. For the topical administration of steroids, it is important to use a preparation that ensures that the steroid will gain access to the squamous cell layer of the epidermis. Lipophilic forms of steroids such as triamcinolone acetonide are many times more effective than pure triamcinolone. Hydrocortisone is absorbed poorly, while hydrocortisone butyrate is an effective topical agent. Systemic absorption may occur

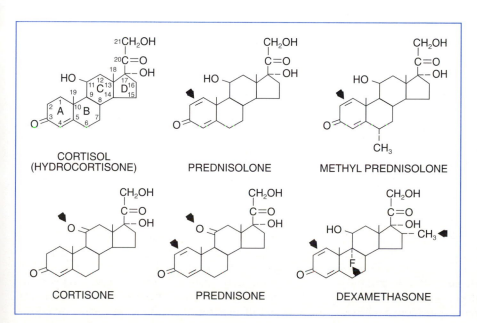

Figure 31.1 Representations of the structures of cortisol and cortisone and some synthetic glucocorticoids. The numbers indicate the conventional numbering of the four benzene rings (A, B, C, D) that make up the steroid molecule with the side chain. The arrows indicate the structural differences between cortisol and the other glucocorticoids. (From Axelrod L. Glucocorticoid therapy. Medicine (Baltimore) 1976;55: 39-65.)

through ulcerated skin. Absorption does vary with the anatomical site even when the skin is intact. Scrotal skin is much more permeable to steroids than is skin of the forearm. The possibility exists of adverse effects of systemic absorption of glucocorticoids using high doses of highly lipophilic preparations, particularly when administered on broken skin. Steroids to be administered intraarticularly should be relatively insoluble to reduce systemic absorption and maintain high concentrations of active steroid within the joint space. Such preparations include hydrocortisone acetate, prednisolone tebutate, and triamcinolone hexacetonide.

Glucocorticoids are an important part of the treatment of asthma. While systemic steroids are effective in promoting bronchodilatation, the accompanying systemic side effects limit the use of glucocorticoids in this way. Because of this, various preparations have been produced that are effective when inhaled. These preparations include beclomethasone dipropionate, budesonide, and fluticasone propionate. Significant systemic absorption may occur with the use of inhaled steroids, but this is rare.

ADVERSE SIDE EFFECTS

In the section dealing with Cushing's syndrome (see also Chap. 29) the clinical picture of glucocorticoid excess is clearly outlined. However, there are some distinct differences between the clinical picture due to endogenous glucocorticoid excess and that occur as a result of exogenous glucocorticoid excess. While most glucocorticoids used in treatment have little if any mineralocorticoid effect and usually no androgen effect, the picture frequently seen in patients with spontaneously arising Cushing's syndrome combines evidence of glucocorticoids, mineralocorticoids, and androgen excess. Thus, with the exception of patients treated with hydrocortisone, the occurrence of hypokalemia and its associated clinical problems are rarely seen in patients using therapeutic glucocorticoids. There may be an increase in non-androgen-dependent fine hair growth on the face and trunk, which, although troublesome, is quite different from the androgen-dependent hirsutism with coarse curling hair in a beard distribution. While centripetal fat distribution, easy bruising, myopathy, osteoporosis, and glucose intolerance are common to both exogenous and endogenous glucocorticoid excess, some features are more typical of, or exclusive to, iatrogenic glucocorticoid effects. These include posterior subcapsular cataracts, pancreatitis, avascular necrosis of bone (typically the femoral head), and increased intracranial pressure. Endogenous glucocorticoid excess is associated with depression, which in rare instances leads to suicide, but euphoria is the more common manifestation of psychiatric disturbances in patients receiving glucocorticoid treatment.

Immunosuppression is associated with the acquisition of new infections and the reactivation of old previously controlled infections. These infections may be bacterial, fungal, or viral. The reactivation or acquisition of tuberculosis is of particular concern. In addition, the usual manifestations of the infective process may be suppressed by the anti-inflammatory effects of glucocorticoids and thus obscure diagnosis. A typical clinical situation that creates particular difficulty is gastrointestinal perforation. The usual clinical manifestation of abdominal pain, tenderness, and fever may be greatly modified in the patient receiving therapeutic glucocorticoids. The non-specific increase in white cells associated with glucocorticoid treatment, even in the uninfected patient, causes greater difficulty in the interpretation.

In children, growth retardation is of profound concern in patients with Cushing's syndrome of any etiology. While withdrawal of steroids is associated with a phase of catch-up growth, bone age usually advances more rapidly so that the final height tends to be significantly less than what is predicted from the genetic endowment.

TREATMENT STRATEGIES

The general treatment strategy is to use the lowest effective dose of glucocorticoid for the shortest period required that is compatible with an acceptable benefit-to-risk ratio. The adverse effects of glucocorticoids may be subdivided into suppression of the HPA axis and other toxic effects. However, glucocorticoid treatment protocols that lessen the likelihood of suppression of the HPA axis are also likely to reduce the emergence of other side effects. There is great variability in the sensitivity of the HPA axis to suppression from one patient to another. The most sensitive patients will demonstrate suppression of the axis when prednisone 10 mg or greater is used more than 2 weeks. When treatment of prednisone 10 mg per day or greater is extended for more than 6 months, suppression of the HPA axis is almost inevitable.

Strategies employed that may lessen the effect of glucocorticoid on the HPA axis are generally dependent on the precise timing of glucocorticoid administration. Because of the diurnal rhythm in ACTH-cortisol secretion, the administration of glucocorticoid in a single dose in the early morning will lessen the likelihood of HPA axis suppression. While the lower the dose of glucocorticoid the less likely it is for clinically significant suppression to occur, in many instances to achieve a good therapeutic effect it is necessary to use pharmacological doses of glucocorticoids at least temporarily, e.g., such as prednisone 20-60 mg per day. There appears to be little loss in therapeutic effectiveness when this amount of glucocorticoid is given as a single dose rather than in divided doses throughout the day, but it may have a beneficial effect by reducing the likelihood of HPA axis suppression. Extending this observation, it has also been found that using alternate day/early-morning glucocorticoid treatment is associated not only with a lesser incidence of suppression of the HPA axis, but also with a lesser incidence of the other side effects of glucocorticoids that occur when a similar amount of glucocorticoid is given in divided doses on a daily basis. Evidence exists to suggest that alternate-day glucocorticoid treatment is effective for the treatment of nephrotic syndrome, asthma, sarcoidosis, ulcerative colitis, and rheumatoid arthritis. Alternate day treatment is particularly useful when the initial therapeutic effect has been achieved with daily or multiple daily doses of glucocorticoids, and when the duration of treatment is expected to exceed several months. Sudden switching from multiple daily treatments to single dose alternate-day treatment may be associated with symptoms of steroid withdrawal and with a worsening of the disease for which the glucocorticoid treatment is indicated. The use of once-daily morning glucocorticoid treatment should precede alternate-day treatment for 1 to 2 weeks. A changeover from once-daily to alternate-day treatment should be gradual. For example, prednisone 5 mg per day or the equivalent may be adjusted on a weekly basis so that after a number of weeks the total dose can be given on alternate days, such as 20 mg per day would change to 40 mg and 0 mg prednisone on alternating days. It is possible that during this time a flare in the underlying disease could occur. It would then be necessary to return to a treatment dose slightly in excess of the last effective dose. When the therapeutic effect has been reestablished, it would be possible to achieve alternate-day treatment using smaller decrements of steroids, such as prednisone 2.5 mg per day undertaken at longer intervals, such as every 2 to 4 weeks. Even following this gentle conversion schedule, it may not be possible to achieve the desired therapeutic result using alternate-day treatment in all patients. When alternate-day treatment is not satisfactory, a daily single dose of glucocorticoid treatment is preferable to multiple doses during the day. When using alternate-day steroids, the optimum results will be achieved by avoiding long-acting glucocorticoids, such as dexamethasone.

Some investigators have suggested that the use of ACTH to stimulate glucocorticoid production from the adrenal rather than exogenous glucocorticoids is associated with less suppression of the HPA axis. While such a treatment will certainly maintain the adrenal in a responsive state, the level of glucocorticoid production achieved is variable from one patient to another. Furthermore, there is little experimental evidence to suggest that for an equivalent glucocorticoid exposure using ACTH and exogenous glucocorticoids there is a different degree of suppression of the entire HPA axis when evaluated as a unit, such as in response to hypoglycemia or metyrapone. While claims have been made that a better therapeutic response is achieved with ACTH than with glucocorticoids in some disorders, such claims have never been confirmed by control trials. ACTH has to be administered as an intramuscular injection. Hypertension and evidence of androgen excess are much more commonly associated with ACTH administration than with exogenous glucocorticoids.

In some circumstances, particularly those associated with the long-term use of glucocorticoid to control the immunological reaction, it may be possible to employ other immunosuppressive agents to achieve a glucocorticoid-sparing affect. For instance, with the combined use of glucocorticoid with azothiaprine or cyclosporin, the dosage can be adjusted to allow the lowest effective glucocorticoid dose to be used. The optimum use of adjunctive treatment for glucocorticoid-responsive disorders, such as the use of theophyllines and inhaled β-adrenergic agonists for asthma, will allow the lowest dose of systemic glucocorticoid necessary to be employed. It may indeed be possible to substitute inhaled glucocorticoid for systemic glucocorticoid in many patients with asthma.

Despite the therapeutic strategies employed, it is not always possible to achieve a glucocorticoid dosage regimen not associated with emergence of long-term complications. Under these circumstances, it may be prudent to use agents that may off-set the likely development of some specific complications. For those patients who appear to be particularly at risk of osteoporosis (i.e., post-menopausal women demonstrating a low bone density or anyone demonstrating an accelerated loss of bone density), the use of vitamin D and calcium supplementations and/or a biphosphonate is probably worthwhile. Evidence exists that there is less loss of bone density and less occurrence of bone fractures in patients treated in this way than in those who have not received supplementation. Similarly, in children for whom long-term high-dose glucocorticoid is indicated, administration of growth hormone should be considered. Such treatment may diminish growth retardation.

PHYSIOLOGICAL REPLACEMENT THERAPY

In primary adrenal insufficiency, the aim of replacement therapy with glucocorticoids is to provide the optimum dose in terms of type of glucocorticoid, amount, and timing of administration. There are estimates for the physiological secretion rate of cortisol, such as 6 mg/m^2 per day, which provides a guide for initiating the dose of glucocorticoid, but individual requirements are assessed on the clinical response. This requires examination to detect any evidence of either under- or over-replacement. The patient with primary adrenal insufficiency should demonstrate normal pigmentation, normal body weight, normal lying and standing blood pressures, and be without evidence of easy bruising, thinning of the skin, or muscle weakness, and have normal potassium, urea, and glucose levels in blood. Short-acting glucocorticoid has traditionally been used in the form of hydrocortisone or cortisone acetate. Since these are not pure glucocorticoid preparations, it is possible to achieve some mineralocorticoid effect that may be adequate, rendering additional use of mineralocorticoid unnecessary, particularly in adults. Furthermore, there is greater flexibility for dosage adjustment using these agents than more potent glucocorticoids, as fewer tablet size options exists for them, making the dosage adjustment more difficult. When using hydrocortisone to simulate the normal diurnal rhythm of cortisol secretion, replacement should be with two doses per day. The second dose should be administered at approximately 12.00-13.00 h, assuming that the morning dose of glucocorticoid is taken at approximately 7.00-9.00 h. Use of short-acting steroid late in the day, such as at 18.00 h, has no physiological counterpart. If it is found that a dosage of dexamethasone such as 0.5

to 0.25 mg provides satisfactory glucocorticoid replacement, then this agent should be used once in the morning only. When using glucocorticoids to replace the deficiency in patients with congenital adrenal hyperplasia, it is also necessary to achieve suppression of the HPA axis so that excess of other adrenal steroids, usually androgens, is corrected. To do this, it is necessary for glucocorticoid to be taken before going to bed each night in order to inhibit the normal surge of ACTH-cortisol secretion prior to waking. In adults this can be best achieved using a long-acting glucocorticoid such as dexamethasone. Inappropriate timing of treatment in patients with congenital adrenal hyperplasia may result in over-replacement with glucocorticoid when the main dose is given in the early morning without suppressing activity of the HPA axis. This causes androgen excess of endogenous origin to not be controlled and is associated with glucocorticoid excess of mixed exogenous and endogenous origins. Merely substituting a physiological replacement dose of long-acting glucocorticoid at night will correct both problems. Similar considerations should be kept in mind when using glucocorticoid treatment to inhibit adrenal androgen secretion, which may be useful in the treatment of some patients with hirsutism/polycystic ovary syndrome.

WEANING PATIENTS OFF GLUCOCORTICOIDS

There are 2 broad categories of situations in which the withdrawal of glucocorticoid treatment is undertaken. Firstly, in conditions where the beneficial effect of long-term use of glucocorticoids is no longer required, such as in patients successfully treated for asthma or rheumatoid arthritis. Secondly, in the situation where endogenous Cushing's syndrome has been corrected. In this case glucocorticoid replacement therapy is necessary until reactivation of the normal HPA axis has been established. It is worthwhile bearing 3 points in mind when considering the weaning process: (1) withdrawal symptoms similar to those appearing in patients with untreated cortisol deficiency may appear when the exposure to glucocorticoids is being reduced, even if still at supraphysiological levels, (2) it is necessary to maintain physiological replacement of glucocorticoids until there is evidence of at least partial reactivation of the HPA axis, and (3) reduction in the dosage of glucocorticoids should be gradual, as a more rapid change in glucocorticoid exposure may bring about disease reactivation or provoke unpleasant withdrawal symptoms.

High-dose glucocorticoid treatment is usually in the form of prednisone or prednisolone. Withdrawal may be undertaken using decrements in dosages of 5 mg every 1 to 4 weeks until a replacement dosage of approximately 5 mg per day is achieved. This should be given once in the morning only to facilitate recovery of the HPA axis. Since hydrocortisone has a shorter half-life than prednisolone, there is some advantage to substituting hydrocortisone for prednisone. Further reduction in glucocorticoid dosage should not be undertaken until the early morning plasma cortisol prior to administration of glucocorticoid on that day is greater than 200 nmol/l. At this point, further gradual reduction in glucocorticoid dosage may be useful, for example, reducing the dosage of hydrocortisone by 5 mg per month until a minimum dosage of 10 mg each morning is achieved and maintained. This should be done until biological evidence for full recovery of the HPA axis is obtained: early morning cortisol plasma levels above 400 nmol/l and/or a normal short ACTH stimulation test are good indicators; yet the former may be obtained late, and the second is not completely reliable (see further). The insulin-induced hypoglycemia is a gold standard, but it is always uncomfortable and sometimes dangerous. Thus, in a patient with normal or subnormal cortisol (200-400 nmol/l) the short metyrapone test is a safe and highly reliable means to assess the full recovery of the HPA axis. Following profound suppression of the HPA axis, up to 9 months may be required to achieve normal reactivation. ACTH levels return to normal and may become supernormal while cortisol levels remain subnormal. Eventually, as adrenal responsiveness improves, cortisol levels rise into the normal range and ACTH levels fall into the normal range, and a normal relationship is re-established. Patients who have received prednisone treatment in excess of 10 mg per day for more than 2 weeks in the preceding 6 months should be advised that under conditions of stress they should take extra glucocorticoid cover. This strategy is particularly important in patients undergoing emergency surgical procedures or in whom significant intercurrent illnesses arises, such as pneumonia. Such a patient should be treated as if they have adrenal insufficiency using a short course of glucocorticoids in dosages approximately two- to threefold greater than physiological replacement in the perioperative period, or until the incidental illness has resolved. Extra glucocorticoids can then be withdrawn over a period of approximately 1 to 2 weeks.

The term "withdrawal syndrome" has been used to indicate the clinical symptoms that arises in some patients while they are undergoing reduction in their doses of glucocorticoid. The condition is also frequently seen in the patient cured of endogenous Cushing's syndrome. Symptoms consist of weakness, lethargy, diffuse body aching, weight loss, headaches, and occasionally fever. The mechanism underlying the development of these symptoms is unknown. Symptoms respond to increasing the dosage of glucocorticoid but may reappear on reduction of the dosage again even when weaning is undertaken very gently. In general, the temptation to maintain treatment with supraphysiological doses of glucocorticoids should be resisted, as it maintains the exposure to glucocorticoid excess without bringing closer the time when glucocorticoids can be discontinued without symptoms. The steroid withdrawal syndrome may persist after the resumption of normal HPA axis activity. As the condition is self-limiting, patients should be reassured that the symptoms will resolve, though this may take 1 to 2 years. The final resolution is usually dramatic, with patients noticing the return of the normal sense of well-being at a particular point. This point will be reached sooner if supraphysiological doses of glucocorticoids are avoided, and when replacement doses of glucocorticoid are withdrawn once reactivation of the HPA axis has been identified.

ASSESSMENT OF THE HYPOTHALAMIC-PITUITARY-ADRENAL AXIS

Plasma cortisol

Early-morning plasma cortisol levels in excess of 400 nmol/l indicate adequate activity of the HPA axis. When this value has been achieved or exceeded, further evaluation of the HPA axis is not warranted. However, when this value is not achieved, additional evaluation is indicated. The strategy recommended for patients whose basal plasma cortisol level is lower than 400 nmol/l, and for whom it is necessary to determine the status of the HPA axis, is to use the metyrapone test since it is safe, simple, and accurate (see below).

Short ACTH stimulation tests

Measurement of plasma cortisol levels in response to the administration of α1-24 ACTH, 250 μg iv, has been promoted as a useful way of determining the status of the HPA axis. However, this test only indicates whether or not the adrenal gland has retained sensitivity to ACTH rather than testing the entire axis. It has been argued that since the hypothalamic-pituitary unit recovers from suppression earlier than the adrenal, that the response to ACTH may be taken as an index of activity in the entire unit. However, approximately 10% of patients who respond normally to ACTH will fail to respond to insulin-induced hypoglycemia. Case reports exist that clearly indicate that the diagnosis of clinically significant adrenal insufficiency was missed when reliance was placed on the ACTH test alone. For this reason this author does not recommend the use of the conventional ACTH stimulation test in the assessment for secondary adrenal insufficiency.

A modification of the ACTH stimulation test has been recommended whereby 1 μg rather than 250 μg of α1-24 ACTH is injected intravenously and the cortisol response evaluated. The occasions for dissociation between the response to low-dose ACTH and the response to hypoglycemia are considerably fewer than those encountered when using the conventional ACTH dosage.

Insulin-induced hypoglycemia

This test has been regarded for many years as the gold standard for the assessment of the HPA axis. However, this test is unpleasant for patients and demanding on medical resources. It requires achieving significant hypoglycemia, that is, blood glucose levels less than 2.2 mmol/l, and requires constant medical attendance. The side effects are those related to hypoglycemia and its reversal. Unfortunately, deaths have been reported as a result of this investigation. While the response to hypoglycemia does provide accurate information on the activity of the entire HPA axis, similar information may be obtained from the metyrapone test, which makes fewer demands on patients and medical resources.

Short metyrapone test

Metyrapone inhibits the conversion of 11-deoxycortisol to cortisol by suppressing the activity of the enzyme 11β-hydroxylase. In all individuals, when metyrapone is given at midnight there is impaired ability of the adrenal to synthesize cortisol the following morning. As a result of this there is increased activity in the hypothalamic-pituitary unit so that the ACTH level rises, which stimulates the adrenal gland and causes the accumulation of 11-deoxycortisol proximal to the metyrapone-induced biosynthetic block. The finding of 11-deoxycortisol levels in excess of 200 nmol/l indicates normal activity in the HPA axis. When values of less than this are found in response to the administration of metyrapone, 30 mg/kg/bodyweight at midnight, it is necessary to confirm that simultaneous plasma cortisol levels are less than 200 nmol/l to establish a diagnosis of adrenal insufficiency. In patients still receiving glucocorticoid therapy, this should be withheld until after blood sampling. This test is associated with only minor side effects, such as occasional light-headedness and vivid dreams, and reported instances of clinical worsening in adrenal insufficiency are extremely rare.

Corticotropin-releasing hormone

The use of corticotropin-releasing hormone to stimulate pituitary-adrenal activity and assess the ACTH and cortisol response has been evaluated in patients undergoing treatment with glucocorticoids. This is probably a useful test. However, it certainly suffers from the theoretical possibility that when suppression of the hypothalamic unit exceeds that of the pituitary and adrenal, a normal response to exogenous corticotropin-releasing hormone may occur while the ability to release corticotropin-releasing hormone endogenously has been impaired.

Suggested readings

ADACHI JD, BENSEN WG, BROWN J, et al. Intermittent etidronate therapy to prevent corticosteroid-induced osteoporosis. N Engl M Med 1997;337:382-7.

ALLEN DB. Growth suppression by glucococrotoid therapy. Endocrinol Metab Clin N Am 1996;25:699-717.

AXELROD L. Corticosteroid therapy. In: Becker KL (ed). Principles and practice. In: Endocrinlogy and metabolism.

2nd ed. Philadelphia: JB Lippincott Company, 1995;695-706.

FIAD TM, KIRBY JM, CUNNINGHAM SK, MCKENNA TJ. The overnight single dose metyrapone test is a simple and reliable index of the hypothalamic-pituitary-adrenal axis. Clin Endocrinol 1994;40:603-9.

GRINSPOON SK, BILLER BMK. Clinical review 62: Laboratory assessment of adrenal insufficiency. J Clin Endocrinol Metab 1994;79:923-31.

GRABER AL, NEY RW, NICHOLSON WE, ISLAND DB, LIDDLE GW.

Natural history of pituitary-adrenal recovery following long term suppression with corticosteroids. J Clin Endocr 1965;25:11-6.

HUREL SJ, THOMPSON CJ, WATSON MJ, HERRIS MM, BAYLIS PH, KENDALL-TAYLOR P. The short Synacthen and insulin stress tests in the assessment of the hypothalamic-pituitary-adrenal axis. Clin Endocrinol 1996;44:141-6.

MOORE GW, LACROIX A, RABIN D, MCKENNA TJ. Gonadal dysfunction in adult men with congenital adrenal hyperplasia. Acta Endorinol 1980;95:185-93.

OELKERS W. Dose-response aspects in the clinical assessment in the hypothalamo-pituitary-adrenal axis and the low dose adrenocorticotropin test. Eur J Endocrinol 1996;135:27-33.

SCHIMMER BP, PARKER KL. Adrenocorticotropic hormone; adrenocortical steroids and their synthetic analogs; inhibitors of the synthesis and actions of adrenocortical hormones. In: Hardman JG, Limbird LE (eds). Goodman and Gillman's The pharmacological basis of therapeutics. 9th ed. New York: McGraw-Hill, 1996;1459-85.

SOULE SG, FAHIE-WILSON M, TOMLINSON S. Failure of the short ACTH test to unequivocally diagnose long-standing symptomatic secondary hypoadrenalism. Clin Endocrinol 1996;44:137-40.

SAMBROOK P, BIRMINGHAM J, KELLY P et al. Prevention of cortiosteroid osteoporosis. A comparison of calcium, calcitriol and calcitonin. N Engl J Med 1993;328:1747-52.

SHAH A, STANHOPE R, MATTHEW D. Hazards of pharmacological tests of growth hormone secretion in childhood. BMJ 1992;304:173-4.

TYRRELL TB. Glucocorticocoid therapy. In: Felig P, Baxter JD, Frohman LA (eds). Endocrinology and metabolism. 3rd ed., New York: McGraw-Hill, 1995;855-82.

WILLIAMS GR, FRANKLYN JA. Physiology of the steroid-thyroid hormone nuclear receptor superfamily. Ballières Clin Endocrinol Metab 1994;8:241-66.

The adrenal medulla: basic concepts

Emmanuel L. Bravo

■ **KEY POINTS** ■

- In the adrenal medulla, most of the synthesized norepinephrine is converted to epinephrine by the enzyme phenylethanolamine-*N*-methyltransferase, which is activated by glucocorticoids secreted by the adrenal cortex.
- In the normal adrenal medulla, the concentration of epinephrine is about four times that of norepinephrine, and the same ratio is found in adrenal venous effluent. In plasma, however, norepinephrine is 8 to 10 times that of epinephrine.
- In adrenal pheochromocytoma – with the rare exception of pure, or predominantly epinephrine-producing, tumors – norepinephrine predominates over epinephrine in adrenal venous effluent.
- Tumors weighing <50 g have *low* concentrations of metabolites relative to free catecholamines in urine, while tumors >50 g have *high* concentrations of metabolites relative to free catecholamines in urine.
- In the normal adrenal medulla, catecholamine secretion is induced by activation of the splanchnic nerve. By contrast, pheochromocytomas do not have any nervous innervation, and the mechanism whereby catecholamines are released remains obscure.

Catecholamine production in the normal adrenal medulla

The biosynthesis, release, and metabolism of norepinephrine in chromaffin cells are essentially the same as that of sympathetic nerves; however, chromaffin cells have the capacity to convert norepinephrine to epinephrine (Fig. 32.1). The initial step in the sequence is the hydroxylation of tyrosine to dihydroxyphenylalanine (L-dopa) by the action of the enzyme tyrosine hydroxylase, and then L-dopa is decarboxylated to dopamine by the enzyme dopa decarboxylase. Dopamine is then actively transported into intracellular vesicles, where it is converted to norepinephrine by dopamine-beta-hydroxylase. Most of the norepinephrine is stored as nondiffusible complexes. In the adrenal medulla most of the norepinephrine leaves the granules, is methylated in the cytoplasm to epinephrine by the enzyme phenylethanolamine-*N*-methyltransferase (PNMT), and then reenters a different group of intracellular granules, where it is stored until released. In mammalian tissue, only the heart, adrenal medulla, brain, and brainstem have measurable amounts of PNMT.

A major factor that controls the rate of synthesis of epinephrine is the level of glucocorticoids secreted by the adrenal cortex. Glucocorticoids are carried in high concentrations by the intra-adrenal portal vascular system directly to the adrenal medullary chromaffin cells, where they induce the synthesis of PNMT, the enzyme that methylates norepinephrine to epinephrine. Thus, any form of stress that invokes enhanced secretion of corticotropin mobilizes the appropriate hormones of both the adrenal cortex (that is, cortisol) and the medulla (that is, epinephrine). This remarkable relationship is present only in certain mammals, including man, where the adrenal chromaffin cells are enveloped entirely by steroid-secreting cortical cells.

The normal adrenal gland is innervated by the splanchnic nerve, which is a preganglionic (cholinergic) portion of the sympathetic nervous systems. Therefore, activation of the splanchnic nerve induces a release of acetylcholine at its nerve terminal, which, in the presence of calcium, causes secretion of catecholamines from the adrenal medulla by exocytosis.

In a normal adrenal medulla, the concentration of epinephrine is about four times that of norepinephrine, and the same ratio is found in the adrenal venous effluent. In plasma, however, norepinephrine is about eight to ten times that of epinephrine. Norepinephrine in plasma is derived almost exclusively (about 98%) from axon terminals of sympathetic postganglionic neurons; the remaining 2% is derived from adrenal medullary secretion. However, all of the circulating epinephrine originates from the adrenal medulla. Centrally synthesized catecholamines do not contribute to the plasma pool of catecholamines.

The catecholamines are metabolized principally by two enzymes (Fig. 32.2): monoamine oxidase (MAO), which is found mainly within adrenergic neurons; and catechol-*O*-methyltransferase (COMT), which is localized for the most part in non-neural tissues. The action of catechol-*O*-methyltransferase results in the formation of the metanephrines; further oxidation of the amines by monoamine oxidase leads to the formation of vanillylmandelic acid. With the use of radioactively labeled norepinephrine, it is estimated that of the circulating norepinephrine, 5% appears in urine as the free form, and 8% is conjugated; 20% appears as free and conjugated normetanephrines; 23% as free and conjugated 3, 4-dihydroxyphenylethyleneglycol; and 30% as vanillylmandelic acid. The free forms, metanephrine, and vanillylmandelic acid are commonly assayed to assess adrenomedullary activity.

Catecholamine production in pheochromocytoma

In pheochromocytoma, the activities of the enzymes involved in catecholamine synthesis are markedly enhanced, whereas the activities of the enzymes involved in catecholamine catabolism are reduced. Therefore, excess amounts of newly synthesized norepinephrine that cannot be stored in the filled catecholamine storage vesicles may not be degraded and could diffuse from the pheochromocytoma into the circulation. This could result in large amounts of circulating norepinephrine with relatively small increases in urinary catecholamine metabolites.

The size of the tumor may be an important determinant of the relative amounts of catecholamine excretory products since small tumors (<50 g) have rapid turnover rates with small catecholamine content. These tumors primarily release unmetabolized catecholamines into the circulation, resulting in low concentrations of urinary metabolites relative to free catecholamines in the urine. Conversely, large tumors (>50 g) have slow turnover rates with a large catecholamine content. These tumors primarily release metabolized catecholamines into the circulation, wich results in high concentrations of metabolites relative to free catecholamines in the urine. These observations have important clinical implications. Because they release free unmetabolized catecholamines into the circulation, small tumors may tend to produce more symptoms and are best diagnosed by the measurement of plasma catecholamines. On the other hand, patients who have large tumors that metabolize most of the secreted catecholamines tend to have fewer symptoms and relatively lower circulating free catecholamines, but high urinary catecholamine metabolites.

Most tumors contain a smaller concentration of epinephrine than does the normal adrenal medulla, or even no epinephrine. Of interest, and of some clinical importance, is the fact that with rare exceptions, pheochromocytomas that secrete at least some epinephrine are located in the adrenal gland. However, since occasionally some extra-adrenal tumors (located, for example, in the hilus of the liver, thorax, urinary tract, bladder, the organ of Zuckerkandl, and other intra-abdominal sites) have been found to contain epinephrine, an epinephrine-secreting tumor is not always invariably of adrenal origin. Also of diagnostic importance is that, unless one is dealing with a pure or predominantly epinephrine-producing adrenal tumor, the adrenal venous concentration of catecholamines will contain mostly norepinephrine, unlike the normal adrenal venous effluent, which contains mostly epinephrine.

The mechanism whereby catecholamine release from pheochromocytoma is triggered remains obscure. There is no evidence that pheochromocytoma have any nervous

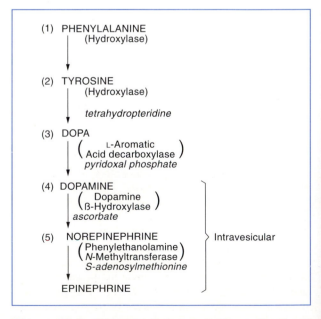

Figure 32.1 Steps in the enzymatic synthesis of dopamine, norepinephrine, and epinephrine.

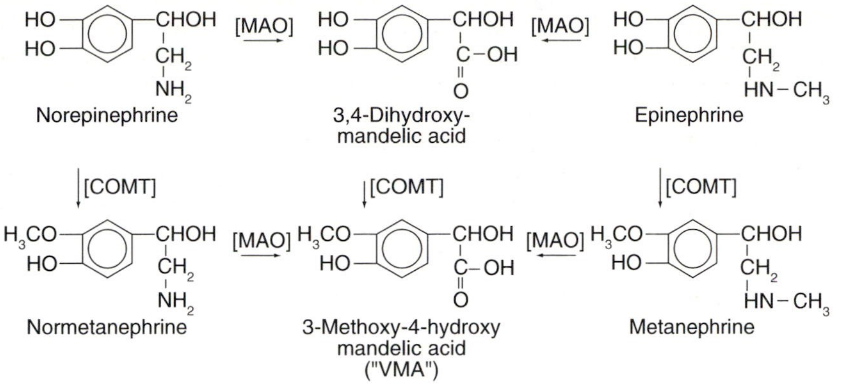

Figure 32.2 Metabolism of norepinephrine and epinephrine. COMT = catechol-*O*-methyltransferase; MAO = monoamine oxidase. (Modified from Mayer SE. In: Goodman LS, Gilman AG, AG, eds. The pharmacolocigal basis of therapeutics, New York: McGraw-Hill, 1980.)

innervation, and studies have demonstrated that activation of the sympathetic nervous system does not result in catecholamine release from a pheochromocytoma. Sudden increases in blood pressure that are sometimes precipitated by emotional upset, hypotension, or anesthesia could result from central sympathetic activation, which induces the release of norepinephrine from sympathetic nerve terminals that have accumulated excessive stores of catecholamines. Therefore, any drug stimulating the sympathetic nervous system directly or in a reflex fashion (such as histamine, tyramine, and glucagon) could release excessive quantities of norepinephrine at effector sites of nerve terminals and produce a hypertensive crisis. This hypothesis draws support from the demonstration that clonidine, a central α_2- agonist that inhibits central sympathetic outflow, decreases blood pressure in patients with pheochromocytoma without detectable changes in circulating norepinephrine.

Suggested readings

AXELROD JO. Purification and properties of pheylethanolamine-N-methyltransferase. J Biol Chem 1962;237:1657-60.

BRAVO EL, TARAZI RC, FOUAD FM, VIDT DG, GIFFORD RW jr. Clonidine-suppression test: a useful aid in the diagnosis of pheochromocytoma. N Engl J Med 1981;305:623-6.

CROUT JR, SJOERDSMA A. Turnover and metabolism of catecholamine in patients with pheochromocytoma. J Clin Invest 1964;43:94-102.

ENGELMAN K, HAMMOND WG. Adrenaline production by an intrathoracic phaeochromocytoma. Lancet 1968;1:609-11.

HERMAN H, MORNEX R. Human tumors secreting catecholamines: Clinical and Physiopathological Studies in Pheochromocytomas. Oxford, New York: Pergamon Press, 1964;207.

JARROTT B, LOUIS WJ. Abnormalities in enzymes involved in catecholamine synthesis and catabolism in pheochromocytoma. Clin Sci 1977;53;529-35.

MAAS JW, LANDIS DH. The metabolism of circulating norepinephrine by human subjects. J Pharm Exp Ther 1971;177:600-12.

SANDERS-BUSH E, MAYER SE. 5-Hydroxytryptamine (serotonin) receptor agonists and antagonists. In: Goodman LS, Gilman AG (eds). The pharmacologic basis of therapeutics. 9th ed. New York: McGraw-Hill, 1996.

VIVEROS OH, ARQUEROS L, KIRSHNER N. Release of catecholamines and dopamine-beta-oxidase from the adrenal medulla. Life Sci 1968;7:609-18.

WURTMAN RJ, POHORECKY LA, BALIGA BS. Adrenocortical control of the biosynthesis of epinephrine and proteins in the adrenal medulla. Pharmacol Rev 1972;24:411-26.

33

Diagnosis and management of pheochromocytoma

Emmanuel L. Bravo

KEY POINTS

- Early recognition and treatment of pheochromocytoma is mandatory. If untreated it can lead to serious cardiovascular complications, and it can become malignant and unresponsive to radiation or chemotherapy.
- When reliably carried out and performed in an appropriate setting, the simultaneous determination of plasma catecholamines and 24-hour urinary metanephrines can establish the diagnosis in about 97% of cases.
- Pharmacologic testing with glucagon (to provoke catecholamine secretion from a tumor with low activity) and/or clonidine (to inhibit central sympathetic outflow) is/are indicated in patients in whom the clinical manifestations are suggestive of pheochromocytoma, but biochemical results are equivocal.
- Magnetic resonance imaging provides the highest sensitivity and metaiodobenzylguanidine scanning the best specificity among current imaging techniques for pheochromocytoma.
- For medical therapy, calcium antagonists with or without specific α1-adrenoreceptor antagonists (e.g., doxazosin) can control symptoms without the side effects associated with non-specific α-adrenoreceptor antagonists (e.g., phenoxybenzamine).

Pheochromocytomas are catecholamine-producing tumors of chromaffin cells present in the sympathetic nervous system that typically represent an uncommon cause of hypertension. They release epinephrine and/or norepinephrine – and sometimes dopamine. In addition to catecholamines, pheochromocytomas have been reported to produce a wide variety of active peptides.

Clinical findings

Symptoms and signs

Priority of evaluation should be given to patients exhibiting any of the following: (1) episodic symptoms of headaches, tachycardia, and diaphoresis (with or without hypertension); (2) family history of pheochromocytoma or a multiple endocrine neoplasia syndrome; (3) incidental suprarenal or abdominal masses; (4) unexplained paroxysms of tachyarrhythmias; hypertension during intubation, the induction of anesthesia, parturition, or prolonged unexplained hypotension after an operation; (5) adverse cardiovascular responses to ingestion, inhalation, or injection of certain drugs; including anesthetic agents, histamine, glucagon, tyramine, thyrotropin-releasing hormone (TRH), adrenocorticotropic hormone (ACTH), antidopaminergic agents, naloxone, succinylcholine chloride, phenothiazine, β-blockers, guanethidine, tricyclic antidepressants, and methacholine; (6) spells or attacks during physical exertion, twisting and turning of the torso, straining (Valsalva's maneuver), coitus, or micturition. Some clinical conditions that are likely to be confused with pheochromocytoma are shown in Table 33.1.

Table 33.1 Clinical conditions likely to be confused with pheochromocytoma

β-adrenergic hyper-responsiveness
Acute state of anxiety
Angina pectoris
Acute infections
Autonomic epilepsy
Hyperthyroidism
Idiopathic orthostatic hypotension
Cerebellopontine angle tumors
Acute hypoglycemia
Acute drug withdrawal
  Clonidine
  β-Adrenergic blockade
  α-Methyldopa
  Alcohol
Vasodilator therapy
  Hydralazine
  Minoxidil
Factitious administration of sympathomimetic
  agents
Tyramine ingestion in patients on monoamine
  oxidase inhibitors
Menopausal syndrome with migraine headaches

(From Bravo EL. The syndrome of primary aldosteronism and pheochromocytoma. In: Schrier RW, Gottschalk CW [eds]. Diseases of the kidney. 5th ed. Boston: Little, Brown & Co, 1993:1475-503.)

Diagnostic procedures

When reliably carried out and performed in an appropriate setting, biochemical testing can establish the diagnosis in over 95% of cases. For example, the demonstration of resting plasma catecholamines (norepinephrine plus epinephrine) >2000 pg/ml, urinary total metanephrines >1.8 mg/24 h, and urinary norepinephrine >156 μg/24 h suggests the diagnosis of pheochromocytoma. Of the various biochemical tests, assays of plasma catecholamines and total urinary metanephrines together have the lowest false-negative rate (7%), assays of urinary norepinephrine and epinephrine the next higher (14%), and assays of urinary vanillylmandelic acid the highest (41%). In our experience, the determination of the combination of resting plasma catecholamines and total urinary metanephrines together gives a false-negative rate of 2.7% (3/109 patients). All three patients not diagnosed by the measurement of plasma catecholamines and urinary metanephrines had multiple endocrine neoplasia syndrome.

The measurement of serum chromogranin A (CgA) (a protein co-released with catecholamines) and plasma catecholamines provides an overall specificity of 95% accuracy, 88% sensitivity, with a positive predictive value of 91%. However, the clinical utility of the test drops significantly in the presence of even mild degrees of renal impairment; at creatinine clearances <80 ml/min, the specificity, accuracy, and positive predictive values are 92%, 86%, and 75%, respectively. In patients with creatinine clearance ≥80 ml/min, the combination gives a speci-

ficity of 98%, accuracy of 89%, and a positive predictive value of 97%.

Certain clinical situations may increase both plasma catecholamines and urinary catecholamine metabolites to levels usually seen in pheochromocytoma. These include: (1) acute clonidine withdrawal, (2) acute alcohol withdrawal, (3) vasodilator therapy with hydralazine or minoxidil, (4) acute myocardial ischemia or infarction, (5) acute cerebrovascular accident, (6) cocaine abuse; and (7) severe congestive heart failure (Classes III-IV). Intravenously administered dopamine (even in small doses), dopaminergic drugs, and acute hypoglycemia produce significant elevations in plasma epinephrine concentrations.

Drugs that inhibit central sympathetic outflow (e.g., clonidine, methyldopa, bromocriptine, and haloperidol) decrease levels of plasma catecholamine secretion in normal and hypertensive patients, but they have little effect on the excessive catecholamine secretion by pheochromocytoma. Drugs that tend to increase levels of plasma catecholamines (e.g., phenoxybenzamine, phentolamine, labetalol, theophylline, β-blockers, and diuretics) do so only slightly, and levels rarely approach those usually encountered in pheochromocytoma.

When the diagnosis is not obvious because of equivocal results, pharmacologic testing should be performed. In such cases, the goal is to separate pheochromocytoma patients with relatively low levels of biosynthetic activity from nonpheochromocytoma patients with increased sympathetic outflow. Tests may be stimulatory (to provoke catecholamine secretion from a tumor with low activity) or suppressive (to inhibit central sympathetic outflow). A provocative test is employed when the clinical findings are highly suggestive of pheochromocytoma, even if the blood pressure is normal or only slightly increased and catecholamine production is near normal (plasma catecholamines between 500-1000 pg/ml). Glucagon is given as an IV bolus of 2.0 mg after an appropriate control. A positive glucagon test requires a clear increase (at least threefold or >2000 pg/ml in plasma catecholamines), 1-3 minutes after drug administration. A simultaneous increase in blood pressure is not essential. Blood pressure should be recorded continuously. If values rise to or exceed 200/120 mmHg, then either phentolamine (5-10 mg iv bolus) or sodium nitroprusside by continuous drip should be initiated. Alternatively, nifedipine XL (30-60 mg orally) can be given 2 hours before the test to prevent the rise in blood pressure without interference with catecholamine release.

Suppressive tests are utilized in patients with moderate increases in plasma catecholamines (i.e., between 1000 and 2000 pg/ml) with or without hypertension. The clonidine suppression test is based on the principle that normal increases in levels of plasma catecholamines are mediated through activation of the sympathetic nervous system, whereas in patients with pheochromocytoma, the increases result from diffusion of excess catecholamines from the tumor into the circulation, thus bypassing normal storage and release mechanisms. Since clonidine suppresses neurogenically-mediated catecholamine release, it should not be expected to suppress the release of catecholamines in patients with pheochromocytoma. This expectation is borne out by studies showing that the release of plasma catecholamines in patients with essential hypertension is suppressed with clonidine, whereas it is unaltered in patients with pheochromocytoma.

Clonidine is given as a single oral dose of 0.3 mg; blood pressure, heart rate, and objective signs of central effects (i.e., sleepiness, thirst, dry mouth) should be recorded before and at 30-minute intervals for 3 hours after clonidine administration. A normal test consists of a fall in the basal values of plasma catecholamines below 500 pg/ml at 2 or 3 hours into the test. A fall in blood pressure and heart rate, and objective signs of central effects, assure adequate absorption of the drug. Marked volume depletion should be avoided, and β-adrenergic blocking agents should be discontinued 48 hours before testing. β-Adrenergic blocking agents tend to augment the vagotonic effects of clonidine, leading to marked bradycardia, decreased cardiac output, and further blood pressure reductions. In addition, β-adrenergic blockers interfere with hepatic clearance of catecholamines and prevent the catecholamine-lowering effect of clonidine in patients with increased neurogenic tone.

Grossman and coworkers assessed the clinical utility of combined glucagon and clonidine testing in 22 patients with and 28 patients without pheochromocytoma. Their study showed that when both tests are negative, a diagnosis of pheochromocytoma is highly unlikely.

From the foregoing discussion, the following approach is suggested for patients clinically suspected of having pheochromocytoma (Fig. 33.1). Initially, resting plasma catecholamines, serum chromogranin A, and serum creatinine levels (for calculation of the creatinine clearance by the Cockroft-Gault equation) should be determined. An increase in both plasma catecholamines (≥2000 pg/ml) and serum CgA (≥70 pg/m) *and* creatinine clearance ≥80 ml/min suggests the presence of pheochromocytoma. This combination has a positive predictive value of 97%. Patients with equivocal increases in plasma catecholamines (between 1000 and 2000 pg/ml) and *normal* serum CgA are likely to have neurogenically-mediated catecholamine release and will require a clonidine suppression test for definitive diagnosis. Patients with plasma catecholamine values ≤1000 pg/ml and serum CgA >70

pg/ml are likely to have creatinine clearance values <80 ml/min; a glucagon-provocative test may be necessary in highly suspect patients. Patients with normal plasma catecholamine and serum CgA values are unlikely to have pheochromocytoma. Clinical judgment will dictate whether additional testing (i.e., use of urinary catecholamines and catecholamine metabolites) should be performed.

Imaging studies

Computerized tomography (CT) and magnetic resonance imaging (MRI) are equally sensitive (98% and 100%, respectively), whereas metaiodobenzylguanidine (^{131}MIBG) scanning has a sensitivity of only 78%. However, ^{131}MIBG has specificity of 100%, whereas CT and MRI have lower specificities of 70% and 67%, respectively.

When biochemical tests suggest pheochromocytoma, MRI provides the highest sensitivity among current imaging techniques (Fig. 33.2). Pheochromocytomas appear hyperintense to the liver on the T_2-weighted image, whereas benign tumors appear isointense (Fig. 33.3). If no tumor is detected, ^{131}MIBG scintigraphy should be employed, followed by vena caval sampling if the scintigraphic finding is negative. Arteriography and/or venous sampling for plasma catecholamines concentrations are rarely indicated. Exceptions to this are situations in which the clinical and biochemical evidence point strongly to pheochromocytoma, yet the noninvasive techniques persistently fail to localize the sites of the tumors. The decision to proceed to ^{131}MIBG scintigraphy in patients with clearly-defined tumors that are hyperintense on the T_2-weighted image by MRI depends on a number of factors. These include a lesion exceeding 5.0 cm in diameter, the familial nature of the disease, the involvement of other endocrine glands (i.e., thyroid, parathyroid, pancreas), and the presence of multifocal disease.

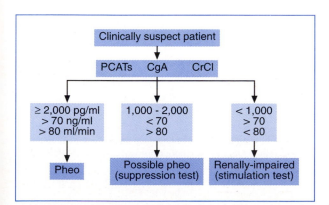

Figure 33.1 Diagnosis of pheochromocytoma. (PCATs = plasma catecholamines; CgA = chromogranin A; CrCl = creatinine clearance.)

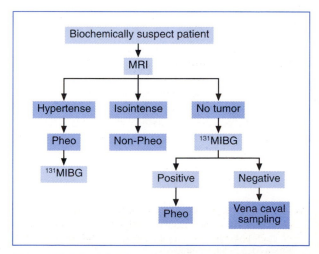

Figure 33.2 Localization of pheochromocytoma. (^{131}MIBG = metaiodobenzylguanidine; MRI = magnetic resonance imaging.)

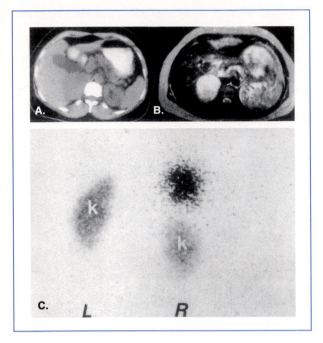

Figure 33.3 Localization of pheochromocytoma in a patient with a tumor in the right adrenal gland by **A**, abdominal CT scan, **B**, MR T2-weighted image, **C**, (131MIBG scintigraphy 72 hours after radioisotope injection. K = kidney, L = left, R = right.) (From Bravo EL. Pheochromocytoma: new concepts and future trends. Kidney Int 1991;40:544-56.)

Treatment

The goal of medical management is to minimize cardiovascular morbidity and mortality. Phenoxybenzamine, a long-acting, non-competitive, non-selective α-blocking agent is the most widely-used agent. There are several disadvantages of α-blockade with phenoxybenzamine. First, it produces marked orthostatic hypotension with tachycardia, sexual dysfunction, and diarrhea. Second, it prolongs and contributes to the hypotension that follows removal of the tumor. Despite adequate α-blockade, total elimination of cardiovascular disturbance is seldom achieved, and significant elevation of blood pressure is to be anticipated during manipulation of the tumor.

β-Adrenergic blocking agents are sometimes needed to control tachycardia or arrhythmias, but only after an α-adrenergic blockade has been established. Labetalol, an α- and β-adrenergic blocker, was reported to be effective in the control of blood pressure and clinical manifestations of pheochromocytoma. The initial dose is 100 mg qid, increased stepwise to a maximum of 800 to 1600 mg per day. However, it has precipitated hypertensive crises in some patients.

The use of more specific α_1-adrenoreceptor antagonists, or one of the calcium antagonists, may be just as effective. Prazosin hydrochloride (Minipres) (in doses of 2-5 mg t.i.d. or q.i.d.) has been shown to reduce blood pressure in pheochromocytoma. The newer α_1-adrenergic blocking agents, terazosin (Hytrin) (1-20 mg/day), and doxazosin (Cardura) (1-16 mg/day), are just as effective. They do not produce reflex tachycardia and have a shorter duration of action, thereby permitting a more rapid adjustment of dosage and decreasing the duration of postoperative hypotension. Calcium antagonists have also been successful in controlling the clinical manifestations of pheochromocytoma. These agents have the advantage of not reducing blood pressure in normotensive patients, and therefore they may be used safely in those who have intermittent hypertension. In addition, these agents do not interfere with biochemical testing. To minimize postoperative hypotension, two or three units of whole blood or another volume expander should be administered within 12 hours preoperatively, and losses during and after surgery should be replaced.

For patients with inoperative, malignant, recurrent, or multicentric pheochromocytoma, long-term medical therapy is the treatment of choice. Calcium antagonists with or without specific α_1-adrenoreceptor antagonists have been used with success. Metyrosine, an inhibitor of catecholamine synthesis, can decrease circulatory catecholamines by 80%. The initial daily dose is 500-1000 mg in divided doses. It may be increased daily by 240 to 500 mg to a maximum of 4000 mg per day. However, control of blood pressure may be incomplete, and serious side effects (extrapyramidal signs, diarrhea, anxiety, and crystalluria) may occur. Partial remission or palliation can sometimes be achieved with 131MIBG, or with a combination of cyclophosphamide, vincristine, and dacarbazine. The results have been disappointing and clinical experience is limited. These therapeutic modalities should be reserved for malignant or inoperable cases who have not responded to other medical regimens. Whenever possible, surgical excision or debulking of accessible tumors should be performed to reduce the mass of tumor tissue. Removal often helps to decrease the levels of circulating catecholamines and provide easier control of blood pressure and other manifestations.

Suggested readings

AVERBUCH SD, STEAKLEY CS, YOUNG RC, et al. Malignant pheochromocytoma: effective treatment with a combination of cyclophosphamide, vincristine, and dacarbazine. Ann Intern Med 1988;109:267-73.

BOUTROS AR, BRAVO EL, ZANETTIN G, et al. Perioperative management of 63 patients with pheochromocytoma. Cleve Clin J Med 1990;57:613-7.

BRAVO EL. Adrenal medulla function. In: Moore WT, Eastman RC (eds). Diagnostic endocrinology. 2nd ed. Philadelphia: BC Decker, 1996;299-309.

BRAVO EL. Pheochromocytoma: new concepts and future trends [clinical conference]. Kidney Int 1991;40:544-56.

BRAVO EL. The syndrome of primary aldosteronism and pheochromocytoma. In: Schrier RW, Gottschalk CW (eds). Diseases of the kidney. 5th ed. Boston: Little, Brown & Co, 1993;1475-503.

BRAVO EL, TARAZI RC, FOUAD FM, et al. Clonidine-suppression test: a useful aid in the diagnosis of pheochromocytoma. N Engl J Med 1981;305:623-6.

CANALE MP, BRAVO EL. Calcium channel entry blockers are effective and safe in the preoperative management of pheochromocytoma [abstract]. Hypertension 1993;21:560-1.

CANALE MP, BRAVO EL. Diagnostic specificity of serum chromogranin-A for pheochromocytoma in patients with renal dysfunction. J Clin Endocrinol Metab 1994;78:1139-44.

GROSSMAN E, GOLDSTEIN DS, HOFFMAN A, et al. Glucagon and clonidine testing in the diagnosis of pheochromocytoma. Hypertension 1991;17:733-41.

JONES NF, WALKER G, RUTHVEN CR, et al. Alpha-methyl-p-tyro-sine in the management of phaeochromocytoma. Lancet 1968;2:1105-9.

SERFAS D, SHOBACK DM, LORELL BH. Phaeochromocytoma and hypertrophic cardiomyopathy: apparent suppression of symptoms and noradrenaline secretion by calcium-channel blockade. Lancet 1983;2:711-3.

SHAPIRO B, SISSON JC, WIELAND DM, et al. Radiopharmaceutical therapy of malignant pheochromocytoma with [131I] metaiodobenzylguanidine: results from ten years of experience. J Nucl Biol Med 1991;35:269-76.

Endocrinology of hypertension

The endocrinology of hypertension: basic concepts and diagnostic procedures

Franco Mantero

Mineralocorticoids are steroid hormones that are secreted by the zona fasciculata (ZF) and the zona glomerulosa (ZG) of the adrenal cortex. Their principal actions are the maintenance of normal electrolyte (sodium and potassium) concentrations and fluid equilibrium in the body. The most powerful mineralocorticoid is aldosterone. Aldosterone is synthesized exclusively in the ZG with its precursor, 18-hydroxycorticosterone, and is mainly regulated by the renin-angiotensin system. Another important mineralocorticoid is deoxycorticosterone (DOC), which is produced in

the ZF together with corticosterone and 18-hydroxydeoxy-corticosterone under the control of adrenocorticotropic hormone (ACTH). As already outlined in Chapter 26, the enzymes involved in mineralocorticoid synthesis are differentially expressed in the ZF and ZG. P450CYP11B1 is mainly a ZF enzyme, but it is also present in ZG and catalyzes the 11-hydroxylation of DOC to corticosterone, while P450CYP11B2 (or aldosterone synthase) is almost exclusively expressed in ZG and is responsible for the three steps leading from DOC to aldosterone (Fig. 34.1).

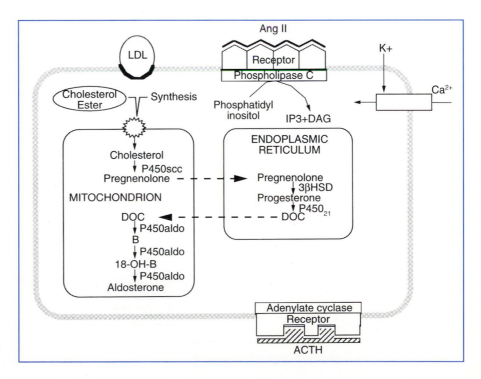

Figure 34.1 Regulation of aldosterone secretion.

Regulation of aldosterone secretion

Aldosterone secretion is regulated by several interacting factors, including circulating and tissue angiotensin II (AII), potassium ion, ACTH, sodium ion, and, to a lesser degree, dopamine, serotonin, natriuretic hormones, and others. AII is an octapeptide that acts principally at two sites, adrenal ZG and vasculature, by binding to specific receptors. At the ZG level AII acutely and chronically stimulates aldosterone production, while at the vessel level it induces arteriolar vasoconstriction. AII is thus the final biologically active product of the cascade of the renin-angiotensin system, the other main components of which are renin, angiotensinogen, angiotensin-converting enzyme, and angiotensin I (AI).

The renin-angiotensin system

Renin is a serine protease enzyme produced by the juxtaglomerular apparatus within the kidney in two main forms, the biologically inactive prorenin, and its product of conversion, active renin. The secretion of renin (Fig. 34.2) is stimulated by decreased perfusion pressure of the afferent arteriole, sodium depletion, increased beta-adrenergic tone, and vasoactive hormones (kallikrein, prostaglandins). Renin acts on its substrate, angiotensinogen, which is a 57 000 dalton liver glycoprotein. Angiotensinogen levels are increased by estrogens and glucocorticoids, and they are decreased in liver cirrhosis and in conditions of chronic high renin. Its variations may influence circulating AII levels (Fig. 34.3). Angiotensinogen releases an amino-terminal decapeptide, AI, converted to AII by the angiotensin-converting enzyme,

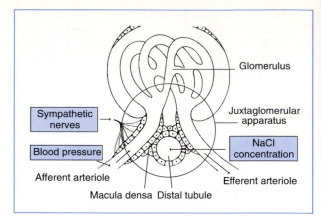

Figure 34.2 Regulation of renin secretion.

which is a zinc-containing enzyme found in several organs, including endothelium. Its main site of activity is the pulmonary vascular bed. This enzyme also acts on different substrates, such as bradykinin, which is inactivated by angiotensin-converting enzyme. Aldosterone regulation by AII thus depends on the same factors involved in renin secretion. A local adrenal renin-angiotensin system acting as a paracrine regulator has also been described. Several subtypes of AII receptors have recently been described as well: the most important are AT1 receptors, which are abundant both on the surface of ZG cells and on vessel walls. The pathways involved in the AII intracellular message transduction leading to aldosterone stimulation are phosphatidyl inositol hydrolysis, calcium mobilization from intracellular storage and extracellular calcium influx, and activation of protein kinase C. The final result is the increased transcription of genes of steroidogenetic enzymes, both in the early steps and the

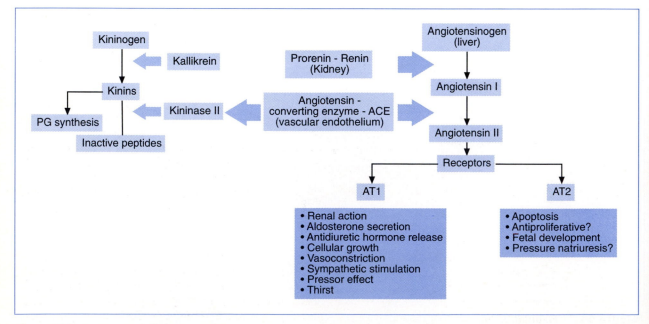

Figure 34.3 The circulating renin-angiotensin system.

late pathway (aldosterone synthase). Angiotensin II acts with a similar mechanism on vascular smooth muscle cells and kidney, inducing general and renal vasoconstriction and sodium reabsorption. While AT1 receptors are present in all organs known to respond physiologically to AII, a second type of AII receptors (AT2) is found primarily during fetal development and in pathological situations involving tissue remodeling and repair. AII, acting through the AT2 receptor, might exert an antiproliferative effect and stimulate apoptosis. Functional cross-talk between the two receptor subtypes is an emerging concept. Important data on the physiological role of AII in aldosterone and blood pressure regulation have become available with the development of angiotensin receptor antagonists and angiotensin-converting enzyme inhibitors. They do not reduce blood pressure in sodium-replete individuals, but they exert a strong hypotensive effect in sodium- or volume-deficient subjects, being active not only in states of renin-dependent secondary forms of hypertension (e.g., renovascular), but also in many patients with "essential hypertension".

The other fundamental aldosterone-regulating factor is potassium ion. Its increase stimulates aldosterone secretion while hypokalemia impairs it. Potassium acts on ZG cells by depolarizing the membrane, thus facilitating the increase of calcium influx. Potassium ion and AII share similar mechanisms of signal transduction that are different from those involved in the action of ACTH on the same cells. ACTH can acutely stimulate aldosterone production via a cAMP-mediated pathway, while in the long-term it may have only a permissive role. Indeed, prolonged stimulation with supraphysiological doses of ACTH may result in suppression rather than stimulation of aldosterone secretion. Among other factors, sodium ions inhibit aldosterone production, but the bulk of its effect is mediated by the renin-angiotensin system. The suppressive role of dopamine and the stimulating effect of serotonin are of uncertain physiological relevance. Atrial natriuretic peptide and brain natriuretic peptide are potent inhibitors of aldosterone (and renin) synthesis; they are secreted by cardiac myocytes and other tissues in response to intravascular volume expansion and may also have a role in the "escape phenomenon", that is, the physiological natriuresis that occurs after prolonged mineralocorticoid surcharge.

Circulating aldosterone and other mineralocorticoids

Sixty per cent of circulating aldosterone is bound to plasma proteins, while DOC is mostly (97%) bound. The half-life of aldosterone is about 15 minutes. It is mainly metabolized by the liver and is excreted in the urine in various forms. The metabolite usually measured as "urinary aldosterone" is 18-glucuronide or acid-labile conjugate (free aldosterone released after acidification at pH 1.0) and accounts for 20% of all aldosterone metabolites. Urinary tetrahydroaldosterone glucuronide accounts for 35% of the metabolites, the free form for less than 1%. Unlike cortisol, the 11β-hydroxyl group of aldosterone undergoes minimal metabolic changes since it is protected by the cyclic 11-18 hemiacetal form. Liver and kidney diseases have minor effects on aldosterone clearance rate, while congestive heart failure may reduce it.

Mechanisms of action of aldosterone and other mineralocorticoids

The action of these steroids on target tissues (kidney, colon, sweat, and salivary glands) is mediated by specific mineralocorticoid receptors (MR). These are similar to glucocorticoid receptors (GR) and differ mainly in binding characteristics, as mineralocorticoids possess greater affinity for MR than GR, while glucocorticoids (especially cortisol) have a similar affinity for both GR and MR. Mineralocorticoid receptors are protected from the mineralocorticoid activity of glucocorticoids by a co-localized enzyme (11β-hydroxysteroid-dehydrogenase), which converts cortisol to the biologically inactive cortisone. The principal sites of mineralocorticoid action are the connecting segments and the distal collecting tubules of the kidney. The steroid enters the tubular cell and binds to a cytosolic receptor protein; the complex is then translocated to the nucleus, where it binds with the hormone-responsive element (HRE) of the DNA in the nucleus. The mRNA transcripts of specific genes generate proteins that mediate the cellular effects of mineralocorticoids (Fig. 34.4). These consist of three mechanisms that stimulate sodium transport: the first could correspond to an increase in apical sodium channels to promote sodium resorption from tubules; then, an effect on the energy-generating systems of the cell (especially on the mitochondrial enzymes involved in ATP generation); and finally, the activation of the Na-K-ATPase of the basolateral membrane subsequent to increased intracellular sodium concentration, which could also be partially responsible for increasing K^+ excretion.

Physiological actions of mineralocorticoids

Aldosterone, the major mineralocorticoid, is the most important regulator of sodium and potassium balance and has a role in the control of the acid-base equilibrium. It acts on several classic mineralocorticoid target organs such as the kidney, gut, and salivary and sweat glands, but

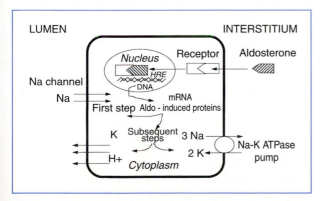

Figure 34.4 Mechanism of action of aldosterone. (HRE = hormone-responsive element.)

it also binds to receptors located in the vascular endothelium, heart, and brain. The kidney connecting segments and cortical and medullary connecting tubules are its sites of action. Even though only 3 to 4% of filtered Na^+ is reabsorbed in response to aldosterone, it is crucial to body sodium balance. The amount of Na^+ reabsorbed depends on the quantity of solute delivered to the kidney. However, in cases of excess mineralocorticoid production, Na^+ retention is limited by the kidney, provided that cardiac and renal function is normal. In fact, after an initial period of positive Na^+ balance and extracellular fluid expansion, the "escape phenomenon" determines a decrease in proximal tubular reabsorption of filtered sodium. This may be partially due to an increase in atrial natriuretic peptide levels following volume expansion. However, an increase in cardiac output, glomerular filtration rate, and peritubular hydrostatic pressure, higher levels of PG and kallikrein, and decreased renal adrenergic activity may also be contributing to the natriuretic response. This "escape" does not occur in patients with secondary hyperaldosteronism due to heart failure, cirrhosis, or nephrosis. The kaliuretic effect of aldosterone depends mostly on the activity of the Na-K-ATPase pump, which exchanges three intracellular Na^+ ions for two extracellular K^+ ions, but also on the amount of sodium intake.

DIAGNOSTIC PROCEDURES OF THE RENIN-ANGIOTENSIN-ALDOSTERONE SYSTEM

The pathophysiological role of the renin-angiotensin-aldosterone system can be evaluated indirectly by case history data, clinical criteria, and the routine biochemical parameters influenced by the system (such as serum and urinary electrolytes, creatinine, and other renal function tests). However, the more specific way is to measure each component of the pathway both in basal condition and in a number of functional tests. One of the major problems in evaluating this system is that patients must meet extremely strict criteria in terms of diet (sodium intake), posture, previous and current pharmacological treatment (diuretics, antihypertensive drugs), time of sampling, and stressful conditions. Each of these points is essential to determine baseline values of renin, angiotensin, and aldosterone and to avoid problems in data interpretation.

Renin-angiotensin system

Renin is routinely measured by radioimmunoassay as AI produced in vitro by its enzymatic activity after incubation of plasma in standardized conditions (plasma renin activity, PRA). Ethylenediaminetetraacetic acid (EDTA) is used as an anticoagulant in plastic tubes to prevent absorption to the walls. Blood samples should be collected and processed at room temperature to avoid the cryo-activation of prorenin and then stored at $-20°$ C. Samples with expected very low PRA levels can be incubated for longer periods of time (up to 12 to 18 hours instead of 1 to 3 hours) to improve sensitivity. The results are expressed as ng/ml/h of AI.

Active renin can now also be measured (in pg/ml) by direct immunometric assay. Alternatively, total renin can be measured with the same assay, plus trypsin activation. The value of inactive renin (prorenin) can be calculated by subtracting active from total renin. Prorenin may be clinically useful as an early marker of vascular complications in diabetic patients. Plasma sampling should be performed in standardized conditions, that is, after overnight (or at least 1 hour) recumbency and with the patient in sitting or standing position for at least 1 hour. The NaCl content of the diet should be monitored by 24-hour urinary sodium excretion analysis. The results should ideally be plotted in a nomogram where urinary sodium is inversely related to normal PRA values. Normal PRA values range from 1 to 2.5 ng/ml/h in the supine position, and from 2 to 5 ng/ml/h in the standing position, assuming a sodium intake of 100 to 150 mEq per day (see Chap. 35).

Renin stimulation test

Acute furosemide administration or chronic salt deprivation can be used to stimulate renin when renin suppression (e.g., mineralocorticoid excess syndrome) is suspected. The most used test is the acute captopril test, where a disruption of the system at the last step is followed by a reactive increase of renin and AI. This test is employed in the screening for renovascular hypertension (where an overreaction is expected) and in primary aldosteronism (where PRA does not increase) (see Chaps. 35 and 36, for further details).

Suppressive maneuvers of renin

Acute (2 l of 0.9% NaCl) sodium load can be used as a suppression test, but there are no major clinical indications for such a test, at least for renin.

Angiotensinogen and angiotensin II assay

Angiotensinogen can be evaluated by measuring the AI formed after the addition of an excess of renin to plasma, or directly by radioimmunoassay or ELISA. There is no clinical diagnostic role for this measure, even though a relationship between a polymorphic pattern of the angiotensinogen gene and increased angiotensinogen levels has recently been described in a subgroup of essential hypertensives and in preeclampsia.

The AII assay is not for routine use mainly due to the methodological difficulties that are encountered in obtaining specific and sensitive assays of the octapeptide, which require high-pressure liquid chromatography (HPLC) separation and radioimmunoassay. A quite specific, direct radioimmunoassay has recently become available.

Aldosterone

Baseline plasma aldosterone concentrations should be measured after 1 hour in the recumbent or standing position, and the values should be compared to the normal range in that specific postural position. Sodium content of the diet should be monitored by 24-hour urinary excretion, and diuretic and antihypertensive drugs should have been withdrawn for a suitable period of time. In cases of severe hypertension, calcium antagonist treatment can be maintained without major consequences on aldosterone levels. Hypokalemia should be corrected. Sampling time and stressful conditions should also be monitored (a simultaneous cortisol assay could be indicated) since aldosterone secretion follows a circadian rhythm parallel to cortisol and is acutely regulated by ACTH. However, in the sitting position, or during deambulation or exercise, the renin-angiotensin system takes over the control of aldosterone except in autonomous aldosterone-producing adenoma. This is why the response of aldosterone to posture is widely used for the differential diagnosis of primary aldosteronism (see Chap. 36). This test is also indicated for other purposes (detection of excessive increments in secondary forms of aldosteronism, in idiopathic aldosteronism, and lack of response in conditions of inadequate or suppressed aldosterone secretion). Normal plasma aldosterone values range from 4 to 12 ng/dl in the supine position and from 10 to 30 ng/dl in the upright position. The ratio between plasma levels of aldosterone and PRA can also be calculated; this is considered a good screening test to diagnose states of primary aldosteronism including cases with non-classic phenotypes (normokalemic). The normal values of this ratio depend on the laboratory and sampling methodology. The widespread use of this test has increased the number of cases of hyperaldosteronism diagnosed per year. Urinary 24-hour aldosterone excretion (18-glucuronide) has been widely used in the past as the gold standard for diagnosing primary aldosteronism. However, limitations due to urine collection and extreme dilution of urine samples make this assay less reliable (normal range: 5-20 µg/24 h).

Suppressive maneuvers

Acute saline infusion Two liters of 0.9% NaCl solution are infused over 4 hours. This test is useful in demonstrating abnormal suppressibility in cases of primary aldosteronism. The fluorohydrocortisone suppression test can be used as an alternative, where 0.4 mg 9α-fluorohydrocortisone per day is administered for 4 days, and plasma aldosterone is measured on the morning of the 5th day.

Captopril test Plasma aldosterone and PRA are measured in baseline conditions (sitting) and 2 hours after 25 mg of captopril administration. A lack of plasma aldosterone decrease (<15 ng/dl) suggests primary aldosteronism.

Dexamethasone suppression test This test is indicated when congenital forms of glucocorticoid-remediable hyperaldosteronism are suspected. It consists of corticosteroid administration (dexamethasone 2 mg/day for 7 days) and subsequent control of blood pressure, serum potassium, and plasma PRA and aldosterone. All of these parameters tend to normalize under ACTH suppression.

In all of the above maneuvers, it is important to obtain a concomitant value of cortisol to distinguish aldosterone changes due to the circadian rhythm or stress.

Adrenal vein sampling

Adrenal vein sampling is indicated in primary aldosteronism when noninvasive tests and CT/MNR or radioisotopic scan are inconclusive for lateralization. Plasma aldosterone and cortisol should be measured in the two adrenal veins and inferior vena cava (below their opening), and the ratios should then be calculated.

Other methods

The assay of other mineralocorticoids, that is, DOC and corticosterone, is indicated in cases of syndromes of mineralocorticoid excess with low aldosterone levels, such as a suspected deficiency of 11β- or 17α-hydroxylase, or DOC-producing tumors. Further useful steroid measurements in these clinical conditions could be urinary free cortisol/free-cortisone assay and related metabolites for the diagnosis of congenital or acquired forms of apparent mineralocorticoid excess (AME).

Suggested readings

BIGLIERI EG, KATER CE, MANTERO F. Adrenocortical forms of human hypertension. In: Laragh JH, Brenner BM (eds). Hypertension pathophysiology, diagnosis and management. 2nd ed. New York: Raven Press, 1995;2145-62.

BOON WC, COGHLAN JP, CURNOW KM, MCDOUGALL JC. Aldosterone secretion. Trends Endocrinol Metab 1997; 8:346-54.

CAMPBELL DJ. Circulating and tissue angiotensin system. J Clin Invest 1987;79:1-8.

CLAUSER E, CURNOW KM, DAVIES E, et al. Angiotensin II receptors: protein and gene structures, expression and potential pathological involvements. Eur J Endocrinol 1996;134:403-11.

FUNDER JW, MANTERO F (eds). The clinical pathophysiology of aldosterone. Journal of Endocrinol Invest (Monothematic issue) 1995;18:492-594.

GIACCHETTI G, OPOCHER G, SARZANI R, RAPPELLI A, MANTERO F. Angiotensin II and the adrenal. Clin Exper Pharm Physiol 1996;3:119-24.

MILLER WL, TYRELL JB. The adrenal cortex. In: Felig P, Baxter JD, Frohman LA (eds). Endocrinology and metabolism. 3rd ed. New York: McGraw-Hill, 1995;580-83,610-4.

SEALEY JE, JAMES GD, LARAGH JH. Interpretation and guidelines for the use of plasma and urine aldosterone and plasma angiotensin II, angiotensinogen, prorenin, peripheral, and renal vein renin tests. In: Laragh JH, Brenner BM (eds). Hypertension pathophysiology, diagnosis and management. 2nd ed. New York: Raven Press, 1995;1953-68.

SEALEY JE, LARAGH JH. The Renin-Angiotensin-Aldosterone System for Normal Regulation of Blood Pressure and Sodium and Potassium Homeostasis. In: Laragh JH, Brenner BM (eds). Hypertension pathophysiology, diagnosis and management. 2nd ed. New York: Raven Press, 1995;1763-96.

WHITE PC. Disorders of aldosterone biosynthesis and action. N Engl J Med 1994;331:250-8.

Renin-angiotensin II-related hypertension

Pierre-François Plouin, Pierre Corvol

KEY POINTS

- Renin determinations may be made indirectly (plasma renin activity) or directly (active renin concentration). Although the plasma renin activity and the active renin concentration are closely correlated, they are expressed in different units (ng/ml per hour and pg/ml, respectively) and their normal ranges differ by one order of magnitude.
- Renin levels are dependent on a patient's age, body position, and sodium intake and are markedly altered by most anti-hypertensive drugs. The determination of renin, frequently coupled with that of aldosterone, is an expensive test. It should therefore be considered only for those few patients with signs of secondary hypertension. Standardized conditions should be used so the values obtained can be compared to those for age-matched normal subjects.
- Peripheral plasma renin and aldosterone levels should be determined in patients with hypertension and hypokalemia to distinguish between primary aldosteronism (suppressed renin with high aldosterone levels), secondary aldosteronism (parallel increase in renin and aldosterone), and primary reninism (extremely high renin levels and high aldosterone).
- Renal vein renin determination may be useful in patients with documented renal artery stenosis. It is an invasive test that helps identify patients who have truly renin-dependent hypertension, who should therefore be offered renal artery percutaneous angioplasty.
- We propose an algorithm using clinical clues, renin determination, and imaging tests for the diagnosis of hypokalemic severe or resistant hypertension.

The renin-angiotensin system (RAS) is a cascade of proteins and peptides – angiotensinogen, renin, angiotensin-converting enzyme (ACE), and angiotensins – which lead to the formation of angiotensin II, the active hormone. Angiotensin II is a vasoconstrictor and a stimulus for the adrenal release of aldosterone. Aldosterone in turn enhances sodium resorption and potassium secretion in the distal nephron. Renin-angiotensin-related hypertension therefore includes a variety of conditions involving high blood pressure, and occasionally alterations in sodium and potassium levels. Assaying the activity of the

RAS in selected cases of hypertension has diagnostic, prognostic, and therapeutic implications.

DOCUMENTING RENIN-ANGIOTENSIN-DEPENDENT HYPERTENSION

Renin-angiotensin-dependent hypertension can be investigated using biochemical or physiological tests. Biochemical tests aim to assess whether plasma levels of RAS components are higher than expected for posture, sodium intake, and age. Physiological tests rely on the blood pressure and hormonal responses to acute administration of angiotensin-converting enzyme inhibitors or angiotensin antagonists.

Biochemical techniques

Angiotensinogen, angiotensin-converting enzyme, and angiotensin II are not routinely determined. Angiotensinogen and angiotensin-converting enzyme are not usually limiting for angiotensin II formation, and angiotensin II concentration is difficult to measure. Techniques for assaying aldosterone are described in Chapter 34. This chapter will only consider the determination of renin, which is rate limiting for the generation of angiotensin II. The standard renin assay is indirect, involving the measurement of renin's enzymatic activity through the in vitro production of angiotensin I. To avoid cryoactivation of the inactive renin precursor prorenin into renin, blood samples are handled and centrifuged at room temperature, and plasma samples are then stored at –20 °C. Angiotensin I is produced by incubating plasma in standardized conditions and is measured using a radioimmunoassay. The result is plasma renin activity (PRA), which is generally expressed in ng/ml per hour. Active renin concentration, expressed in pg/ml, can also be measured directly using an immunometric assay.

Conditions for a valid assessment of renin levels

The RAS is finely tuned by posture and sodium balance and is affected by age. Walking for 1 hour induces a twofold increase in plasma renin. Renin secretion is stimulated by sodium deprivation and suppressed by sodium loading. Renin measurements should therefore be related to sodium intake. Sodium intake and urinary sodium excretion are presumed to be equal if a patient's diet is stable. In patients on a free sodium diet, the renin-sodium profile is based on a nomogram relating PRA to urinary sodium excretion. Alternatively, patients are instructed to ingest 75-150 mmol sodium/day, and sodium excretion is determined over a 24-hour period to confirm that sodium output is within this range. Renin levels are not markedly influenced by variations in sodium intake within these limits. Plasma levels of renin and aldosterone are markedly higher in children than in adults. In normal adults, they fall by half between the ages of 30 and 70. Values obtained from patients should therefore be compared with those of age-matched normal subjects studied under the same conditions. In our laboratory, 49 normal volunteers (21 men) aged 40±13 years (mean±SD) had a urinary sodium excretion of 137±57 mmol/day. Blood sampling was performed between 8:00 and 10:00 a.m. after 1 hour of supine rest and then after 1 hour of walking. Values for supine PRA and plasma renin concentration averaged 1.33±0.64 ng/ml per hour and 16.9±6.5 pg/ml, respectively. After walking, PRA averaged 2.78±1.75 ng/ml per hour and plasma renin concentration 31.6±16.8 pg/ml, respectively.

Most anti-hypertensive agents influence renin release. This is done either directly, or through counter-regulations in response to blood pressure decrease or the suppression of renin-angiotensin II negative feedback. Renin release is increased by diuretics, ACE inhibitors, angiotensin receptor antagonists, and vasodilators; and decreased by beta-blockers and centrally-acting agents. Treatment with these drugs should be discontinued before assessing renin levels, although this may be difficult in patients with severe hypertension. In such cases, alpha-blockers and calcium antagonists may be continued because they have little influence on renin release.

Acute renin-suppression tests

Acute renin-suppression tests interrupt the RAS, demonstrating its involvement in hypertension. Although suppression tests using angiotensin II receptor antagonists have been reported, oral administration of the ACE inhibitor captopril is generally used due to its rapid onset of action (20 minutes) and maximum action (1 to 3 hours). The fall in blood pressure in response to captopril should be proportional to pre-test RAS activation. A consistent drop in blood pressure is predicted to occur in renin-dependent hypertension. The blood pressure and hormonal response to the captopril test has been widely studied in patients with hypertension and renal artery stenosis (see below).

Guidelines for renin measurement

In patients with essential hypertension, renin determination may help select the most effective first-line drug therapy (Tab. 35.1). Patients in the highest renin index quartile have the greatest response to beta-blockers, and those in the lowest quartile have a greater response to diuretics. In addition, the renin-sodium index is independently related to the risk of myocardial infarction in hypertensive patients. However, considering the fluctuations of renin levels in individual patients and the relatively high cost, the therapeutic and prognostic value of measuring plasma renin during routine investigation of mild to moderate essential hypertension are limited. Renin should be determined in patients prone to secondary hypertension. Such patients may be identified by their history, signs and symptoms, by the presence of hypokalemia, hyperazotemia, or asymmetrical kidneys. Renin should also be determined in the small proportion of patients with severe, untreated hypertension, or whose hypertension is resistant to conventional treatment. In such cases, an unsuspected form of secondary hypertension or a pronounced drug-induced stimulation of the RAS may be found. Such findings may indicate that additional etiologic evaluation is required, or that either an ACE inhibitor or a beta-blocker should be added to the previous regimen.

INVESTIGATION OF RENIN-ANGIOTENSIN-DEPENDENT FORMS OF HYPERTENSION

Table 35.2 summarizes the presentation and key findings in cases with high renin and primary or secondary hypertension. Figure 35.1 suggests a practical approach to the analysis of these conditions.

RENIN-ANGIOTENSIN II-RELATED HYPERTENSION • 357

Essential hypertension

Approximately 1 out of 6 patients with benign essential hypertension has a high renin level. The purpose and efficiency of screening high renin hypertension in this setting is discussed above. Most cases with malignant hypertension have high renin levels. Renin concentration is very high in the hyponatremic hypertensive syndrome, leading to hyperangiotensinemia with thirst, polyuria, and hyponatremia; and to secondary aldosteronism with potassium wasting and hypokalemia. Malignant hypertension may be primary or, as in 45% of cases, the consequence of an underlying renal or adrenal disease.

Renal artery stenosis

Renal ischemia associated with renal artery stenosis is the most frequent condition occurring with renin-angiotensin-dependent hypertension. Uni- or bilateral renal artery stenoses can cause renovascular hypertension, a form of hypertension reversible with nephrectomy or renal revascularization. About two-thirds of stenoses are due to atherosclerosis, usually in patients over the age of 50. One-third are due to fibromuscular dysplasia, mostly in young female patients. The standard procedure for diagnosing renal artery stenosis is arteriography. For screening use, this invasive procedure can be replaced by intravenous subtraction angiography or Duplex Doppler sonography. These techniques estimate the frequency of renal artery stenosis at 1% in unselected patients with hypertension,

and 10 to 30% in drug-resistant hypertensive patients. The standard for defining renovascular hypertension is that the blood pressure outcome is favorable following revascularization. This definition is retrospective. The actual frequency of the condition is unknown because hypertension reversal is dependent on various parameters such as the patient's age, hypertension duration, stenosis etiology and grade, parenchymal consequences of hypertension, the feasibility of revascularization, and the risk of restenosis. Initial failure or subsequent restenosis are more frequent in ostial than in truncal stenoses.

Considering the risks associated with renal artery surgery or percutaneous angioplasty, efforts have been made to design tests for selecting patients with renal artery stenosis who have truly renin-dependent hypertension. In such patients, the captopril test is expected to induce a sharp drop in blood pressure. The captopril test with concurrent determination of plasma renin levels is predicted to induce a homeostatic increase in renin secretion from the stenotic kidney. Although there have been numerous analyses of the captopril test in patients at risk of harboring renovascular hypertension, a complete analysis is not possible because of multiple inconsistencies in patient selection, standards, test procedures, and cut-off points. Simultaneous determination of renin in both renal veins has been used to predict blood pressure outcome following revascularization in patients with unilateral renal artery stenosis. If the renal vein renin ratio (i.e., the ratio between the renal vein renin levels at the stenotic and non-stenotic sides) exceeds 1.5, the stenosis is

Table 35.1 Guidelines for measuring renin

Condition	Purpose	Comment
Mild or moderate untreated hypertension	Determination of renin subgroup for prognostic or therapeutic purposes	Classification of individual patients into low or high renin subgroups probably not cost-effective in this setting
Severe untreated hypertension (diastolic BP consistently above 110 mmHg) and/or hypokalemic hypertension	Guidance for subsequent etiologic work-up	High renin levels suggest performing a captopril test, renal scintigraphy, or angiography (Fig. 35.1), whereas low renin levels suggest adrenal investigations (Chaps. 34 and 36)
Drug-resistant hypertension	Guidance for anti-hypertensive treatment adaptation	Discontinue current treatment (calcium channel antagonists and α-blockers may be continued) and determine plasma renin. High renin levels suggest adding a β-blocker, an ACE inhibitor, or an angiotensin II receptor antagonist to previous regimen
Hypertension with renal failure	Guidance for anti-hypertensive treatment adaptation	Low or normal renin levels suggest increasing loop diuretic daily dose; high renin levels suggest adding small doses of an ACE inhibitor
Hypertension with renal artery stenosis or unilateral small kidney or kidney tumor	Evaluation of asymmetrical renin secretion before nephrectomy or renal artery angioplasty	A RVR ratio ≥1.5 is generally associated with a favorable BP outcome following nephrectomy or renal artery angioplasty

(ACE = angiotensin-converting enzyme; BP = blood pressure; RVR ratio = renal vein renin ratio [affected to non-affected side].)

Table 35.2 Etiology, presentation and key findings in renin-angiotensin II-related forms of hypertension

Underlying disease	Usual presentation	Key tests and findings
Primary hypertension		
Benign	Non specific. 10-15% of patients with primary hypertension belong to the high renin subgroup	Larger than average response to beta-blockers or ACE inhibitors
Accelerated or malignant	Headache, thirst, weight loss, diastolic BP usually >140 mmHg with hypokalemia, azotemia, proteinuria	Funduscopy: hemorrhages, exudates, papilledema. An underlying renal disease is present in −50% of cases
Renal ischemia		
Renal artery stenosis	Recent, progressive and/or severe hypertension, hypertension in young females (fibromuscular dysplasia) or in patients with angina or arteritis (atherosclerosis), hypertension with ACE inhibitor-induced rise in plasma creatinine	Renal angiogram: renovascular (curable) hypertension is probably present if reduction in artery diameter (i) exceeds 75% or (ii) ranges 50-75% with a positive captopril test, a lateralized captopril renography or a RVR ratio ≥1.5
Renal infarction	Hyponatremic hypertensive syndrome: lumbar pain and hematuria followed by acute hypertension, polyuria, hypokalemia, hyponatremia and extremely high renin concentrations	Segmental renal infarction is detected by CT scan and its cause by renal angiogram (embolism, thrombosis, renal artery dissection or occlusion)
Polyarteritis nodosa	Systemic necrotizing vasculitis	Widespread microaneurysms on renal angiogram
Systemic scleroderma	Skin thickening, Raynaud's phenomenon, progressive hypertension and azotemia	Clinical presentation. ACE inhibitors greatly improve scleroderma crisis
Renal tumors and cysts		
Juxtaglomerular cell tumor	Severe hypokalemic hypertension with very high prorenin and active renin levels	Normal renal angiogram with a small cortical tumor on CT scan. BP returns to normal after tumor removal
Other renal renin-producing tumors	Hypertension with renal cell carcinoma	Primary reninism is present and BP returns to normal following nephrectomy in about 5% of cases
Compressive cysts and tumors	Hypertension with ultrasound scan evidence of a large cyst or tumor	Improvement in BP following cyst drainage or tumor resection may be expected if RVR ratio exceeds 1.5
Polycystic kidney	Family history of renal cysts, hypertension and azotemia	Ultrasound scan evidence of >3 bilateral cysts in a person with a positive family history
Unilateral non-vascular small kidneys	Hypertension with asymmetrical kidneys; often a history of recurrent urinary tract infection	Pyelographic or ultrasound scan evidence of pyelonephritic scarring, reflux nephropathy and/or segmental hypoplasia
Extrarenal tumors		
Pheochromocytoma	Paroxysmal hypertension with vasomotor symptoms	High urinary catecholamine metabolites, adrenal tumor
Ectopic primary reninism	Malignant tumor with hypertension and/or hypokalemia	Rare cases of cancers (lung, liver, pancreas, ovary) present with a paraneoplastic secretion of prorenin or active renin

(ACE = angiotensin-converting enzyme; BP = blood pressure; RVR ratio = renal vein renin ratio [affected to non-affected side].)

assumed to cause a renin-dependent hypertension amenable to surgical or angioplastic cure. The test may be performed after acute oral captopril administration. Captopril enhances the renin gradient between the stenotic and non-stenotic sides, but it is unknown whether this improves the predictive value of the test. Post-captopril renal scintigraphy is a less invasive alternative to renal vein renin determination and is more accurate than the

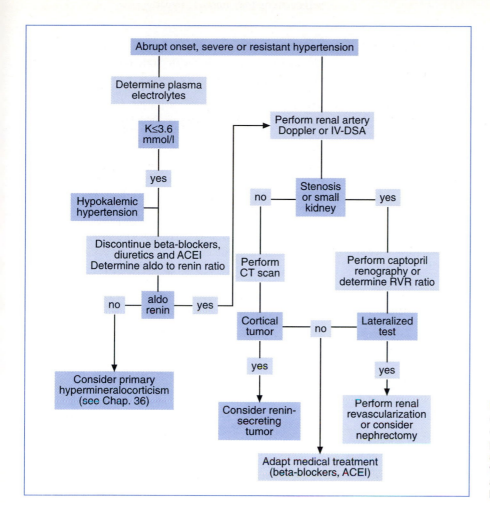

Figure 35.1 An algorithm for diagnosing renin-angiotensin-dependent hypertension. (K = plasma potassium; aldo = aldosterone; IV-DSA = intravenous digitized substraction angiography; ACEI = ACE inhibitors.)

captopril renin test. Post-captopril scintigraphy is the most appropriate test in unilateral renal artery stenosis. Renal vein renin determinations should only be performed in complex cases such as branch stenoses or renovascular disease associated with focal renal parenchymal infarction. The management of patients at risk from renovascular hypertension is shown in Figure 35.1.

Other conditions with renal ischemia

A few conditions with chronic or acute intrarenal ischemia may also induce renin-dependent hypertension. These include systemic diseases such as polyarteritis nodosa and scleroderma, in which blood pressure and renal outcomes are greatly improved by ACE inhibitors, and segmental renal infarction. Segmental renal infarction may result from renal embolism, renal artery thrombosis or dissection, or in situ thrombosis in cases with coagulation disorders. It usually presents as an abrupt-onset malignant hypertension with hyponatremic hypertensive syndrome. The condition may revert spontaneously to normotension. This occurs because the ischemic renal tissue, which releases large amounts of renin – causing

renin-angiotensin-dependent hypertension – may subsequently evolve to a silent renal scar.

Renal tumors and cysts

Primary reninism is a purely renin-dependent form of hypertension. It may be caused by juxtaglomerular cell tumors, malignant kidney tumors (nephroblastoma, adenocarcinoma), epithelial (broncho-pulmonary, ovarian, fallopian, pituitary) or soft tissue (alveolar and epithelioid sarcoma, leiomyosarcoma, hemangiopericytoma) tumors. This rare condition causes severe hypertension with hypokalemia. Such signs are usually investigated by renin determination, which would reveal very high plasma renin concentrations, and by renal angiogram, which would depict no renal artery stenosis or intrarenal ischemia. The presence of a small, hypodense renal cortical tumor (juxtaglomerular cell tumor) or of a larger renal tumor would be detected by CT-scan (Tab. 35.2 and Fig. 35.1). Blood pressure usually drops during angiotensin-converting enzyme inhibition. Hypertension is cured by tumor resection, although it may recur if metastasis develops in malignant cases.

Some large non-renin-secreting cysts and tumors may present as renin-dependent hypertension, with the mechanism of RAS stimulation being renal artery compression. In selected cases with a lateralized renal vein renin ratio, cyst drainage or tumor resection may improve or cure hypertension. Activation of the RAS also occurs in hypertensive patients with polycystic kidney disease, presumably because the stretching of intrarenal vessels around cysts causes areas of intrarenal ischemia (Tab. 35.2).

Unilateral non-vascular small kidneys

Pyelonephritic scarring associated with urinary tract infection and vesicoureteric reflux can cause childhood hypertension and the progressive degradation of renal function. Plasma renin activity is often high, and RAS activation has been implicated as a cause of hypertension. High renin concentrations may also occur in cases of renal hypoplasia. In cases with a very small unilateral kidney and a lateralized renal vein renin ratio, unilateral nephrectomy may improve hypertension.

Extrarenal tumors

Pheochromocytoma is a catecholamine-secreting neoplasm of adrenal or extra-adrenal chromaffin tissue. Patients with pheochromocytoma usually have sustained or paroxysmal hypertension with headache, palpitations, and excessive sweating. Diagnosis relies on the determination of plasma catecholamine levels or urinary excretion of catecholamine metabolites. The tumor is located using CT-scan and metaiodobenzyl guanidine scintigraphy (Chap. 33). The high blood pressure levels associated with pheochromocytoma are caused by high plasma catecholamine levels via the stimulation of vascular α-adrenergic receptors. They are also caused indirectly through RAS activation, which is mediated by the adrenergic stimulation of juxtaglomerular cells and renal vasoconstriction. Consequently, angiotensin-converting enzyme inhibition may be used to control blood pressure before surgery.

Rare cases of primary reninism may be due to renin-secreting extrarenal tumors.

Suggested readings

ALDERMAN MH, MADHAVAN S, OOI WL, COHEN H, SEALEY JE, LARAGH JH. Association of the renin-sodium profile with the risk of myocardial infarction in patients with hypertension. N Engl J Med 1991;324:1098-104.

BLAUFOX MD, LEE HB, DAVIS B, OBERMAN A, WASSERTHEIL-SMOLLER SD, LANGFORD H. Renin predicts diastolic blood pressure response to nonpharmacologic and pharmacologic therapy. JAMA 1992;267:1221-5.

CORVOL P, PINET F, PLOUIN PF, BRUNEVAL P, MÉNARD J. Renin-secreting tumors. Endocrinol Metab Clin North Am 1994;23:255-70.

DERKX FHM, SCHALEKAMP MADH. Renal artery stenosis and hypertension. Lancet 1994;344:237-9.

ELKIK F, CORVOL P, IDATTE JM, MÉNARD J. Renal segmental infarction: a cause of reversible malignant hypertension. J Hypertens 1984;2:149-56.

GABOW PA. Autosomal dominant polycystic kidney disease. N Engl J Med 1993;329:332-42.

GAUL MK, LINN WD, MULROW CD. Captopril-stimulated renin secretion in the diagnosis of renovascular hypertension. Am J Hypertens 1989;2:335-44.

GOONASEKERA CDA, SHAH V, WADE AM, BARRATT TM, DILLON MJ. 15-year follow-up of renin and blood pressure in reflux nephropathy. Lancet 1996;347:640-3.

LÜSCHER TF, WANNER C, HAURI D, SIEGENTHALER W, VETTER W. Curable renal parenchymatous hypertension: current diagnosis and management. Cardiology 1985;72:33-45.

PICKERING TG, SOS TA, VAUGHAN ED JR, et al. Predictive value and changes of renin secretion in hypertensive patients with unilateral renovascular disease undergoing successful angioplasty. Am J Med 1984;76:398-404.

PLOUIN PF, CORVOL P, GUYENE TT, MÉNARD J. Clinical investigation of the renin-angiotensin-aldosterone system. In: Davison AM, Cameron S, Grunfeld JP, Kerr DNS, Ritz E, Winearls CG (eds). Oxford Textbook of clinical nephrology. Oxford: Oxford Medical Pub, 1997;1425-32.

Mineralocorticoid-related hypertension

Michel B. Vallotton

▮ KEY POINTS ▮

- A great variety of tumoral or genetic causes of the syndrome of hypermineralo-corticoid present with the same chief features of hypertension with hypokalemic alkalosis.
- Most of these conditions are curable by either removal of the adrenal tumor, by specific pharmacological treatment (most often dexamethasone suppression of ACTH), or by withdrawal of causative substances.
- Physicians caring for hypertensive patients should first suspect such conditions when spontaneous or diuretic-induced hypokalemia is present, in cases of resistance to antihypertensive treatment, and when distinct biological and clinical features are present (described below), particularly when familial.

Pathophysiology

Mineralocorticoid-related forms of hypertension consist of a family of secondary forms of arterial hypertension that share many pathophysiological mechanisms of clinical presentation and biological features. As for all forms of secondary hypertension, a physician should be alerted when a patient presents with hypertension of recent-onset or that is resistant to common antihypertensive treatment. Features of mineralocorticoid-related hypertension can occur at any age and in both sexes. In view of the specific medical or surgical types of treatment they require, the physician should always keep in mind such a possibility.

Mineralocorticoids represent a family of corticosteroid hormones synthesized in either the zona glomerulosa or the zona fasciculata of the adrenal cortex (see Fig. 26.3). They all act upon the same intracellular receptor, the type I or mineralocorticoid receptor (MR). These receptors are primarily present in the distal tubules and cortical collecting tubules of the kidneys. Upon binding to these receptors, mineralocorticoids act to increase sodium resorption from, and potassium excretion into, the urine (Fig. 36.1). They do so by increasing the synthesis of Na^+/K^+-ATPase located in the basolateral cell membrane, thereby increasing the electromechanical gradient that drives diffusion through the sodium and potassium channels. Mineralocorticoids also increase the number of the potassium channels or the percentage of time each channel remains open. Thus, sodium diffuses passively through these sodium-permeable channels in the apical membranes into the cells and is then actively transported out of the cells along with water into the extracellular fluid at the basolateral membrane. Increased volemia ensues, together with a loss of urinary potassium. As a consequence of these disorders, hypertension supervenes, accompanied by a tendency toward hypokalemia (Fig. 36.1). A further consequence of hypervolemia is suppressed plasma renin activity due to an inhibition of renin synthesis and release from the juxta-glomerular apparatus in the kidney. As a consequence of chronic hypokalemia, hydrogen ions are lost into urine, causing metabolic alkalosis. Chronic hypokalemia is also responsible for muscle weakness or

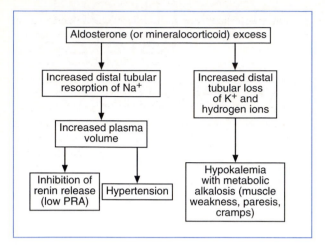

Figure 36.1 Simplified scheme of the pathophysiology of primary aldosteronism.

even paresis or tetanic cramps, as well as mild glucose intolerance with a tendency toward hyperglycemia secondary to defective insulin release.

In humans, the major mineralocorticoid is aldosterone, which is synthesized in the zona glomerulosa. Aldosterone has been the subject of the most extensive mineralocorticoid studies concerning its mode of action, regulation of synthesis, and physiological and clinical roles. Other minor mineralocorticoids of weaker action play a role in rarer forms of mineralocorticoid excess in selective disorders or under special conditions.

The most characteristic presentation of excess mineralocorticoids, mainly hyperaldosteronism, is that of hypertension of every grade accompanied by chronic hypokalemia (Tab. 36.1), metabolic alkalosis, and suppressed plasma renin activity (PRA) unresponsive or poorly responsive to stimulating maneuvers. Suspicion is further raised if the patient has presented with episodes of paresis or tetanic cramps and is mildly hyperglycemic. However, hypokalemia may be absent or can be hidden by treatment with antihypertensive drugs, which tend to raise plasma potassium, such as

Table 36.1 Causes of hypertension accompanied by hypokalemia

1. All forms of hypertension (essential or secondary) treated with diuretic agents
2. Secondary hyperaldosteronism:
   a. reno-vascular hypertension
   b. hypertension accompanied by heart failure or cirrhosis
   c. reninoma (or renin-secreting tumor)
3. Mineralocorticoid-related hypertension:
   a. Primary aldosteronisms (see Tab. 36.3)
   b. Pseudoaldosteronism (see Tab. 36.4)
   c. Systemic or topic administration of steroids with mineralocorticoid action
4. Cushing's syndrome

angiotensin-converting enzyme inhibitors (ACEI), potassium-sparing diuretics (amiloride, triamterene), or the specific aldosterone antagonist, spironolactone.

In view of the fact that 20 to 30% of patients with essential hypertension fall into the category of "low-renin hypertension", a thorough search for an unidentified mineralocorticoid has been launched, though with little success. Diabetic patients with autonomic failure may present with low plasma renin activity, but generally this is accompanied by hyperkalemia and not hypokalemia. In addition, some drugs inhibit renin release and can thus falsely induce in error. Those drugs are primarily beta-blocking agents and nonsteroidal anti-inflammatory agents (NSAIDs), which both tend to raise kalemia. Since potassium is, along with angiotensin II, one of the major stimuli of aldosterone synthesis, severe hypokalemia tends to lower the production of aldosterone and thus partly conceals the degree of excessive synthesis. It is thus mandatory, when an excess of aldosterone is suspected, to perform diagnostic procedures after correcting for hypokalemia and after ceasing potentially interfering treatments. There are no specific studies that address the time required for a return to basal conditions after stopping such treatment, but empirically and on the basis of pharmacokinetic data, a few days are sufficient for angiotensin-converting enzyme inhibitors (possibly also for angiotensin II antagonists) and NSAIDs, whereas for beta-blocking agents 2 to 3 weeks are required and even more for spironolactone.

PRIMARY ALDOSTERONISM

Epidemiology

Among the forms of mineralocorticoid-related hypertension, the syndrome of primary aldosteronism is the most frequently encountered. However, its true prevalence is difficult to assess, since most reports originate from referral centers that recruit a high percentage of secondary forms of hypertension. Furthermore, depending on the alerting threshold values of hypertension and hypokalemia, the percentage may vary considerably. In large series, the occurrence rates of primary aldosteronism varies from 0.01% among 25 589 patients from the Mayo Clinic to 2.7% among 4429 cases consecutively referred to the SUNY Health Science Center in Syracuse, New York, when a diastolic value >100 mmHg was taken as a selection criterion. In most textbooks a prevalence of 0.5 to 2.0% is indicated. Normokalemic primary aldosteronism was recognized as early as 1965 by Conn, and up to 27.5% of proven cases of primary aldosteronism presenting with a plasma potassium value of >3.5 mmol/l have been reported. In addition, as indicated in the introduction, the current widespread use of antihypertensive drugs that raise plasma potassium concentration such as angiotensin-converting enzyme inhibitors tend to conceal underlying aldosteronism by correcting the hypokalemia. No longer considering hypokalemia as a prerequisite to search for aldosteronism, Gordon et al. (1994) even proposed the amazing prevalence of 12% of primary aldosteronism in their population of hypertensive patients.

Other than the common biological characteristics that should alert the physician as indicated above, patients with primary aldosteronism present with no peculiar features. Both sexes are almost equally represented in all decades of age - from ages 18 to >70 years - and in all races. The severity of hypertension extends from mild to severe. Neurological complications from transitory paresis to hemiplegia are often encountered. Renal insufficiency or cardiac failure are rarer occurrences at the time of diagnosis.

Diagnostic procedures

For the sake of simplicity and clarity, diagnostic procedures can be divided into three stages (Fig. 36.2). The first step is aimed at confirming the diagnosis of primary hyperaldosteronism. Joint determination of plasma renin activity (PRA) and plasma aldosterone (PA) concentration permits the distinction of three groups of conditions (Tab. 36.2): (1) Secondary forms of aldosteronism when both PRA and

plasma aldosterone are elevated, (2) primary aldosteronism when PRA is suppressed and plasma aldosterone elevated with a PA/PRA ratio abnormally high, and (3) syndromes of pseudoaldosteronism when both PRA and plasma aldosterone are suppressed. These determinations are best performed when all antihypertensive treatment has been stopped, a normal sodium diet has been followed, and plasma potassium concentration has been corrected. However, depending upon the condition of the patient and the severity of the hypertension, this is not always feasible. When antihypertensive treatment must be maintained, it is best to use calcium antagonists that least affect the values of plasma potassium concentration, PRA, and aldosterone biosynthesis. Determining singly either PRA or plasma aldosterone is of little use, particularly under antihypertensive treatment, since many agents can affect the value of PRA (Fig. 36.3) and secondarily plasma aldosterone. Patients with essential hypertension falling into the category of

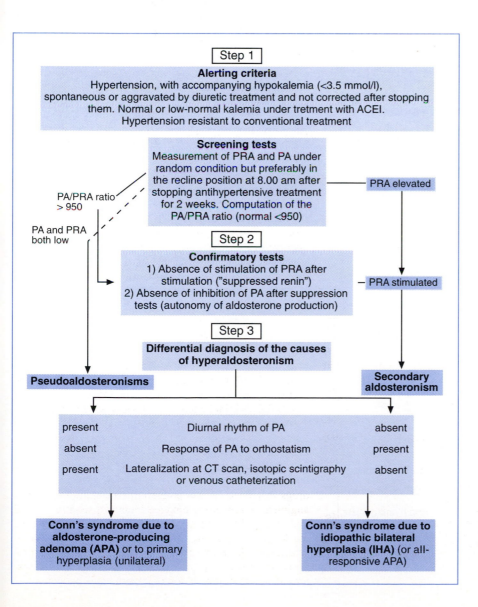

Figure 36.2 The plan of investigation of patients suspected of hypermineralocorticism with the three main steps to ascertain diagnosis, and differentiating between secondary aldosteronism and the various forms of primary aldosteronism and pseudoaldosteronism.

Table 36.2 Plasma renin activity and plasma aldosterone values in the differential diagnosis of the various forms of aldosteronism

	PRA	PA
Secondary aldosteronism	Elevated	Elevated
Primary aldosteronism	Suppressed	Elevated
Pseudoaldosteronism	Suppressed	Suppressed

(PRA = plasma renin activity; PA = plasma [or serum] concentration of aldosterone.)

"low-renin hypertension" – and the observed fact that plasma aldosterone, even in cases of primary aldosteronism, varies considerably from day to day and can be subjected to diurnal variation – represent additional confounding factors. The position of the patient (reclining or upright), to which the renin-aldosterone system is normally responsive, must always be monitored as well. Therefore, since in cases of primary aldosteronism PRA and plasma aldosterone are modified in opposite directions, it has been proposed to compute the ratio PA/PRA which sensitizes the procedure and allows for the performance of these tests under random conditions. Depending on the unit used for plasma aldosterone concentration reporting and on the experience of various centers, different cut-off values of this ratio have been proposed (as indicated in Figure 36.2, we used a cut-off point of 950 when plasma aldosterone concentration is expressed in pmol/l and plasma renin activity in ng, angiotensin I formed per ml per hour).

The value of a 24-hour urinary aldosterone excretion measurement has been variously evaluated, from being of little or no value to having a high sensitivity (96%) and specificity (93%) to essential hypertension, when considering a threshold value of 14 µg (38.5 nmol) per 24 hours after a high sodium intake for 3 days. It is always best evaluated by comparison with a 24-hour sodium excretion measurement using a nomogram. Aldosterone excretion measurement can thus support the diagnosis of excess aldosterone production but does not differentiate between secondary and primary aldosteronism and does not distinguish between the various subsets of primary aldosteronism.

The second stage (Fig. 36.2) of the diagnostic procedure is aimed at confirming the diagnosis of primary aldosteronism and consists of dynamic tests to demonstrate the chronic suppression of renin release and the autonomy of aldosterone production.

Stimulatory tests of PRA

Combined stimulation by furosemide and upright posture This is the easiest test. It can be performed on an ambulatory basis and consists of administering 40 mg furosemide in the evening and the morning of the next day and drawing blood for PRA after 2 hours of ambulation. After this combined hypovolemic and orthostatic stimulation, PRA remains suppressed below 1.5 ng/ml/h in cases of primary aldosteronism.

Sodium deprivation test After measuring PRA after 3 to 5 days of normal dietary sodium, the determination is repeated after 4 days of sodium deprivation, preferably in the upright position. Essential hypertension displays a stimulated PRA value of 5 ± 1 ng/ml/h (n = 40) under those conditions. However, according to the experience of Bravo et al. (1994), some 35% of cases with primary aldosteronism displayed a PRA value of 2 ng/ml/h or above, rendering a sensitivity and a specificity of 64% and 83%, respectively.

Captopril test Blood for PRA determination is drawn 2 hours after administering 25 mg of captopril. A rise of PRA above 2 ng/ml/h is observed in all normotensives,

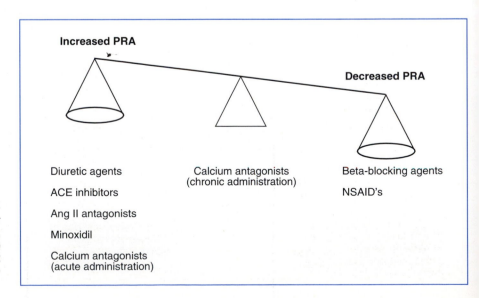

Increased PRA

Decreased PRA

Diuretic agents

ACE inhibitors

Ang II antagonists

Minoxidil

Calcium antagonists
(acute administration)

Calcium antagonists
(chronic administration)

Beta-blocking agents

NSAID's

Figure 36.3 The effect of antihypertensive agents and other drugs on plasma renin activity, which must be taken into account to obtain a correct interpretation of abnormal values.

while in primary aldosteronism it remains below this threshold. However, the distinction from hypertensive patients is poor, and thus this test cannot be recommended.

Inhibitory test of plasma aldosterone

Saline infusion test Patients with primary aldosteronism, after an initial period of salt retention, are in a phase of renal sodium escape. No lowering of plasma aldosterone is expected from the sodium loading that results from the infusion of 2 l of 0.9% saline over a time period of 4 hours. However, two confounding factors can result in false-positive tests: plasma aldosterone, in patients with aldosterone-producing adenoma (APA), follows a diurnal rhythm, such that a decrease in these cases could be interpreted as a response to sodium loading; whereas patients with one of the subsets of primary aldosteronism, either idiopathic adrenal hyperplasia or angiotensin II-responsive adrenal-producing adenoma (AII-responsive APA) may respond during the 4 hours of the reclining position and sodium loading with a decrease of plasma aldosterone. Furthermore, in elderly patients or patients with severe forms of hypertension, sodium loading may be contraindicated.

Fludrocortisone suppression This test consists of the administration of 0.1 mg fludrocortisone daily 6-hourly for 4 days, along with supplemental sodium chloride (20-30 mmol NaCl three times daily and a supplement of potassium to prevent aggravation of hypokalemia, which should be monitored carefully). The absence of a significant lowering of plasma aldosterone by this excess of another mineralocorticoid is considered as the definitive test. The same restriction, as in the preceding test, applies to the elderly or the severely hypertensive patient.

Captopril test with plasma aldosterone as end-point
Plasma aldosterone, or better the PA/PRA ratio, is determined 2 hours after administration of 25 mg captopril. Two groups consider this test to be extremely powerful: (1) according to Lyons et al. (1983), all normotensive and the vast majority of essential hypertension patients present with plasma aldosterone values <15 ng/ml (<0.41 nmol/l) or a PA/PRA ratio <50 (PA being expressed in ng/ml); according to Thibonnier et al. (1982), this test assured the correct diagnosis of all patients with aldosterone-producing adenoma, versus hypertensive subjects, when a cut-off plasma aldosterone value of 665 pmol/l was selected 3 hours after administering 1 mg per kg body weight of captopril. Of note, all cases of idiopathic adrenal hyperplasia were missed by this procedure.

Differential diagnosis

The goal of the third step is to distinguish between the various anatomical abnormalities leading to excessive aldosterone production (Fig. 36.4). Five forms of primary aldosteronism have been described thus far. By and large, the most frequent ones (Tab. 36.3) are represented by the aldosterone-producing adenoma (APA) and idiopathic hyperaldosteronism due to bilateral hyperplasia, together encompassing 95% of all forms of aldosteronism. They

are important to distinguish, since only aldosterone-producing adenoma patients benefit from surgical removal.

Two physiological characteristics distinguish them. In the case of the vast majority of aldosterone-producing adenomas, aldosterone production is insensitive to stimulation by angiotensin II, and plasma aldosterone displays a diurnal rhythm similar to that of plasma cortisol. On the contrary, when IHA is present, aldosterone production is sensitive to an angiotensin II rise, even if very modest, such as during the orthostatic test in the face of low PRA. Although there are exceptions, these two simple tests are worth being performed by measuring PRA and plasma aldosterone in the recumbent position at 8 hours and again after 2 hours, ambulating at 10 hours, along with plasma cortisol, and then measuring plasma aldosterone and plasma cortisol in samples drawn at noon and 4:00 p.m. A rise of plasma aldosterone after orthostatism and an absent diurnal rhythm favors IHA, while no response to orthostatism (or even a decrease) and a continuous decline of

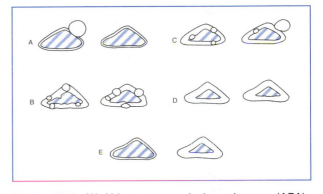

Figure 36.4 (A) Aldosterone-producing adenoma (APA); (B) idiopathic, micro-macronodular, bilateral hyperplasia (IHA); (C) idiopathic, micronodular, bilateral hyperplasia (IHA); (D) idiopathic, bilateral, simple adrenal hyperplasia (IHA); (E) primary, unilateral adrenal hyperplasia (PAH).

Table 36.3 Relative prevalence among the various anatomical forms of the syndrome of primary aldosteronism

	Prevalence
Aldosterone-producing adenoma (APA)	50-64%
Aldosterone-producing/AngII-responsive adenoma (AP-RA)	1.7-3%
Idiopathic hyperaldosteronism (IHA)	32-44%
Primary adrenal hyperplasia (PAH)	0.8-5%
Glucocorticoid-remediable aldosteronism (GRA)	<2%
Aldosterone-producing carcinoma	<1%
Total number of cases	115-154

(Range of values taken from three large series: Irony et al. [1990]; Mantero et al. [1991]; Young and Hogan [1994].)

plasma aldosterone throughout the day suggests aldosterone-producing adenoma. However, a subset of aldosterone-producing adenoma was found to present with a rise of plasma aldosterone following orthostatism (or angiotensin II infusion) and has been termed either aldosterone-producing renin-responsive adenoma (AP-RA) or AII-R APA. Thus, caution should be exerted when a diagnosis of IHA is made on the basis of these tests in view of the risk to miss the diagnosis of surgically correctable AII-R APA.

Imaging procedure

The next procedure consists of demonstrating the presence of a unilateral production of aldosterone that is consistent with the findings of imaging techniques. The discovery by computed tomography of a one-sided adrenal tumor, once the biological tests performed have been shown to favor primary aldosteronism due to aldosterone-producing adenoma, is strong evidence of a surgically correctable form of primary aldosteronism. These tumors are usually of small size (between 0.5 and 5 cm). However, two confounding factors are represented by the frequent occurrence in the general population of non-functioning incidentalomas and of visible macronodules in cases of multinodular bilateral hyperplasia in IHA (Fig. 36.4 b or c). In this situation, one feels more comfortable if the nor-[131]iodo cholesterol scintigraphy reveals unilateral uptake of the tracer on the same side or if sampling of adrenal veins for plasma aldosterone and plasma cortisol determination, during catheterization, indicates a unilateral excessive production of aldosterone on the same side.

An even rarer form of primary aldosteronism should be mentioned that behaves as an aldosterone-producing adenoma but is actually unilateral primary adrenal hyperplasia (PAH). Although the number of these occurrences is very limited, patients appear to also benefit from surgical removal and therefore should be dealt with as patients of aldosterone-producing adenoma. Only a few instances of aldosterone-producing adrenal carcinoma have been reported.

Treatment

Medical treatment

In all forms of idiopathic bilateral hyperplasia, surgery is contraindicated, since both electrolytic abnormalities and hypertension have been found to persist in all cases. Thus, in those forms and in cases of aldosterone-producing adenomas where surgery is not possible or contraindicated for medical reasons or refused by the patient, medical treatment should be selected. It consists of the administration of the aldosterone antagonist spironolactone at a dose of 50 to 100 mg orally qd. In view of the fact that a chronic dose of over 50 mg of this compound frequently induces the development of gynecomastia in male patients, which can be painful, it is recommended to administer no more

than 50 mg spironolactone combined with another potassium-sparing diuretic such as amiloride or triamterene. A new aldosterone antagonist that would not induce gynecomasty is currently in the phase of clinical assay.

Surgical treatment

Unilateral adrenalectomy is the treatment of choice in cases of solitary aldosterone-producing adenomas. It is generally followed by curing of the electrolytic abnormalities; hypertension, albeit of a milder degree, is easily manageable with few hyperantihypertensive drugs, and persists in about 40% of the cases. In recent years the technique of adrenalectomy through laparoscopy has been introduced in a few centers.

GLUCOCORTICOID-SUPPRESSIBLE HYPERALDOSTERONISM (GSH) OR GLUCOCORTICOID-REMEDIABLE HYPERALDOSTERONISM (GRA)

Glucocorticoid-suppressible hyperaldosteronism (GSH), or glucocorticoid-remediable hyperaldosteronism (GRA), is a familial, non-tumorous, glucocorticoid-remediable form of hyperaldosteronism that was described by 1966, and since then many isolated cases and kindreds have been reported. This fascinating and unique genetic disorder, which leads to the excessive production of aldosterone, was discovered by Lifton and Dluhy in 1993. An unequal crossing-over results in the fusion on chromosome 8q of the 5'-regulatory region of 11β-hydroxylase to the coding sequence of the complex of aldosterone synthase. Normally 11β-hydroxylase is expressed in both the zona glomerulosa and the zona fasciculata, but aldosterone synthase is expressed uniquely in the zona glomerulosa. Through this fusion, aldosterone synthase is also expressed in the zona fasciculata and falls, just as cortisol, under the control of adrenocorticotropic hormone (ACTH). Aldosterone is thus constantly synthesized in excessive quantity and, just as for cortisol, its production can be inhibited by ACTH suppression with dexamethasone. Along with aldosterone, 18-oxocortisol and 18-hydrocortisol are produced. This familial genetic disorder is autosomal dominant, thus a familial form of primary aldosterone should alert the physician to the possibility of this genetic disorder. As in cases of aldosterone-producing adenoma, plasma aldosterone does not respond to the orthostatic test and presents a diurnal rhythm parallel to that of cortisol.

FORMS OF HYPERMINERALOCORTICISM MIMICKING PRIMARY ALDOSTERONISM (PSEUDOALDOSTERONISMS)

Forms of hypermineralocorticism mimicking primary aldosteronism are a group of genetic syndromes and enzymatic disorders of the adrenal glands or kidneys involving cortisol, deoxycorticosterone (DOC), and some of their derivatives, or involving a genetic mutation of the genes coding for some subunits of the sodium channel in the distal renal tubule. Most of those disorders can in the present day and age be diagnosed by molecular genetic testing (Tab. 36.4).

Genetic disorders affecting the adrenal gland

Hypertensive forms of congenital adrenal hyperplasia

11β-hydroxylase deficiency syndrome (see Fig. 26.3 in Chap. 26). The enzymatic defect of 11β-hydroxylase results in the reduced production of cortisol, corticosterone, and aldosterone with a concomitant overproduction of DOC (the cause of mineralocorticoid hypertension with hypokalemia) and androgenic steroids, dehydroepiandrosterone (DHEA), and Δ4-androstenedione, which are responsible for virilization in genetically female patients and for isosexual precocious puberty in males. This excessive production of the steroids upstream from the enzymatic block is due to the counter-regulated increased secretion of ACTH in the face of decreased plasma concentration of cortisol.

The diagnosis is confirmed by increased basal or ACTH[1-18]-stimulated levels of 11-deoxycortisol (substance S); and by increased levels of 17α-OH-progesterone, DHEA, and Δ4-androstenedione and their urinary metabolites tetrahydro-S and 17-ketosteroids, which can be suppressed by dexamethasone. Genetic demonstration of the mutations of the gene coding for CYP11B1 located on chromosome 8q21-q22 has been achieved, where about 20 causative mutations have now been identified.

The treatment consists of inhibiting the excessive ACTH secretion by glucocorticoids, either cortisol or dexamethasone.

17α-hydroxylase/17,20-lyase deficiency syndrome (see Fig. 26.3 in Chap. 26). In the adreno-genital syndrome of 17α-hydroxylase/17,20-lyase deficiency, the enzymatic deficiency at the level of 17α-hydroxylase results in a marked decrease or absent biosynthesis of 17α-OH-progesterone and the distal steroids, in both the pathways leading to cortisol and to all the gonadal and adrenal sexual steroids. The latter defect is responsible for a hypergonadotropic hypogonadism so severe that, if undiagnosed at birth, genotypic males can be unknowingly raised as females. In female subjects (and in males raised as females) the syndrome is characterized by absent puberty, primary amenorrhea, and eunuchoid body proportions with long limbs. In both sexes axillary and pubic hairs are absent. Due to the low or absent production of cortisol, ACTH is overproduced, which in turn stimulates the intact deoxy-steroid pathway and thus the production of deoxycorticosterone (DOC), corticosterone, 18-OH-deoxycorticosterone, and 18-OH-corticosterone. The excessive, uncontrolled production of DOC is responsible for hypertension, with salt and water retention accompanied by a loss of potassium and hypokalemia and by suppression of renin release and aldosterone production. This characteristic profile of steroid production establishes the diagnosis. Treatment is similar to all of the other forms of adreno-genital syndromes and consists of the administration of glucocorticoids (either cortisol or dexamethasone) to suppress ACTH release. The initiation of this treatment should be progressive to allow time for the renin-aldosterone axis to resume its activity, otherwise severe natriuresis with weight loss, hypotension, and hyperkalemia could endanger the patient.

Approximately 18 mutations of several types have been localized in the coding region of the CYP17 gene,

Table 36.4 Syndromes of pseudoaldosteronism mimicking primary aldosteronism

Syndromes	Genetic defect	Enzymatic or protein defect	Steroid(s) involved	Suppression treatment with
Syndrome of apparent mineralocorticoid excess:				
SAME type 1	Yes	11β-HSD2	Cortisol	Dexamethasone
SAME type 2	Yes	11β-HSD2 +5a-reductase?	Cortisol	Dexamethasone
Liquorice abuse	No	11β-HSD2 inhibition	Cortisol	Suppression of liquorice intake
Cushing's syndrome	No	11β-HSD2 overwhelmed by the excess of cortisol	Cortisol	Surgery, chemical
Congenital adrenal hyperplasia (CAH):				
11β-OHase deficiency	Yes	CYP11B1	11-deoxy-cortisol, DOC	Dexamethasone or cortisone
17α-OHase deficiency	Yes	CYP17	19-nor-DOC, DOC	Dexamethasone or cortisone
Liddle's syndrome	Yes	β or γ subunit of the amiloride-sensitive epithelial Na+ channel	None	Amiloride or triamterene
Syndrome of general resistance to cortisol	Yes	Decrease number or affinity of cortisol receptor	DOC	Dexamethasone
DOC-producing adrenal tumour	No	Unknown	DOC	Surgery or spironolactone

which is located on chromosome 10q24-25 and codes for the 17α-hydroxylase/17,20 lyase enzyme complex.

Cushing's syndrome Although Cushing's syndrome is always a candidate in the differential diagnosis of hypertension accompanied by hypokalemia, it is rare that these signs are not accompanied by all of the other features resulting from cortisol excess herald the actual disease (truncal obesity, rounded plethoric face, purple striae, atrophic skin with bruising, muscle wasting and weakness, osteoporosis, hirsutism, amenorrhea, carbohydrate intolerance, and emotional disturbances). This is particularly true for the central pituitary form of Cushing's disease, which is due to the excessive production of ACTH stimulating all of the various steroid pathways, including those leading to glucocorticoids, mineralocorticoids, and androgens. The rarer form of Cushing's syndrome caused by an adrenal benign adenoma classically produces exclusively cortisol and is therefore not accompanied by marked signs of mineralocorticoid excess. The particular form of Cushing's syndrome caused by ectopic production of ACTH is addressed below.

Rare adrenal tumors exclusively secreting DOC that mimic primary aldosteronism have been described. Adrenal carcinomas with disorderly production of many steroids and their precursors – including mineralocorticoids such as DOC and androgens leading to virilization – are more frequent. All of these tumors are generally of large size and malignant and become apparent due to their mass effect.

Genetic disorders affecting the kidneys

Liddle's syndrome

This syndrome mimics primary aldosteronism in all aspects but with the following diagnostic characteristics: (1) aldosterone production is suppressed and the clinical and biological features do not respond to the aldosterone antagonist spironolactone, indicating that it is not due to another mineralocorticoid, and (2) antagonists of the epithelial sodium channel such as triamterene and amiloride correct all of the abnormalities. Furthermore, the prismatic case was later cured by kidney transplantation after terminal renal failure had developed, which indicated that the defect was in the nephron. Recently the cause of the syndrome was found to be the result of a mutation on chromosome 16 (introducing a stop codon or a frameshift) in the gene coding for the β or the γ subunit, which results in a truncation of the carboxy-terminus of one or the other subunit of the amiloride-sensitive epithelial sodium channel. As a consequence of these mutations, this channel – which is normally controlled by aldosterone – is constitutively activated. About 50 cases in large kindreds have now been described. Treatment is amiloride administration, which corrects all of the clinical abnormalities.

Syndrome of generalized, inherited glucocorticoid resistance (GIGR), or cortisol resistance

The patients with the syndrome of generalized, inherited glucocorticoid resistance (GIGR) present the usual features of mineralocorticoid excess; however, due to excessive DOC production, primary aldosteronism is simulated. An excess of adrenal androgens are also produced, causing hirsutism, virilization, menstrual irregularities, and/or isosexual precocity.

This syndrome is caused by either one of two different genetic disorders: (1) a spliced-site germline deletion that results in a decreased number of the human glucocorticoid receptor, or (2) various missense mutations in the ligand-binding domain, causing decreased binding affinity for cortisol. As a result of the defective, negative retroaction exerted by cortisol on the hypothalamo-pituitary axis, ACTH is overproduced and stimulates DOC and adrenal androgens in excess, accounting for the characteristic clinical features.

Syndromes of apparent mineralocorticoid excess

Syndromes of apparent mineralocorticoid excess mimic primary aldosteronism; the mineralocorticoid type I receptors are constantly activated by cortisol instead of their usual agonist, aldosterone. These receptors are normally protected from activation by cortisol (to which they would potentially be exposed to much larger amounts than to aldosterone within the kidneys) because a locally active custodial enzyme, 11β-hydroxysteroid dehydrogenase (11β-HSD), converts cortisol – with its high-binding affinity to type I mineralocorticoid receptors – into cortisone, which has much less affinity for the receptors. These patients, who are otherwise indistinguishable from patients with primary aldosteronism, respond to treatment by suppressive doses of dexamethasone that inhibit endogenous ACTH and thus cortisol production, which results in natriuresis and the correction of hypertension and electrolyte abnormalities, including hypokalemia. Since the local renal excess of cortisol activates type I mineralocorticoid receptors, the patients also respond to mineralocorticoid antagonists such as spironolactone, and also to amiloride, the antagonist of the epithelial sodium channels activated by mineralocorticoids.

This syndrome is either acquired or genetically transmitted. The *acquired form* is caused by inhibition of the 11β-HSD enzyme. The most common culprits are liquorice-containing laxatives, non-alcoholic beverages, chewing tobacco, and a variety of candies and breath fresheners. Liquorice is an extract from the root of the plant *Glycyrrhiza labra*, which contains glycyrrhetinic and glycyrrhizic acids that inhibit 11β-HSD. Flavonoids have also been found to be inhibitors of the 11β-HSD; they include gossypol from cotton seed, which can be found in Chinese preparations of oral contraceptives and cause hypokalemia; and naringenin and naringin, which are found in grapefruit juice. A derivative of glycyrrhetinic acid, carbenoxolone was used for treating peptic disease in the sixties and is still used today in some countries. It inhibits both 11β-HSD and 11-oxoreductase, which converts cortisone back to cortisol. Therefore, a careful history of the eating habits of patients is mandatory in attempting to identify this acquired form of pseudoaldosteronism.

Cushing's syndrome due to ectopic production of ACTH

Cushing's syndrome due to ectopic production of ACTH is a form of hypercorticism that, in contrast to other causes of Cushing's syndrome, is often characterized by early and marked signs of mineralocorticoid excess with hypertension and severe electrolyte disorders, including hypokalemia. One possibility is that ACTH in excess is able to inhibit 11β-hydroxysteroid dehydrogenase and thus raises the cortisol/cortisone ratio, which accounts for the occurrence of apparent mineralocorticoid excess in addition to that which results from the stimulation of aldosterone and DOC production. Another, more likely possibility is that the 11β-HSD enzyme is overwhelmed by the excess of cortisol. The most frequent source of ectopic production of ACTH is the anaplastic or oat-cell bronchial carcinoma. In this disease, this ectopic production of ACTH usually confers a rapidly fatal course to the patient.

The 11β-HSD gene has been cloned and two isoforms of the gene described. The second, (11β-HSD K, B2 or type II) is NAD-dependent and more tissue-specific than type I and has been isolated from the kidney. Its gene, HSD11B2, is located on chromosome 16. It is the second isoform of 11β-HSD that is defective in the congenital/familial type of apparent mineralocorticoid excess, and many

mutations have been reported in HSD11B2 that are causative of this disease.

In both the acquired and the inherited forms of apparent mineralocorticoid excess, the biological characteristics consist of a reduced ratio of tetrahydrocortisone to tetrahydrocortisol, the respective urinary metabolites of cortisone and cortisol, and a prolonged half-life of plasma cortisol, whose concentration is otherwise within the normal range.

The treatment can include withdrawal of the substances inhibiting 11β-HSD in the acquired forms of apparent mineralocorticoid excess, removal of the source of ectopic ACTH production if feasible, or pharmacological adrenalectomy with aminoglutethimide, ketoconazole, and/or mitotane. In the congenital or familial forms, inhibition of the hypothalamo-pituitary-adrenal axis with a suppressive dose of dexamethasone corrects all of the abnormalities.

Iatrogenic causes of mineralocorticoid excess

Long-term topical abuse of the fluorinated derivatives of steroids 9α-fluoroprednisolone on the skin or as nasal spray, or excessive use of 9α-fludrocortisone for the treatment of orthostatic hypotension or as substitution for adrenal insufficiency or adreno-genital syndromes, may lead to severe hypertension with hypokalemia.

Suggested readings

Anderson GH, Blakeman N, Streeten DHP. The effect of age on prevalence of secondary forms of hypertension in 4429 consecutively referred patients. Journal of Hypertension. 1994;12:609-15.

Bravo EL. Secondary hypertension: adrenal and nervous system, in atlas of heart diseases. In: Braunwald E (ed). Hypertension mechanisms and therapy. Vol. 1. Hollenberg NK. Philadelphia: Current Medicine, 1995;1-15.

Gordon RD, Stowasser M, Klemm SA, Tunny TJ. Primary aldosteronism and other forms of mineralocorticoid hypertension. In: Swales JD (ed). Textbook of hypertension. London: Blackwell Scientific Publications, 1994, 865-92.

Irony I, Kater CE, Biglieri EG, Shackleton CHL. Correctable subsets of primary aldosteronism. Primary adrenal hyperplasia and renin responsive adenoma. Amer J of Hypertension. 1990;3:576-82.

Lifton RP, Dluhy RG. Glucocorticoid-remediable aldosteronism. Current Op Endocrinol Diabetes. 1994;1:117-22.

Lyons DF, Kem DC, Brown RD, Hanson CH, Carollo ML.

Single dose captopril as a diagnostic test for primary aldosteronism. B Clin Endo Metab 1983;57:892-6.

Mantero F, Armanin D, Boscaro M, et al. Steroids and hypertension. J Steroid Biochem Molec Biol 1991;40:35-44.

Thibonnier M, Sassano P, Joseph A, Plouin PF, Corvol P, Ménard J. Diagnostic value of a single dose captopril in renin- and aldosterone-dependent, surgically curable hypertension. Cardiovascular Rev Reports 1982;3:1659-67.

Tucker RM, Labarthe DR. Frequency of surgical treatment for hypertension in adults at the Mayo Clinic from 1973 through 1975. Mayo Clinic Proceedings 1977;52:549-55.

Vallotton MB. Primary aldosteronism. Part I Diagnosis of primary hyperaldosteronism. Clin Endo 1996;45:47-62.

Vallotton MB. Primary aldosteronism. Part II Differential diagnosis of primary hyperaldosteronism and pseudoaldosteronism. Clin Endo 1996;45:53-60.

White PC. Inherited forms of mineralocorticoid hypertension. Hypertension 1996;28:927-36.

Young WF, Hogan MJ. Renin-independent hypermineralocorticoidism. Trends Endocrinol Metab 1994;5:97-106.

Hypertension related to other diseases

Franco Mantero

██ **KEY POINTS** ████████████████

- Hypertension is present in approximately 50% of acromegalic patients.
- Hypercalcemic primary hyperparathyroid patients are hypertensive in 50% of cases. Hypertension persists in most patients after surgical removal of a parathyroid tumor.
- Thyroid disorders (hypo- and hyperthyroidism) are frequently accompanied by hypertension, although with different hemodynamic patterns.
- Several hormonal or hormone-like drugs may induce hypertension in susceptible patients.

VOLUME-RELATED HYPERTENSION

Apart from the classical forms of endocrine-dependent hypertensive syndromes described in the previous chapters, high blood pressure levels may be encountered in variable percentages and degrees as part of the clinical picture of several other endocrine diseases. The underlying physiopathogenetic mechanisms are more subtle and indeterminate in the latter than in the typical forms. Furthermore, hypertension may be the consequence of treatment with hormonal substances in susceptible patients, or when used in excess.

ACROMEGALY

An increased prevalence of hypertension occurs with acromegaly, especially in female and aged patients (approximately twice the control population), which is due to one or more mechanisms that depend on excessive growth hormone secretion.

Acromegalic patients have increased plasma volume, total body water, and exchangeable sodium and potassium, irrespective of the presence of high or normal blood pressure, although some correlations do exist with exchangeable sodium. These abnormalities are present both in normotensive and hypertensive patients, indicating that these factors may be more effective in inducing high blood pressure in some acromegalics than in others. The volume and electrolytic effect are thought to be due to a direct effect of growth hormone on tubular resorption since growth hormone receptors have been found along the nephron by in situ hybridization, but other endocrine systems may intervene (e.g., renin-angiotensin-aldosterone system).

In rare cases aldosterone is elevated, and adrenal nodular enlargement or aldosterone-producing tumors have been described. A direct trophic effect of growth hormone or insulin-like growth factor 1 (IGF1) on the adrenal could explain some of these cases, although the possibility of multiple endocrine neoplasia (MEN I) cannot be excluded.

An important factor, recently confirmed, is a direct trophic role of growth hormone and related growth factors on the cardiovascular tissues, which may favor the onset of hypertension in predisposed subjects.

MISCELLANEOUS

HYPERPARATHYROIDISM

The prevalence of hypertension in patients with primary hyperparathyroidism is approximately 50%. This association is difficult to explain, in part because parathyroid hormone acts as an acute vasodilating agent with a blood pressure-lowering effect. The understanding of the pathogenetic role of parathyroid hormone in hypertension is further complicated by its effect on several factors (ions such as Ca^{2+}, Mg^{2+}, PO_4), and other hormones that may affect the vascular smooth muscle tone. It is possible that a portion of patients with primary hyperparathyroidism have pre-existing or concomitant essential hypertension. Furthermore, an association between renal functional impairment – due to primary hyperparathyroidism, calcium deposition within the kidney, and hypertension – may exist. Sustained hypercalcemia may change the sensitivity of vascular smooth muscle cells to parathyroid hormone (desensitization to its vasodilating activity).

The picture is further complicated by the controversial blood pressure variation results obtained following surgical removal of parathyroid hormone-producing adenomas. Several reports showed a range of no changes to approximately 50% improvement of hypertension, while a high proportion of reversals of hypertension was found in a series of patients when those with renal insufficiency were excluded. In general, the evidence of a therapeutic effect on high blood pressure is still lacking, and hypertension per se is not an indication for surgery.

THYROID DISORDERS

Thyroid hormones have significant effects on the cardiovascular system and on blood pressure. It is well-known that hypertension may be present both in patients with hypothyroidism and in those with hyperthyroidism, although the hemodynamic abnormalities differ significantly between the two conditions.

Hypothyroidism

In patients with primary hypothyroidism of varying etiology, hypertension is more common than in control age-matched populations, with a prevalence ranging from 11 to 26% of cases.

Diastolic hypertension may be associated to the degree of thyroid dysfunction. The hemodynamic features of this form of hypertension include a low cardiac index and stroke volume, as well as of total volume, although some controversy exists on the latter. An increase in peripheral vascular resistance accounts for the consistent finding of high diastolic pressure.

The role of the sympathetic nervous system has attracted much attention, with high levels of plasma norepinephrine being a consistent finding in hypothyroid patients.

Hyperthyroidism

The prevalence of increased systolic levels of blood pressure in patients with overt hyperthyroidism is high, although the criteria for systolic hypertension are seldom consistent. Diastolic blood pressure is nearly always normal or reduced, leading to the well-known increase of differential pressure. Hypertension is more frequently found in patients with toxic adenoma, probably because patients with toxic adenoma tend to be older.

This blood pressure pattern normalizes quite rapidly, as the thyrostatic treatment becomes effective in reducing heart rate as well. The hemodynamic basis of this form of hypertension consists of increased cardiac output, stroke volume, heart rate, and ejection fraction; the peripheral vascular resistances are decreased.

In spite of overt symptoms of hyperadrenergic status, no increase of catecholamines or of muscle-nerve sympathetic activity has been demonstrated, whereas increased β-receptor density in various tissues (heart, leukocytes) has been found. This could explain the efficacy of beta-blockers upon the hemodynamic features of hyperthyroidism.

GONADAL STEROIDS

It is well-known that oral estroprogestin contraceptives, especially those of relatively high dosages, can induce hypertension in a small fraction of women. The early alarming data on the hypertensive effects of oral contraceptives were related to the use of compounds with high levels of both estrogens (ethinylestradiol or mestranol, about 50 to 100 µg) and various types of progestins. Hypertension occurred in 5% of women taking these pills.

The subsequent reduction of the estrogen content (which was also suspected for the relatively high incidence of thromboembolism) to 20 to 30 µg, accompanied by a reduction of the progestins, lowered the incidence of hypertension to approximately 1% of women treated over periods of 4 months to 3 years.

The mechanism underlying the effect of oral contraceptives on blood pressure, as well as the respective roles of estrogens and progestins, are still partially unclear.

Most of the investigative attention has been directed at the renin-angiotensin system, since estrogens stimulate angiotensinogen production by the liver. Plasma renin activity tends to be slightly increased, while immunoreactive renin is lower. This last phenomenon may occur as a feedback mechanism due to angiotensinogen increase and subsequent increased angiotensin II formation. One could speculate that this feedback is less active in women developing hypertension, that increased sensitivity to angiotensin II is present in some subjects genetically predisposed to develop hypertension, or in older ones, or in patients with increased body mass index or with some pre-existing renal disorder aggravated by the reduction of renal blood flow.

Progestins seem not to significantly influence blood pressure in most studies, whether they are used alone or in increasing amounts in the face of a constant low dose of estrogens.

Sympathomimetic drugs

A dose-related increase in blood pressure may be consequent to the treatment of conditions associated with hypotension or, more frequently, an adverse reaction to the treatment of clinical conditions not related to blood pressure disturbances.

Sympathomimetic agents such as ephedrine, phenylpropanolamine, and phenylephrine, which are used in the treatment of orthostatic hypotension, may induce supine hypertension. More frequently, sympathomimetic-induced hypertension occurs as a secondary effect of nasal decongestives, anorectics, or central nervous system stimulators, when used in excessive amounts or over prolonged periods of time (Tab. 37.1).

Other imidazolinic sympathomimetics, primarily used as topical nasal or ocular vasoconstrictors, may sometimes, though rarely, induce systemic cardiovascular effects.

Other drugs

As shown in Table 37.1, the list of substances that may be responsible for hypertension as an unexpected event includes monoamine oxidase inhibitors, ergot alkaloid, and nonsteroidal anti-inflammatory drugs. Some monoamine oxidase inhibitors interact with tyramine present in food (such as alcohol, cheese, and chocolate) and increase its effect on blood pressure, which is mediated by noradrenaline release.

Ergot alkaloids (ergotamine and dihydroergotamine), mostly used in hemicrania, are also partially adrenergic and 5-hydroxy-tryptamine (5-HT) receptor agonists. Indomethacin and other more recently identified *nonsteroidal anti-inflammatory drugs* may act on blood pressure by their effect on prostaglandins, thus reducing the antihypertensive effects of some drugs.

The immunosuppressive drug *cyclosporine* has unexpectedly revealed the appearance of hypertension in a percentage of patients. The mechanism is still under debate: nephrotoxicity, renal or peripheral direct vasoconstriction, changes in prostaglandin metabolism, direct endothelial damage (increased release of endothelin, or nitric oxide release impairment) have been advocated.

Human recombinant *erythropoietin* is widely used in the treatment of anemia in advanced renal insufficiency. The percent incidence of hypertension or of its worsening is about 20%. Although the increase of red cell counts may contribute to the increased peripheral vascular resistance in these subjects, other factors are likely to be involved (such as changes in the renin-angiotensin system or disorders of autonomic regulation of blood pressure).

Glucocorticoids are widely used in a number of diseases for their anti-inflammatory and immunosuppressive action. Both systemic and topical use of these steroids may cause, when chronically administered and/or in high doses, symptoms and signs of hypercortisolism, including hypertension. The mechanism of glucocorticoid-induced hypertension is still not completely understood; it is possibly related not only to salt and water retention, but also to an increase of vascular sensitivity to endogenous vasoactive substances (noradrenaline, angiotensin II), decreased prostaglandin synthesis, a direct vascular effect, endothelial dysfunction, impairment of renal metabolism of steroids, and so on.

Fluorinated steroids may have a high mineralocorticoid-like activity, as demonstrated by the occasional presence of hypokalemia. The same is true for exogenous adrenocorticotropic hormone (ACTH)-induced hypertension and patients treated with long-acting ACTH preparations.

Hypertension due to chronic synthetic steroid treatment may persist for a long period of time after withdrawal of the drug since vascular organic damage is likely to occur in such cases.

The common steroid used in orthostatic hypotension or as replacement therapy in adrenal insufficiency is 9α-fluorohydrocortisone. When supraphysiological doses (0.5 to 1 mg) are employed for an adequate period of time, hypertension may occur, persisting in the recumbent position, accompanied by sodium retention and, subsequently, by hypokalemia. This remains, however, an unusual finding. More frequently, at least in some countries, is the discovery of such cases due to chronic abuse of topical preparation (for nasal, mucosal, or cutaneous application in cases of rhinitis or dermatitis), of mixtures of vasoactive amines and some fluorinated anti-inflammatory steroids such as 9α-fluoroprednisolone, which also presents potent mineralocorticoid activity.

Another form of mineralocorticoid-like iatrogenic hypertension is consequential to the use of the anti-ulcer drug *carbenoxolone*. Its mechanism of action is similar to that of *liquorice*, being itself a derivative of glycyrrhizic acid (see Chap. 36). Carbenoxolone blocks the activity of 11β-hydroxysteroid dehydrogenase, which converts cortisol to cortisone, thus leaving the kidney mineralocorticoid receptors unprotected from the mineralocorticoid activity of cortisol.

Table 37.1 Drug-induced hypertension

Sympathomimetics
  Ephedrine
  Phenylpropanolamine
  Phenylephrine, etc.

Monoamine oxidase inhibitors
  Tyramine
  Sympathomimetics
  Ergot alkaloids
  Nonsteroidal anti-inflammatory drugs
  Cyclosporine
  Erythropoietin
  Glucocorticoids
  Mineralocorticoids
  Estrogens

Suggested readings

BRICKMAN AS, NYBY MD. Parathyroid disease and hypertension. In: Laragh JH, Brenner BM (eds). Hypertension pathophysiology, diagnosis and management. 2nd ed. New York: Raven Press, 1995;2263-80.

CHUA SS, BENRIMOI SI. Non-prescription sympathomimetic agents and hypertension. Med Toxicol Adverse Drug Exp 1988;3:387-417.

DAVIES DL, CONNELL JMC, REID R, FRASER R. Acromegaly: the effects of growth hormone on blood vessels, sodium homeostasis and blood pressure. In: Robertson JIS (ed). Handbook of hypertension. Vol.15. Clinical hypertension. Amsterdam: Elsevier, 1992;545-75.

HERLITZ H, JONSSON O, BENGTSSON BA. Effect of recombinant human growth hormone on cellular sodium metabolism. Clin Sci (Colch) 1994;86:233-7.

MANTERO F. Exogenous mineralocorticoid-like disorders. Clin Endocrinol Metab 1981;10:465-78.

MANTERO F, OPOCHER G, ARMANINI D, PAVIOTTI G, BOSCARO M, MUGGEO M. Plasma renin activity and urinary aldosterone in acromegaly. J Endocrinol Invest 1979;2:13-8.

PANG PK, SHAN JJ, LEWANCZUK RZ, BENISHIN CG. Parathyroid hypertensive factor and intracellular calcium regulation. J Hypertens 1996;14:1053-60.

SAITO I, SARUTA T. Hypertension in thyroid disorders. Endocrinol Metab Clin North Am 1994;23:379-89.

SWALES JD. Textbook of hypertension. Oxford: Blackwell Science, 1994.

ANONYMOUS. The WHO multicentre trial of the vasopressor effects of combined oral contraceptives: 1. Comparison with IUD. Task Force on Oral Contraceptives. WHO Special Programme of Research, Development and Resarch Training in Human Reproduction. Contraception 1989;40:129-45.

Male reproductive system

Pathophysiology of sex determination and differentiation

Alessandra De Bellis, Mario Serio

NORMAL SEX DETERMINATION AND SEX DIFFERENTIATION

Sex determination and differentiation are sequential events that successively involve the establishment of the genetic sex in the zygote from the moment of conception, the determination of gonadal sex by the genetic sex, and the regulation by gonadal sex of the differentiation of the genital apparatus and thus the phenotypic sex. At puberty, the development of secondary sexual characteristics provides more visible phenotypic manifestations of the sexual dimorphism.

Both male and female embryos possess indifferent, common primordia that have an inherent tendency to feminize unless there is an interference by masculinizing factors. The embryonic gonad develops into an ovary unless it is diverted by a testis-determining factor regulated by the Y chromosome; female differentiation of the somatic sex structures occurs independently of gonadal hormones and will take place in the absence of fetal testes whether ovaries are present or not. Thus, the sexual dimorphism in phenotype in mammalians is mediated by the fetal testis and not by the ovary.

MAMMALIAN SEX DETERMINATION

It has been know since 1959 that the Y chromosome in humans is male-determining. Individuals with a normal Y chromosome, regardless of the number of X chromosomes, develop as males; the presence of only one X chromosome leads to female development. The Y chromosome has since been subjected to extensive molecular genetic analysis in an effort to clarify which genes are involved. Over the past 15 years, a series of candidate genes have been proposed as the testis-determining factor (TDF), which is now known to be located on the distal Y short arm (Yp) just below the pseudoautosomal boundary. Since 1990, consensus exists that the sex-determining region

(SRY) is identical to the TDF. The SRY product belongs to a newly recognized family of DNA-binding proteins. These proteins do not function as traditional transcription factors but rather bend the DNA (DNA-bending proteins), possibly facilitating an interaction between proteins bound on either side that subsequently alters transcription. Although SRY is clearly the major testis-determining factor, additional genes must be involved in testicular differentiation, though the exact role that autosomal loci play in the normal testicular cascade is unclear.

Genes that are possibly regulated by SRY, either directly or indirectly, or that alternatively work independently of SRY include the gene for anti-müllerian hormone (AMH). The anti-müllerian hormone, also know as müllerian inhibiting factor, is a glycoprotein hormone secreted by Sertoli cells. The gene for AMH encodes a 560-amino acid protein and is located on the short arm of chromosome 19. Male and female mice and humans express AMH well after the müllerian ducts have regressed or differentiated. In human males, immunoreactive AMH peaks at age 3 to 6 months and declines to background levels at puberty. In females AMH is essentially undetectable until puberty and continues to be expressed into adulthood. In addition, the levels vary during follicular development, which implies that it has a role in oocyte development. After puberty the serum concentrations are similar in both sexes. AMH inhibits aromatase activity in granulosa cells of the ovary and possibly also inhibits steroidogenesis by the Leydig cells of the testis, since mice in which the gene for müllerian inhibiting substance has been inactivated have Leydig cell hyperplasia. The AMH receptor, a serine-threonine kinase with a single transmembrane domain, is expressed around the fetal müllerian duct and in Sertoli and granulosa cells. Its gene has been cloned and mapped to chromosome 12. Measurements of serum AMH have been proposed as an indicator of testicular function. This assay might be helpful for identifying the presence of testicular tissue in prepubertal boys with nonpalpable gonads and in patients with intersexual disorders who have no palpable gonads.

Steroidogenic factor-1 (SF-1), a member of the nuclear hormone receptor superfamily, has been also implicated in gonadal development. The protein has been identified as a regulator of steroidogenic enzymes in the adrenals and gonads. The finding that SF-1-deficient mice lack adrenals and gonads suggests a role for SF-1 in the early stages of development of these organs.

Another gene involved in gonadal development and differentiation is WT-1, the Wilms' tumor suppressor locus at 11p13. Wilms' tumors are childhood kidney cancers that, in a small number of cases, are associated with genitourinary defects (cryptorchidism and hypospadias) and gonadoblastomas in the contiguous gene syndrome WAGR (Wilms' tumor, aniridia, genitourinary anomalies, mental retardation). Such an association between gonadal abnormalities and renal neoplasms and disease is not surprising given the intimacy of gonadal and renal morphogenesis. However, studies in both SF-1-deficient and WT-1-deficient mice indicate that the expression of the two genes is not dependent upon one another.

NORMAL SEX DIFFERENTIATION

Gonadal differentiation

Factors controlled by the genetic sex initiate a process in which the undifferentiated bipotential gonad is converted into a testis or an ovary. The differentiated gonad then secretes the hormonal signals that direct internal and external genital development. The primitive gonad, often called the genital ridge, develops at day 32 as a thickening of the celomic epithelium covering the ventral side of the cranial mesonephros, near the dorsal mesentery. Shortly thereafter these gonadal ridges shorten and project into the celomic cavity. The normal development of the gonad is dependent upon the migration of primordial germ cells from an extragonadal location (yolk sac) to the gonadal ridge, aided by active ameboidal movements. The irregular profile and cytoplasmic pseudopodia of these germ cells, as well as their alkaline phosphatase activity, identify them throughout their journey. Not all arrive at their final destination, as some are trapped in the adrenal cortex while others may undergo tumoral development in ectopic sites. Failure of the migration of primordial germ cells into the gonadal ridge causes lack of gonadal development (gonadal agenesia), and only a fibrous streak develops. Once incorporated into the primitive gonad, the germ cells are enveloped by epithelial cells, which are precursors of granulosa-Sertoli cells. At 6 weeks of fetal life the gonad is undifferentiated and bipotential, possessing both cortical and medullary areas and being composed of primordial germ cell mesenchyme and a covering layer of epithelium.

Testicular differentiation Testicular differentiation can be detected in a human fetus between 43 and 50 days. The initial event appears to be differentiation of seminiferous tubules and tunica albuginea; however, more sensitive techniques of investigation show that the first sign of primary male differentiation is the appearance of a new cell type, the Sertoli cell, which is characterized by an abundant, clear cytoplasm with abundant rough endoplasmic reticulum and complex membrane interdigitations. These aggregate to form seminiferous tubes and begin to secrete anti-müllerian hormone (AMH). Soon after the differentiation of the seminiferous tubules, the testis become rounded and blood vessels appear at the surface, allowing easy macroscopical recognition. At the same time, at approximately 8 weeks in the human fetus, Leydig cells differentiate in the intertubular compartment and start to synthesize testosterone under human chorionic gonadotropin (hCG) stimulation. These large eosinophilic polyhedral cells contain an abundant smooth endoplasmic reticulum and numerous mitochondria, but they lack Reinke crystalloids typical of adult Leydig cells. From the 12th to the 18th fetal weeks they crowd the interstitium, at which point degeneration sets in. Only a few cells are still visible at birth.

Descent of the testis from its pararenal position to its terminal location in the scrotum is a complex process that has been subdivided into several stages. Transabdominal movements bring the testis to the internal inguinal ring at 12 weeks. As the testis approaches the inguinal ring, the epididymis is pulled into the canal, serving as a wedge for opening it. The actual passage of the testis through the inguinal canal into the scrotum does not occur until after the 7th month and may be delayed until the immediate postnatal period. The mechanism of testicular descent is not completely understood and probably results from a combination of mechanical and endocrine factors. The gubernaculum testis, a jelly-like structure extending from the caudal pole of the testis to the inguinal ring, precedes the testis into the inguinal canal and reaches the scrotum at 150 days. The gubernaculum is believed to play a critical role in testicular descent, but testicular factors controlling its growth and differentiation are not yet completely elucidated. Androgens are involved, though probably not exclusively.

Ovarian differentiation Mingled cells and somatic cells are arranged in stacks, often called ovigerous cords, which are separated by mesenchyme and blood vessels. They extend to the periphery of the gonad and are confluent with the surface epithelium, whereas in males, epithelial cells are excluded from the gonadal surface by the differentiation of the tunica albuginea. During the 9th week the rete ovarii arise from the hilar mesonephric tubules and infiltrate the gonad as a syncytium of tubules and cords. About the 11th to 12th week, long after differentiation of the testis in the male fetus, germ cells begin to enter meiotic prophase, which characterizes the transition of oogonia and marks the onset of ovarian differentiation. The oogonia in the most central part of the ovary are the first to come in contact with the rete ovarii and the first to enter meiosis. The formation of primordial follicles reaches a maximum during the 20th to 25th weeks of gestation; during this period the plasma concentrations of fetal pituitary follicle-stimulating hormone (FSH) attains its peak and the first primary follicles are formed. Hence, by the 20th to 25th week, the gonad has the morphological characteristics of a definitive ovary. The maximum number of the cells decreases from a peak of between 6 to 7 million to 2 million at term. The last oogonia enter meiosis at 7 months' gestation.

Differentiation of the genital ducts

At the 7th to 8th week of gestation, the human internal reproductive tract consists of unipotential wolffian and müllerian ducts and of bipotential sinusal and external genitalia primordia. Wolffian ducts, the primordia for the male sex accessory organs, are originally the excretory canals of the mesonephros or primitive kidney, and they are incorporated into the genital system when renal function is taken over by the metanephros or definitive kidney. Müllerian or paramesonephric ducts (the primordia for the female internal reproductive organs) arise from a cleft line by celomic epithelium, which originates between the gonadal ridge and the mesonephros, grows caudally, parallel to pre-existing wolffian ducts, and then crosses it ventrally to join with the duct on the opposite side. At 8 weeks the paired ducts reach the dorsal part of the urogenital sinus where they cause an elevation, the müllerian tubercle.

Male differentiation: müllerian ducts regress and wolffian ducts persist

The first step of somatic male differentiation is müllerian duct regression. Testis-mediated müllerian regression begins at 8 weeks, however, in vitro experiments have demonstrated that human müllerian ducts will undergo regression only if exposed to testicular tissue prior to that time and cannot be rescued beyond that period when removed from testicular influence. In the human, müllerian ducts have nearly completely disappeared by 10 weeks. The second aspect of inertial male differentiation is the integration of wolffian ducts in the genital system and their subsequent development into epididymes, vasa deferentia, and seminal vesicles.

Female differentiation: müllerian ducts develop and wolffian ducts degenerate

As described above, female differentiation of the genital tract lags behind male organogenesis. It is characterized essentially by the stabilization of müllerian ducts and their differentiation into fallopian tubes and the uterus. Wolffian ducts begin to degenerate at 10 weeks, and their obliterated remnants are incorporated into müllerian derivatives.

Sex differentiation of the urogenital sinus and genitalia

The müllerian tubercle separates the cranial vesicourethral canal from the caudal urogenital sinus. The fused tips of the müllerian ducts are separated from the dorsal wall of the urogenital sinus by a solid mass, the vaginal plate. As the corpora cavernosa and glans differentiate, the genital tubercle elongates to form the phallus, whose ventral surface is depressed by a deep furrow, the urethral groove. No sex difference is detectable in human fetuses prior to 9 to 10 weeks.

Male differentiation

Male orientation of the urogenital sinus is characterized by prostatic development and the regression of vaginal development. Prostatic buds appear at approximately 10 weeks at the side of the müllerian

tubercle and grow into solid branching cords. Maturation of the prostatic glands is accompanied by the development of the prostatic utricles. Two buds of epithelial cells called the sino-utricular bulbs in the male develop from the urogenital sinus near the opening of the wolffian ducts and grow inward, fusing with the medial müllerian tubercle to form the sino-utricular cord, which joins with the caudal tip of the fused müllerian ducts. The sino-utricular cord is enclosed within the prostate gland at 12 weeks and canalizes at 18 weeks to form the prostatic utricle, the male equivalent of the vagina. Masculinization of the internal genital organs begins in 10-week-old human fetuses with the lengthening of the anogenital distance, followed by fusion of the labioscrotal folds and closure of the rims of the urethral groove. This leads to the formation of a perineal and penile urethra. Penile organogenesis is completed at 80 days gestation, but until the 16th week, the penis and clitoris are more or less the same size. Paradoxically, the major period of penile growth occurs, with no evidence of deceleration in rate, at the same time serum testosterone levels sharply decline in the male.

Female differentiation

Female differentiation of the urogenital sinus is characterized by the formation of the vagina. The developmental origin of the vagina is a highly controversial subject in embryology. The most likely hypothesis is that müllerian, wolffian, and sinusal structures all contribute. At 11 weeks the vaginal primordium is formed by the caudal tip of the müllerian ducts and by outgrowths of the posterior sinusal wall, the sino-vaginal bulbs laterally, and the müllerian tubercle medially. At 15 weeks these structures fuse to form the vaginal plate, which acquires a lumen approximately halfway through prenatal life. The major differences between male and female organogenesis lies in the downgrowth of the vaginal plate. In males, the prostatic utricle (the male equivalent of the vagina) opens just beneath the bladder neck. In females the vaginal cord proliferates, and its caudal end slides down the urethra to acquire a separate opening on the perineum (Fig. 38.1).

ENDOCRINE REGULATION OF SEX DIFFERENTIATION

Male sexual differentiation is mediated by two different substances produced by the fetal testis: AMH produced by the Sertoli cells are responsible for the regression of the müllerian ducts, and testosterone is responsible for the maturation of the wolffian ducts and for the virilization of the urogenital sinus and external genitalia.

Testosterone

Testosterone is directly responsible for the maintenance of wolffian ducts and their differentiation into vasa deferentia and seminal vesicles. After reduction into dihydrotestosterone (DHT), testosterone accounts for the viril-

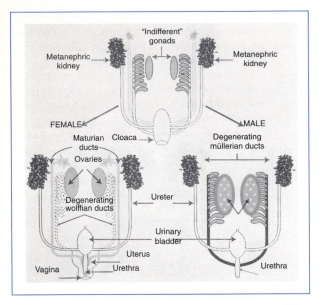

Figure 38.1 Sexual differentiation. *Female*: the wolffian ducts give rise to the female reproductive tract. *Male*: the Müllerian ducts degenerate, and the wolffian ducts give rise to the male reproductive tract. (From Garcia-Castro et al. Sex differentiation. Topical Endocrinology, May 1996.)

ization of external genitalia and for the growth of the prostate and the repression of vaginal development. Testosterone secretion by the fetal testis is detectable shortly after the time Leydig cells form the interstitium at approximately 9 weeks in the human fetus. There is a rise in serum and testicular testosterone concentrations to a peak at approximately 15 to 18 weeks, then a decline, which is in close correlation with the histological pattern of fetal Leydig cell development. Fetal testes and ovaries acquire endocrine function at approximately the same time, each producing its own characteristic hormone. The rate-limiting enzyme for testosterone synthesis is 3β-hydroxysteroid dehydrogenase, which is approximately 50 times higher in the fetal testis than in ovaries at similar ages. Conversely, aromatase activity is higher in the fetal ovary. In the human fetus, testicular and serum levels of testosterone are closely correlated with chorionic gonadotropin concentration. When hCG declines in the third trimester, the fetal hypothalamo-pituitary axis gains control over testicular functional activity. Chorionic gonadotropin and then luteinizing hormone (LH) act on target cells through interaction with a specific receptor located on the cell surface. The LH receptor belongs to the large family of seven transmembrane domain receptors coupled with the G protein (guanine nucleotide) system. Binding of LH to its receptor activates increased production of cyclic adenosine monophosphate (cAMP).

Steroidogenic factor-1

All cytochromes of the P450 family that participate in the steroidogenesis pathway exhibit a consensus-binding sequence for SF-1 in the promoter region of their gene. This nuclear transcription factor is involved in steroidogenic cell differentiation and stimulates the expression of P450 genes.

Locally produced factors

Many locally produced factors, peptides, and steroid hormones have been implicated in the activation or inhibition of testosterone production in the testis. These include: (1) activators, such as insulin-like growth factor I (IGF-I), paracrine and autocrine activators of the Leydig cells; and inhibin, which increases LH-stimulated testosterone production; and (2) inhibitors, such as transforming growth factor alpha (TGF-α); epidermal growth factor (EGF); fibroblast growth factor (FGF), which inhibits Leydig cell function; activin, which decreases LH-stimulated testosterone production; interleukin 1 (IL-1), which reduces hCG-stimulated production; and other substances.

5α-Reductase

Testosterone can be converted to DHT inside the cell by the enzyme 5α-reductase when this enzyme is present. The conversion of testosterone to DHT amplifies the androgenic signal through several mechanisms. Since DHT cannot be aromatized to estrogen, its effects are purely androgenic. DHT also binds to the androgen receptor with greater affinity and stability than does testosterone. Therefore, in tissues equipped with 5α-reductase at the time of sex differentiation, such as at prostate, urogenital sinus, and external genitalia formation, DHT is the active androgen. However, at high concentrations, testosterone interacts with the androgen receptor in a manner similar to DHT. The wolffian ducts do not form DHT prior to sex differentiation because they are exposed to high concentrations of testosterone, which acts as a paracrine factor rather than a circulating hormone, though they virilize nevertheless. At least two steroid 5α-reductase enzymes exist in humans (designated type I and type II). Type I is expressed in nongenital skin, is optimally active at an alkaline pH in cultured genital skin fibroblasts, and is encoded by a gene located on chromosome 5. Type II is expressed in male genitalia, is optimally active at an acid pH, and is encoded by a gene on chromosome 2. Type II has a high affinity for the specific inhibitor, finasteride. Gene deletion and point mutation studies have demonstrated that the type II gene is the locus for 5α-reductase deficiency, a rare cause of male pseudohermaphroditism.

The alkaline enzyme, human steroid 5α-reductase 1, was cloned first; however the predominant enzyme in fetal sex differentiation is acid 5α-reductase 2, for which more than 20 mutations have been identified in patients with defective 5α-reductase activity.

The androgen receptor: molecular biology and molecular mechanisms of androgen action

A functional androgen receptor (AR) is absolutely required to mediate the actions of both testosterone and DHT in inducing the expression of androgen-dependent genes necessary for internal and external genitalia masculinization. The AR is a member of the group of four closely related steroid receptors sometimes referred to as the GR-like receptors, the other members of which are the glucocorticoid receptor (GR), the mineralocorticoid receptor (MR), and progesterone receptor (PR). Like other members of this family, the androgen receptor, as a hormone receptor complex, interacts directly with its target genes to regulate their transcription. Failure of the receptor to activate its target genes in the presence of hormone results in target organ resistance to the hormone.

The androgen receptor gene and protein The androgen receptor gene and encoded protein are structurally and functionally similar to those of other steroid hormone receptors. Studies of the promoter for the human AR gene have determined that there are different sites of transcription initiation (TIS I and TIS II). Other sequences have recently been identified to be important for steroid hormone regulation of AR mRNA expression.

Androgen receptors encode a receptor protein of an apparent molecular weight of 110 to 114 kDa, comprised of 900 to 919 amino acids. The carboxy-terminal third of the AR makes up the steroid-binding domain. The amino acid sequence of this region displays about 50% identity with the corresponding residues in glucocorticoid, mineralocorticoid, and progesterone receptors. A principal function of the steroid-binding domain is the specific high affinity binding of androgens.

Molecular mechanisms of androgen action Androgens are transported to target tissues largely in a protein-bound state. They dissociate from carrier proteins, diffuse into target cells, and bind to the intracellular androgen receptor protein. Androgen binding induces a conformational change in the AR that facilitates receptor dimerization, nuclear transport, and interaction with target DNA, culminating in the regulation of target gene transcription. A variety of androgens and other steroids are bound by AR. The AR has highest affinity for DHT, followed by testosterone, primarily because testosterone dissociates from AR more rapidly than DHT. Receptor activation is ligand-specific, since functional activity of the receptor correlates with binding activity of the ligand. Androgen binding stabilizes the receptor, resulting in higher levels of immunoreactive receptors and higher levels of binding.

The AR is believed to be cytoplasmic before binding to the androgen, although the precise intracellular location is currently uncertain. Once bound by androgen, the androgen receptor is clearly a nuclear protein. The binding of the receptor to its response elements results in the regulation of the rate of transcription of target genes, probably through interactions with other components of the transcription complex near the transcription start site of the gene (Tab. 38.1).

DISORDERS OF CHROMOSOMAL SEX

KLINEFELTER'S SYNDROME AND ITS VARIANTS

Klinefelter's syndrome is the most frequent major abnormality of sexual differentiation, with an incidence of

Table 38.1 Classification of errors in sex differentiation

Disorders of chromosomal sex
   Klinefelter's syndrome
   Turner's syndrome
   Mixed gonadal dysgenesis
   True hermaphroditism

Disorders of gonadal sex
   Pure gonadal dysgenesis
   Anorchia

Disorders of phenotypic sex
   Female pseudohermaphroditism
      Congenital adrenal hyperplasia
      Nonadrenal female pseudohermaphroditism
      Developmental disorders of müllerian ducts

   Male pseudohermaphroditism
      Leydig cell hypoplasia
      Abnormalities in androgen synthesis
      Abnormalities in androgen function
      Persistent Müllerian duct syndrome

approximately 1 in 1000 men. The characteristic features are a variable degree of eunuchoidism, small atrophic testes with hyalinization of the seminiferous tubules, azoospermia, gynecomastia, and increased urinary excretion of gonadotropin. The sex chromosome constitution in these men is characterized by the presence of at least two X chromosomes and a Y chromosome. Various other sex chromosome variants, including mosaicism, have been described.

Pathophysiology

47,XXY males may arise by nondisjunction of the sex chromosomes during either the first or second meiotic division in either parent or, less commonly, by mitotic disjunction in the zygote at the time of or after fertilization. These abnormalities of meiosis almost always occur in patients with normal sex chromosome constitutions. The most important factor imputed in the etiology of Klinefelter's syndrome is advanced maternal age. The maternal age effect on chromosome abnormalities may be a consequence of the long diplotene stage of human ova. Ova remain suspended in prophase of the first meiotic division from birth to ovulation, which may not occur for years. The defective segregation of the two X chromosomes could be caused, at least in part, by reduction of the length of the chiasma between certain chromosomes as the length of the diplotene stage increases.

Clinical findings

Prepubertally, patients have small testes but are otherwise apparently normal. As a group they have lower birth weights, smaller mean head circumferences, a slightly increased incidence of major and minor congenital abnormalities (particularly clinodactyly), height percentiles that increase with age, a lower verbal IQ than normal boys, delayed emotional development, and poor motor control. There is a higher than average incidence of problems with speech development and learning. These subjects tend to be taller than average, mainly because of a disproportionate length of legs. Prepubertally, the basal plasma concentrations of FSH and LH and the response to gonadotropin-releasing factor (GnRH) are within the normal range. With the onset of puberty, progressive histological changes and a decreased capacity of the Leydig cells to synthesize testosterone become apparent. Thus, in postpubertal patients, the concentration of testosterone tends to be low, the levels of plasma estradiol are normal or increased, and gonadotropin levels are elevated. Testosterone responses to hCG appear to be normal in childhood and early adolescence as opposed to those in adults.

After puberty the disorder manifests as infertility and signs of androgen deficiency, such as diminished facial and body hair, a small phallus, poor muscular development, diminished potency, and a further increase in the disproportion between leg and body length. The testicular failure in Klinefelter syndrome appears to progress with age. The testes are characterized by small dysgenetic tubules with arrested development and often early fibrosis and hyalinization. The result is that testes are small in size and firm in consistency. Peritubular elastic tissue is usually absent or diminished in the small dysgenetic tubules. Gynecomastia, which occurs in about 90% of patients, is probably secondary to an increased ratio of serum estradiol to testosterone. Abnormalities in thyroid function — including a diminished response to thyrotropin and decreased uptake of radioactive iodine — are described, although clinically significant thyroid disease is uncommon. The frequency of diabetes mellitus is increased, and chronic pulmonary disease and varicose veins may also be more prevalent in adults with Klinefelter's syndrome.

Subjects with Klinefelter's syndrome with gynecomastia have an increased predisposition to breast cancer, the risk being about 20 times that of normal men.

Variant forms of the Klinefelter's syndrome

46,XY/47,XXY Mosaicism

Mosaicism is defined as the presence of two or more cell lines with different karyotypes in the same individual derived from a single zygote. 46,XY/47,XXY is the second-most common karyotype in phenotypic males with X chromatin-positive patterns. The presence of a normal XY cell line in these patients can modify the clinical expression of the 47,XXY cell line. Thus, in general, these patients manifest a lesser degree of gynecomastia, androgen deficiency, and testicular pathology. Symptoms of decreased libido and potency may not appear until the fourth or fifth decade, secondary sexual characteristics are

less impaired than those of patients with 47,XXY karyotype, and seminiferous tubules exhibiting spermatogenesis are more common than in 47,XXY patients.

Other karyotypic varieties of Klinefelter's syndrome have been described: 48,XXYY is usually associated with mental retardation, tall stature, gynecomastia, and delinquent behavior; 48,XXXY and 49,XXXYY are also associated with mental retardation. With the increase in the number of X chromosomes, the severity and frequency of somatic abnormalities such as a short neck and epicanthal folds also increases.

46,XX Males

The incidence of a 46,XX karyotype in phenotypic males is approximately 1 in 20 000 male births. These subjects have a male phenotype and psychosocial orientation, and they are similar clinically and endocrinologically to individuals with classic Klinefelter's syndrome except for minor differences. Postpubertally, as in the Klinefelter's syndrome, they have varying degrees of testosterone deficiency, gynecomastia, and small testes with azoospermia. There is a 10% incidence of hypospadia in prepuberal 46,XX males that can be attributed to a deficiency of testosterone secretion by the fetal Leydig cells. 46,XX males with genital abnormalities tend to lack evidence for Y chromosomal DNA in their genome and to manifest a greater prevalence and degree of gynecomastia than their counterparts in whom a Y to X chromosome translocation is present. In comparison to males with a 47,XXY karyotype, 46,XX males have a lower frequency of intellectual and psychosocial problems, and they are shorter and have abnormal skeletal proportions. In a few subjects, 46,XX maleness is associated with other congenital abnormalities such as cardiac malformation. All 46,XX males are infertile. Molecular genetic analysis suggests that most of the 46,XX males result from an anomalous Y to X translocation during meiosis. The amount of Y material translocated to the X chromosome is variable.

Diagnosis and treatment

The diagnosis of Klinefelter's syndrome in the postpubertal male is suggested by typical phenotype and hormonal changes, and it is confirmed by the finding of a 47,XXY karyotype. Treatment should be directed toward androgen replacement therapy where there is evidence of androgen deficiency. Prepubertally diagnosed patients with Klinefelter's syndrome should be treated with testosterone at 11 to 12 years of age to initiate puberty and to prevent both the physical and psychological problems of hypogonadism.

THE SYNDROME OF GONADAL DYSGENESIS: TURNER'S SYNDROME AND ITS VARIANTS

The term "gonadal dysgenesis" was coined to describe all subjects with female genitalia, normal müllerian structures, and streak gonads. While many of these subjects have the typical features of Turner's syndrome, others have none. The condition of these patients without

Turner's stigmata has been referred to as "pure gonadal dysgenesis". When karyotype analysis became available, it was observed that most of the patients with gonadal dysgenesis have a 45,X karyotype or a variant that can be considered part of the spectrum of this syndrome.

The absence of an X chromosome is associated with the female phenotype, short stature, sexual infantilism, and a variety of associated abnormalities. These features may be modified by the presence of lesser degrees of sex chromosome deficiency. It is therefore useful to consider the syndrome of gonadal dysgenesis and its variants as a continuum of features ranging from those of the typical 45,X karyotype to a normal female or male.

Typical Turner's syndrome (45,X gonadal dysgenesis)

Pathophysiology

About half of all Turner's syndrome patients have a 45,X karyotype, one-fourth have mosaicism with no structural abnormality, and the remainder have a structurally abnormal X chromosome with or without mosaicism. The 45,X variety may arise through a variety of chromosomal errors. It may be a consequence of nondisjunction or chromosome loss during gametogenesis in either parent that results in a sperm or ovum lacking a sex chromosome; it could also be the result of a mitotic error during one of the early cleavage divisions of the fertilized zygote. Short stature and other somatic features result when genetic material is missing from either the long or the short arm of the X. There is probably a locus important for stature on the distal short arm (Xp) in the pseudoautosomal region; the long arm (Xq) appears to carry one or more genes important for fetal viability; and both Xp and Xq appear to contain loci necessary for normal ovarian function. A gene from a region of the Y chromosome whose homologue on the X chromosome is in the region of the X inactivation center has been cloned. This gene, called RP54, codes for a ribosomal protein. A role of this protein in the Turner's phenotype is suggested. In individuals with mosaicism or structural abnormalities of the X chromosome, phenotypes are intermediate in severity between that seen in 45,X and the normal.

Clinical findings

The incidence of the typical Turner's syndrome is estimated to be 1 in 2500 newborn females. There is, however, a considerable loss of 45,X embryos and fetuses. About 10% of all clinically recognizable spontaneous abortuses have a 45,X constitution, and perhaps as many as 1 to 2% of all human conceptions do. The diagnosis is made either at birth because of the associated abnormalities, or more frequently, at puberty when amenorrhea and failure of sexual development are noted in conjunction with the associated abnormalities. The typical patient is often recognizable by the distinctive facies in which micrognathia, epicanthal folds, prominent ears, a fish-like mouth, ptosis, and strabismus are present with varying

degrees of frequency. The neck is short, and webbing of the neck is present in 25 to 40% of the patients. Additional abnormalities include cubitus valgus, congenital lymphedema of the feet and hands, short fourth metacarpal, renal abnormalities, various skeletal anomalies, and abnormal nails. The incidence of mental retardation is not increased over normal. Cardiovascular abnormalities such as coarctation of the aorta, bicuspid aortic valves, and partial anomalous venous drainage are described. Thus, all patients with gonadal dysgenesis should have a cardiac evaluation in infancy and at adolescence. Associated conditions also include renal malformations, such as rotation of the kidney and duplication of the renal pelvis and ureter. Abnormal differentiation of the kidneys and upper collecting system are so common that a renal sonogram should be routinely obtained. Skeletal maturation is normal or slightly delayed in childhood but lags in adolescence secondary to gonadal steroid deficiency. In addition to the shortening of the fourth metacarpal, an abnormality of the wrist (bayonet deformity) is also described; cubitus valgus occurs in half of the patients.

Short stature is an invariant feature in 45,X individuals. The mean final weight of patients ranges from 142 to 147 cm. Intrauterine growth retardation is common, and the average birth weight and length are 1 standard deviation (SD) below the mean for normal infants of comparable gestational age. For the first 3 years of life, growth velocity is usually within the normal range. Subsequently, velocity decelerates so that by a bone age of 9 the difference in mean height between patients and normal individuals is close to that of maturity. Hence it appears that there is a little additional loss of height relative to normal individuals after a bone age of 9, in spite of a lack of a pubertal growth spurt. The short stature in this syndrome is not due to a deficiency of growth hormone, insulin-like growth factor I (IGF-I) or insulin-like growth factor II (IGF-II), or adrenal or gonadal steroids. The etiology of short stature is not yet known.

Sexual infantilism is a typical feature in 45,X subjects. The external genitalia and genital ducts are female, but immature. Typically, fibrous streaks of connective tissues located in the mesosalpinges are present and lack primordial follicles. However, exceptions have been documented. Primary follicles have been described in some of these subjects, which correlates with the rare occurrence of menarche and a variable period of regular menses. Occasionally enough ovarian function remains for spontaneous puberty, and very rarely for pregnancy; but infertility is the rule in Turner's syndrome. Both basal and LHRH-evoked gonadotropin secretion demonstrate a lack of feedback inhibition of the hypothalamic-pituitary axis by the dysgenetic gonads in infants and young children with gonadal dysgenesis. Plasma FSH levels are elevated between 2 and 4 years of age and decrease to high-normal values at 5 to 10 years of age. After 10 years the plasma FSH levels rise again into the castrate range. The pattern of changes in LH levels is similar. Patients with gonadal dysgenesis experience adrenarche with a normal rise in adrenal androgen production in childhood and develop sparse axillary and pubic hair. After age 15 years, the levels of dehydroepiandrosterone, testosterone, and androstenedione are lower than normal, reflecting absence of the gonadal contribution.

Associated disorders. There is an increased incidence of autoimmune disorders in patients with gonadal dysgenesis, the most prevalent being Hashimoto's thyroiditis. An increased frequency of hypothyroidism is documented. Carbohydrate intolerance and diabetes mellitus are common.

Treatment

Therapy is directed toward augmenting stature, correcting somatic abnormalities, and inducing secondary sexual characteristics. Although the short stature in Turner's syndrome does not seem to be related to a deficiency of growth hormone, IGF-I, or adrenal or gonadal steroids, data on the effect of the treatment with GH or oxandrolone are encouraging. Because these patients lose most of their height between the ages 3 and 9, therapy should be started early in childhood. Estrogen therapy should be instituted at around age 15 considering that a treatment at an earlier age could lead to rapid skeletal maturation.

Rarely, patients with 45,X develop a gonadoblastoma when there is a mosaicism involving the Y chromosome. Consequently, streak gonads should be removed in patients with evidence of virilization or a Y-containing cell line.

Clinical variants of the syndrome of gonadal dysgenesis

Approximately 30 to 40% of patients with the typical syndrome of gonadal dysgenesis are X-chromatin positive. This group usually has a structurally abnormal X chromosome, or more commonly sex chromosome mosaicism involving a 45,X cell line. In patients with sex chromosome mosaicism, the ratio in each gonad of 45,X primordial germ cells and blastemal components to those with a normal 46,XX or 46,XY constitution is probably the major determinant of whether the ultimate gonadal structure is a streak dysgenetic or hypoplastic ovary or testis, or whether it is a relatively normal gonad.

X chromatin-positive variants of gonadal dysgenesis

45,X/46,XX mosaicism is the most common finding in patients with chromatin-positive gonadal dysgenesis and is second in frequency only to 45,X. Patients with this form of mosaicism exhibit fewer of the associated somatic abnormalities; they are not invariably short, and some may menstruate. One gonad may be of the streak type and the contralateral gonad may be either a hypoplastic or normal ovary; alternatively, ovaries may be either normal or hypoplastic. Deletions of the short arm of the X chromosome (Xp-) are rare and frequently associated with 45,X mosaicism. Deletions of the long arm of the X chromosome are rarely described. Patients with the isochromosome for the long arm of the X (X chromosome that consists of two long arms and lacks a short arm) are invariably short and have streak gonads, and the somatic stigmata of Turner's syndrome are usually less severe than in 45,X0 patients.

Controversies exist regarding the existence of an isochromosome for the short arm of the X chromosome.

X chromatin-negative variants of gonadal dysgenesis

45,X/46,XY; 45,X/47,XYY; 45,X/46,XY/47,XYY mosaicism usually results in individuals who are phenotypic females or phenotypic males or who have ambiguous genitalia. The differentiation of the gonads varies from bilateral streaks in the phenotypic female to bilateral dysgenetic testes. The propensity of patients with this mosaicism to develop gonadal tumors is high, and therefore removal of the streak gonads or of the dysgenetic undescended testes is indicated. Gonadoblastoma is the neoplasia most often found. The presence of functional testicular elements can be detected before puberty by the rise in concentration of serum testosterone above prepubertal values, upon hCG test.

Diagnosis and treatment

The diagnosis is established by the demonstration of 45,X/46,XY mosaicism in blood, skin, and gonadal tissue. The decision of sex rearing should be based upon the potential for normal functioning of the external genitalia. In patients assigned to the female gender, the gonads should be removed and the external genitalia should be repaired. Estrogen therapy should be performed at puberty to induce female secondary sexual characteristics. In affected infants for whom a male gender is assigned, all gonadal tissue except that which appears functionally and histologically normal and is in the scrotum should be removed, and prosthetic testes should be placed in the reconstructed scrotal sac.

Mixed gonadal dysgenesis

Mixed gonadal dysgenesis is an entity in which phenotypic males or females have a testis on one side and a streak gonad on the other. Most have a 46,X/46,XY mosaicism, but the clinical entity is not confined to that chromosomal pattern. However, most of the clinical features are similar. It is postulated that in 46,XY gonadal dysgenesis there is a normal amount of sex-determining region (SRY) protein, while in 45,X/46,XY subjects there is a decreased amount of normal SRY protein. The majority of patients have ambiguous genitalia, including some degree of phallic enlargement, a urogenital sinus, and varying degrees of labioscrotal fusion. In most the testes are located in the abdomen; a uterus, vagina, and at least one fallopian tube are almost invariably present. The prepubertal testes appear relatively normal, the postpubertal testes contain abundant mature Leydig cells and secrete testosterone, and the streak gonads are composed of ovarian stroma.

The diagnosis of mixed gonadal dysgenesis is suspected in a child with ambiguous genitalia, a 46,XY karyotype, and a subnormal plasma level of testosterone but no abnormal accumulation of plasma precursors of testosterone. The diagnosis is confirmed by gonadal histology. If gender assignment is female, gonadal tissue and wolffian structures should be removed and estrogen therapy should be performed at puberty. When gender assignment is male, removal of dysgenetic gonads is also recommended if they cannot be brought into the scrotum to prevent the occurrence of malignancy, and testosterone replacement therapy is begun at puberty.

TRUE HERMAPHRODITISM

The diagnosis of true hermaphroditism requires the presence of both ovarian and testicular tissues in either the same or opposite gonads. The ovarian tissue must include follicles as well as stroma, and the testicular tissue must contain well-differentiated tubules. True hermaphroditism, which occurs in a number of animal species, is the most rare form of intersexuality in humans: it has been reported in approximately 400 cases worldwide, with the highest incidence in the black population in southern Africa. Various classification schemes have been proposed based on all of the possible combinations of gonadal findings. The ovotestis is the most common gonad in true hermaphroditism, the ovary is the next most common, and the testis is the least common. Interestingly, the ovaries occur on the left side more commonly than on the right. Conversely, testicular tissue is found on the right side more frequently than on the left. The reason for this finding is not known. The ovotestis may be located in the ovarian position, in the labioscrotal folds, in the inguinal canal, or at the internal inguinal ring. The ovotestis can usually be diagnosed by gross appearance: the ovarian and testicular tissues are typically connected end to end and are usually separated by connective tissue. While approximately 50% of ovotestes show evidence of ovulation, the testicular tissue is frequently abnormal, and histological examination reveals no evidence of spermatogenesis. In true hermaphroditism, the ovary is usually located in its normal position, although occasionally it is located in the left inguinal scrotal area. The testis is most commonly located in the scrotum, and it may also be found in the normal position of the ovary.

The ductal system, which is adjacent to an ovary or a testis, corresponds in its development to the sex of the gonad. Most patients with ovotestes have predominantly female development of the genital ducts. The relationship between gonadal structure and differentiation of the genital tract provides added evidence for the essentially local effect of AMH secreted by the Sertoli cells of the embryonic and fetal testes. The external genitalia of true hermaphrodites are ambiguous in the vast majority of cases. Most of them have in the past been raised as males, despite the presence of incomplete labioscrotal fusion or severe hypospadias. Even when the sex of rearing was female, the external genitalia were often ambiguous. Cryptorchidism is common, and an inguinal hernia, which may contain a gonad or a uterus, is present. Breast development is frequent during puberty in true hermaphrodites, and the occurrence of menstruation is more common in the XX genotype.

The etiology of ovarian and testicular formation in the same individual remains unclear. Genetic chimerism appears to be the etiology in patients with a 46,XY/46,XX karyotype. Chimerism may be the result of several events, such as postzygotic mitotic errors and double fertilization. Autosomal factors are thought to play a role in the etiology of true hermaphroditism. The diagnosis of true hermaphroditism should be considered in all patients with ambiguous genitalia. A 46,XX/46,XY karyotype in a patient with ambiguous genitalia strongly suggests the diagnosis, and a 46,XX or a 46,XY karyotype does not exclude the diagnosis. The diagnosis of true hermaphroditism should be confirmed by gonadal biopsy that indicates the presence of testicular and ovarian tissues.

The management of true hermaphroditism is contingent upon the age at the diagnosis and upon a careful assessment of the functional capacity of the internal and external genitalia. In infants in whom gender identity has not already been established, either a male or female assignment of sex can be made. If a male gender role is assigned, all müllerian and ovarian structures should be removed. The testes or testicular component of an ovotestis is usually dysgenetic, and the risk of malignant transformation is increased. Thus, in 46,XX true hermaphrodites raised as males, gonadectomy and hormone replacement therapy are recommended at puberty. In true hermaphrodites raised as females, all testicular tissue should be removed. Normal ovarian function and in rare instances pregnancy have been reported. In older subjects, gender identity is the main consideration; typically the identity conforms to the sex of rearing. The discordant gonad and dysgenetic gonadal tissue should be removed, and plastic repair of the external genitalia should be carried out. Appropriate gonadal hormone replacement therapy is also recommended at puberty.

DISORDERS OF GONADAL SEX

Disorders of gonadal sex result when chromosomal sex is normal but differentiation of the gonads is abnormal. Thus gonadal and phenotypic sex do not correspond to chromosomal sex.

PURE GONADAL DYSGENESIS

This term has been applied to phenotypic females with a 46,XX or 46,XY karyotype who have rudimentary streak gonads and remain sexually infantile but are of normal or tall stature and lack the somatic stigmata of Turner's syndrome. At puberty they exhibit the usual effect of prepubertal castration, and plasma and urinary gonadotropin values are increased. 46,XX gonadal dysgenesis is characterized by normal stature, sexual infantilism, bilateral streak gonads, normal female internal and external genitalia, primary amenorrhea, elevated gonadotropin levels, and an absence of the somatic stigmata of Turner's syndrome. Familial 46,XX gonadal dysgenesis has been associated with sensorineural deafness, and sporadic cases of 46,XX gonadal dysgenesis have also been described. In contrast to 46,XY gonadal dysgenesis, gonadal neoplasms are rare in 46,XX gonadal dysgenesis. The diagnosis of 46,XX gonadal dysgenesis is based upon identifying a normal karyotype in a sexually infantile phenotypic female with hypergonadotropic hypogonadism. Replacement therapy with estrogen is similar to the regimen recommended for patients with 45,X gonadal dysgenesis.

46,XY gonadal dysgenesis is characterized by a female phenotype, normal to tall stature, sexual infantilism with primary amenorrhea, and a 46,XY karyotype. The internal structures are female, clitoral enlargement is not uncommon, and the prevalence of gonadal neoplasms – especially gonadoblastoma and germinoma – is high. Familial aggregates as well as sporadic cases have been described. In sum, deletions and/or mutations of the Y chromosome, the X chromosome, and downstream autosomal genes involved in the testes-determining cascade have all been implicated. There is high prevalence of gonadal tumors, and they can occur bilaterally in childhood, hence bilateral prophylactic gonadectomy is indicated. The sex of rearing of these patients is determined by the extent of genital ambiguity and the age at diagnosis.

Patients raised as females should be treated with estrogen therapy; and in patients raised as males, testosterone replacement therapy is begun at the age of puberty.

ANORCHIA

Various terms have been proposed to describe the spectrum of genital anomalies that result from the cessation of testicular function during the middle phase of male sexual differentiation at 8 to 14 week of gestation. These patients have 46,XY karyotype. Gonadal elements are absent, and the differentiation of the genital ducts, urogenital sinus, and the external genitalia is variable. At one end of the spectrum are the patients with female external and internal genitalia in whom the deficiency of testicular function must have occurred before week 8 of gestation. Lack of deficient testicular function between weeks 8 and 10 of gestation would lead to ambiguous genitalia and variable development of genital ducts. Loss of testicular function after the critical phase of male differentiation (12 to 14 weeks) results in anorchia, a syndrome characterized by the finding of normal male differentiation but no gonadal tissue. Sporadic and familial forms of monolateral and bilateral anorchia have been described. The nature of the underlying defect is not known.

The diagnosis of anorchia can be suspected in normally differentiated males with cryptorchidism and elevated gonadotropin levels. It has been proposed that the finding of elevated FSH levels in conjunction with lack of plasma testosterone response to hCG establishes the diagnosis of anorchia and obviates the need of laparotomy.

DISORDERS OF PHENOTYPIC SEX

MALE PSEUDOHERMAPHRODITISM

A male pseudohermaphrodite is an individual with testes but absent or incomplete masculinization of the genitalia. Male pseudohermaphroditism results when testosterone biosynthesis or response of the tissues to testosterone or dihydrotestosterone is impaired. The causes of male pseudohermaphroditism are listed in Table 38.2.

Leydig cell hypoplasia

A rare cause of male pseudohermaphroditism is hypoplasia, or agenesis of Leydig cells of the testis, resulting in inadequate testosterone production. The mode of inheritance of this condition fits a male-limited autosomal recessive pattern.

Most affected 46,XY subjects have a predominantly female phenotype with mild posterior labial fusion, although there is a report indicating that a form with ambiguous genitalia may occur. A urogenital sinus is present with an interior urethra and a blind vaginal pouch. Wolffian duct structures are usually present, although they may be hypoplastic. It is postulated that these effects might be due to low levels of local testosterone secretion associated with inadequate circulating levels in early gestation. Müllerian duct structures are absent due to the normal secretion of AMH by the Sertoli cells, indicating that Leydig cells are not required for this Sertoli function. Small testes are located in the inguinal canals or the abdomen. Absence of labeled hCG binding to testicular membrane preparations raises the possibility of a luteinizing hormone (LH)/hCG receptor defect. Alternatively, the binding could reflect absent Leydig cell precursors.

Table 38.2 Causes of male pseudohermaphroditism

Conditions resulting in decreased testosterone production

  Leydig cell hypoplasia
  Defects of testosterone biosynthesis
    congenital lipoid adrenal hyperplasia
    3β-hydroxysteroid dehydrogenase deficiency
    17α-hydroxylase deficiency
    17,20-lyase deficiency
    17β-hydroxysteroid dehydrogenase deficiency

Conditions resulting in decreased androgen response

  Androgen insensitivity syndromes
  5α-reductase deficiency

Persistent Müllerian duct syndrome

The diagnosis of Leydig cell hypoplasia is suggested by low levels of testosterone and a lack of response to hCG stimulation in an infant 46,XY. The lack of abnormal elevation of testosterone precursors argues against a testosterone biosynthetic defect. The diagnosis is confirmed by histological examination of hCG stimulated testis showing absence or paucity of Leydig cells with relatively well preserved seminiferous tubules.

Defects of testosterone biosynthesis

A block in any of the enzymatic steps of testosterone biosynthesis can cause ambiguous genitalia due to insufficient testosterone production during male sexual differentiation. Depending on the location of the enzymatic defect in the steroidogenetic pathway, these disorders may also affect glucocorticoid and mineralocorticoid biosyntheses. The pattern of inheritance in each of these defects indicates an autosomal recessive mode of transmission. The biochemical heterogeneity within each defect and the subsequent variability of the testosterone biosynthetic block make it impossible to distinguish these enzyme disorders based on the appearance of the external genitalia alone. The clinical presentation varies from normal female external genitalia to ambiguous genitalia with incomplete labioscrotal fusion and a clitoris-like phallus. Milder forms may be manifested by hypospadias, chordee, or cryptorchidism. The testes may be located within the labioscrotal folds, inguinal canals, or peritoneal cavity. Wolffian derivatives may be normal or hypoplastic, depending on the severity of the testosterone biosynthetic block. Müllerian structures are absent because secretion of AMH by the Sertoli cells is unaffected. The following section describes specific features of each of these defects.

Congenital lipoid adrenal hyperplasia

The first and rate limiting step in gonadal and adrenal steroidogenesis is the conversion of cholesterol to pregnenolone, which involves three different biochemical reactions: the 20α-hydroxylation, 22-hydroxylation, and side chain cleavage of cholesterol. A defect in the conversion of cholesterol to pregnenolone causes the rare condition of congenital lipoid adrenal hyperplasia. Infants with this disorder often present in the first weeks of life with severe adrenal insufficiency, accumulation of lipids in the cells of both the adrenal cortex and the gonads, and salt-wasting. Affected 46,XY males usually have female external genitalia, although minimal masculinization has been reported. The testes are in the abdomen or high in the inguinal canal. The P450 scc gene is located in chromosome 15 (q23-q24 region). Although a defect in this enzyme has been implicated in the pathology of this disorder, no deletion or mutation has been identified in the P450 scc genes of five affected individuals. Causes other than a defect in the conversion of cholesterol to pregnenolone could include a defect in the transcript of cholesterol to the mitochondria and in the binding of cholesterol to cytochrome P450 within the mitochondrial membrane.

Congenital lipoid adrenal hyperplasia should be considered in the differential diagnosis of any newborn male pseudohermaphrodite (or phenotypic female) with adrenal insufficiency. Laboratory studies show decreased serum and urinary levels of all adrenal and gonadal steroids and their metabolites, even after adrenocorticotropic hormone (ACTH) or hCG stimulation. Elevated ACTH levels, hyponatremia, hyperkalemia, and metabolic acidosis indicate salt-wasting adrenal insufficiency. CT or MRI scan of the abdomen shows very large, lipid adrenal glands due to the accumulation of cholesterol and cholesterol esters. Adrenal insufficiency in these patients must be treated with glucocorticoid and mineralocorticoid replacements.

3β-Hydroxysteroid dehydrogenase deficiency

3β-Hydroxysteroid dehydrogenase (3β-HSD) catalyzes the conversion of 3β-hydroxy-Δ^5-steroids (pregnenolone, 17-OH pregnenolone, dehydroepiandrosterone) to the 3-keto-Δ^4-steroids (progesterone, 17OH progesterone and Δ^4-androstenedione). A deficiency of 3β-HSD in steroidogenic tissues impairs both adrenal and gonadal steroidogenesis. Affected 46,XY individuals present with various degrees of incomplete masculinization due to a block in testosterone biosynthesis and with salt-wasting adrenal insufficiency due to decreased synthesis of aldosterone and cortisol. The fact that less severe forms of 3β-HSD exist with no salt-wasting and more complete masculinization suggests genetic heterogeneity. The inheritance of this disorder is consistent with an autosomal recessive trait. In affected 46,XX individuals there is clitoral hypertrophy, sometimes with mild posterior labial fusion. This has been interpreted as due to peripheral conversion of high plasma concentration of dehydroepiandrosterone (DHEA) to androstenedione and testosterone. Males with 3β-HSD deficiency exhibit partial masculinization of the external genitalia: a small phallus with hypospadia and partial fusion of the labioscrotal folds. The testes are usually in the scrotum, and müllerian structures are absent. Two genes, encoding isoenzymes 3β-HSDI and 3β-HSDII, have been identified. The human 3β-HSD genes are located on chromosome 1 at locus p11-p13. Type I appears to be expressed in peripheral tissues, for example liver and placenta, and type II is expressed in adrenals and gonads. The fact that steroidogenesis is intact in peripheral tissues of these patients correlates with the finding that the type I 3β-HSD gene is normal. The first missense mutations in the human type II 3β-HSD gene were described in a study of two male compound heterozygotes with severe salt-losing 3β-HSD deficiency.

The diagnosis of 3β-HSD deficiency should be considered in any 46,XY infant with ambiguous genitalia and/or adrenal insufficiency. The classic hormonal profile is an elevated concentration of the (5 steroids and their metabolites in the serum and urine. However, the conversion of Δ^5 to Δ^4 steroids due to intact 3β-HSD activity in peripheral tissues can result in an elevation of $\Delta4$ steroids as well, potentially confusing the diagnosis.

Despite the peripheral conversion, the ratio of Δ^5 to Δ^4 steroids and their metabolites should still be abnormally elevated in this disorder. Salt-wasting adrenal insufficiency is treated with glucocorticoid and mineralocorticoid replacements.

17α-hydroxylase deficiency and 17,20-lyase deficiency

17α-Hydroxylase catalyzes the conversion of pregnenolone to 17-hydroxypregnenolone and progesterone to 17-hydroxyprogesterone in adrenal and gonadal steroidogenesis. This enzyme activity is mediated by cytochrome $P450_{17\alpha}$, which is bound to the smooth endoplasmic reticulum. A deficiency of 17α-hydroxylase blocks the synthesis of the precursors necessary for the production of testosterone by the testes. Affected 46,XY subjects usually have female external genitalia with complete lack of masculinization. Wolffian duct derivatives are absent or hypoplastic, and müllerian duct derivates are absent. However, several reported patients have had slight masculinization of the external genitalia, ranging from labioscrotal fusion to perineal hypospadius with micropenis. A deficiency of 17α-hydroxylase activity also impairs cortisol production, which causes ACTH hypersecretion and results in the accumulation and secretion of deoxycorticosterone (DOC), corticosterone, and 18-hydroxycorticosterone in the zona fasciculata of the adrenal glands. These compounds possess mineralocorticoid activity, and their excess causes salt and water retention, hypertension, and hypokalemia. The high concentrations of DOC, corticosterone, and 18-hydroxycorticosterone suppress aldosterone production. Despite cortisol production, evidence of glucocorticoid deficiency is unusual, possibly because corticosterone has weak glucocorticoid activity. At puberty, appropriate steroid replacement therapy is indicated, as well as gonadectomy, in 46,XY patients who have been assigned a female sex of rearing.

The same cytochrome $P450_{17\alpha}$ that catalyzes the 17α-hydroxylation reaction in the adrenals and gonads catalyzes the 17,20-lyase reaction. 17,20- Lyase (17,20-desmolase) activity cleaves the side chains of 17-hydroxypregnenolone and 17-hydroxyprogesterone to form DHEA and androstenedione, respectively. A deficiency of this activity results in testosterone deficiency due to decreased synthesis of the precursors DHEA and Δ^4-androstenedione. Glucocorticoid and mineralocorticoid production remain normal because the enzymatic block is distal to these pathways. The phenotypic appearance of affected 46,XY individuals varies from female, with a blind vagina pouch, to male, with perineal hypospadius and chordee. The human $P450_{17\alpha}$ cDNA from 46,XY individuals with 17α-hydroxylase deficiency includes small duplications, point mutations, and a large deletion. Theoretically, different mutations in the $P450_{17\alpha}$ gene could result in either 17α-hydroxylase deficiency, 17,20-lyase deficiency, or both. Protein expression of mutant genes in individuals with a clinical diagnosis of 17α-hydroxylase deficiency has generally revealed the presence of combined enzyme deficiencies. However, a conversion from pure 17,20-desmolase to combined 17,20-desmolase/17α-hydroxylase deficiency has been shown in one patient. The factors leading to this change are unknown. It is conceivable that, for unknown reasons, fetuses, infants, and children with a deficiency of the cytochrome P450 C17α present signs of pure 17,20-desmolase deficiency, whereas adults show signs of the combined defect.

The diagnosis of 17α-hydroxylase deficiency should be considered in a male pseudohermaphrodite (or any phenotypic female) with hypertension. Laboratory studies show elevated serum levels of progesterone, DOC, corticosterone, 18-hydroxycorticosterone, and ACTH. Hypokalemic alkalosis develops due to increased mineralocorticoid activity. Serum concentrations of cortisol, 17-hydroxyprogesterone, DHEA, androstenedione, testosterone, aldosterone, and renin are decreased.

Treatment with physiological doses of glucocorticoids suppresses ACTH production, thus reducing levels of DOC, corticosterone, and 18-hydroxycorticosterone and resolving the hypertension and hypokalemia.

The diagnosis of 17,20-lyase deficiency is made by finding an increased ratio of 17-hydroxy-C21-steroids (17-hydroxyprogesterone and 17-hydroxypregnenolone) to C_{19} steroids (DHEA and Δ^4-androstenedione) after hCG stimulation. Cortisol and aldosterone concentrations remain normal, which indicates clinically intact 17α-hydroxylase activity.

17β-hydroxysteroid dehydrogenase deficiency

17β-Hydroxysteroid dehydrogenase (17β-HSD) catalyzes the conversion of Δ^4-androstenedione to testosterone, DHEA to Δ^5-androstenediol, and estrone to estradiol. This enzyme catalyzes the only reversible step in the steroid biosynthetic pathway. A deficiency of 17β-HSD in affected 46,XY individuals results in phenotypically female external genitalia or a mild to moderate degree of masculinization characterized by a clitoris-like phallus with chordee. Indirect evidence of 17β-HSD deficiency in these patients has been shown by the measurement of elevated ratios of Δ^4-androstenedione to testosterone and estrone to estradiol in spermatic venous samples. This defect appears to be isolated to the gonads of affected individuals because other tissues have normal 17β-HSD activity.

Two contiguous 17β-HSD genes, 17β-HSDI and 17β-HSDII, located in the chromosome 17(q11-q12) have been cloned. Mutations of these genes in patients with 17β-HSD have not been reported.

A striking feature of this disorder is the marked virilization that occurs at puberty. Affected subjects develop a male body habitus with abundant body and facial hair. The phallus and testes enlarge to the normal adult range, and labioscrotal folds become pigmented and rugated. Gynecomastia is variably present. A majority adopt the male gender role, have penile erections and ejaculate. These clinical observations correlate with normalization of peripheral and spermatic vein testosterone levels. This effect appears to be related to increased LH secretion and Leydig cell hyperplasia rather than recovery of enzymatic activity because Δ^4-androstenedione levels remain markedly elevated. However, this enzyme deficiency has also been reported to cause mild ambiguity of female genitalia and affected subjects are raised as girls. These subjects during puberty develop male secondary sexual characteristics and some patients spontaneously develop male identity. This change from female to male resembles that of 5α-reductase deficient patients even though the hormonal pattern is quite different.

The diagnosis of 17β-HSD deficiency should be suspected in 46,XY male pseudohermaphrodites if the ratios of Δ⁴ androstenedione to testosterone and of estrone to estradiol are markedly elevated after hCG stimulation. DHEA may be normal or only mildly elevated due to the preference for the Δ⁵-biosynthetic pathway and increased 3β-HSD activity in this condition. Glucocorticoid and mineralcorticoid synthesis remains normal because the enzymatic block is distal to these pathways.

Those 46,XY patients with complete female external genitalia should be raised as girls and gonadectomized before puberty, thus avoiding significant virilization. Male sex rearing should be considered if a patient presents with ambiguous genitalia that can be surgically corrected. If the diagnosis is made during or after puberty gender identity should be determined through psycosexual evaluation before considering any therapy.

Androgen insensitivity syndromes

Androgen insensitivity syndromes (AIS) referred by some authors as testicular feminization has been suggested to be the most common cause of male pseudoermaphroditism. Affected individuals classically have a 46,XY karyotype, normally developed, incompletely descended and a female or partially masculinized external genital phenotype. AIS has traditionally been classified into clinical subgroups based on the genital phenotype (complete AIS, partial AIS, Reifenstein syndrome, infertile male syndrome) or into biochemical subgroups according to the presence or absence of specific high affinity androgen binding in cultured genital skin fibroblasts. Molecular analysis of the AR gene in individuals with AIS revealed that the various clinical forms of AIS and their associated AR defects form a continuum resulting from mutations of variable type and severity in the AR gene which cause a defective function of the androgen receptor.

Complete AIS is a relatively rare disorder (prevalence of approximately 1:60 000 males). Individuals with complete AIS present at various stages of life: a few affected individuals are diagnosed before or soon after birth, the diagnostic evaluation having resulted from the discrepancy between the finding of a 46,XY karyotype on amniocentesis and the presence of a female phenotype on prenatal ultrasound examination at birth. A more common presentation is with the development of inguinal herniae often bilateral during infancy. Infants with the complete form of AIS present with unambiguously female external genitalia, complete absence of sexual hair, and, because testicular differentiation and AMH secretion are normal there is a blind-ending vagina and no uterus (Fig. 38.2). However, Müllerian remnants may be present in as many as 35% of cases, suggesting that a functional AR may be involved in mediating the effects of AMH, and remnants of Wolffian structures such as vestigial vas deferens or epididymis may also been found. At puberty subjects with complete AIS have excellent feminization resulting from high estrogen levels due to testicular estrogen secretion and periph-

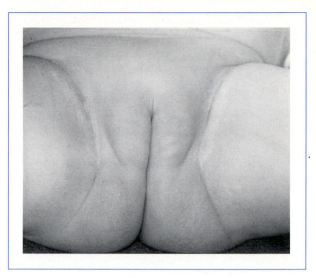

Figure 38.2 Subject with complete androgen insensitivity syndrome.

eral aromatization of testosterone. A proportion of individuals, undiagnosed throughout childhood, present after puberty with primary amenorrhea. Women with complete AIS are taller than average for females, their adult heights generally falling between those of normal males and females. The clinical findings in complete AIS and the recently reported case of estrogen resistance suggest that androgens alone have little direct action on epiphyseal fusion and prevention of osteoporosis and that initial conversion to estrogens is required. The normal bone maturation reported in women with complete AIS supports the concept that sex hormone effects on bone are mediated by the estrogen receptor. In contrast, delayed onset of puberty of 46,XY girls with complete AIS (and some 46,XX carriers) suggests a direct role of androgens in the induction of pubertal hypothalamic-pituitary-gonadal axis activity (Fig. 38.2).

Partial AIS or an incomplete form of androgen insensitivity comprise a wide spectrum of clinical phenotypes. Because of the variability of clinical manifestations and the existence of subtle or atypical forms of androgen resistance such as the infertile male syndrome, the prevalence of the partial form is unknown. The clinical spectrum of partial or incomplete AIS varies from an essentially female phenotype with mild clitoromegaly or slight labial fusion to significant genital ambiguity (Fig. 38.3). Partial development of wolffian structures can also occur, producing epididymes and vasa deferentia. The degree of virilization at puberty would likely be consistent with the degree of masculinization at birth. In some cases, particularly in those patients referred to as having Reifenstein syndrome, there is more extensive masculinization; the affected individuals have an essentially male but severely undermasculinized phenotype with micropenis, perineal hypospadias, and cryptorchidism. A smaller number of studies also suggest that in the mildest form of expression, partial AIS may be manifest simply by uncomplicat-

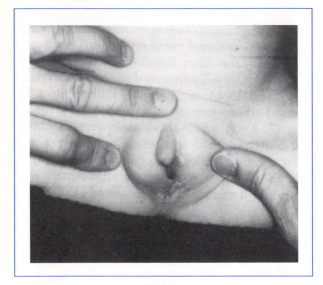

Figure 38.3 Subject with partial androgen insensitivity syndrome (From De Bellis et al. J Clin Endrocrinol Metab 1994;78:513-22.)

ed hypospadias, by infertility in a phenotypically normal male, or even by gynecomastia and androgen binding abnormalities in a fertile male. It is important to note that affected individuals with quite different phenotypes may be present within a single family. Although many studies in adolescents and adults with AIS indicate that serum testosterone, DHT, and gonadotropins are normal or mildly elevated, there have been no definitive studies in newborns or young infants. In the normal male, LH and testosterone increase during the first 2 months of postnatal life, reaching a peak between 6 and 8 weeks.

A disturbance at any level in the pathway of androgen action – from androgen production and secretion, to androgen binding, nuclear localization of androgen receptors, binding of AR to target DNA or transcriptional activation of target genes – could result in failure of response to androgen. The AR is encoded by an X-chromosomal gene, thus the syndromes of AIS follow an X-linked recessive pattern of inheritance. At the functional level, two types of AR defects underlying AIS have been described: abnormalities of androgen binding and abnormalities such as thermolability of binding, increased binding dissociation, or altered binding specificity (Fig. 38.3).

A variety of molecular defects causing androgen resistance have been described and characterized in more than 200 individuals with various forms of AIS. Broadly, they can be classified as: (1) major structural defects of the AR gene (complete and partial deletions); (2) minor structural defects of the AR gene (one to four base pair deletions or insertions); (3) single base mutations that introduce a premature termination codon or alter the splicing of mRNA; (4) single base mutations that result in amino acid substitutions in the receptor protein; and (5) expansion of a trinucleotide repeat.

Deletions are uncommon, representing only about 10% of AR gene mutations reported to date. No deletion has been reported in a subject with partial AIS. Complete deletion of the AR gene results in total absence of the AR protein and represents the null phenotype of AIS. Deletions of exons encoding the androgen-binding domain or DNA-binding domain also result in complete AIS. A number of single base changes have been found in various locations within the coding region of the AR gene that convert a codon for an amino acid into a premature termination codon. Numerous point mutations that alter a single amino acid have been described in AR genes of subjects with both complete and partial AIS. About one-third of the reported mutations have been reported only once to date, while the remainder have been reported in two or more apparently unrelated individuals. The rate of mutations appears unusually high at four codons, and these locations may be considered mutational "hot spots."

Mutations occurring in the exons encoding the androgen-binding domain cause disturbances of androgen binding, while those in exons encoding the DNA-binding domain disturb the interaction of the receptor with its target DNA. Alterations in receptor function range from complete loss to subtle qualitative changes. In vitro studies indicate that the final common pathway in molecular defects such as those described above is failure of the AR to stimulate transcription of androgen-dependent target genes.

It is of interest that the normal AR gene contains a polymorphic stretch of CAG triplets in exon 1, which is repeated an average of 21±2 times. This repeat segment was found to be expanded to 40 to 52 repeats in 35 patients with Kennedy's disease, a neurologic disease characterized by progressive atrophy of the spinal and bulbar muscles.

The relationship between the genital phenotype of individuals with AIS and the characteristics of androgen binding in their cultured skin fibroblasts has been inconsistent. Therefore with the advent of molecular analysis of the AR, it has been of interest to determine whether correlations exist between the molecular defects and the external genitalia phenotypes of affected individuals. Individuals with complete AIS have AR defects ranging from complete deletion of the gene to a wide array of amino acid substitutions in the DNA – or steroid binding domains that disrupt DNA binding or androgen binding of the receptor to a greater or lesser degree, depending on the location and nature of the substitution. Individuals with partial AIS have an almost equally varied collection of AR defects, although deletions are extremely rare. Amino acid substitutions in the DNA or steroid binding differ somewhat from those associated with complete AIS, tending to be more conservative in nature and less often affecting highly conserved residues, features that are reflected by retention of some degree of DNA- or steroid-binding function of the receptor. However, there are now a number of studies demonstrating that different amino acid substitutions at the same site can produce quite disparate effects on androgen binding and genital phenotype and that identical amino acid substitutions may produce different phenotypes in different kindreds or even within the same family. For these reasons it has not been possible to establish any clear correlation between genotype and phenotype to date. Moreover, in a number of subjects with clinical evidence consistent with AIS, it has not been possible to detect a mutation within the coding region of the AR gene. While in some cases this may be due to technical problems, this apparent absence of mutation in the AR-coding region raises the possibility of defects in other regions of the AR gene not yet examined, such as the promoter region or in other genes involved in sex differentiation.

5α-Reductase deficiency

5α-Reductase is a microsomal enzyme that catalyzes the conversion of testosterone to dihydrotestosterone (DHT). A deficiency of 5α-reductase in the indifferent fetal external genitalia and urogenital sinus results in inadequate DHT concentrations, causing incomplete masculinization of these structures. The resulting ambiguous genitalia are characterized by a clitoral-like phallus with hypospadias and chordee, a bifid scrotum, a persistent urogenital sinus that opens on the perineum, and a blind vaginal pouch. Because normal male differentiation of the gonads and wolffian ducts is not dependent upon DHT, the testes, epididymes, vasa deferentia, and seminal vesicles develop normally. Testes are located in the labioscrotal folds or inguinal canals. Müllerian structures are absent because AMH is produced normally by the Sertoli cells. Studies in two large kindreds in the Dominican Republic and Turkey indicate that the pattern of inheritance in 5α-reductase deficiency is autosomal recessive. Clinical manifestations are not present in heterozygous males or homozygous females, however carriers of the trait can be detected by showing a decreased concentration of urinary C_{19} and C_{21} steroid 5α-metabolites. Cultured genital skin fibroblasts of affected individuals have reduced 5α-reductase activity. Furthermore, differences in enzyme stability and affinity for testosterone and NADPH have suggested genetic heterogeneity of the enzyme defect between kindreds. This enzyme heterogeneity reflects different gene mutations. In fact, two genes have been cloned and identified as 5α-reductase I and II. The 5α-reductase II gene is located on chromosome 2. Molecular analysis of the 5α-reductase II gene in different families with this disorder has identified at least 35 different mutations. Expression of mutant proteins has shown alterations in both substrate and NADPH binding. The 5α-reductase I gene localized on chromosome 5 is normal in male pseudohermaphrodites with inherited 5α-reductase deficiency. The enzyme is active at an alkaline pH, is expressed in low levels in the prostate; its distribution and function in human physiology is under investigation.

At puberty a variable degree of virilization occurs in affected males due to an increased production of testosterone, although DHT levels are relatively low. The voice deepens, the body habitus becomes more muscular, the scrotum becomes hyperpigmented, and the phallus enlarges as well as the testes. However, acne, facial hair, temporal hair recession, and enlargement of the prostate do not occur, suggesting that these processes are dependent upon relatively high levels of DHT. In a study of 18 affected subjects in the Dominican Republic, 17 of 18

changed to a male gender during or after puberty. Although testosterone exposure of the brain has a greater effect in determining male gender identity than sex of rearing, the influence of cultural factors in this homogeneous population may have been significant.

The diagnosis of 5α-reductase deficiency in infancy is based on finding a normal to elevated plasma testosterone level with low plasma DHT and an increased testosterone to DHT ratio, decreased conversion of testosterone to DHT in cultured genital skin fibroblasts of the affected subjects, decreased production of urinary 5α-reduced metabolites of testosterone, and decreased urinary 5α-reduced metabolites of C_{19} and C_{21} steroids.

Treating infants with DHT cream to enlarge the phallus and facilitate hypospadias repair is a useful therapy prior to surgery. The cream has also been used following puberty to promote growth of facial and body hair. Treatment of 5α-reductase deficient individuals beyond infancy and early childhood involves consideration of the physical and psychosexual orientation of the patient. Development of strong male secondary sexual characteristics at puberty supports male sex of rearing. Management of the condition is problematic when diagnosed in the peripubertal and early postpubertal periods.

Persistent Müllerian duct syndrome (PMD)

In subjects affected by persistent Müllerian duct syndrome, müllerian derivates, the uterus and fallopian tubes, persist in otherwise normal boys. External genitalia, wolffian derivates, and testes develop as expected, and pubertal virilization occurs. Infertility is common, and about 5% of reported individuals develop a seminoma or other germ cell tumor. In the more prevalent form, there is a hernia in which a partially descended testis is present. In addition, the uterus and tubes are in the hernia or they can be brought down by traction. In the other form, the uterus and tubes as well as the testes are in the pelvis. Perturbations of the gene encoding AMH have been identified. Both AMH positive and negative cases of PMD have been reported. When AMH is absent, a mutation can usually be demonstrated. AMH gene mutations have been identified and the first three exons are more consistently involved. The same group has also reported mutations of the AMH receptor in other patients with PMD. In most familial cases, inheritance is consis-

---

Table 38.3 Causes of female pseudohermaphroditism

Congenital adrenal hyperplasia
  21-hydroxylase deficiency
   11β-hydroxylase deficiency
   3β-hydroxysteroid dehydrogenase deficiency
Drug exposure
Maternal hyperandrogenism
Nonhormonal causes

tent with a sex-limited, autosomal recessive trait. Care must be exercised in the repair of the cryptorchidism and resection of the müllerian structures because of the proximity of the vasa deferentia and epididymes to the female duct derivates. Examination of testicular biopsy specimens has revealed normal germ cell populations, and the risk of malignancy does not appear to be higher than in other patients with cryptorchidism.

Diagnosis and management

Ambiguous genitalia in the newborn period requires evaluation by an experienced team that should include a pediatric endocrinologist and urologist. Rapid diagnosis and early sex assignment are essential to minimize psychosocial problems. A prompt diagnosis is also critical for the right management of adrenal insufficiency associated with congenital lipoid adrenal hyperplasia and 3β-HSD deficiency and mineralocorticoid excess associated with 17α-hydroxylase deficiency. The presence of hyperpigmentation, dehydration, hypertension, or electrolyte disturbances would suggest these possibilities. A family history may indicate individuals with ambiguous genitalia, infertility, amenorrhea, and/or lack of pubertal development. Measuring serum steroids before and after hCG stimulation will help to determine the presence of testosterone synthetic defect. If testosterone DHT and steroid precursors are normal, AIS is the most likely diagnosis. Molecular analyses for mutations in the AR gene, 5α-reductase gene, and certain genes involved in testosterone biosynthesis are available at specialized research centers.

The most important consideration in determining the sex of rearing is the potential to achieve an unambiguous appearance of the external genitalia and normal sexual functions after surgical reconstruction and hormonal therapy. The consideration of a male sex assignment depends primarily on whether the phallus is large enough for the reconstruction of the phallic urethra. Administration of testosterone and subsequent measurement of penile growth may be necessary to determine androgen responsiveness. Reconstructive surgery should be initiated as early as medically and surgically feasible to reduce the psychological stress on the family and patient. If a female gender assignment has been made, it is recommended to proceed with gonadectomy at the time of the initial repair. Gonadectomy is important for preventing the potential virilization that may occur at the time of puberty. At the time of puberty, estrogen replacement is required to induce secondary sexual development.

If a male gender assignment has been made, the testes should remain in situ to induce as much spontaneous masculinization as possible at the time of puberty. If the testes are not descended into the scrotum and a trial with hCG therapy fails to induce their descent, orchiopexy is indicated to reduce the risk of gonadoblastoma. Testosterone replacement therapy is required to support masculinization at puberty.

FEMALE PSEUDOHERMAPHRODITISM

A female pseudohermaphrodite is defined as an individual with ovaries, an XX karyotype, and masculinized genitalia. The clinical presentation may range from isolated clitoromegaly to complete masculinization of the external genitalia with scrotal development and the presence of a phallic urethra. The degree of fetal masculinization is determined by the stage of differentiation at the time of exposure. The causes of female pseudohermaphroditism are listed in Table 38.3.

Approximately 1 in 2000 newborns have ambiguous external genitalia. Among genetic females with ambiguous genitalia, congenital adrenal hyperplasia (CAH) is the most common cause, with an incidence between 54 and 85%. 21-Hydroxylase deficiency is the most frequent diagnosis in CAH. 11β-Hydroxylase and 3β-hydroxysteroid dehydrogenase deficiency are identified less frequently. The clinical presentation and characteristics of CAH are discussed elsewhere. Other causes of masculinization are rare but must be considered in the differential diagnosis. Masculinization of the female fetus has also been observed after maternal ingestion of testosterone or synthetic progestational agents during the first trimester of pregnancy. Danazol, a derivate of 17α-ethinyl testosterone, used for the treatment of endometriosis, has been noted to cause female pseudohermaphroditism. Suppression of ovulation is not universal and pregnancy may occur during danazol therapy. Clitoromegaly, labial fusion, and formation of the urogenital sinus have been variably noted in virilized females. Masculinization with prenatal progestin exposure is rare but has been reported. Masculinization of the female fetus may rarely occur if the mother has a virilizing tumor (usually arrhenoblastoma or Krukenberg tumor) or adrenal tumor. Luteoma during pregnancy, an ovarian pseudotumor composed of hyperplastic luteinized thecal cells that regress post partum, has been associated with masculinization of the external genitalia of female infants, especially when there has been maternal virilization. Ovarian lutein cysts in pregnancy, considered by some to be a cystic form of luteoma, are less frequently associated with maternal virilization and only rarely with fetal masculinization.

Nonhormonal causes of female pseudohermaphroditism are rare. Hormonal causes always should be excluded before nonhormonal causes are considered. A vaginal urethra, prominent clitoris, and accessory phallic urethra are seen in the syndrome of idiopathic female pseudohermaphroditism. Only a few causes of this syndrome have been described in the literature. Genital abnormalities can be associated with imperforate anus, renal agenesis, and other congenital malformations of the lower intestine and urinary tract, such as bladder outlet obstruction. Treatment in patients with idiopathic female pseudohermaphroditism is directed at correcting the masculinized appearance of the genitalia and correcting urinary obstruction when present.

Diagnosis

The presence of ambiguous genitalia in a newborn is a social and potentially medical emergency. Rapid and organized evaluation must be initiated to assign the appropriate gender, identify a possible life-threatening medical condition, and begin necessary medical, surgical, and psychological intervention. The first step must be eliciting a thorough family history. The mother should be interviewed regarding illness and ingestion of drugs, alcohol, or hormonal agents during pregnancy.

Evaluation of the infant should begin with a careful physical examination. If palpable gonads are present, they are assessed for symmetry and their position, and each gonad is examined to evaluate size, consistency, and for the presence of an epididymis. The phallus length should be precisely measured; standards of newborn penile length are available as well as of normal penile diameter. The position of the urethral meatus should be noted, whether at the tip of the phallus, along the shaft, or on the perineum. Hypospadias is almost always accompanied by chordee (ventral curvature of the penis resulting from a shortened urethra). The labioscrotal folds are assessed for degree of fusion. The spectrum of phenotypes seen with varying degrees of labioscrotal fusion includes labia majora (normal female), labia majora with posterior fusion, bifid scrotum, and fully fused scrotum (normal male). The perineum should be further examined for the presence of a vagina, vaginal pouch, or urogenital sinus. A rectal examination should be included in an attempt to palpate a uterus.

Clinical evaluation should include the examination of areolar or genital hyperpigmentation; signs of dehydration, which may be present in patients with congenital adrenal hyperplasia; the stigmata of Turner's syndrome; and the finding of dysmorphic features that may indicate the presence of a complex malformation syndrome that includes genital ambiguity.

All patients with ambiguous genitalia require a pelvic ultrasound, as it can detect ovaries and undescended testes. A genitogram with retrograde injection of contrast media via the urogenital orifice is also required to detect the presence of a uterus. Blood leukocytes should be cultured for karyotype analysis in all newborns with sexual ambiguity. Laboratory evaluation, which should be instituted immediately, include the measurement of serum androgens, 17-OH progesterone, as well as serum electrolytes and glucose levels since salt-wasting adrenal crises may occur secondary to several enzyme deficiencies regardless of the karyotype.

The determination of palpable gonads (testes), the presence or absence of a uterus, and the karyotype allows for the placement of the patient into one of the categories of abnormal sex differentiation. Female pseudohermaphrodites with no history of maternal androgen exposure will almost certainly have one of the three forms of CAH that cause virilization.

The diagnosis of 21-hydroxylase deficiency is confirmed by the finding of an elevated serum level of 17-OHP. Elevated levels of 11-deoxycortisol are found in 11β-hydroxylase deficiency, while 17-hydroxypregnenolone and dehydroepiandrosterone levels are high in 3β-hydroxysteroid dehydrogenase deficiency. All three disorders are characterized by elevated levels of ACTH.

The differential diagnosis of male pseudohermaphroditism includes testosterone biosynthetic errors (see the paragraph "male pseudohermaphroditism"). In particular, the testosterone biosynthetic errors that cause genital ambiguity (17,20-lyase deficiency and 17β-HSD deficiency) involve enzymes that are not required for mineralocorticoid and glucocorticoid synthesis. The diagnosis is confirmed by measuring testosterone precursors before and after hCG stimulation. Elevated levels of 17-OH pregnenolone and 17-hydroxyprogesterone are found in newborns with 17,20-lyase, while infants with 17β-hydroxysteroid dehydrogenase deficiency have elevated androstenedione and dehydroepiandrosterone levels. An elevated ratio of testosterone to DHT after hCG test suggests the diagnosis of 5α-reductase deficiency. Male pseudohermaphrodites with normal ACTH and normal hCG tests should be evaluated for partial androgen insensitivity. The diagnosis is made detecting an androgen receptor mutation and showing abnormal androgen binding in genital skin fibroblasts. The diagnosis of true hermaphroditism or gonadal dysgenesis is confirmed by finding the presence on gonadal biopsy of normal ovarian and testicular tissue or dysgenetic testicular tissue, respectively. Gender assignment is a complex issue that requires consideration of the potential for (1) an unambiguous appearance of the genitalia before and after puberty; (2) adequate sexual functioning; and (3) fertility.

Decisions regarding gender assignment in an infant with a 46,XX karyotype tend to be easier. A 46,XX individual who has been virilized by elevated androgens associated with adrenal hyperplasia or exogenous sources has a normal uterus, fallopian tubes, and ovaries, hence a female gender assignment is the most obvious choice. With appropriate perineal reconstruction and medical therapy, they will have female appearing external genitalia, spontaneous puberty, and fertility. Gender assignment in an infant with a 46,XY karyotype is more complex. Few individuals with genital ambiguity and a male karyotype are fertile, and so the primary question is whether or not the patient will be able to grow into a psychologically normal adult. Phallus size is usually very important for gender assignment. A phallic length of 1.9 cm is 2.5 SD below the mean for a normal newborn boy and may be considered the lower limit in assessing future function. If phallic size cannot be brought into the normal range even after a trial with androgen therapy, a male sex assignment is not advisable. In male pseudohermaphrodites with 5α-reductase deficiency, a course of topical DHT rather than parenteral testosterone may be more successful. In patients with gonadal dysgenesis and Y chromosomal material, dysgenetic testes and internal anatomy usually preclude fertility. A female sex is usually assigned due to small phallus size. True hermaphrodites with a unilateral ovary and müllerian structures may have spontaneous puberty and normal fertility and should therefore be raised as females. Although most true hermaphrodites are assigned a female sex because of external anatomy, an individual with a predominantly male phenotype and a normal size penis may be raised as a male.

Treatment

Surgical repair of the female pseudohermaphrodite consists of clitoral reduction, labioscrotal reduction, and vaginoplasty. Individuals with CAH require glucocorticoid therapy to prevent adrenal insufficiency and to suppress the production of virilizing adrenal androgens.

Male pseudohermaphrodites who are assigned a female sex of rearing undergo clitoral reduction, vaginoplasty, gonadectomy, and removal of wolffian structures. Estrogens are provided at puberty and in adulthood, at which time they initiate and maintain secondary sex characteristics and optimize bone mineralization. In individuals raised as males, surgical correction of hypospadias is usually initiated at one year but will usually require a second-stage procedure later. Testes are placed in the scrotum if necessary. Testosterone therapy is initiated at the time of puberty to induce and maintain secondary sex characteristics. Male pseudohermaphrodites with congenital adrenal hyperplasia will require glucocorticoid therapy.

In gonadal dysgenesis syndromes associated with Y chromosome material, the dysgenetic gonads are prone to neoplastic transformation and should be removed. In patients raised as females, surgical reconstruction consists of clitoral reduction, labioscrotal reduction, vaginoplasty, removal of wolffian structures, and gonadectomy. In patients raised as males, müllerian structures and dysgenetic gonads are removed and any hypospadius is surgically corrected. Secondary sex characteristics are induced with parenteral testosterone at the time of puberty. If the gonadal biopsy indicates that one of the testes in an individual with 45,X/46,XY gonadal dysgenesis is normal, the testes may be left in the scrotum in the hope that spontaneous puberty will occur. However, it should be noted that the normal-appearing testis may contain dysgenetic elements and is therefore susceptible to gonadoblastoma formation.

In patients with true hermaphroditism raised as females, ovarian tissue should be preserved and testicular tissue should be removed. Measurement of testosterone after hCG stimulation may be indicated to verify complete removal of testicular tissue. Surgical reconstruction is completed with müllerian structures preserved and wolffian structures removed. In patients raised as males, ovarian tissue and müllerian structures are removed and wolffian structures are preserved. The testicular tissue in true hermaphroditism is usually dysgenetic and should be removed. Exceptions may be made when a normal-appearing testis is located in the scrotum.

The psychosocial issues that accompany the findings of ambiguous genitalia should be addressed in parallel with medical and surgical evaluations. Parents require education with respect to sex differentiation and the specific disorder of the child. Normal psychosocial development is dependent upon parents' confidence in their ability to raise their child according to the assigned sex.

Suggested readings

BERKOVITZ GD, ROCK JA, URBAN MD, et al. True hermaphroditism. John Hopkins Med J 1982;151:290-7.

CAROTHERS AD, FILIPPI G. Klinefelter's syndrome in Sardinia and Scotland: comparative studies of parenteral age and other etiological factors in 47,XXY. Hum Gent 1988;81:71-5.

DE BELLIS A, QUIGLEY CA, MARSCHKE KB, et al. Characterization of mutant androgen receptors causing partial androgen insensitivity syndrome. J Clin Endocrinol Metab 1994;78:513-22.

EVANS RM. The steroid and thyroid hormone receptor superfamily. Science 1988;240:889-95.

FOREST M. Serum Mullerian inhibiting substance assay-a new diagnostic test for disorders of gonadal development. New Engl J Med 1997;336:1519-21.

GRUMBACH MM, CONTE FA. Disorders of sexual differentiation. In: Wilson JD, Foster DW (eds). Williams Textbook of endocrinology. Philadelphia: Saunders, 1985; 312-401.

GUBHAY J, COLLIGNON J, KOOPMAN P. A gene mapping to the sex determining region of the mouse Y chromosome is a member of a novel family of embryonically expressed genes. Nature 1991;346:245-50.

HSUCH WA, HSU TH, FEDERMANN DD. Endocrine features of Klinefelter's syndrome. Medicine 1978;57:447-61.

JENKINS EP, ANDERSON S, IMPERATO-MC GINLEY J, et al. Genetic and pharmacological evidence for more than one human steroid 5(-reductase. J Clin Invest 1992;89:293-300.

KUPFER SR. QUIGLY CA, FRENCH FS. Male pseudohermaphroditism. Seminars in Perinatology 1992;16:319-31.

LUBAHN DB, JOSEPH DR, SULLIVAN PM, et al. Cloning of human androgen receptor complementary DNA and localization to the X chromosome. Science 1988;240:327-30.

NEW MI, WHITE PC, PANG S, et al. The adrenal hyperplasia. In: Scriver CR, Beudet AL, Sly WS, et al. (eds). The metabolic basis of inherited disease. 6th ed. New York: McGraw-Hill, 1989; 1881-1917.

QUIGLEY CA, DE BELLIS A, MARSCHKE KB, et al. Androgen receptor defects: historical, clinical and molecular perspectives. Endocr Rev 1995;16:271-321.

WILSON JD, GRIFFIN JOE, RUSSELL DW. Steroid 5α-reductase 2 deficiency. Endocr Rev 1993;14:577-93.

Testicular physiology

Mario Serio, Mario Maggi

The human testes are paired organs, each measuring approximately 3 to 5 cm across and containing a volume ranging from 15 to 30 ml. They are, in normal conditions, located in the scrotum with a temperature lower (about 2 °C) than other abdominal tissues. The temperature of the testes is kept rather constant by the retraction or relaxation of the cremasteric muscle, and by the peculiar testicular circulation with shunts among the testicular arteries and veins. Arterial blood to the testis is supplied by the internal spermatic, cremasteric, and vas deferential arteries; venous blood drains into the pampiniform plexus and then into the internal spermatic vein, which on the right enters into the inferior vena cava and on the left drains into the renal vein.

The testis has two compartments: the interstitial compartment devoted to testosterone production, and the tubular compartment devoted to production of spermatozoa.

THE INTERSTITIAL COMPARTMENT

The Leydig cells of the testis are specialized in testosterone synthesis and secretion. Under light microscopy these cells are polygonal, measure 10 to 25 μm in diameter, and represent approximately 5% of the total testicular volume. Clusters of Leydig cells are interspersed in the space adjacent to seminiferous tubules. They are contiguous to capillaries and deliver the steroids into the testicular vein, and, to a lesser extent, into the lymphatic vessels.

The Leydig cells contain lipid droplets, and they have a high ratio of cytoplasm to the nucleus and prominent nucleoli.

THE TUBULAR COMPARTMENT

The spermatogenetic tubules are composed of the germinal epithelium and Sertoli cells.

The seminiferous tubules measure approximately 0.12 to 0.30 cm in diameter and up to 70 cm in length. These structures provide a continuous pathway for delivery of sperm from the testis to the rete testis, epididymis, and vas deferens. The human testis produces $123 (\pm 18) \times 10^6$ sperms daily. Tight junctions between the Sertoli cells form a diffusion barrier that divide the testis into two functional compartments. The basal compartment consists of Sertoli cells and the other portion of the tubules that includes spermatogonia. The adluminal compartment contains the inner two-thirds of the tubules and includes primary and secondary spermatocytes and round and elongated spermatids. The Sertoli cells line the spermatogenetic tubules, and their inner portion consists of an arborized cytoplasm, such that spermatogenesis takes place within a network of Sertoli cell cytoplasm.

TESTOSTERONE SYNTHESIS AND SECRETION

The lipid droplets in the Leydig cells contain both esterified cholesterol (derived from circulating lipoproteins) and locally-synthesized cholesterol. Following hydrolysis, free cholesterol moves to mitochondria where the side chain is cleaved to form pregnenolone, which in turn is converted to testosterone in the endoplasmic reticulum.

Five enzymatic processes are involved in the conversion of cholesterol to testosterone: cholesterol side-chain cleavage ($P450_{SCC}$), 3β-hydroxysteroid dehydrogenase/isomerase (3β-HSD), 17α-hydroxylase ($P450_{17\alpha}$), 17,20-lyase ($P450_{17\alpha}$), and 17β-hydroxysteroid oxidoreductase (17β-HSOR) (see Chap. 26).

The testosterone synthesis is under luteinizing hormone (LH) control. The Leydig cells contain specific membrane receptors that bind LH with high affinity.

The LH receptor contains an extracellular domain of approximately 340 amino acids and a 330 amino acid residue C-terminal region containing seven transmembrane spanning elements. The extracellular domain shows a structural relative specificity for LH, whereas the transmembrane portion displays sequence similarity to other members of the G-protein-coupled receptor gene, such as follicle-stimulating hormone (FSH) receptor and β-adrenergic receptor.

Exposure to a high concentration of LH over several hours reduces the LH receptor content, a process generally termed down-regulation. Experiments in men treated by human chorionic gonadotropin (hCG) suggest the potential physiological relevance of LH receptor suppression. After 1- to 2-day exposure to high doses of hCG, there is a disproportional rise in 17α-hydroxyprogesterone in comparison with testosterone, which seems to be correlated with the increment of 17β-estradiol (17β-E$_2$) in plasma. Receptor down-regulation explains why men with choriocarcinoma secrete reduced amounts of testosterone.

The major androgen secreted by the testis is testosterone; approximately 7 mg per day enters the peripheral circulation. As a consequence of LH pulsatile secretion due to the luteinizing hormone-releasing hormone (LHRH) pulse generator, testosterone is secreted in a pulsatile manner.

The secretion rate can be obtained using the formula "spermatic vein-peripheral vein gradients x testicular blood flow." A comparison of the calculated values of the testosterone secretion rate when using this approach with those of the testosterone production rate obtained using continuous infusion of radioactive testosterone has clearly demonstrated that in adult man the circulating testosterone is coming almost completely from testicular secretion. The testes are also found to secrete a significant amount of 17α-hydroxyprogesterone, androstenedione, and pregnenolone, and a small amount of 5α-dihydrotestosterone (69 μg/24-hour). They secrete an even smaller amount of 17β-estradiol (10 μg/24-hour), which in man is produced almost entirely by peripheral conversion from testosterone.

A small percentage of testosterone (approximately 2%) circulates in the free state in plasma, and the remainder is bound either to sex hormone-binding globulin (SHBG) or to albumin. The affinity of sex hormone-binding globulin for testosterone (1.6×10^{-9} M) is several orders of magnitude higher than that of albumin (4×10^{-4} M).

The levels of sex hormone-binding globulin can be reduced (such as in obesity, hyperprolactinemia, and hypothyroidism) and increased (such as in aging, hyperthyroidism, and chirrosis), and they can affect the total amount of circulating testosterone. Sex hormone-binding globulin is synthesized in the liver. Estrogens stimulate, and testosterone and dihydrotestosterone inhibit its synthesis.

Testosterone serves as a circulating precursor or prehormone for two types of metabolites, which in turn mediate several androgen actions. Some biological effects, however, can be mediated directly by testosterone (Fig. 39.1).

Testosterone can be converted to 5α-reduced steroids, principally dihydrotestosterone, which mediates many differentiative actions in fetal life (see chapter on sexual differentiation) and some functional actions in adulthood. Alternatively, androgens can be aromatized in the extraglandular tissue to estrogens that act independently (such as in breast growth) or in concert (such as the negative feedback of LH) with androgens.

Dihydrotestosterone formation is mediated by two widely-distributed membrane-bound 5α-reductase isoenzymes (called I and II). The isoenzyme I is prevalently

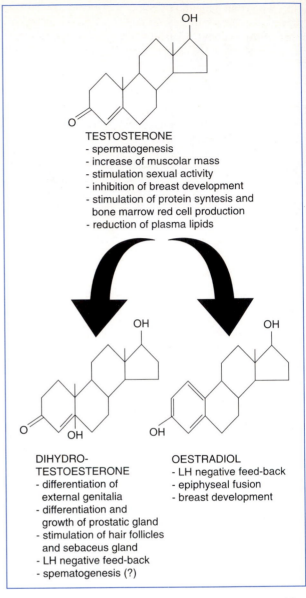

Figure 39.1 Biological effects of testosterone and its metabolites.

present in the liver, the scalp, and the non-genital skin, while the isoenzyme II is prevalently distributed in the prostate, in the genital skin, and in the genital tubercle and swelling (fetal life). The majority of circulating dihydrotestosterone is produced in androgen target tissues.

Aromatization of androgens also occurs in many tissues, the most important being the adipocytes.

HYPOTHALAMIC-PITUITARY-LEYDIG CELL AXIS

An integrated, highly-complex system regulates the level of circulating androgens within a relatively narrow range in man.

The hypothalamus plays a fundamental regulatory role by the release of LHRH, which controls both LH and FSH secretion from the pituitary. Luteinizing hormone binds to specific receptors in Leydig cells and stimulates testosterone production. Circulating testosterone, through negative feedback, regulates LHRH and LH secretion.

Hypothalamic pulse generator

The release of luteinizing hormone-releasing hormone is controlled by peptidergic neurons, which are highly concentrated in the arcuate nucleus.

A characteristic property of LHRH neural function is an intrinsic functional pulsatility with variable amplitude and frequency modulation. Consequently, LHRH is secreted in a series of pulses with variable amplitude and frequency. The pituitary responds with pulsatile secretion of LH (at intervals of 90 to 120 minutes) and to a lesser extent into peripheral circulation. Sex steroids, catecholamines, opiates, galanin, and neuropeptide Y can alter the amplitude and frequency of LHRH pulses.

Pituitary

The determinant factor controlling the LH release by the pituitary is LHRH.

This decapeptide binds to specific receptors on cells that synthesize both LH and FSH. Luteinizing hormone-releasing hormone stimulates the mobilization of ionized calcium within the cells and induces LH release. In response to a LHRH bolus, the pituitary promptly releases LH into peripheral circulation. On the contrary, with the exposure to constantly infused LHRH, after an initial burst of LH secretion, the levels of this gonadotropin decrease progressively and loses pulsatility. This phenomenon is called desensitization.

Luteinizing hormone is a glycoprotein with a molecular weight of 28000 kD and is composed of two separated subunits. The α subunit contains 92 amino acids and is identical to the α subunits of TSH, FSH, and hCG; the β subunit contains 115 amino acids and is specific for LH. The hCG β subunit shows analogy with the 115 amino acids of β-LH, but it has 30 additional amino acids in addition to the β-LH peptide sequence.

The pituitary gonadotropin-secreting cells independently synthesize both α and β subunits of LH, which are coded by separate genes. After transcription and translation are completed, these subunits join to form a native LH molecule. Later, a variable amount of carbohydrate is inserted into the molecule. These complex phenomena explain the micro-heterogeneity of circulating LH.

A reduction in the carbohydrate content of LH enhances its clearance rate and reduces its biological potency. The metabolic clearance rate of LH is in the range of 35-25 ml/min.

LH in the testis binds to a specific membrane receptor (i.e., LH receptor).

The negative feedback of gonadal steroids

Two steroids, testosterone and estradiol, independently control luteinizing hormone secretion at the hypothalamic and pituitary level. An elevation of sex steroid circulating values causes a reduction of LH secretion and, in the pituitary, a reduction in mRNA levels for the LH subunits. The negative feedback effects can be mediated either by a reduction in the frequency or by a decrease of amplitude of LH pulses. Testosterone exerts negative feedback effects through interactions with the androgen receptor or after aromatization to estradiol. Several lines of evidence support the independent action of testosterone on LH secretion.

For example, non-aromatizable androgens such as dihydrotestosterone inhibit LH. Similarly, patients affected by the complete form of 5α-reductase II deficiency and total androgen resistance have elevated LH levels in spite of the secretion, and the metabolism of estradiol is normal. Vice versa, patients affected by estrogen resistance have elevated LH levels, in spite of the normal testosterone circulating values.

Based on these data, current opinion is that two negative feedback systems, one mediated by androgens and the other by estrogens, operate independently. Both systems exert rapid effects on LH secretion within a few hours.

The negative feedback effects of androgens appear to be mediated through an opiatergic system. The inhibitory effects of testosterone can be blocked by naloxone (an opiate receptor antagonist). Consequently, naloxone stimulates LH and testosterone secretion.

HYPOTHALAMIC-PITUITARY-GERM CELL AXIS

Germinal function of the human testis is controlled by FSH as well as by intratesticular androgens. Follicle-stimulating hormone binds to specific receptors located in Sertoli cells and consequently induces adenylate cyclase activation. Follicle-stimulating hormone induces synthesis and secretion of several Sertoli cell proteins such as transferrin, androgen-binding protein (ABP), and inhibins. Androgen receptors are also primarily located in Sertoli cells.

The physiological roles of transferrin and ABP in man has not yet been demonstrated. Inhibins seem to be involved in the FSH feedback. A specific feedback interaction between the germ cell compartment of the testis and FSH was first suggested by the observation that isolated FSH increases in patients with germ cell failure. In addition, irradiation of testes of animal and man induces germ cell arrest and FSH elevation without altering LH and testosterone levels. These observations initially suggested that the germinal cell compartment, specifically the Sertoli cells, secretes a substance that inhibits FSH. Such a factor has been identified and called inhibin. Inhibins (as well activins) are part of a family of peptides that includes transforming growth factor β (TGF β). Inhibin consists of a 31 kD heterodimeric protein with α and β subunits connected by a disulfide bridge. Homodimers of the β subunit form the activin A (B_A-B_B) and B (B_B-B_B). The biological activity of activin is tenfold more potent than LHRH in stimulating FSH secretion.

The relative roles of activins and inhibins in the feedback regulation of FSH is incompletely understood, and even the biological role of inhibin in the negative loop of the feedback mechanism to reduce FSH secretion is controversial. However, a significant inverse relationship between FSH and inhibin B has been recently reported in oligozoospermic men. Both activins and inhibins share homology with many growth factors and are present in many tissues, such as the brain, adrenal, pituitary, kidney, and bone marrow. These peptides most likely exert local regulatory effects in many tissues in addition to the testis.

ANTI-MÜLLERIAN HORMONE

Anti-Müllerian hormone (AMH) is a chimerical glycoprotein encoded by a gene located in the short arm of chromosome 19. It has interesting structural homologies with TGF β and the β chain of inhibin. Its secretion begins at the seventh week of gestation, at the same time as Sertoli cell differentiation. In boys, the circulating AMH is higher the earliest month of life, but significant levels remain throughout their childhood. While the physiological action of AMH is to induce the regression of the Mullerian ducts during fetal life, its functional significance in postnatal life is still unknown.

Suggested readings

DYM M. Basement membrane regulation of Sertoli cells. Endocr Rev 1994;15:102-15.

GNESSI L, FABBRI A, SPERA G. Gonadal peptides as mediators of development and functional control of the testis: an integrated system with hormones and local environment. Endocr Rev 1997;18:541-609.

HAMMOND GL, RUAKONEN A, KONTTURY M, KOSKELA E, VIHKO R. The simultaneous radioimmunoassay of seven steroids in human spermatic and peripheral venous blood. J Clin Endocrinol Metab 1977;45:16-21.

PETERSON RE, IMPERATO-MCGINLEY J, GAUTIER T, STURLA E. Male pseudoermaphroditsm due to steroid 5α–reductase deficiency. Am J Med 1977;62:170-80.

REYES-FUENTES A, VELDHUIS JP. Neuroendocrine physiology of normal male gonadal axis. Endocrinol Metab North Am 1993;22:93-124.

SMITH EP, BOYD J, FRANK GR, et al. Estrogen resistance caused by a mutation in the estrogen-receptor gene in a man. New Engl J Med 1994;331:1056-61.

SAEZ JM. Leydig cells: endocrine, paracrine and autocrine Regulation. Endocr Rev 1994;15:574-626.

SCALFAN SC, WEINSTEIN H, MILLAR RP. Molecular mechanism of ligand interaction with gonadotropine releasing hormone receptor. Endocr Rev 1997;18:180-205.

YING SY. Inhibins, activin and follistatin: gonadal proteins modulating the secretion of FSH. Endocr Rev 1988;9:267-93.

Male hypogonadism

Stephen J. Winters

███ **KEY POINTS** ███

- Measurement of plasma levels of testosterone, luteinizing hormone, and follicle-stimulating hormone are used to distinguish men with primary testicular failure from those with hypogonadotropic hypogonadism.
- Men with hypogonadotropic hypogonadism require a thorough endocrine and radiographic evaluation for hypothalamic or pituitary disease before beginning androgen replacement therapy.
- Systemic illnesses frequently disturb testicular function.
- With very few exceptions, hypogonadal men should receive androgen replacement therapy.
- There are effective methods to stimulate spermatogenesis in most gonadotropin-deficient men.

The testes are the site of sperm production as well as the source of testosterone for fetal male sexual differentiation, pubertal development, adult sexual function, and spermatogenesis. Leydig cell clusters and seminiferous tubules are in near proximity within the testis and the compartments are functionally interrelated. Therefore, hypogonadism usually involves both the sperm-forming and androgen-producing functions of the testis.

Differential diagnosis

The identification of male hypogonadism begins with a thorough medical history and a complete physical examination. The clinical presentation of male hypogonadism depends upon the age and developmental state at which disease first occurs. A convenient conceptual approach is to divide disorders causing hypogonadism into those that begin during fetal life, in childhood, or in adulthood. Accordingly, the presence of ambiguous genitalia signifies an in utero androgen disorder. Growth disturbance and abnormal pubertal development may result from congenital or childhood-acquired disorders. When mild, these disorders may escape detection in childhood, and instead may present in adulthood.

Clinical findings

The clinical features of adult male hypogonadism may be similar when the pathological process affects the testis (primary testicular failure) or impairs gonadotropin secretion (hypogonadotropic hypogonadism). The most common complaint among hypogonadal adult men is a decrease in libido. By contrast, the impaired erectile function characteristic of elderly men is usually accompanied by a preserved libido. Other common presenting complaints among hypogonadal men are incomplete sexual maturation, gynecomastia, sexual dysfunction, and infertility. There may be symptoms of a sellar or suprasellar mass such as headaches, visual disturbance, or panhypopituitarism. The diagnosis of hypogonadism in men is often delayed because the symptoms are subtle, or because of denial.

A complete physical examination is needed for all hypogonadal men because many systemic disorders may present with testicular dysfunction. Pubertal staging is the basis for classifying the physical features of normal and abnormal pubertal development (see Chap. 9). Measurement of the testes is easily accomplished by aligning the testis with a ruler, or by comparing the volume of the testes with the beads of an orchidometer. The median testis length among normal adult men is 5 cm, equivalent to a volume of 25 ml. Testes that are 4 cm in length or less are usually abnormal, and the right testis is often slightly larger than the left. Prepubertal Leydig cell insufficiency causes eunuchoidism characterized by a juvenile voice; scant facial, axillary, pubic and body hair; smooth skin; poorly developed musculature; increased fat accumulated in the hips and lower abdomen; a small prostate and phallus; and failure of epiphyseal closure, which leads to an arm span that exceeds the height by more than 6 cm and to disproportionately long legs. Physical characteristics regress slowly in adult hypogonadal men. The presence of soft, smooth skin, reduced body hair, and decreased musculature suggest long-standing and pronounced androgen deficiency. Gynecomastia is a common finding among hypogonadal men, but galactorrhea is rare.

Diagnostic procedures

The laboratory evaluation of hypogonadism begins with the measurement of testosterone in plasma. Circulating testosterone levels vary slightly from moment-to-moment due to pulsatile release from the testis, and values are about 15% higher in the early morning than in the evening. Testosterone levels on consecutive days are quite reproducible. The total testosterone concentration is influenced considerably by the plasma level of sex hormone-binding globulin (SHBG). For example, total testosterone levels are frequently low in obese hyperinsulinemic men because SHBG levels are reduced. To control for changes

in SHBG, the non-SHBG-bound (bioavailable) testosterone, or the percentage of free testosterone by equilibrium dialysis or ultrafiltration, can be determined. Direct free testosterone assay kits that use radiolabeled testosterone analogs may be less accurate.

The screening evaluation should include measurement of luteinizing hormone (LH), follicle-stimulating hormone (FSH), and prolactin, as well as testosterone, since total testosterone may be normal in men with testicular failure or with hyperprolactinemia. Because of the pulsatile pattern of LH secretion, one approach is to draw three blood samples at 20 minute intervals and pool the samples for measurement of LH. By measuring the plasma levels of LH and FSH with the new generation of sensitive two site-assays as well as testosterone, it is possible to make the important distinction between primary testicular failure and hypogonadotropic hypogonadism (Fig. 40.1).

Dynamic tests of the hypothalamic-pituitary-Leydig cell axis are rarely necessary. The testosterone response to human chorionic gonadotropin (hCG) stimulation is used to examine Leydig cell function before puberty, but it is nonspecific in adults. The response of LH to gonadotropin-releasing hormone (GnRH) stimulation is likewise nonspecific in adult men, and the peak value correlates positively with the basal level. Follicle-stimulating hormone levels are often elevated with seminiferous tubular dysfunction, and the FSH response to GnRH stimulation is exaggerated. Inhibin-B levels are reduced in both primary and secondary hypogonadism. The routine semen analysis provides useful information concerning testicular function, but it is less able to distinguish fertile from infertile men.

GONADOTROPIN DEFICIENCY

Congenital hypogonadotropic hypogonadism

Patients with congenital hypogonadotropic hypogonadism (HH) fail to enter into or progress normally through puber-

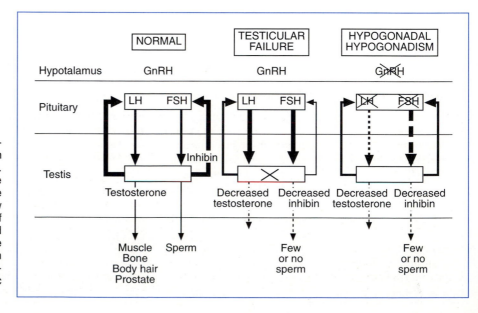

Figure 40.1 Hypothalamic-pituitary testicular function in normal and hypogonadal men. Hypogonadal men often have small testes, low testosterone and inhibin-B levels, and a low sperm count. Measurement of luteinizing hormone (LH) and follicle-stimulating hormone (FSH) is used to distinguish between primary testicular failure and hypogonadotropic hypogonadism.

ty because gonadotropin secretion is insufficient to stimulate testosterone production into the range typical of normal adult men. The disorder is quantitatively and qualitatively heterogeneous. Some patients present with sexual infantilism. Other men present later in life often with infertility or osteoporosis. They relate a history of partial pubertal development and are found to have idiopathic gonadotropin deficiency. Because these men have had some testicular growth, it was formerly called the "fertile eunuch syndrome." Most men with congenital gonadotropin deficiency have selective gonadotropin deficiency, although gonadotropin deficiency can also occur together with growth hormone, thyroid-stimulating hormone, and/or adrenocorticotropic hormone (ACTH) deficiency.

Patients with congenital HH are often divided into those with anosmia or other midline defects (Kallmann's syndrome), those in whom HH is associated with other disorders, and those with isolated gonadotropin deficiency (Tab. 40.1).

Male hypogonadism with anosmia was first described in 1856 by Maestre de San Juan and was called olfacto-genital dysplasia. Familial male hypogonadism with anosmia was reported by Kallmann in 1944, but many other congenital defects may be present (Tab. 40.2). Anosmia results from hypoplasia of the olfactory nerves and tracts.

Most cases of Kallmann's syndrome seem to be sporadic mutations, though in approximately 25% a family history of either midline defects or hypogonadism is present. Although the association of anosmia and familial HH in the kindred described by Kallmann appeared to be an X-linked trait, other kindreds suggest autosomal recessive or dominant inheritance with incomplete penetrance. The X-linked form of Kallmann's syndrome was recently mapped to Xp22.3. The candidate gene encodes a 680 amino acid protein, KAL, which is thought to be processed on the cell membrane and to function in the migration and targeting of GnRH neurons and other axons during development, providing an explanation for the neurological and somatic abnormalities. Most cases of Kallmann's syndrome may not have this etiology, however. The coding region sequence of the GnRH gene has been uniformly normal.

Congenital HH is occasionally associated with congenital adrenal hypoplasia, an association that has provided insight into the control of gonadotropin subunit gene expression. Congenital adrenal hypoplasia is characterized by neonatal hypotension, hyponatremia and hyperkalemia, and it is generally fatal if untreated with glucocorticoids and mineralocorticoids. Congenital HH and adrenal hypoplasia are now known to be mechanistically related. Congenital adrenal hypoplasia was found to result from mutation of the gene for the transcription factor DAX-1. A second transcription factor, steroidogenic factor-1 (SF-1), is also required for adrenal and gonadal organogenesis, and it regulates the promoters for the GnRH receptor and the gonadotropin α- and LH-β subunit genes. Current evidence suggests that DAX-1 and SF-1 form a nuclear protein complex that regulates GnRH and LH gene expression, such that DAX-1 mutations result in HH because the pituitary is unable to respond to the GnRH signal. GnRH production may also be impaired.

Men with HH due to mutations of the GnRH receptor gene have also been recently identified.

Acquired hypogonadotropic hypogonadism

Gonadotropin deficiency may result from a pathological process within the sella that compresses or destroys the

Table 40.2 Congenital defects associated with hypogonadotropic hypogonadism

Neurological defects	Genital defects	Somatic abnormalities
Anosmia	Microphallus	Cleft lip
Nystagmus	Cryptorchidism	Cleft palate
Synkinesias		Malformed incisors
Sensorineural hearing loss		Arched palate
Cerebellar ataxia		Unilateral renal agenesis
Seizures		Horseshoe kidney
Color blindness		Pes cavus
		Digital deformity

Table 40.1 Syndromes associated with congenital hypogonadotropic hypogonadism

Syndrome	Clinical findings
Kallmann's syndrome	Anosmia and other midline defects
Congenital adrenal hypoplasia	Neonatal adrenal failure
Congenital ichthyosis (Rud's syndrome)	Steroid sulfatase deficiency, seizures
Prader-Willi syndrome	Hypotonia, obesity, small hands and feet, retardation
Moebius syndrome	Oculofacial paralysis, seizures, limb anomalies, retardation
Lowe syndrome	Lenticular opacities, hypotonia, renal tubular acidosis
Multiple lentigines (LEOPARD) syndrome	Lentigines (EKG conduction defects, ocular hypertelorism, pulmonic stenosis, growth retardation, deafness)
Carpenter's syndrome	Obesity, acrocephaly, craniosynostosis, limb agenesis
Septo-optic dysplasia	Absent septum pellucidum, optic nerve hypoplasia
Partial- or pan-hypopituitarism	Cranial-facial abnormalities, growth hormone, thyroid-stimulating hormone and ACTH deficiency, diabetes insipidus, birth trauma

normal pituitary gland, via pathology in the suprasellar space that interrupts the axons transporting GnRH to the hypophysial-portal capillaries, or by other mechanisms. Various mass lesions, infectious and infiltrative processes, head trauma and X-irradiation may produce HH (Tab. 40.3). Tumors and other lesions of the pituitary and suprasellar regions are discussed in Chapter 6. Unique aspects of those disorders that produce hypogonadism are discussed in the following paragraphs.

Men with prolactin-producing pituitary adenomas generally present with symptoms of hypogonadism such as a decline in libido and decreased sexual potency, and tender gynecomastia. Prolactinomas in teenagers result in delayed pubertal development. Testosterone levels are reduced, and the pulsatile pattern of LH secretion is attenuated. In spite of high prolactin levels, galactorrhea is rare in men with prolactinomas, presumably because circulating estradiol levels are too low to stimulate mammary gland growth and development. With microadenomas, the decrease in LH secretion results from GnRH deficiency, because pulsatile GnRH treatment restores LH and testosterone levels to normal. Studies in rats with experimental hyperprolactinemia indicate that GnRH mRNA levels are reduced. Successful lowering of prolactin levels with dopamine agonists most often normalizes testicular function. Unfortunately, many men with prolactin-producing pituitary tumors continue to present later in the course of their disease with macroadenomas that have destroyed the gonadotrophs. These men require testosterone replacement or gonadotropin treatment to restore fertility.

Hypogonadism is common, and it may be the presenting complaint in men with Cushing's syndrome. Serum testosterone levels are low, and basal and GnRH-stimulated LH concentrations are reduced in men with either ACTH-producing pituitary tumors or with adrenal adenomas. Increased cortisol production is responsible for the gonadotropin deficiency since adrenalectomy, treatment with the steroidogenesis inhibitor mitotane, or the glucocorticoid receptor antagonist mifepristone (R1881) can restore LH and testosterone secretion. Furthermore, high-dose glucocorticoid treatment of men with otherwise normal testicular function also suppresses gonadotropin

secretion. Experimental studies with GnRH-producing hypothalamic cell lines reveal that activated glucocorticoid receptors bind to the promoter region of the GnRH gene and repress its transcription.

Autoimmune (lymphocytic) adenohypophysitis is an autoimmune disorder of the anterior pituitary that occurs most often in women, frequently in the peripartum period. Approximately 10% of the cases have been in men who have presented with headaches and HH, other anterior pituitary hormone deficits and diabetes insipidus, and were found to have enlargement of the pituitary gland on magnetic resonance images. The disorder cannot be distinguished readily from a pituitary tumor, but it is suggested by the coexistence of other autoimmune endocrine disorders such as thyroiditis. Surgery is needed to confirm the diagnosis.

Gonadotropin insufficiency may also occur with estrogen-producing tumors of the adrenals or gonads. Patients present with gynecomastia, infertility, decreased libido and impotence, or with a testicular or adrenal mass. Plasma levels of estradiol and/or estrone are often elevated, and testosterone, LH, and FSH levels are reduced or normal. The overexpression of a G-protein by the tumor may activate adenylate cyclase and stimulate steroidogenesis. ACTH and hCG may further increase the production of estrogens by adrenal and testicular tumors, respectively. Ketoconazole was reported to decrease estrogen production by an adrenal tumor. Testicular tumors may be palpable, or may require ultrasonography for detection. Adrenal tumors are usually identified by computed tomography scan. These uncommon tumors may be benign or malignant, and treatment is surgical. Testis tumors may be composed of Leydig cells or of Sertoli cells in tubular structures resembling seminiferous tubules. Androgen-producing adrenal and testicular tumors go undetected in adult men but produce precocious puberty in boys. Hormone-producing testicular tumors may occur as part of the Carney complex (cardiac myxomas, cutaneous lesions, primary pigmented nodular adrenocortical hyperplasia, growth hormone-producing pituitary adenomas).

Rarely, men present with HH in adult life with a history of normal and complete sexual development, and no explanation for acquired HH is found. Careful follow-up of these men with magnetic resonance scans is necessary since tumors and infiltrative lesions of the hypothalamus are sometimes difficult to diagnose initially. Some patients with adult onset idiopathic HH give a history of remote head trauma.

Selective deficiency of luteinizing hormone or follicle-stimulating hormone

Gonadotropin deficiency generally involves both LH and FSH, because GnRH stimulates the synthesis and secretion of both gonadotropins and both hormones are produced by pituitary gonadotrophs. However, more recently, sensitive two-site assays suggest that there is a component of FSH secretion that is less dependent on GnRH stimulation. Thus, men with complete GnRH deficiency, absent LH, and plasma testosterone levels in the castrate range,

Table 40.3 Causes of acquired hypogonadotropic hypogonadism

Pituitary adenoma	Acute and chronic
Prolactinoma	systemic illness
Cushing's syndrome	Weight loss
Suprasellar tumors	Hemochromatosis
Craniopharyngioma	Autoimmune hypophysitis
Germinoma	Head trauma
Histiocytosis	X-irradiation
Sarcoidosis	Polyarteritis
Tuberculosis	Estrogen-producing
	adrenal and testicular tumors
	Idiopathic

have measurable plasma levels of FSH identical to puri-fied FSH by size exclusion chromatography. Similarly, FSH is often present in excess of LH in plasma of patients with GnRH deficiency due to prolactin-producing pituitary microadenomas. Studies in rats indicate that activin produced within the pituitary functions to sustain FSH production, but to what extent these findings are applicable to humans is presently unknown. LH and testosterone deficiency with elevated FSH levels suggests an FSH-producing pituitary tumor.

Mutations of the genes encoding LH and FSH have been identified. A series of case reports have described an adult male with sexual infantilism who demonstrated a low plasma testosterone and an elevated plasma LH level. The LH produced was devoid of bioactivity in vitro. This man was shown to be homozygous for a missense mutation of the coding region of the LH-β gene. A second kindred with a similar, but incompletely evaluated, syndrome has been reported. As many as 3.6% of the Finnish population produce an LH molecule that was not detected by a two-site immunometric assay. In these subjects, among whom reproductive function is normal, point mutations of the LH-β gene are believed to alter the carbohydrate structure of LH, obscuring the epitopes detected by the highly specific two-site assay used. Other two-site assays also recognize the variant LH.

Normally virilized infertile men are occasionally encountered with normal LH but persistently low plasma FSH levels. Most of these cases were identified using older double antibody radioimmunoassays in which plasma FSH levels in normal men were sometimes undetectable. Thus the significance of "isolated FSH deficiency" in these infertile men was controversial. Women with primary amenorrhea and FSH deficiency who harbor mutations in the coding region of the FSH gene have recently been reported, as has one male who had unexpected testosterone deficiency as well as hypospermatogenesis.

Patients with mutations of the LH and FSH-receptor genes have also recently been reported. Missense mutations of the LH receptor in males cause Leydig cell hypoplasia with ambiguous genitalia, whereas activating mutations cause gonadotropin-independent precocious puberty. Men homozygous for inactivating mutations of the FSH receptor have small testes, oligospermia, and poor sperm motility but are not azoospermic. Inhibin-B levels were reduced and plasma FSH was increased. Whether these men were completely unresponsive to FSH was not entirely clear. Activating mutations of the FSH receptor may produce a normal phenotype in men, since the only case so far reported was of a man with hypopituitarism following hypophysectomy and radiotherapy for a pituitary adenoma. His sperm count was unexpectedly normal in the absence of measurable levels of LH or FSH during treatment with testosterone.

Delayed puberty

Delayed pubertal development is a relatively common clinical problem in boys, which is generally defined as a lack of sexual development by age 14 years. This age rep-resents a delay of 2 SD beyond the mean age for the onset of testicular growth, the first event in male puberty, which occurs at age 11.2 to 11.9 years, depending on the population studied. Visible pubic hair growth (Tanner stage 3) does not occur until age 13.5 to 13.9 years in normal boys, however, and it is a lack of pubic hair growth and other signs of androgenization that generally prompt referral to an endocrinologist.

Most boys with delayed puberty have constitutional delay, which represents an abnormally slow but otherwise normal pubertal process. Many patients have been shorter than their peers throughout their school-age years; growth hormone deficiency should be excluded by measuring the plasma level of insulin-like growth factor-I (IGF-I) and IGF-binding protein 3. There may be a family history of delayed puberty. A normal medical history and a physical examination demonstrating testis growth are often all that is required to confirm early pubertal development and to alleviate the anxieties of the parent and patient. On the other hand, visible pubic hair growth in the absence of testis enlargement suggests gonadotropin deficiency since simple delayed puberty is generally accompanied by delayed adrenarche. Tumors of the hypothalamic-pituitary unit, including craniopharyngioma and prolactinoma, nutritional deprivation, and chronic diseases such as cystic fibrosis and inflammatory bowel disease, as well as primary testicular failure, should also be considered in boys with delayed puberty.

The hypothalamic-pituitary-gonadal axis before puberty is normally quiescent, so that low levels of LH and testosterone are characteristic of both simple delayed puberty and gonadotropin deficiency. Accordingly, differentiating these disorders in the endocrine laboratory has been problematic. During early puberty, however, LH secretion increases during nocturnal sleep, and testosterone levels rise in the early morning. Hourly blood sampling from 8 p.m. to 8 a.m. can be used to demonstrate normal pubertal changes in plasma LH and testosterone levels even before testis growth is observed. Because this approach to diagnosis is costly, the difference between a single early morning and evening testosterone level can instead be calculated. An increase from evening to morning values suggests early puberty. The plasma LH and testosterone response to GnRH-analog administration can also be examined. The LH response to GnRH stimulation increases during puberty. Although the LH response to native GnRH is attenuated or absent in GnRH-deficient men, it overlaps with the responses among prepubertal boys. GnRH analogs have a longer half-life than does native GnRH, and in delayed puberty GnRH-analog stimulation often produces a sustained LH rise for several hours followed by an increase in testosterone levels, but it produces no change in LH and testosterone in patients with complete HH. The responses in patients with incomplete GnRH deficiency will be similar to delayed puberty, however, and only longitudinal observation can presently distinguish these two conditions if no midline markers or other clinical findings are present.

PRIMARY TESTICULAR FAILURE

The many disorders that can damage the testis are subdivided into congenital and acquired disorders in Table 40.4. The symptoms and signs of primary testicular failure are usually gradual in onset, with the exception of orchitis, which like orchidectomy or GnRH-analog treatment, can produce vasomotor symptoms like those in menopausal women. The most constant physical finding in men with primary testicular failure is a decrease in the size of the testes.

Plasma levels of FSH and LH are characteristically elevated in men with primary testicular failure, and the testosterone concentration is usually reduced. Total testosterone levels are sometimes normal, however, because SHBG levels are increased. Bioavailable or free testosterone levels should be measured if the clinical findings suggest androgen deficiency, but the total testosterone level is normal. Because the seminiferous tubules are more sensitive to damage than are Leydig cells, tubular dysfunction with normal testosterone production may occur. Testosterone production may be sustained by increased LH concentrations, or both LH and testosterone may be normal, and FSH levels may be increased selectively. Decreased testosterone production results in elevated gonadotropin concentrations. LH concentration profiles in men with primary testicular failure are characterized by an increased number and amplitude of LH (and presumably GnRH) secretory episodes, indicating an effect on the GnRH pulse generator. Experiments in monkeys and cross-sectional studies in men have shown that a deficiency in the production of inhibin-B by the testes is responsible for the rise in FSH in selective seminiferous tubular failure.

Klinefelter's syndrome

Klinefelter's syndrome (KS) results from the presence of an extra Xchromosome that causes seminiferous tubular sclerosis and Leydig cell insufficiency. KS occurs in 1 per 500 to 1 per 2000 live male births. Meiotic nondisjunction leads to the formation of 23,XY sperm or to 23,XX ova. Fertilization results in a 47,XXY karyotype. The additional X is as likely to be of maternal as of paternal origin, but only advanced maternal age is a risk factor for the development of the syndrome. Nearly 20% of KS patients are 46,XY/47,XXY mosaics in whom the clinical abnormalities are less pronounced. Other reported sex chromosomal abnormalities include 48,XXYY, 48,XXXY and 49,XXXXY. In addition to testicular failure, these men are often short, dysmorphic, and mentally retarded.

Clinical findings

The clinical features of KS are summarized in Table 40.5. KS is sometimes diagnosed in teenagers who present with incomplete pubertal development, gynecomastia, or small testes. The remaining cases are detected in adulthood due to infertility and azoospermia. The testes are usually 1 to 2 ml in volume or <2 cm in length, and are somewhat firm. The amount of body hair is often reduced, especially if the patient is compared to male siblings, but hirsutism and frontal balding may occur. Gynecomastia is present in 30 to 75% of cases. The phallus may be slightly reduced in size but is normally formed, and cryptorchidism is unusual.

Virtually all men with KS are azoospermic. If sperm are present in the ejaculate, the karyotype is usually 46,XY/47,XXY. Testicular biopsy reveals that most seminiferous tubules are sclerotic, but a few tubules may contain Sertoli cells. The testis of the newborn with KS is believed to be normal, but the mean seminiferous tubule diameter and germ cell number is reduced slightly in prepubertal boys with KS. Extensive testicular damage occurs with the rise in gonadotropin production in puberty. Although there is an appearance of Leydig cell hyperplasia, the Leydig cell mass is normal. It remains to be determined whether Leydig cell dysfunction is a consequence of Sertoli cell or germ cell damage, or if it occurs through some other mechanism.

Men with KS are at increased risk for many pathological conditions (Tab. 40.6). There is a tendency to develop testicular or extragonadal germ cell tumors, particularly in the mediastinum. Accordingly, a chest X-ray should be performed if pulmonary symptoms occur in KS patients. Most of the cancers are nonseminomatous. There is an increased incidence of immune disorders such as systemic

---

Table 40.4 Causes of primary testicular failure

Congenital

Klinefelter's syndrome and variants
Cryptorchidism
Noonan's syndrome
Laurence-Moon-Bardet-Biedl syndrome
Congenital anorchia
Myotonic dystrophy
Sickle cell disease

Acquired

Orchitis: e.g., mumps, leprosy
Trauma
Torsion
Spinal cord injury
Retroperitoneal fibrosis
Cancer chemotherapy
X-irradiation

Table 40.5 Clinical features of Klinefelter's syndrome

Childhood	Adulthood
Small testes and penis	Small testes
Increased leg and arm length	Infertility
Decreased head circumference	Gynecomastia
	Long extremities
	Reduced body hair

Table 40.6 Disorders associated with Klinefelter's syndrome

Germ cell tumors: mediastinum, brain, testis
Immunological disorders: scleroderma, lupus, rheumatoid
  arthritis
Varicose veins and leg ulcers
Diabetes mellitus
Restrictive lung disease
Osteopenia
Hypopituitarism

lupus and scleroderma in KS patients. Hormonal factors may be responsible for this predisposition since immune disorders are far more common in normal women than in men. Leg ulcers sometimes begin in young adulthood, and varicose veins may be present. Platelet hypercoagulability or increased plasminogen activator inhibitor have been proposed to cause leg ulcers in KS. Bone density is lower than normal in KS. Reduced levels of osteocalcin and increased ratio of urinary hydroxyproline/creatinine suggest that bone formation is reduced and that absorption is increased. A few cases of coexistent Klinefelter's syndrome and hypopituitarism have been reported. As in other forms of long-standing untreated primary testicular failure, pituitary hyperplasia may occur, simulating a pituitary tumor. Massive obesity may contribute to reduced gonadotropin secretion in KS as well.

Treatment

Treatment of KS with testosterone is currently individualized based on the judgment and attitude of the physician. Testosterone replacement is generally recommended for adult men with symptomatic androgen deficiency. A case can be made for uniform testosterone replacement beginning in adolescence, however. The endocrine function of the hypothalamic-pituitary-testicular unit in KS is similar to that of post-menopausal women, and the organic and psychophysiological components of menopause may apply to teenagers with KS as well. Personality traits often noted in adolescents as well as adult men with KS include shyness, fatigability, low self-esteem, and learning and language disorders, which may all be improved by androgen replacement therapy. Moreover, low bone density in adult men with Klinefelter's syndrome is prevented by testosterone treatment prior to age 20 years, and other complications may benefit from androgen replacement as well. Further controlled studies of androgen replacement therapy in KS are needed.

Cryptorchidism

Cryptorchidism is a congenital anomaly with multiple causes, but most cases are idiopathic. Its prevalence is 2.5 to 5% at birth but declines to 1% by age 1 year because of delayed testicular descent. Approximately 10% of cryptorchid testes are intra-abdominal, 20% are within the inguinal canal, and the remainder are high in the scrotum. Many high scrotal testes are retractile; that is, a reflex pulls them out of the scrotum due to cold temperature or other stress, but they are scrotal when the patient is relaxed. The disorder is bilateral in 10 to 15% of cases. Recognized causes of cryptorchidism are listed in Table 40.7. Cryptorchidism occurs in androgen-deficient men with GnRH deficiency or androgen biosynthetic defects, and in androgen resistance syndromes. The persistent Müllerian duct syndrome is sometimes associated with undescended testes, as are structural anomalies of the abdominal wall and neurological defects such as meningomyelocele. This heterogeneity of pathophysiology and gonadal location leads to variable testicular function.

The most important clinical consequences of cryptorchidism are infertility and malignancy. Gonocytes in the cryptorchid testis degenerate in early childhood rather than undergo normal transformation to type A spermatogonia. Accordingly, orchidopexy is almost always performed in early childhood. The percentage of married men with a history of unilateral cryptorchidism who report fathering children has ranged from 60 to 90%, whereas only 13 to 60% of men with bilateral cryptorchidism are fertile. There does not appear to be any relationship between the age of orchidopexy and fertility. Plasma FSH levels are generally increased in those men with severe oligospermia and small testes. Plasma LH and testosterone levels are usually normal, but mean basal and peak GnRH-stimulated LH levels are slightly higher than normal, suggesting subtle Leydig cell dysfunction.

Cryptorchidism is the most important risk factor for germ cell carcinoma of the testis, with approximately 10% of testicular cancer patients reporting a history of an undescended testis. Estimates of the increased risk of developing testicular cancer with unilateral cryptorchidism have ranged from 2.7- to 5.8-fold above that of the general population, whereas the cancer risk with bilateral cryptorchidism is substantially greater. From another perspective, however, surveillance data suggests that only 1% of patients who undergo orchidopexy subsequently develop a testicular neoplasm. Approximately 80% of the testicular cancers occur before age 40 years. The pathophysiology of testicular cancer with cryptorchidism is uncertain, since at times the tumor develops in the scrotal testis, and case reports of extra-gonadal germ cell cancers

Table 40.7 Causes of cryptorchidism

Gonadal dysgenesis
Hypogonadotropic hypogonadism
Testosterone biosynthesis defects
Androgen resistance syndromes
Abdominal wall defects
Multiple congenital malformations
Meningomyelocele

in men with cryptorchidism have also been published. Orchidopexy below age 10 years may reduce the subsequent cancer risk.

Germinal aplasia

Germinal aplasia is a histological finding that was first described by Del Castillo in 1947 in azoospermic men. The subjects of that report were well-virilized, healthy men with scrotal testes that were reduced in size, although the size of the testes may have been normal. Testicular biopsies may reveal foci of preserved spermatogenesis, even though by definition most tubules contain only Sertoli cells. Germinal aplasia is a syndrome with multiple etiologies (Tab. 40.8). The most common cause is presently cancer chemotherapy. Approximately 10% of men with germinal aplasia have mutations of genes on the Y chromosome that are required for normal spermatogenesis. Serum FSH levels are almost always elevated, but LH and testosterone levels are generally within the normal range.

Miscellaneous causes of testicular failure

Testicular failure involving both the seminiferous tubules and Leydig cells occurs in patients with orchitis. Clinical infection of the testis occurs in 15 to 35% of adult men with mumps. In severe cases, distension of the testes with leukocytes is followed by necrosis and atrophy. Epididymo-orchitis is a recognized complication of gonorrhea. Leprosy, tuberculosis, brucellosis, nocardia, salmonella, schistosomiasis, filariasis and syphilis may affect the testes as well. Torsion of the testes in adolescents and testicular trauma may result in testicular atrophy. Autoimmune testicular failure may occur in polyendocrine deficiency types 1 and 2, although males are much less frequently affected than are females. Testicular failure has also been reported in men with idiopathic retroperitoneal fibrosis or scleroderma.

SYSTEMIC DISORDERS PRODUCING HYPOGONADISM

Critical illness

Hypogonadism is common in critical illness. Surgery with general anesthesia, head trauma, burn trauma, and myocardial infarction have been associated with suppressed plasma LH and testosterone levels within 24 hours, and the magnitude of suppression is related to disease severity. In fact, among intensive care unit patients, a very low testosterone level is a predictor of mortality. Stress-induced increases in corticotropin-releasing factor, cortisol, opioid peptides, and prolactin may decrease GnRH secretion. Pain, drugs, and nutritional factors may also contribute to gonadotropin suppression. Recent experimental studies indicate that the testicular level of

Table 40.8 Causes of germinal aplasia
Cancer chemotherapy
Chronic renal failure
Y chromosome mutations
Cryptorchidism
Androgen insensitivity syndromes
Testicular irradiation
Idiopathic

steroidogenesis acute regulatory protein (StAR), a protein thought to transport cholesterol to the inner mitochondria for conversion to pregnenolone, is rapidly decreased following endotoxin injection, providing a testicular mechanism for low testosterone levels observed in acute illness.

Chronic illnesses including cancer, AIDS, inflammatory bowel disease, and anorexia nervosa may produce male hypogonadism. In addition to the stress-related mechanisms discussed above, relative caloric deprivation is likely to play a role in the hypogonadism of chronic illness. Fasting for 48 hours lowers plasma testosterone and LH levels in normal men. The LH response to GnRH stimulation is preserved or enhanced with short-term fasting, indicating GnRH deficiency. The secretory pattern of GnRH deficiency remains controversial, however, since a decrease in LH pulse amplitude and a decrease in LH pulse frequency have been alternatively reported. Neuropeptide Y, which stimulates feeding and gonadotropin secretion, gut peptides such as cholecystokinin, leptin, as well as glucose and insulin are each candidates for the nutrition signal to GnRH release.

Exercise

Intense exercise is an established cause of reproductive dysfunction in women, but abnormalities also occur in men. Short-term intensive exercise is associated with a rise in testosterone levels, which appears to be due to hemoconcentration and to a decrease in testosterone clearance. Several hours after heavy exercise serum testosterone levels decline, however the fall can be prevented by treatment with a GnRH analog, suggesting decreased GnRH production. With prolonged intensive physical exercise associated with weight loss and sleep deprivation, very low testosterone and reduced LH levels are observed. On the other hand, testosterone levels are generally normal in trained marathon runners, although men who develop an abnormally low body mass index (<20 kg/m^2) may develop HH.

Obesity

Testosterone levels are frequently reduced in obese men. Much of the decrease is due to low SHBG levels, but free and non-SHBG-bound testosterone concentrations are also reduced in massive obesity. LH levels are normal in moderate obesity but may be low in the massively obese.

The limited information available suggests that sperm production is normal in obese men. Hyperinsulinemia due to peripheral insulin resistance with visceral obesity is believed to suppress SHBG production, but the explanation for gonadotropin deficiency is less certain. With dieting and weight loss, estrone levels decline as testosterone levels increase, suggesting that increased estrogen production could play a role in the gonadotropin suppression, although individual cases have not demonstrated an inverse relationship between testosterone and estrone levels. Because testosterone treatment reduces triglyceride production, and may decrease the waist-to-hip ratio reducing the cardiovascular risk in obese men, some authors have advocated testosterone replacement therapy for massively obese men.

Thyroid disease

Hyperthyroid men sometimes develop gynecomastia, depressed sperm count and/or sperm motility, and a decline in libido and potency. Thyroxine stimulates SHBG gene expression, and therefore hyperthyroxinemia increases plasma SHBG levels. Elevated levels of SHBG may increase the total plasma testosterone sufficient to produce hypertestosteronemia. Plasma LH levels are also elevated, and FSH levels may rise. Increased production of SHBG may produce a transient decline in circulating bioavailable (free + albumen-bound) testosterone levels, which results in increased LH secretion. With this resetting in negative feedback control, an increased LH drive restores the bioavailable testosterone level to normal. An alternative explanation for elevated LH and FSH levels in hyperthyroid men is mild Leydig cell dysfunction. The blunted testosterone response to hCG stimulation in hyperthyroid men is consistent with this interpretation of the hormone profile.

The increased LH drive in hyperthyroid men also stimulates the aromatase gene in Leydig cells to increase estradiol production. Plasma estradiol levels in hyperthyroid men may be as high as those of normal women in the mid-follicular phase of the menstrual cycle. Peripheral aromatization of androstenedione to estrone, and testosterone to estradiol, were also found to be increased in men with hyperthyroidism. Abnormal values normalize with treatment of hyperthyroidism.

Testicular dysfunction may occur more commonly among men with untreated primary hypothyroidism than in the general population. In addition, case reports describing pituitary enlargement, hyperprolactinemia, and hypogonadism in men with severe long-standing hypothyroidism have been published, although most cases have been in women.

Alcoholic liver disease

Hypogonadism is common in men with chronic alcoholic liver disease. Among the symptoms and signs often observed are a decline in libido and potency, infertility, reduced body hair, testicular atrophy, oligo- or azoospermia, and gynecomastia. Several factors contribute to the hypogonadism in alcoholic liver disease. Serum levels of testosterone are reduced, and LH and FSH are generally elevated. This primary testicular failure has been attributed to a toxic effect of alcohol on the testes, perhaps via a decrease in steroidogenic enzyme activity. SHBG levels are elevated, further reducing the bioavailable testosterone level and contributing to the rise in LH and FSH. Increased estradiol secretion through LH stimulation of testicular aromatase, together with increased production of corticotropin-releasing factor-ACTH, and androstenedione from the adrenal, which can be converted in peripheral tissues to estrone and estradiol, lead to feminization. Sick and nutritionally deprived alcoholic men may develop severe hypogonadism due to superimposed gonadotropin deficiency. Hyperprolactinemia may also occur. Cessation of drinking or liver transplantation improves the endocrine status of these men.

Non-alcoholic liver disease

Testicular dysfunction occurs in men with non-alcoholic liver disease as well. Low testosterone and normal LH levels suggest hypothalamic-pituitary dysfunction. Unlike most cases of alcoholic liver disease, LH pulsatile secretion is blunted. Increased SHBG is believed to reflect hepatic injury, but the precise mechanism is unknown. The extent of the disturbance correlates with the severity of the liver disease. The hypogonadism of hemochromatosis may be particularly severe, with testosterone levels as low as those of male castrates. In fact, decreased libido is an early symptom of hemochromatosis that may precede skin changes, diabetes mellitus, cardiomyopathy, or liver disease. Iron deposition in the hypothalamus and pituitary is the presumed cause of HH in these men. SHBG and estradiol levels tend to be normal, and gynecomastia is uncommon. These findings are applicable to chronic iron overload from multiple transfusions as well as to the heredofamilial disorder. Intensive phlebotomy may reverse the hypogonadism but results are conflicting. Partial improvement occurs following liver transplantation. The consequences of hypogonadism in men with liver disease, such as loss of muscle mass, osteopenia and anemia, are pronounced.

Chronic renal insufficiency

Testicular dysfunction is common in men with chronic renal insufficiency even with effective dialysis. The extent of the hypogonadism is variable, and the disorder is multifactorial. Impotence, infertility, testicular atrophy, hypospermatogenesis, and gynecomastia are common in these men, and delayed puberty is generally observed in teenage boys with the same disorder. Chronic illness and the medications used to treat chronic renal insufficiency contribute to the endocrine disturbance. Primary testicular failure is suggested in some men by low testosterone and elevated LH and FSH concentrations, and by a blunted rise in testosterone levels following hCG stimulation. Decreased gonadotropin clearance may contribute to these findings, however. Selective elevation in LH levels may have reflected cross-reactivity of gonadotropin α-subunit in double antibody LH assays. The gonadotropin α-subunit and inhibin α-subunit accumulate in plasma in chronic renal insufficiency because these polypeptides are predominantly cleared by renal mechanisms. In other men, reduced total and free testosterone and normal LH levels, or spontaneous LH secretory episodes of reduced amplitude, suggest impaired gonadotropin secretion. Hyperprolactinemia may be present. Hypogonadism can be reversed by successful transplantation, but with prolonged dialysis and the use of chemotherapeutic drugs, hypospermatogenesis may be permanent.

Neurological disorders

Myotonic muscular dystrophy is an autosomal disorder characterized by weakness, myotonia, frontal baldness, cataracts, cardiac arrhythmias, insulin resistance, and primary testicular insufficiency. Mean serum FSH and LH levels are increased and testosterone is reduced, but many affected men have normal testicular function. The disease results from an expansion of CTG trinucleotide repeats in the 3' untranslated region of the myotonin protein kinase (Mt-PK) gene on chromosome 19, leading to reduced Mt-PK gene expression. Mt-PK is presumed to participate in a signal transduction pathway, but the relevance of this abnormality to reduced testicular function remains unknown.

Spinal and bulbar muscular atrophy (Kennedy disease) is an X-linked disorder in which men present with progressive muscular fasciculations, weakness, and atrophy, beginning at age 20 to 40 years. Although fertile as young adults, affected men develop gynecomastia, hypospermatogenesis, and androgen deficiency as they grow older. The observation that both serum LH and testosterone levels are elevated suggest androgen resistance. Affected patients have an expansion of the CAG trinucleotide repeat, which codes for glutamine, in the first exon of the 5' flanking region of the androgen receptor gene. Normal alleles have 17 to 26 CAG repeats, whereas patients with spinal and bulbar muscular atrophy have 40 to 52 repeats. Earlier onset and severity of disease, as well as extent of androgen resistance, correlate positively with longer CAG repeats. The expansion of the glutamine region of the AR amino terminus leads to impaired transactivation of androgen responsive genes. AR are present in spinal and bulbar motor neurons, but the link between the AR abnormality and the neurological disease is presently unknown.

Adrenomyeloneuropathy is a peroxisomal disorder in which very long chain fatty acids accumulate in plasma and in various tissues including the spinal cord and peripheral nerves, and in endocrine cells. The disorder is X-linked, and presents in late adolescence or early adulthood, usually with spasticity. Primary adrenal failure and testicular failure may occur.

Respiratory insufficiency

Patients with sleep apnea have daytime sleepiness and episodes of nighttime breathing cessation followed by heavy snoring. Obstructive sleep apnea, characterized by narrowing of the hypopharynx, is often observed in obese men, and it is associated with sexual dysfunction. Several studies found low total and free testosterone but normal LH levels in these men, and they concluded that the hormonal findings cannot be explained entirely by obesity. Moreover, continuous positive airway pressure treatment may improve testosterone deficiency not only in men with sleep apnea, but also in men with chronic obstructive pulmonary disease of other etiologies, although the link between hypoxia and testosterone deficiency is unclear. There is a suggestion that testosterone treatment worsens sleep apnea by increasing oxygen consumption or reducing hypoxic respiratory drive.

Delayed sexual maturation is common in patients with cystic fibrosis in whom hypoxia, poor nutrition, malabsorption, and hypercortisolemia may decrease GnRH secretion. Obstructive azoospermia, due to congenital bilateral agenesis of the vas deferens (CBAVD) is a common clinical finding in adult men with cystic fibrosis. Genetic testing of healthy men with CBAVD may also reveal cystic fibrosis. The cystic fibrosis transmembrane regulator gene (CFTR), which codes for a phosphorylation activated calcium channel, is expressed in the epithelium of the epididymis and vas deferens, and in germ cells, although the pathogenesis of male genital tract damage is uncertain. Obstructive azoospermia also occurs in patients with mucociliary transport disorders producing bronchitis and bronchiectasis (Young's syndrome) and in the immotile cilia (Kartagener's) syndrome.

Diabetes mellitus

Erectile and ejaculatory function are often abnormal in men with diabetes mellitus, but these long-term complications of diabetes are thought to be due to neuropathy and to vascular disease. The majority of men with well-controlled insulin-dependent diabetes mellitus (IDDM) have normal endocrine testicular function, although some men have elevated FSH and LH levels of uncertain etiology. Low testosterone levels in men with IDDM during ketoacidosis, which presumably result from the stress of acute illness, normalize within a few days of insulin treatment. Insulin suppresses plasma SHBG, and men with non-insulin-dependent diabetes mellitus (NIDDM) may have low total testosterone levels due to reduced SHBG, whereas free or bioavailable testosterone levels are generally in the normal range. In fact, low total testosterone and SHBG levels together with hyperinsulinemia predict the development of NIDDM. Secondary diabetes may be associated with hypogonadism in hemochromatosis, polyglandular endocrine failure, Prader-Willi syndrome, Laurence-Moon-Bardet-Biedl syndrome, acromegaly, Cushing's syndrome, myotonic dystrophy, and alcohol-related pancreatitis.

Congenital adrenal hyperplasia

Deficiency of steroid 21-hydroxylase leads to increased androgen production by the adrenal cortex. Some men with inadequate treatment for this congenital adrenal hyperplasia have presented with infertility, small testes, oligo- or azoospermia, and reduced circulating LH and FSH levels. Chronic suppression of gonadotropin secretion by adrenal androgens is the likely explanation for this condition. Adequate replacement with gluco- and mineralocorticoids may restore spermatogenesis to normal. Interestingly, other male patients with 21-hydroxylase deficiency who receive inadequate hormone replacement maintain normal sperm production.

Bilateral testicular tumors may also occur with inadequate treatment of 21-hydroxylase deficiency. These tumors are in the form of multiple irregular hard nodules, measuring 1 to 2 cm in diameter, that develop from adrenal rests within the testes. Spermatic vein levels of adrenal-specific 11β-hydroxysteroids, including cortisol, are increased, indicating functional adrenal fasciculata within the testis. If replacement therapy remains insufficient, the normal architecture of the testis may be destroyed, which would result in an elevated plasma FSH level and infertility. Bilateral testis tumors have also been reported in men with ACTH-producing pituitary adenomas following bilateral adrenalectomy (Nelson's syndrome).

GYNECOMASTIA

Gynecomastia, the enlargement of the male breast, results from an increase in glandular tissue, stroma, and fat. Transient gynecomastia is common in newborn and pubertal males in whom it presents as a small firm subareolar mass that may be tender. Enlargement of the breast is also common among elderly men. Gynecomastia is most often bilateral but asymmetrical. Unilateral breast enlargement in older men could represent a malignancy, and a biopsy should be performed. Breast enlargement occurs if estrogens are increased, or with androgen deficiency, even if estrogens are normal. Breast enlargement is generally a benign condition but rarely is the first sign of an aggressive hCG-producing neoplasm. The conditions associated with gynecomastia are listed in Table 40.9.

Medications often cause gynecomastia. Some drugs such as hCG, clomiphene, and antiandrogens such as flutamide and spironolactone increase estrogen production. Antineoplastic agents, which damage the testis and increase gonadotropin secretion, may produce gynecomastia via this mechanism. Antiandrogens may also directly block the inhibitory effect of androgens on breast tissue. Other drugs have estrogenic properties or contain estrogens as a contaminant, such as lotions used by morticians. Ketoconazole reduces testosterone production. Case reports describing breast enlargement with a variety of other drugs have been published, but the mechanisms are uncertain.

The gynecomastia of adolescence, which most often resolves, sometimes persists into adulthood without apparent cause, and is termed pubertal or idiopathic gynecomastia. A few patients have a mild testosterone biosynthesis defect or androgen insensitivity syndrome leading to an imbalance between estrogens and androgens but without ambiguous genitalia. Obesity may also con-

tribute to pubertal gynecomastia because fat tissue expresses the aromatase gene. Some authors have proposed that exposure to environmental toxins with estrogenic or antiandrogenic properties leads to pubertal gynecomastia.

Treatment of long-standing gynecomastia, which is embarrassing to the patient, is surgical. The results of plastic surgery using liposuction are generally excellent, with no skin depression or nipple deformity. Even when an etiology can be identified and corrected, breast enlargement may not regress. Medical management of recent-onset gynecomastia using antiestrogens, the progestin danazol, the aromatase inhibitor testolactone, or the non-aromatizable dihydrotestosterone may be effective, but reports are conflicting.

Treatment of hypogonadal men

Androgen replacement therapy

With very few exceptions, all hypogonadal men should receive androgen replacement therapy. Parenteral, oral,

Table 40.9 Conditions associated with gynecomastia

Physiological
  Newborn
  Puberty
  Aging
Neoplasms
  Steroid-producing (testis and adrenal)
  hCG-producing (germ cell tumors and hepatomas)
Primary testicular failure
Hypogonadotropic hypogonadism
Refeeding after starvation
Chest wall injury
Testosterone biosynthetic defects
Androgen resistance syndromes
True hermaphroditism
Systemic disorders
  Thyrotoxicosis
  Alcoholic liver disease
  Hepatitis
  Chronic renal insufficiency
Medications
  Hormones: estrogens, androgens, hCG
  Antiestrogens: clomiphene, tamoxifen
  Androgen antagonists or inhibitors, flutamide, cyproterone, spironolactone, ketoconazole
  Antiulcer drugs: cimetidine, *omeprazole*
  Cardiovascular drugs: amiodarone, *captopril*, digitoxin, *diltiazem, enalapril, methyldopa, nifedipine, reserpine*
  Chemotherapeutic agents: alkylating agents, methotrexate
  Psychoactive drugs: *haloperidol, phenothiazines, tricyclic antidepressants*
  Street drugs: *opiates, marijuana*, alcohol
Idiopathic

(For drugs in italics, the link to gynecomastia is incompletely established.)

and transdermal androgens are currently available, and other products are under investigation.

The most commonly used androgen replacement therapy is intramuscular depot injections of testosterone esters. Esterification increases the lipid solubility of testosterone producing a depot. The esters are converted to free testosterone in the circulation. Testosterone enanthate and testosterone cypionate are available in an oil suspension and have equivalent pharmacokinetics. Although it is important that dosages be adjusted to meet the needs of the individual patient, the usual dosage for adults is 150-200 mg administered every 10 to 14 days. Pediatric patients generally receive 50-100 mg monthly initially, increasing to 50-100 mg every 2 weeks. This is followed by further gradual increases to the adult dose. Testosterone propionate has a short duration of action of 2 to 3 days, and has limited clinical usefulness. In some countries a mixture of testosterone esters composed of 30 mg of propionate, 60 mg of phenylpropionate, 60 mg of isocaproate, and 100 mg of decanoate per 250 mg is available.

The clinical response to intramuscular injections is quite good. Drawbacks of the intramuscular route of administration are the pain and discomfort of intramuscular injections, and the high levels of serum testosterone and estradiol for several days after injection, which fall to subnormal levels at the end of the dosing interval. This pharmacokinetic profile may be accompanied by a fluctuation in sexual function, energy level, and mood. High levels of testosterone may predispose a patient to acne and polycythemia, and may adversely affect the lipid profile. Elevated estradiol levels may cause gynecomastia. Many patients can be taught to self-administer depot androgens. Other patients do not choose this option, but instead travel to a physician's office or clinic for their treatment, which is both expensive and inconvenient.

Methyltestosterone and fluoxymesterone are alkylated derivatives of testosterone for oral or sublingual use. Alkylated androgens are more slowly metabolized by the liver than is natural testosterone, but like testosterone these androgens interact directly with androgen receptors. Although their oral route of administration is advantageous, the clinical response is variable, and plasma levels cannot be determined because alkylated androgens are not recognized by most testosterone assays. These drugs are no longer used in certain countries because of the potential for hepatotoxicity. Moreover, alkylated androgens increase low density lipoprotein (LDL) and suppress high density lipoprotein (HDL) cholesterol levels.

Testosterone undecanoate is absorbed from the gastrointestinal tract into the circulation via the lymphatic system because of the aliphatic side chain and encapsulation with arachnois oil. It is de-esterified in the circulation to testosterone. Peak levels are achieved 4 to 6 hours after dosing with a return to baseline by 12 hours. Usual clinical doses are 80-240 mg/day in two divided doses. Absorption of testosterone undecanoate is quite variable and may depend upon the fat content of the diet. Flatulence may occur, but hepatotoxicity is rare.

The skin absorbs drugs, including steroid hormones, into the systemic circulation at a controlled rate, avoiding the high and low levels observed with long-acting testosterone esters. Scrotal skin was selected initially for use because it is at least five times more permeable to testosterone than are other skin sites. High levels of dihydrotachysterol (DHT), the need to shave scrotal skin regularly, deattachment with exercise and hot weather have limited the use of this product.

Nonscrotal transdermal systems for the delivery of testosterone have now been developed. Each system delivers approximately 5 mg of testosterone over 24 hours. The systems produce continuously normal plasma levels of both testosterone and estradiol. Patients using these systems report substantially improved sexual function, including the achievement of potency, and an improvement in sense of well-being, mood, and energy. With the product containing an enhancing vehicle, mild to moderate redness, blisters, and pruritus may occur in approximately 50% of men. A generalized allergic contact dermatitis may also develop. The tendency toward skin irritation can be reduced by applying the system to the lower back, thigh, lower abdomen, and upper arm, and avoiding areas of bony prominence and less subcutaneous tissue. Applying 0.1% triamcinolone cream to the application site before applying the patch may also reduce skin irritation.

Testosterone pellets, which are currently in use in the United Kingdom and in Australia, consist of 3-6 200 mg testosterone pellets that are implanted subcutaneously every 4 to 6 months. Pellets do not produce the bimonthly swings in plasma testosterone levels and mood changes that some patients find objectionable. The need to introduce the pellets with a trocar, and the occurrence of pellet extrusion in 5 to 10% of patients limit the acceptability of this approach.

In addition to the marketed formulations for androgen replacement therapy discussed above, other formulations are under investigation. Testosterone has been complexed with 2-hydroxypropyl-β-cyclodextrin, to be administered sublingually at a dosage of either 2.5 or 5.0 mg 3 to 4 times per day. Two long-acting intramuscular formulations of testosterone are also currently under investigation. Testosterone microspheres, consisting of unmodified testosterone encapsulated in a biodegradable copolymer, are injected every 11 to 12 weeks, resulting in near zero-order release of testosterone at a rate of about 6 mg per day. Testosterone buciclate, a long-acting 17β-hydroxyl ester of testosterone, is administered intramuscularly at a dosage of 600 mg every 12 weeks.

Adverse effects of androgen treatment Androgen replacement therapy is straightforward and almost always successful, and it is usually very well tolerated. Some adverse effects of androgen replacement therapy occur, however. Most side-effects are dose-dependent, and a few are formulation-specific. Acne results when sebum production by sebaceous glands is increased by testosterone and the sebum is ingested by bacteria, leading to inflammation. Sebum production is upregulated in part through dihydrotestosterone produced locally by type 1 5α-reductase. Weight gain and edema may occur with androgen treatment, especially in patients with underlying edematous states, such as congestive heart failure, hepatic cirrhosis, and nephrotic syndrome, although the mechanism for androgen-induced salt and water retention is poorly understood. Androgens stimulate erythropoiesis, occasionally resulting in polycythemia. In many instances, men who develop erythrocytosis have a second disorder, such as sleep apnea or polycythemia vera. Testosterone treatment may also predispose to sleep apnea by decreasing hypercapnic ventilatory drive. Androgen-stimulated prostate growth may lead to prostatism, including urinary obstruction. Priapism, a prolonged painful erection, is a urological emergency that often leads to life-long erectile dysfunction. Priapism is a rare complication of high-dose testosterone treatment; patients with sickle cell disease are predisposed to this condition. Some patients receiving injections of testosterone esters experience emotional lability and excessive stimulation of libido. Because injected testosterone is converted to estradiol, gynecomastia occurs in testosterone-treated men.

Male breast cancer and known or suspected prostate carcinoma are contraindications to androgen replacement therapy. Before beginning androgen treatment, after 3 and 6 months of therapy, and yearly thereafter, the possibility of prostate carcinoma should be evaluated by digital rectal examination and a serum prostate-specific antigen level. If an abnormality is detected, the patient should undergo a transrectal sonogram and a biopsy of suspicious regions. Follow-up studies of hypogonadal men undergoing androgen replacement therapy reveal that prostate volume and prostate-specific antigen levels are stimulated from the depressed level associated with the hypogonadal state to levels comparable to those of age-matched normal men.

Androgen derivatives are potentially hepatotoxic. Cholestasis with mild elevations of transaminases occurs in 2 to 3% of patients treated with methylated androgens and is usually reversible after androgens are discontinued. Clinical jaundice has occurred. Peliosis hepatis, the development of blood-filled spaces within the liver, presents with hepatic enlargement and tenderness. Rupture of the cysts can result in death. Hepatocellular adenoma and carcinoma occur much more often than expected with 17-alkylated androgen use.

HDL cholesterol is reduced and LDL cholesterol is increased in patients treated with 17α-alkylated androgens. Both the oral route of administration and the lack of bioconversion of these androgens to estradiol contribute to these changes. The reduction in HDL cholesterol may result from an increase in hepatic triglyceride lipase to stimulate HDL catabolism. By contrast, physiologic replacement doses of natural testosterone do not produce clinically significant effects on lipid levels, although higher doses also suppress HDL cholesterol.

Anabolic-androgenic steroid use and abuse Androgens in high doses are used illegally for their anabolic actions by professional athletes, body builders and others because they increase muscle size and strength, although for many years the medical and scientific community thought otherwise. Various combinations of testosterone and its deriva-

tives and hCG are used (stacking), and the drugs are administered intermittently (cycling) with intervals of non-treatment timed to coincide with competitions, since detection in plasma or urine would cause disqualification from the athletic event (see Chap. 73). Because the androgens are used in very high dosage, there are many sideeffects, including edema, acne, and gynecomastia. Spermatogenesis is reduced. Cycling may cause emotional lability and fluctuating libido. The prevalence of long-term adverse effects such as hepatocellular carcinoma and coronary artery disease because of suppressed levels of HDL cholesterol levels remains to be established.

Gonadotropin therapy

The standard treatment to stimulate sperm production in gonadotropin-deficient men is with human chorionic gonadotropin (hCG) alone or in combination with human menopausal gonadotropins (hMG) as a source of FSH. There are few large series reported, and fewer controlled studies, so that treatment guidelines are subjective. Because of the higher cost and need for frequent injections with hCG, virilization is usually accomplished with testosterone, and hCG is employed when fertility is desired. Prior treatment with testosterone does not adversely affect responsiveness to hCG.

Human chorionic gonadotropin is used to stimulate Leydig cells, since high levels of intratesticular testosterone and perhaps other hCG-stimulated Leydig cell products are required for quantitatively normal spermatogenesis. Human chorionic gonadotropin, rather than LH, is used because it has a longer circulating half-life. The preparations of hCG in clinical use have been purified from pregnancy urine, although recombinant hCG is currently being evaluated. Doses of 1000 to 1500 U 2 or 3 times weekly subcutaneously or intramuscularly will usually maintain serum testosterone levels within the range of normal. Some patients find the former route of administration to be less painful. Side effects such as acne and weight gain are similar to those of testosterone. Gynecomastia is more common than with testosterone because hCG stimulates Leydig cell aromatase. Therefore, the plasma level of estradiol as well as testosterone is monitored. Rarely, an allergic response to hCG occurs, or neutralizing antibodies develop. To prevent these complications, the usual recommendation is to avoid intermittent treatment. Human chorionic gonadotropin stimulates growth of the testes, and careful monitoring of the testis size is helpful in predicting the spermatogenic response to treatment. Selected patients with hypogonadotropic hypogonadism may produce sperm and successfully impregnate their partners when treated with hCG alone, including men with adult onset HH (e.g., pituitary tumor patients), and those with congenital partial GnRH deficiency (pretreatment testis size >4 ml). Human chorionic gonadotropin may also maintain spermatogenesis in men in whom spermatogenesis was initiated with the combination of hCG and FSH. If the patient remains azoospermic after 12 months of hCG treatment, however, FSH should be added to the regimen.

Most men with complete HH (pretreatment testis size <4 ml) require the combination of hCG and FSH. Human chorionic gonadotropin is begun first in these men to increase the intratesticular level of testosterone and Leydig cell proteins, and the plasma levels of testosterone and estradiol are monitored. Generally, if after 6 months of hCG treatment the size of the testes remains <10 ml and the subject remains azoospermic, FSH is added to the regimen. The usual beginning dose of FSH is 75 IU every other day. To minimize the number of injections, hCG and FSH can be mixed in the same syringe. FSH alone does not stimulate spermatogenesis. Although FSH has been produced from the urine of post-menopausal women (hMG), recombinant human FSH is now available in selected markets, and it should soon be widely available. Because the maturation of spermatogonia to sperm takes about 70 days in men, sperm generally do not appear in the ejaculate for 3 to 6 months. If after 6 months of combination treatment the patient remains azoospermic, the dose of FSH can be increased to 150 IU. FSH is generally well-tolerated. The mixture of hCG and FSH may produce higher plasma levels of testosterone and estradiol than does hCG alone, permitting a reduction in the dose of hCG.

The sperm output among hCG/FSH-treated men is quite variable, ranging from 1 to 60 million/ml, with an average value of about 5 million/ml. Lower values are observed in men with complete GnRH deficiency. The inability to stimulate quantitatively normal spermatogenesis in these patients has been proposed to result from gonadotropin deficiency during the newborn and prepubertal periods of life resulting in impaired Sertoli cell development. The sperm quality (motility and morphology) is usually normal during treatment with hCG/FSH. If not, a secondary cause for infertility may be present.

Overall the pregnancy rate ranges from 50 to 80% with gonadotropin therapy, but patients with a history of cryptorchidism tend to respond less well. If pregnancy occurs, FSH can be discontinued, but hCG is maintained until delivery since miscarriage could occur. Thereafter if the couple does not want to conceive additional children, hCG is discontinued and testosterone replacement is resumed. Otherwise hCG treatment is maintained.

Gonadotropin-releasing hormone

Pulsatile GnRH therapy can be used to stimulate spermatogenesis in men with GnRH deficiency and normal pituitary function. This approach is more physiological because it reproduces the normal pulsatile pattern of LH and FSH release from the pituitary. A starting dose of 4 μg per pulse delivered every 2 hours into the subcutaneous tissue of the abdomen is often used, with increases of 2 μg every 2 weeks if LH secretion does not rise, up to a maximum dose of 20 μg per pulse. Serum testosterone levels are usually normal within 1 to 2 months, and the testes increase in size within 3 to 6 months after beginning therapy. Up to 2 years of treatment may be needed before sperm appear in the ejaculate, however. Similar to hCG/hMG therapy, the final testicular volume and sperm count are greater, and the time to first appearance of sperm in the ejaculate is less, among men with partial GnRH deficiency compared to those with complete GnRH deficiency. The sperm density generally increases to 1 to 10 million/ml in complete and 50 to 100 million/ml in partial GnRH deficiency. The data available suggest that GnRH-treatment stimulates spermatogenesis more rapidly than does gonadotropins, but that the maximum sperm output is similar for both therapies among GnRH-deficient men. Elevated estradiol levels and gynecomastia are less common with pulsatile GnRH than with hCG. Given the complexity and inconvenience of pulsatile GnRH, however, it is recommended as initial therapy only for highly motivated patients, and it is used for hCG/FSH non-responders.

Suggested readings

BRAUNSTEIN, GD. Gynecomastia. N Engl J Med 1993;328:490-5.

BAGATELL CJ, BREMNER WJ. Androgens in men - uses and abuses. N Engl J Med 1996;334:707-14.

CHILVERS C, DUDLEY NE, GOUGH MH, JACKSON MB, PIKE MC. Undescended testis: the effect of treatment on subsequent risk of subfertility and malignancy. J Pediatr Surg 1986;21:691-6.

CLAYTON RN. Molecular genetics, hypogonadism and luteinizing hormone. Clin Endocrinol 1992;37:201-2.

CONWAY GS. Clinical manifestations of genetic disorders affecting gonadotrophins and their receptors. Clin Endocrinol 1996;45:657-63.

GIAGULLI VA, KAUFMAN JM, VERMEULEN A. Pathogenesis of the decreased androgen levels in obese men. J Clin Endocrinol Metab 1994;79:997-1000.

HABIBY RL, BOEPPLE P, NACHTIGALL L, SLUSS PM, CROWLEY WF JR, JAMESON JL. Adrenal hypoplasia congenita with hypogonadotropic hypogonadism: evidence that DAX-1 mutations lead to combined hypothalamic and pituitary defects in gonadotropin production. J Clin Invest 1996;98:1055-62.

HASLE H, MELLEMGAARD A, NIELSEN J, HANSEN J. Cancer incidence in men with Klinefelter syndrome. Br J Cancer 1995;71:416-20.

LUTZ B, RUGARLI EI, EICHELE G, BALLABIO A. X-linked Kallmann syndrome. A neuronal targeting defect in the olfactory system? FEBS Lett 1993;325:128-34.

SCHOPOHL J. Pulsatile gonadotropin releasing hormone verus gonadotrophin treatment of hypothalamic hypogonadism in males. Hum Reprod 8 Suppl 1993;2:175-9.

SEMPLE CG, GRAY CE, BEASTALL GH. Male hypogonadism – a nonspecific consequence of illness. Quart J Med 1987;64:601-7.

STYNE DM: Puberty and its disorders in boys. Endocrinol Metab Clin North Am 1991;20:43-69.

WHITCOMB RW, CROWLEY WF JR. Male hypogonadotropic hypogonadism. Endocrinol Metab Clin North Am 1993;22:125-43.

WINTERS SJ, BERGA SL. Reproductive disorders in thyroid disease. The Endocrinologist 1997;7:167-73.

Male infertility

Giovanni Forti

▌ KEY POINTS ▌

- Medical history, physical examination, and testicular volume assessment are the keystones of the clinical evaluation of the infertile male. The measurement of plasma follicle-stimulating hormone is the most important hormonal parameter, as it is significantly related to the entity of seminiferous tubule damage. Recent data suggest that inhibin B levels seem to be inversely related with follicle-stimulating hormone levels.
- Several studies demonstrated that in 5 to 15% of men with tubular azoospermia or severe oligozoospermia, microdeletions of the long arm of the Y chromosome are present.
- The congenital bilateral absence of the vas deferens can now be considered a mild form of cystic fibrosis, and testing for cystic fibrosis transmembrane conductance regulator gene mutations should be performed in men with this disorder.
- As medical treatments for idiopathic male subfertility are usually not effective, assisted reproductive techniques are now widely used with very good results. These techniques should be chosen according to the specific situation. In moderate oligozoospermia, intrauterine insemination can be of some help, particularly if coupled to the induction of multiple ovulation. In vitro fertilization is a more complex technique with results similar to those obtained when a female factor is present. Intracytoplasmic sperm injection is a more aggressive but effective technique, which is usually indicated both in severely oligozoospermic and azoospermic men using spermatozoa retrieved by needle aspiration or open biopsy from the epididymis (obstructive azoospermia) or the testis (tubular azoospermia).
- In counseling a couple, it should be noted that with most assisted reproductive techniques the average delivery rate per cycle of treatment is around 10 to 15%, and the cumulative delivery rate after six cycles is approximately 50%.

Infertility is a condition that affects a couple: both male and female infertility cannot be considered in isolation. The prevalence of infertile couples differs according to the definition of couple infertility. If we accept the most commonly used definition, that is, the lack of pregnancy after one year of unprotected regular intercourse, infertile couples represent approximately 10% of all couples. According to the definition of the European Society for Human Reproduction and Embryology, that is, the lack of pregnancy within 2 years by regular coital exposure, the prevalence of infertile couples in Europe and North America is approximately 5 to 6%. When a woman is in her 20s, the average time to pregnancy is 6 months. This time frame reflects not only the limited few days in the middle of the menstrual cycle when ovulation occurs and conception is possible, but also the fact that most embryos are not viable and are lost before the woman's next menstrual period. In addition, spontaneous miscarriage occurs in about 15% of couples with an established clinical pregnancy. An important determinant of the man's ability to induce a pregnancy is related to the woman's age, since the length of time required to obtain a pregnancy increases with advancing maternal age, as fertilization of human oocytes is more difficult and embryonic losses are more frequent in women of older reproductive age.

The causes of infertility can be divided into four major categories: (1) the female factor, (2) the male factor, (3) combined factors, and (4) unexplained infertility. Although the approximate percentages of each of these categories vary with different authors, according to a recent report of the European Society for Human Reproduction and Embryology, approximately 35% of cases are due to a female factor, 30% to a male factor, 20% to abnormalities detected in both partners, and in 15% of cases no diagnosis can be made after a complete investigation (Tab. 41.1). In some couples there is no possibility of natural conception because of sterility of the male (azoospermia or lack of ejaculation) or of the female (ovarian failure, tubal occlusion, or absence of the uterus). Minor degrees of fertility impairment are not necessarily associated with infertility when present in only one partner, but they may become important when present in both partners.

According to data reported in Table 41.1 in 100 infertile couples, 6% of men are sterile (i.e., with azoospermia or aspermia), and 24% are subfertile (i.e., with oligo-astheno-teratozoospermia; see below).

In contrast with women's infertility, many conditions with male infertility cannot be adequately medically treated. However, in the last few years dramatic progress has been made in the diagnostic assessment and treatment of the infertile male, and significant hope can be offered today to many couples for whom hope could not have been offered in the past.

SPERMATOGENESIS

Physiology

The human testis has the following important functions: (1) during fetal life, by the production of testosterone and of the Müllerian inhibiting hormone, the testis induces the differentiation of both the internal and external genitalia (for which 5α-reductase activity type II must be present); (2) during adult life, the testes produces approximately 200 to 250 million mature spermatozoa and 5 to 6 mg of testosterone per day, thus ensuring the fertilizing potential and the normal sexual behavior of the human male.

The testis is divided into two compartments: the seminiferous tubule and the interstitial compartment. The seminiferous tubule compartment represents approximately 85% of the testicular volume. Each adult human testis contains approximately 100 tubules, each of 70 to 80 cm of length and of 0.3 to 0.4 mm of diameter. All of the tubules end in the rete testis, from which originate the tubuli efferentes, which join the testis to the epididymis. The interstitial compartment, representing approximately 15% of the testicular volume, contains blood and lymphatic vessels, macrophages, fibroblasts, and Leydig cells.

Seminiferous tubules contain the somatic Sertoli cells and the developing germ cells. Each tubule is surrounded by the peritubular lymphatic endothelium and by the peritubular myoid cells. The seminiferous tubule compartment is divided into a basal and an adluminal portion by the so-called "gap junctions" between the Sertoli cells. The Sertoli cells limit the movement of nutrients, hormones, and growth factors toward the adluminal portion of the tubule where the developing germ cells live in a special biochemical environment. This anatomical and functional barrier, known also as the blood-testis barrier, is probably aimed to ensure this environment and to protect the more mature, haploid germ cells from the immune system. Spermatogonia and early spermatocytes reside in the basal compartment and are exposed to the same biochemical environment of the interstitium. The blood-testis barrier is very selective and some molecules, such as glucose and testosterone, enter the tubules very quickly, while others, such as peptide hormones and gonadotropins, are almost completely excluded.

Spermatogenesis is a very complex process in which undifferentiated stem cells (spermatogonia) divide and differentiate into mature spermatozoa. Four distinct phases can be recognized in the spermatogenetic process: (1) the *mitotic phase*, characterized by proliferation and differentiation of spermatogonia; (2) the *meiotic phase*, in which spermatocyte development occurs; (3) the *spermiogenesis phase*, in which spermatids differentiate in mature spermatozoa; and (4) the *spermiation phase*, in which testicular spermatozoa are released into the lumen of the seminiferous tubule.

Mitotic phase. There are three types of spermatogonia in the human testis: type Ap (pale), type Ad (dark), and type B. Type Ap spermatogonia are considered to be renewing stem cells: they can generate both type Ap and type B spermatogonia. Type B spermatogonia subsequently differentiate into spermatocytes. Type Ad spermatogonia are considered to be quiescent stem cells. The spermatogonia are joined by intercellular bridges that probably contribute to the synchronous maturation of germ cells, as these bridges are severed just prior to the release of the spermatozoa into the tubular lumen.

Table 41.1 Percentage distribution of diagnosis in infertile couples

Diagnosis	Both partner (%)	Only female (%)	Only male (%)
Sterile	–	10	6
Subfertile	20	25	24
Unexplained	15	–	–

(From Crosignani PG, Rubin B. The ESHRE Capri Workshop. Guidelines to the prevalence, diagnosis, treatment and management of infertility. Hum Reprod 1996;11:1775-807.)

Meiosis. Type B spermatogonia detach from the basal membrane of the tubule and start their differentiation into primary spermatocytes, which in an initial phase (prophase) of the *first meiotic division* undergo the duplication of their DNA content (*preleptotene* stage). Condensation of chromatin into thin filaments then occurs, and the *leptotene stage* is identified. In the *zygotene* stage pairing of homologous (paternal and maternal) chromosomes occurs. Each pair of chromosomes then shortens and thickens in the *pachytene stage*, where each pair of chromosomes is made up of four bivalent chromatids. During this stage the exchange of genetic material between homologous chromosomes occurs by crossing over. After the *pachytene* stage, which has a duration of approximately 15 to 16 days in the human, partial separation of homologous chromatids at the chiasmata occurs in the *diplotene* stage. The chromosomes then shorten and lose contact with the nuclear membrane at the *diakinetic* stage, which is characterized by the disappearance of the nuclear membrane and the formation of the spindle. At this time the primary spermatocytes complete the first meiotic division through the metaphase, anaphase, and telophase, during which separation and migration of homologous chromosomes occurs. The two resulting *secondary spermatocytes*, with a haploid number of chromosomes but a diploid DNA content, still connected by the intercellular bridges, undergo the *second meiotic division*, thus generating four spermatids that have both a haploid number of chromosomes and a haploid DNA content.

Spermiogenesis. The round spermatids originating from the second meiotic division undergo a complex process of differentiation characterized by several phases: (1) Formation of the *acrosomal vesicle* resulting from the transformation of the Golgi complex. The acrosomal vesicle flattens and associates with the nucleus, which rotates toward the basement membrane, thus establishing the cranial pole of the spermatid; (2) Development of the *flagellum*, beginning from the centrioles, which move to the nuclear membrane opposite to the acrosomal vesicle in the caudal pole of the spermatid; (3) *Condensation* of the nuclear chromatin and elongation of the nucleus and the cell. In this phase nuclear DNA becomes cross-linked, most non-histone nuclear proteins are lost, and gene transcription is ultimately suppressed.

Recently the important role of the transcriptional activator CREM (cyclic AMP-responsive element modulator), which is highly-expressed in postmeiotic germ cells, has been demonstrated in CREM-mutant mice generated by homologous recombination. In homozygous mice, the weight of the testes was reduced by 20 to 25%, the seminal fluid completely lacked spermatozoa, and analysis of the seminiferous epithelium revealed postmeiotic arrest at the first step of spermiogenesis. Late spermatids were absent, and there was a significant increase in apoptotic germ cells.

Spermiation. After the separation of most of the cytoplasm from the head and the tail, which is phagocytosed by the Sertoli cells, the mature spermatid is displaced toward the lumen of the tubule. After detachment from surface specializations between the spermatid acrosome and the Sertoli cells, it is released into the lumen of the tubule.

Hormonal and paracrine control of spermatogenesis

Follicle-stimulating hormone and testosterone

Along the seminiferous tubules, the germ cells are associated in morphologically-distinct groups of cells called "stages." The number of stages is different from species to species, such as 14 in the rat, 12 in the monkey, and 6 in man. In most mammals the spatial arrangement of the spermatogenetic process occurs about a radial axis, such that in a cross-section of a tubule only one stage is evident. In the human the spatial arrangement of the different stages of spermatogenesis follows a helical pattern, such that in a cross-section of a tubule several stages occur adjacent to each other.

An important role in the coordination of spermatogenesis is played by the Sertoli cells. The Sertoli cells are tall, columnar cells extending from the basal membrane to the lumen of the tubule, with many cytoplasmic branches surrounding the developing germ cells. As already mentioned before, due to their tight junctions, the Sertoli cells create a unique biochemical environment in which completion of meiotic maturation and spermiogenesis occur. The interactions between the Sertoli cells, the germ cells, and the interstitium are only partially known. However, it is known that the Sertoli cells are the target and have the receptors for the two the main regulators of spermatogenesis, that is, *follicle-stimulating hormone (FSH)* and *testosterone*. Sertoli cells in fact have the capacity to bind FSH, and they contain mRNA for the FSH receptor, which is expressed stage-dependently during spermatogenesis. The presence of FSH receptors on spermatogonia has been reported but not confirmed, and hence it is generally accepted that the action of FSH on spermatogenesis is mediated through the Sertoli cells. In immature Sertoli cells in vitro, FSH stimulates mRNA synthesis and the secretion of many proteins such as androgen-binding protein, transferrin, and inhibin. The effects of FSH on the adult testis have been difficult to demonstrate, however the stage-dependent expression of the FSH receptor mRNA suggests a specific action. Follicle-stimulating hormone is also probably involved in the distribution and remodeling of cell structural proteins such as actin, vinculin, and associated Sertoli-germ cell junctions. In the prepubertal animal, FSH induces the division of Sertoli cells; therefore, conditioning the future spermatogenic output of the adult testis as the number of germ cells that can be nursed by a Sertoli cell is limited. Several data suggest that FSH is necessary for spermatogenesis: (1) in monkeys with suppressed spermatogenesis by a gonadotropin-releasing hormone (GnRH) antagonist treatment, FSH administration completely maintained the number of spermatogonia, and it maintained at 50% of control the number of spermatocytes and spermatids; (2) in men in whom spermatogenesis was suppressed by testosterone-induced reduction of gonadotropin secretion, FSH treatment could partially restore sperm counts, whereas the total quantitative restoration was obtained only by the combined administration of FSH and hCG (purified human chorionic gonadotropin extracted from the urine of pregnant women, which has luteinizing hormone [LH] action). Luteinizing hormone acts through the stimulation of testosterone secretion by the Leydig cells where LH receptors are present.

The presence of androgen receptors on germ cells has not been reported, whereas they are abundant on Sertoli, myoid peritubular, and Leydig cells. A stage-dependent expression of androgen receptors in Sertoli cells has also recently been demonstrated. According to this data it is clear that testosterone produced by the Leydig cells can affect spermatogenesis, acting both on peritubular myoid cells or directly influencing Sertoli cells. High levels of intratesticular testosterone are necessary for normal spermatogenesis. The reason why the testis requires a testosterone concentration that in other target tissues (such as the prostate) is clearly supraphysiologic is unclear. The androgen receptor binds testosterone with an affinity constant 1 to 10 nM, and the intratesticular testosterone concentrations are approximately 500 nM. Therefore the androgen receptor operates in the presence of saturating concentrations of testosterone. The role of dihydrotestosterone in spermatogenesis is unclear, however the failure of 5α-reductase inhibitors to influence spermatogenesis suggests that testosterone is the predominant ligand for the androgen receptor.

The molecular mechanisms involved in the action of testosterone to spermatogenesis are unknown. Several effects on Sertoli cell protein synthesis and secretion have been reported both by testosterone withdrawal and administration. In the rat the stages of spermatogenesis influenced by testosterone are stages VII-VIII. Testosterone seems to facilitate the transformation of round to elongated spermatids by maintaining the ectoplasmic junctional area that surround the spermatid head between Sertoli cells and round spermatids. In testosterone-deficient animals, spermatid adhesion to Sertoli cells is lost, and further maturation of spermatids does not occur. Restoration of spermatogenesis by testosterone alone has been reported in hypophysectomized rats, however data obtained in primates and humans suggests that both FSH and testosterone are necessary for the initiation and maintenance of full spermatogenesis.

The role of FSH in human spermatogenesis has been recently questioned because in 5 males homozygous for an inactivating point mutation of the FSH receptor (and therefore lacking FSH action), variable degrees of spermatogenic failure have been observed. Surprisingly, however, two of them had fathered children, and variable degrees of oligozoospermia were present in the other three.

Other factors

The requirement of *vitamin A* for normal spermatogenesis was demonstrated by germ cell arrest at the preleptotene stage in rats fed a vitamin A-deficient diet. Replacement of vitamin A to deficient animals restores normal spermatogenesis.

A recent advance in understanding the regulation of spermatogenesis was the discovery of the testicular interaction between *stem cell factor (SCF, or steel factor)*, encoded by the *Sl* locus and its receptor *c-kit*, encoded by the *W* locus. Mice with homozygous mutations in the *Sl* locus or the *W* locus are deficient in hematopoietic cells, germ cells, and melanocytes. In the testis, *SCF* is produced mainly by the Sertoli cells, whereas the *c-kit* receptor is present in spermatogonia and Leydig cells. Mice with mutations in both *SCF* and *c-kit* receptor genes have abnormal spermatogenesis, suggesting that a normal interaction between *SCF* and *c-kit* is necessary for a normal development of germ cells.

Many other oncogenes are expressed in spermatogenic cells during their proliferation and differentiation, however, very little is known about their function (Tab. 41.2).

The *c-fos* nuclear proto-oncogene is a member of a ubiquitous gene family whose products mediate protein-protein interactions. Several stimuli (physical, growth factors) can induce a fast transcriptional activation of *c-fos* in many tissues. Homozygous mutant mice with mutations of the *c-fos* locus usually survive and grow normally until 10 to 12 days of age. At that time the mice develop lymphopenia, osteopetrosis, and abnormal testicular development. In the small testes spermatogonia are present, but progression through meiosis is impaired. These findings suggest that the expression of *c-fos* is not necessary for normal development and the function of most tissues, but that it is essential for the physiologic maturation of spermatogenesis.

Cell-to-cell interaction in the seminiferous tubule

Growth and differentiation factors are exchanged among Leydig, peritubular, and Sertoli cells. Within the seminiferous tubule, however, the only cell-to-cell communications that can occur are between the Sertoli and the germ cells and between the germ cells themselves. Although the mechanisms of these interactions are not well-understood, it is generally accepted that the Sertoli cells provide the nutrients, growth factors, and the ultrastructural environment necessary for germ cell development. Several proteins such as transferrin, *stem cell factor*, activin, insulin-like growth factors (IGF)-I, -II, and -BP3 are produced by the Sertoli cells and have corresponding receptors (transferrin receptor, *c-kit* receptor, IGF-I receptor, and activin A receptor) in the germ cells. In contrast, several factors produced by testicular germ cells such as nerve growth factor, proenkephalin and pro-opiomelanocortin, basic fibroblast factor, and growth hormone-releasing hormone have the corresponding receptors (nerve growth factor receptor, opioid receptors, basic fibroblast receptor, and growth hormone-releasing hormone receptor) on the Sertoli cells. Finally, there is a consistent number of Sertoli cell ligands for which the corresponding receptors have not been yet identified: interleukin-1, plasminogen activator, ceruloplasmin, testins, Sertoli-cell-secreted growth factor, Müllerian inhibitory substance, transforming growth factors α and β, seminiferous growth factor, and sulfated glycoproteins 1 and 2 (SGP-1 and SGP-2).

Finally we must remember that several classes of cell adhesion molecules have been reported to be present in the testis: (1) *integrins*, (2) *Ca²⁺-dependent cadherins*, (3) *Ca²⁺-independent cell adhesion molecules (CAM) of the immunoglobulin-like superfamily*, and (4) *selectins*. Fibronectin and laminin, both present in the seminiferous tubular wall, are each recognized by several different integrin heterodimers and by nonintegrin receptors. The intracellular domain of integrins binds to cytoskeletal elements and transduces structural information from the extracellular matrix to the cell interior. An integrin-mediated adhesion mechanism between developing germ cells and Sertoli cells has been recently suggested. An antiserum against N-cadherin has been reported to inhibit the attachment of spermatogenic cells to Sertoli cells in vitro. Several CAMs have been reported in the testis. Leydig cells in vivo and in vitro express neural CAM (N-CAM). Similar to CD4, a member of the CAM immunoglobulin-like superfamily and a receptor for the human immunodeficiency virus; and D2, an interneuronal adhesion molecule homologous to N-CAM; have been detected by immunocytochemistry and immunoblotting in the human testis. In particular D2 has been observed in the head region of rat late spermatids but is absent in spermatogonia, mature sperm, and Sertoli cells. Galactosyl receptor, a selectin-like molecule, and galactosyltransferase have been observed on the surface of Sertoli cells, spermatocytes, and spermatids.

In conclusion, the two main regulators of spermatogenesis are testosterone and FSH, which act on the receptors present in the Sertoli cells. Follicle-stimulating hormone stimulates Sertoli cell division, maturation, secretion, and cytoskeletal modifications. Stimulation of spermatogonial multiplication and meiosis also occur through signals originating from the Sertoli cells. Testosterone seems to exert its main effect at the level of spermiogenesis: this effect is also mediated by Sertoli cells that receive signals from the germ cells and show several secretory, shape, and cytoskeletal modifications during the stages of the cycle of the seminiferous epithelium. As already mentioned above, the role of FSH has recently been questioned due to the finding that men with an inactivating mutation of the FSH receptor – leading to absent or dramatically reduced FSH action – show very low to normal sperm concentration, thus suggesting that testosterone could variably be compensating for the missing action of FSH. The complex network of paracrine, autocrine, juxtacrine phenomena, which are still poorly known, probably have the role of fine-tuning and coordinating one of the most complex processes of cellular differentiation occurring in the human body.

EPIDIDYMAL TRANSPORT AND MATURATION OF SPERMATOZOA

Testicular spermatozoa are immotile and devoid of the ability of fertilizing the human oocyte. These abilities are acquired during their transit into the epididymis. The epididymis is an androgen-dependent organ constituted by a convoluted tubule approximately 5 to 6 meters long, which can schematically be divided in three portions: the *caput*, the *corpus*, and the *cauda*. The epididymal functions are: (1) the transport of spermatozoa, (2) the storage of spermatozoa, and (3) the maturation of spermatozoa.

Table 41.2 Cell distribution of proto-oncogene mRNAs in the seminiferous epithelium

Type of cell	Proto-oncogene mRNA	Encoded product
Sertoli cell	Steel factor	c-kit ligand
Spermatogonia	*c-fos*	Nuclear transcription factor
	c-jun	Nuclear transcription factor
	c-kit	Tyrosine kinase receptor
	c-raf	Ser-threonine protein kinase
	c-ras	GTP-binding protein
Spermatocytes	*c-abl*	Tyrosin protein kinase
	c-fos	Nuclear transcription factor
	c-jun	Nuclear transcription factor
	c-raf	Ser-threonine protein kinase
	c-ras	GTP-binding protein
Spermatids	*c-abl*	Tyrosin protein kinase
	Wnt-1	Secretory protein
	c-mos	Ser-threonine protein kinase
	plm-1	Ser-threonine protein kinase
	c-raf	Ser-threonine protein kinase
	c-ras	GTP-binding protein

(From Kierszenbaum AL. Mammalian spermatogenesis in vivo and in vitro: a partnership of spermatogenic and somatic cell lineages. Endocr Rev 1994;15:116-34.)

The epididymal transport of spermatozoa, which is estimated to occur in 2 to 6 days, is due to (1) the testicular secretions flowing from the testis, (2) the ciliary activity of the luminal epithelium, and (3) the contraction of myoid elements of the duct walls. The contractile activity of the epididymis is probably regulated by adrenergic fibers, which are more represented in the distal tract of this organ. Recently we demonstrated in the human epididymis the presence of endothelin-1 and endothelin-converting enzyme in the epithelial compartment. We also demonstrated the presence of specific ET receptors in the smooth muscle cell layer mediating epididymal contractility, suggesting that, in the human, endothelin-1 could be a paracrine factor involved in sperm transport through the epididymis.

The number of spermatozoa stored in the epididymis depends on the testicular sperm production rate, the age, and the frequency of ejaculation. In men 20 to 30 years old, the number of spermatozoa in the epididymis is around 200 million, 50% of which are in the cauda. A reduction of approximately 25% is observed in men 40 to 50 years old. The fate of unejaculated spermatozoa is different from species to species (reabsorption, passage in the urinary tract). In the human, phagocytosis of spermatozoa has been observed, but there are no data suggesting reabsorption or passage in the urinary tract.

Sperm maturation in the epididymis is a very complex, poorly understood phenomenon. During their epididymal transit, spermatozoa undergo physico-chemical modifications of their sperm plasma membrane and acquire progressive motility and the ability to bind the zona pellucida of the oocyte. The epididymal fluid, which is hyperosmotic and very different from plasma, probably has an important – though not well-known – role in the maturation process.

SEX ACCESSORY GLANDS

The sex accessory glands of the human male genital tract are specialized, androgen-dependent secretory organs that produce two different types of fluids. These fluids mix at the moment of ejaculation and ensure the transport of the spermatozoa into the female genital tract. It is generally accepted that the seminal fluid probably has other functions as well, though they are not yet fully understood.

Seminal vesicles

The seminal vesicles are convoluted glandular sacs about 5 to 6 cm in length, arising from the vas deferens below the ampulla and lining the dorsal face of the bladder. They secrete a yellowish, viscous, alkaline fluid that is the last fraction of the ejaculated semen and represents approximately 60 to 70% of the total ejaculate volume. The vesicular fluid contains proteins that are responsible for the coagulation of the semen, as well as high concentrations of fructose, prostaglandins, ascorbic acid, inorganic phosphorus, and potassium. In physiologic condi-

tions the seminal vesicles are not a site of storage of spermatozoa.

Prostate

The prostate is a gland weighing approximately 20 g in the adult male and completely surrounds the urethra below the neck of the bladder. The prostate secretes a slightly acidic fluid (pH 6.8), which becomes alkaline (pH 7.5-8.0) in men with prostatitis. Prostatic fluid contributes approximately 30% to the total ejaculate volume and constitutes the first fraction of the ejaculate that contains most of the spermatozoa. In the prostatic fluid, which does not coagulate, fibrinolytic enzymes responsible for the liquefaction of coagulated vesicular secretion are present. One of these enzymes is the prostatic-specific antigen. Prostatic fluid also contains high levels of citric acid, zinc, and acid phosphatase.

Bulbourethral glands and other minor accessory glands

The bulbourethral glands (or Cowper's glands) are two small, lobulated glands located at the base of the penis. Their excretory ducts open into the penile urethra. The fluid secreted by these glands is rich in sialoprotein and probably has the function of lubricating the urethra and neutralizing any acidic urinary residue in the urethra before ejaculation.

Other small, poorly studied glands are the ampullary, urethral (Littre's), and preputial (Tyson's) glands.

SPERM CAPACITATION AND ACROSOME REACTION

Immediately after the ejaculation spermatozoa are not able to fertilize an oocyte. This ability is acquired during their transit in the female genital tract and is called capacitation, which can be considered the final stage of the maturation of spermatozoa. Capacitation is a complex phenomenon during which spermatozoa undergo several modifications, such as removal of cholesterol from the plasma membrane, exhibit increased intracellular calcium concentration, increased tyrosine phosphorylation of proteins, and express a distinct motility pattern called hyperactivation. Upon completion of capacitation, spermatozoa are able to undergo the acrosome reaction, an exocytotic process involving localized fusions between the outer acrosomal and sperm plasma membranes that results in the formation of vesicles. The enzymes contained in the acrosome (hyaluronidase, acrosin, and many others) are then released through the holes between the vesicles. The acrosome reaction is supposed to occur after the binding of the spermatozoon to the glycoprotein component of the oocyte zona pellucida (called ZP3). Progesterone, which is present in high concentrations in the matrix of the cumulus oophorus, has also been shown to induce both calcium entry and acrosome reaction in human spermatozoa through a nongenomic mechanism and is considered a physiologic stimulator of sperm activation.

The main causes of male infertility and their approximate percentage incidence are reported in Table 41.3.

Erectile dysfunction is a very frequent disorder that is usually due, in young males, to psychosexual problems. It is an infrequent cause of infertility and can also be due to endocrine, neural, and vascular causes. *Failure of semen emission* can be due to psychosexual disorders, and also to spinal cord injury, pelvic surgery, and neural diseases such as multiple sclerosis and diabetic neuropathy. *Retrograde ejaculation* can be due to injury to the lumbar sympathetic nerves, to surgery that damages the neck of the bladder, and diabetic neuropathy.

The most common form of *isolated hypogonadotropic hypogonadism* is congenital hypogonadotropic hypogonadism and its variant, the Kallmann's syndrome, which are associated with anosmia or hyposmia and are due to deficient hypothalamic secretion of GnRH. Kallmann's syndrome can occur sporadically or in a familial setting. Three modes of transmission have been documented: X-linked, autosomal dominant with variable penetrance, and autosomal recessive. The incidence of Kallmann's syndrome is 1:10 000 male births. The affected males are fivefold more than the affected females, suggesting that the X-linked form is the most frequent. The X-linked form of Kallmann's syndrome is a developmental disorder that results from the failure of olfactory nerves to penetrate the forebrain with consequent arrested migration of

GnRH cells. It has been recently demonstrated to be due to deletion/mutations of the KAL gene, a 14-exon gene spanning approximately 210 kb and located on chromosome Xp22.3. The KAL gene encodes a putative protein factor with high homology to molecules important in cell adhesion and axonal guidance, which is probably involved in the migration of olfactory axons and GnRH neurons from the olfactory placode to the forebrain and thereafter to the hypothalamus. It is assumed that a similar pathological process underlies autosomal Kallmann's syndrome. However, the pathophysiology of GnRH deficiency in isolated hypogonadotropic hypogonadism without olfactory deficit remains unresolved. An impairment of gonadotropin secretion (alone or combined with other pituitary defects) can also be caused in the adult male by adenomas of the pituitary, metastases, hemochromatosis, or traumatic lesions of the pituitary stalk. In these patients, in contrast to the congenital form, normal virilization is present and only accurate history-taking can give information on testosterone deficiency.

Among the *genetic forms of primary testicular failure*, the 47,XXY karyotype of the Klinefelter's syndrome is one of the most important chromosome abnormalities, which are approximately eight- to tenfold more frequent in infertile males than in the general population. The incidence of the 47,XXY karyotype in newborns is 1:500. The extra X chromosome is generally due to a meiotic non-dysjunction, which can occur with a similar frequency both in the paternal or maternal gametes. Men with the 47,XYY karyotype (1:750 newborns) have various degrees of spermatogenic impairment, ranging from normal spermatogenesis to spermatogenic arrest and the Sertoli-cell-only pattern. Autosomal chromosome rearrangements, including Robertsonian translocations and other types of translocations, can also be found in infertile males, and the pattern is also heterogeneous.

Our improved knowledge of genetic sequences of the Y chromosome has recently shown that not only macroscopic but also microscopic deletions of the Y long arm can be associated with azoospermia or severe oligozoospermia. Recently microdeletions of three regions of the Y chromosome were found in a large sample of severely oligozoospermic and azoospermic men, and the regions were named azoospermia factor (AZF) a, AZFb, and AZFc. Within the AZFc region a gene family termed DAZ (deleted in azoospermia) has been identified. AZFa and AZFb deletion intervals include members of a related gene family (RBM, for RNA binding motif) which, like DAZ, are predicted to encode testis-specific ribonucleoproteins. The frequency of microdeletions of these regions of the Y chromosome, reported by several authors in azoospermic and severely oligozoospermic males, ranges between 3 and 18%. Men with deletions in peripheral blood lymphocytes also have the deletions in ejaculated sperm.

A history *of unilateral or bilateral undescended testis* is rather frequent in infertile males (7-8%). Undescended testis occur in up to 4 to 5% of males at birth, but less

Table 41.3 Causes of male infertility

Type of disorder	% Incidence
Erectile dysfunction	4
Disorders of the ejaculation	5
Failure of emission	
Retrograde ejaculation	
Hypogonadotropic hypogonadism	5
Primary testicular impairment	25
Genetic (Klinefelter, Y microdeletions)	
Cryptorchidism	
Chemotherapy	
Heat	
Radiation	
Infections (orchitis)	
Vascular causes (varicocele)	16
Immunologic	4
Sex accessory gland infections	?
Impaired sperm transport	2
Epididymis	
Congenital	
Infective	
Vas deferens	
Congenital (cystic fibrosis)	
Idiopathic	39

than one-fourth (approximately 1%) of these still have an abnormality by 6 to 12 months. In the last 30 to 40 years the frequency of undescended testis at one year of age appears to have increased in some countries, but there are few reliable studies with sufficient population numbers and standardized methods of assessment. As spermatogenesis is also impaired in contralateral testis, in patients with unilateral maldescent deficiency of spermatogenesis in undescended testis is considered congenital. However, in recent years evidence has accumulated that also supports a secondary, temperature-induced, degeneration of germ cells.

Semen quality can be affected by several *drugs*, such as sulfasalazine, nitrofurantoin, anabolic steroids, and cytotoxic drugs, particularly the alkylating agents. Impaired semen quality has also been observed in men occupationally exposed to *toxicants* such as the nematocides dibromodichloropropane and chlordecone, pesticides such as carbaryl and ethylenedibromide, and glycol ethers, lead, cadmium, and mercury.

Occupational exposure to heat has also been known to have an adverse effect on male fertility. Orchitis (infectious, post-mumps, and post-trauma) can also obviously affect spermatogenesis.

Even if the role of *varicocele* in male infertility is controversial, the presence of left varicocele in men attending an infertility clinic is nearly double compared with that of the general population. The mechanism(s) by which varicocele impairs spermatogenesis is/are not known. Several theories have been proposed, such as reflux of adrenal metabolites, increased testicular temperature, hypoxia and stasis, but no demonstration exists of their validity. As many men with varicocele have normal semen quality, varicocele is likely to have adverse effects on the spermatogenesis of susceptible men.

The presence of *antibodies coating the head of spermatozoa* can be an isolated cause of infertility in approximately 4 to 5% of infertile males. Circulating sperm antibodies can be present in men with obstructions of the male genital tract and with sex accessory gland infections. The percentage of spermatozoa coated with antibodies must be high (>50%) to be clinically relevant. The presence of sperm autoantibodies can be due to sex accessory gland infection. The mechanism responsible for the induction of antibodies is unknown. Inflammation may lead to the migration of immune cells into the genital tract that then react to spermatozoa, which may be trapped in excurrent ducts.

Sex accessory gland infections are a controversial cause of male infertility (see question mark in Table 41.3). There is no doubt that acute inflammation of the sex accessory gland can be a cause of infertility, both because of the possible extension of the infection to the epididymis (where spermatozoa are stored) and because of the possible obstructive sequelae at the level of the epididymis or of the ejaculatory ducts. The relevance of subclinical sex accessory gland infection to male fertility is less certain, although the expanding use of rectal ultrasound indicates that a large number of men with poor sperm quality have non-symptomatic, chronic prostatovesiculitis.

Impaired transport of spermatozoa can occur at the epididymal level both for congenital malformations of the epididymis (lack of connection with the testis, agenesis or hypoplasia), which often occur, for example, in patients with undescended testes. Another possibility is that sexually transmitted diseases may cause epididymitis and lead to blockage of the ductal system, resulting in permanent azoospermia.

Congenital bilateral absence of vas deferens (CBAVD) is present in approximately 1% of infertile males. Recently CBAVD has been reported in about 95% of male patients with cystic fibrosis, a disorder characterized by chronic pulmonary disease, exocrine pancreas insufficiency, and elevated concentrations of electrolytes in sweat. In patients with cystic fibrosis, several types of mutations have been found in the cystic fibrosis transmembrane conductance regulator (CFTR) gene, which encodes a cAMP-regulated chloride channel. Patients with the severe form of the disease have severe mutations in each copy of the CFTR gene, whereas patients with a less severe or mild form of the disease have a severe mutation in one copy of the gene and a mild mutation in the other, or mild mutations in both copies. Mutations of the CFTR gene have been found in 60 to 80% of patients with isolated CBAVD, thus suggesting that this condition is a primary, genital mild form of cystic fibrosis.

In a group of 102 patients with CBAVD, 19 patients had mutations in both copies of CFTR (one severe and one mild mutation in 16 patients, two mild mutations in 3); 54 patients had mutations in only one CFTR allele; and in 29 patients no CFTR mutations were found. In 34 patients (63%) with only a mutation in one copy of the CFTR, a specific DNA sequence of thymines in intron 8 of CTFR gene called *5T*, which causes reduced levels of normal CFTR mRNA, was found in the other allele. These data suggest that the combination of the *5T* allele in intron 8 with a cystic fibrosis mutation of the CFTR gene in the other copy is the most common cause of CBAVD. However, other undetected mutations of the CFTR gene may be involved in CBAVD. CTFR mutations have also been found in patients with congenital unilateral absence of vas deferens (CUAVD), a condition in which azoospermia or low-normal sperm concentration can be found. Therefore, CUAVD could be an incomplete form of CBAVD.

Unfortunately, in many patients the presence of azoospermia or poor semen parameters cannot be related to any cause. Therefore *idiopathic infertility* still represents a significant percentage of male infertility, ranging from 30 to 50% of cases according to different authors.

Clinical findings

The cornerstones of evaluation of the infertile male include a careful comprehensive history, physical examination, and semen analysis. According to the results, additional testing (endocrine evaluation, scrotal and/or rectal ultrasound, genetic assessment, testicular biopsy, tests of sperm function) may also be indicated, taking into account the therapeutic strategy counseled to the couple.

Symptoms and signs

Important anamnestic data are a history of drug abuse, occupational exposure to toxicants (lead, arsenic, pesticides), excess alcohol consumption, ongoing medical treatments (anabolic steroids, cancer chemotherapy, sulfasalazine, nitrofurantoin), high fever in the past 6 months, history of sexually transmitted disease, epididymitis, urinary infection, surgery for varicocele, cryptorchidism or any other inguinal surgery, testicular injury, mumps or post-traumatic orchitis.

Reduced levels of testosterone due to the impairment of Leydig cell function might explain some symptoms such as reduced libido, reduction of the volume of ejaculate, and reduction of beard growth. General physical examination should be focused on body proportions (normal or eunuchoid), body hair distribution, and the presence of gynecomastia. If features of hypogonadism are present, the sense of smell (which is defective in Kallmann's syndrome) should also be tested. At the genital level, the penis should be inspected and palpated to detect hypospadias, surgical or traumatic scars, induration plaques, or other pathology. As seminiferous tubules account for 85 to 90% of the testicular mass, testicular volume should be carefully evaluated with a Prader's orchidometer. A reduced testicular volume is usually found in patients with severe oligospermia or tubular azoospermia. Small testes, 3 to 4 ml in volume, are usually found in men with Klinefelter's syndrome. For Caucasian men a bilateral testicular volume of less than 15 ml is indicative of damage to the seminiferous epithelium. In a man with azoospermia, a normal testicular volume may indicate impairment of sperm transport. During scrotal palpation, the epididymis and the vas deferens on each side should be gently palpated to check for signs of inflammation such as thickening, nodules, and/or pain. The presence of varicocele and hydrocele should also be evaluated. Examination of the prostate gland by digital rectal examination must be performed if there is a history, physical signs, or indications from urine or semen analysis that the patient may have inflammation of the sex accessory glands.

Diagnostic procedures

Semen analysis Normal semen is an admixture of spermatozoa suspended in secretions from the testis and epididymis that are mixed, at the time of ejaculation, with secretions of the prostate, seminal vesicles, and bulbourethral glands. The relative contribution of seminal vesicles and prostate secretions to the volume of the ejaculate is about 65 to 70% and 25 to 30%, respectively. The volume of spermatozoa and of the secretions coming from the testis and the epididimis, as well as the bulbourethral glands, is no more than 5% of the total ejaculate volume.

Semen analysis should be performed according to the World Health Organization (WHO) recommended procedure (1992). The manual provides normal values (Tab. 41.4) as well as nomenclature for normal and pathological findings (Tab. 41.5). Normal values help to identify patients who should have no difficulty in inducing a pregnancy, however, unless there is a severe oligozoospermia or azoospermia, the predictive value of subnormal semen variables is limited. It must be remembered that conception can also occur if one or more of the semen characteristics is under the lower limit of the normal range, especially if the low fertilizing ability of the spermatozoa of the male is compensated by the high fecundability of a young fertile woman. The introduction of computer-assisted semen analysis, which needs expensive and sophisticated equipment, has not yet lead to any substantial improvement in diagnosis and must still be considered primarily a research tool.

If the first semen analysis is normal, there is generally no need for a repeat analysis. In all other circumstances in which an abnormal semen sample is obtained, an additional semen sample should be examined after a 6 to 8 week interval because of the large variability of semen parameters. In azoospermia, after centrifugation of the semen sample, a careful analysis of the pellet is also necessary because, with the new micromanipulation techniques (see below), the presence of a few spermatozoa

Table 41.4 Normal values of semen parameters

Standard tests	Normal value
Volume	$\geq$2 ml
pH	7.2–8.0
Sperm concentration	$\geq$20 x 10^6 spermatozoa/ml
Total sperm count	$\geq$40 x 10^6 spermatozoa per ejaculate
Motility	$\geq$50% with forward progression (categories 'a' and 'b') or $\geq$25% with rapid progression (category 'a') within 60 minutes of ejaculation
Morphology	$\geq$30% with normal forms
Vitality	$\geq$75% or more live, i.e., excluding dye
White blood cells	<1 x 10^6/ml
Immunobead test	<20% spermatozoa with adherent particles
Mixed agglutination reaction test	<10% spermatozoa with adherent particles

Optional tests

α-Glucosidase (neutral)	$\geq$20 mU per ejaculate
Zinc (total)	$\geq$2.4 µmol per ejaculate
Citric acid (total)	>52 µmol per ejaculate
Acid phosphatase (total)	>200 U per ejaculate
Fructose (total)	$\geq$13 µmol per ejaculate

(From WHO Laboratory manual for the examination of human semen and sperm-cervical mucus interaction. 3rd ed. Cambridge, UK: Cambridge University Press, 1992; 44-5.)

Table 41.5 Nomenclature for normal and pathological findings in semen analysis

Definition	Explanation
Normozoospermia	Normal ejaculate (as defined in Tab. 41.2)
Oligozoospermia	Sperm concentration <20 x 10^6/ml
Asthenozoospermia	<50% spermatozoa with forward progression (categories 'a' and 'b') or <25% spermatozoa with category 'a' movement
Teratozoospermia	<30% spermatozoa with normal morphology
Oligo-astheno-terato-zoospermia	Signifies disturbance of all three variables (combination of only two prefixes may also be used)
Azoospermia	No spermatozoa in the ejaculate
Aspermia	No ejaculate

(From WHO laboratory manual for the examination of human semen and sperm-cervical mucus interaction. 3rd ed. Cambridge, UK: Cambridge University Press, 1992;44-5.)

(cryptozoospermia) can substantially change the prognosis and the therapeutic approach.

When azoospermia is present, obstruction should be distinguished from seminiferous tubular damage. A reduced bilateral testicular volume (<10-12 ml) with normal volume ejaculate (>2 ml) and high FSH is indicative of damaged spermatogenesis, which can be confirmed by testicular biopsy (see below). Obstructive azoospermia is usually characterized by a normal testicular volume and normal FSH levels. In these patients very simple semen parameters such as lack of coagulation, low volume of the ejaculate, and acidic pH can suggest CBAVD. In such cases, as well as in the rare cases of acquired ejaculatory duct obstruction, seminal fructose, which is produced by seminal vesicles, is usually very low. Low levels of seminal α-gluosidase, the most used epididymal marker, are present in these men, in men with epididymal obstruction, and have also been found in several men with azoospermia due to tubular damage.

The percentage of motile spermatozoa coated by antisperm antibodies has to be >50% before the test is considered to be clinically significant. Additional tests, such as the sperm-cervical mucus penetration test or titration of sperm antibodies in serum, will add weight and confirm the diagnosis.

If more than 10^6 leukocytes/ml are present in the ejaculate, the possibility of accessory gland infection (prostatitis or prostatovesiculitis) must be kept in mind, however the clinical significance of leukocytospermia as well as the role of subclinical genital infections in male infertility is controversial (see above). Some authors suggest that the presence of symptoms of genital infections (perineal pain, dysuria) as well as ultrasound evidence of prostatitis or prostatovesiculitis must be present to confirm the diagnosis. Reduced seminal levels of acid phosphatase, citric acid, and zinc are also usually associated with prostatitis.

Hormone levels The measurement of gonadotropins, testosterone and prolactin can be of value only when primary or secondary congenital (Kallmann's syndrome) or acquired (pituitary tumor) hypogonadism is suspected. In normally virilized, infertile males the only hormonal measurement important both from the diagnostic and prognostic point of view is serum FSH. High FSH levels are present in the majority of men with sperm concentration lower than 5×10^6/ml and are usually related with the entity of spermatogenetic damage. In subjects with normal testicular volume and obstructive azoospermia, FSH levels are usually normal. Due to methodological problems, immunoreactive inhibin serum levels were of difficult interpretation until recently, when reliable methods for the measurement of the different isoforms of inhibin (inhibin A and inhibin B) have been published. Serum inhibin B levels have been reported to be inversely related with FSH in infertile men, suggesting that inhibin B reflects Sertoli cell function. However, the diagnostic value of inhibin B measurement in the routine assessment of male infertility must still be evaluated.

Imaging studies

Testicular ultrasonography Testicular ultrasonography is routinely suggested by several authors in infertile males because such patients show a high rate of abnormalities (hydrocele, epididymal pathology, spermatocele, tumors) that can be missed at physical examination. In particular testicular tumors (which appear as hypoechoic images) can be diagnosed at an early stage before they become clinically evident. Rectal ultrasound can give further information concerning the presence of chronic inflammation in the prostate and seminal vesicles. The following ultrasound criteria are usually considered indicative of chronic prostatitis: (1) glandular asymmetry, (2) hypoechogenicity associated with edema, (3) hyperechogenicity associated with areas of calcification, and (4) dilation of the periprostatic venous plexus. Vesiculitis is characterized by (1) enlargement and asymmetry, (2) thickening and calcification of the glandular epithelium, and (3) areas of encapsulation. Usually evidence of chronic inflammatory changes are present both in the prostate and in the seminal vesicles.

Other diagnostic tests

Genetic assessment Genetic assessment can be useful for a more accurate diagnosis of the cause of male infertility and must be considered necessary for genetic counseling, in particular if the couple is planning to undergo in vitro fertilization by intracytoplasmic sperm injection (ICSI, see below).

Karyotype is indicated in males with severe oligozoospermia or azoospermia because of the relative frequency of chromosome abnormalities in such patients.

In men with azoospermia due to CBAVD, testing for

CFTR gene mutations must be considered for the male partner; if mutations of the gene are found, the female partner must also be screened due to the high frequency of heterozygote carriers of mutations in the Western populations (1:25).

Assessment of Y microdeletions by polymerase chain reaction amplification of genomic DNA using specific oligonucleotide primers for the AFZa, AZFb and AZFc locus is possible only in a limited number of laboratories, but it should be considered an obligatory genetic assessment in all couples undergoing ICSI. This is due to the fact that men with deletions in peripheral blood lymphocytes also have the deletions in ejaculated sperm, and the couple must be informed of the risk of giving birth to infertile male progeny.

Testicular biopsy Until recently testicular biopsy was a procedure aimed to confirm a normal spermatogenesis in patients with suspected obstructive azoospermia (with normal FSH and normal testicular volume) in whom reconstructive microsurgery was planned. Today testicular biopsy can be considered both a diagnostic and therapeutic procedure. Testicular sperm can be obtained from testicular biopsies of men with azoospermia caused by impaired sperm transport, maturation arrest or Sertoli-cell-only syndrome and can be successfully used for ICSI treatment. Open testicular biopsy seems to be more successful for sperm retrieval than the fine needle testicular aspiration technique. Cryopreservation of retrieved spermatozoa or of a portion of testicular biopsy is suggested to avoid further bioptic procedures if other ICSI cycles will be attempted.

Sperm function tests Routine semen analysis provides little information on sperm fertilizing ability, and the percentage of fertilization failure in assisted reproductive techniques is rather high in cases where the male partner is subfertile. Therefore the possibility of predicting the sperm fertilizing ability would be of great help in defining the best therapeutic strategy for the infertile couple. Several sperm function tests have been reported to have a good predictivity of the sperm ability to fertilize human oocytes in vitro. As shown in Table 41.6, the best results are obtained with the hemizona assay, which compares the ability of spermatozoa of the patient and of a fertile control subject to bind to the zona pellucida of two halves of a human oocyte, but the scarceness of human oocytes makes this test unlikely to be used for routine purposes. A good alternative option seems to be the sperm responsiveness to progesterone. Progesterone is able to induce, through a non-genomic mechanism, both intracellular calcium increase and acrosomal reaction in human spermatozoa. We have recently reported, in a large group of unselected couples, that both acrosomal reaction and intracellular free calcium concentration increases in response to progesterone and were good predictors of the in vitro fertilization rate of human oocytes.

Treatment

Medical treatment

As reported before in 30 to 50% of infertile males, no definite etiology can be found. However, even in men in whom the reason of infertility is known, it is very difficult to develop a rational treatment because pathogenetic mechanisms leading to poor semen parameters are far

Table 41.6 Sperm function tests: correlation (r value) with in vitro % fertilization rate of oocytes, sensitivity, specificity, positive and negative predictive values (PPV and NPV)

Test	Correlation with % fertilization rate r value	Sensitivity %	Specificity %	PPV %	NPV %
Morphology by strict criteria	0.31	94	40	22	98
Hemizona assay	0.75	100	94	85	100
AR induction by A_{23187}	0.30	85	58	87	53
AR induction by follicular fluid	0.39	55	71	75	49
AR induction by progesterone	0.49	89	69	91	64
$[Ca^{2+}]i$ induction by progesterone	0.44	96	53	89	77

(AR = acrosome reaction; $[Ca^{2+}]i$ = intracellular free calcium concentration.)

from being understood. Therefore many therapeutic options are empirical and/or lack proven efficacy.

Elimination of factors known to interfere with spermatogenesis (medicaments, illicit drugs, toxicants, heat) is the first step.

In men with *failure of emission* because of pelvic surgery, spinal cord injury, multiple sclerosis, or diabetic neuropathy, medical treatments include α-adrenergic agonists (ephedrine sulfate 25-50 mg qid, ephedrine hydrochloride 25 mg bid, pseudoephedrine hydrochloride 60 mg qid) that facilitate ejaculation by stimulating peristalsis in the vas deferens and closing the neck of the bladder. Alpha-adrenergic agonists have a better effect if given for several days before the collection of the sperm specimen. In some cases failure of emission can be transformed in retrograde ejaculation (see below). If the drugs have no effect within two weeks, external vibratory stimulation or rectal-probe electroejaculation may be tried, which is successful in 60 to 75% of cases. The obtained specimens can be used for artificial insemination or other assisted reproductive techniques.

Retrograde ejaculation, which can be confirmed by the detection of spermatozoa in the urine after orgasm, can also be treated with α-adrenergic agonists. If such therapy has no effect, sodium bicarbonate (0.65-1.30 g qid) should be given to alkalinize the urine. Increased fluid intake should also be suggested to make the urine isotonic. Spermatozoa can be recovered from voided urine and used for intrauterine insemination or other assisted reproductive techniques.

Hypogonadotropic hypogonadism due to impaired pituitary function, an infrequent cause of infertility, can be effectively treated by parenteral administration of preparations of urinary gonadotropins: purified human chorionic gonadotropin (hCG), which is extracted from the urine of pregnant women, is usually started in a dose of 2000 IU im or sc 2 to 3 times per week for 4 to 8 weeks to induce development of Leydig cells. Thereafter, while hCG is continued at the same dosage, injections of 75-150 IU of purified human menopausal gonadotropin (hMG) with FSH action are added, which is extracted from the urine of menopausal women. Recombinant FSH, which by principle should be preferable but is very expensive, has effects comparable to extractive FSH. In hypogonadotropic hypogonadism due to GnRH deficiency such as in Kallmann's syndrome, endogenous gonadotropins can be stimulated by the pulsatile administration of GnRH using small portable infusion pumps connected to butterfly needles into the abdominal wall. Usually GnRH pulses are administered every 2 hours, and doses range between 5-20 μg GnRH/pulse according to the circulating levels of FSH, LH, and testosterone. If the patient is not concerned with getting his partner pregnant, the treatment of hypogonadotropic hypogonadism can first be performed with testosterone depot preparations, a simpler and less expensive way of treatment, to induce and/or maintain virilization, libido, and sexual drive. When pregnancy is desired, treatment has to be switched either to gonadotropins or to GnRH according to the etiology. Testosterone treatment does not reduce the effectiveness of gonadotropin or GnRH treatment. However, as spermatogenesis is more responsive to treatment once it has initiated, GnRH or gonadotropin treatment, which are equally effective, can be suggested at the beginning of treatment in young patients. This can be suggested even if pregnancy is not desired such that a faster response will be possible in the future. The length of gonadotropin and pulsatile GnRH treatment necessary to obtain a significant number of sperm in the ejaculate is usually in the range of 6 to 18 months. A large variability of responses is observed in individual patients, and the presence of a history of undescended testis is a negative prognostic factor for the treatment outcome. However, pregnancy can occur in these patients with sperm counts as low as 1 to 5 million/ml.

If *infection of the sex accessory glands* is diagnosed in an infertile male, therapeutic doses of antibiotic agents that are selected on the basis of in vitro sensitivities should be performed for 8 to 10 days. The difficulty of getting effective concentrations of antibacterial agents in the prostate should also be considered, and the choice is usually limited to trimethoprim-sulfamethoxazole, doxycycline, erythromycin, and chinoleine derivatives such as ciprofloxacin or norfloxacin. Treatment of the female partner is also recommended, particularly if infection with *Chlamydia trachomatis, Mycoplasma hominis* or *Ureaplasma urealyticum* are documented or suspected.

If *high levels of antisperm antibodies* coating the head of spermatozoa are present, high doses of glucocorticoids can be used. However, both efficacy and lack of efficacy have been reported for this treatment in controlled studies. Furthermore, the patients should be informed of the risk of aseptic necrosis of the head of femur, which is estimated to be at least 1:300.

Empirical treatment. In patients with idiopathic oligozoospermia or azoospermia, different kinds of empirical pharmacological treatments have been tried: testosterone rebound therapy, mesterolone, gonadotropins (hCG/hMG), pulsatile GnRH, antiestrogens, aromatase inhibitors, bromocriptine, and kallikrein. None of these treatments, however, has been demonstrated to be effective in controlled, double-blind randomized studies, and the improvements in semen parameters occasionally seen are likely to be due to spontaneous oscillations.

Surgical treatment

In patients with varicocele, the effectiveness of treatment (surgical or by embolization under radiologic control) is a controversial issue. Recently, four published, controlled, prospective randomized trials have been reviewed, and improved fertility by treatment was reported in two and no effect in the other two. However, there is some consensus that, in view of the apparent progressive nature of this condition, intervention should be suggested in adolescence as a preventive measure. It should also be suggested in young infertile couples (both partners <30 years) with a duration of infertility less than 3 years, if the male partner has subnormal semen analysis. There is some evidence that response to treatment may take up to 2 years, and couples should be counseled in light of this information.

In men with the *obstruction of the epididymis* due to congenital abnormalities or infections, microsurgical vasoe-pididymostomy can be performed by an expert surgeon. There are different techniques, and the results are better if the anastomosis is done at the level of the distal epididymis. The vas deferens is anastomosed end-to-end or end-to-side to the epididymal tubule. The success rate of microsurgery depends on the skill of the surgeon and the level of obstruction: congenital obstructions are usually more proximal and have a less favorable outcome than obstructions due to infections, which usually are more distal.

In patients with CBAVD (in whom no reconstruction can be obtained by surgery), as well as in congenital or acquired obstruction of the epididymis, microsurgical sperm aspiration from the epididymis coupled to ICSI is another effective form of treatment.

Other measures

Expectant management If there are no obvious treatable male factors, the therapeutic approach to the couple with a subfertile male must also take into account the woman's fecundability, which could compensate the male subfertility. If the woman has regular menstruation and is very young (i.e., less than 25 years), even if the male sperm concentration is lower than 5 million/ml, expectant management can be counseled for at least 2 years, because the spontaneous cumulative live birth rate after 36 months in untreated couples with a male partner having less than 5 million motile sperm/ejaculate has been reported to be approximately 30%.

Assisted reproductive techniques As medical treatments for idiopathic male subfertility are usually not effective, attempts have been made to increase the chances of sperm-egg interaction by bringing the spermatozoa closer to the oocyte. *Intrauterine insemination* (IUI) by itself with motile sperm selected by swim-up techniques can be more effective than natural intercourse if timed by the LH surge. The chances of sperm-egg interaction (and therefore the pregnancy rates) can be increased, coupling IUI to multiple ovulation by clomiphene citrate or hMG in the female partner. Intrauterine insemination can be performed only if a minimum number of motile spermatozoa (ranging between 1 000 000 and 2 000 000) can be obtained with sperm preparation techniques.

In vitro fertilization (IVF) and embryo transfer (ET) have become increasingly popular for male factor infertility and, in a recent worldwide survey, approximately 20% of IVF cycles were performed for male factor only infertility. The available data, however, demonstrate that fertilization and pregnancy rates in IVF are lower when performed for male than for tubal infertility. Gamete intra-fallopian transfer and zygote intra-fallopian transfer, two variants of IVF that require laparoscopy for visualization of fallopian tubes, are no more effective than IVF. The number of motile spermatozoa necessary for IVF are lower than for IUI because the number of motile sperm necessary for the in vitro fertilization of an oocyte is usually 50 to 100 000.

In severe oligozoospermia, however, too few sperm are available for IVF. In these cases the *ICSI* procedure is the only therapeutical option. The microinjection of a single spermatozoon in the oocyte is a form of microsurgical fertilization that is more invasive but also more effective than subzonal insertion of spermatozoa or partial zona dissection. Both of these techniques can in fact be considered techniques of historical importance only. After the first demonstration of fertilization and live births with the ICSI procedure in 1993, ICSI has been extensively used in many centers to treat patients with severe male factor infertility, as well as to treat patients with obstructive azoospermia with spermatozoa retrieved from the epididymis or from the testis. Furthermore, it has been recently demonstrated by several authors that in men with azoospermia due to testicular damage and high FSH levels, small islands of tubules with complete spermatogenesis can be found, and for these men testicular spermatozoa can be obtained by a testicular biopsy and then successfully used for ICSI in 50 to 70% of cases. The pregnancy rates/cycle obtained by ICSI range between 17 and 41% in different centers, with the increasing age of the female partner being a negative prognostic factor. The results obtained with ejaculate, epididymal, or testicular spermatozoa do not differ. There is no general agreement on ICSI indications, however it can be reasonably proposed as a therapeutic option in the following situations: (1) Sperm concentration <1 million/ml; (2) Sperm motility <5%; (3) Normal sperm morphology by strict criteria <4%; (4) Obstructive and tubular azoospermia with surgically retrieved fresh or cryopreserved spermatozoa (5) Failure of fertilization in a previous IVF cycle.

International registry studies demonstrate that the risk of malformation after conventional IVF is not increased. Some reports suggest that incidence of congenital major and minor malformations are not increased in children born following ICSI. However, the rate of sex chromosome anomalies in ICSI fetuses has been reported to be around 1% in approximately 600 prenatal diagnoses, a frequency four times increased if compared with naturally conceived liveborn babies. ICSI by-passes the physiological selection of spermatozoa, which occurs at the level of the testis, epididymis, in the female reproductive tract as well as at the sperm-oocyte interface, and it should be considered an effective but still experimental procedure.

In conclusion, assisted reproductive techniques, and in particular ICSI, can offer to the couple with male factor infertility an effective therapeutical approach that could not be offered a few years ago. However in counseling the couple, it must be kept in mind that with most assisted reproductive techniques, the average delivery rate per cycle is approximately 10 to 15%, and the cumulative delivery rate after six cycles is approximately 50%. In other words, at the present time, assisted reproductive techniques can reach no more than 50% of positive results in terms of live births in couples who come to the decision of facing the direct costs, and the emotional and social burden of these procedures. Further research is therefore needed in the future to improve the effectiveness of assisted reproductive techniques, and also to reduce the need of assisted reproductive techniques altogether. In particular, research should be focused on: (1) the identification of regulatory mechanisms of spermatogenesis, spermiation, and epididymal function; (2) the identification of sperm receptors that react with oocyte ligands and of the signaling cascades that lead to sperm activation (acrosome reaction, hyperactivated motility); and (3) the examination of sperm factors involved in oocyte activation and molecules that mediate sperm-egg interaction after penetration, and their relationship with early embryo development.

Suggested readings

ANAWALT BD, BEBB RA, MATSUMOTO AM, GROOME NP, ILLINGWORTH PG, McNEILLY AS, BREMNER WJ. Serum inhibin B levels reflect Sertoli cell function in normal men and men with testicular dysfunction. J Clin Endocrinol Metab 1996;81:3341-5.

BALDI E, KRAUSZ CS, FORTI G. Non genomic actions of progesterone in human spermatozoa. Trends Endocrinol Metab 1995;6:198-205.

CHILLON M, CASALS T, MERCIER B, et al. Mutations in the cystic fibrosis gene in congenital absence of the vas deferens. N Engl J Med 1995;332:1475-80.

COLLINS JA, BURROWS EA, WILLAN AR. The prognosis for live birth among untreated infertile couples. Fertil Steril 1995;64:22-8.

CROSIGNANI PG, RUBIN B. The ESHRE Capri Workshop. Guidelines to the prevalence, diagnosis, treatment and management of infertility. Hum Reprod 1996;11:1775-807.

HUTSON JM, HASTHORPE S, HEYNS CF. Anatomical and functional aspects of testicular descent and cryptorchidism. Endocr Rev 1997;18:259-80.

KIERSZENBAUM AL. Mammalian spermatogenesis in vivo and in vitro: a partnership of spermatogenic and somatic cell lineages. Endocr Rev 1994;15:116-34.

KRAUSZ CS, BONACCORSI L, MAGGIO P, et al. Two functional assays of sperm responsiveness to progesterone and their predictive values in in vitro fertilization. Hum Reprod 1996;11:1661-7.

McLACHLAN RI, WREFORD NG, ROBERTSON DM, DE KRETSER DM. Hormonal control of spermatogenesis. Trends Endocrinol Metab 1995;6:95-101.

NIESCHLAG E. Care for the infertile male. Clin Endocrinol 1993;38:123-33.

PESCOVITZ OH, SRIVASTAVA CH, BREYER PR, MONTS BA. Paracrine control of spermatogenesis. Trends Endocrinol Metab 1994;5:126-31.

PURVIS K, CHRISTIANSEN E. Infection in the male reproductive tract. Impact, diagnosis and treatment in relation to male infertility (review). Int J Androl 1993;16:1-14.

TAPAINEN JS, AITTOMAKI K, MIN J, VASKIVUO T, HUHTANIEMI IP. Men homozygous for an inactivating mutation of the follicle-stimulating hormone (FSH) receptor gene present variable suppression of spermatogenesis and fertility. Nature Genet 1997;15:205-6.

VOGT PH, EDELMANN A, KIRSCH S, et al. Human Y chromosome azoospermia factors (AZF) mapped to different subregions in Yq11. Hum Mol Genet 1996;5:933-43.

World Health Organization. 1992 WHO Laboratory manual for the Examination of Human Semen and Sperm-Cervical Mucus Interaction. 3rd ed. Cambridge, UK: Cambridge University Press, 1992; 44-5.

42

Reproductive function in elderly men

Jean-Marc Kaufman, Alex Vermeulen

Andropause, defined as the male equivalent of menopause, does not occur in healthy aging men. When considering men as a group, however, advancing age is accompanied by many changes in the reproductive system: a progressive decline of Leydig cell function and increased prevalence of subnormal serum testosterone levels, a markedly increased prevalence of impotence, and more subtle alterations of spermatogenesis. There is, however, a striking interindividual variability in the degree to which aging affects reproductive function in men.

Age-related decline of Leydig cell function

Cross-sectional studies in healthy men have shown an age-related decline of mean total serum testosterone levels. This becomes clearly apparent after the age of 50 years and amounts to an approximately 30% decline between ages 25 and 75 years. The biologically active free (or bioavailable) testosterone fraction in serum is reduced by as much as 50% over the same period, a significant decrease being demonstrated at a younger age than is the case for total serum testosterone (Fig. 42.1). The steeper decline of the serum free testosterone fraction is the consequence of an age-associated progressive increase of the serum sex hormone-binding globulin (SHBG) binding capacity. Circadian rhythmicity of serum testosterone is markedly blunted in the elderly, so that the age-related differences in serum testosterone are most clearly demonstrated when blood sampling is performed in the morning (before 10:00 a.m.). More recently, the occurrence of an age-related decline of Leydig cell function has also been confirmed in longitudinal studies.

The normal range for serum testosterone levels in healthy men is generally considered to lie between 11 and 40 nmol/l (320 and 1160 ng/dl) for total testosterone and between 0.21 and 0.70 nmol/l (6 and 20 ng/dl) for free testosterone (which may vary according to assay methods). Prevalent serum testosterone levels in elderly men are characterized by a high degree of interindividual variability, so that even at very old age some men have values

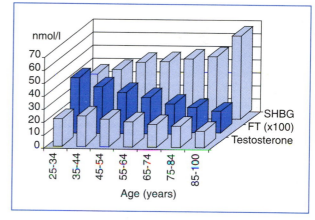

Figure 42.1 Mean serum levels of testosterone, free testosterone (FT), and sex hormone-binding globulin (SHBG), according to age in a cross-sectional study of 300 healthy men (According to Vermeulen A, et al., J Clin Endocrinol Metab 1996;81:1821.)

that fall well within the range for young adults, while others present with levels corresponding to a frankly hypogonadal state. With advancing age, a progressively larger proportion of men present with subnormal testosterone levels (more than 20% after age 60 years). However, limits of normality in the elderly are rather arbitrary, as the sensitivity threshold for androgens might vary from tissue to tissue and possibly also according to age. Awaiting the results of more systematic studies, male hypogonadism in the elderly is usually defined, from a biochemical point of view, as a serum (free) testosterone below the normal range for young men.

Constitutional, physiological, and life-style related factors, which account for part of the wide range of normal values observed in healthy men, are summarized in Table 42.1. Moreover, both acute critical illness and chronic disease states, as well as their treatment, may transiently or more permanently accentuate the age-associated decrease of (free) testosterone levels.

Table 42.1 Factors contributing to the interindividual variability of serum testosterone and/or free testosterone levels

Factor	Comment
Heredity	Genetic influences documented for total T and SHBG
Ultradian rhythm	Episodic mode of T secretion
Circadian rhythm	Less prominent in the elderly
Circannual variations	Seasonal variations with amplitude of 25% of annual mesor
Serum albumin	Influences total T (20-40% albumin-bound)
Insulin levels	Inversely correlated to SHBG and total T
Body mass index	Inversely correlated with SHBG and total T; FT affected mainly if BMI>35
Growth hormone/insulin-like growth factor-1 levels	Inversely correlated with SHBG and total T
Thyroid hormone levels	Positive correlation with SHBG and total T
Diet	Lower SHBG in western-type diet; higher SHBG in fiber-rich, vegetarian diets; lower total T and FT after acute fat intake
Prolonged fasting	Transient decrease T secretion
Smoking	5-15% higher T and FT in smokers
Stress	Decrease of (F)T possible with both physical and psychological stress
Alcohol abuse	May accentuate age-associated changes

(T= testosterone; FT = free testosterone; SHBG = sex hormone-binding globulin; BMI = body mass index.)

Pathophysiology

Testicular factors

That primary testicular dysfunction is implicated in the age-related decline of Leydig cell function is suggested by a decreased absolute testosterone response upon human chorionic gonadotropin (hCG) stimulation. The anatomical substrate for this impaired response appears to be a decreased number of Leydig cells, but vascular changes and functional alterations of Leydig cell function may also be involved. In accordance with the existence of primary testicular deficiency, moderate increases of basal levels of gonadotropins were observed in many studies in elderly men. This increase involves both immunoreactive- and bioactive forms of the gonadotropins.

Neuroendocrine regulation

The observed testosterone response to hCG challenges in elderly men indicates that the secretory reserve of the Leydig cells, albeit diminished, should still be sufficient to allow for normalization of testosterone plasma levels if the endogenous drive by pituitary luteinizing hormone (LH) were adequate. Serum LH levels in elderly men, although moderately elevated, thus remain inappropriately low in the face of persistently decreased testosterone levels, notwithstanding the fact that the pituitary secretory capacity for LH is well-preserved or even increased in the elderly.

Several observations have confirmed the existence of changes in neuroendocrine control of Leydig cell function in aging men. The circadian variations of serum LH and testosterone are markedly blunted in elderly men. As to the pulsatile pattern of LH release, mean LH pulse amplitude is decreased in the elderly. Taken that the responsiveness of the pituitary gonadotrophs to "physiologic" doses of gonadotropin-releasing hormone (GnRH) is maintained, this decrease of LH pulse amplitude most probably reflects a reduction of the amount of GnRH intermittently released into the pituitary portal circulation.

The negative feedback action of testosterone on LH secretion is exerted essentially through a deceleration of the frequency of the hypothalamic GnRH pulse generator, and hypoandrogenism is expected to result in an increased frequency of LH pulsatility. The unchanged LH pulse frequency in elderly men, as observed by most investigators, should thus probably be considered as inappropriately low in the face of a prevailing relative hypoandrogenism. This may, in turn, be related to the observation that the hypothalamo-pituitary compartment of the gonadal axis in elderly men is clearly more sensitive to the negative feedback effects of sex hormones than is the case in young adults. Furthermore, the LH response to opioidergic blockade is markedly reduced in elderly men, as opioidergic receptor blockades fail to produce the expected increase in frequency and amplitude of LH pulses.

Sex hormone-binding globulin levels

A third aspect of the age-related changes in circulating testosterone levels consists of a progressive increase of plasma SHBG binding capacity. In the presence of an inadequate neuroendocrine response to decreased testosterone levels, this increase of serum SHBG binding capacity results in an even sharper fall of the biologically active serum free testosterone fraction. The age-related increase in SHBG serum levels is remarkable, as it occurs in the face of an increase of body mass index and insulin levels, which are known to be accompanied by a decrease in SHBG levels. The mechanisms responsible for the elevated SHBG levels in the elderly remain unclear, but neither the reduced serum testosterone per se nor changes in serum estradiol seem to be implicated. A possible role of the age-related decline of growth hormone and insulin-like growth factor-1 levels remains to be confirmed.

Testosterone metabolites and tissue levels

Although some investigators have reported a small decrease in 5α-androstan-17β-ol-3-one (5α-dihydrotestosterone, DHT) plasma levels in elderly men, most investigators failed to observe a significant age-related decline of serum DHT levels. There is, however, great uncertainty about the clinical significance of plasma DHT levels, as only a small fraction of the peripherally formed DHT reaches the general circulation. In contrast to the findings for DHT, plasma levels of 5α-androstane 3α-, 17β-diol and its glucuronide, considered to be indices of androgenicity, are decreased to about the same extent as the free testosterone serum levels. Moreover, studies of age-related changes in androgen tissue concentrations have shown a highly significant decrease in both testosterone and DHT in different tissues.

Clinical findings

The clinical changes that generally accompany aging in men include a decrease in general well-being and energy; a decrease in virility, sexual pilosity, and skin thickness; a decrease in muscular mass and strength; an increase in upper and central body fat; osteopenia; a decrease in sexual drive; and an increased prevalence of impotence. As these changes are reminiscent of the clinical picture of hypogonadism in younger individuals, it seems plausible that they may be at least in part the consequence of a (relative) androgen deficiency resulting from the age-related decline of Leydig cell function. A causal link between decreased testosterone production and clinical changes in aging men has, however, not been formally established.

In any case, decreased androgen levels can at best be responsible for part of the clinical changes in aging. Impotence seldom has an endocrine origin. Moreover, the testosterone levels required to sustain sexual activity seem to be rather low. Low testosterone levels appear to be accompanied by an increase of biochemical risk factors for cardiovascular disease, that is, an atherogenic lipid profile and increased insulin resistance. However, the low testosterone levels may be either the cause or the consequence of these biochemical changes, and they are apparently not associated with an increase of cardiovascular death. Bone density has been reported to be positively correlated to androgen levels in elderly men, but this association is rather weak. Nevertheless, hypogonadism has been identified as a risk factor for hip fracture in elderly men. The cause of the decrease in muscle mass and strength in elderly men is most likely multifactorial; possible contributing factors include the decline of testosterone secretion, the diminished activity of the somatotropic axis, and the decrease of physical activity.

Clearly, there is a need for more definitive data on the possible clinical implications of the age-related decline of androgen production in men. One key issue in need of clarification is what testosterone plasma levels are required for the maintenance of adequate end-organ androgen response in most elderly subjects.

Treatment

The observation that a substantial proportion of elderly men (>20% of men older than 60 years) present with testosterone serum levels in the hypogonadal range for young adults raises the question of whether these men should be substituted with androgens. Unfortunately, to date only few controlled trials of rather short duration and involving a limited number of subjects have assessed the risks and benefits of androgen replacement in elderly men.

Although it has been reported that androgen replacement may improve mood and sense of well-being, libido, and spatial cognition; the findings are not consistent and are too limited to be regarded as conclusive. Impotence in elderly men usually has a multifactorial origin, and the effects of androgen treatment have generally been disappointing. In elderly men with low serum testosterone, androgen treatment has a positive effect on lean body mass and muscle strength, with a more modest decrease of fat mass. Preliminary data indicate possible favorable effects of androgen replacement on bone density in elderly men, while limited data on the induced changes in biochemical indices of bone turnover have been inconsistent.

A significant proportion of men may develop polycythemia and androgen treatment has been reported to exacerbate sleep apnea syndrome. The possibility of water retention should be taken into account in subjects with pre-existent cardiovascular pathology.

The reported effects of androgen treatment on lipoprotein profiles in elderly men have been rather inconsistent, but when unfavourable changes are reported they are usually of modest amplitude and hence are probably not a safety issue of major concern. Elderly men may develop gynecomastia during androgen treatment. Hepatotoxicity is not an issue of real concern for treatment with substitutive doses of androgens, particularly for the non-oral forms of treatment.

Androgen treatment may exacerbate pre-existent malignant or benign prostatic disease, which are known to be androgen sensitive. To date most studies in elderly men failed to demonstrate clinically significant changes at the level of the prostate, either in terms of prostatic volume or serum levels of prostate-specific antigen. It should be pointed out, however, that only a limited number of subjects have been followed prospectively for only short periods of time (up to one year) in controlled trials. Moreover, although there is presently no indication that androgen substitution may activate subclinical prostatic carcinoma, which is present in more than half of the men over 70 years, this possibility cannot be definitively ruled out and is awaiting the results of larger-scale controlled trials of long duration.

In view of the paucity of reliable data on both the consequences of the relative hypoandrogenism of the elderly and the risks and benefits of androgen replacement therapy, it would certainly be unwise to propose a strategy of systematic androgen supplementation in elderly men who present with only marginally or moderately decreased plasma testosterone levels. Any change of attitude on this issue should be supported by a favorable risk-benefit balance for androgen substitution with clear benefits in terms of quality of life that are demonstrated in carefully controlled prospective trials of sufficient duration. Meanwhile, there is also no reason to withhold androgen treatment from selected patients presenting with biochemically and clinically manifest hypogonadism, after careful screening for contra-indications. A possible approach to the evaluation of elderly men with suspected hypogonadism is proposed in Figure 42.2.

The practical modalities for androgen substitution in hypogonadal men are discussed in another section of this book (Chap. 40). Due to the lack of relevant controlled clinical trials, it is presently not possible to propose an ideal therapeutic regimen for elderly men, but based on the current state of our knowledge, it seems advisable to aim for substitutive doses of testosterone, achieving serum levels not much higher than the mid-normal range for young men. Given that gonadotropin secretion in elderly men is exquisitely sensitive to the negative feedback effects of androgens, administration of even modest doses of androgens can be expected to suppress residual endogenous testosterone production. Thus, one should logically select a therapeutic regimen that would ensure full androgen substitution. Regular monitoring of the treatment by an experienced physician seems mandatory.

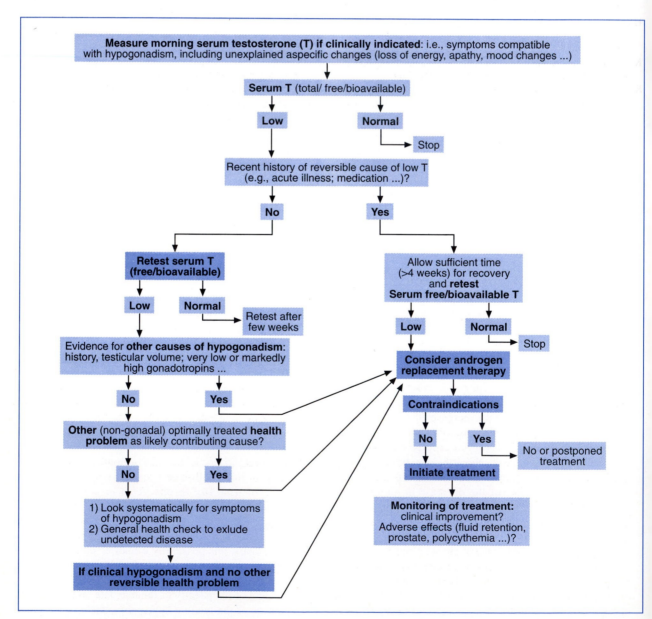

Figure 42.2 Flow chart for a possible approach to clinical decision making regarding androgen replacement therapy in elderly men.

Spermatogenesis and sperm quality

In aging men, there is no abrupt loss of fertility, and although there have been no systematic studies addressing this issue, it is clear that fertility can be preserved until old age in at least some men. Reported age-related changes in the quality of the ejaculate include a reduced ejaculatory volume with unchanged sperm concentration, a decreased motility of the spermatozoa, and a decreased proportion of spermatozoa with normal morphology. A decline of the ejaculatory frequency may be a confounding factor when interpreting these age-related changes.

The observation of a decrease in the number of Sertoli cells constitutes a morphological basis for an age-related decrease of spermatogenesis, which is in accordance with the observation of an age-related increase of follicle-stimulating hormone (FSH) serum levels. Nevertheless, there have been reports of similar fertilizing capacity of sperm of young and elderly men under in vitro conditions.

Suggested readings

DESLYPERE JP, VERMEULEN A. Leydig cell function in normal men. Effect of age, life style, residence, diet and activity. J Clin Endocrinol Metab 1984;59:955-61.

HAJJAR RR, KAISER FE, MORLEY JE. Outcomes of long-term testosterone replacement in older hypogonadal males: a retrospective analysis. J Clin Endocrinol Metab 1997;82:3793-96.

KAUFMAN JM, VERMEULEN A. Declining gonadal function in elderly men. Baillière Clin Endoc 1997;11:289-309.

ROLF C, BEHRE HM, NIESCHLAG E. Reproductive parameters of older compared to younger men of infertile couples. Int J Androl 1996;19:135-42.

SIH R, MORLEY JE, KAISER FE, PERRY III HM, PATRICK P, ROSS C. Testosterone replacement in older hypogonadal men: a 12-month randomized controlled trial. J Clin Endocrinol Metab 1997;82:1661-59.

TENOVER JS. Androgen administration to aging men. Endocrin Metab Clin 1994;23:877-92.

TSITOURAS PD, BULAT T. The aging male reproductive system. Endocrin Metab Clin 1995;24:297-315.

URBAN RJ, BODENBURG YH, GILKISON C, et al. Testosterone administration to elderly men increases skeletal muscle strength and protein synthesis. Am J Physiol 1995;269:E820-6.

VERMEULEN A. Androgens in the aging male. J Clin Endocrinol Metab 1991;73:221-4.

Female reproductive system

Basic concepts of the female reproductive system

NEUROENDOCRINOLOGY OF FEMALE REPRODUCTION
Cornelis B. Lambalk

For the normal function of the ovary with respect to developing puberty and reproduction, pituitary gland luteinizing hormone (LH) and follicle-stimulating hormone (FSH) secretion are required in a well-organized way (Fig. 43.1). Both hormones are glycoproteins with a common α-chain and different β-chains. The half-life of both hormones depends on the level of glycosylation and

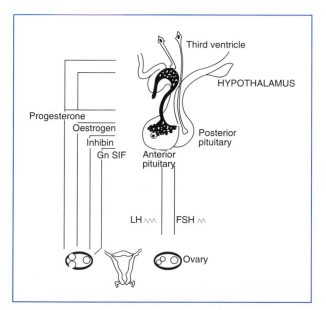

Figure 43.1 Diagrammatic presentation of the interplay between the hypothalamus, pituitary, and ovary in the regulation of the reproductive axis (see text for explanation).

varies between 20 to 60 minutes for LH and between 120 to 240 minutes for FSH. In absence of these hormones, puberty will not develop and menstrual cycles will not occur. The secretion of these hormones is entirely dependent upon regulation by luteinizing hormone-releasing hormone (LHRH), which is often referred to as gonadotropin-releasing hormone (GnRH).

A monthly variation in LH and FSH occurs in adult premenopausal women that is related to the stage of their menstrual cycle (Fig. 43.2). Highlights are the subtle perimenstrual increase in FSH levels for the induction of follicle growth; and the high mid-cycle elevation of LH (the LH surge) for the induction of (1) termination of meiosis I of the oocyte, (2) luteinization of granulosa, and (3) ovulation.

Gonadotropic hormones are secreted episodically at intervals that vary between 1 to 4 hours, closely related to the synchronous episodic release of LHRH, which is often referred to as the hypothalamic "pulse generator". This pulsatility is considered to be a key feature of gonadotropin secretion. During the normal ovarian cycle of the human, plasma LH shows pulses about every hour in the follicular phase of the cycle and about every 4 hours during the luteal phase. FSH is also secreted in a pulsatile way throughout the menstrual cycle. After menopause, LH and FSH pulses occur every 1 to 2 hours.

Regulation of gonadotropin secretion at the pituitary level

Releasing hormones LHRH is the only known direct activator of pituitary secretion of both gonadotropins. The hormone is identical for all mammals and has a plasma half-life of about 4 minutes. The interaction of LHRH with its plasma membrane receptor is the first step leading to gonadotropin release. The receptor belongs to the family of G protein-coupled receptors and is probably coupled

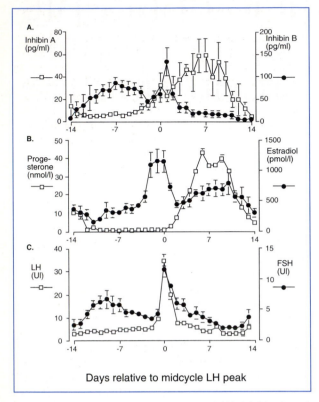

Figure 43.2 Plasma concentrations of (**A**) inhibin A and inhibin B, (**B**) estradiol and progesterone, and (**C**) LH and FSH during the female menstrual cycle. (From Groome NP et al. Measurement of dimeric inhibin B throughout the human menstrual cycle. J Clin Endocrinol Metab 1996;81:14015. Reproduced with permission of the Endocrine Society.)

to a calcium ion channel. The influx of Ca^{2+} from the extracellular space in response to LHRH stimulates a cellular response through the binding of Ca^{2+} to calmodulin. The LHRH receptor also activates the phosphatidyl inositol and diacylglycerol (DAG) pathway, thus further stimulating the intracellular Ca^{2+} mobilization. Despite many efforts, no separate releasing hormone for FSH has been found. LHRH is a crucial hormone, since both the induction of puberty as well as the initiation of ovulation can result from the administration of LHRH alone. As already mentioned, this hormone is secreted episodically into the portal vessels by neurons of the hypothalamus, resulting in the pulsatile nature of pituitary LH release. In the absence of LHRH, no LH secretion will occur. The direct role of LHRH in the synthesis and release of FSH is less clear. However, in the absence of pulsatile LHRH stimulation, no adequate FSH secretion will occur.

Self-priming and gonadotropin surge-inhibiting factor (GnSlF) The binding of LHRH to its receptor also stimulates the formation of cyclic adenosine monophosphate (cAMP), which through the activation of a protein kinase stimulates the synthesis of a factor that increases the cel-

lular response to LHRH. This phenomenon is called the self-priming action of LHRH. The mechanism by which priming occurs remains unknown. Under normal circumstances, the FSH-stimulated ovary produces a nonsteroidal, noninhibin factor referred to as gonadotropin surge-inhibiting factor (GnSlF), which prevents this pituitary priming process for LHRH and thus maintains a relatively low responsiveness. It is hypothesized that only during the LH surge, the pituitary temporarily turns into a highly primed, responsive state by a decline of ovarian GnSlF secretion prior to ovulation.

Desensitization The pulsatile nature of LHRH secretion is important for the generation of a normal pattern of LH and FSH release. Continuous stimulation, by infusion of natural LHRH with its short half-life or by the administration of LHRH agonistic analogues with longer half-lives, initially results in the secretion of large amounts of LH and FSH; however, after a while gonadotropin secretion begins to decline despite the presence of LHRH (the so-called desensitization phenomenon). Eventually plasma gonadotropin concentrations become equal to or fall below normal values. The response of plasma LH and FSH concentrations to a test dose of LHRH at this stage is much smaller than before the LHRH treatment. Desensitization also occurs to a certain extent to pulses of LHRH. Immediately following a pulse stimulus of LHRH, a sharp decline in the pituitary responsiveness to a subsequent LHRH pulse occurs for a few minutes.

The hypothesized molecular mechanisms of desensitization include: (1) down-regulation of LHRH receptors; (2) internalization of receptors after LHRH binding; (3) depletion of LH and FSH stores; and (4) post-receptor mechanisms, yet to be defined. It is currently believed that the homologous desensitization by LHRH (i.e., desensitization by the same substance that caused the stimulation earlier) is different from the desensitization mechanism after stimulation of other members of the G protein-coupled receptor family.

Estradiol At the level of the pituitary, estradiol exerts complex inhibitory and augmentative effects on the LH and FSH pituitary responsiveness to LHRH. The first few hours after exposure of the pituitary gland to estradiol, secretion of LH and FSH decreases and the pituitary does not release gonadotropins if LHRH is injected. After a period of about 6 to 24 hours, the pituitary enters a state in which high responsiveness to LHRH exists and large amounts of LH and FSH are secreted in its presence. This augmentative mechanism is thought to underlie in part the estradiol-induced preovulatory gonadotropin surge. Both in the human and in the rat, prolonged exposure to estradiol also results in a decline of the responsiveness to LHRH.

Progesterone Progesterone alone does not have an "intrinsic" influence on the pituitary responsiveness to LHRH, but it amplifies the effects of estradiol on gonadotropin secretion. Just prior to ovulation in primates there is a small rise of plasma progesterone, and there is increasing evidence that this preovulatory rise may facilitate the preovulatory surge.

Regulation of FSH All of the regulatory mechanisms discussed above concern modulation of pituitary LH or combined LH/FSH secretion. The secretory regulation of LH and FSH have much in common. About 50% of FSH pulses occur synchronously to LH pulses in pre- and postmenopausal conditions. This implies that LHRH has an important role in FSH secretion as well. Presumably all gonadotropic cells can synthesize and release both LH and FSH upon stimulation with LHRH. It has been shown that these cells contain either LH or FSH or both hormones. However, during stimulation with LHRH, more cells start to produce both hormones. This increase in cells that produce both hormones results from the transformation of cells that first produced only a single hormone rather than from newly formed cells that produce both. LH and FSH in these cells are stored in different regions of the cell.

FSH pulses and their duration are important determinants for the final number of follicles that will continue to grow until ovulation. In the human, the concentration of serum FSH must be maintained at levels such that one follicle will continue to grow for final ovulation. In view of the direct involvement of FSH levels in determining litter size, it is probably not surprising that additional regulatory mechanisms are available in order to maintain these levels within narrow limits. Ovarian estradiol is probably the most active FSH suppressive factor throughout the menstrual cycle. Recently, however, several peptides (inhibin, follistatin, and activin) have been identified that are specifically involved in the regulation of FSH secretion. Among these recently discovered peptides, probably only ovarian inhibin plays a role as a classical hormone by selective suppression of pituitary FSH secretion, while activin and follistatin modulate by auto/paracrine mechanisms. As the final result of the different regulatory mechanisms, the course of FSH throughout the cycle is in general characterized by a persistently low level but with a subtle early follicular rise for induction of follicular growth and a mid-cycle surge. The periods with low levels, ensuring periodical monofollicular growth, correlate closely with estradiol and inhibin levels (Fig. 43.2).

Regulation of hypothalamic LHRH release

The secretory pattern of pituitary gonadotropins is the consequence of synchronous discharges from LHRH-producing neurons that are directed by a neural signal generator (the pulse generator), which likely resides within the mediobasal hypothalamus. The LH pulse pattern is closely related to that of LHRH. Thus, in human studies, investigators of the LHRH pulse generator have relied on information from episodically measured LH in peripheral blood.

Peptidergic, monoaminergic, excitatory amino-acid, nitric oxide and steroidal regulation Despite many efforts, no clear insight exists in the regulation of the cyclic activity of LHRH-secreting neurons. In vitro cultured LHRH neurons secrete the hormone in episodes; most likely under in vivo conditions a high grade of synchronous activation may be responsible for distinct episodes of LHRH release into the hypophyseal portal

vessels. In the adult human, only about 1500 neurons constitute the LHRH pulse generator. The isolated mediobasal hypothalamus is able to secrete LHRH episodically. All together, this suggests that the episodic release is an autonomous system. One of the mechanisms underlying the synchronization is the neuropeptide LHRH modulating its own secretion via an ultra-shortloop negative feedback mechanism, probably via presynaptic innervation. Many neuroregulatory systems are directly or indirectly connected with the pulse generator to enable the transmission of information meant to adjust its activity in relation to internal and environmental conditions. From the experimental evidence, the picture that evolves is of a highly complicated system with β endorphins, γ-aminobutyric acid (GABA), and galanin as direct inhibitors and excitatory amino acids (NMDA), neuropeptide Y and nitric oxide as direct excitators; all with individual interconnections (Fig. 43.3). The inhibitory action of estradiol at the hypothalamic level primarily results in a reduced amplitude of LH pulses, while progesterone and testosterone markedly inhibit the LH pulse frequency. This would suggest that estradiol preferentially lowers the LHRH pulse amplitude and that the other two steroids considerably lower the frequency of the "LHRH pulse generator". These effects are probably all mediated mainly via intermediate neurons such as opiodergic and GABA-ergic neurons, since LHRH neurons in the medio-basal hypothalamus do not have receptors for gonadal steroids.

The origin of the mid-cycle LH surge

The mid-cycle LH surge is induced by signals from the ovary. Most likely the strong increase in levels of estradiol, produced by the dominant ovarian follicle, exerts a

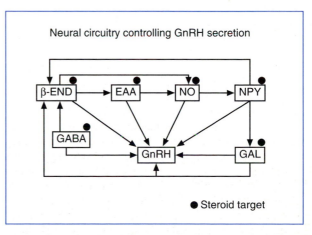

Figure 43.3 The interactive circuitry governing hypothalamic LHRH secretion. (β-END = β-endorphin, NO = nitric oxide, EAA = excitatory amino acids, NPY = neuropeptide Y, GAL = galanin, GABA = γ-aminobutyric acid.) (From Kalra SP et al. The interactive language of the hypothalamus for the Gonadotropin Releasing Hormone (GnRH) system. J Neuroendocrinol 1997;9:569-76. Reproduced with permission of the publisher Blackwell Science.)

positive feedback and elicits changes at the level of the pituitary, thus causing the massive release of LH. Whether the mid-cycle LH surge is also the result of mid-cycle hyperactivity of the LHRH pulse generator remains unclear. While in humans and in the nonhuman primate, in the absence of LHRH no LH surge occurs even when high levels of estradiol are reached, a mid-cycle increase in hypothalamic LHRH release is not necessary for occurrence of the LH surge. Indeed, treatment with exogenous pulses of LHRH by means of a pump in patients who lack endogenous LHRH pulsatility (patients with anorexia nervosa or Kallmann's syndrome) does not require a mid-cycle adjustment of the LHRH pulse-dose or frequency to obtain an ovulatory LH surge. Episodic LHRH secretion can probably be considered as a permissive factor for the occurrence of the mid-cycle LH surge. On the other hand, there is evidence suggesting an increase in mid-cycle activity of the LHRH pulse generator in normal women, and an increased pituitary responsiveness to LHRH. The latter is caused by estradiol, but in addition, this higher responsiveness may be the result of a decline of the peptide GnSIF, which normally maintains the pituitary in a state of low responsiveness. The surge is characterized by a sudden increase of LH with levels that double every 2 hours, with maximum values of about 10 times that of basal and lasts for 24 to 48 hours.

The endocrine hallmark of ovulation is luteinization of the granulosa cells and subsequent increase in production of progesterone, probably as a result of a combination of an increase in available substrate (low-density lipoprotein particles containing cholesterol) and required enzymes for rapid conversion of cholesterol via pregnenolone into progesterone. The LH surge most likely comes to an end by exhausting the pituitary LH reserve. Furthermore, the progesterone, in combination with estrogen feedback, results in a decrease in the frequency of the LHRH pulse generator. As a final result, a low frequency of LH pulses with large amplitudes can be observed throughout the luteal phase. In parallel to the LH surge, a threefold rise of plasma FSH levels also occurs. The role of this mid-cycle rise in FSH remains unclear. The underlying mechanism is probably the same as with the LH surge, but a temporary decline in inhibin is involved as well.

Intermediate influences

It is generally assumed that good health is a prerequisite in an organism's ability to procreate. Most of the severe nonendocrine disorders influence the reproductive axis by disrupting the function of the LHRH pulse generator and thus cause anovulation. This is almost always mediated via effects exerted on higher brain systems that in turn adjust the input of one or more of the factors that were discussed above, which determine the activity of the pulse generator.

The adrenal axis   The most important determinants of adequate functioning of the adrenal gland are the hypothalamic hormone corticotropic hormone-releasing hormone (CRH), the adrenocorticotropic hormone (ACTH), and cortisol. Whether appropriate secretion of cortisol is a premise for a normal hypothalamic-pituitary-ovary (HPO)-axis function is probably best illustrated by patients who develop Addison's disease. Only 25% of these patients develop menstrual dysfunction, which is often the result of premature ovarian failure based on autoimmune destruction of ovarian tissue. This suggests only a limited role for adrenocortical hormones. On the other hand, patients with adrenal enzyme deficiencies causing low levels of glucocorticoids and/or mineralocorticoids are often amenorrheic but normalize abruptly upon corticosteroid treatment. The latter would suggest that normal secretion of cortisol is of importance. Almost 70% of patients with nonpituitary Cushing's syndrome experience cycle disturbance and sexual dysfunction, implicating that either overexposure to adrenal steroids and/or absence of CRH and ACTH are involved in the function of the regulation of the HPO axis. LH and FSH levels and responses to LHRH are normal, suggesting that changes are due to a disturbance of the generation of the mid-cycle LH surge. CRH has an inhibitory influence on LH secretion if any. Therefore, an appropriate presence of CRH and ACTH are probably not permissive for adequate gonadotropin secretion. All together it appears that a reduced *and* increased production of adrenal steroids are involved in disturbing the normal function of the HPO-axis, without clear proof of direct involvement. Concurrent alterations in ovarian and adrenal sex steroid activity are most likely the underlying mechanism. The importance of appropriate adrenocorticoid hormone activity for the function of the reproductive axis is to ensure normal sex steroid activity.

The thyroid axis   Normal functioning of the thyroid gland is important for the HPO axis. Primary hypothyroidism could lead to anovulation and amenorrhea. Compensatory increased levels of thyrotropin-releasing hormone (TRH) induce hyperprolactinemia, which interferes with the regulation of gonadotropin secretion. Furthermore, hypothyroidism reduces sex hormone-binding globulins (SHBG) and subsequently the metabolic clearance rate of the weak androgens and estrogens such as androstenedione and estrone. Aromatase activity is also increased. Overall estrogen activity is increased, which in turn may also interfere with the function of the reproductive axis. In hyperthyroid conditions, the alterations in sex hormone activity play a more prominent role in disturbing the balance via a marked increase in SHBG with a substantial decrease of the metabolic clearance of the relatively strong androgens and estrogens. In particular, the hyperandrogenic status often leads to anovulatory conditions via disturbances of pituitary gonadotropin secretion.

Growth hormone axis   Growth hormone deficiency in adult females is often associated with disturbances of the menstrual cycle, which indicates some role for growth hormone (GH) in the function of the HPO axis. In patients with Laron type dwarfism, a condition characterized by the absence of GH receptor function, menstrual cyclicity is normal. GH exerts direct effects on the human ovary and synergizes the effect of FSH in inducing follicle growth. Lower levels of FSH are required to obtain monofollicular growth when GH is given to GH-deficient patients. It is currently unclear whether this effect is mediated via GH receptors present in the ovary or via insulin-like growth factors 1 and/or 2 (IGF-1, IGF-2). Amenorrhea often occurs in acromegalic patients. This may result from hyperprolactinemia due to dual secretion of GH and prolactin by some pituitary adenoma or due to pituitary stalk disconnection with subsequent lack of prolactin-inhibiting factor dopamine.

There seems to be a direct relation between the size of the adenoma and the degree of menstrual disturbance. An adverse direct effect of the high GH levels on the reproductive axis is the appearance of polycystic ovaries, which may be related to the anti-apoptotic property of the IGF that is hypersecreted. Blocked apoptosis in the ovary indicates diminished atresia, and this probably plays a role in the cystic appearance of the ovaries.

Adipose tissue   Adipose tissue is a major factor in determining the normal function of the HPO axis. Adipose tissue is a major source of aromatase, converting testosterone into estradiol and androstenedione into estrone. Furthermore, the enzyme 5α-reductase converts testosterone into the very active androgen 5α-dihydrotestosterone. Adipose cells also secrete leptin, the so-called fat cell reporter hormone, which is also involved in the function of the hypothalamus and pituitary.

Loss of weight is one of the most frequent causes of hypogonadotropic hypogonadism. This involves a direct inhibition of the LHRH pulse generator, thus causing an arrest of pituitary secretion of LH and FSH. A critical fat mass exceeding the 10th percentile is necessary to allow ovulation in women. Leptin is the key player in this mechanism. Leptin deficiency is associated with inactivation of LHRH neurons. A further physiological role for leptin may be in the initiation of puberty. Leptin may also play a role in the typical disturbances of the HPO axis associated with obesity: the polycystic ovary syndrome (PCO). In obese persons, hypersecretion of leptin occurs on the basis of a state of leptin resistance. Perhaps the hypersecretion of LH in PCOS is mediated by the high leptin levels. On the other hand, it may be possible that high levels of leptin have direct deleterious effects on ovarian function in the patients. Adipose tissue is regulated by insulin. Under relative unresponsiveness (insulin resistance), which is associated with many disorders, hyperinsulinism occurs, which probably interferes with the function of cytochrome P450 complex enzymes involved in adrenal androgen synthesis. This may thus have implications for the function of the reproductive axis.

Regulation of prolactin and lactation

Prolactin is a hormone produced by the pituitary lactotrophic cells and is structurally related to growth hormone (GH) and human placental lactogen (hPL). Other, extra-pituitary sources are the placental membranes and the endometrium. Several forms of prolactin can be distinguished: the most common form is a peptide of 198 amino acids with a molecular weight of 22 000 kilodalton (kD). Glycosylation produces larger forms, such as "big" prolactin with a molecular size of 50 000 kD and "big-big" prolactin of 100 000 kD. The larger molecules have the least biological activity. The half-life of prolactin is approximately 60 minutes.

Regulation of prolactin   A key feature in the regulation of prolactin is that it is one of the few pituitary hormones that undergoes active inhibition by hypothalamic dopamine reaching the anterior pituitary via the portal vessels (Fig. 43.4). Under normal circumstances this inhibition is constantly present, thus only minimal amounts of prolactin are synthesized and secreted. The process is mediated by dopamine receptors on the surface of the lactotroph. In addition, GABA may be involved in direct inhibition of prolactin secretion. No releasing hormones for prolactin have been identified so far. Importantly, the hypothalamic-releasing hormone TRH directly induces prolactin secretion via specific TRH receptors on the prolactin cells. Another significant stimulatory influence on prolactin secretion is due to estrogens and is mediated by nuclear estrogen receptors in the lactotroph and by stimulation of the number of TRH receptors. Prolactin secretion occurs throughout life in both sexes. An acceleration occurs at puberty but only in the female. Many physiological events such as nocturnal sleep and food intake are stimulatory and thus determine the typical 24-hour pattern of serum prolactin, with a nocturnal and post-prandial elevation (Fig. 43.5). Furthermore, physiological elevations occur upon exercise, nipple stimulation, coitus, pregnancy, lactation, and psychological stress. Finally, a number of nonphysiological factors cause high prolactin levels, among which are hypothyroidism, medications (psychiatric drugs, estrogens, serotoninergic drugs, dopamine-blocking agents), irritation of the thoracic wall by scars, esophageal reflux, anesthesia, hypoglycemia, and hypovolemia. Most of these effects are mediated through dopamine secretion.

The role of prolactin in the nonpregnant and nonlactating human female is unclear. The hormone is not required for the normal menstrual cycle. In its absence, such as in patients with panhypopituitarism, substitution with FSH and LH only is necessary for the normal functioning of the reproductive axis. Remarkably, in the rodent, prolactin instead of LH is the hormone for the maintenance of the corpus luteum and is thus already of crucial importance in an early stage of the reproductive process. In the human, pituitary prolactin has important functions with respect to the physiology of lactation, which will be discussed below.

Pregnancy and lactation   Even at a very early stage of pregnancy, tremendous changes in the anatomy of the breast occur. These changes are entirely due to the increase of serum, placental-derived estrogens and progesterone and pituitary prolactin. Estrogen induces growth of the

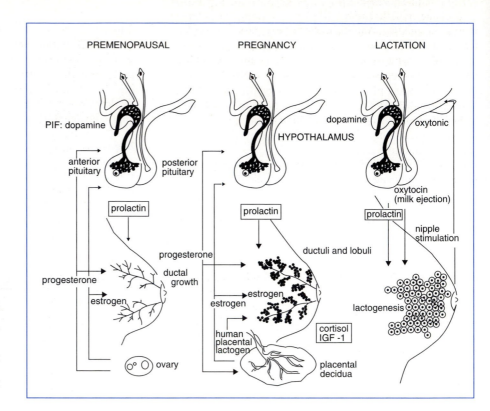

Figure 43.4 Diagrammatic representation of the neuroendocrine regulation of prolactin secretion in premenopausal nonpregnant women, during pregnancy, and during lactation (see text for explanation).

ductal system; and a combination of estrogens, prolactin, and progesterone causes growth of the lobuli and alveoli (Fig. 43.4). Insulin-like growth factor 1 (IGF-1) and cortisol also attribute to growth of the mammary gland. Lactogenesis during pregnancy is minimal or absent because estrogen and, mainly, progesterone inhibit prolactin-induced synthesis of casein and a lactalbumin. The increase of prolactin secretion is the result of the increase in the number and size of pituitary lactotrophs, which in turn are affected by the high estrogenic stimulation. This process causes a doubling of pituitary size during pregnan-

cy. After parturition, a rapid decline of the placenta-derived serum estrogen and progesterone levels occur, and thus the continuous inhibition of prolactin-induced lactogenesis disappears. This leads to a rapid induction of milk production. The milk ejection occurs via pituitary oxytocin release, which is caused by a neuroendocrine reflex upon nipple stimulation. Several weeks after parturition, prolactin levels have returned to normal pre-pregnancy values, however regular suckling causes sufficient periodic elevations of prolactin to maintain lactogenesis.

The hypothalamic pituitary reproductive axis during lactation The course of the reproductive hormones during the period of lactation is characterized by very low levels of LH, estradiol, and inhibins. Initially, FSH is also far below the range of normal values of the follicular phase; but it increases above the highest range of follicular phase values around 60 days after parturition, at a time when serum estrogen has reached its lowest levels. Lactational amenorrhea is a highly hypoestrogenic state because of an absence of any ovarian follicular activity. Some breastfeeding women even experience hot flushes, and the hypoestrogenic state may be one of the factors involved in temporary postpartum loss of libido and the occurrence of vaginal discomfort during intercourse, as experienced by some.

The ovarian quiescence is the result of the absence of adequate stimulation of LH and FSH by the pituitary.

The most important factors involved in causing absence of adequate pituitary LH and FSH secretion are:

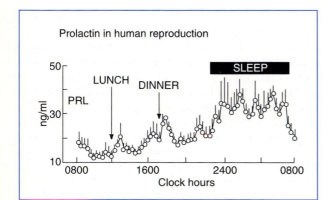

Figure 43.5 Prolactin levels over a 24-hour period in normal women. (From Yen SSC. Prolactin in human reproduction. In: Yen SSC, Jaffe RB [eds]. Reproductive endocrinology. 3rd ed. Philadelphia: Saunders, 1991;369.)

(1) diminished activity of the LHRH pulse generator, and (2) low pituitary responsiveness to LHRH. The suppression of the hypothalamic LHRH results from inhibitory inputs via suckling. Administration of exogenous pulsatile LHRH induces LH and FSH secretion and produces ovulation in lactating women. It seems that the impaired pituitary responsiveness to LHRH only plays a secondary role in the early stage of the lactational period. It is probably the result of a previously prolonged arrest of gonadotropic synthesis in the absence of adequate pulsatile LHRH.

FEMALE PUBERTAL DEVELOPMENT
Henriette A. Delemarre-van de Waal

The term puberty is derived from the Latin "pubes", meaning hair. Puberty can be defined as a maturational process of the hypothalamo-pituitary-gonadal axis resulting in growth and development of the genital organs and concomitantly in physical and psychological changes toward adulthood, leading to the capacity to reproduce. Puberty presents with breast enlargement in girls at a mean age of 10.5 years in the Netherlands and with testicular growth in boys at a mean age of 11.3 years. Breast development is the result of increasing levels of circulating estrogens, while testicular growth depends upon FSH stimulation.

Development of the external sex characteristics

The external sex characteristics include development of the breasts, pubic and axillary hair, the vulva, a change of fat composition, and changes in the vocal cords. The first sign of puberty is "budding" of the breasts, which may start at one side only and can be temporarily painful. As a result of enhancing estrogen activity, breast development increases, and other estrogen effects such as changes of the vulva, vaginal epithelium, and fat distribution occur. Androgens produced by the ovaries and adrenal glands induce growth of the clitoris and labia minora, as well as the development of pubic and axillary hair, and they are responsible for the change of voice. In prepuberty the labia majora covers the labia minora, while during puberty the labia minora grow and become visible. Androgens are also responsible for acne, body odor, and lowering of the voice.

According to Tanner, development of the breast can be divided into five stages (Fig. 43.6) and that of pubic hair into six (Fig. 43.7 and Tab. 43.1). Growth of pubic hair begins at about 3 months after the onset of first breast development (mean age 10.8 years). Duration of pubertal development is about 3 to 3.5 years, but it may vary from 2 to 6 years. Menarche occurs on the average 2.7 years after the onset of breast development. Menarche does not imply fertility. In general, there is a considerable period of irregular, anovulatory menstrual cycles. A regular pattern of ovulatory cycles is established within 5 years after menarche in most adolescents. Pubertal development is accompanied by a pubertal growth spurt. The increased height velocity occurs during the first half of puberty in girls, starting at the onset of breast development. At

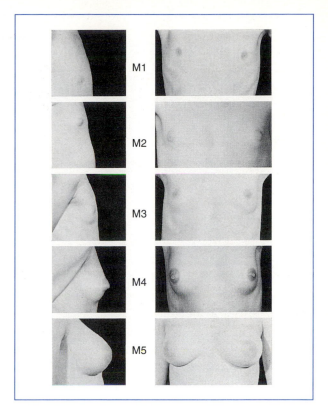

Figure 43.6 Breast development from the prepubertal stage B1 to the adult stage B5. (From Wieringen van JC, et al. In: Groeidiagrammen Nederland 1965. Groningen: Wolters- Noordhoff n.v., 1968; 41.)

menarche, growth is in the end phase, although height gain may be another 6 to 8 cm.

Development of the internal genital organs

The ovary In the third month of gestation, germ cells have multiplied and formed small groups of oogonia surrounded by a layer of mesenchymal cells. The oogonia further develop into primary oocytes; meiosis begins, but it soon arrests in the prophase stage of cell division. The conglomerate of one oocyte with two to three surrounding spindle-shaped cells, which will develop into granulosa cells, is the primordial follicle. From the fifth to sixth month follicular growth and atresia occur. At this time the ovaries contain a maximum number of oocytes of 6 million. Due to continuous atresia, 1 to 2 million are left at birth, and at menarche there are only about 400 000 primordial oocytes left. Maturation of primordial follicles into pre-antral follicles occurs, whereby the oocyte grows and the granulosa cells multiply, resulting in several layers of cells with fluid in between. Around the granulosa cells surrounded by a basal membrane, theca cells differentiate. The pre-antral follicle may further develop into the antral follicle, with a mature oocyte embedded in granulosa cells and a cavity filled with follicular fluid.

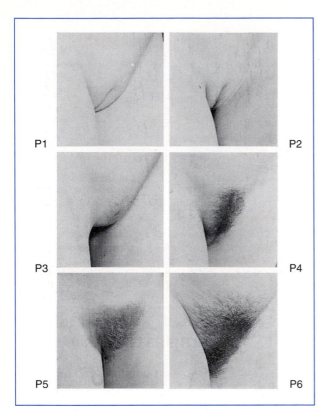

Figure 43.7 Developmental stages of pubic hair in female puberty, from the prepubertal stage indicated as P1 to the adult stage P5. Stage P6 is present in 10% of adult women. (From Wieringen van JC, et al. In: Groeidiagrammen Nederland 1965. Groningen: Wolters- Noordhoff n.v., 1968; 40.)

Table 43.1 Tanner classification of breast and pubic hair development

Breast

Stage B1	Prepubertal stage
Stage B2	Budding stage (of one or both sides); elevation of the breast and papilla, enlargement of the areolar diameter
Stage B3	Further enlargement of breast and areola, a clear breast contour
Stage B4	Increasing distribution of fat tissue; areola is above the level of the breast
Stage B5	Mature stage; recession of the areola to the general contour of the breast

Pubic hair

Stage P1	Prepubertal, i.e., no pubic hair
Stage P2	Sparse growth of slightly pigmented, straight or slightly curled hair, appearing chiefly along the labia
Stage P3	Increase of dark, strongly curled hair, which is spread sparsely over the junction of the pubes
Stage P4	Adult type of hair, but the area is considerably smaller than in adults
Stage P5	Hair is distributed as an inverse triangle of the classic feminine pattern
Stage P6	Further distribution of pubic hair in width across the linea inguinales and upwards to the linea alba. This hair type is present in 10% of adult women

The diameters of these antral follicles may vary between 2.5 and 6.5 mm. Large pre-ovulatory follicles with a diameter of 15 to 25 mm only develop in the fertile phase of life. At birth, the ovary contains all of the different stages of follicle development. In childhood the maturation process also continues, in spite of low gonadotropin stimulation. Therefore, the presence of ovarian follicles during infancy and childhood, often defined as cysts, is a physiologic event due to the persistent growth followed by atresia of primordial follicles. At puberty as a result of increased stimulation by luteinizing hormone, the ovary starts to produce estrogens. With the progression of puberty, the alternating growth and atresia of follicles results in a cyclic estrogen production. A fall of estrogens is responsible for the first vaginal bleeding, the menarche.

With progression of puberty, the ovary and uterus show a parallel volume increase. The myometrium thickens and a cavum becomes visible by sonography. The corpus and cervix develop into an adult shape. The vulva and vagina also undergo estrogen effects: the epithelium thickens and the cells change from mostly parabasal cells at the onset of puberty into mainly cornified cells at menarche. The mucosa color changes from red to pinkish. The mucosal changes result in vaginal secretion.

Endocrine control of the onset of puberty

The endocrine axis regulating puberty consists of the hypothalamic factor gonadotropin-releasing hormone (GnRH) and the pituitary hormones, LH and FSH. GnRH is a 10-amino acid peptide. It is present in the fetal hypothalamus at about 9 weeks of gestation. The hypothalamic GnRH content increases with gestation, with highest levels at mid-gestation. Pituitary content as well as blood levels of both gonadotropins show a similar increasing pattern. After mid-gestation LH and FSH pituitary content remain at about the same level, while the plasma gonadotropin levels decrease from high ("castrate") levels to a very low range at term. After birth, gonadotropin levels show a transient increase, which may last much longer in girls than in boys (Fig. 43.8). This incomplete suppression of GnRH release is probably responsible for the frequently seen premature thelarche in infancy. After the "prepubertal silence", gonadotropin levels increase until adult values have been reached; in pubertal girls the hypothalamus, the pituitary, and the ovaries will harmonize the secretion of their products in order to orchestrate the mature endocrine cycle.

LH levels show a pulsatile secretion pattern, which is a result of a pulsatile stimulation of the gonadotrophs by GnRH. FSH is secreted in a pulsatile fashion as well, but because of a longer half-life of about 2 hours versus 20 minutes for LH, a pulsatile pattern is less outspoken. This

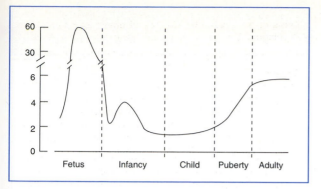

Figure 43.8 Changing pattern of gonadotropin plasma levels from the fetal period into adulthood. (Adapted from Winter et al. Pituitary-gonadal relations in infancy: 2. Patterns of serum gonadal steroid concentrations in man from birth to two years of age. J Clin Endocrinol Metab 1976;42:679.)

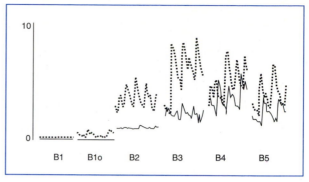

Figure 43.9 The changing pattern of LH plasma levels during female puberty. The first LH increase appears only during the night (broken lines) in the prepubertal phase, indicated as B1o (stage B1 onset), when there is no breast development yet. With the progression of puberty, the LH pulse frequency increases as well as the LH pulse amplitude. The day-night rhythm for LH is a characteristic pubertal phenomenon, which disappears during the last pubertal stage. (Adapted from Wennink JMB. Pulsatile hormone patterns in human puberty, thesis. Amsterdam: VU University Press, 1990.)

pulsatile pattern can already be demonstrated during the transient gonadotropin rise in infancy. The pulsatile stimulation is essential for an appropriate gonadotropin release, since continuous infusion results in desensitization of the GnRH receptor and therefore decreased secretion of both LH and FSH. This phenomenon is used in patients to suppress gonadotropin secretion by long-acting GnRH analogs. These analogs have a short-term GnRH-like effect. Due to prolonged occupation of the receptor, desensitization will occur.

Puberty is the result of increasing GnRH activity both in frequency and amplitude. The first endocrine change in pubertal development is the appearance of an LH elevation during the night, with low frequency LH pulses. This LH increase is followed by an estrogen elevation early in the morning. During puberty GnRH secretion increases, which is reflected by an increase in LH levels in both LH pulse amplitude and pulse frequency (Fig. 43.9). In the adult state, the day-night rhythm has disappeared. However, in the early follicular phase, an opposite pattern can be observed, with lower LH levels and a slowing pulse frequency during the night.

In adult men, as well as in women in the follicular phase, LH pulses have a frequency of one pulse every 90 to 120 minutes, while in the luteal phase the LH pulse frequency is about one pulse every 4 hours. Since qualitative and quantitative differences in the pulsatile patterns of LH have been demonstrated between the different phases of the menstrual cycle as well as between subjects with and without ovarian function, it is concluded that ovarian steroids modulate the episodic release of gonadotropins.

At the onset of puberty, LH first increases during the night. Regarding diurnal levels, the FSH increase tends to precede the LH increase. The GnRH-stimulated gonadotropin response increases with the progression of puberty. This response depends upon the previous stimulation of the gonadotrophs by endogenous GnRH. In the prepubertal stage, the GnRH silent period, a gonadotropin release barely occurs in response to a GnRH challenge

(Fig. 43.10). The response increases during puberty for LH. FSH has a similar trend, although the highest FSH response is present when GnRH release has just started, in pubertal stage 2. This high FSH response is also observed during infancy, just prior to complete suppression of the GnRH axis.

One of the important factors modulating gonadotropin secretion are the sex steroids. A sex steroid negative feedback develops during the second half of pregnancy. Estrogens suppress gonadotropin secretion, presumably at both the hypothalamic and pituitary levels. In the absence of estrogens, such as in Turner patients, gonadotropin levels are extremely high (castrate levels). This is seen in infancy and from puberty onwards. In prepuberty, gonadotropin levels in agonadal girls can be indistinguishable from those of normal children. During puberty an LH positive feedback of estrogens develops. This positive feedback depends upon GnRH stimulation as well as on the increase in the plasma estrogen level. The positive feedback is indispensable for the LH surge and therefore for the ovulatory cycle. Other factors modulating gonadotropin release are catecholamines, opioids, and melatonin. Dopamine exerts an inhibiting effect, with reduction of both pulse frequency and amplitude of LH secretion being observed; the mechanisms are still unknown. One possibility is a direct action on the GnRH-producing neurons at the median eminence, since dopamine does not cross the blood-brain barrier. Opioids suppress gonadotropin release. Opioid-containing neurons are present in the hypothalamus. These opioid neurons appear to play a role in the feedback action of sex steroids, whose effects are presumably mediated by catecholaminergic neurons. This indicates that the opiate

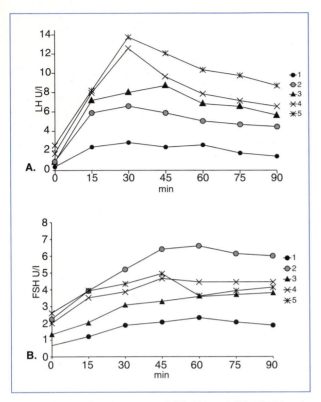

Figure 43.10 The increase of (**A**) LH and (**B**) FSH levels in response to 100 μg GnRH during the various stages of puberty. (Adapted from Dickerman et al. Response of plasma LH and FSH to synthetic LHRH in children at various pubertal stages. Am J Dis Child 1976;130:634.)

receptor antagonist is able to interfere with the opioid system only in the presence of sex steroids, which results in increased LH and FSH plasma levels. Melatonin inhibits gonadotropin secretion. Its physiologic role is uncertain, but tumors of the pineal gland are associated with precocious puberty.

Adrenarche

Adrenarche includes an increased secretion of the adrenal androgens dehydroepiandrosterone (DHEA) and androstenedione, produced by the zona reticularis. Adrenarche starts several years before the onset of puberty at 6 to 8 years of age and continues until late puberty. Since in normal development adrenarche and puberty are closely linked in time, it has been suggested that the adrenal is involved in the process of pubertal development as a "puberty triggering" factor. However, patients with premature adrenarche have a normal age of puberty, patients with gonadal failure have a normal adrenarche, and patients with primary adrenal insufficiency do not necessarily show a delay in pubertal development. Adrenarche will initiate the start of pubic hair growth in girls. Ovarian androgens will strengthen this process.

The mechanisms of the control of puberty

The "gonadostat" theory is based upon the concept of a changing sensitivity of the GnRH-releasing hypothalamus to the negative feedback of gonadal steroids. This negative feedback, developed during the fetal period, has the strongest potential during prepuberty: small doses of estrogens are able to suppress gonadotropin secretion in this period. According to this concept, at the onset of puberty this sensitivity decreases, which results in increasing GnRH release until adulthood when a new equilibrium between the sex steroids and gonadotropin secretion is reached. Growing evidence contradicts this concept, such as gonadotropin patterns of agonadal patients (Turner patients) that are similar to those in normal girls. Further, anti-estrogens do not result in an increase of gonadotropin levels as expected when a negative feedback is highly operative, but the low estrogen activity of these anti-estrogens appears to suppress gonadotropin levels, suggesting that there is no or hardly any negative feedback action during prepuberty. It is possible there is continued development of neurons, concomitant with an increase in terminal arborization and synapsing with neurons elaborating GnRH. The changing innervation of the GnRH neurons is responsible for the pattern of gonadotropin secretion from the fetal period into adulthood. There is increasing evidence that the prepubertal GnRH silence is the result of a GnRH restraint: the so-called "intrinsic restraint" concept. At the onset of puberty the influence of this mechanism is decreasing or becomes overruled.

GnRH is secreted in a pulsatile fashion. The prepubertal hypothalamus contains the same amount of GnRH as the adult hypothalamus. The prepubertal lack of release may be due to desynchronization of the "firing" of GnRH neurons. In vitro studies in immortalized GnRH neurons revealed that these neurons may be coupled electrically through cap junctions, which leads to the coordination of the secretion between separate cells. According to this concept, synchronization of the GnRH neuronal network will result in the onset of puberty.

The most recent concept involves excitatory neurotransmitters playing a key role in signaling the hypothalamic control of GnRH release. Glutamate neurons are present in the hypothalamus of the monkey. The GnRH neuronal network receives axodendritic synaptic input from this neurotransmitter. Glutamate as well as N-methyl-D-aspartate (NMDA), a synthetic analog of aspartate, stimulate GnRH release directly. Since NMDA antagonists inhibit the pulsatile release of LH, it is suggested that the glutamate receptors of the NMDA subtype are involved in the physiology of GnRH release. Based on studies in the rat, Bourguignon postulated three potential mechanisms that may be involved in the increase of GnRH pulsatility (Fig. 43.11): (1) The increase in the frequency of pulsatile GnRH release is the result of an increased rate of restoration of the releasable pool of glutamate by glutaminase (A); (2) Increased GnRH release may involve a reduction in the potency of competitive antagonism by GnRH (1-5) at NMDA receptors (B); and (3) Increasing GnRH release is achieved by the disappearance of inhibitory interneurons activated through NMDA receptors (C).

All of these concepts suggest that puberty is an ongoing developmental process, beginning during the fetal period and dynamically continuing to at least the last stage of puberty.

STRUCTURE AND FUNCTION OF THE OVARY

Jock K. Findlay

The human ovary is a multifunctional, dynamic organ essential for fertility and secondary sex characteristics (Fig. 43.12). Its primary functions are to release fertiliz-

able oocytes and produce the sex steroids and other protein hormones in a timely manner. It has the unique role of housing oocytes at a resting stage of meiosis from before birth to beyond 40 years of age.

The ovaries are slightly flattened, oblong bodies 2.5 to 4 cm in length and about 1.5 to 2 cm wide during the fertile years, but they can vary in size according to the stage of the menstrual cycle, the reproductive status of the individual (e.g., prepubertal, pregnant, or menopausal), and whether or not they are under stimulation by exogenous hormones. The change in size reflects primarily the number and size of large follicles and corpora lutea.

The massive hormone output and constant tissue remodeling required to accommodate its functions endow the ovary with some distinctive properties. These include cyclic episodes of angiogenesis and mitosis, a very high blood flow rate per gram of tissue, rapid tissue remodeling and repair, and extensive programmed cell death or apoptosis. Perhaps not surprisingly given these activities, the ovary is the site of the most common form of gynecological cancer, with a lifetime incidence rate of 1 in 90, the majority occurring in postmenopausal women.

Finally, the ovary is the "Zeitgeber" of the menstrual cycle. The ebb and flow of the hormones produced by the ovary, particularly by the larger follicles and corpora lutea, determine the length of the cycle, the time of ovulation, and consequently the fertile period and the time of menstruation.

The major ovarian cell types

The outer surface of the ovary exposed to the abdominal cavity consists of a *germinal epithelium*. Although it is not appropriately named since it has no germinal capabilities, this cell layer expresses many differentiated activities. For example, it expresses relatively high levels of steroid receptors, indicating it is a site of steroid action. The germinal epithelium is breached at every ovulation, which requires activation of tissue remodeling enzymes, the matrix metalloproteinases, and reestablishment of the epithelial integrity after release of the oocyte.

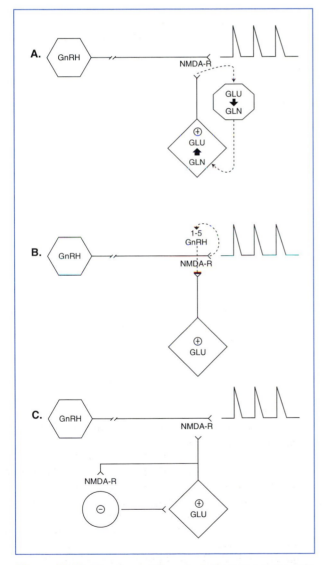

Figure 43.11 The three different mechanisms in the role of excitatory amino acids on the increase of GnRH release at the onset of puberty. (From Bourguignon JP, et al. The role of excitatory amino acids in triggering the onset of puberty. In: Plant TM, Lee PA [eds]. The neurobiology of puberty. Bristol: Society for Endocrinology, 1995;129.)

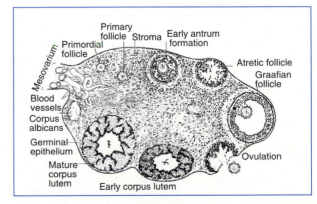

Figure 43.12 The human ovary in cross section. (From CIBA collection of medical illustrations: the reproductive system. 4th ed. New York: CIBA, 1970.)

The *oocytes* begin as primordial germ cells, which originate in the endoderm of the yolk-sac. They migrate from there along the dorsal mesentery of the embryonic hindgut, and across the coelomic angle to the genital ridge by a combination of amoeboid movements of the primordial germ cells, the influence of chemotactic agents, or association of the primordial germ cells with mesodermal cell movements during embryogenesis, although the precise mechanisms of migration are not known. It is known that primordial germ cells cannot survive outside the genital ridge, and induction of genital ridge development is dependent upon the presence of primordial germ cells. By 5 weeks of intrauterine life, the premeiotic primordial germ cells – now known as oogonia in the genital ridge – undergo intense mitosis and increase to 10 000 by 6 to 7 weeks and 600 000 by 8 weeks. At around 8 weeks, the onset of meiosis and degeneration of oogonia compete with mitosis, such that the number of oogonia peaks at 6 to 7 million at about 20 weeks and thereafter declines as more oocytes enter meiosis and remaining oogonia are depleted. The oogonia that enter the prophase of the first meiotic division are called primary oocytes, and they persist in this phase of meiosis until the time of ovulation (if that is ever reached) when meiosis resumes and they become secondary oocytes. The mechanisms underlying meiotic arrest are not known, but available evidence points to a role for an inhibitory factor(s) originating from the granulosa cells, which are in intimate cellular contact with each oocyte. The number of primary oocytes declines further such that at birth, there are between 1 to 2 million in the human ovary. This represents the maximum germ cell endowment of the postnatal human female; this number will decline continuously and irreversibly from birth until age 38, following which the rate of decline increases until the supply is exhausted at menopause. By the onset of puberty there are about 400 000 follicles containing primary oocytes, of which it can be calculated only about 400 to 500, or <1%, *will ovulate.*

The *granulosa cells* form an avascular syncytium around the oocyte. They have intimate contacts with the oocyte and between themselves through specialized gap junctions. Recent gene deletion studies in mice have shown that failure to express connexin 43, a component of gap junctions between the oocyte and granulosa cells, results in abrogation of follicular development. The granulosa cells are believed to derive from cells of the rete ovarii, a microtubular network within the genital ridge. These cells surround the primary oocyte to become squamous or flattened pre-granulosa cells. When the follicle recommences growth, they assume a cuboidal shape and begin mitosis and differentiation. There has been speculation about the existence of stem cells that could give rise to either granulosa or theca cells, or to other granulosa cells, but this has never been clearly demonstrated. The granulosa cells are functionally very heterogeneous, differentiating into mural and antral forms located near the basement membrane and antrum of the follicle, respectively, and into cumulus cells that surround the oocyte and

are released with it at ovulation. The mural granulosa cells express higher levels of steroidogenic enzymes and other proteins than the antral cells, which show signs of atresia before the mural cells. The cumulus cells, on the other hand, are often described as having higher mitotic rates than the other granulosa cells, and they have specialized gap junctions with the oocyte. Follicular growth consists partly of mitosis of the granulosa cells. It has been hypothesized that granulosa cells undergo a finite number of divisions before terminally differentiating into luteal cells (twelve such divisions in the case of the rat). This sets the final number of granulosa cells in an ovulatory follicle and determines the size of the ensuing corpus luteum. The granulosa layer is functional throughout folliculogenesis, implying that when not dividing the granulosa cells, or a subpopulation of them, produce hormones, as the remainder proceed through the mitotic divisions. Little is known about the factors that determine whether or not a granulosa cell will divide or differentiate.

Those cells that lie outside the basement membrane of the granulosa-oocyte complex form the interstitial compartment and are made up of a heterogeneous mixture of different cell types. They include theca interna and externa cells, leukocytes, endothelial cells of blood and lymph vessels, and vascular smooth muscle cells. The *theca interstitial cells* are the androgen-producing cells of the ovary. Four types have been identified: transient primary interstitial cells in the medulla of the fetal ovary, theca cells associated with developing follicles, secondary interstitial cells made up of the remnants of hypertrophied theca interna after the demise of a follicle, and hilar interstitial cells that look like Leydig cells and contain crystals of Reinke. Theca interstitial cells first become apparent as concentric layers adjacent to the basal lamina of follicles that have two to three layers of granulosa cells. They derive from cells of unknown identity in the interstitium, presumably as a result of a factor produced locally by the granulosa-oocyte unit, although its identity is not known. Theca cells undergo mitosis and differentiate into an interna and an externa layer endowed with rich lymphatic and vascular supplies. Theca cells are characterized structurally by the presence of organelles and lipid droplets associated with steroidogenesis. Cells with characteristics of smooth muscle cells that are not part of the vasculature have also been identified in the theca externa layer. Their function remains speculative but could be important at ovulation to assist extrusion of the oocyte.

The ovary, unlike the testis, is not a privileged immune site. Consequently, a wide range of *leukocytes* is always present in the ovary, but the numbers of neutrophilic granulocytes and activated macrophages increase considerably around the time of ovulation. It is hypothesized that the leukocytes resident in the ovary at the time of ovulation play a paracrine modulatory role akin to an inflammatory reaction to facilitate the actions of gonadotropins and growth factors.

The vasculature and lymphatics

The ovarian artery arises from the abdominal aorta below the level of the renal vessels and enters the ovary at the mesovarian border, at the hilus. There can be a considerable degree of coiling of the ovarian artery before it enters the ovary, and there are extensive spiraling, branching, and anastomoses with ovarian veins within the ovary. The growth and maintenance of the spiral arteries are estrogen-dependent. A secondary source of arterial blood supply to the ovary comes from the uterine artery.

Primordial follicles do not have their own blood supply. Once the theca interna forms it becomes vascularized, but the vessels do not cross the basement membrane until after ovulation occurs. The granulosa syncytium and a layer called the macula pellucida that develops at the site of follicular rupture remain avascular. Capillaries from follicles drain into veins in the theca externa, and the ovarian veins emerge from the ovary at the hilus. Blood flow to the ovary changes across the cycle, with an average in the ovarian vein of 21 ml per minute, which increases around the time of ovulation. The ovary has an extensive lymphatic system that contains high concentrations of ovarian steroids and inhibin. The lymphatic vessels can be seen around follicles with several layers of granulosa cells and in the corpus luteum, and they are characterized by the discontinuity of the endothelial layer of the vessels. The ovarian lymphatic channels follow the course of blood vessels and drain into the middle lumbar nodes and through uterine anastomoses to the sacral nodes.

Morphology of follicles

Follicles can be divided into two broad categories, preantral and antral, based on the absence or presence, respectively, of a fluid-filled cavity in the granulosa compartment. Preantral follicles may be either primordial, primary, or secondary, whereas antral follicles are either tertiary or Graafian follicles (large tertiary follicles of which preovulatory follicles are the most advanced). The percentage distribution of each type of follicle will vary primarily with the age of the individual, due to the depletion of the pool of primordial follicles. For example, women in their twenties have 92% primordial, 6% primary, 1.7%

secondary, and 0.3% tertiary follicles. By comparison, women over 45 years of age have 78% primordial, 16% primary, 5% secondary, and 1% tertiary follicles. The absolute number of all growing follicles – that is, primary, secondary, tertiary, and Graafian – remains relatively constant at 20 to 25 up to the age of 38 to 40 years. *Primordial follicles* are formed during the fourth month of fetal life in the human and consist of a primary oocyte in its arrested meiotic prophase, surrounded by a single layer of squamous or flattened pre-granulosa cells and no recognizable basal lamina. These follicles are nongrowing or quiescent, with an average diameter of 35 μm, an oocyte diameter of 32 μm, and approximately 7 to 23 pre-granulosa cells (average 13) (Tab. 43.2). An intermediary form of very small follicles has been identified as having a mixture of flattened and cuboidal granulosa cells (average 28; range 9-20), but no significant change in follicle or oocyte diameter. *Small primary follicles* are surrounded by a single layer of cuboidal granulosa cells with an outer basal lamina and a zona pellucida surrounding the oocyte that is traversed by the cytoplasmic processes of the granulosa cells. These follicles have an average diameter of 46 μm due to increase in the size and number of granulosa cells (average 76; range 23-223) but with no change in oocyte diameter. The transition from primordial to small primary follicle is thought to be a very slow maturation process rather than a growing process. The earliest *growing primary follicle* is recognizable by an increase in follicle diameter to 77 μm, an increase in the diameter of the oocyte (from 32 to 48 μm), and a fivefold increase in the number of granulosa cells (average 360; range 60-990) as a result of mitotic activity. *Secondary preantral follicles* are between 60 to 120 μm in diameter and consist of the primary oocyte with its zona pellucida surrounded early in development by several layers of granulosa cells (≤600 cells), a basal lamina, and a theca layer that forms when follicles have two to three layers of granulosa cells. This

Table 43.2 Morphometric characteristics of very small follicles in the human ovary

Follicle	Follicular diameter (μm)	Oocyte diameter (μm)	Oocyte nuclear diameter (μm)	Granulosa mean (No)	Cells range
Primordial (408)	35.4 ± 0.3	32.1 ± 0.3	16.1 ± 0.3	13 ± 6	7 - 23
Intermediary (409)	37.8 ± 0.4	31.7 ± 0.4	16.3 ± 0.2	28 ± 6	9 - 50
Small primary (153)	46.0 ± 0.5	32.6 ± 0.4	16.7 ± 0.2	76 ± 27	23 - 223
Early growing (30)	77.2 ± 2.0	47.8 ± 2.2	20.9 ± 0.6	360 ± 34	60 - 990

(Diameters in μm expressed as mean ± SEM, and number of granulosa cells expressed as mean ± SD for the number of follicles given in parentheses.)
(From: Gougeon A. In: Filicori M, Flamigni C [eds]. The ovary: regulation, dysfunction and treatment. Amsterdam: Elsevier Sciences, 1996.)

stage of folliculogenesis is marked by a rise in the mitotic activity of theca and granulosa cells and formation of the blood capillary and lymph networks in the theca layer. By the end of the secondary stage, oocyte diameter stabilizes at around 80 µm, and there has been a 600-fold increase in the granulosa cell number and a 15-fold increase in the follicle diameter. The appearance of a central fluid-filled cavity or antrum signals the formation of a *tertiary follicle*. The oocyte assumes an acentric position within the cavity surrounded by several layers of specialized granulosa cells known as cumulus oophorus cells, which maintain their connections via gap junctions with the oocyte. The cumulus cells are contiguous with the mural granulosa cells lining the antral cavity, and there is still mitotic activity in the granulosa and theca cell layers, although this begins to decline in the later stages. An increase in antral fluid volume contributes significantly to follicle growth in the tertiary stages. *Graafian follicles* are large tertiary follicles at the preovulatory stage.

Atresia is the process by which oocytes are lost other than by ovulation and is the fate of more than 99% of primary oocytes. Atretic follicles are thought to be incapable of ovulating and, once initiated, the process cannot be reversed. Atresia has been defined as the commitment of the oocyte and granulosa cells within a growing follicle to the state of *apoptosis* or programmed cell death. Apoptosis is a physiological process in which mammalian cells are triggered to express a genetic program that leads to cell death. Unlike necrosis – which is characterized by membrane disruption, hypoxia, cell swelling and rupture – apoptosis is an active, energy-dependent process consisting of nuclear and cytoplasmic condensation that leads to a decrease in cell volume and organelle compaction, except that the mitochondria are spared (Tab. 43.3). Nuclear and cytoplasmic fragmentation occur, which contribute to the formation of characteristic apoptotic bodies that eventually are shed from the cell surface and are phagocytosed by neighboring cells or macrophages. It can be viewed as the process reciprocal to mitosis, to ensure a stable cellular population. Biochemically, apoptosis is associated with an increase in Ca^{+2}, Mg^{+2}-dependent endonuclease activity and DNA fragmentation shown by a characteristic pattern of DNA laddering on agarose gel electrophoresis. A number of genes have been identified in the cascade, including members of the bcl-2 family, which code for survival factors. Although the trigger to apoptosis remains elusive, tumor necrosis factor-α and the Fas ligand/ Fas antigen system are strong contenders. All the morphological and biochemical markers of apoptosis also apply to atresia, such as nuclear pyknosis of granulosa cells, breakdown of the basement membrane, and fragmentation of DNA. Like apoptosis, the trigger to atresia is not known. Atresia occurs in all follicle classes throughout life and in a sense, predetermines the time of menopause. Teleologically, it can be viewed as a wasteful process. However, growing follicles at all stages contribute to the production of hormones essential for the maintenance of fertility and secondary sex characteristics.

Table 43.3 A comparison of the characteristics of apoptosis and necrosis

Characteristics	Apoptosis	Necrosis
Stimuli	Physiologic[1]	Pathologic
Inflammation	Absent	Present
Cell adhesion	Lost early	Lost late
Cell size	Shrinkage	Swelling
Intracellular macromolecules	Retained	Lost by leakage
DNA breakdown	Internucleosomal	Random
Phagocytosis	Present	Absent
Scar formation	Absent	Present

[1] May be a programmed event in some development processes. Biological agents, including hormones, can be stimuli. Loss of trophic signals may initiate apoptosis.
(From: Stouffer RL. In: Adashi EY, Rock JA, Rosenwaks Z [eds]. Reproductive endocrinology, surgery, and technology. Vol 1. Philadelphia: Lippincott-Raven, 1996, Chap. 12.)

Furthermore, if growing follicles were not turned over through atresia, it would have been necessary to evolve a process to hold ovulatory follicles for long periods of time to ensure the ready availability of a fertile oocyte in the event of a failed pregnancy.

Production and regulation of hormones and growth/inhibitor factors by follicular cells

Steroid hormones The human ovary actively secretes pregnenolone, progesterone, 17α-hydroxyprogesterone, dehydroepiandrosterone, androstenedione, testosterone, estrone, and 17β-estradiol. Studies have shown compartmentalization of production and regulation of these steroids. Granulosa cells principally produce progesterone, estrogens, and 17α-hydroxyprogesterone, but not androgens; whereas theca cells produce progesterone, 17α-hydroxyprogesterone, and androstenedione/testosterone, and secrete relatively little estrogen. Theca cells are regulated by luteinizing hormone (LH), whereas granulosa cells are regulated by follicle-stimulating hormone (FSH), and subsequently by FSH and LH. Both cell types are subject to paracrine and autocrine regulation by locally produced factors.

As a consequence of this compartmentalization, it becomes necessary for granulosa and theca cells to cooperate in the synthesis of *estrogens*. This was first recognized by Falck in 1959 and led to the two-cell/two-gonadotropin hypothesis, which states that LH stimulates the P450 side chain cleavage (scc) enzyme and 17α-hydroxylase activity in theca cells to produce aromatizable androgen (testosterone or androstenedione), which traverses the basal lamina and is converted to estrogen by P450 aromatase (arom) activity in granulosa cells under the influence of FSH (Fig. 43.13). At later stages of follicular development when granulosa cells acquire LH receptors, aromatase activity may be LH-driven. Follicular fluid contains micromolar concentrations of androgens, sufficient to drive the P450arom at maximum, and estradiol at concentrations 1000-fold above that found in peripheral blood. However, the presence of steroid-binding proteins in follicular fluid may render much of this steroid unavailable for metabolism or secretion. It is hypothesized that the mural granulosa cells, which are in close contact with the thecal vasculature across the basal lamina, act as the major site of synthesis of estrogen secreted by the ovary. The preponderance of 17β-estradiol over estrone is maintained by 17β-hydroxysteroid dehydrogenase activity in granulosa cells. The actions of both FSH and LH are mediated by adenylate cyclase in the cell membrane and the consequent production of cAMP. A corollary of the two-cell/two-gonadotropin hypothesis is that estrogen production cannot begin before the late primary stage because follicles must acquire a theca layer with LH receptors to activate androgen synthesis. IGF-1 increases and IGF-binding proteins (IGFBP) decrease the ability of theca cells to respond to LH by modulating the LH receptor, the cAMP response to LH, and the concentration of P450scc. At the stage of theca formation, the granulosa cells already have P450arom activity, which is stimulated via the FSH receptor-signaling system. The level of P450arom can be up-regulated in the presence of FSH by IGF-1, activin, and transforming growth factor-β (TGF-β), and down-regulated by follistatin, IGFBP, luteinization, and atresia. Furthermore, estrogen production increases as healthy follicles grow due to an increase in cell number and in production per cell by virtue of enhanced production of cAMP in response to gonadotropin stimulation. It has been hypothesized that follicular growth and differentiation, including the capacity to produce steroids, depends on the level of the cAMP tone in the follicle. A decrease in estrogen production is characteristic of atretic follicles, such that a fall in the estrogen/androgen ratio in follicular fluid below 1 is used as a marker of atresia.

Progestins can be synthesized by both theca and granulosa cells, and production is limited by the availability of cholesterol within the cell and the activity of P450 scc. Cholesterol used as a substrate for steroidogenesis is preferentially derived from circulating serum lipoproteins such as low density lipoprotein (LDL), which enters the cell by receptor-mediated endocytosis. There is evidence that this process may be facilitated by IGF-1. After fusing with lysosomes, the cholesterol esters are hydrolyzed and the free cholesterol is either taken up by the mitochondrial membrane with the assistance of steroidogenic acute regulatory protein (StAR) for metabolism by P450ssc through to pregnenolone, or re-esterified for storage in the cytoplasmic lipid droplets. The StAR proteins are a class of 30 kilodalton molecules localized in the mitochondria and induced by trophic hormones. The promoter region of the StAR gene contains sites for the transcription factor, steroidogenic factor-1, which can also regulate a number of steroidogenic enzyme genes. Theca cells have LH-dependent P450scc and ready access to serum LDL, making them a major site of progestin production in follicles. Production of progestins by follicular granulosa cells is limited by their avascular location, the very low levels of LDL in follicular fluid, and late acquisition of LH receptors to stimulate P450scc activity. Overall, progestin release by healthy follicles is low until after the preovulatory surge of gonadotropin, because most of the steroid is diverted to androgen and estrogen, whereas atretic follicles that lose their P450arom activity have a higher output of progestin and androgen until that too declines in advanced atresia.

The human theca interstitial cell is the major site of androgen production in the follicle. The process is LH-dependent and relies upon activation of the 17α-hydroxylase/17-20 desmolase activity, which in follicles is only found in theca interstitial cells. This enzyme converts Δ^5 and Δ^4 progestin precursors such as pregnenolone and progesterone, respectively, to C19 androgens. Its activity can be up-regulated in the presence of LH by insulin, IGF-1, and inhibin, and down-regulated by activin, bFGF and IGFBP.

Protein hormones The follicle makes a major contribution to the circulating levels of inhibin in the human. Although the follicle also synthesizes activin and follistatin, which act as intraovarian regulators, the extent of its contribution to circulating activin and follistatin is uncertain. There is preliminary evidence for a gonadotropin-surge inhibitory factor, which is found in follicular fluid, but its molecular nature has not been described.

Inhibin is a glycoprotein hormone made up of two dissimilar, disulfide-linked subunits termed α and β. It is particularly involved in the suppression of pituitary FSH. There are two forms of inhibin, called A and B, based on the nature of the β-subunit. Both forms have FSH-suppressing activity and are differentially regulated. The

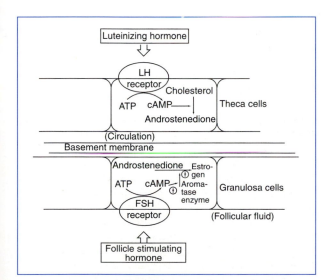

Figure 43.13 The two-cell/two-gonadotropin hypothesis of follicular estrogen production. (From Adashi EY. In: Adashi EY, Rock JA, Rosenwaks Z [eds]. Reproductive endocrinology, surgery, and technology. Vol. 1. Philadelphia: Lippincott-Raven, 1996;214.)

three subunits are coded by separate genes, members of the TGF-β superfamily, and they are synthesized as pre-pro molecules that undergo post-translational processing, giving rise to various free and dimeric molecular weight forms ranging from 105 to 14 kilodaltons. A 31 to 32 kilodalton inhibin dimer with one or two N-linked glycosylation sites is the smallest form with biological activity. Both inhibins are products of the granulosa cells. The β-subunit is expressed in all follicle classes examined except primordial follicles. Expression of the β-subunit is differentially regulated, with the βB form being prevalent before the βA form, implying that inhibin B is produced by late secondary-early tertiary follicles and inhibin A in late tertiary-Graafian follicles. This requires verification. Inhibin production by granulosa cells is FSH-dependent and LH-dependent in FSH-primed cells, and can be up-regulated by activin, TGF-β, and IGF-1, and down-regulated by follistatin, IGFBP, and epidermal growth factor (EGF)/TGF-α. Inhibin is present in human follicular fluid at concentrations 100 to 200-fold higher than in peripheral blood and is thought to be secreted by the ovary down this concentration gradient. The relative importance of lymphatic fluid and the ovarian vein as routes of secretion has not been resolved.

Intraovarian regulators The concept of local gonadal regulators is based on the fact that a number of well-established phenomena involving follicle growth and atresia could not be explained by altered gonadotropin profiles. Some phenomena can occur in the absence of gonadotropin while others can be modified while under gonadotropin control. Broadly, local regulation can be paracrine, involving diffusion of the regulator between two different cell types, or autocrine, involving one cell type self-stimulating with its own product. To qualify as a local regulator, there should be evidence of regulated local production, local action via specific receptors, a mechanism of inactivation, and some in vivo evidence of indispensability to the ovary. Many growth factors, cytokines, and neuropeptides are under investigation as potential intraovarian regulators, however relatively few meet all or most of these criteria.

Activin is a homo- or heterodimer of the inhibin β-subunits, joined by disulfide bonds. It was originally identified as three forms viz. activin A, AB, and B, on the basis of its FSH-stimulating activity, but it is now recognized as a pleiotropic growth factor that is present in many tissues. The significance to the ovary of the recently identified C and D forms of activin is not known. The mature form of activin is 24 kilodaltons and has no N-linked glycosylation sites. Activin is a product of the granulosa cells. It is up-regulated by FSH and further stimulated by IGF-1 and activin itself, and it is down-regulated by follistatin and EGF/TGF-α. The relative production rates and physiological significance of the different activin forms are not known, though on the basis of expression of the subunit genes it would be expected that activin B would be produced in the follicles before activin A. Activin has both autocrine and paracrine actions in follicles. Receptors for activin have been identified on granulosa cells and primary oocytes, and by implication on theca cells. Activin bound to follistatin is biologically inactive and very difficult to recover; it is also bound to α2-macroglobulin, which may provide an alternative avenue of clearance. Evidence is lacking for the absolute indispensability of activin for follicular growth.

Follistatin was first identified as an FSH-suppressing protein, structurally different from inhibin. It is the product of a single gene and consists of a number of isoforms ranging in size from 31 to 42 kilodaltons, which arise by a combination of alternative splicing of the mRNA and post-translational processing involving proteolysis and glycosylation. A major finding was the observation that follistatin is an activin-binding protein. It is produced by granulosa cells and stimulated by FSH, and by LH in FSH-primed cells. Its production is up-regulated by activin; down-regulated by EGF; is not influenced by IGF-1, prolactin, or growth hormone; and it appears to increase as follicles increase in size. While there is no evidence for follistatin receptors, some forms of follistatin bind strongly to heparan sulfates on the surface of granulosa cells whereas other forms are not bound. The significance of this binding is not understood and does not appear to be necessary to facilitate activin action.

Insulin-like growth factor-1 (IGF-1) is strongly implicated as an intraovarian regulator. Evidence has been obtained that a complete IGF-1 intrafollicular system exists in the rat. It is produced by granulosa cells, but not theca cells, under the influence of FSH and acts via IGF-1 receptors on granulosa and theca cells, where it amplifies gonadotrophic hormone action. The indispensability of IGF-1 for ovarian function is supported by recent studies with null mutant mice in which it was shown that inactivation of the IGF-1 gene resulted in gonadotropin resistance and follicular arrest at the early antral stage. Its production is reduced in atretic follicles and its activity is neutralized by IGFBPs (principally 4 and 5), which are also synthesized by granulosa cells, particularly in atretic follicles. FSH suppresses production of IGFBPs by granulosa cells. In women, IGF-2 and IGF-1 may be responsible for amplifying gonadotrophic action, because theca cells express IGF-1 and granulosa cells express IGF-2. IGFBP 1, 3, and 6 are probably the more important binding proteins for ovarian function. However, IGFs may be dispensable for fertility in women, because Laron dwarfs who have an IGF gene defect can become spontaneously pregnant.

Transforming growth factor-β (TGF-β) is a pleiotropic growth factor originally recognized by its ability to cause acute, reversible phenotypic transformation of mammalian cells. It is a homodimeric polypeptide of 25 kilodaltons and is associated with a carrier protein derived from the prepro precursor molecule. Activation of TGF-β requires separation from the carrier protein, and it is cleared following binding to α2-macroglobulin. There are multiple forms of TGF-β expressed in the human ovary (type 1 in oocytes, theca cells, and granulosa cells; type 2 only in theca cells), but very little is known about its level and regulation of production. In vitro studies have shown profound effects of TGF-β on proliferation and differentiation of granulosa cells and on oocyte maturation. Nevertheless, the physiological significance of TGF-β for follicular physiology is not yet known.

Epidermal growth factor (EGF) was originally identified by its capacity to induce precocious eyelid opening and eruption of the incisors in mice. It was identified as urogastrone in humans. It is a single polypeptide chain of 5 kilodaltons present in human follicular fluid, however evidence for its production by human follicular cells is limited. *Transforming growth factor-α (TGF-α)* is the same size as EGF and was identified for its ability to stimulate anchorage-independent growth of cells in soft agar. In the ovary, it is a product exclusively of theca cells and shares common activities and receptors with EGF. Both factors are generally inhibitory on gonadotropin-induced differentiation of granulosa and theca cells and can induce proliferation of granulosa cells where EGF receptors can be found. There is no evidence of an absolute necessity for the factors for normal ovarian function.

Basic fibroblast growth factor (bFGF) is a member of a large family of heparin-binding growth factors that can induce chemotactic, mitogenic, or angiogenic activity in a variety of cell lineages. bFGF has been identified in the granulosa, theca, and luteal cells. Increased expression of bFGF in the ovulating follicle has been associated with induction of plasminogen activator activity involved in follicular rupture and angiogenesis in the newly forming corpus luteum. bFGF has also been reported to exert inhibitory effects on FSH-induced steroidogenesis of granulosa cells and to facilitate mitotic division of these cells.

Tumor necrosis factor-α (TNF-α) induces cytolytic or cytostatic actions on a broad range of malignant and non-malignant cells. It has been implicated as an atretogenic and luteolytic agent and as a proinflammatory cytokine essential for ovulation. It is a product of macrophages, may also be produced by granulosa cells, and is found in human follicular fluid. It attenuates the differentiation of granulosa cells, stimulates progesterone and prostaglandin production, and facilitates LH-induced ovulation in ovarian perfusion models. TNF-α acts on granulosa cells via specific receptors, which in other cell types are linked to the apoptotic cascade of programmed cell death genes. More work is needed to establish the true role of TNF-α in ovarian function.

Interleukin 1 (IL-1) was originally discovered as an immunomodulatory cytokine product of monocytes and macrophages. It was shown to inhibit FSH-induced differentiation of granulosa cells, especially progesterone production, and to stimulate production of 20α-hydroxyprogesterone and prostaglandins. For this reason it has been postulated to also function as a luteinization inhibitor. It can also inhibit androgen production by theca cells. These actions are confined to IL-1 and not IL-2 or -3, with IL-1β being more potent than IL-1α. IL-1 is present in human follicular fluid, but its cellular origin in the ovary remains controversial. Ovarian macrophages are a likely site of production, but the possibility that follicular cells may also contribute has not been resolved.

Hormone receptors and signaling systems

Gonadotropin receptors The gonadotropin receptors are members of the G protein-coupled receptor superfamily containing 7 transmembrane regions and a relatively long extracellular ligand binding domain (Fig. 43.14). They are encoded by large genes (>70 kb) in the human with 11 (LHR) or 10 (FSHR) exons. The last exon encodes the transmembrane and intracellular regions of each receptor. The mRNA for each receptor is alternately spliced, encoding truncated forms with unknown biological significance. Mutations in the FSHR and LHR lead to constitutively activated and inactivated forms, explaining certain pathologies of gonadal function. Changes in the synthesis and degradation of the respective receptor mRNA are thought to be a qualitatively important mechanism for regulating the receptor number. Most actions of FSH and LH on their respective receptors can be attributed to activation of the adenylate cyclase/protein kinase A pathway via stimulation of Gs proteins. High levels of both ligands can also activate the phospholipase C/protein kinase C pathway under certain circumstances.

Expression of the FSHR is confined exclusively to granulosa cells and is first detected when the cuboidal

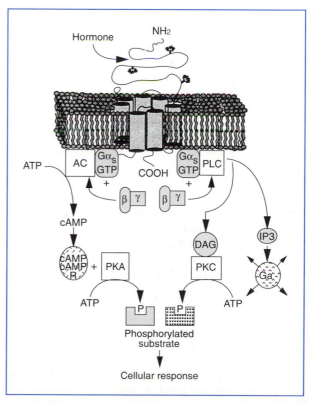

Figure 43.14 Structural features of the G protein-coupled gonadotropin receptor and some of its potential signaling pathways. (From Park-Sarge OK, Mayo KE. In: Findlay JK [ed]. Molecular biology of the female reproductive tract. San Diego: Academic Press, 1994;157.)

granulosa cells of primary follicles begin mitosis. Studies in neonatal rodents suggest that the truncated forms of FSHR are produced early in folliculogenesis and followed later by full length transcripts. There are relatively few factors known to influence the expression of FSHR. The identified factors include FSH itself (in synergy with estradiol), cAMP and its analogs, EGF, TGF-β, and activin, but not IGF-1. Activin increases transcription of the FSHR gene and stabilizes the mRNA, which results in an increase in FSH binding sites on granulosa cells. The relative importance of activin and TGF-β in up-regulating FSHR has not been resolved. Transgenic mice with a null mutant gene for the FSHR and women with inactivating mutations in the FSHR gene are infertile.

While FSHRs are expressed on the granulosa cells of all growing follicles, LHRs first appear on the theca cells of primary follicles, and subsequently on differentiated granulosa cells of tertiary follicles. Little is known about regulation of the isoforms of LHR. Receptor number is tightly correlated with changes in LHR mRNA, suggesting that synthesis and degradation of LHR mRNA are important points of regulation. IGF-1 augments the ability of theca cells to respond to LH by increasing the number of LHR and augmenting the intracellular response to LH. Expression of LHR on granulosa cells is FSH-dependent and is further amplified by IGF-1, estradiol, and activin. FSH increases transcription of the LHR gene and may also stabilize LHR mRNA.

Steroid receptors Steroids act via receptors that are a family of nuclear transcription factors. These molecules consist of a C-terminal domain involved in ligand binding and ligand-dependent transactivation, a highly conserved central domain responsible for dimerization, nuclear localization, and DNA binding, and a hypervariable domain at the N-terminal end that contributes to the transactivation function. When bound with ligand, the receptor undergoes a conformational change, allowing it to bind with high affinity to specific responsive elements in the regulatory region of steroid responsive genes and to modulate gene transcription. *Progesterone receptors (PR)* have been detected in nuclei of theca cells and surrounding stroma of growing follicles but not in granulosa cells of preantral or tertiary Graafian follicles in women and rhesus monkeys. After a mid-cycle gonadotropin surge or an ovulatory bolus of hCG, there is intense expression of PR in luteinizing granulosa cells. This corresponds with evidence for a role of progesterone in the ovulatory process. *Androgen receptors (AR)* in the primate ovary are found in both theca and granulosa cells, which is consistent with a modifying action of androgens on gonadotropin-induced functions of these cells. However, the ontogeny of expression of AR is not resolved. In several studies, AR were not detected in primordial or primary follicles of women or macaques, but they were present in theca and granulosa cells of secondary and tertiary follicles, with expression becoming more intense in granulosa cells of Graafian follicles. In another study, AR expression was most intense

in granulosa cells of secondary and early tertiary follicles of nonhuman primates and decreased as the follicle matured. *Estrogen receptor (ER)* expression in follicular cells of the primate ovary has been controversial. There is a consensus that ER are not detectable in primordial or growing primary and secondary follicles of women or macaques. However, it is not clear what the case is in tertiary and Graafian follicles. Some report intense localization of ER in granulosa cells, but not theca cells, which disappear after the gonadotropin surge. Others are unable to detect ER in these follicle types. Resolution of this problem may lie with the recent identification of a second ER gene (ER-β), which is strongly expressed in granulosa cells of the ovary.

REGULATION OF FOLLICULAR DEVELOPMENT

A morphological model of folliculogenesis and atresia

A morphological model for folliculogenesis in the human ovary has been proposed by Alain Gougeon. It is based on the size of the oocyte, the shape and number of granulosa cells, the presence of a theca layer and antrum, and the diameter and health status of the follicle (Fig. 43.15). This model defines a growth path for healthy follicles and identifies stages from quiescence to initiation/maturation, growth, selection, maturation, dominance, and ovulation or atresia. The growth stages are divided into eight classes, beginning arbitrarily at the secondary preantral stage and preceded only by the primordial to the maturing primary stages. It also defines the time taken for follicles to proceed through the growth trajectory based on mitotic indices and doubling times (Fig. 43.16). The period in which a primordial follicle matures into a primary follicle is very long, >150 days, followed by another 120 days to become a Class 1 secondary preantral follicle, totalling >270 days or nine menstrual cycles. Growth from Class 1 to Class 8 (ovulatory) requires 85 days or approximately three menstrual cycles, with the last 4 Classes requiring only 20 days.

A functional model of folliculogenesis and atresia

The functional processes that occur during growth – differentiation and atresia of follicles, and how these are controlled by local factors and gonadotropins – are becoming better understood. This has led to the development of follicle classification systems based on functional rather morphological criteria. A major problem with models based solely on morphological criteria, particularly size, is the grouping of cohorts of follicles that may be functionally quite distinct. Some of the sequential physiological changes critical for growth and development can occur within a single morphological stage, which masks both the significance of these changes and the uniqueness of each follicle.

One functional model proposed recently consists of five groups of follicles based upon their dependency on and sensitivity to gonadotropins (Fig. 43.17). Follicles

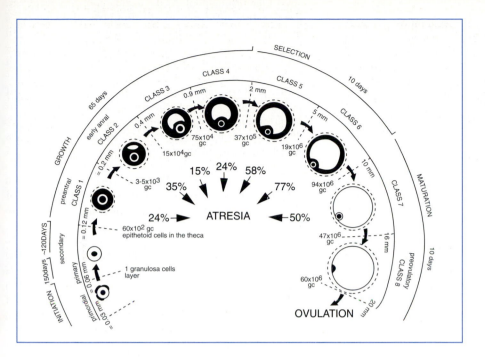

Figure 43.15 Classification of follicles in the human ovary. (From Gougeon A. Dynamics of follicular growth in the human: a model from preliminary results. Human Reproduction 1986;1:1-87.)

can be quiescent (i.e., primordial), committed to growth (preantral and antral), ovulatory, or atretic. Committed follicles become responsive to gonadotropin but do not have an absolute dependence on gonadotropin for growth until a later stage. At advanced stages of growth, committed follicles may be gonadotropin-sensitive, requiring an appropriate balance of LH and FSH to maintain growth, or else atresia occurs. These five follicle groups are not

regarded as absolutely discrete because folliculogenesis is considered to be a continuous process with a hierarchy among follicles according to their developmental status. Put another way, no two follicles are identical in their functional properties, which may have implications at the time of commitment to the growth of primary follicles and selection of ovulatory follicles. The assumptions of this model also include: the quiescent nature of primordial

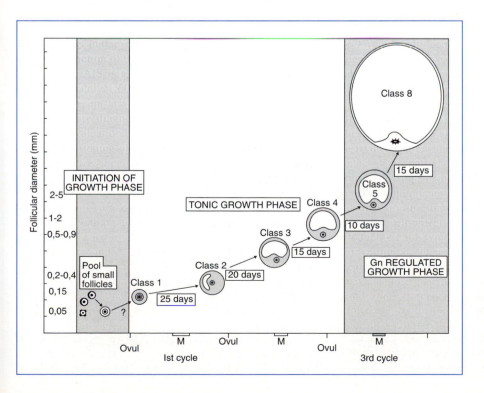

Figure 43.16 The follicular growth trajectory in the human ovary. (From Gougeon A, cited by Adashi EY. In: Adashi EY, Rock JA, Rosenwaks Z [eds]. Reproductive endocrinology, surgery, and technology. Vol. 1. Philadelphia: Lippincott-Raven, 1996;30.)

follicles until they become committed, follicles that are committed to grow either ovulate or become atretic, functional atresia is an irreversible process that can occur at all stages, FSH and LH are the only pituitary hormones essential for growth and development, and autocrine and paracrine factors are essential for folliculogenesis. The validity of this model is the subject of current research.

Initiation of commitment to growth

When follicles leave the primordial pool, they become irreversibly committed to growth or atresia. Growth is said to begin in small primary follicles in the human ovary when the oocyte nuclear diameter reaches 19 μm and there are >15 granulosa cells in the largest cross section of the ovary. Biochemical markers of growth, such as thymidine incorporation and proliferating cell nuclear antigen, have not been applied to the human ovary in the same way as rodents. The mechanisms that control the initiation of follicular growth are not known, though several models have been proposed. It has been suggested that follicles commence growth in the order in which they were formed and in relation to their association with the rete ovarii. In a second related model, it is hypothesized that follicles initiate growth independent of influences from outside the follicle, that the number that begin growth at any one time is fixed by the size of the pool, and that the reduction in the size of the pool that occurs with aging does not alter the proportion that begin growth per unit time. In the third model, entry of follicles into the growing pool is hypothesized to be regulated by intra- or extraovarian factors, and a reduction in the size of the nongrowing pool is accompanied by a compensatory increase in the proportion of follicles beginning to grow. Evidence to date favors the last model, at least up to 38 years of age, supporting a role for local or extraovarian (endocrine) factors. It is possible that there is a negative influence of primordial and early primary follicles on

themselves, the magnitude of which is proportional to the size of the resting pool. As the resting pool size decreases, the negative influence would diminish, allowing for a larger proportion of follicles to commence growth until the pool is exhausted. Several intracellular proteins have been implicated in this negative influence, including Wilms' tumor suppressor transcription factor, retinoblastoma protein, and *myc* oncoprotein. The role of gonadotropins, FSH in particular, in the initiation of follicle growth in primates is complex and may be age-dependent. Whereas hypophysectomy of adults does not block initiation, anencephalic fetuses lack early growing follicles. The increase in the disappearance rate of nongrowing and early growing follicles in aging women has been linked to the increase in circulating concentrations of FSH. Gougeon concluded that, "rather than initiating follicle growth per se, gonadotropins may act on resting follicle maturation by transforming their granulosa cells, thereafter making possible for these follicles to enter the growth phase in response to an unknown signal." This implies a presence of functional FSHR on pre-granulosa cells, for which there is no evidence as yet. A number of other factors has been suggested to influence initiation, including nerve growth factor, c-kit ligand via c-kit receptor, bFGF, EGF and TGF-α, based largely on their appearances in early growing follicles. More recently, growth/differentiation factor 9 has been implicated in oocyte growth in mouse primary follicles.

Growth of committed follicles

Tonic growth phase Follicles in Classes 1 to 4 in the Gougeon model are in a slow tonic growth phase lasting 65 days (Fig. 43.16). Cell proliferation and atresia rates are low and independent of the cyclic hormonal changes. Judging from observations on ovaries from prepubertal girls, pregnant women, and patients with Kallmann's syndrome, all of whom have reduced gonadotropin output, these follicles require tonic levels of gonadotropins to be quantitatively normal and form antra by Class 2. Atresia in these early growing follicles is low (15-35%) compared

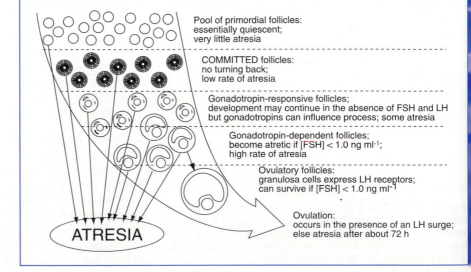

Figure 43.17 A functional model for follicular growth based on the dependence and sensitivity of the ovine follicles to gonadotropins. (From Scaramuzzi RJ, et al. Reproduction fertility and development 5. p. 465, Fig. 4, 1993.)

Pool of primordial follicles: essentially quiescent; very little atresia

COMMITTED follicles: no turning back; low rate of atresia

Gonadotropin-responsive follicles; development may continue in the absence of FSH and LH but gonadotropins can influence process; some atresia

Gonadotropin-dependent follicles; become atretic if [FSH] < 1.0 ng ml⁻¹; high rate of atresia

Ovulatory follicles: granulosa cells express LH receptors; can survive if [FSH] < 1.0 ng ml⁻¹

Ovulation: occurs in the presence of an LH surge; else atresia after about 72 h

ATRESIA

to larger follicles (>50%) and is characterized by degeneration of the oocyte before the somatic cells. The granulosa cells are relatively undifferentiated with a low steroidogenic capacity and an increasing proliferative potential. The mitotic index of the granulosa layer increases from around 0.4 in Class 1 to 0.8 in Class 4 follicles. Although they are responsive to FSH, the granulosa cells express low levels of P450arom, make very little estrogen or progestin, and lack LHR expression. Theca cells are LH responsive and synthesize androgen; consequently, the intrafollicular androgen to estrogen ratio is high. Local regulatory factors such as activin, IGF-1, inhibin, TGF-β, and EGF/TGF-α, which can be identified in follicular cells and shown to be capable of acting during this time, could be important for minimizing the responses to gonadotropin.

Gonadotropin-regulated growth phase Follicles in Classes 5 to 8 are heavily dependent on gonadotropin for their exponential growth (Fig. 43.16), and their growth and atresia rates are related to the hormonal fluctuations of the menstrual cycle. It is from these Classes that the follicle destined to ovulate will be selected and become the dominant Graafian follicle over a 25-day period. The

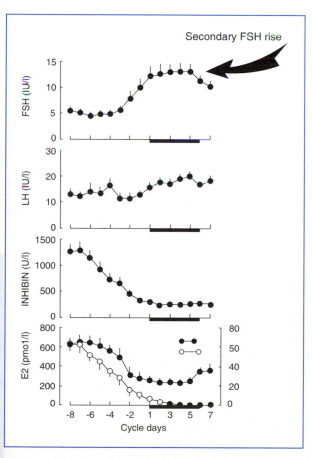

Figure 43.18 The hormonal changes at the time of the luteal-follicular transition when the dominant follicle is selected in women. The inhibin form shown in the late luteal phase is likely to be inhibin A. (From Roseff SJ, et al. J Clin Endocrinol Metab 1989;69:1033-9.)

dominance established by this follicle persists into the secretory phase of the cycle in the form of the corpus luteum. Atresia in these follicle classes can be as high as 70% and is first characterized by nuclear pyknosis in the granulosa layer and by the irregular shape of the follicle or oocyte. Follicles in Class 5 with a follicular diameter of 2 to 3 mm are said to be selectable and require a rise in FSH to sustain them (Fig. 43.18). This is accompanied by an up to two-to threefold increase in the mitotic index, and up-regulation in the capacity of the follicle to synthesize estrogen through an increase in FSH-dependent P450arom in the granulosa cells. There is also enhanced LH-dependent androgen synthesis by the theca cells. All of these activities are likely to be influenced by local regulators. For example, activin at low doses in conjunction with FSH promotes proliferation of granulosa cells and inhibits LH-stimulated androgen synthesis by theca cells. At higher doses activin increases the FSHR number and the responsiveness of granulosa cells to FSH. IGF-1 (or -2) plays a key role during these stages by amplifying gonadotrophic-dependent differentiation of follicular cells.

The first indication that a Class 5 follicle has been selected as a result of an FSH rise is that its diameter reaches 5 mm and the high mitotic index in the granulosa layer is maintained, whereas the mitotic rate in the remainder of the cohort of follicles of similar size falls and they eventually become atretic. FSH is the survival factor for the healthy selected follicles, preventing them from undergoing atresia and promoting their growth and differentiation. The granulosa cells become more responsive to FSH, assisted by local regulators such as IGF-1 and activin, which results in a large increase in P450arom activity and increased production of inhibin, probably the B form. Comparison of the follicular fluid contents of selected and nonselected follicles reveals higher FSH and estradiol concentrations, similar androstenedione concentrations, and an androgen/estrogen ratio <1 in the newly selected follicle.

The follicle continues to increase dramatically in size due to an increase in granulosa cell number and an expansion of the antral fluid volume, and it eventually becomes dominant. The dominant follicle is characterized by its size (>10 mm) and its capacity to produce estradiol (200 times that of follicles before selection), 99% of which is made by the granulosa cells. It continues to secrete inhibin, although the A form may now predominate. A higher concentration of estradiol in the ovarian vein on the side of the dominant follicle can be detected by the mid-follicular phase. The dominant follicle also expresses LHR induced on the granulosa cells by FSH and amplified by local regulators such as IGF-1 and activin. Not only is the presence of LHR important to allow the dominant follicle to respond to the mid-cycle ovulatory surge of gonadotropin, it also enables granulosa cell function to be driven by LH pulses late in the follicular phase when FSH concentrations may be limiting. The FSH/LH ratio may be important for the future survival of a follicle under some circumstances, especially if the LH is too high. The fractional area of the thecal layer occupied by blood vessels also increases in a dominant follicle, presumably due to the influence of angiogenic factors such as estrogen, FGF, and vascular endothelial growth factor made by granulosa cells.

Follicles are thought to maintain dominance in two ways. The first is by endocrine starvation of the nondominant cohort of follicles by virtue of the increased estradiol production and continuing inhibin secretion by the dominant follicle suppressing the output of FSH below a point critical for survival of subordinate follicles. The dominant follicle protects itself in these circumstances of low FSH by producing local factors such as IGF-1 and activin that amplify the actions of FSH and LH, and by increasing its capacity to respond to rising levels of LH. The second is by production of local factors by the dominant follicle that inhibit growth of smaller and nondominant follicles and their responsiveness to gonadotropin. Evidence for this second hypothesis is not substantial. Follicles in Class 4 (2-5 mm) become less responsive to human menopausal gonadotropin stimulation as ovulation approaches, and there is in vitro evidence for production of factors such as TGF-α that inhibit estradiol production by the ovary.

OVULATION

Ovulation is the process by which the ovum is released from the follicle in response to the mid-cycle surge in gonadotropins. The interval between the onset of the LH surge or administration of an ovulatory dose of LH or hCG and ovulation is 36 to 42 hours in women. The cascade of morphological and biochemical events initiated by the gonadotropin surge can be conveniently divided into the resumption of oocyte meiosis, follicular rupture, and the onset of luteinization. It is critical that ovulation is timely to allow for the maximum opportunity for the mature ovum to be fertilized after its release, and that the ovum is released outside, not within, the ovary.

Resumption of meiosis

Resumption of meiosis in the oocyte of the dominant follicle is associated with chromatin condensation, disintegration of the nuclear membrane or germinal vesicle breakdown (GVB), chromosome segregation, and shortly before ovulation appearance of the first polar body. This ability to resume meiosis is called meiotic competence and is acquired only at the later stages of oocyte growth during advanced folliculogenesis. Meiotic competence appears to be regulated by FSH and involves follicular estradiol. The local factors involved in meiotic arrest and its resumption after the LH surge are not well understood. The arrest of meiosis is related to the integrity of the gap junctions between the cumulus cells and the oocyte, and it has been suggested that cAMP could serve as the inhibitory signal that is transferred to the oocyte via the gap junction system of the granulosa and cumulus cells and the oocyte. It should not be inferred, however, that the break-

down of the gap junctions between the oocyte and cumulus cells per se allows for the resumption of meiosis to take place. Although the LH surge causes the cumulus cells to undergo a characteristic disaggregation and expansion and a breakdown in these gap junctions, this may still be preceded by resumption of meiosis. Nevertheless, it has been hypothesized that decreased cAMP production within the follicular unit by the granulosa-cumulus layers after the LH surge and a consequent fall in intra-oocyte cAMP levels allows for the resumption of meiosis. A maturation promoting factor or M-phase promoting factor (MPF) has been described that presumably controls the transition from the G2- to M-phase of the cell cycle in mitosis and meiosis. M-phase promoting factor activity is present in mammalian oocytes and may control meiosis once it resumes. However, the identity of M-phase promoting factor and its mechanisms of action in the human oocyte remain elusive.

Follicular rupture

Characteristic structural changes occur in the wall of the follicular apex during the interval between the LH surge and follicular rupture. The oocyte-cumulus unit must pass through the granulosa layer, the basal lamina, the theca interna and theca externa layers, and the tunica albuginea and germinal epithelium. The outer germinal epithelium on the apex of the ovulatory follicle begins degradation by apoptosis several hours before rupture such that there is increased transillumination through the wall. Perforations eventually develop in the deep collagenous layers, allowing follicular fluid and single cells to escape. There is a decrease in blood flow to the apical area, and eventually a sticky, translucent exudate accumulates on the site of the follicle stigma. Release of the oocyte-cumulus unit occurs over a period of 2 to 5 minutes once degradation of the apical wall is sufficiently advanced.

Follicular rupture has been likened to acute inflammation, which has been a helpful analogy to unravel the mechanisms involved. Rupture includes collagen and extracellular matrix breakdown, which weakens the follicle wall, and involves increased blood flow and vascular permeability and edema to deliver substrates and maintain a positive intrafollicular pressure. A number of inflammatory substances, inflammatory cells, and steroids are involved in the ovulatory cascade. The LH surge is believed to cause an increase in the level of these mediators and cells within the ovary that lead to rupture and release of the ovum. An element of redundancy exists in these mediator pathways, which must ensure that ovulation occurs.

Progesterone is one steroid for which there is strong evidence of a role in ovulation in women and rodents, most recently in mice with a mutant PR gene. The effects of progesterone have been connected with proteolysis of the follicle wall and plasminogen activator activity. Progesterone production increases dramatically as a result of the LH surge luteinizing the granulosa and theca cells.

Members of the eicosanoid family can also have multiple effects on the cascade. Eicosanoids are polyunsaturated, hydroxylated fatty acids derived from arachidonic acid, grouped into cyclooxygenase or COX products (prostaglandins and thromboxanes) and lipoxygenase products (leukotrienes and lipoxins). The gonadotropin surge induces the expression of a COX 2 enzyme in granulosa cells, resulting in high prostaglandin levels in follicular fluid of the ovulatory follicle. Similarly, lipoxygenase activity in granulosa cells is increased by hCG. Experimental inhibition of COX 2 or lipoxygenase activities can block or suppress ovulation, supporting a role for these products in the ovulatory process. There is accumulating evidence that they are involved in activating procollagenase and increasing vascular permeability. Site-directed proteolysis must take place at the follicular apex for ovulation to occur; and plasminogen activators (PA) and matrix metalloproteinases (MMP), which include collagenases and gelatinases, are implicated. The plasminogen activators include tissue-type (tPA) and urokinase-type plasminogen activators (uPA), which convert plasminogen in follicular fluid and derived from serum into active plasmin, which in turn activates latent matrix metalloproteinases into active forms. Coordinate regulation of these protease activities in a time- and cell-specific manner is achieved by an increase in the level and activity of the protease and the presence of specific inhibitors, plasminogen activator inhibitor-1 (PAI-1) and tissue inhibitors of matrix metalloproteinases (TIMPs). The cytokine interleukin 1 has been implicated in the ovulatory cascade. Although usually a product of leukocytes, IL-1 is synthesized by theca cells in response to LH and amplifies the ovulatory response induced by LH; including promotion of matrix metalloproteinases, and synthesis of progesterone, prostaglandins, and nitric oxide (NO). The presence of NO synthase in the theca compartment, presumably due to the presence of endothelial cells and leukocytes, has implicated NO in ovulation. Evidence to date suggests that it influences blood flow. There is evidence for a *renin-angiotensin* system in the ovary that has been connected to ovulation, however, the data is limited, particularly for the human ovary. *Bradykinin* is a nonapeptide generated locally in the ovary from plasma kininogen by kallikrein enzymes that become particularly active after the LH surge. Bradykinin mediates increased vascular permeability and vasodilation. Of the wide range of lymphohemopoietic cells found in the ovary, only *neutrophilic granulocytes* and *activated macrophages* increase at ovulation. There is evidence for a role of leukocytes and macrophages in ovulation in rodents.

CORPUS LUTEUM

The corpus luteum is formed from the cellular wall of the ovulated follicle and continues the endocrine dominance that follicles established in the previous follicular phase. Its lifespan depends upon the fate of the oocyte released at ovulation. If fertilization and implantation are successful, the corpus luteum lifespan will be prolonged under the influence of hCG, at least until the time of the luteoplacental shift at around 2 to 3 months in women. If there is no pregnancy, the corpus luteum lifespan is about 2

weeks, after which it undergoes regression or luteolysis, loses its dominance, and menstruation follows.

Formation and structure

In 1911, Meyer divided the life history of the corpus luteum into 4 phases, which we now know as proliferation and hyperemia, vascularization, maturity, and regression or luteolysis. After rupture of the ovulating follicle, the stigma is sealed off by coagulation of follicular fluid and blood. There is disruption of the basement membrane between the granulosa and thecal compartments, which allows the vasculature of the theca layer to enter the newly forming corpus luteum, followed by proliferation of endothelial cells as the vessels extend throughout the corpus luteum. The endothelial cells are the predominant cell type in the mature corpus luteum, which is highly vascularized and has one of the highest blood flow rates per gram of tissue of all organs excluding the brain. An extensive lymphatic system also develops in the corpus luteum, which in domestic species carries high concentrations of steroids from the ovary, the physiological significance of which is uncertain. At the same time as the basement membrane breaks down, the granulosa cells luteinize, during which they hypertrophy and acquire increased quantities of lipid droplets and organelles associated with steroidogenesis. The fate of the theca cells in the human follicle after ovulation is controversial, although it is clear that some of the cells luteinize to become paraluteal cells, which are clustered around the periphery and along infoldings of the corpus luteum. K cells (believed to be ketosteroid-rich) derived from the theca interna have also been described in the newly-forming human corpus luteum, but their precise origin and function remain unclear. Nevertheless, the primate corpus luteum is compartmentalized into granulosa-luteal and paraluteal segments, which may cooperate to produce the steroids of the corpus luteum (see below). Large and small luteal cell types that show differential function have been isolated from primate ovaries and may correspond to granulosa luteal and paraluteal cells, respectively. Several types of leukocytes have been identified in the human corpus luteum, including macrophages and T-lymphocyte subsets, and the cytokine products of these cells have been postulated to influence steroidogenesis and to have a role in luteolysis. The final size and therefore functional capacity of the corpus luteum is governed primarily by the number of granulosa and theca cells comprising the ovulatory follicle from which it formed.

Functional changes at luteinization

The LH surge has multiple actions on the ovulating follicle and newly forming corpus luteum that constitute luteinization, the process whereby the somatic cells of the follicle wall differentiate into functional luteal cells. This is thought to be the terminal differentiation step of the granulosa cells. Changes occur in the cell-specific expression of genes that may be transient at the time of ovulation and luteinization or be stably expressed in the luteal phenotype. The actions of the LH surge include promotion of angiogenesis, increased provision of substrate for steroidogenesis, and induction of enzymes in the steroid and polypeptide biosynthetic pathways. Several factors of granulosa-luteal origin have been implicated in the angiogenic response induced by LH, including bFGF and vascular endothelial growth factor(s). Studies in the rat by Joanne Richards and her colleagues demonstrated a shift from hormone-dependent to hormone-independent constitutive expression of P450scc in granulosa cells, a decline in expression of P450arom and P450-17α, with a transient increase in COX-2 enzyme mRNA and protein and plasminogen activator activity during the ovulatory period. Similar changes occur in the primate corpus luteum, except that they reflect species differences that occur with respect to hormone production. For example, unlike the rat, the primate corpus luteum produces estrogen and inhibin. Consequently, the LH surge induces an increase in the mRNA and protein of P450scc and 3β-hydroxysteroid dehydrogenase (3β-HSD), and after a transient decline around ovulation, an increase in P450arom, P450-17α, and the inhibin genes. Unlike the rat, these activities are not constitutive and require continued stimulation by LH. The LH surge also induces the expression of PR in luteinizing granulosa cells. There is mounting evidence that progesterone is critical for events at the time of ovulation and corpus luteum formation, leading to the proposal that the LH surge not only turns on production of progesterone but also facilitates its local action by induction of PR.

Function and regulation of luteal cells

The major hormonal products of the human corpus luteum, for which there is evidence for an endocrine role, are progesterone, 17β-estradiol, inhibin A, and relaxin. There are other factors made in the corpus luteum such as oxytocin, growth factors, cytokines, and eicosanoids that, together with steroids and inhibin-related peptides, may have autocrine or paracrine actions within the corpus luteum. Pituitary LH appears to be the only luteotrophin essential for maintaining the function of the primate corpus luteum, although its precise roles are ill-defined.

The LDL-cholesterol pathway and the expression of steroidogenic enzymes responsible for progesterone synthesis are both up-regulated by LH in the luteal cells. Small (paraluteal) and large (granulosa) luteal cells synthesize and secrete progesterone, but the large cells appear to have over twice the capacity, at least in vitro. It has been hypothesized that estrogen production results from an extension of the two-cell, two-gonadotropin mechanism established in follicles, which remains compartmentalized in the primate corpus luteum (Fig. 43.19). In this case it is the paraluteal (ex-theca) cells under the influence of LH that convert progesterone to androgen by

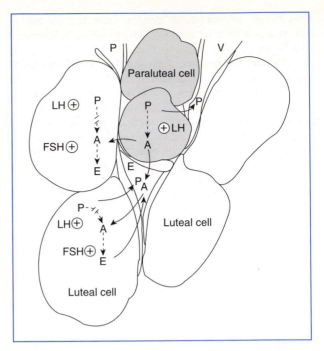

Figure 43.19 The two-cell/two-gonadotropin hypothesis for estrogen production by the primate corpus luteum. (From Brannian JD, Stouffer RL. Seminars in reproductive endocrinology. 1991;9:341-51.)

virtue of their P450-17α activity, whereas the P450arom is confined to the large (granulosa) luteal cells, which convert the androgen to estrogen. Despite some controversy, both the small and large luteal cells of the primate corpus luteum have been shown to respond to LH, which could therefore control estrogen production. The corpus luteum is not traditionally considered a target for FSH, however there is indirect evidence that FSH may facilitate aromatization by luteal cells, which deserves more research.

Inhibin is a product of the primate ovary, including the human. The genes for inhibin α-, βA- and βB-subunits are expressed in human and monkey corpus luteum, and the respective protein subunits have been localized immunocytochemically to the large luteal cells. The small paraluteal cells stained only faintly or not at all for any subunit. These observations localizing inhibin to the corpus luteum are supported by in vitro studies in which inhibin was shown to be produced by luteal cells under the influence of hCG. The main form of circulating inhibin produced by the human corpus luteum would appear to be inhibin A (Fig. 43.2). Experiments involving the use of GnRH agonists and LH/hCG replacement argue that the control of inhibin A production by the primate corpus luteum is LH-dependent. However, it is of interest that FSH is capable of increasing the circulating concentrations of immunoactive inhibin in the human luteal phase, though the form of inhibin released is not known. The extent to which the primate corpus luteum synthesizes and secretes inhibin B and the activins is not clear. The corpus luteum does not appear to be a major source of circulating follistatin, since the concentrations in peripheral plasma do not change across the menstrual cycle and there is relatively little expression of follistatin in mature luteal tissue.

Relaxin is a product of the paraluteal and true luteal cells of the primate corpus luteum, but it is a hormone of pregnancy, and its production is first detected simultaneously with hCG. Oxytocin has also been detected as a product of large luteal cells, particularly in domestic animals. However, in the human corpus luteum the concentrations are low (100- to 300-fold lower than in corpus luteum of domestic species), suggesting that if oxytocin plays a role in the primate corpus luteum, it is more likely to be as a local regulator than as a circulating hormone.

There is mounting evidence that substances produced by the corpus luteum can have autocrine or paracrine actions to modulate or mediate the actions of LH on the corpus luteum, and in some cases act independently of LH. These substances include steroids (progesterone, estrogen, androgen), activin, oxytocin, growth factors, cytokines, prostaglandins, and leukotrienes. Much of the evidence is based on in vitro studies in animal models and requires verification, particularly using primate corpus luteum. One substance for which there is substantial evidence of a local role is progesterone, originally proposed by Irving Rothchild as a universal luteotrophin in the mammalian corpus luteum. It is hypothesized that the luteotrophic action of LH is direct and acute to produce progesterone and indirect and chronic via the local effects of progesterone on luteal cell structure and function. The cytokine products of leukocytes, which are present in large numbers, are also known to influence luteal function, particularly around the time of regression, however the physiological significance of these actions is unclear.

Regression of the corpus luteum

Luteolysis is the process whereby the corpus luteum regresses toward the end of a nonfertile menstrual cycle and involves the gradual destruction of the corpus luteum. Functional luteolysis in women is characterized by a fall in the circulating concentrations of progesterone, 17β-estradiol, and inhibin A, beginning about 10 days after the mid-cycle LH surge and reaching its nadir by about 14 days at the time of menstruation (Fig. 43.2). Structurally, the luteal cells become atrophic, blood flow declines, the surrounding connective tissue disintegrates, and fibroblasts invade the corpus luteum, which is transformed into a corpus albicans.

The identity of the luteolysin in primates is not known. The fact that women continue regular ovarian cycles after hysterectomy indicates that, unlike ruminants, the uterus is not essential for luteolysis and is therefore probably not the source of the luteolysin. Attempts to show that either diminishing levels or pulses of LH, or intraovarian estradiol or prostaglandin-F2α are the physiological luteolytic signals in the primate corpus luteum have not been convincing. Other intriguing hypotheses yet to be substantiated include a role for lymphokines and monokines produced by macrophages and T-lymphocytes, and the generation of reactive oxygen species normally suppressed by enzyme-catalyzed degradation of superoxides and scavenging by antioxidant vitamins, all of which are present in the corpus luteum.

Another possibility involves cell dynamics and apoptosis. Animal studies support the idea of small cells transforming to large cells as the corpus luteum matures. There is also a decrease in the responsiveness of small and large luteal cells of the primate ovary to LH and PGE$_2$ as the corpus luteum ages. Taken together, these observations could reflect the terminal differentiation of the luteal cells, which in the absence of a continuing influence of hCG, ends in apoptosis. The morphological and biochemical indices of apoptosis have been demonstrated in ruminant luteal cells undergoing luteolysis. Similar studies relating apoptosis to luteolysis are needed on the primate corpus luteum. One problem with this hypothesis is that luteal cell apoptosis is correlated with the structural disintegration found at latter stages of luteal demise and not with early functional luteolysis when progesterone production is decreased.

THE OVARIAN ACTIVITY AND MENSTRUAL CYCLES

Approximately 70 days or over two menstrual cycles are required for a Class 1 preantral follicle to become a Class 5 selectable antral follicle. Furthermore, another 15 days are required for the selected follicle to become the dominant ovulatory follicle, and that period coincides with the follicular phase of a menstrual cycle, implying that the process of selection takes place at about the time of menstruation of the preceding cycle. Based on this information, it is possible to track the growth trajectory of an ovulatory dominant follicle from its preantral stage in relation to stages of the intervening menstrual cycles. (Fig. 43.16) It can be calculated that the Class 1, preantral secondary follicle enters the growth trajectory several days after ovulation in a cycle designated as cycle 1. Some 25 days later in the late follicular phase of cycle 2, the follicle becomes early antral Class 2. After a further 20 days during the latter part of the luteal phase of the same cycle 2, the follicle becomes Class 3. During the late follicular phase of cycle 3, 15 days later, the follicle has become Class 4. A further 10 days is required to transform the follicle to Class 5, corresponding to the late luteal/menstrual phase of cycle 3: the time of selection. Up to this point in time, folliculogenesis is responsive to and eventually requires gonadotropins, FSH for granulosa cell function, and LH for theca cell function; however, it is not dependent on the cyclic fluctuations in FSH and LH occurring during cycles 1 to 3 and has relatively little influence on those gonadotropin levels. After selection and establishment of follicular dominance, the hormone products of these Class 5-8 follicles have a major influence on circulating hormone concentrations.

A rise in plasma FSH is critical for selection of the Class 5 follicle. This rise begins a few days before plasma progesterone reaches basal levels at the end of cycle 3 and continues into the first 7 days of the follicular phase of cycle 4. The FSH rise is the result of a decline in the negative feedback influence of steroids and inhibin A produced by the regressing corpus luteum (Fig. 43.2) of cycle 3, and its extent and duration is probably determined by the output of inhibin B and estradiol by the selected follicle during the early follicular phase of cycle 4 (Fig. 43.2). By day 7 of cycle 4, the selected follicle becomes dominant by virtue of its size and functional capacity, particularly estradiol production. At this time it is possible to detect more estradiol secretion in the vein draining the ovary containing the dominant follicle, inhibin B is declining, inhibin A is rising in the circulation, and FSH concentrations are declining (Fig. 43.2). The dominant follicle now determines the circulating concentrations of estradiol and inhibin and regulates the levels of FSH and LH by negative feedback and will continue to do so until the end of cycle 4, either as the dominant follicle or as the ensuing corpus luteum with the added assistance of progesterone. In the late follicular phase of cycle 4, LH pulse frequency increases under the influence of increasing output of estradiol by the dominant follicle. These LH pulses take over from FSH as the drive to the dominant follicle. The dominant follicle has now acquired LHR on the granulosa cells as well as the theca cells, is more responsive to trophic stimulation through the influence of local factors, and has an increased blood supply to the theca layer. In the face of declining FSH and rising LH, and possibly by a direct intraovarian influence of the dominant follicle, all other follicles reaching Class 5 become atretic (Fig. 43.5). Estradiol production by the dominant follicle finally reaches concentrations sufficient to trigger the mid-cycle surge of gonadotropins, and the follicle that entered the growth trajectory 4 cycles earlier is induced to ovulate.

Rapid and profound changes occur in hormone output by the ovary across the mid-cycle period before the corpus luteum takes over as the dominant structure (Fig. 43.2). There is a transient fall in the levels of estradiol and inhibin A following the mid-cycle surge as ovulation and luteinization occur, but the output of both hormones rise again as the corpus luteum becomes fully functional. Inhibin B levels continue to decline at the time of the mid-cycle surge and remain low for the remainder of the cycle. In contrast, progesterone rises at mid-cycle as luteinization occurs and reaches peak levels by around day 7 to 8 of the luteal phase, coincident with peak levels of estradiol and inhibin A. These three hormones are all products of the primate corpus luteum and allow it to maintain its dominance over the circulating concentrations of FSH and LH, which are suppressed to their lowest levels during the luteal phase. As a consequence, follicular development is suppressed during the luteal phase. In the absence of hCG from an implanting blastocyst, the corpus luteum will regress and progesterone, estradiol, and inhibin A output will decline (Fig. 43.2), followed by menstruation. At the same time, FSH and LH levels rise, and a new Class 5 follicle will be selected to ovulate in the next cycle.

CLIMACTERIC AND POSTMENOPAUSE: BASIC CONCEPTS

Peter Kenemans

For a woman, the reproductive period is demarcated by two main events: the menarche and the menopause. Traditionally, *menopause* has been defined as the point in time of the last menstrual bleeding in a woman's life. In most industrialized countries, natural menopause occurs on average around the age of 51, but there is a large variation in age at natural menopause (mean age: 51 yrs; range: 39 to 59 yrs). Menopause and the last ovulatory bleeding are not identical in many cases. Although a menopause age of 57 and over is regularly reported, the age of the oldest woman becoming pregnant in a natural way ever reported was 56 years (Guinness Book of Records).

By definition, menopause occurring before the age of 40 is called precocious or premature menopause. Today, the term premature ovarian failure is also used. The incidence of premature menopause is approximately 1%.

Typically the date of menopause is established in retrospect, following a full year of amenorrhea. In a woman around 50 years of age, periods of secondary amenorrhea shorter than 12 months do not guarantee that menopause has been passed.

Although the "one year amenorrhea"-criterium seems primitive, all other methods of diagnosing menopause earlier are less accurate. It should be remembered that elevated FSH and LH levels and severe vasomotor symptoms can be present long before menopause is reached, while even ovarian biopsies without follicles can be false-negative. In some instances it can be difficult to establish the moment of menopause accurately, for instance after hysterectomy or in case of oral contraceptive use.

The *postmenopause* is the period of life after the menopause. Increasingly, the term menopause is used in a different sense than its original meaning. The term menopause has come to refer to the total postmenopausal period and thus is synonymous to the term postmenopause. The World Health Organization defines menopause as the permanent cessation of menstruation resulting from the loss of ovarian follicular activity.

Early menopause is a term sometimes used to denote the first few years directly after menopause, in which still considerable, endogenous estradiol activity can be present. Late menopause is the period thereafter.

The *perimenopause* can be defined as the period of time around the menopause in which marked menstrual cycle changes occur, often in conjunction with vasomotor symptoms and in which no period of 12 consecutive months of amenorrhea has yet occurred. The median length of the perimenopause is 4 to 5 years (range: 1 to 9 years).

The term *climacteric* refers to the period of menopausal transition. During this period, many profound changes take place in a woman's life (Tab. 43.4). Many, but not all, are directly related to the aging process of the ovaries. Body changes and mood swings are intermingled with changes in family and social environment. All of these factors together can have a profound influence on the psycho-social functioning and general well-being of the climacteric woman.

There is great variability in climacteric complaints and symptoms, both between cultures as well as between individuals within a culture. In Western society, for many women the menopausal experience with transient climacteric effects is minimal, for others the impact is severe. Climacteric and perimenopausal women should not be regarded as a homogeneous group.

Ovarian physiology

The onset of menopause is determined by the ovary. All other functional body changes are secondary to this change in ovarian function. This also includes changes in hypothalamic and uterine functioning. The primary event is the loss of the capacity of the ovary to sustain the process of ovulation as a direct consequence of the (nearly complete) loss of ovarian follicles. It has been estimated that in the ovaries a minimum of around 1 000 follicles must be present for ovulation to still occur. Natural menopause occurs when this stage of near-depletion of oocytes and follicles is reached.

Normally, at birth, a few million primordial follicles are present, each containing an oocyte. After the time of menarche, around 250 000 follicles are still present in the ovaries. During the fertile period, there is continuing loss of follicles, of which only a maximum of about 500 will reach the stage of a Graafian follicle and then disappear by ovulation. All other follicles – including the nongrowing primordial follicles and those in which growth has been initiated – disappear spontaneously, probably via a process of apoptosis and atresia, which is only partly understood. After the age of approximately 38 years, the disappearance of follicles becomes even more accelerated. Additionally, a further increased loss of follicles can also be the result of damage to the ovary through surgery, radiation, chemotherapy, a virus, or other factors such as smoking (Tab. 43.5).

Idiopathic premature menopause will be increasingly shown to be, at least in part, genetic in origin. Both X chromosome micro-deletions as well as auto-chromosomal abnormalities can be a cause.

Surgery, not only surgical castration per se, can bring down the age of menopause substantially. Early removal of one ovary or a substantial part of a functional ovary (e.g., by a large wedge resection) can provoke menopause by reducing the actual amount of follicles still present. Hysterectomy with uni- or bilateral conservation of the ovary can also advance menopause, possibly through disturbance of the ovarian circulation.

Radiation therapy in the pelvic area (particularly in women with cervical cancer or Hodgkin's disease) can lead to irreversible damage to the ovary that results in permanent amenorrhea, especially in older premenopausal women who have a limited follicular reserve.

Chemotherapy may do the same, however the possibility of a temporary hyper- gonadotrophic amenorrhea (during treatment and months or years thereafter, but with a full recovery of the ovulatory cycle) is also frequently seen, especially where cytotoxic drugs damage the theca and granulosa cells and not primarily the oocytes.

Viral infections (e.g., mumps) and other exotoxins might impair follicular function. Cigarette smoking can accelerate follicular loss. Heavy smokers reach menopause significantly earlier than nonsmokers, on average 1 to 2 years earlier.

Premature menopause, on the basis of premature permanent ovarian failure, with a fair amount of follicles still present has also been described. These irresponsive follicles (the "resistant ovary syndrome") can be found in various conditions such as auto-immune diseases and

Table 43.4 The climateric: the period of transition from fertility to sterility

	Transition from	Via	To
Reproductive capacity	Fertility	Subfertility	Sterility
Ovarian folliculogenesis	Regular recruitment and maturation	Accelerated loss of follicles after 38 yrs of age	Total depletion of follicles
Ovarian cycles	Ovulatory	Increasingly anovulatory with luteal phase defects	Anovulatory
Menstrual periods	Regular periods	Initial shortening of the cycle; thereafter longer, irregular cycles	Amenorrhea
Hormonal profile	Ovulatory cycle profile	Increase in early follicular FSH; often low progesterone levels in second half; decreasing inhibin; LH, E2, and androgen levels stay long stable	Hypogonadotropic, hypoestrogenic status with low androgen levels and undetectable inhibin
Needs, complaints, and risks	Contraception needs	Contraception needs and climacteric complaints	Increased risk of osteoporosis and cardiovascular disease
Family life	Active family life; professional career	"Empty nest" situation; midlife crisis	Re-orientation; re-integration

Table 43.5 Factors associated with early onset of menopause

Genetic factors

e.g., microdeletions X-chromosome, mosaic 45X0/46XX
e.g., mutation in FSH receptor gene

Viral factors

e.g., mumps

Iatrogenic factors

surgery (e.g., oophorectomy, hysterectomy)
chemotherapy (e.g., for breast cancer, lymphoma)
radiotherapy (e.g., for cervix cancer, morbus Hodgkin)

Lifestyle factors

e.g., cigarette smoking, vegetarian diet

Other factors

e.g., autoimmune diseases (myasthenia gravis)
e.g., low body weight

genetic mutations affecting the FSH receptor and its function.

Ovarian failure secondary to conditions such as diabetes mellitus, thyroid disease, and anorexia nervosa is, in principle, transient, and ovarian function should be restored by treatment directed to the underlying disease. Therefore, these conditions do not belong to the premature ovarian failure syndrome. Race, socioeconomic status, age of menarche, and prior use of oral contraceptives are all factors not affecting the age of menopause. Increased parity may be associated with a later onset of the menopause.

Ovarian function and perimenopausal cycle changes

The last ovulation is a milestone event, heralding a new phase in a woman's life. Generally, this final ovulation is the end result of a long process over many years of gradual changes in reproductive and endocrine functions of the ovaries, that long before menopause cause anovulatory cycles, menstrual disorders, and subfertility. From the mid-thirties, the duration of the menstrual cycle gradually and continuously declines up to approximately 4 to 6 years before menopause. At that time many women start to notice changes in their menstrual cycle, sometimes accompanied by night sweats, hot flushes, and vaginal dryness, all long before the actual time of menopause.

Generally, the ovulatory cycle remains intact until the mid-forties, with 17β-estradiol and progesterone secretion unchanged, however, with a gradual increase of FSH levels. Thereafter, cycles may get longer due to disturbed folliculogenesis and impaired corpus luteum function, causing very low luteal phase progesterone serum levels and periods characterized by irregular bleeding.

In the last 5 years before menopause, in three-quarters of all women, mean cycle length gradually increases from 28 days (range 26 to 32 days) to 60 days (range 35 to >100 days).

Individual hormone levels may fluctuate and can be highly variable between cycles in this climacteric period. Where an increasing frequency of low luteal progesterone levels can be seen during the climacteric years, estradiol tends to stay within the normal fertile range (400-600 pmol/l), but it may fluctuate considerably over time, decreasing sharply in the few months directly before and after the moment of menopause, to reach levels below 200 pmol/l at one year after menopause. Although estradiol levels will decline further with increasing menopausal age, detectable levels of circulating estradiol will be present long after natural (and also after surgical) menopause.

Postmenopausally, non-ovarian tissues such as fat, liver, and kidney produce small amounts of estrogens by peripheral conversion of androgens. Obese postmenopausal women have higher circulating estradiol levels therefore, with less estrogen bound to the rather low SHBG concentrations found in adipose women.

After natural menopause, estrone may rise. The secretion of androgen by the ovary is reduced, resulting in a decline of peripheral androgen levels by 20 to 40%. After menopause, an increased androgen to estrogen ratio can be related to an androgen-associated facial hair pattern and a deepening of the voice that can be seen in some postmenopausal women.

The hypothalamic-pituitary-ovarian axis

From the mid-thirties on, for many years, a diminishing ovarian potential for normal folliculogenesis is counterbalanced by a growing hypothalamic-pituitary stimulation, as is evident from early follicular phase FSH levels (cycle day 3 FSH) that start to rise typically 10 years before the menopause. Finally, although FSH (essential for maturation and survival of the follicle after the preantral stage) and LH (important for ovulation, corpus luteum development, and steroidogenesis) reach high serum levels, ovarian follicle stimulation becomes ineffective.

In the perimenopausal period, the ovaries also become progressively less responsive to exogenous gonadotropins. At the time of menopause, the small population of follicles still present has been shown to be refractory to stimulation with exogenous gonadotropins as well.

Partially independent from GnRH control, secretion of FSH is influenced by various substances, of which estradiol and inhibin are the most important. Both of these substances are products of the ovarian granulosa cells and both suppress the pituitary secretion of FSH, each in its own way. As LH serum levels remain remarkably unchanged during the climacteric period, it can be hypothesized that increasing serum FSH levels result from decreasing serum inhibin levels that follow the decline in a number of ovarian follicles.

Acknowledgements

J.K. Findlay wishes to thank Sue Panckridge, Faye Coates, and Judy Forsyth for editorial assistance; Professors Henry Burger and Aaron Hsueh for critically reading the manuscript; and the National Health & Medical Research Council of Australia (RegKey 943208) for supporting his Fellowship and a Program Grant.

Suggested readings

ADASHI EY, ROCK JA, ROSENWAKS Z (eds). Reproductive endocrinology, surgery and technology. Vol. 1. Philadelphia: Lippincott-Raven Press, 1996.

BURGER HG (ed). Inhibin and inhibin-related proteins. Rome: Ares-Serono Symposia Publications, 1994.

BURGER HG, EC DUDLEY, JL HOPPER, et al. The endocrinology of the menopausal transition: a cross-sectional study of a population-based sample. J Clin Endocrinol Metab 1995;80:3537-45.

CONN PM, CROWLEY WFJ. Gonadotropinreleasing hormone and its analogues (see comments). N Engl J Med 1991;324:93-103.

CONTE FA, GRUMBACH MM, KAPLAN SL, REITER EO. Correlation of luteinizing hormone and follicle stimulating hormone release from infancy to 19 years with the changing pattern of gonadotropin secretion in agonadal patients: relation to the restraint of puberty. J Clin Endocrinol Metab 1980;50:163-8.

CROWLEY WF JR, FILICORI M, SPRATT DI, SANTORO NF. The physiology of gonadotropinreleasing hormone (GnRH) secretion in men and women. (Review) (48 refs). Recent Prog Horm Res 1985;41:473-531.

DE KONING J. Gonadotropin surgeinhibiting/attenuating factor governs luteinizing hormone secretion during the ovarian cycle: physiology and pathology. Hum Reprod 1995;10:285-461.

FADDY MJ, RG GOSDEN. A mathematical model of follicle dynamics in the human ovary. Human Reprod 1995;10:770-5.

FILICORI M, FLAMIGNI C (eds). The ovary: regulation, dysfunction and treatment. Amsterdam: Elsevier Science, 1996.

FINDLAY JK (ed). Molecular biology of the female reproductive system. USA: Academic Press, 1994.

GRUMBACH MM, SIZONENKO PC, et al. Control of the onset of puberty. Baltimore: Williams and Wilkins, 1990.

HARDELIN JP, LEVILLIERS J, YOUNG J, et al. Xp22.3 deletions in isolated familial Kallmann's syndrome. J Clin Endocrinol Metab 1993;76:827.

HSUEH AJW, SCHOMBERG DW (eds). Ovarian cell interactions. New York: Springer-Verlag, 1992.

LAMBALK CB, SCHOEMAKER J, VAN REES GP, et al. Shortterm pituitary desensitization to luteinizing hormonereleasing hormone (LHRH) after pulsatile LHRH administration in women with amenorrhea of suprapituitary origin. Fertil Steril 1987;47:385-90.

RANNEVIK G, S JEPPSSON, O JOHNELL, et al. A longitudinal study of the perimenopausal transition: altered profiles of steroid and pituitary hormones, SHBG and bone mineral density. Maturitas 1995;21:103-13.

44

Precocious puberty

Henriette A. Delemarre-van de Waal

KEY POINTS

- The diagnosis of central precocious puberty is best made from the growth curve of a patient, the skeletal age, and a gonadotropin-releasing hormone test.
- In cases of central precocious puberty in boys, if at diagnosis the cerebral evaluation revealed no abnormalities, this investigation should be repeated after several years.
- When considering the discontinuation of GnRH analog treatment in central precocious puberty, the achieved height is an important issue, since growth after gonadotropin-releasing hormone treatment is minimal.
- The diagnosis of pseudoprecocious puberty in boys is best made using the growth curve of the patient, a physical examination, the skeletal age, and by exceptionally small testes.

Precocious puberty is defined as the early appearance of sex characteristics, that is, at an age less than 2.5±SD from the mean age when pubertal development generally starts. For example, for Dutch children, this is before the age of 8 years in girls and before 9 years in boys. Two forms of precocious puberty exist: (1) central precocious puberty due to premature activation of the gonadotropin-releasing hormone (GnRH) system, resulting in gonadotropin secretion and gonadal stimulation (also known as true or gonadotropin-dependent precocious puberty); and (2) pseudoprecocious puberty, whereby gonadotropins, or more frequently sex steroids, initiate development of the sex characteristics without activation of the GnRH axis (also known as peripheral or gonadotropin-independent precocious puberty). Incomplete precocious puberty exists clinically in the appearance of only thelarche or only pubic hair, premature thelarche or premature pubarche, respectively (Tab. 44.1).

CENTRAL PRECOCIOUS PUBERTY

Etiology

The incidence of central precocious puberty in a general Caucasian population is about 0.6%. The idiopathic form is

Table 44.1 Classification of precocious puberty in girls

Central precocious puberty

Idiopathic
CNS tumors
Other CNS disorders: e.g., hydrocephalus, developmental abnormalities, head trauma, cranial irradiation
After previous long- term exposure to sex steroids: e.g., adrenal and ovarian tumors, congenital adrenal hyperplasia, exogenous sex steroids

Pseudoprecocious puberty

Estrogen-secreting tumors
Exogenous estrogens
McCune-Albright syndrome
Gonadotropin-secreting tumors (LH, hCG)

Incomplete variant of precocious puberty

Premature thelarche
Premature pubarche
Isolated vaginal bleeding

(CNS = central nervous system; LH = luteinizing hormone; hCG = human chorionic gonadotropin.)

more common in girls (80 to 90%) than in boys. This may, at least in part, be explained by the fact that in girls the period of complete suppression of the GnRH axis is shorter, as well as that the gonadotropin-gonadal axis is easier to activate. During the prepubertal period girls have higher estrogen levels than boys, which is a possible explanation for the physiologic earlier start of puberty, as well as for the accelerated bone maturation in girls compared to boys. Sex steroids seem to bring on central pubertal development at an earlier age. Evidence for this is found in patients with congenital adrenal hyperplasia and in patients with ovarian tumors, who are exposed to sex steroids for long periods; these children will experience an early puberty, often in conformity with advanced skeletal age.

The risk for central precocious puberty is increased in disorders of the brain such as a cerebral tumor, hydrocephalus, neonatal encephalopathy, and when there was irradiation of the skull at a young age. The mechanisms by which central nervous system (CNS) tumors induce central precocious puberty is unknown, but it may be related to interference of the neurogenic influences suppressing the GnRH pulse generator. In hypothalamic hamartoma, the tumor imitates the GnRH pulse generator by a pulsatile release of GnRH. In contrast to the idiopathic form, there is no sex difference in incidence rate in the other causes of central precocious puberty.

In central precocious puberty, breast development is associated with an increased growth velocity and an advanced bone age. Clinical signs of central precocious puberty start before the age of 6 years in about 50% of the affected children. Girls with an onset of puberty between 6 and 8 years of age may show a slow progression of breast development associated with only slightly accelerated growth and moderately advanced bone maturation. A familial history of early puberty onset is common in these children. This form of central precocious puberty – a premature start of puberty that is not very progressive and often has a family history – defines a gray area between normal, early puberty and true precocious puberty.

In "premature thelarche," breast development is the isolated symptom. It is common at infancy, but it may also occur later. The breast development is inconsistent, not progressive. Endocrine evaluation reveals low pubertal estrogen levels associated with pubertal follicle-stimulating hormone (FSH) levels, while luteinizing hormone (LH) levels are low. The GnRH test shows an early pubertal response with an exaggerated FSH and a low LH response. At infancy, the underlying mechanism is an incomplete suppression of the GnRH axis. Since inhibition of the GnRH release is continued, breast development will regress spontaneously.

Transient central precocious puberty has been described in girls aged 2.0 to 5.7 years. After a period of 7 to 15 months of clinical symptoms, breast development regressed, as did the pubertal GnRH response.

Girls adopted from developing countries have an increased incidence of idiopathic central precocious puberty. Puberty starts at an earlier age of either their original country or their adoptive country. In general these girls have a greater height at prepuberty, through which

final height prediction is promising. Due to the early pubertal start (according to the definition of precocious puberty), final height is less than predicted, although it is not significantly different from the final height of girls in the country of origin.

In summary, central precocious puberty defined as premature activation of the hypothalamic GnRH pulse generator is seen in girls mostly in the absence of a demonstrable central nervous system lesion (idiopathic form). Since the first clinical signs of idiopathic central precocious puberty begin in about 55% between ages 7 and 8, they may be caused by a physiologic variability of the onset of puberty.

Clinical findings

Clinical features of central precocious puberty, besides the appearance of breast development, are an increased height velocity and advanced skeletal maturation, and sometimes vaginal bleeds. Pubic hair growth is an inconsistent finding. The early start of the pubertal growth spurt means that the period of prepubertal growth is insufficient. Since bone maturation is accelerated, final height will be reduced. The early pubertal development may lead to psychosocial problems such as social isolation or aggressive behavior, while intellectual function and school performance are appropriate.

The progression of pubertal development in idiopathic central precocious puberty is faster than normal puberty, which indicates that central precocious puberty is not only the result of premature GnRH reactivation but also of faster central development.

In central precocious puberty secondary to other anomalies, symptoms of the underlying disease will be prominent, although precocious puberty may be a first symptom.

Diagnostic procedures

The endocrine status in central precocious puberty reveals pubertal levels of luteinizing hormone (LH), follicle stimulating hormone (FSH), and estrogens. The GnRH test is within the pubertal range or may even show an exaggerated response. In idiopathic central precocious puberty, both the LH and FSH responses to GnRH are increased, even more than in adult women, possibly due to the more rapid development of the GnRH pulse generator with a delayed equilibrium of the hypothalamic-pituitary-gonadal axis. In idiopathic central precocious puberty, the 24-hour pattern of LH has pubertal characteristics: a day-night rhythm for LH with increased levels during the night. There is increased growth hormone secretion resulting in increased IGF-1 levels. The skeletal age will be advanced.

Imaging studies

Ultrasound evaluation shows developmental changes seen in normal puberty. Endometrial thickening indicates estrogen exposure. With an endometrium of 5 mm or more, menarche can be expected soon. The ovaries will be enlarged and contain multiple follicles with a diameter > 4 mm.

In order to locate cerebral defects, a neuroradiologic examination is needed. In cases of central precocious puberty secondary to other defects, specific diagnostic evaluations should be performed.

Treatment

Options to treat must take into consideration the psychosocial problems of premature pubertal development, as well as the accelerated growth in association with an advanced bone age, which will otherwise result in a compromised final height. The aim of treatment is to suppress sex steroid production and to bring the patient back into a prepubertal state.

Long-acting GnRH agonists are the first choice treatment. They induce desensitization of the gonadotropin-secreting cells. The GnRH analog treatment will result in a complete suppression of gonadotropin secretion as well as of sex steroid levels, resulting in an arrest of pubertal development. Breast development may even regress to a certain extent. Vaginal bleeds will disappear, although shortly after the start of treatment, estrogen withdrawal bleeding may still occur. Height velocity decreases into a prepubertal range. Skeletal maturation slows down, which results in an improvement of predicted adult height during treatment, though the ultimate results on final height are more disappointing than these predictions promise. The fact that after the discontinuation of gonadotropin suppression treatment the resumption of endocrine activity can be explosive may play a role in the minimal height gain. While gonadotropin secretion is inhibited, the central GnRH pulse generator will continue its maturation. Therefore, at the discontinuation of the GnRH agonist treatment, the hypothalamus may have reached its adult mature state and will soon stimulate the gonadotrophs in an adult way. This indicates that under GnRH agonist treatment, puberty is not postponed. In female puberty, most pubertal height gain is achieved in the first half of puberty when estrogen levels are not as high as in late puberty. Therefore, when girls with central precocious puberty discontinue GnRH analog treatment, estrogen levels soon reach the adult range, and a physiologic pubertal growth spurt cannot be expected anymore.

In most girls, vaginal bleeding will resume within about one year. Since these patients are too young to be reproductively active, no data on fertility are available yet. However, based on endocrine data and on ultrasound studies of the internal genitalia, there is no evidence for fertility problems to be expected for them in the future.

Patients with early or precocious puberty associated with short stature have been treated with a combination of a GnRH agonist and growth hormone. The results on final height, however, are not convincingly better. In these patients, ultrasound of the ovaries revealed follicular cysts similar to the polycystic ovary syndrome. After discontinuation of treatment, these abnormalities disappeared.

In conclusion, long-acting GnRH agonist treatment appears to be a feasible and safe approach to suppress gonadotropin and sex steroid levels in girls with central precocious puberty. The effect on growth remains debatable. In estimating the time to discontinue the GnRH agonist treatment, the present height as well as the psychosocial development of the patient should be considered.

PSEUDOPRECOCIOUS PUBERTY

Etiology

Pseudoprecocious puberty, or gonadotropin-independent puberty, is the result of sex steroid production independent of the GnRH axis (Tab. 44.1). In girls, benign estrogen-producing tumors located in the ovary are the most common cause. Sometimes these tumors are gonadotropin dependent. The granulosa cell tumor is the most common feminizing ovarian neoplasm. These tumors may produce human chorionic gonadotropin as well. Usually the granulosa cell tumor is benign.

Exogenous estrogens – ingested via food contaminated with artificial estrogens, through contraceptive pills, and through the use of estrogen-containing creams – can cause precocious puberty as well.

The McCune Albright syndrome is characterized by precocious puberty, café-au-lait pigmentations in nevi that have an irregular border, and polyostotic fibrous dysplasia. The syndrome may occur in an incomplete form without cutaneous lesions or bone abnormalities or even with isolated sexual precocity alone. The disorder is predominantly seen in girls and is considered to be the opposite of testotoxicosis in boys. The ovarian stimulation in McCune Albright syndrome is gonadotropin-independent. Immunoreactive LH and FSH are not detectable. Ovarian stimulation is the result of a somatic activating mutation in the subunit-α of the G protein that couples transmembrane receptors to adenyl cyclase. The follicle cysts function autonomously.

Other endocrine disorders, which can be present in this syndrome, are pituitary adenomas secreting LH, FSH, growth hormone, and/or prolactin. Patients may have Cushing's syndrome and hyperthyroidism caused by autonomous multinodular hyperplasia.

Gonadotropin (usually hCG)-producing tumors are a rare cause for precocious puberty. They can be hepatoblastomas and teratomas, but they can also be an intracranial tumor such as a pineal germ cell tumor or a teratoma.

Clinical findings

The pubertal development in pseudoprecocious puberty can be similar to that seen in central precocious puberty, although the progression may be more advanced.

High levels of estrogens associated with low, suppressed gonadotropin levels are found. In case of an hCG-producing tumor, the hCG may cross-react in the LH assay. In addition, the tumor marker α-fetoprotein may be increased.

Ultrasound and radiological investigations are needed to find underlying causes.

Treatment

Treatment of tumors is by surgical resection. When the underlying cause of elevated sex steroid levels cannot be corrected surgically, medical treatment can be prescribed in order to antagonize the sex steroid biologic activity.

Cyproterone-acetate is an antiandrogen, which blocks the androgen receptor, as well as having progestogenic properties. Before GnRH analogs were available, cyproterone-acetate was also used to suppress gonadotropin secretion. Nowadays it is used predominantly to inhibit skeletal maturation in cases of untreatable sex steroid exposure, among others in McCune Albright syndrome.

Testolactone inhibits the aromatization of testosterone into estradiol. It is also used in girls with McCune Albright syndrome.

Suggested readings

BRIDGES NA, BROOK CGD. Disorders of puberty. In: Brook CGD (ed). Clinical paediatric endocrinology. Oxford: Blackwell Science, 1995;253-73.

EHRHARDT AA, MEYER-BAHLBURG HFL. Psychosocial aspects of precocious puberty. Horm Res 1994;41(Suppl. 2):30-5.

KAPLAN SL, GRUMBACH MM. Pathophysiology and treatment of sexual precocity: a clinical review. J Clin Endocrinol Metab 1990;71:785-9.

KLEIN KO, BARON J, COLLI MJ, McDONNELL DP, CUTLER GB JR. Estrogen levels in childhood determined by an ultrasensitive recombinant cell bioassay. J Clin Invest 1994;94:2475-80.

INCOMPLETE VARIANT OF PRECOCIOUS PUBERTY

It is important to differentiate premature thelarche from central precocious puberty, since in most patients premature thelarche does not require treatment.

The most common cause of premature pubarche is premature adrenarche. Adrenarche includes maturation of presumably the zona reticularis with an increased production of 17-ketosteroids. As a result, the blood dehydroepiandrosterone (-sulfate) levels increase. Premature adrenarche is often associated with axillary hair, acne, and sweating. There is hardly any increase of height velocity or an advanced bone age. When growth is distinctly increased, one should consider other endocrine disorders. Five to 10% of cases of premature adrenarche are caused by late-onset congenital adrenal hyperplasia.

In general, isolated vaginal bleeds are not due to an endocrine disorder. The underlying causes are a foreign body, sexual abuse, or tumors of the genital tract. A bad smell is highly suggestive of a foreign body.

PESCOVITZ OH, HENCH KD, BARNES KM, LORIAUX DL, CUTLER GB JR. Premature thelarche and central precocious puberty: The relationship between clinical presentation and the gonadotropin response to luteinizing hormone-releasing hormone. J Clin Endocrinol Metab 1988;67:474-9.

SCHROOR EJ, WEISSENBRUCH VAN MM, DELEMARRE-VAN DE WAAL HA. Pathophysiology of central precocious puberty. In: Plant TM, Lee PA (eds). The neurobiology of puberty. Bristol: J Endocrinology Ltd, 1995;199-208.

SONIS WA, COMITE F, BLUE J, et al. Behavior problems and social competence in girls with true precocious puberty. Pediatrics 1985;106:156-60.

Primary amenorrhea

Winfried G. Rossmanith

KEY POINTS

- Primary amenorrhea is the lack of experiencing spontaneous menstrual bleedings by the age of 16 years, while growth and pubertal development are otherwise undisturbed.
- Primary amenorrhea is not a clinical entity by itself; it represents a symptom and not a disease.
- Genetic disorders, anatomic abnormalities, minor and severe endocrinopathies, and tumorous and nontumorous diseases may present with the common clinical feature of primary amenorrhea.
- It is advised to first rule out anatomic defects in the genital tract before endocrinopathies and genetic disorders are considered.
- The principle of treating patients with primary amenorrhea should be to initiate or preserve full reproductive capacity.
- If fertility cannot be restored, appropriate surgical and medical management should be given, thus allowing adequate physical development and normal sexual relationships.

The term *amenorrhea* indicates an absence of menstruation for a time period of at least 6 months. Amenorrhea is *primary* if the spontaneous onset of menstrual periods has not occurred by the age of 16 years. *Secondary* amenorrhea relates to the cessation of menstruation after a period of spontaneous menstruation. Stringent adherence to the clinical definition of *primary amenorrhea* may often result in delayed treatment. Thus, any patient presenting with amenorrhea and the following criteria should be evaluated:
- if no spontaneous periods have occurred by the age of 14 years and secondary sexual characteristics are absent or inappropriately developed for the age;
- if no spontaneous menses have occurred by the age of 16 years, in the presence or absence of normal growth and development of secondary sexual characteristics.

It is usually considered appropriate for a girl to have a clinical evaluation for primary amenorrhea by the age of 16 years if menstruation has not begun, but if other clinical signs indicate a possible disturbance of puberty at an earlier age, there is no reason to postpone the evaluation and treatment.

Etiology

Amenorrhea is a *symptom* related to a variety of physiological and pathological conditions. The majority of patients with amenorrhea have problems that can generally be diagnosed and managed by the primary physician. Occasionally amenorrhea presents as an early symptom of an underlying serious disease, severe genetic disorder, or endocrinopathy for which early diagnosis and treatment may be essential. The following classification depicts the cascade of events upon which regular menstrual cyclicity depends:

- intact function of the central nervous system and the hypothalamic control of reproduction;
- time-appropriate secretion of stimulatory hormones by the anterior pituitary;
- secretory responses by the ovaries;
- intact uterus as the target organ and intact vagina as the outflow tract.

Classification of primary amenorrhea is best achieved in clinical categories (Tab. 45.1). Even when evaluating a patient for primary amenorrhea, it is important to also consider the physiological causes that are generally associated with secondary amenorrhea. Therefore, exclusion of pregnancy is essential even with primary amenorrhea. Several etiological causes of amenorrhea are exclusively related to primary amenorrhea, such as genetic defects or anatomic malformations, adding up to about half of all causes for primary amenorrhea (Tab. 45.2).

Pathophysiology

The average European girl experiences her first menstrual period (menarche) at about the age of 12 years. Bleeding may be irregular with prolonged periods of amenorrhea for several years after the onset of menstruation. The time within which an adolescent girl should have regular menstrual cycles is usually 4 years after menarche. Feedback systems interact between the central nervous system (the hypothalamus and pituitary) and the peripheral target organs (ovaries with sex steroid production). This maintains the time- and quantity-appropriate secretion of hormones as messengers for folliculogenesis, ovulation, and corpus luteum formation. The maturation of the follicles is governed by the sequence and magnitude of the secretion of the gonadotropins, luteinizing hormone (LH), and follicle-stimulating hormone (FSH) from the anterior pituitary. This gland is, in turn, dependent on the intermittent stimulation by gonadotropin-releasing hormone (GnRH). The presence of a menstrual flow also depends on the existence of a functionally intact endometrial lining within the uterus. This tissue is stimulated and transformed by the sex steroids estradiol and progesterone from the ovaries. For menstruation to occur, the outflow tract with the vaginal orifice, the vaginal canal, and the endocervical os is required to be patent.

Clinical findings

The complaint of primary amenorrhea is occasionally the first opportunity to uncover anatomical malformations or serious endocrine and genetic abnormalities in a young woman (Tab. 45.2). Evaluation is comprised of a careful medical history and physical examination and also performing a few laboratory tests. Additional investigation directed towards systemic disorders or psychic disturbances is required only if indicated by specific findings or complaints (Fig. 45.1).

Table 45.1 Classification of primary amenorrhea, based on its etiologic origin

Disorders of the central nervous and hypothalamic control of menstruation

Anatomical destruction
Tumor, irradiation, surgical intervention
Idiopathic hypogonadotropic hypogonadism
Congenital agenesis of GnRH-containing neurons (Kallmann's Syndrome)
Psychogenic causes of primary amenorrhea
Psychosis, anorexia nervosa, pseudocyesis
Constitutional factors
Malnutrition, obesity, diabetes, thyroid dysfunctions, consuming diseases (tuberculosis, malignancies, drug addiction)

Disorders of anterior pituitary function

Anatomical abnormalities
Adenoma, craniopharyngioma, tumors, cysts, empty sella syndrome
Isolated gonadotropin deficiency
Mixed deficiencies
Basophilic and eosinophilic adenomas
Panhypopituitarism
Tumors, destructive lesions, surgical interventions

Disorders of ovary function

Genetic abnormalities
Ovarian dysgenesis: 46,XX – 46,XY (Swyer's syndrome), 45,X0-mosaics, hermaphroditism
Functional resistance of the ovaries
Resistant ovary syndrome (Savage syndrome)
Hypofunctional states
Polycystic ovaries, congenital adrenal hypoplasia, persisting functional cysts, irradiation, chemotherapy
Functioning and non functioning ovarian tumors
Arrhenoblastoma, hilus cell tumors, germinoma

Disorders of the uterus and vagina

Congenital anomalies of the uterus
Mayer-Rokitansky-Küster syndrome
Destruction of the endometrium
Irradiation, trauma, disease
Malformations of the vagina
Congenital absence of the vagina, hymen imperforatum, vaginal septa

Physiologic circumstances

Prepubertal period
Delayed menarche
Pregnancy

(GnRH = gonadotropin-releasing hormone.)

The medical history consists of a concise follow-up of regular development and growth, and looking for other signs of pubertal development and evidence for physical problems such as malnutrition, obesity, or excessive exercise. It should also include questions relating to a family history of apparent genetic abnormalities or regarding frequent occurrence of amenorrhea in the family. The physician should refer to potential underlying endocrinopathies by asking about unusual changes in body weight, loss of hair or hirsute changes,

Table 45.2 Distribution of the causes of primary amenorrhea

Hypergonadotropic hypogonadism	43%
Anatomical anomalies	20%
Normogonadotropic hypogonadism	16%
Hypogonadotropic hypogonadism	14%
(Pseudo-)Hermaphroditism	7%

galactorrhea, or signs of thyroid dysfunction. Lastly, a history of current medications or drugs is taken, and the intactness of the central nervous system is thoroughly assessed.

A thorough physical examination includes searches for clinical signs of a possible genetic disorder or derangements in the somatic development, such as extremely short or tall stature. Endocrine stigmata should be looked for, such as abnormal hair growth, missing or underdeveloped pubic hair, abnormal deposition of body fat, absence of breast development, and enlargement of the clitoris. A gynecological work-up includes inspection of the external genitalia and palpation of the pelvic organs to detect gross anatomic abnormalities and exclude genital pathology (Fig. 45.1). A transabdominal ultrasound of the pelvic organs should be performed to detect the absence of the ovaries or any changes in their appearance (multifollicular, polycystic) to rule out a uterine abnormality and to evaluate the endometrial thickness.

When a complete physical and gynecological examination excludes specific clues for primary amenorrhea, including pregnancy, the next step in the evaluation of an amenorrheic patient is the endocrinological examination (Fig. 45.1). A comprehensive work-up should entail the determination of levels of the following: thyroid-stimulating hormone (TSH); thyroxine (T_4) and triiodothyronine (T_3) levels and their free concentrations; prolactin; estradiol; androgens: testosterone, dehydroepiandrosterone sulphate, and androstenedione; gonadotropins (LH and

FSH); and urinary free cortisol (to exclude the rare case of a beginning Cushing's syndrome).

Based on the determination of the serum levels of the gonadotropins and of estradiol, amenorrhea as the prevailing symptom of hypogonadism can be endocrinologically classified as: (1) *hypergonadotropic hypogonadism*. This is invariably encountered in primary ovarian failure (such as in gonadal dysgenesis or resistant ovary); or (2) *normogonadotropic and hypogonadotropic hypogonadism*. If the central stimulation of the ovaries by the hypothalamus and/or pituitary is insufficient, low serum concentrations of ovarian sex steroids with normal or low levels of LH and FSH are observed. This form also comprises other dysfunctions in endocrine systems in their projection to reproduction (i.e., hyperprolactinemia, thyroid disturbances, pancreatic or adrenal dysfunctions).

In endocrine terms, primary amenorrhea is characterized by: (1) low or normal serum concentrations of estradiol; (2) low progesterone levels; (3) normal or elevated levels of ovarian and adrenal androgens; (4) normal, low, or high levels of the gonadotropins LH and FSH; (5) normal or elevated levels of prolactin; (6) normal or low levels of total T_4 and T_3; and (7) normal urinary free cortisol excretion.

The diagnostic repertoire may be further enlarged if any hormone within the basal evaluation diagram indicates pathology and requires further evaluation.

- Progesterone challenge test: This provocative test is useful to determine the levels of endogenous estrogens and the endometrial responsiveness. Following a course of synthetic progesterone (10 mg medroxyprogesterone PO for 5 to 8 days), if bleeding occurs within 2 to 7 days after administration, it establishes the presence of a functional outflow tract and a uterus with reactive endometrium. With additional normal TSH and prolactin levels, further endocrinological evaluation is unnecessary. However, if bleeding does not occur in response to progesterone administration, then the estro-

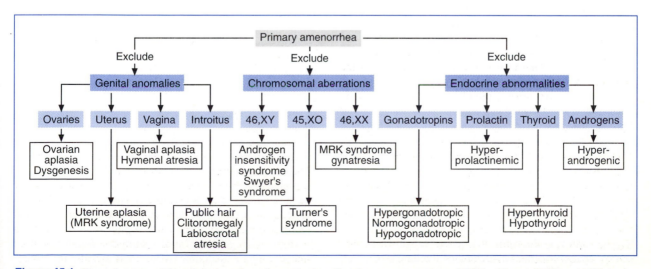

Figure 45.1 Flow diagram of the clinical work-up for patients with primary amenorrhea. (MRK = Mayer-Rokitanski-Küster.)

genic stimulation of the endometrium is ineffective, and various causes need to be considered. Therefore, the exact serum levels of estrogens should be determined, because this does not only help to classify amenorrhea into its clinical form, but it may also facilitate the planning of further treatment.

- TSH-stimulation test by TRH (200 μg iv): if TSH levels are elevated in patients with amenorrhea and/or galactorrhea, this test helps to distinguish a subclinical form of hypothyroidism. It also helps to discern a subclinical (latent) form of hyperprolactinemia, since TRH is a potent stimulator of prolactin secretion.
- GnRH stimulation test (25 μg GnRH iv): this test is advised in patients with low gonadotropins to determine the pituitary gonadotropin responsiveness and reserve. This test may also be used to distinguish a hypothalamic from a pituitary form of amenorrhea, but its results should be interpreted with caution.

The following diagnostic steps are recommended only when pathological findings from the basic endocrine work-up or the physical examination indicate it.

- Genetic analysis: determination of the karyotype using the patient's lymphocytes. This procedure has replaced the buccal smear in most centers. Patients with a normal female appearance and who are suspected to have ovarian failure (based on elevated gonadotropins) must have their karyotype determined.
- Radiological evaluation: CT scan of the adrenals (if a tumorous lesion or congenital hyperplasia is suspected). This is usually indicated if the basal testosterone levels are elevated; increased concentrations of dehydroepiandrosterone sulphate indicate an adrenal source of hyperandrogenemia.
- CT scan of the sella with intravenous contrast enhancement: this is advised in patients with suspected pituitary adenomas (prolactinomas are rarely seen with prolactin levels <40 ng/ml) or intrapituitary lesions, such as craniopharyngioma. Magnetic resonance imaging (MRI) is even more sensitive than the CT scan. Due to the high costs of these procedures, the physician should select only those few patients who indeed require the scans.
- Psychiatric counseling: when a profound psychogenic disturbance is suspected or signs of psychosomatic deviations with known severe progress (such as anorexia nervosa) are noted, psychiatric consultation is advised. A neurological consultation is recommended in cases of suspected pituitary tumors or when hypogonadotropic hypogonadism is assumed on the base of amenorrhea in association with anosmia (Kallmann's syndrome).

Differential diagnosis

Hypogonadism in the form of amenorrhea can be mimicked by anatomical malformations or functional derangements of the outflow tract (aplasia of the vagina and/or uterus, hymen imperforatus, nonresponsive endometrium). Amenorrhea may be associated with general and endocrine diseases or conditions of various origins: hypo- or hypercortisolism, thyroid dysfunction, diabetes, weight loss, obesity, irradiation, and chemotherapy. Amenorrhea may be based on immunological disorders rendering the ovary unresponsive: resistant ovary syndrome, immunologic thyroid dysfunction, or in rare cases autoimmune Addison's disease.

Treatment

If the cause of the primary amenorrhea is established, effective treatment can be specifically designed. Otherwise the treatment is considered symptomatic and is directed toward the individual needs and complaints of the patient.

Medical treatment

Progesterone supplementation When amenorrhea is associated with a lack of progesterone, administration of a progestational agent such as medroxyprogesterone acetate (5-10 mg daily PO for 14 days) will induce cyclic withdrawal bleedings. This can be produced by the use of oral progestin alone if endogenous estrogens sufficiently stimulate the endometrial proliferation. Progestational compounds are required to prevent the progressive changes of the endometrial tissue turning from a normal appearance into atypia and cancer.

Estrogen treatment When endogenous estrogen levels are inappropriately low, the essential requirement is hormonal replacement with estrogens (estradiol valerate 1-2 mg daily, equine estrogens 0.3-1.25 mg daily, micronized estradiol 1-2 mg daily, transdermal estradiol 25-100 μg/day). Whenever the primary cause of amenorrhea cannot be eliminated and young women present with an endogenous deficit of estrogens, estrogen therapy is mandatory to prevent the atrophy of the sexual secondary characteristics and, most importantly, to prevent osteoporosis and vascular changes as the sequelae of longstanding hypoestrogenism. Administration of estrogens alone can be advised only in the absence of the uterus, and the cyclic addition of progesterone can prevent atypical proliferation and cancer in the estrogen-stimulated endometrium.

Cyclic estrogen and progesterone treatment This cyclic type of replacement will produce a menstrual flow, but the bleeding is unaccompanied by ovulation and occurs only in response to repeated courses of hormonal therapy. Therefore, a young woman with a history of hypoestrogenic amenorrhea exceeding a period of half a year must be supplemented with estrogens. The loss of trabecular bone substance is most rapid in the first few years, which emphasizes the need for early replacement. In women with primary gonadal failure, hormone replacement of long duration is undoubtedly essential. Besides the somatic demand for hormone replacement and the facilitation of the development of sexual characteristics, these women feel psychologically relieved, even though the underlying problem of a missing menstruation cannot be directly resolved. If young women under heavy exercise or with anorexia nervosa do not desire menstrual bleeding, a continuous estrogen-progestin administration regimen may be an option.

Oral contraceptives Patients with hypothalamic forms of primary amenorrhea must be advised that hormone replacement therapy will not protect against pregnancy, since normal reproductive function may return without the patients' awareness. If a patient wishes safe contraception, it is feasible to prescribe oral contraceptives. Administration of low-dose contraceptives would certainly replace the missing estrogens and provide contraceptive safety. It is essential to note that oral contraceptives are likely to suppress the endogenous system, and therefore spontaneous recovery may be delayed.

Clomiphene citrate, exogenous gonadotropins, and GnRH When amenorrhea is associated with infertility, treatment is directed toward establishing ovulatory cycles. Administration of clomiphene citrate, a potent anti-estrogen (at 50-100 mg daily for 5 days), is of great value in the treatment of anovulatory women in whom residual production of gonadotropins and estrogen is found (normogonadotropic patients). This drug activates negative feedback at hypothalamic and pituitary sites and thus increases gonadotropin secretion for the stimulation of follicular growth and ovulation. Administration of human chorionic gonadotropin (hCG) at a dose of 5000-10 000 units at midcycle is often required to enhance the LH surge and induce ovulation. Both clomiphene and human menopausal gonadotropin may overstimulate the ovaries, which could lead to multiple pregnancies, considerable ovarian enlargement, and ascites. To circumvent this problem, the synthetic analogue of GnRH has been administered to patients with amenorrhea who have the desire to conceive. This compound, administered in an intermittent fashion at intervals of every 60 to 90 minutes with doses of 5-20 µg, can often successfully stimulate FSH and LH release in patients with normo- or hypogonadotropic amenorrhea.

Bromocriptine Hyperprolactinemia with and without pituitary adenomas is rarely associated with primary amenorrhea. When this is the underlying cause of amenorrhea, a specific treatment with a dopamine agonist (such as bromocriptine 5-10 mg daily orally) or with long-acting derivates (such as cabergoline) can be offered. All these compounds are highly effective in correcting hyperprolactinemia, with a subsequent restoration of normal reproductive cycles.

Anti-androgens Anti-androgens are only used in patients with considerable hirsutism associated with hyperandrogenic anovulation and amenorrhea. Occasionally the hirsutism in peripubertal patients with polycystic ovaries can be extreme. In these instances, specific progestins with anti-androgenic properties (cyproterone acetate, chlormadi-

none acetate) or compounds with anti-androgenic side-effects (spironolactone, dienogest) are useful and may be added as progestins to estrogens in hormone replacement regimens or as components of oral contraceptives.

Growth hormone In the rare event that a patient with growth hormone deficiency complains about primary amenorrhea as the predominant syndrome, treatment with growth hormone should be initiated to allow for a growth spurt before estrogen-progestin therapy is commenced, and sex steroid replacement should be delayed until growth is gained because of the rapid closure of the epiphyseal clefts.

Surgical treatment

Surgery is required for the correction of malformations of the genital tract. This approach can be considered curative when obstructions in the vagina are removed by very simple procedures, such as the incision of an imperforate hymen or the correction of a cervical stenosis. However, occasionally extensive abdominal and transperineal surgery may be required if preservation of fertility is the aim. Surgical correction is not possible in uterine aplasia. Remnants of the Müllerian duct need to be removed when functional endometrium is present.

When pathological changes in the ovaries are evident, such as tumors or cysts, operative procedures are indicated. Due to the high risk of developing a malignancy, gonads should be removed by laparotomy or laparoscopy if the abnormal chromosomal pattern contains either a Y or a marker chromosome. Since most women prefer to have menstrual bleeding, the uterus may be preserved. This approach should also be considered in view of future fertility, as it would be possible to transfer fertilized ova into an intact uterus in an agonadal woman.

Neurosurgery is indicated in patients with craniopharyngiomas and pituitary lesions. Prolactinomas unresponsive to dopamine agonist treatment or that are expanding extensively into adjacent brain areas should be removed by the transsphenoidal or transfrontal approach. Microsurgical techniques allow for the removal of pituitary tumors with a high margin of safety. However, medical treatment should be the first choice and tried in most cases, with the aim of shrinking the tumor and rendering it hormonally less active.

General measures

Patients suffering from diseases such as tuberculosis or diabetes require specific therapy for these conditions. Most amenorrheic patients will benefit from measures directed toward the improvement of their general health. One important consideration is the restoration of adequate nutrition. When obesity or underweight are found associated with amenorrhea, weight correction may be the primary aim.

Psychotherapy is particularly advisable for those patients with psychogenic amenorrhea. Explanation of the findings and a realistic approach to the patient's problems are essential in the management. Most patients will adequately comply with their symptoms if they understand that the failure to menstruate implies an underlying disorder with potentially serious consequences. In a group of women with exercise-induced amenorrhea, supportive treatment and the persuasion to reduce the work-load were useful. Patients are often unwilling to give up their routine of exercising or dieting, in which case somatic intervention is required to support their vitality. Hormone replacement therapy is advised for hypoestrogenic patients since the lack of estrogen is not compensated for by heavy exercise in terms of preservation of bone mass.

DISORDERS OF THE CENTRAL NERVOUS SYSTEM AND HYPOTHALAMIC CONTROL OF MENSTRUATION

Failure of hypothalamic stimulation is a very common cause of amenorrhea. In the absence of clearly localized destruction, it is often difficult to distinguish between dysfunction of the hypothalamus and the pituitary. It may even be impossible to demonstrate the potential function of the anterior pituitary without prior priming with GnRH for several days. The common feature in amenorrhea of hypothalamic and pituitary dysfunction is the reduced pulsatile secretion of the gonadotropins. These changes, albeit subtle, represent a continuous spectrum ranging from a hypogonadotropic state to minor abnormalities of the cycle.

IDIOPATHIC HYPOGONADOTROPIC HYPOGONADISM

Etiology

Idiopathic hypogonadotropic hypogonadism is due to the suppression or absence of pulsatile GnRH secretion. It is a diagnosis by exclusion, when no other cause for amenorrhea is identified. Hypothalamic hypogonadotropic amenorrhea may be inferred when any organic hypothalamic lesion is absent. The hypothalamic GnRH drive may be inappropriate to intermittently stimulate the pituitary. Patients with amenorrhea without galactorrhea who present with normal imaging of the sella and adjacent brain areas are referred to as having hypothalamic amenorrhea.

An idiopathic delay of menarche in a young woman with otherwise normal pubertal development represents the result of delayed hypothalamic maturation. Although weight loss has long been recognized in terms of its close relationship with secondary amenorrhea, it has gained increasing importance as a source of primary cycle disturbances. Anorexia nervosa rarely occurs before the time of puberty, but it may then be associated with primary amenorrhea. Far more common is a decrease in body fat mass in girls who are heavily exercising and/or ballet dancing. On the other hand, adolescent girls with massive exces-

sive weight may also present with amenorrhea as the same clinical endpoint.

Clinical findings

Patients presenting with complaints of primary amenorrhea are usually of normal height, and unlike those with hypogonadotropic hypogonadism they have well-developed secondary sexual characteristics. Endocrine findings in these patients are compatible with those of hypogonadotropic hypogonadism, and they are characterized by low or normal serum levels of gonadotropins in association with low concentrations of estrogens. Occasionally, in patients with anorexia nervosa or weight loss-related problems, subclinical hypothyroidism with low total T_4 and T_3 levels is noted. There is no clinical or biochemical evidence for hyperandrogenemia or hyperprolactinemia.

Treatment

Specific treatment of this hypothalamic form of amenorrhea is available and consists of the pulsatile administration of GnRH to these patients. This treatment mode is employed if pregnancy is desired. In all other instances, hormone replacement is given to the patients. In the presence of sufficient endogenous estrogen (which is rarely the case), progesterone is given alone (MPA 5-10 mg for 14 days followed by a free interval of 14 days). In hypoestrogenic states, therapy with estrogens and cyclical progestins is the treatment of choice. The patient should be advised that the spontaneous resumption of menstrual cyclicity may occur, and that hormonal replacement therapy is not contraceptive. If contraception is a concern, low-dose contraceptives are recommended, but spontaneous recovery of the endogenous system is then delayed. After a period of 6 to 9 months, hormone replacement may be stopped to allow for endogenous activity to resume. Sporadic bleeding under a replacement regimen may indicate a resumption of endogenous hormone production.

KALLMANN'S SYNDROME

Etiology

A rare hypothalamic form of primary amenorrhea is the syndrome of hypogonadotropic hypogonadism associated with amenorrhea, anosmia, and infantile sexual development: these combined symptoms are referred to as Kallmann's syndrome. Kallmann's syndrome represents an isolated deficiency of GnRH-containing neurons along the remnants of the olfactory placode. It relates to the hypoplasia of the rhinencephalon with hypoplastic or absent olfactory sulci. GnRH-containing neurons are also missing, as they are derived from this identical anatomical structure.

Clinical findings

Women with this defect present with complaints about primary amenorrhea and under-developed secondary sexual characteristics. They occasionally present with cranio-facial deformities and normal or increased height. These patients are found to have a normal female karyotype and are unable to perceive odors. A pelvic examination is normal, although the uterus and ovaries may be smaller in size due to a lack of continuous estrogen stimulation. The serum gonadotropins are found in the low range, but LH and FSH are released by GnRH administration. Estradiol concentrations in the serum are virtually undetectable, though they can be stimulated to reach the normal range by intermittent GnRH administrations.

Treatment

Since the defect is based on an organic deficit in GnRH-containing neurons, the most specific treatment is the pulsatile administration of GnRH. Indeed, the gonads can readily respond to gonadotropins, and therefore induction of ovulation by means of a miniature pump delivering GnRH in a pulsatile fashion is highly successful. However, since such treatment is quite costly and impracticable in longer time-frames, only amenorrheic patients with the desire to conceive are treated in this way. All other patients need to be supplemented by cyclical administration of estrogens and progestins for a life-long period in order to avoid bone loss due to hypoestrogenism.

FUNCTION DISORDERS OF THE ANTERIOR PITUITARY

Because normal functioning of the ovaries depends on intact stimulation by the anterior pituitary, any defect in this organ leads to a breakdown of cyclic menstruation. The degree of failure of the pituitary may range from total to minor deficiencies in gonadotropin secretion.

ISOLATED GONADOTROPIN DEFICIENCY

Etiology

The etiology of isolated gonadotropin deficiency is not known at the present time, but it may be due to a lack of gonadotropin-producing and storing cells in the anterior pituitary.

Clinical findings

Patients usually present with normal stature and a female appearance, but the development of secondary sex characteristics is impaired or absent. Endocrinological evaluation reveals hypogonadotropic hypogonadism. The finding of abnormally low gonadotropins in association with primary amenorrhea can be referred to lesions or functional deficits in both the hypothalamus and the pituitary. Differential diagnosis between these two possibilities can be extremely difficult. If repetitive pituitary stimulation

by GnRH does not release gonadotropins in measurable amounts, gonadotropin deficiency is more likely, although a hypothalamic deficit cannot be entirely excluded. Radiological imaging does not reveal any lesions at the level of the pituitary.

Treatment

Therapy is aimed at restoring the estrogen deficit. Therefore, cyclical hormonal therapy is advised and should be indefinitely continued, unless fertility is desired. In this case, treatment with exogenous gonadotropins (human menopausal gonadotropin, human chorionic gonadotropin) appears to be the treatment of choice and is usually successful, since the ovaries readily respond to gonadotropin stimulation with regular folliculogenesis.

PITUITARY TUMORS

Etiology

Prolactin-secreting adenomas are the most common pituitary tumors in association with primary amenorrhea. High prolactin levels are found in about one-third of women who do not complain of amenorrhea. Conversely, only one-third of women with hyperprolactinemia would complain about simultaneous galactorrhea. With the use of serum prolactin assays of increased sensitivity and the availability of new radiological techniques, the association of amenorrhea and small intrapituitary tumors has become apparent.

Clinical findings

The clinical symptoms do not necessarily correlate with the degree of prolactin elevation and the extension of the pituitary tumor. Diagnosis is based on the determination of prolactin levels, which are invariably increased. Extremely high prolactin concentrations are always associated with amenorrhea and galactorrhea. In the presence of normal or low gonadotropin serum concentrations, estrogen levels are low and indicate inappropriate stimulation of the ovary as the target organ of gonadotropins. Radiological imaging reveals an intrasellar or suprasellar mass.

Treatment

Even in the presence of macroadenomas, the treatment of first choice is to use dopaminergic compounds. The clinical availability of dopaminergic drugs such as bromocriptine permits specific suppression of prolactin secretion. While on this treatment, the determination of serum prolactin levels can be used to control the inhibition of prolactin hypersecretion. Conversely, shrinkage of tumors may require weeks or months of treatment, and the treatment period is best followed by MRI scans. The enhanced ability to detect pituitary tumors and the development of surgical techniques have enabled surgeons to remove small tumors with a high margin of safety (transsphenoidal approach).

PANHYPOPITUITARISM

Etiology

If a considerable part of the anterior pituitary is damaged, various functions of the pituitary, including the secretion of gonadotropins, are impaired. Occasionally such pituitary hypofunction is found in association with a hydrocephalus related to events around the time of birth or in the postnatal period, such as a carotid aneurysm or obstruction of the aqueduct. A similar deficit may be encountered after a severe head injury or in Sheehan's syndrome, presumably resulting from combined damage to the pituitary and the hypothalamus. Not uncommonly, an endocrinologically inert tumor of the pituitary, such as a craniopharyngioma or a malignant cerebral tumor, may be found. These tumors affect gonadotropin secretion in that they either disrupt the hypothalamic-pituitary connections via a blockade of the portal circulation or they directly destroy the cells of the anterior pituitary.

Clinical findings

Patients with panhypopituitarism will frequently present with short stature and signs of sexual infantilism. Since vital pituitary functions are destroyed or severely impaired, patients may present with cachexia and dehydration. This condition must be differentiated from anorexia nervosa, as the psychiatric problem of anorexia nervosa begins with hypogonadism and ends as a threatening physical state, and it may resemble the conditions found in panhypopituitarism. Diagnosis of panhypopituitarism is confirmed with measurements of low gonadotropins, low levels of TSH and prolactin, and low or undetectable peripheral levels of sex steroids and glucocorticoids. Radiological imaging of the sella may demonstrate lesions in this area.

Treatment

The immediate replacement of vital hormones such as glucocorticoids, thyroxine, and mineralocorticoids is mandatory. Hormone replacement with cyclical estrogen-progestin preparations is required to protect against estrogen-deficient consequences and to prevent atrophy of the secondary sexual characteristics. In children or adolescents, frequent administration of growth hormone is required to restore their full capacity to grow. Although

not mandatory for adults, clinical experience shows that growth hormone substitution results in an increased sense of well-being. If fertility is desired, the only way to stimulate the ovaries is by the exogenous administration of gonadotropins. This should be monitored by ultrasound in order to avoid ovarian hyperstimulation.

DISORDERS OF THE NORMAL FUNCTION OF THE OVARIES

Any of the causes of premature ovarian failure (onset of failure before the age of 40 years) that may present with secondary amenorrhea may also present with primary amenorrhea. An association between castrate levels of gonadotropins and extremely low or undetectable levels of estrogens indicates ovarian failure. It is important to emphasize the need for a karyotype in patients presenting with primary amenorrhea as a symptom of primary ovarian failure. The likelihood of a secondary malignant tumor to occur during reproductive life is very high, with a probability of 25% in women with gonadal dysgenesis and a chromosomal pattern containing a Y or a marker chromosome. Therefore, if the karyotype is abnormal, containing a Y or a marker chromosome, the ovaries of such women should be surgically removed. Ovarian failure is diagnosed by repeatedly elevated gonadotropin levels.

OVARIAN DYSGENESIS (46,XX GONADAL DYSGENESIS; 45,X0 AND MOSAICS – TURNER'S SYNDROME; 46,XY – SWYER'S SYNDROME; TRUE HERMAPHRODITISM)

Etiology

Genetic abnormalities present with primary and complete ovarian failure. In the presence of a normally developed uterus and vagina, the ovaries appear elongated and whitish, with streaks on the broad ligaments (see Fig. 45.2 in Color Atlas). In conditions of genetic abnormalities, even though the fetal ovary may begin normal development, it ends up completely depleted of primordial follicles long before the age of normal puberty. Patients with Turner's syndrome present with a deletion of the second X-chromosome (45,X0) and are therefore chromatin-negative. The chromosomal constitution of other patients may show mosaicism such as X0/XX or X0/XXX. While the chromosomal number of the majority of Turner's patients is 45, some have chromosomal counts of 46 (46,XX) or even 47. Some other individuals with primary amenorrhea present with a 46,XY chromosomal constitution (XY females). They have a palpable Müllerian system, but show true gonadal dysgenesis and a lack of sexual development (Swyer's syndrome).

Clinical findings

Clinical features of ovarian dysgenesis include webbing of the neck, low-set ears, cubitus valgus, short stature, and sexual infantilism. Other malformations such as congenital heart disease, coarctation of the aorta, and renal abnormality may also be observed. The complete picture of the syndrome is relatively rare, and some women, particularly those with chromosomal mosaicism, may even present with a normal female appearance. Female patients with the XY karyotype present with primary amenorrhea, gonadal dysgenesis, and normal or increased stature, and they resemble those with 46,XX dysgenesis in their sexual infantilism. Diagnosis is confirmed by determination of the chromosomal constitution of 45,X0 or any mosaic variant of this, and by the detection of high gonadotropin levels and low estrogen concentrations. A laparoscopic approach reveals ovaries in a streak-like appearance, and biopsies of these ovaries show stroma tissue without primordial follicles. In XY gonadal dysgenesis, patients present with partially or fully developed derivates of the Müllerian system, streak gonads, and normal female testosterone levels.

Treatment

Since patients with Turner's syndrome are devoid of any endogenous estrogens, estrogenic hormonal replacement should not be delayed until growth is completed. Cyclical therapy using estrogens and progesterone is used to induce menstrual cycles and secondary sex characteristics and to prevent osteoporosis. Surgical removal of streak gonads is particularly advised in those individuals presenting with a Y or marker chromosome, since a high percentage of these patients develop malignancies such as gonadoblastoma or germinoma. Prognosis for the resumption of fertility is very poor, but patients can be offered the transfer of a fertilized donor ovum into the uterus after appropriate hormonal preparation of the endometrial receptivity. In patients with Swyer's syndrome, extirpation of the gonadal streaks should be performed as soon as the diagnosis is established.

PREMATURE OVARIAN FAILURE

Etiology

Premature ovarian failure resides primarily in the ovaries and represents a rare clinical condition in which the karyotype is normal female and the gonads, although present, are immature and do not respond adequately to stimulation by gonadotropins. This defect may be genetically predetermined or acquired through diseases such as oophoritis during mumps. More likely it is the result of an immunological autoaggressive disorder, which may also occur before the age of menarche. The most common causes are physical insults such as irradiation of the gonads or exposure to cytotoxic drugs. Ovarian failure is more common if chemotherapy is radical or whole body irradiation is given. Finally, rare conditions associated with high gonadotropins and ovarian failure include galactosemia and enzymatic deficits in the ovaries and adrenal glands, such as the 17α-hydroxylase deficiency.

Clinical findings

Patients present with a normal female appearance, but the development of secondary sexual characteristics may be delayed or absent. Patients with 17α-hydroxylase deficiency present with hypertension and high blood levels of progesterone. Serum titers of gonadotropins are high, whereas estrogen levels are extremely low or undetectable. On ultrasound, the ovaries are rather flat and show minimal or no evidence of follicular growth. The endometrium demonstrates atrophic changes with little glandular development. The diagnosis is of great consequence for the patient and should only be made with caution after repeated analysis of serum levels of gonadotropins and of ovarian hormones. Because a number of cases of ovarian failure have been reported in association with autoimmune disorders, a few selected tests are recommended for further analysis, including the detection of thyroid antibodies, rheumatoid factor, and antinuclear antibodies. Ovarian resection by laparoscopy is of no value, whereas determination of the karyotype is essential to exclude genetic disorders. However, when future fertility is a concern, ovarian biopsy by laparoscopic means should be done to distinguish between the condition of ovarian dysgenesis and that of a resistant ovary, in which case the ovaries contain primordial follicles. If the levels of FSH are grossly elevated, the ovaries are virtually deprived of oocytes, and irreversible ovarian failure has ensued.

Treatment

Since the clinical condition is in general irreversible, replacement therapy with cyclical estrogen and progestin is indicated in these patients. Hormone replacement will prevent genital atrophy and other effects of hypoestrogenism. Recently some cases of normal menstrual cyclicity resumption have been reported; this has occurred preferentially with the use of hormone replacement therapy, suggesting that estrogen may activate the gonadotropin receptor formation of follicles. Although the chances of conceiving are extremely rare, the patient needs to also be informed of the unlikely possibility of a future pregnancy. Even if restoration of fertility is impossible, the feasibility of pregnancy with the transfer of a fertilized donated ovum could be considered.

RESISTANT OVARY SYNDROME (SAVAGE SYNDROME)

Etiology

The very rare (<1%) clinical condition of Savage syndrome is encountered when a patient presents with elevated levels of gonadotropins despite the presence of ovarian follicles. Gonadotropin receptors are absent on the follicles, or alternatively, the cause is a post-receptor defect.

Clinical findings

The occurrence of a resistant ovary syndrome may be assumed on the basis of findings of hypergonadotropic hypogonadism and the existence of follicle-like structures in the ovaries. A definitive diagnosis is established by laparoscopic ovarian biopsy. This diagnostic step is not recommended for patients with amenorrhea and high gonadotropins who do not desire pregnancy, since no apparent immediate consequence for treatment options can be drawn. Histological evaluation of ovarian biopsies can demonstrate the presence of primordial follicles (in contrast to ovarian failure) and the absence of lymphocytic infiltration as an indicator of non immunological origin. Genetic karyotyping is recommended even in a normal-appearing adolescent woman with this condition, since several forms of mosaicism are encountered.

Treatment

In patients with hypergonadotropic hypogonadism, treatment should be aimed at replacing the lack of sex steroids in the form of cyclic estrogen-progestin therapy. This treatment modality may be continued life-long for protection against hypoestrogenic long-term sequelae. If a patient wishes to conceive and follicles are outlined on ultrasonography, one could consider exogenous gonadotropin stimulation to induce ovulation. It is appropriate to offer the choice between laparoscopic ovarian biopsy and empirical treatment, since even in the presence of follicular residual activity, the response to exogenous gonadotropins is very limited. Suppression of gonadotropins by steroids or GnRH analogues for several months may help in the induction of ovulation. However, the chances of achieving pregnancy are very rare even with large doses of exogenous gonadotropins. The only treatment alternative is oocyte donation and embryo transfer into the uterus.

DISORDERS OF THE UTERUS AND VAGINA

CONGENITAL ANOMALIES OF THE MÜLLERIAN DUCT (MAYER-ROKITANSKY-KÜSTER SYNDROME)

Etiology

The lack of Müllerian duct development is a frequent cause of primary amenorrhea (about 20% of all patients), since it is accompanied by no apparent development of the uterus or upper part of the vagina. This syndrome is often referred to as Mayer-Rokitansky-Küster syndrome and represents a relatively common cause of primary amenorrhea. Patients presenting with this syndrome have an absent or hypoplastic uterus, which lacks a continuous outflow to the introitus or may merely be rudimentary in the form of bicornuate cords. In addition, the upper parts of the vagina are either completely absent or hypoplastic. These parts of the reproductive system are derived from the Müllerian duct system and are atretic or incompletely developed in these women.

Clinical findings

If a partial endometrial cavity is present, cyclic patterns of lower abdominal pain in the absence of any menstrual flow may be a complaint. However, most patients become clinically apparent when they present with primary amenorrhea. They are normally developed females with no evident disturbance of the pubertal development, growth, or sexual characteristics. The clinical picture gets manifested on clinical inspection and examination, when a vaginal pouch of variable length is found and not any or just a rudimentary uterus can be palpated. When the presence of uterine remnants is suspected, ultrasound can be utilized to depict the size and symmetry of the structure. Ovarian function is normal and can be documented by normal basal body temperature charts or normal peripheral levels of sex steroids. Attention should be paid to renal and skeletal abnormalities, which are frequently found in these patients.

Treatment

Unless Müllerian remnants are causing lower abdominal pain, hematometra, or uterine fibroids, there is no need to surgically excise them. One way of reconstructing the vagina may be the progressive dilatation of the pouch, which is conducted upwards for a period of 6 to 12 weeks. Operative treatment may be carried out by several transabdominal and perineal methods, including that of Vecchietti, in which the vaginal pouch is lengthened by constant traction via an extraperitoneally applied tractor. Since complications experienced during surgical procedures are encountered, reconstruction of the vagina is usually planned when the patient wishes to have a sexual relationship. Restoration of fertility is impossible. No hormonal substitution is required, since these patients have normal ovarian function.

ANDROGEN INSENSITIVITY SYNDROME (MALE PSEUDOHERMAPHRODITISM)

Etiology

The syndrome of testicular feminization is characterized by androgen insensitivity. The target tissues are unable to respond to endogenous androgens. This clinical condition is caused by either a lack of the cytosolic androgen receptor or the inability to convert testosterone into the biologically active form of dihydrotestosterone (5α-reductase deficiency). The karyotype of these patients is 46,XY, but they lack androgenization to varying degrees. Male pseudohermaphroditism means that the external genitalia have the opposite appearance of the gonads; the individual is phenotypically female, with normal breast development, but scanty or absent pubic or axillary hair. The uterus and the upper vagina are absent because of the production of Müllerian inhibiting factor by the testes. The testes secrete normal male amounts of testosterone and estradiol and are retained within the abdominal cavity or the inguinal canal.

Clinical findings

Patients with testicular feminization represent up to 5% of all patients with primary amenorrhea and are frequently recognized only at puberty, as they are born with equivocal external genitalia. Occasionally, testes are found in inguinal hernias of a small girl, and thus the syndrome gets discovered. Growth and development are normal, although the overall height is usually greater than average. The diagnosis should be suspected in a patient with primary amenorrhea, normal female development, and scanty or absent pubic and axillary hair. On pelvic examination, the labia minora are usually underdeveloped, the vagina is less deep than usual and ends blindly in a pouch, while the uterus and ovaries are absent. Diagnosis is confirmed by the finding of a male karyotype (46,XY) and by male levels of testosterone in plasma. Occasionally increased levels of LH and FSH are found, while estrogen levels correspond to those found in males.

Treatment

Individuals with testicular feminization are psychologically and morphologically female and should be confirmed in their gender identity. These patients are normal in their role as females, except that they are amenorrheic and infertile. Since the inguinal and intra-abdominal testes are more likely to develop malignant tumors, they should be surgically removed as soon as the diagnosis is established. To maintain the female secondary sex characteristics and prevent estrogenopenic consequences, substitution with continuous estrogens is required after bilateral gonadectomy.

DESTRUCTION OF THE ENDOMETRIUM OR STENOSIS OF THE CERVICAL OS

Etiology

Very rarely, an intercurrent infectious disease may destroy the endometrium to produce primary amenorrhea. Dependent on the dose employed, irradiation of the pelvis may result in either permanent or temporal amenorrhea. This is probably a very rare cause of primary amenorrhea, since the endometrium is non proliferative during the prepubertal period and protected against traumas.

Clinical findings

Although very rare, such conditions should be considered when there is a history of irradiation or intercurrent disease that could have destroyed the endometrium. Diagnosis is confirmed by hysteroscopy, when no functional endometrium can be discerned.

Treatment

Once the endometrium is destroyed, no specific interaction can be offered to restore menstrual function and fertility. In the case of post-infectious synechiae that may partially or completely obliterate the uterine cavity, they may be dissected by hysteroscopic instruments and the cavity distended until healed by the insertion of a Foley catheter or an intrauterine device. Endometrial scarring usually occurs in the hypo-estrogenic state as in the prepubertal period, and therefore it may be valuable to stimulate the endometrium with high doses of cyclical estrogens and progestins.

MALFORMATIONS OF THE VAGINA (CONGENITAL ATRESIA OF THE VAGINA, HYMEN IMPERFORATUM, VAGINAL SEPTA)

Etiology

Etiological causes for the finding of several forms of uterovaginal agenesis are unknown. The existence of an anatomical defect as a rare cause for primary amenorrhea underscores the importance of a complete physical and gynecological examination of a girl in the evaluation of amenorrhea. In these patients, the absence of menstruation results from an anatomical obstruction of the outflow tract. The most frequent congenital abnormality is an imperforate hymen. Since the ovaries and endometrium are functionally intact in these girls, the discharge from the uterus at the time of menstruation is retained and hidden in the vagina. This process leads to a progressive distension of the vagina, which is filled with blood (hematocolpos). When this condition is long-standing and untreated, menstrual blood drains back to the uterus and the fallopian tubes (hematometra, hematosalpinx). Similar observations are encountered with a partial or complete atresia of the vagina.

Clinical findings

Characteristic of partial or complete vaginal atresia, a transverse vaginal septum, or imperforate hymen in the presence of an intact uterus are the periodic episodes of pain in the lower abdomen, occurring at the same time as expected menstruation. Inspection of the vagina and a rectal examination reveals this condition. Transverse septa of the vagina may be distinguished from an imperforate hymen by their lack of distension at the introitus on Valsalva's maneuver. The karyotype in these patients with vaginal atresia is 46,XX, and all hormones indicate normal pituitary and ovarian function. This clinical entity is to be differentiated from vaginal and uterine agenesis in patients with testicular feminization. Ultrasonography may confirm the appearance of a hematocolpos or hematometra. Magnetic resonance imaging has been utilized to accurately delineate the degree of anatomical abnormality.

In all instances, the obstacle must be incised and drained from below. Even in more complex malformations, the continuity of the outflow tract can usually be achieved surgically. Treatment of an imperforate hymen or a transverse septum is relatively easy: a cruciate incision of the hymen, either by laser or by knife, will correct it. This procedure should be done under antibiotic protection. When a partial or complete vaginal atresia is found, surgical correction with restoration of the continuity of the tract is essential. A passage between the urethra and the rectum is dissected and a skin graft is placed over a mold. Other approaches have used vaginal dilators to which firm pressure is applied.

Suggested readings

BAIRD DT. Amenorrhea, anovulation, and dysfunctional uterine bleeding. In: DeGroot L (ed). Endocrinology. Vol. 3. Philadelphia: Saunders, 1995;2059-79.

PADILLA SL. Primary amenorrhea. In: Schlaff WD, Rock JA (eds). Decision making in reproductive endocrinology. Oxford: Blackwell Scientific Publishing, 1993;49-55.

ROSSMANITH WG. The basic physiology of the hypothalamo-pituitary-gonadal axis. In: Grossman A (ed). Clinical endocrinology. Oxford: Blackwell Scientific Publications, 1997;655-65.

SPEROFF L, GLASS RH, KASE NG (eds). Clinical gynecologic endocrinology and infertility. Baltimore: Williams and Wilkins, 1994;401-56.

WOOD DF, FRANKS S. Hypogonadism in women. In: Grossman A (ed). Clinical endocrinology. Oxford: Blackwell Scientific Publications, 1992;667-83.

Secondary amenorrhea

- The presence of secondary versus primary amenorrhea renders serious underlying abnormalities (such as congenital defects) less likely. The prevalence of secondary amenorrhea is between 3 to 8%, dependent upon age.
- Secondary amenorrhea is associated with low serum estradiol levels, combined with either reduced (central origin of ovarian dysfunction) or elevated follicle-stimulating hormone (FSH), (ovarian origin) concentrations. Whether additional hormone assays such as luteinizing hormone or androgens are required for endocrine evaluation should depend upon clinical signs and symptoms and upon serum estradiol and FSH levels.
- Environmental problems, including psychogenic stress or lifestyle issues such as diet or exercise patterns, are frequently involved in hypothalamic amenorrhea. Radiologic assessment of the sella turcica and suprasellar region by CT scan or MRI should be performed to exclude occult hypothalamic-pituitary defects in patients presenting with hypogonadotrophic hypo-estrogenic amenorrhea. Hormone replacement therapy should be considered in hypo-estrogenic conditions that extend for a 6-month period or longer to prevent increased fracture and cardiovascular risks.
- The incidence of hyperprolactinemia in secondary amenorrhea is approximately 20%.
- Premature ovarian failure represents 10 to 20% of women with secondary amenorrhea. Ovarian failure is considered to be premature in case it occurs before the age of 40 years.
- The heterogenous group of patients diagnosed with polycystic ovary syndrome is part of the spectrum of amenorrheic women with normal serum FSH and estradiol levels (World Health Organization, Group 2). Diagnostic criteria used, as well as short- and long-term consequences of the syndrome, are poorly validated.
- Induction of ovulation is the complete process of the stimulation of follicular growth, stimulation of the final maturation of the follicle and oocyte, and the ultimate rupture of the dominant follicle. This treatment strategy should only be applied in anovulatory infertility.
- Making a diagnosis before starting ovulation induction is of great importance for the choice of therapy.
- Treatment of an underlying disease or cause is the preferential treatment for anovulation.
- Clomiphene citrate is the drug of choice (in a maximum dose of 200 mg per day for 5 days) in ovulation induction, except in hypergonadotropic and hyperprolactinemic anovulation.
- If a patient fails to ovulate on the maximal dose, or if a patient has had 12 ovulatory cycles on clomiphene citrate and is still unable to conceive, treatment should be continued with either gonadotropin-releasing hormone in hypogonadotropic anovulation, or FSH in normogonadotropic anovulation.

- Gonadotropin-releasing hormone, administered in a pulsatile fashion, is the treatment of choice in severe hypogonadotropic hypogonadism. Treatment should be started with a low dose, because multiple ovulation and hence multiple pregnancies primarily occur during the first treatment cycle.
- FSH is the drug of choice in clomiphene citrate-resistant normogonadotropic anovulation. The drug should preferably be applied according to the so-called low-dose step-up schedule.
- Multiple pregnancies and the hyperstimulation syndrome are the major complications of inducing ovulation. In particular, the hyperstimulation syndrome should be treated in a center with ample experience with this disorder.
- Dopamine agonists are the drug of choice for the treatment of hyperprolactinemic anovulation

HYPOTHALAMIC, PITUITARY, OVARIAN AND UTERINE DEFECTS
Bart C.J.M. Fauser

A so-called normal menstrual cycle is characterized by bleeding intervals, varying between a total of 21 and 35 days. Uterine bleeding occurs in response to the withdrawal of sex steroid hormones due to the demise of the corpus luteum in the preceding cycle. Therefore, normal menstrual patterns require a careful orchestration of various organs, including the hypothalamus, pituitary, and ovary, as well as the uterus. Consequently, defects underlying a deviation from normal cyclicity can occur at various levels. Amenorrhea is arbitrarily defined as an absence of vaginal bleedings for at least 6 months, and oligomenorrhea as bleedings occurring at intervals between 35-42 days and 6 months.

Amenorrhea can be primary (absence of previous bleedings). In this case a thorough investigation of potential structural congenital abnormalities, such as genetic genital tract anomalies, is mandatory. The diagnosis of secondary amenorrhea renders such severe abnormalities less likely since the reproductive system has been operative before. Menstrual bleeding indicates proliferation of the endometrium due to exposure to at least some estrogens. Therefore, as a rule, oligomenorrheic patients present with serum estradiol levels within the normal range. Continued endometrial exposure to estrogens may also give rise to metrorrhagia. In contrast, low estradiol levels - suggesting a total absence of ovarian activity - are associated with amenorrhea. The prevalence of secondary amenorrhea in women during the reproductive years is reported to be between 3 and 8%, depending on age.

Clinical findings

The purpose of an extended evaluation of patients presenting with secondary amenorrhea is threefold (Tabs. 46.1 and 46.2). First, to recognize patients with potential

(future) health risks. For instance, patients may suffer from pituitary tumors such as prolactinomas. In rare cases, gonadal or adrenal malignancies may be diagnosed

Table 46.1 Practical guidelines for the evaluation of patients presenting with secondary amenorrhea

History
  Dietary history, weight changes
  Psychological and physical stress factors
  Galactorrhea, changes in body hair, use of drugs, family history
  Climacteric symptoms

Physical examination
  Body weight, body composition, body hair, acanthosis nigricans
  Breast and thyroid palpation
  Gynecological investigation

Hormone assays in peripheral blood
  First line: serum FSH, estradiol, and prolactin
  Second line: serum LH, cortisol, SHBG, TSH testosterone, androstenedione, DHEAS 17-hydroxyprogesterone

Additional endocrine tests (dynamic organ function tests)
  Pulsatile GnRH
  Dexamethasone suppression test
  ACTH stimulation test

Pelvic ultrasound
  Detection of polycystic ovaries
  Detection of ovarian mass (malignancies)
  Endometrial thickness
  Obliteration uterine cavity

Other relevant tests
  Progestogen challenge test
  Endometrial biopsy
  Assessment of bone density
  Investigation of sella turcica and suprasellar region (CT scan/MRI)
  Visual fields
  Chromosomal/genetic investigation

Table 46.2 Goals of evaluation of amenorrheic patients

Recognize patients with potential (future) health risks
Tumors
Endometrial hyperplasia
Osteoporosis
Cardiovascular disease ?
Diabetes ?

Choice of therapeutic options
Surgery
Estrogen replacement
Progestogen withdrawal
Dopamine agonist
Ovulation induction (anti-estrogens, gonadotropins, GnRH)
In vitro fertilization (oocyte donation)

Detection of patients at risk for low success rates and high complications during ovulation induction (polycystic ovary syndrome?)

in patients presenting with secondary amenorrhea. Moreover, long-term hypo-estrogenic conditions may give rise to osteoporosis, whereas extended endometrial exposure to normal estrogen levels may result in hyperplasia, eventually leading to endometrial carcinoma. Additional risks in polycystic ovary syndrome (PCOS) patients may include increased chances for cardiovascular disease and diabetes. Secondly, appropriate therapy may be chosen on the basis of previous considerations being either surgery/radiation or dopamine agonist medication in cases of hypothalamic-pituitary abnormalities. Estrogen replacement therapy should be considered in women suffering from long-term hypo-estrogenic conditions, whereas the induction of withdrawal bleedings by progestin administration is required in normo-estrogenic amenorrheic conditions. If patients wish to conceive, further screening may be helpful in selecting the appropriate drug for inducing ovulation. Thirdly, more and more attention is focused toward the detection of patients at risk during the induction of ovulation. These patients should be monitored more intensively, and stimulation should be prudent.

Hence, for reasons of safety, a clear diagnosis may in some cases be mandatory. On the other hand, a distinct etiological diagnosis may not be possible in the majority of patients, and attention is shifted from diagnosis toward prognosis. Classification may be helpful, particularly in infertile amenorrheic patients where it is necessary to decide whether inducing ovulation is useful. An appropriate drug must be chosen, and hopefully we can predict treatment outcome in terms of chances for success and complications.

Symptoms and signs

Since menstrual bleeding and ovarian function are intimately related, a thorough history and physical examination focusing on gonadal activity should be the first step in the assessment of amenorrheic patients. Physiologic causes of amenorrhea such as pregnancy and lactation should be excluded before further investigation is performed. Special attention should be focused toward dietary history and related weight changes, psychological stress or strenuous physical exercise, galactorrhea, family history of cycle abnormalities or early menopause, an increase in body hair, and the use of certain psychotropic drugs. Complaints of climacteric symptoms such as sweating and hot flashes suggest low estradiol levels in these patients.

An assessment of secondary sex characteristics may be of limited value in cases of secondary amenorrhea. Recording a patient's body weight (preferably body mass index [weight divided by square height] or waist-to-hip ratio as an indication of body fat distribution), scoring the distribution and amount of body hair and other signs of virilization (such as clitoris enlargement), breast palpation in search of galactorrhea, and thyroid palpation should be included in the routine work-up of amenorrheic patients. Acanthosis nigricans (localized hyperpigmentation of the skin) (Fig. 46.1) may be observed in insulin-resistant patients. In addition, measuring blood pressure may sometimes be useful. A gynecologic investigation should be performed. The presence of vaginal atrophy by inspection and a small uterus by palpation suggests low estradiol levels, whereas clear cervical mucus suggests exposure to normal estradiol concentrations. Enlarged ovaries may sometimes be detected, which may suggest polycystic ovaries.

Diagnostic procedures

For the practical evaluation of amenorrheic patients, hormone assays in peripheral blood may be helpful in the determination of the level of abnormality. Classification of amenorrheic patients on the basis of ovarian steroids and gonadotropins has been adopted by the World Health Organization (WHO). In brief, low gonadotropin levels

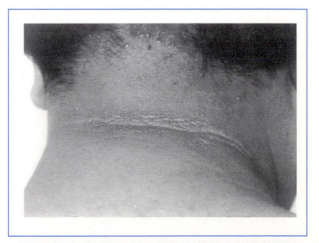

Figure 46.1 Acanthosis nigricans. (Courtesy of Mr. Van der Stek, Dijkzigt University Hospital, Rotterdam, The Netherlands.)

are usually associated with low estradiol concentrations due to absent ovarian stimulation. This condition suggests a central origin of ovarian dysfunction. Primary defects in ovarian function are characterized by low estradiol output in combination with high gonadotropin levels due to reduced steroid feedback. Again, both of these conditions present with amenorrhea because estradiol levels are low. However, the great majority of patients present with serum gonadotropin and estradiol levels within normal limits. Despite "normal" stimulation of ovaries, ovulation does not occur for reasons not completely understood (Tab. 46.3). These patients may present with either oligomenorrhea or amenorrhea. In addition, serum prolactin levels should always be assayed. Therefore, it is proposed that serum follicle-stimulating hormone (FSH), estradiol, and prolactin levels should be assayed as a first step in all patients (Tab. 46.1).

The determination of serum thyroid-stimulating hormone (TSH) levels may be considered as an indication of thyroid dysfunction. Although both hypo- and hyperthyroidism have been associated with cycle abnormalities, it is uncertain as yet what the incidence of abnormal thyroid hormones is in amenorrheic patients without obvious clinical signs of thyroid dysfunction.

Additional assays of serum luteinizing hormone (LH) levels, ovarian and adrenal steroids (testosterone, androstenedione, dehydroepiandrosterone-sulphate [DHEAS], 17-hydroxyprogesterone, and cortisol), and sex-hormone binding globulin (allowing for the assessment of the amount of unbound biologically active testosterone) should be dependent upon results from first-step hormone assays and on clinical signs and symptoms (see also the section on PCOS). DHEAS is a weak androgen

but is derived exclusively from the adrenals. The remaining steroids are both from adrenal and ovarian origin, and therefore they do not allow for the discrimination between hyperfunction of both organs. On the basis of fasting early morning cortisol levels, adrenal hyperfunction (Cushing's syndrome) or hypofunction (Addison's disease) may be suspected. Fasting levels of glucose and insulin may be assessed as a measure for insulin resistance occurring in some PCOS patients.

The role of dynamic organ function tests, such as gonadotropin-releasing hormone (GnRH) stimulation of pituitary function, FSH/human chorion gonadotropin (hCG) stimulation of ovarian activity, or steroid feedback tests by estrogen administration are for research purposes only and should not be included in routine screening programs.

Adrenocorticotropic hormone (ACTH) stimulation or dexamethasone suppression of adrenal function should be performed when cortisol levels outside of the normal range or elevated DHEAS levels are found. Finding increased cortisol levels following ACTH stimulation is a common screening test for primary or secondary adrenal insufficiency. In contrast, dexamethasone suppression assesses the integrity of the cortisol feedback system of the hypothalamic-pituitary-adrenal axis. It can therefore exclude Cushing's disease (adrenal hyperfunction due to augmented ACTH production by pituitary tumors), and it can also differentiate between adrenal or ovarian origin of hyperandrogenemia.

Endometrial exposure to estradiol may also be tested by the so-called progestogen challenge test. Vaginal bleeding subsequent to progestogen administration only occurs in patients previously exposed to estrogens. However, the reliability of this test has recently been questioned. Endometrial biopsy may be performed to exclude the presence of endometrial hyperplasia in normo-estrogenic women presenting with long-standing amenorrhea.

Imaging studies

Ultrasound examination of the ovaries and uterus may be helpful in the detection of polycystic ovaries, endometrial thickness (as a measure for endometrial proliferation in response to estradiol), and obliteration of the uterine cavity. Unfortunately, sonographic criteria for polycystic ovary diagnosis are poorly defined, and it is uncertain as yet whether this information is clinically useful. The presence of polycystic ovaries (PCO) (Fig. 46.2) may or may not coincide with clinical and endocrine features associated with polycystic ovary syndrome. Therefore, a clear distinction should be made between these two entities.

HYPOTHALAMIC DEFECTS

Functional hypothalamic amenorrhea

The pulsatile secretion of GnRH from neurons in the hypothalamus into the portal capillary system is responsible for the maintenance of pituitary gonadotropin secretion. Hypothalamic amenorrhea is characterized by low

---

Table 46.3 Classification of secondary amenorrhea on the basis of hormone assays in peripheral blood

Low gonadotropin, low estradiol levels (WHO, Class 1)

Hypothalamus
 Functional
 Brain tumors (craniopharyngioma)
 Injury, systemic illness

Pituitary
 Pituitary adenomas (prolactinomas, nonfunctional, endocrine active [secreting for instance FSH, TSH, ACTH, growth hormone])
 Empty sella
 Following surgery or radiation
 Hemorrhage, necrosis

Normal gonadotropin (FSH), normal estradiol levels (WHO, Class 2)
 Polycystic ovary syndrome
 Other forms of normogonadotropic anovulation
 Endocrine ovarian / adrenal tumors

High gonadotropin, low estradiol levels (WHO, Class 3)
 Premature ovarian failure (true early menopause)
 Resistant ovary syndrome (follicular form)

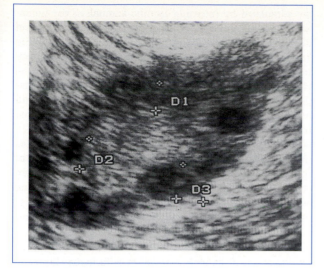

Figure 46.2 Polycystic ovary diagnosed by transvaginal ultrasound. (Courtesy of Dr. Imani, Dijkzigt University Hospital, Rotterdam, The Netherlands.)

serum gonadotropin and estradiol concentrations (WHO, Class 1) due to decreased hypothalamic secretion of GnRH. Such patients have small ovaries with few early antral follicles, which is due to insufficient stimulation by gonadotropic hormones. Discrimination between normal and reduced hormone levels is not always clear, and patients may present with low estradiol concentrations in combination with FSH levels within the normal range. Due to the short half-life of GnRH, this releasing hormone cannot be assessed in the general circulation. Measurement of changes in amplitude and frequency of pulsatile LH concentrations in peripheral blood is impractical and should be used for research purposes only. The common hypothesis is that increased corticotropin-releasing hormone directly or through augmented β-endorphin secretion suppresses GnRH pulsatility. Radiologic assessment of the sella turcica and suprasellar region by computerized tomography (CT scan) or magnetic resonance imaging (MRI) may be performed to exclude occult hypothalamic-pituitary defects in patients presenting with hypogonadotrophic hypo-estrogenic amenorrhea. Tumors arising from surrounding tissue (such as craniopharyngiomas) of the hypothalamus are extremely rare.

The term functional suggests a nonorganic genesis. This condition in principle should be considered to be reversible. Frequently environmental problems – including psychogenic stress or lifestyle issues such as changes in diet, exercise, or sleeping patterns – are involved in hypothalamic amenorrhea. Patients who are underweight due to severe chronic illness present with similar endocrine features. Most patients are intelligent and highly motivated. They usually have a history of normal-onset menarche. Sporting activities that frequently induce hypothalamic amenorrhea include long-distance running, ballet dancing, and gymnastics. Young women with a low body weight (over 10% below ideal body weight) or reduced body fat distribution (below 20% of body fat) are at increased risk for developing amenorrhea. The onset of

amenorrhea is usually abrupt. It is of interest to note that loss of weight is much more frequently associated with ovarian dysfunction as compared to overweight, where approximately 50% of women remain ovulatory.

Classical anorexia nervosa patients are usually adolescents, over-achievers, hyperactive, and frank regarding their diet habits. These women suffer from a disturbed body perception and are usually obsessively concerned about becoming overweight. Psychiatric counseling is desirable. Other symptoms include constipation, hypotension, and hypothermia. Cortisol secretion and thyroid function may be altered in these patients. Bulimic behavior is often secretive, and artificial means such as vomiting or laxatives may be used. Bulimia may coincide in anorectic patients, though body weight may also remain normal. Reproductive dysfunction is thus less frequent in these patients. A careful history including other compulsive behaviors and associated physical findings (such as swollen parotic glands, tooth decay, and cramps of hands) may be helpful for proper diagnosis. Although hypothalamic dysfunction is reversible, these women frequently remain amenorrheic even when their weight changes are corrected. Reduced bone density due to long-term hypo-estrogenic conditions and related increased risk for bone fractures may occur. Bone density can easily be assessed by dual energy X-ray absorptiometry (DEXA). Hormone replacement therapy should be considered unless inducing ovulation is required for fertility therapy. This form of amenorrhea can be treated effectively with pulsatile GnRH administration. However, attention should first be focused on potential stress factors underlying this functional hypothalamic disturbance.

Other causes

Significant injury (especially following head-on car collision), as well as systemic illnesses and shock, may also result in hypothalamic-pituitary dysfunction.

PITUITARY DEFECTS

Amenorrhea due to hypothalamic or pituitary dysfunction are both characterized by low serum gonadotropin and estradiol levels. Differentiation may be possible by the pulsatile administration of GnRH. Normal secretion of LH can only be restored when pituitary function is intact. Assessment of the sella turcica and suprasellar region by CT scan or MRI (Fig. 46.3) should be performed.

Pituitary tumors

Pituitary adenomas – the most common intracranial neoplasia – usually originate from the anterior lobe. A prolactinoma (which will be discussed separately) is the most common pituitary tumor, constituting approximately 40% of pituitary adenomas. Nonfunctional tumors may eventually give rise to pituitary dysfunction by compressing

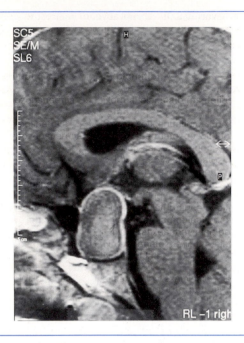

Figure 46.3 Magnetic resonance imaging of the sella turcica and suprasellar region showing a macroprolactinoma. (Courtesy of Dr. Tanghe, Dijkzigt University Hospital, Rotterdam, The Netherlands.)

adjacent structures and subsequent endocrine abnormalities. Pituitary adenomas may in rare cases secrete growth hormone (giving rise to acromegaly), adrenocorticotropic hormone (leading to hypercortisolism, also known as Cushing's disease), TSH, or gonadotropins (mostly FSH or free α-subunits). Exact mechanisms by which reproductive function is affected remains unclear for most hormonally active adenomas.

Patients with pituitary tumors usually require transphenoidal surgery. Radiation therapy may be required in instances of incomplete surgery or inoperable tumors. Hypopituitarism is often a complication of surgery or radiation, and multiple substitution of endocrine function is indicated.

Prolactinoma (prolactin-producing pituitary adenoma). Hyperprolactinemia can be diagnosed by a single morning serum prolactin measurement. It may be associated with galactorrhea. It should be realized that a distinct diurnal variability exists for prolactin secretion, with the highest levels occurring at night. Therefore, the best time for adequate assessment is late in the morning before lunchtime. This should be considered when levels appear to be elevated. The incidence of increased prolactin output in anovulatory patients has been reported to be around 7% in oligomenorrheic patients and 20% in women with secondary amenorrhea. Prolactin secretion by the lactotroph cells of the adenohypophysis is under tonic inhibitory control of dopamine from the hypothalamus and tuberoinfundibular neurons. In contrast, all other pituitary hormones are stimulated by releasing factors. Lesions of the central nervous system or the use of drugs (Tab. 46.4) that affect dopamine secretion also influence prolactin levels. Other known causes of hyperprolactinemia include hypopituitarism, liver cirrhosis, and adrenal insufficiency. Hypothalamic GnRH output is inhibited in these patients through increased dopamine secretion and β-endorphin activation. Hyperprolactinemia is thus usually accompanied by hypogonadotrophic hypo-estrogenic amenorrhea. In addition, prolactin may exert direct effects at the adrenal or ovarian level. Hyperprolactinemia may also be associated with hypothyroidism, since thyrotropin-releasing hormone stimulates both TSH and prolactin release. Radiologic assessment of the sella turcica and suprasellar region (Fig. 46.4) is mandatory to exclude the existence of a macroprolactinoma (arbitrarily defined as an adenoma of 10 mm in diameter or larger). Macroprolactinomas are more likely to be diagnosed in patients presenting with higher prolactin levels. In patients with macroadenomas, careful assessment of other endocrine pituitary function to exclude pituitary compression, as well as visual field testing to exclude optic chiasmatic compression, is mandatory. An "empty sella" may also be found in hyperprolactinemic patients.

Dopamine agonist medication (bromocriptine, pergolide, cabergoline, and quinagolide) is the therapy of choice, and surgical resection – even in cases of macroadenomas – is rarely needed. Due to potential serious side effects such as fatigue, dizziness, nausea, and vomiting, initial doses should be low, with slow incremental steps with weekly intervals thereafter. Recently released drugs are targeted more specifically to D2 receptors located in the pituitary, and therefore side effects of these compounds are reduced. Prolactin levels are usually normalized within several weeks. Doses should be increased until serum prolactin levels are within normal limits and a regular bleeding pattern is recovered. In patients with microprolactinomas, medication should be discontinued in cases of pregnancy. Little is known regarding the natural course of the disease, but it seems that lifelong medication is not required. If it is decided to stop medication in these patients, the menstrual pattern and serum estradiol levels should be monitored, because distinctly decreased bone density has been reported in untreated hyperprolactinemic patients. Estrogen replacement therapy should be considered under these conditions. It is believed that steroid contraception should not be prescribed in these patients because prolactinomas may grow due to augmented estrogen exposure. Patients suffering from macroadenomas should be monitored carefully,

Table 46.4 Medication that may induce hyperprolactinemia due to depletion of central stores of catecholamines or through action as dopamine receptor blockers

Phenothiazines
Tricyclic antidepressants
Haloperidol
Methyldopa
Metoclopramine
Verapamil
Cocaine

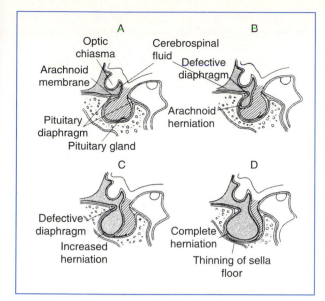

Figure 46.4 Schematic representation of the empty sella syndrome. (From Shoupe M. Hyperprolactinemia, diagnosis and treatment. In Infertility, contraception, and reproductive endocrinology. Lobo et al. Blackwell Science 1997; 323-41.)

including visual field testing. Medication should be continued even during pregnancy. The tumor may grow during pregnancy due to high levels of estrogens.

Empty sella syndrome The sella may sometimes appear empty due to incomplete development of the sellar diaphragm, allowing the subarachnoid space to extend to surround the pituitary gland to a variable degree (Fig. 46.4). This may also be found in patients after pituitary surgery or radiation. Pituitary function can remain normal, but hyperprolactinemia may occur.

Other forms of hypopituitarism In rare cases, severe postpartum hemorrhage may result in pituitary necrosis (Sheehan's syndrome), hypocortisolism, and failure to initiate lactation because of deficient prolactin secretion. Other causes of hypopituitarism include pituitary apoplexia; pituitary or suprasellar tumors following pituitary surgery or radiation; infection (tuberculosis, mycosis); metastasis of the breast; prostate, lung or colon cancer; and granulomatous disease such as sarcoidosis. Complaints are related to the failure of adrenals, thyroid, or gonads. Substitution therapy – in particular cortisol, thyroxin, and gonadal steroids – is indicated.

Pituitary-ovarian imbalance

An imbalance in the pituitary-ovarian axis is proposed in anovulatory patients presenting with serum FSH and estradiol levels within normal limits. However, these normal limits are not clearly defined, and substantial individual variability in FSH and estradiol concentrations as well as distinct changes during the follicular phase have been observed in regularly cycling women. It is difficult to understand why these patients with an essentially intact pituitary-ovarian axis remain acyclic. Endocrine signaling appears intact. Therefore, attention has focused in recent years on potential abnormalities in intra-ovarian modification of gonadotropin (especially FSH) action. This implicates a shift from endocrine to auto/paracrine regulation. Different growth factor systems may be involved.

Polycystic ovary syndrome In the original publication by Stein and Leventhal in 1935, the presence of bilaterally enlarged ovaries exhibiting multiple follicle cysts was described in seven women presenting with sterility, amenorrhea, and masculinization. Ovarian wedge resection was considered to be the therapy of choice, providing ovarian tissue allowed for microscopic confirmation of the diagnosis of Stein-Leventhal disease. Characteristic morphologic features include enlarged ovaries with a thickened cortex, a marked increase in stroma with nests of luteinized cells, and an increased number of antral follicles beneath the ovarian surface (Fig. 46.5). Certain signs and symptoms (such as infertility, hirsutism, amenorrhea, and obesity) are frequently associated with polycystic ovaries upon surgery. Complaints typically start early in life, shortly after menarche. PCOS patients may also present with oligomenorrhea.

Endocrine studies have shown that serum LH concentrations and androgen levels are frequently elevated in these patients. However, the interpretation of a single LH estimate is not without difficulties because of the pulsatile nature of LH release, differences in specificity between immunoassays, and timing of blood withdrawal. Some oligomenorrheic patients may occasionally ovulate. In case serum LH concentrations are assessed during or shortly after corpus luteum activity, actual LH levels may be underestimated due to progestin negative feedback actions. Moreover, there is no consensus regarding which androgen should be assessed, whether it be total testosterone, free testosterone, testosterone/SHBG ratio, or

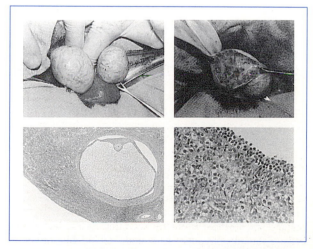

Figure 46.5 Macroscopic and microscopic characteristics of polycystic ovaries.

androstenedione. Elevated DHEAS or 17-OH progesterone levels are generally excluded from PCOS diagnosis, although phenotype expression of late onset adrenal
hyperplasia is very similar. Alternatively, this condition
could be viewed as a separate entity within the overall
spectrum of this heterogeneous syndrome. Serum FSH
and estradiol levels are normal. Therefore these patients
should be classified as a WHO Group 2, despite the fact
that serum LH levels may be elevated.

The term PCOS or polycystic ovary syndrome was
introduced and diagnosis has been largely based on clinical and endocrine criteria, suggesting that this syndrome
involves a heterogeneous group of patients. Since the
mid-eighties pelvic ultrasonography has enabled the noninvasive examination of ovaries on a large scale, allowing for the re-examination of ovarian abnormalities in
these patients. Despite the fact that ultrasound criteria
used for polycystic ovary diagnosis (see Fig. 46.2) (such
as increased follicle number, increased amount or density
of stroma, or augmented ovarian volume) have not been
carefully evaluated, many clinical investigators apply
ultrasound as an important if not only criterion for PCOS
diagnosis. A distinction has been made by some investigators between polycystic and multicystic ovaries,
depending on the amount of ovarian stroma. At the present time, there is major controversy regarding criteria
used for PCOS diagnosis. Studies from our own group in
350 WHO Group 2 anovulatory infertile patients suggest
that criteria used to diagnose PCOS overlap considerably.
However, ultrasound diagnosis of PCO is a poor predictor of PCOS, and over 30% of these patients exhibit normal LH and androgen levels (Fig. 46.6). It is of interest
to note that only 20% of patients score positively for both
ultrasound and endocrine criteria. Although it is generally believed that PCOS patients perform poorly during
induction of ovulation and that complication rates are
high – especially following the use of exogenous
gonadotropins – little prospective data are available in

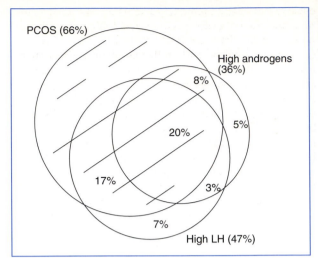

Figure 46.6 Distribution of diagnostic features associated
with PCOS (polycystic ovaries, elevated serum LH, or
androgen levels) in 330 normogonadotropic anovulatory
infertile women. (From van Santbrink EJP, Hop WC,
Fauser BCJM. Classification of normogonadotropic infertility: polycystic ovaries diagnosed by ultrasound versus
endocrine characteristics of polycystic ovary syndrome.
Fertil Steril 1997;67:4528.)

the literature. Observations from our own group suggest
that being overweight, hyperandrogenemia, and the
severity of the cycle disturbance are good predictors for
ovarian response following anti-estrogen medication.
Again, during initial screening, attention may shift from
the search for criteria for proper diagnosis toward prognosis (of fertility therapy) (Tab. 46.5).

Clustering of the disease within families has been
established by several investigators. Indeed, single gene
mutations resulting in the PCOS phenotype have been
reported. Patients suffering from gene mutations that only
partially reduce 21-hydroxylase enzyme activity involved
in the conversion of progestins to adrenal steroids
(referred to as "late-onset adrenal hyperplasia") may be
diagnosed as PCOS. In addition, cytochrome P450C17
enzyme (involved in the conversion of progestins to
androgens) defects have also been implemented in these
patients on the basis of abnormal steroid profiles following ovarian stimulation by the flare effect of GnRH agonists. Several investigators have shown that insulin resistance is present in a proportion of PCOS patients.
Multiple mutations of the insulin receptor have been
described in insulin resistant (obese) PCOS patients.
Although hyperinsulinemia has been proposed to underlie
hyperandrogenemia at the ovarian level, important questions regarding a potential causal relationship remain to
be answered. Acanthosis nigricans (hyperpigmentation)
may be observed in PCOS patients with severe insulin
resistance.

It is difficult to comprehend how these women fail to
ovulate despite "normal" circulating FSH and estradiol
concentrations. However, it should be realized that FSH
and estradiol levels vary greatly during the follicular
phase of the menstrual cycle. Moreover, during the inter-

Table 46.5 Polycystic ovary syndrome: overview of diagnostic criteria

Clinical presentation
Obesity
Hirsutism
Early onset of oligo-/amenorrhea
Infertility

Hormone assays
Normal FSH and estradiol levels
Elevated androgen levels (testosterone, free
  testosterone, or androstenedione)
Elevated LH levels
(Altered glucose/insulin ratio)

Pelvic ultrasound
Polycystic ovaries

cycle rise in FSH, serum levels surpass the threshold value for stimulation of ovarian activity, and follicle recruitment is subsequently initiated. FSH levels in PCOS women are certainly below these early follicular phase concentration maximums. Recent observations support the concept of abnormal intra-ovarian modification of the FSH signal. Alternatively, FSH bioactivity, FSH receptor interaction, or post-receptor signal transduction in granulosa cells may be affected. Elevated intra-ovarian androgen levels have long been implicated in inducing follicle atresia in PCOS. However, the mechanism of action is not entirely clear, and studies on steroid levels in follicle fluid failed to show augmented intrafollicular androgen levels in individual PCOS follicles. Data generated recently by ovarian ultrasound, assays of hormones, and growth factors in follicle fluid, cultures of human granulosa cells in vitro, as well of ovarian morphology all suggest that early antral follicle development is normal but that dominant follicle selection is disrupted in PCO. As more information becomes available regarding autocrine and paracrine intra-ovarian regulators (such as insulin-like growth factor, epidermal growth factor and the inhibin/activin system) of dominant follicle selection under normal conditions, more will be understood from ovarian abnormalities in PCOS.

As previously mentioned, evidence has accumulated to suggest that long-term exposure of endometrium to unopposed estrogens in amenorrheic patients may lead to endometrial carcinoma. Therefore, for safety reasons, regular withdrawal bleedings should be recommended in these patients, induced either by the transient administration of progestins or by combined steroid contraception. Complaints of hirsutism can be alleviated with anti-androgens such as cyproterone acetate or spironolactone. However, local treatment will remain the cornerstone of effective therapy for hirsute patients. Clinicians should explain to patients that being overweight is a crucial factor in maintaining PCOS and that much attention should therefore be focused toward weight reduction. If successful, ovulation induction outcome will improve and future health risks may decrease. Induction of ovulation strategies in these patients (anti-estrogens and gonadotropins) will be discussed below. Long-term health risks in PCOS patients may include increased chances for cardiovascular disease, diabetes, and possibly breast cancer. Few data are available at the present time that allow for the assessment of the true future risks for individual patients.

Other forms of normogonadotropic anovulation A group of women remain when PCOS patients are excluded from WHO Group 2 anovulation. The size and profile of this heterogeneous group of patients is heavily dependent upon PCOS criteria used by various investigators (Fig. 46.6). Little if anything is known regarding characteristics and pathophysiology involved in these anovulatory patients.

Endocrine tumors Virilizing ovarian or adrenal tumors may cause amenorrhea and signs of severe androgen excess such as rapidly developing hirsutism, clitoris enlargement, and male pattern baldness (alopecia adrogenetica). These conditions are extremely rare, but they should always be considered in patients presenting with signs of hyperandrogenemia. Feminizing malignancies such as granulosa cell tumors are more likely to present with dysfunctional uterine bleeding rather than amenorrhea.

OVARIAN DEFECTS

Amenorrhea caused by defective ovarian function is characterized by low serum estradiol concentrations and elevated FSH and LH levels due to absent steroid feedback at the hypothalamic-pituitary unit (WHO, Class 3). This group represents approximately 10 to 20% of women with secondary amenorrhea. Pregnancy can only be achieved in these patients with in vitro fertilization of donor oocytes. Special attention should be given to the prevention of decreasing bone density due to long-term hypoestrogenic conditions. Again, estrogen replacement therapy should be recommended, and therapy should be initiated soon after diagnosis.

Premature ovarian failure

The number of oocytes present in the ovaries is maximal at approximately 5 months of fetal life. Thereafter, a continuous loss of follicles occurs throughout life. Absence of follicles results in low estrogen output (estradiol is synthesized by granulosa cells surrounding the oocyte) and amenorrhea. The last menstrual period (menopause) coincides with exhaustion of the follicle pool and usually occurs around the age of 51 (Fig. 46.7). However, a major variability in menopausal age exists, ranging between 40 and 60 years of age. Menopause is preceded by 2 decades of gradually declining ovarian reproductive function. Every woman is virtually infertile 10 years before menopause. Imminent ovarian failure (also referred to as ovarian aging) is characterized by regular but shortened menstrual cycles and elevated early follicular phase serum FSH concentrations. Reduced cycle length seems to be caused by a shortening of the follicular phase, whereas

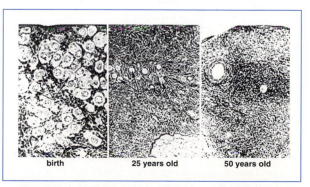

Figure 46.7 Morphology impression of a number of primordial follicles present in the ovary at birth and at 25 and 50 years of age.

luteal function remains unaltered. It is unknown as yet which mechanisms underlie this altered relationship between FSH and follicle development in women of advanced reproductive age. Diminished ovarian feedback by estradiol or inhibin B to the hypothalamic-pituitary unit may be involved. The likelihood for conception is clearly compromised in these patients with seemingly normal menstrual cycles, presumably due to reduced oocyte quality. The chances of successful fertility therapy are low.

By definition, ovarian failure is referred to as premature in cases of secondary amenorrhea characterized by high FSH and low estradiol levels before 40 years of age. Familial occurrence is clearly established in some cases. Recent observations also suggest that early menopause is associated with a reduced life expectancy. It may be hypothesized that early depletion of the follicle pool is due to a reduced number of follicles during early fetal development or accelerated exhaustion. Chromosomal abnormalities are reported in these patients and may involve mosaic Turner's syndrome (45 X), fragile X syndrome, and others. Two or more cell lines may exist. The risk of malignant degeneration of streak gonads containing a Y chromosome is high (up to 25%), and this tissue should therefore be removed. It is generally recommended that screening for chromosomal abnormalities should be performed in women presenting with ovarian failure before the age of 40. However, it is uncertain whether chromosome studies are cost-effective as routine clinical evaluation. Other causes of premature ovarian failure include gonadal exposure to radiation or chemotherapy (especially alkylating agents used for the treatment of various malignancies such as Hodgkin's disease) due to direct depletion of the follicle pool, or surgical removal of ovarian tissue, extensive coagulation or laser surgery of the ovaries, or extensive pelvic infection due to a substantial decrease in the number of remaining primordial follicles. It has been suggested that suppression of ovarian activity using a GnRH agonist during chemotherapy may provide some protection against gonadal damage. However, clinical data to support this notion are poor. Some inherited enzyme defects such as 17α-hydroxylase or 17-ketoreductase deficiency and galactosemia (decreased galactose-1-phosphate uridyltransferase activity) may also be associated with premature ovarian failure.

Resistant ovary syndrome

It is estimated that approximately 10 to 20% of women presenting with hypergonadotropic hypo-estrogenic amenorrhea do have follicles present in their ovaries. This condition is referred to as the "follicular form" of premature ovarian failure, or resistant-ovary syndrome. It is largely unknown why these follicles do not respond to stimulation by high FSH levels; and several factors such as anti FSH antibodies, FSH receptor-binding inhibitors, and FSH

receptor defects have been implicated. Several Finnish families presenting with ovarian dysgenesis have recently been described with a specific mutation in the gene encoding for the FSH receptor. In addition, autoantibodies directed against antigens present in ovarian or adrenal cells have been reported to be present in most of these patients. Unfortunately, testing for these autoantibodies is complex and nonspecific. Certainly other autoimmune disorders such as thyroiditis, adrenal insufficiency, myasthenia gravis, rheumatoid arthritis, and hemolytic anemia occur more frequently in these patients, strongly suggesting an autoimmune genesis of ovarian failure in at least a proportion of these patients suffering from early menopause. It has been known for a long time that ovarian failure may precede the onset of Addison's disease. Testing for thyroid and adrenal function should therefore be performed. It is uncertain as yet whether clinical screening should include both endocrine and autoimmune parameters, how frequent screening should be performed, and for how long.

Ovarian biopsy may confirm the presence of ovarian follicles. However, this procedure is traumatic and unreliable and should not be performed in the routine evaluation of these patients. If follicles are present, they usually reach the antral stage, and their presence can be detected by less invasive techniques such as transvaginal ultrasound. Pregnancies have been reported following transient suppression of gonadotropin levels as well as following corticosteroid medication. However, these empirical observations have recently been disproved in proper randomized trials, and therefore they should not be recommended.

UTERINE DEFECTS

In rare cases, secondary amenorrhea may occur in women with completely normal ovarian function combined with

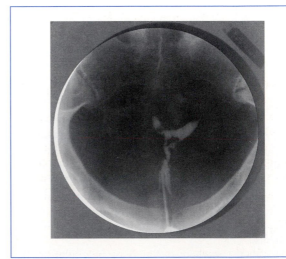

Figure 46.8 Partially obliterated uterine cavity (Asherman's syndrome) as demonstrated by hysterosalpingogram. (Dijkzigt University Hospital, Rotterdam, The Netherlands.)

uterine pathology. Hormone testing or basal body temperature will indicate ovulatory cycles in these patients.

Asherman's syndrome

This form of amenorrhea is caused by traumatic obliteration of the endometrial cavity following myomectomy or vigorous curettage for postpartum bleeding or abortion. Incomplete obliteration (Fig. 46.8) is more common than complete, which may cause reduced menstrual bleeding, dysmenorrhea, or infertility. If possible, hysteroscopy and removal of synechiae is recommended.

Genital tract tuberculosis

Genital tract tuberculosis is an extremely rare cause of endometrial destruction in developed countries. It may result in the complete loss of functional endometrial tissue. Diagnosis is made by culturing menstrual blood.

INDUCTION OF OVULATION
Joop Schoemaker

In this chapter, induction of ovulation is defined as the complete process of stimulation of follicular growth, as well as the stimulation of final maturation of the follicle and oocyte, and the ultimate rupture of the dominant follicle. The technique of follicular stimulation as practiced in *controlled ovarian hyperstimulation* in assisted reproduction is discussed elsewhere (see Chap. 50).

Induction of ovulation is the therapy for infertility caused by anovulation. This implies that anovulation as such does not need to be treated by ovulation induction. It either does not need treatment at all or can be treated by substitutional therapy, such as the oral contraceptive pill (see chapter on secondary amenorrhea). It also implies that infertility must be a complaint.

It is the aim of inducing ovulation to either restore a patient's own menstrual cycle, as done by treating with placebo or by treating a possible underlying disease, or to stimulate follicular growth and induce final maturation of the follicle and actual follicle rupture, thus setting the oocyte free to be fertilized. It is the ultimate goal with this therapy to obtain monofollicular growth, single follicle rupture, and the achievement of a singleton pregnancy.

Ovulation induction is usually performed by one of four groups of drugs: anti-estrogens, gonadotropin-releasing hormone (GnRH), gonadotropins, or dopamine receptor agonists. Each of those has its own specific indications.

Indications and contraindications

As described elsewhere in this book, anovulation may have a variety of different causes and can be classified into different categories, such as:

- Anovulation due to congenital defects of either central or ovarian origin; the former patients lacking the pituitary gonadotropins and therefore being *hypo*gonadotropic, the latter patients lacking the ovarian factors (steroids as well as peptides), which feed back to the central system to suppress gonadotropin secretion and therefore are *hyper*gonadotropic.
- Anovulation due to dysfunction of the hypothalamus due to rapid or excessive weight loss, anorexia nervosa, emotional or physical stress, excessive exercise, and so on. To this group also belong patients who are anovulatory due to the fact that they are suffering from another underlying disease. Patients who suffer from hypothalamic dysfunction usually are *hypo*gonadotropic as well.
- A special group of women with hypothalamic dysfunction are those with hyperprolactinemia, because high levels of prolactin suppress hypothalamic GnRH secretion and therefore indirectly suppress pituitary gonadotropin secretion
- A group of disorders in women who complain of either oligo- or amenorrhoea, which usually had begun at puberty, who are usually overweight and often also complain of hirsutism. To this latter group belong the patients with polycystic ovary syndrome (PCOS), if in fact not all of them should be classified as such. In this chapter they will be designated as women with PCOS. Although they often have elevated LH levels, they are usually called *normo*gonadotropic. A better designation would be women with inappropriate gonadotropin secretion.

Women with hypergonadotropic amenorrhea cannot be treated with induction of ovulation because their ovarian defect is such that a further increase of gonadotropins will not lead to follicular growth, if follicles are still present in the ovaries. Usually, however, the ovaries are depleted of follicles and thus of oocytes.

As many of the amenorrheas are of psychogenic origin, it is not surprising that placebo demonstrates good potential in treating anovulation. In a classic study, it was shown that 40.3% of women had spontaneous ovulations after placebo therapy and a further 18.5% established ovulatory cycles after they had been treated with cyclical estrogen/progesterone therapy; 19.3% of the total group became pregnant under placebo therapy and another 14.5% of the total group under cyclical hormone therapy. Hence, it may sometimes be worthwhile to use either cyclical or placebo therapy first.

A number of more general diseases and illnesses are accompanied by cycle disturbances, some of which are anovulatory. Examples are infectious mononucleosis, Cushing's disease, debilitating diseases such as tuberculosis, and malignant diseases such as Hodgkin's disease and the leukemias. In addition, thyroid disease, either hypo- or hyperthyroidism, may lead to anovulatory cycle disorders; however, the pattern may vary from patient to patient. It seems logical that these types of anovulation should be handled by treating the underlying disease, but one of the most often-made mistakes is that they are not. This illustrates how a good and sound diagnosis should always be obtained before deciding what type of ovulation induction will be used in each patient. Alleviating the symptom of anovulation first with clomiphene citrate, without a diagnosis, leads to missing an underlying disease of which anovulation may be the first and, at that moment, still the only symptom.

The first choice of treatment in hypogonadotropic and normogonadotropic anovulation is clomiphene citrate; its success will greatly depend on the severity of the hypogonadotropic state and particularly on the amount of estradiol that is still being produced by the ovaries. Therefore, some authors advise performing a progesterone provocation test first. Such a test would be carried out by prescribing the patient a short course of progesterone or a progestative, such as 100 mg of progesterone im or medroxyprogesterone acetate 10 mg per os per day for 5 to 7 days. If the patient's endometrium is developed well enough under the endogenously secreted estradiol, a few days after the discontinuation of progesterone, a withdrawal bleed will follow. If withdrawal bleeding does not take place, this should be taken as evidence that little endogenous estradiol is available to make successful induction of ovulation with an anti-estrogen likely. Some of the patients who do not bleed after progesterone may still have a positive response to clomiphene citrate, but the number of failures is certainly high. In patients with primary amenorrhea on the basis of a congenital abnormality, such as in idiopathic hypogonadotropic hypogonadism or in Kallmann's syndrome, clomiphene citrate is useless.

Hypogonadotropic patients who are resistant to clomiphene citrate are ideal patients for pulsatile GnRH treatment. Hypogonadotropic patients who have had twelve ovulatory cycles of clomiphene induction and have not become pregnant are also possible candidates for this type of treatment. However, when the latter patients are normogonadotropic, and in general fit the picture of PCOS, pulsatile GnRH is not the treatment of choice. Another indication for the use of pulsatile GnRH is the hyperprolactinemic patient who does not properly respond to dopamine receptor agonists.

The use of gonadotropins is indicated in normogonadotropic anovulation when the patient appears to be clomiphene resistant. Furthermore, gonadotropins must be used in the rare hypogonadotropic patient whose defect is at the pituitary level. Lastly, gonadotropins can be used as a last resort for every type of anovulation when other methods have failed.

Dopamine agonists have only one indication, which is anovulatory infertility caused by hyperprolactinemia. The use of this drug is an exception to the rule that it should only be used to induce ovulation in case of infertility. Galactorrhea or severe hypo-estrogenism, leading to a decreased incorporation of calcium in bone or even loss of bone mineral density, can also be a good indication. Moreover, dopamine agonists have a strong power to restrict further growth of prolactinomas or even cause regression of the tumor, particularly macroadenomas. For this reason, they are also used during pregnancy when a macroadenoma with suprasellar extension compromises the optic chiasm.

There are few contraindications for the induction of ovulation. The first is pregnancy itself. Thus, a course for ovulation induction, regardless of the drug regimen, should always be begun with an unequivocal ruling out of pregnancy. Furthermore, one should always consider whether the patient is able to carry a pregnancy to term without undue complications. For instance, a woman should not undergo ovulation induction when her health would be seriously harmed by a pregnancy, such as in the case of severe anorexia nervosa. A patient who is underweight more than 10% of her ideal weight should have this and the implications discussed with her before starting therapy. Being overweight also bears important risks, such as an increased risk of gestational diabetes; hypertensive disease of pregnancy; and thrombosis during pregnancy, delivery, or postpartum; in addition to problems that, due to obesity, could arise during delivery if a caesarean section would be necessary. Ovarian cysts should always be considered a contraindication when the cyst is larger than 3 cm in diameter because of the risk of excessive enlargement of the ovary under stimulation. If a cyst is present, it should either be allowed to disappear with time, or to suppress ovarian function for a period of time, such as by prescribing the use of an oral contraceptive for one month, or by puncturing the cyst via the transvaginal route under sonographic guidance. One important contraindication for ovulation induction is a macroprolactinoma of the pituitary. While the pituitary further enlarges during pregnancy under the influence of massively produced estrogens; the risk for eye complications, compression of the optic chiasm with subsequent defects in the eye fields, as well as involvement of other cranial nerves that pass by the sella turcica (such as the oculomotor, trochlear, and abducens nerves) is not to be underestimated. Pituitary apoplexia due to bleeding in the tumor can also acutely deprive the patient of all pituitary hormones for the rest of her life, subsequently making lifetime substitutional therapy necessary.

A model for follicular stimulation and selection

To comprehend the mechanism of action of the different ovulation inducing agents, a thorough understanding of the initiation of follicular growth and selection is of great importance. The model is based on the FSH threshold concept for follicular growth. This means that growth of follicles under stimulation of FSH is not ruled by a simple linear dose/response relationship, but the FSH plasma concentration must surpass a certain threshold level before a follicle will start to respond. This threshold level is different for each follicle: the more sensitive a follicle is to FSH, the lower its threshold level is. The threshold level of the most sensitive follicle at the beginning of stimulation is the threshold level for that particular woman.

At the end of the luteal phase of a menstrual cycle or when a patient is anovulatory, at any given time the ovaries contain a number of early antral follicles that are 2 to 5 mm in diameter and all sensitive to FSH. This group of potentially stimulable follicles is called the cohort. With respect to follicle sensitivity, the cohort can be compared to a conically shaped bag, a cornet, filled with follicles. In the lower tip of the bag is the follicle with the highest sensitivity, or the lowest FSH threshold (Fig. 46.9 *A*). This follicle determines the threshold of the cohort and thus the threshold of the patient. Every other follicle has a lower sensitivity to FSH, that is, has a higher threshold. When the FSH concentration rises during the luteal/follicular transition, or due to exogenous stimulation by an ovulation-inducing agent, the concentration at a certain moment will surpass the threshold level of the most sensitive follicle. When the rise in FSH concentration would stop here, that one single follicle would be the only one to be stimulated and resume further development. However, in general the FSH concentration will rise somewhat higher, also selecting the next most sensitive follicles. Depending on how high the FSH concentration rises, more or fewer follicles will start to grow. During the initial development, follicles – whether they have already been or are not yet selected – increase their sensitivity to FSH. This means that when the FSH concentration remains the same, more follicles drop their threshold levels under the actual FSH concentration, thereby also becoming selected (Fig. 46.9 *B*). During a normal menstrual cycle, and also during ovulation induction, FSH concentration will decrease due to feedback of steroidal and nonsteroidal factors secreted by the developing follicles, such as estradiol and inhibin B, provided that no desensitization has been initiated, such as by the use of GnRH analogues. This decrease of FSH levels brings the concentration under the threshold of a number of follicles again, resulting in their growth arrest and ultimate atresia. Only those follicles that have been able to increase their sensitivity to FSH to such an extent that they can still cope with the falling FSH levels will continue to develop and finally become Graafian follicles, ready to ovulate (Fig. 46.9 *C*). This phenomenon of losing follicles to atresia because of declining FSH levels is particularly made use of in the step-down induction technique.

The increase in sensitivity to FSH during follicular development is limited to the first few days. Thus, if follicles have not been selected after the first few days of stimulation, they rapidly lose their sensitivity to FSH and cannot be selected anymore, not even with high doses of FSH (Fig. 46.9 *D*).

How many follicles ultimately develop depends upon how high the FSH rises in initial stimulation, how long the FSH level stays above the threshold level, the threshold level of the most sensitive follicle, the density of the cohort, that is, the number of follicles that will start to develop with a given increase in FSH concentration, and the slope of the decreasing FSH level after initial selection.

Methods

Anti-estrogens

Anti-estrogens have an estrogen receptor blocking effect. Most of these drugs are competitive receptor antagonists, meaning that they have a high affinity for the estrogen receptor but cause only a low postreceptor signal, which leads to only a small effect.

If normal estrogens are available on the receptor sites, the estrogen receptor agonist will replace the estrogen from its receptor and have an anti-estrogenic effect, however, if no estrogen is present on the receptors, the anti-estrogen will have a week estrogenic effect. Although several of those drugs are available and all have been derived from triphenylethylene – a molecule from which stilbestrol has also been derived – the only one that has gained much popularity in ovulation induction is clomiphene, commercially available as clomiphene cit-

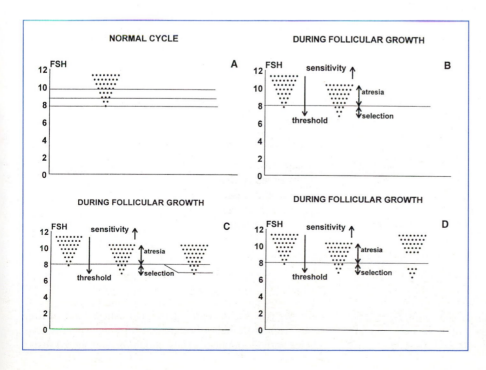

Figure 46.9 A model of follicular selection. See text for explanation.

rate. Other derivatives, such as tamoxifen, has gained popularity in cancer treatment, particularly for breast cancer, and further derivatives, such as raloxifene, are now grouped under the name of selective estrogen receptor modulators (SERMs) and are used in hormone replacement therapy for postmenopausal complaints, particularly in the prevention of osteoporosis. Clomiphene is marketed as a racemic mixture of two stereoisomers, that is, a zu- (cis) and an en-(trans)form. Of these, the en-form possesses most of the biological activity. It has a much shorter half-life than the zu-form. Clomiphene acts primarily at the level of the hypothalamus, where it occupies estrogen receptors, probably on catecholaminergic neurons. It is through these neurons that the effect of the blockade of the estrogen feedback is transmitted to the neurons that regulate the pulse generator in the hypothalamus. Through this pathway the blockade of the estrogen receptors leads to an increase in the pulse frequency with which GnRH is secreted, which in turn leads to an increase in both LH and FSH secretion. This is not to say that there are no effects of clomiphene on other estrogen target tissues. The effect on the pituitary is not well-known. A direct effect on the ovary is likely because of an accumulation of clomiphene there, but what the exact effect is is unclear. A direct effect of clomiphene on the oocyte or the early embryo is likely since fewer oocytes lead to pregnancies in clomiphene-treated rats as compared to non-treated rats, and this effect can be counteracted by simultaneous treatment of the rats with estradiol. The effect of clomiphene suppressing the secretion of cervical mucus is well-documented. The effect on the endometrium may be the cause for a higher than normal rate of luteal phase defect, as determined by endometrial biopsy in clomiphene-treated individuals.

It is the rise in FSH levels that initiates the further growth of one or more follicles from the cohort, depending on how high the FSH concentration rises in comparison to the threshold levels of the most sensitive follicles. This rise is dependent on how severely hypogonadotropic the patient is and on the dose of clomiphene. Once the follicle begins growing, it will also secrete more factors that feed back on the pituitary and hypothalamus. Initially this is inhibin B, but later on inhibin A and estradiol will also be included. Moreover, the growing follicles will increase their sensitivity to FSH. FSH levels will now start to decrease, but as long as the threshold of the follicle remains under the decreasing FSH plasma concentration, the follicles will continue to grow. When the follicle has come to a size where its estradiol secretion leads to rising plasma concentrations high enough to induce a midcycle LH surge, ovulation will follow as in a normal menstrual cycle. At the end of that cycle, however, FSH levels, in general, will not (through the falling concentrations of estradiol, progesterone, and inhibin A) rise to such an extent that the threshold of the most sensitive follicle of the next cohort will be surpassed again. Generally, a new short course of clomiphene will be necessary to initiate a following cycle.

One should realize that if clomiphene would be given continuously, a continuous block of the positive feedback of estradiol would prevent the occurrence of an LH surge, and thus would prevent ovulation. It is therefore essential that clomiphene is given in short courses.

Technique Clomiphene is given in courses of 5 days, either from day 3 to day 7 or from day 5 to day 9 of the menstrual cycle. If a patient is amenorrheic, usually a withdrawal bleeding is induced with either progesterone alone or a short sequential course of estrogen and progesterone. Before starting, one should determine definitively that no pregnancy exists, particularly because clomiphene is potentially teratogenic. If no spontaneous bleeding or withdrawal bleed occurs, which can be taken as signs that a pregnancy might exist, a pregnancy test that is as sensitive as possible should be performed. A first course is always performed with a dose of 50 mg daily. In the beginning the patient only needs to register her basal body temperature for monitoring. If her temperature is biphasic, giving evidence of ovulation, the patient should be seen approximately 7 days after the temperature rise for a bimanual or ultrasound evaluation of the size of her ovaries. If these are not enlarged, the following course of the same dose can be given after her period. If no period follows, a pregnancy test should be performed 18 days after the rise of the basal body temperature. As the incidence of luteal phase defects under clomiphene treatment has been reported to be high by several authors in the literature, it is advised that if pregnancy has not been established after three ovulatory cycles, an endometrial biopsy be done to rule out this defect.

If the basal body temperature does not show a rise within 21 days from the last clomiphene tablet, this is evidence that the dose has been insufficient, and a withdrawal bleeding should be induced again before beginning the next cycle with a dose of 100 mg daily. Unless the withdrawal bleeding is induced by dydrogesterone, a progestative that does not result in a temperature rise, the progesterone provocation can show whether a specific patient is sensitive to progesterone with respect to inducing a temperature rise. This can thus rule out whether the patient is ovulatory and still has a monophasic basal body temperature. It is therefore wise to have the patient taking her temperature during the progestative intake as well. If a patient does not ovulate on a dose of 150 mg per day, a new cycle with 200 mg daily should be monitored by determination of estradiol every 7 days after clomiphene intake and a progesterone determination 3 and 4 weeks after the last tablet. Moreover, regular ultrasound scans will also give evidence of follicular growth. If the latter is adequate and the patient still does not ovulate, the therapy can be combined with 5 000 IU of human chorionic gonadotropin (hCG), administered when the largest follicle reaches a diameter of 20 mm.

Based on epidemiologic data, it has been established that women who have been treated for more than twelve cycles with clomiphene without becoming pregnant are at a higher risk for developing ovarian cancer later in life. Thus women should not be treated for longer than twelve cycles with clomiphene. They should be considered resistant, and therapy should be changed to either pulsatile GnRH or gonadotropins, depending on the classification of their anovulation (see above).

Results Approximately 70 to 80% of women treated by clomiphene will ultimately ovulate. The number of dominant follicles under clomiphene treatment is 2.4 on average versus 1.2 on average in spontaneous cycles, leading to an increased incidence of multiple ovulations and multiple pregnancies, the latter being 8% (7% twins and 1% higher order multiple births). Even a sextuplet has been reported. However, only 50 to 55% of the treated patients will become pregnant within one year after data are corrected for loss to follow-up during treatment by life-table analysis. In a retrospective analysis encompassing all patients in whom all other infertility factors had been ruled out and who were treated with clomiphene in the author's unit from 1982 till 1986, the average monthly fecundity rate for the first 6 months of treatment was 14%. This relatively low percentage could be caused by a deterioration of cervical mucus under clomiphene treatment, as well as by the detrimental effect of clomiphene on the oocyte or early embryo (see above).

Side effects and complications Side effects are relatively common. Hot flushes, occurring in about 10% of women taking clomiphene are due to the anti-estrogenic effect, causing the same effect as actual withdrawal of estrogens in the climacteric period. Visual symptoms are reported occasionally, particularly in the form of scintillating scotomas. Discontinuation of clomiphene treatment leads to a rapid disappearance of symptoms. Although not often mentioned, a number of women complain of temporary accelerated hair loss.

The increased incidence of multiple pregnancies has been mentioned above. Pregnancy outcome does not reveal an increased incidence of congenital anomalies. Controversy exists regarding a possibly increased incidence of early abortion under clomiphene treatment. Although such an increased incidence has been reported, this may well be completely accounted for by the increased incidence of early pregnancy loss associated with infertility as such.

Gonadotropin releasing hormone

For a detailed description of the action of GnRH at the pituitary level, the reader is referred to Chapter 43, "Neuroendocrinology of Female Reproduction." Gonadotropin-releasing hormone (GnRH) when administered either iv or sc acts directly on the pituitary, in very much the same way as endogenously secreted GnRH does. GnRH therapy is therefore a substitutional therapy. Native GnRH is a decapeptide that has a short half-life of only 4 minutes. Moreover, GnRH desensitizes the pituitary very rapidly. In fact it has been shown that each iv shot, which leads to a physiological release of LH, already desensitizes the pituitary to a certain extent. A continuous infusion of GnRH will thus lead to an initial release of LH and FSH but will very rapidly completely desensitize the pituitary, decreasing to a minimum the amount of

gonadotropin secreted. It is therefore essential that GnRH be administered in a pulsatile manner, such that the pituitary can recover from its desensitization after each injection of a GnRH dose. It is clear that such a therapy could mimic the endogenous pulsatile secretion of GnRH in patients who lack any activity of the hypothalamic pulse generator. However, even when endogenous secretion of GnRH is still present to a certain extent, the pulsatility of the exogenously applied GnRH overrules the pulsatility of the endogenous secretion because the endogenous pulses come at a time when the pituitary is partially desensitized by the exogenous pulses. Further, in pulsatile GnRH therapy, the effect on the initiation of follicular growth is brought about by the rise in FSH, which is brought about by the pulsatile stimulation of the gonadotrophs in the pituitary. Under this therapy feedback action of ovarian factors, estradiol, progesterone, and inhibins A and B remain intact only at the pituitary level. However, it appears that under a fixed pulse-dose and pulse-frequency regime, the endocrine events of a normal menstrual cycle – including the occurrence of a normal LH surge – are orchestrated. No hypothalamic feedback appears to be necessary to bring about monofollicular ovulation.

Technique GnRH is administered, either iv or sc in small doses (usually between 5 and 20 µg) in a pulsatile fashion: one dose every 60 to 120 minutes. These small doses are infused by a portable infusion pump approximately the size of a pack of cigarettes, via a catheter and a needle placed either in a forearm vein or subcutaneously under the skin of the abdomen. The pump can be worn on the belt of a skirt or trousers. A wide shirt, sweater, or blouse with long sleeves will hide the pump as well as the catheter and the needle. Pumps are very often provided by either the hospital or by the pharmaceutical company that sells the GnRH. Depending on the pump used, the amount of GnRH dissolved in the amount of solution appropriate for the syringe is calculated on the basis of the volume the syringe will inject with every pulse and on the pulse-dose required. A small amount of heparin is added when treatment is administered intravenously in order to prevent clotting at the tip of the needle.

A first induction cycle is begun after a withdrawal bleeding has been induced. On day 2 or 3 of the bleeding, an iv needle is placed in a forearm vein and connected to a catheter and the pump. The first cycle is always started with a pulse-dose of 5 µg and a pulse-frequency of one pulse every 2 hours. The pulse-dose of 5 µg is chosen because it is known that the first cycle carries the highest risk of multiple ovulation and multiple pregnancy. In a second cycle the pulse-dose is always increased to 10 µg because a pulse-dose of 5 µg in subsequent cycles has a significantly lower ovulation frequency. An alternative to this is to not increase the pulse-dose but to reduce the pulse-interval to 90 or even 60 minutes in the second and subsequent cycles. If therapy is interrupted for more than one month, the starting pulse-dose should be 5 µg again.

The pump will usually contain enough GnRH for at

least 8 days, even with a pulse-dose of 10 µg. It is convenient to have the patient record her basal body temperature in order to have a simple method to verify ovulation. Little monitoring is necessary because ovarian cysts are not frequently seen. It is advisable, however, to perform a bimanual examination once a month in the middle of the luteal phase. Treatment can go on uninterrupted during the follicular and the luteal phases. For a better cost/benefit ratio, it is possible to reduce the pulse-frequency to one pulse every 4 hours after ovulation has been established. At the time of menstruation, the pulse-frequency is returned to the one used during the follicular phase.

Subcutaneous treatment is also possible. A slightly higher pulse-dose is used: in general 10 to 20 µg. No heparin should be added to the solution, as this may lead to subcutaneous hematomas. The subcutaneous treatment may be more convenient for the patient because she can be taught to replace the needle herself, however failure cycles are more frequent.

If a cycle is anovulatory, treatment should be discontinued after 28 days of continuous administration. The pulse-dose may then be increased to 20 µg and/or the pulse-interval may be reduced to a minimum of 60 minutes. If anovulation persists, one should reconsider first whether this patient is actually hypogonadotropic. If the patient appears to be normogonadotropic with inappropriate gonadotropin secretion, and particularly when the LH appears to be elevated (PCOS), the therapy should be shifted to gonadotropins. If the patient is hypogonadotropic and still remains anovulatory under pulsatile GnRH treatment, a small amount of gonadotropins such as one ampule per day could be added to the treatment. When ultrasound monitoring in such a case shows adequate follicular growth, such as a follicle over 12 mm in diameter, gonadotropins can be discontinued again.

An alternative treatment during the luteal phase is to remove the pump shortly after ovulation has been established. The luteal phase is then supported by hCG:10 000 IU every third day for 12 days.

Results The results of pulsatile GnRH treatment are excellent with respect to ovulation as well as to pregnancies in patients with hypogonadotropic amenorrhea of hypothalamic origin. The combined results from a literature survey showed an ovulation rate of 83% and a pregnancy rate of 23% per cycle, or 27% per ovulatory cycle. Figure 46.10 shows the cumulative pregnancy rate calculated by life-table statistics from the author's own group, divided in patients with and without additional infertility factors. The fecundity rate, that is, pregnancy rate per cycle, appears not to change per cycle number. Thus the pregnancy rate over cycles 7 to 12 appeared not to differ from those over cycles 1 to 6. The pregnancy rate was 78% after 6 cycles and 93% after 12 cycles. The results in patients with inappropriate gonadotropin secretion have been disappointing. Although several authors achieved very reasonable ovulation rates, the pregnancy rates were low. Pulsatile GnRH treatment in this group after a period of pituitary suppression by GnRH agonists appeared hopeful initially, but the treatment takes approximately 8 weeks per cycle and because of this has not gained much popularity. This may also have been caused by the recent improvement in the technique of ovulation induction by gonadotropins.

The frequency of spontaneous abortion and congenital anomalies in the offspring born after pulsatile GnRH induction in hypogonadotropic patients are comparable with those in spontaneous pregnancies. Multiple pregnancy rate, however, is higher. In initial studies this was around 15% per cycle. After this report it appeared that the multiple pregnancy rate was dependent on dose as well as on the cycle number. First cycles showed a much higher incidence than subsequent cycles. For this reason it is advised to start with a smaller dose in the first cycle (see above). No recent data are available on the multiple pregnancy rate.

Side effects and complications In general the side effects of treatment are minor. The main side effect is infections at the needle site. Signs of local infection should immediately lead to replacement of the needle at a different site, and the patient should be instructed likewise. Although rare, sepsis has been reported and requires immediate removal

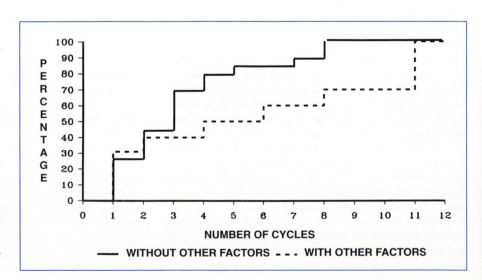

Figure 46.10 Cumulative pregnancy rate, as calculated by life-table statistics, for the induction of ovulation by clomiphene citrate in women with (interrupted line) and without (uninterrupted line) other infertility factors.

of the needle and a course of antibiotics. It is therefore of utmost importance that the patient is always able to reach her physician, 24 hours a day and 7 days a week. Hyperstimulation of the ovaries has not been reported. Some rare incidents of urticaria and even one case of anaphylactic shock in response to GnRH treatment have been reported. Occasionally the formation of antibodies has been reported, but only in subcutaneous treatment.

Gonadotropins

Preparations available For ovulation induction, three human gonadotropins play a major role: follicle-stimulating hormone (FSH), luteinizing hormone (LH), and human chorionic gonadotropin (hCG).

At the time this chapter is written, we are in a transitional period in gonadotropin therapy. Until 1985 the only preparations available were gonadotropins extracted from human urine, collected either from pregnant women for hCG, or for a mix of FSH and LH (HMG) from elderly women. Traditionally the latter was distributed in ampules containing approximately 75 IU of FSH and 75 IU of LH. These preparations were far from pure, containing only a few percentages of gonadotropins in a mix of all kinds of other proteins that were extracted at the same time from the urine. In 1985 a first preparation became available that only contained FSH, so-called purified FSH (pFSH). This preparation contained less than 0.5 IU of LH per ampule, and it was still contaminated with more than 95% of other proteins. In the early nineties an even more purified FSH preparation, the so-called highly purified urinary FSH (FSH-HP), became available, which was devoid of the foreign protein contamination. Ninety-eight percent of the protein in the ampule was now FSH. A further step in the development of new gonadotropins was the adaption of the gene transfer technology and molecular biology to produce not only recombinant FSH (rFSH), but also rLH and rhCG. Recombinant FSH became commercially available in 1995 from two different companies, one marketing the drug in the conventional 75 IU per ampule (Ares Serono, Aubonne, Switzerland) and one marketing it in ampules containing 50 IU (Organon, Oss, The Netherlands). There is now good evidence that rFSH has a higher potency than the urinary preparations, meaning that the same dose in IU, on average, leads to more follicles and more oocytes. There seems to be no difference between the two commercially available preparations. rLH and rhCG are not yet available on the market but will be shortly. Given this development, it seems logical to use the recombinant preparations since they are more pure, have a higher potency, and have a great deal of consistency from batch to batch. However, pricing and different government health policies have so far prevented a general switch from urinary to recombinant preparations. It looks as if this will be a matter of time and that in the end, only recombinant preparations will be available.

Mode of action For a detailed description of the effect of gonadotropins on the ovary, the reader is referred to the chapter on structure and function of the ovary (Chap. 43).

When inducing ovulation, a distinction between the functions of FSH and LH is important, because preparations are now available that contain either FSH exclusively or a combination of FSH and LH. In the future LH will also become available in a pure form.

FSH exerts a number of actions on the ovary. It stimulates follicular growth and differentiation, primarily by stimulating the multiplication of granulosa cells. In addition, FSH induces the action of the cytochrome P450-aromatizing enzyme, which converts the androgens androstenedione and testosterone (diffusing from the theca cells to the granulosa cells) into estrone and estradiol, respectively. Moreover, FSH induces the synthesis and secretion of several peptide factors that are either important for growth and differentiation, such as the IGFs; or for controlling negative feedback on FSH secretion from the pituitary, such as inhibin A by growing follicles and corpus luteum, and inhibin B by the small growing follicles.

LH stimulates secretion of androgens by the theca cells during follicular growth. For this action, very little LH is needed: a plasma concentration of 2 IU/l is probably enough for full production of androgens as substrate for estradiol production. During ovulation induction, enough endogenous LH is usually available to take care of theca cell androgen production. Only women who are severely hypogonadotropic (such as women with severe anorexia nervosa or psychogenic amenorrhea) or women with primary amenorrhea of hypothalamic origin (that is, idiopathic hypogonadotropic hypogonadism or with Kallmann's syndrome) need exogenous administration of LH to properly produce androgens. In general, however, these women should be treated with pulsatile GnRH (see above). Thus, the only indications for additional LH are for women who cannot be treated with pulsatile GnRH or for women with pituitary hypogonadotropic hypogonadism.

Other functions of LH are chiefly involved in the actual ovulation process and in the maintenance of progesterone synthesis during the luteal phase.

Technique Over the last 10 years there has been great change in the technique of ovulation induction by gonadotropins. In 1987 David Polson from the group of Stephen Franks in London introduced the low-dose step-up treatment protocol, which has since become popular in reproductive endocrinology because it greatly reduced the undesirable side effects of multiple pregnancies and the ovarian hyperstimulation syndrome (OHSS). In 1992, Schoot from Fauser's group in Rotterdam introduced the step-down regime, which after some alterations and modifications has since been worked into a regime that also has much reduced side effects than in the past. Both techniques have a high percentage of monofollicular cycles. Both will be discussed here. Although the step-down regime has the advantage of a shorter stimulation cycle, closer monitoring must take place. It is probably for this reason that the technique has not gained considerable popularity until now.

Low-dose step-up. This technique is based upon the principle that the number of follicles being selected can be restricted when the FSH threshold level of the most sensitive follicles is slowly approached by gradually increasing the FSH plasma concentration. Stimulation is performed *without* previous desensitization of the pituitary by GnRH agonists

Stimulation with this technique is begun on the third day of a spontaneous menstrual cycle or a progesterone-induced withdrawal bleeding, with either 50 or 75 IU FSH per day. FSH is administered SC if rFSH or FSH-HP is used and IM when pFSH or HMG is used. This dose is maintained for the first 10 days while the patient is monitored every 3 days by ultrasound and later on also by daily rapid estradiol determinations. When no follicular growth is observed by the end of the first 10 days, that is, when no follicle of 12 mm in diameter has been observed, the dose is increased by half an ampule of 75 IU per day, which is then maintained for 7 days. If at the end of these 7 days again no follicular growth is seen, the dose is again increased by half an ampule for 7 days, and so on. If follicular growth is observed, the dose will not be further increased, ultrasound monitoring will be increased from once every 3 days to once every other day until the largest follicle is 16 mm in diameter. From there on, ultrasound monitoring is performed daily, as are plasma estradiol measurements. When the largest follicle is 18 mm in diameter, 10 000 IU of hCG are administered im for final maturation of the follicle and the oocyte, as well as for induction of actual ovulation. Usually no support of the corpus luteum or the luteal endometrium with either progesterone or further administration of hCG is necessary.

No hCG is given if at the time that the largest follicle is 18 mm, more than three follicles are greater than 15 mm or more than six follicles are greater than 13 mm. No hCG is given if the plasma estradiol concentration is greater than 4000 pmol/l.

Alternative treatments in these instances could be reducing the number of follicles by ultrasound-guided puncturing of a number of follicles, or diverting to a full-scale IVF procedure. If no such possibilities are available, the cycle should be completely abandoned, discontinuing all medication and waiting for the follicles to disappear. The patient should be monitored, however, to see if she ovulates spontaneously, and if so, observed to see if she develops a hyperstimulation syndrome. Moreover, she should be advised to abstain from intercourse until the danger of spontaneous ovulation is over. When all follicles present are clearly in regression, a withdrawal bleed is once again induced and treatment is resumed.

The second and subsequent cycles are induced in much the same way as the first cycle, taking advantage of the experience of the first cycle. In such a cycle, the starting dose is one-half an ampule less than the dose at which adequate follicular growth was obtained in the previous cycle. This first dose is then maintained for only 7 days. The rest of the induction is the same as described above for the first cycle.

If no menses has appeared 18 days after the hCG injection, a pregnancy test should be performed.

Step-down. In the step-down technique for ovulation induction, use is made of the fact that follicles, once being selected, lose their ability to further develop if at any time during their development the FSH concentration falls below the threshold level of that follicle. In other words, follicles become atretic if insufficient FSH is present to support their further development.

In the step-down technique, stimulation is also begun on the third day of a bleeding, whether it is either spontaneously occurring or induced. Stimulation is performed *without* previous desensitization of the pituitary by GnRH agonists. The starting dose is 2 ampules of FSH per day. This dose is increased by half an ampule if no clear response of the ovary is obtained after 5 days. The patient is monitored by ultrasound every 2 or 3 days. If an ovarian response is obtained, the FSH dose is decreased by one-half an ampule as soon as the first follicle with a diameter of 10 mm is observed. Subsequently the dose is reduced by half an ampule every 3 days until a minimum dose of one ampule per day is reached. From there, the dose is maintained until the largest follicle has surpassed a diameter of 18 mm. Criteria for the time at which hCG is given, cancellation criteria, and alternatives for completing the cycle or complete cancellation are the same as described under the low-dose step-up regime. No luteal support is given.

Results Results of the low-dose step-up technique have been reported by several large groups over a couple of hundred cycles. A summary of those is presented in Table 46.6.

The percentage of 70% uniovulatory cycles is consistent throughout the literature thus far. The pregnancy and, more importantly, the fecundity rate, are quite acceptable in ovulation induction because it is close to the natural overall fecundity rate in fertile women. It certainly is not worse than results obtained with the now outdated techniques of gonadotropin ovulation induction. The main advantage of the new techniques is the very low ovarian hyperstimula-

Table 46.6 Combined results from 6 studies published on low-dose step-up treatment outcome in women with polycystic ovary syndrome compared to step-down results

	Low-dose step-up	Step-down
Patients	464	82
Cycles completed	1131	234
Clinical pregnancies (n)	221	37
Clinical pregnancies (%)	48	47
Fecundity per cycle (%)	19.5	17
Uniovulatory cycles (%)	70	62
Ovarian hyperstimulation syndrome (%)	< 0.1	1.7
Multiple pregnancies (%)	6	8

(Data from Homburg R. Low dose therapy with FSH: endocrine aspects and clinical results. In: Filicori M, Flamigni C, eds. Ovulation induction: Update '98. London/New York, and van Santbrink EJ, Donderwinkel PF, van Dessel TJ, Fauser BC. Gonadotropin induction of ovulation using a step-down dose regimen: single-centre clinical experience in 82 patients. Hum Reprod 1995; 10:1048-53.)

tion rate as well as the low multiple pregnancy rate, with a virtual absence of high order multiple births.

Much less is known about the results of the step-down technique; they are virtually only from the one center where the technique was developed. The results are presented in Table 46.6. There seem to be few differences between the two treatment regimens.

Side effects and complications The major side effects of gonadotropin therapy are multiple gestations and the ovarian hyperstimulation syndrome. In addition, primarily due to the high multiple pregnancy rate in the past, the early and late spontaneous abortion rate has been reported to be high. On the other hand, most patients treated with ovulation induction suffer from PCOS, a disease that is notorious for its high abortion rate after pregnancy has been induced regardless of technique.

Multiple pregnancies have been a major problem, with rates of up to 35% being reported in the past. With the new induction protocols, as described in this chapter, prevention of multiple births is accomplished by strict adherence to the cancellation rules. In no circumstance should these rules be broken. The ovarian hyperstimulation syndrome (OHSS), also a major problem in the past, is now a problem in assisted reproduction more so than in ovulation induction. For a discussion of the syndrome, the reader is referred to the chapter 50. Because the condition is potentially life-threatening, if the patient develops an OHSS, it is important to note that she should be referred to a center with ample experience with the problem.

Surgical

Mode of action The surgical approach to ovulation induction is the oldest method employed. In 1935 Stein and Leventhal already advocated ovarian wedge resection as a form of treatment for women with PCOS, and in fact this was the only form of treatment for this ailment until the end of the fifties when clomiphene citrate, and shortly thereafter gonadotropins, became available. The surgical approach has been revived by Gjonnaes, a Norwegian clinician who reported excellent results of laparoscopic ovarian cautery in patients with PCOS. This therapy was in later years brought up to modern standards by replacing ovarian cautery by laser evaporation of surface areas of the ovary.

The mechanism of action of this therapy has been unknown until today. Recent findings suggest that PCOS has a tendency to disappear as a clinical entity with age, and it might well be that the pathogenesis of PCOS can partly be explained by the existence of a cohort of available follicles too large to be stimulated by FSH. If FSH levels rise, too many follicles would develop, generating a negative feedback too large for the level of the pituitary, probably via inhibin B. This negative feedback excess would than suppress FSH to a level that no follicles would continue to develop at because the FSH plasma concentration drops under the threshold level of all follicles. With age the size of the cohort will diminish and the overshoot in negative feedback will disappear, which leads to spontaneous, ovulatory, and often regular menstrual cycles in older PCOS women. It is possible in wedge resection or other forms of partial ovarian destruction that part of the cohort is destroyed and so the patients attain a regular menstrual pattern.

Technique The modern technique is through laser evaporization of several small areas at the ovarian surface, usually the size of 3 to 8 mm. However, the laser equipment is very expensive, and the much cheaper ovarian electro-cautery is a good alternative. Ten to fifteen small holes, approximately 3 to 5 mm in diameter and approximately 5 mm deep are drilled into the ovarian surface.

Results It has been reported that 80 to 90% of the clomiphene-resistant PCOS patients will resume ovulation after electrocautery. Conception rates are in the range of 45 to 65% within 6 to 12 months. It is reported that in 30 to 40% of patients treated, a relapse of PCOS will occur. It is therefore mandatory that the technique should only be used when infertility is a concern.

Side effects and complications The complications of these techniques are those directly related to similar surgical techniques in which either laser evaporation or electro-cautery are used in laparoscopy. Careful administration of the procedure should avoid those complications. The major complication to occur is adhesion formation around the ovary, which could ultimately cause infertility from adhesions once infertility due to anovulation has been cured. Adhesion formation was one of the main reasons why wedge resections were abandoned when medical therapy became available. The modern techniques have not been successful in nullifying this problem.

Dopamine receptor agonists

Dopamine receptor agonists are not ovulation inducers in the strictest sense. That is, they are not only used for the treatment of infertility but also have indications in tumor reduction, restoration of normal estrogenization in order to prevent premature bone loss, the treatment of galactorrhea, and the discontinuation of breast feeding. They are also used outside of reproduction, such as in the treatment of Parkinson's disease. Hence, treating hyperprolactinemia for fertility purposes can also be regarded as the treatment of an underlying disease, causing anovulation.

Mode of action Dopamine, locally secreted in the hypothalamus, acts as a prolactin-inhibiting factor once it is transported via the long portal vessels of the pituitary stalk to the anterior pituitary and the lactotroph cells. Pituitary prolactin-producing tumors, whether they are micro- or macroadenomas, for the most part maintain their sensitivity to dopamine, at least to a certain extent. This makes dopamine a good drug to control pathological prolactin secretion. However, dopamine as such, due to its short half-life and its generalized effects, is unsuitable for this purpose. In the early seventies bromocriptine became available, which has a selective effect on D2 dopamine receptors, the receptor that is present on the membrane of the prolactin-secreting cell of the anterior pituitary, the lactotroph. Bromocriptine has a much longer half-life and so appeared to be a very suitable drug to suppress both physiologically, that is, in breast feeding or pathologically elevated prolactin levels. Bromocriptine and other classes of D2 receptor agonists (e.g., pergolide, quinagolide, cabergoline), which have been developed in the meantime, have a direct effect on the D2 receptor on the lactotroph membrane. There is some difference between the different compounds because, even though they all manifest similar side effects, some patients who do not tolerate one drug will be able to tolerate another.

Anovulation in hyperprolactinemia is caused in the first place by the feedback system controlling prolactin secretion. Prolactin is normally released spontaneously from the lactotrophic cells of the anterior pituitary, although there is evidence for prolactin-releasing factors such as thyroid-stimulating hormone (TRH) and vasoactive intestinal protein (VIP). Prolactin secretion is inhibited by a prolactin-inhibiting factor, dopamine, secreted in the median eminence by the arcuate ventromedial nucleus of the hypothalamus. Prolactin has a positive feedback on this dopamine secretion. Therefore if a prolactinoma produces prolactin more or less autonomously, the arcuate nucleus will respond with an increased endogenous dopamine output. This increased dopamine turnover will, at the level of the median eminence, suppress secretion of GnRH, diminishing the amplitude of the GnRH pulses. The decreased GnRH output will then lead to anovulation in a basically hypogonadotropic state. Plainly, suppression of the increased prolactin secretion from the prolactinoma will not only restore normal dopamine secretion but also allow for normal GnRH secretion to begin again, which will restore normal ovulatory menstrual cycles.

Technique Women with microadenomas can be treated with dopamine receptor agonists without restriction. They typically have very few complications during pregnancy. Women with a macroadenoma confined to the boundaries of the sella turcica can also be treated unrestrictedly. Women with a macroadenoma that extends beyond the sella turcica should be treated for a prolonged period of time before they be allowed to conceive. Ideally this only happens when the adenoma has decreased so much in size that it is within the sellar boundaries again. Despite such a result, treatment with dopamine receptor agonists in these women (preferably bromocriptine) should not be discontinued during pregnancy. Any other situation should be judged by the treating physician, but it should be realized that in such patients severe complications may occur (see below).

All pregnant women who carry a prolactinoma, be it a micro- or a macroadenoma, should be monitored during pregnancy for pituitary/tumor enlargement. Full eye examinations, including eye fields, should be done every

6 weeks, and if indicated an MRI scan should be made during pregnancy, such as in women in whom the distance of the tumor to the optic nerve is very small.

Dopamine receptor agonists are usually given orally, although a long-acting bromocriptine preparation, to be given im, is also available in some countries. As most of the drugs have side effects of nausea and orthostatic hypotension, which disappear with time but may recur with every increase in dose, it is advisable to start with a small dose and only when the patient is well-adjusted to the dose increase further in small steps, guided by prolactin normalization. Usually after normalization of prolactin levels, ovulation will be restored within 4 weeks, although in some macroadenomas it may take considerably longer. As stated above, side effects are often related to a particular compound in a particular patient. Changing preparations will therefore sometimes solve the problem. When side effects, particularly nausea, do not disappear, bypassing parenteral resorption can be accomplished by vaginal administration, which often gives better results. Total resistance to dopamine receptor agonists occurs. In these cases ovulation can be induced by pulsatile GnRH administration (see above).

As soon as pregnancy is established, medication is discontinued in cases of microadenomas and macroadenomas that are and always have been within the boundaries of the sella turcica.

Results Ovulation returns after prolactin levels have been normalized within 4 weeks in 80 to 90% of cases. After ovulation has returned fecundity (the monthly conception rate) is the same as in fertile women. Pregnancy outcome as well as the incidence of congenital anomalies are also normal.

Side effects and complications The direct side effects of nausea and orthostatic hypotension have been mentioned above. Indirect side effects are the risks of complications of prolactinoma growth during pregnancy. The tremendously increased secretion of estrogens during pregnancy stimulates growth of the normal pituitary as well as of the prolactinoma, leading to extension outside the boundaries of the normal or even already enlarged sella turcica. Surrounding structures such as the optic nerve above the sella and the oculomotor, the trochlear, and the abducens nerves on either side of the sella may thereby become compromised by pressure of the tumor. This will result in either visual defects in cases of compression of the optic nerve or in disturbances in the control of eye movements in cases of compression of the other nerves.

A final complication is a hemorrhage in the tumor, which leads to a very acute situation with excruciating headache and compression of the surrounding structures, resulting in symptoms as described above, or even in sudden blindness. The bleeding will in a short time lead to destruction of the tumor and often of the pituitary, leading to an acute deprivation of all pituitary hormones.

Treatment of symptoms of tumor growth during pregnancy can be treated in the following ways: Medical treatment is to be preferred at all times. Bromocriptine is the drug of choice in such cases because there has been a great deal of data collected on the use of this drug during pregnancy. There is no indication that the drug will harm the fetus in any way, either given early, late, or during the whole of pregnancy. At the time of this writing, the experience with other drugs is not convincing yet. Medication should be restarted as soon as symptoms occur and the patient should be carefully monitored by MRI for tumor shrinkage. Eye field defects will be tolerated for at least some weeks before permanent damage is irreversible, but it is not known exactly how long. Termination of pregnancy is the second choice if gestational age is such that a

viable fetus would be born. This should seriously be considered from 34 weeks onward. Surgical treatment is the third choice and should not necessarily aim at complete removal of the tumor but primarily at decompression. Surgery at this stage is difficult, particularly because of the increased vascularization of the pituitary and its surroundings during pregnancy. Pituitary apoplexia always necessitates surgical decompression.

Suggested readings

ADASHI EY. Ovulation induction: clomiphene citrate. In: Adashi EY, Rock JA, Rosenwaks Z (eds). Reproductive endocrinology, surgery, and technology. Philadelphia-New York: Lippincott-Raven Publishers, 1996.

BAIRD DT. Amenorrhoea, anovulation and dysfunctional uterine bleeding. In: de Groot LJ (ed). Endocrinology. New York: Saunders, 1995; 2059-79.

EVANS J, TOWNSEND L. The induction of ovulation. Am J Obstet Gynecol 1977;125:321-7.

FAUSER BCJM, HSUEH AJW. Genetic basis of human reproductive endocrine disorders. Hum Reprod 1995;10:826-46.

FAUSER BCJM, VAN HEUSDEN AM. Manipulation of human ovarian function: physiological concepts and clinical consequences. Endocr Rev 1997;18:71-106.

FILICORI M, FLAMIGNI C (eds). Ovulation induction: update '98. London-New York: The Parthenon Publishing Group, 1998.

HOEK A, SCHOEMAKER J, DREXHAGE HA. Premature ovarian failure and ovarian autoimmunity. Endocr Rev 1997;18:107-34.

LUNENFELD B, INSLER V. Classification of amenorrheic states and their treatment by ovulation induction. Clin Endocrinol (Oxf) 1974;3:223-37.

REBAR RW. Disorders of menstruation, ovulation, and sexual response. In: Becker KL (ed). Principles and practice of endocrinology and metabolism. Philadelphia: Lippincott, 1990;798-814.

VAN SANTBRINK EJP, HOP WC, FAUSER BCJM. Classification of normogonadotropic infertility: polycystic ovaries diagnosed by ultrasound versus endocrine characteristics of polycystic ovary syndrome. Fertil Steril 1997;67:452-58.

YEN SSC. Chronic anovulation due to CNS hypothalamic pituitary dysfunction. In: Yen SSC, Jaffe RB (eds). Reproductive endocrinology. Philadelphia: Saunders, 1991;631-88.

SCHOEMAKER J, BRAAT DDH. Pulsatile gonadotropin-releasing hormone therapy. In: Adashi EY, Rock JA, Rosenwaks Z, (eds). Reproductive endocrinology, surgery, and technology. Philadelphia-New York: Lippincott-Raven Publishers, 1996.

WHITE DM, POLSON DW, KIDDY D, et al. Induction of ovulation with low-dose gonadotropins in polycystic ovary syndrome: an analysis of 109 pregnancies in 225 women. J Clin Endocrinol Metab 1996;81:3821-4.

Dysfunctional uterine bleeding, luteal phase defect

Beverley Vollenhoven, Henry Burger

▰ KEY POINTS ▰

- Dysfunctional uterine bleeding is defined as excessive uterine bleeding with no organic cause and is a diagnosis of exclusion. It is a common reason for women to seek medical consultation.
- Over 80% of cases are due to anovulation. The problem is more common in the adolescent years and in the years leading up to menopause.
- The treatment of anovulatory dysfunctional uterine bleeding is undertaken hormonally, with the oral contraceptive pill being the treatment of choice provided there are no contraindications to its use.
- The treatment of ovulatory dysfunctional uterine bleeding can be undertaken either hormonally using the oral contraceptive pill or the levonorgestrel-releasing intrauterine contraceptive device, or non-hormonally using cyclo-oxygenase inhibitors or anti-fibrinolytic agents.
- Luteal phase defect is a condition with a multifactorial etiology that may occur as a result of poor follicular development or from hypothalamic-pituitary abnormalities, and it is often difficult to diagnose.
- Luteal phase defect causes loss of pregnancy.
- Luteal phase defect may be treated by stimulating folliculogenesis, therefore stimulating luteal function or by luteal phase support.

The normal menstrual cycle has a duration of 23 to 35 days. If bleeding occurs at less than 23- or greater than 35-day intervals, the cycle is regarded as possibly anovulatory. The usual duration of blood flow is 4 to 6 days, with most blood loss occurring in the first 3 days. Bleeding for longer than 7 days is considered abnormal. The more rapid the loss, the shorter the duration of flow. If there is incomplete initial shedding, there is a heavier and prolonged period.

The normal menstrual blood loss is 30 ml. Loss of greater than 80 ml is defined as menorrhagia. Regular loss of this magnitude will cause iron-deficiency anemia. The amount of blood loss is determined by (1) the total area of the endometrial cavity, (2) the vascularity of the uterus and the structure of the uterine vessels, (3) the balance between vasoconstrictor and vasodilator substances released by the endometrium, (4) the balance between coagulator and fibrinolytic substances released by the endometrium, (5) the responsiveness of the spiral arterioles, and (6) the rate of regeneration of the endometrium.

Blood accounts for 50 to 75% of the menstrual flow. The remainder consists of endometrial tissue and tissue fluid, desquamated vaginal epithelium, and mucus. Blood loss ceases because of prolonged vasoconstriction, vascular stasis, tissue collapse, and a resumption of estrogenic activity that leads to clot formation.

The most physiological menstrual pattern occurs following estradiol priming of the endometrium for 1 to 2 weeks, followed by estradiol and progesterone for 2 weeks. Any substantial departure from this pattern leads to menstrual disturbance. The removal of progesterone alone will cause bleeding if the endometrium has been primed by estrogen. If estrogen therapy continues while progesterone therapy stops, bleeding will still occur. Only if estrogen levels are increased by 10 to 20 times will progesterone withdrawal bleeding be prevented.

DYSFUNCTIONAL UTERINE BLEEDING

Dysfunctional uterine bleeding (DUB) is defined as excessively heavy, prolonged, or frequent bleeding of uterine origin that is not due to recognizable pelvic, pregnancy-related, generalized medical disease or iatrogenic causes (Tab. 47.1). It is therefore excessive uterine bleeding with no organic cause. It is a diagnosis of exclusion. Over 80% of DUB cases result from anovulation, which may occur for a number of different reasons. The most common complaint is of excessive irregular bleeding.

Epidemiology

Ten percent of women attending a gynecological outpatient clinic have dysfunctional uterine bleeding as their

Table 47.1 Differential diagnosis of abnormal uterine bleeding

Pelvic	Fibroids
	Adenomyosis
	Endometrial/endocervical polyps
	Functional ovarian tumors
	Cervical or vaginal lesions
	Genital tract malignancies
	Endometritis
Pregnancy-related disease	Threatened/incomplete/ missed abortion
	Ectopic pregnancy
	Gestational trophoblastic disease
Generalized medical disease	Blood dyscrasias
	Thyroid dysfunction
	Hepatic dysfunction
Iatrogenic	IUD
	Oral/injectable contraceptives
	Rifampicin
	Anti-epileptics
	Spironolactone

diagnosis. It is more common in the adolescent years and in the 10 years leading up to menopause.

Etiology

Anovulatory bleeding

An anovulatory bleeding pattern consists of prolonged and excessive irregular bleeding, associated with prolonged and unopposed endometrial stimulation by fluctuating and sometimes excessively elevated levels of estradiol. The endometrium displays abnormal height without concomitant stromal support. It is therefore weak and fragile and suffers spontaneous superficial breakage that leads to bleeding. As one site heals another may breakdown.

The proliferative endometrium may evolve to cystic or simple glandular hyperplasia. There may also be a change to adenomatous hyperplasia and possibly to atypical hyperplasia, which may progress to neoplasia, although this remains controversial. It has been proposed that endometrial hyperplasia without atypia and endometrial hyperplasia with atypia are different biological entities and that the former is not a precursor of neoplasia.

Ovulatory bleeding

An ovulatory bleeding pattern consists of regular menstrual loss that is heavy and/or prolonged. It is more common in the mid-reproductive years. There may be a local corpus luteum abnormality, an abnormality within the uterus related to an abnormal ratio of prostaglandins ($PGF_{2\alpha}/PGE_2$), or possibly a disturbance in the estrogen/progesterone balance.

Clinical findings

As over 80% of dysfunctional uterine bleeding is due to anovulation, especially in adolescence and perimenopause, the diagnosis is made by demonstrating anovulation either clinically or biochemically and excluding other causes for the bleeding (Tab. 47.1). A detailed history, examination including speculum examination and a bimanual pelvic examination, and a cervical Papanicolaou smear are mandatory in all patients. Some women will require pregnancy to be excluded. Anovulation may be demonstrated clinically in a woman who has a cycle outside the range of 23 to 35 days and, biochemically, by demonstrating a low serum progesterone concentration (< 10 nmol/l or < 3 ng/ml) in the mid-luteal phase of the cycle (7 ± 3 days prior to the next the menses).

If there is suspicion of a coagulation defect, a clotting screen should be performed. Thyroid function should be assessed depending on clinical suspicion. A complete blood count will be required to diagnose anemia.

Transvaginal ultrasonography is an effective tool as a first step procedure to select those for hysteroscopy and biopsy. If an intrauterine abnormality is seen or the endometrium is irregular in diameter with abnormal blood flow on ultrasound examination, hysteroscopy and biopsy under vision should be undertaken. The hysteroscopy and biopsy may be performed as an office procedure in which a cervical block anesthetic or no anesthetic is used. Alternatively, hysteroscopy and dilatation and curettage (D & C) can be performed under light general anesthesia. The performance of blind D & C is no longer an acceptable treatment.

Treatment

The mode of treatment depends on the woman's age, her desire for future fertility, the amount of blood loss, and if it is acute or chronic in nature (Tab. 47.2). The aim of treatment is to stop the acute episode, and to prevent recurrence and therefore prevent long-term complications.

ACUTE TREATMENT

Surgical treatment

If blood loss is life-threatening or if signs of hypovolemia are displayed, D & C is the treatment of choice. The endometrium (the site of the bleeding) is removed and the bleeding stops. The patient may require transfusion.

Medical treatment

If the blood loss is not as severe as to be life-threatening but is still very heavy, Premarin 25 mg intravenously

every 4 hours until the bleeding ceases can be used (up to 3 doses may be given). The loss will cease within 4 to 24 hours in 70% of patients. If there is no change in the blood flow, a D & C will need to be performed. Premarin acts rapidly and has effects on clotting factor levels. Once blood loss has ceased, a change to oral Premarin 10 mg is made, slowly decreasing to 2.5 mg daily. At this stage 10 mg medroxyprogesterone acetate for 10 days is added to produce an orderly maturation of the endometrium. Norethisterone at a dose of 2.5 mg for 10 days may also be used instead of medroxyprogesterone acetate. Both medications (Premarin and either medroxyprogesterone acetate or norethisterone) are then withdrawn, and the endometrium will be shed. The patient should be warned that the subsequent withdrawal bleed will be heavy and may be painful. Patients treated with Premarin often require an antiemetic.

Acute bleeding can also be stopped using 100 µg ethinyl estradiol daily for 5 to 7 days. A heavy cramping withdrawal bleed will subsequently occur within 5 days of therapy cessation. The oral contraceptive pill can then be started on the 5th day after withdrawal bleeding occurs.

Oral medroxyprogesterone acetate is also effective in stopping bleeding when starting at a dose of 30 mg daily (60 mg if obese) for 3 days, reducing to 20 mg daily for 3 days, then 15 mg daily for 3 days, and finally to 10 mg daily for 5 days. Alternatively, oral norethisterone may also be very effective in causing bleeding cessation. The initial dose is 15 mg daily for 3 days, reducing to 10 mg daily for 3 days, then 7.5 mg daily for 3 days, and finally to 5 mg daily for 5 days.

CHRONIC TREATMENT

Surgical treatment

Dilatation and curettage is rarely therapeutic unless a polyp is removed. The first 1 to 2 cycles after D & C may be better, but invariably the abnormal bleeding returns.

Total abdominal hysterectomy is the most commonly used surgical modality for dysfunctional uterine bleeding. Whether bilateral salpingo-oophorectomy should be routinely carried out in women over 40 years of age remains controversial.

Endometrial ablation is an alternative surgical procedure that is permanent and effective. The goal of treatment is to destroy the basal layers of endometrium, thereby causing uterine synechiae. Treatment can be carried out using the laser Neodymium yttrium aluminum garnet (Nd:YAG), using electrosurgical resection with a cutting loop or by using a roller-ball to produce coagulation. It often requires pre-treatment using luteinizing hormone-releasing hormone analogs (LHRHa) for 2 to 3 months to ensure endometrial atrophy. This medication is often more effective than danocrine (800 mg daily) or medroxyprogesterone acetate. Alternatively, the procedure may be car-

---

Table 47.2 Treatment modalities for dysfunctional uterine bleeding

Acute	Surgical	D & C
	Medical	Premarin iv
		Premarin oral
		Ethinyl estradiol
		MPA
		NET
Chronic	Surgical	TAH
		Endometrial ablation
	Medical-hormonal	OCP
		MPA
		NET
		Depot MPA
		LNG- IUD
		Danocrine
		LHRHa
		Clomiphene citrate
	Medical-non-hormonal	Cyclo-oxygenase inhibitors
		Anti-fibrinolytic agents
		Hemostatic agents

(MPA = medroxyprogesterone acetate; NET = norethisterone; TAH = total abdominal hysterectomy; OCP = oral contraceptive pills; LNG-IUD = levonorgestrel releasing intra-uterine contraceptive device; LHRHa = luteinizing hormone releasing hormone analogs.)

ried out in the very early follicular phase. Endometrial ablation is effective in 90% of women (50% will become amenorrheic and 40% will have decreased bleeding). The remaining 10% will not improve and, rarely, may be worse. More than 1 procedure may be carried out. O'Connor and Magos (1996) followed 525 women for up to 5 years after endometrial resection and reported that 9% subsequently underwent hysterectomy. There were no reported long-term complications of the procedure. However, a potential complication is the development of endometrial adenocarcinoma, which is masked by the endometrial ablation (due to adhesion formation) many years after the procedure has been performed. To try to minimize this risk, a progestin in an adequate dose for at least 10 days each month must always be added to estrogen therapy when these women reach menopause and request treatment of symptoms. The advantages of endometrial ablation over total abdominal hysterectomy are that the former is a day surgical procedure, and recovery is rapid because of the absence of an incision; and not removing the uterus is of psychological benefit to some women.

Historically, radium implants have been placed in the uterus to "ablate" the endometrium.

Medical treatment

The medical treatment options are reported in Table 47.3. If the patient is anovulatory, hormonal therapy is the treatment of choice. If the patient is having regular heavy periods and is therefore likely to be ovulating, either hormonal or non-hormonal medical treatment may be undertaken.

Table 47.3 Medical treatment of chronic dysfunctional uterine bleeding

Anovulatory	OCP
	MPA
	NET
	Depot MPA
	LNG-IUD
	LHRHa
	Clomiphene citrate
Ovulatory	OCP
	MPA
	NET
	Depot MPA
	LNG-IUD
	Danocrine
	LHRHa
	Cyclo-oxygenase inhibitors
	Anti-fibrinolytic agents
	Hemostatic agents

(MPA = medroxyprogesterone acetate; NET = norethisterone; OCP = oral contraceptive pills; LNG-IUD = levonorgestrel releasing intra-uterine contraceptive device; LHRHa = luteinizing hormone releasing hormone analogs.)

The oral contraceptive pill is a valuable drug in the treatment of dysfunctional uterine bleeding, especially if contraception is also required. It reduces menstrual flow by at least 60% in a normal uterus, as well as reduces dysmenorrhea. It can be used for both anovulatory and ovulatory bleeding.

Alternatively, medroxyprogesterone acetate 10 mg or norethisterone 1.25-2.5 mg both for 10 to 12 days each month can be used to replace progesterone. A withdrawal bleed will occur within 7 days of the last tablet. Some women may ovulate on these drugs; therefore they are not the treatment of choice if contraception is needed. If the patient is ovulatory and has regular heavy menstrual blood loss, medroxyprogesterone acetate 10 mg or norethisterone 1.25-2.5 mg both for days 5 to 25 of the cycle are possible choices. This treatment may decrease blood loss by 20%.

Depot medroxyprogesterone acetate (150 mg every 3 months) is an acceptable alternative if the patient is non-compliant with oral medication. The levonorgestrel releasing intrauterine contraceptive device (LNG-IUD) may also be used in women who desire contraception. This device releases 20 µg LNG per day and is effective for 5 years. It has been reported to reduce menstrual blood loss by 50%. Both depot medroxyprogesterone acetate and the LNG-IUD can be used for anovulatory and ovulatory DUB. Progestins act by diminishing the estrogen effects on target cells by decreasing the production of estrogen receptors. Therefore, there is an antiproliferative, antimitotic action that leads to endometrial atrophy.

Other hormonal agents that can be used include danocrine 100 to 200 mg daily. With this dose of danocrine there are few androgenic side effects, but it is not a contraceptive. It is used for regular heavy periods. Luteinizing hormone-releasing hormone analogs are also effective but in the long-term (greater than 6 months) will produce osteoporosis and therefore will need to be combined with add-back hormone replacement therapy. The oral contraceptive pill is a better and cheaper alternative.

If the patient desires pregnancy and is anovulatory, clomiphene citrate is the treatment of choice.

Non-hormonal therapy for ovulatory DUB includes the cyclo-oxygenase inhibitors, antifibrinolytic agents, and hemostatic agents, all of which are taken during menstruation. Cyclo-oxygenase inhibitors include mefenamic acid, ibuprofen, and naproxen. These will decrease blood loss by 30% but only while treatment is continued, and if used for over 6 months the therapy loses its effectiveness. The inhibition of cyclo-oxygenase in the prostaglandin pathway causes a reduction in prostacyclin and thromboxane levels. Because prostacyclin levels are inhibited more effectively, there is blood vessel contraction and platelet aggregation. These drugs are contraindicated in those with peptic ulcer disease, liver or renal disease, and in those who develop bronchospasm with aspirin or who have an aspirin intolerance.

Antifibrinolytic agents include amino caproic acid and tranexamic acid, which are effective in 50% of women with DUB. The minor side effects of these drugs include nausea, abdominal pain, diarrhea, dizziness, and headache.

The major but rare side effect of thrombosis is a potentially life-threatening problem.

Hemostatic agents include ethamsylate. Their effectiveness in the treatment of excessive menstrual blood loss is questionable. In a randomized trial Bonnar and Shepppard (1996) compared the efficacy of mefenamic acid (500 mg 8 hourly), ethamsylate (500 mg 6 hourly), and tranexamic acid (1g 6 hourly) in 76 women with regularly heavy DUB. The treatment began on day 1 of the cycle and continued for 5 days, and the treatment continued for 3 consecutive cycles. They reported that ethamsylate did not reduce blood loss, mefenamic acid reduced loss by 20%, and tranexamic acid reduced blood loss by 50%. They concluded that tranexamic acid was a safe and effective treatment for DUB.

Iron supplementation may be required. Counseling regarding the cause for bleeding is also extremely important.

LUTEAL PHASE DEFECT

A defective corpus luteum leading to inadequate progesterone secretion, termed luteal phase defect (LPD), was first proposed by Jones (1976) as a significant cause of subsequent reproductive failure. It is clear that LPD is a condition with a multifactorial etiology. The diagnosis is often difficult to substantiate and the treatment options are for the most part empirical and unproven.

Further complicating this issue is the inclusion of a short luteal phase, that is, one that is less than 11 days duration based on basal body temperature chart testing, under the umbrella of LPD. In these latter women, there may be a greater incidence of subclinical abortions.

Luteal phase defect may be the result of poor follicular development that leads to subsequent poor corpus luteum function and subnormal progesterone secretion. Luteal phase defect may also be the result of hypothalamic-pituitary abnormalities, including mild and often transient hyperprolactinemia, and inadvertent surgical removal of the corpus luteum before the 8th week of pregnancy. In addition, LPD may be present in elite athletes, those with extreme weight loss, those under stress, women at the extremes of their reproductive lives (adolescent and perimenopausal years), women who commence cycling after breast feeding, and in some women treated with clomiphene citrate.

In general, LPD causes pregnancy loss, which may be recurrent. The production of progesterone by the corpus luteum is critical for pregnancy maintenance in the first 7 to 9 weeks of gestation. However, the minimum serum concentration of progesterone that is required for pregnancy maintenance is unknown.

Luteal phase defect is implicated as a cause for infertility. It remains a somewhat controversial concept because of the difficulty of formulating anything other than a somewhat arbitrary definition. It is conventionally defined by the finding of endometrial histology (on biopsy) that is more than 2 days "out of phase" with the expected appearance, in 2 successive cycles.

Epidemiology

Luteal phase defect has been variously described as occurring in 15-20% to 23-60% of couples with recurrent pregnancy loss, and in 27% of cycles in fertile women who have no history of recurrent pregnancy loss. It has also been variously reported to occur in 3 to 20% of cycles in infertile couples.

Clinical findings

A day-26 (12 days post-ovulation on luteinizing hormone testing) endometrial biopsy is said to be the gold standard for the diagnosis of LPD. Luteal phase defect is arbitrarily diagnosed if the biopsy is out of phase by more than 2 days in 2 consecutive cycles. The stipulation of 2 successive cycles is made because of the high incidence of out-of-phase biopsies in the normal fertile population. The histological dating must be compared with the day of ovulation rather than the day of the next menstrual period for greater accuracy.

A mid-luteal progesterone (7 ± 3 days prior to next menses) less than about 10 ng/ml, or less than 30 nmol/l, is also conventionally taken to be diagnostic of LPD. However, some claim that this is inadequate for diagnosis, as progesterone is secreted in a pulsatile fashion that leads to variable serum concentrations of progesterone when samples are obtained at random. The condition of a short luteal phase may be suspected if the basal body temperature chart reveals a luteal phase of less than 11 days duration. However, the basal body temperature will not diagnose other forms of LPD. Jordan et al. (1994) evaluated the sensitivity and specificity of the various diagnostic tests available for LPD. They reported that the most sensitive and specific test for the diagnosis of LPD was a single mid-luteal progesterone < 10 ng/ml. An endometrial biopsy was marginally acceptable, but basal body temperature, luteal phase length, and preovulatory follicle diameter were not acceptable for making a diagnosis of LPD. The major advantage of mid-luteal progesterone is that it is a non-invasive test.

Treatment

Luteal phase defect may be treated by luteal phase support or by stimulating folliculogenesis and thus stimulating luteal function. There are advocates for each of these treatments, but none is based on randomized controlled trials.

Luteal phase support is undertaken using progesterone beginning on day 16 of the cycle and continuing until 8 weeks gestation. The progesterone may be administered in the form of vaginal suppositories at a dose of 25 mg twice daily or alternatively as intramuscular injections at a dose of 12.5 mg daily. The only studies that showed a benefit from progesterone therapy were retrospective.

There have been no randomized controlled studies that have shown that progesterone therapy is effective in the treatment of recurrent abortion. In fact, a meta-analysis of 6 trials by Goldstein et al. (1989) in which progesterone was administered after conception showed no treatment benefit. Daya (1989), in a meta-analysis of 3 trials, showed that progesterone therapy was effective in women with recurrent pregnancy loss not necessarily due to LPD. Large, randomized, prospective double-blind trials are required to assess the use of progesterone therapy for the treatment of LPD, which causes recurrent pregnancy loss as well as infertility.

Luteal support may also be undertaken using human chorionic gonadotropin 1500-5000 IU every 2 to 5 days after the luteinizing hormone surge and continuing until 8 weeks gestation. This therapy has not been definitely shown to be effective.

The stimulation of follicular function and hence improved luteal function is undertaken using clomiphene citrate or human menopausal gonadotropin therapy. The rationale is to stimulate better folliculogenesis in these women. It must be remembered, however, that some women may develop an "out-of-phase" endometrium on clomiphene citrate therapy due to its potential anti-estrogenic effects on the endometrium, thus leading to the diagnosis of LPD. Therefore, it has been advocated that women who have a diagnosis of LPD and are treated with clomiphene citrate have an endometrial biopsy in treatment cycles. It may be just as adequate to perform a mid-luteal progesterone.

Bromocriptine therapy is recommended if luteal dysfunction is thought to be due to an elevated serum prolactin concentration.

Suggested *readings*

Dysfunctional uterine bleeding

BONNAR J, SHEPPARD BL. Treatment of menorrhagia during menstruation: randomized controlled trial of ethamsylate, mefenamic acid, and tranexamic acid. BMJ 1996;313:579-82.

O'CONNOR H, MAGOS A. Endometrial resection for the treatment of menorrhagia. N Eng J Med 1996;335:151-66.

SPEROFF L, GLASS RH, KASE NG (eds). Dysfunctional uterine bleeding. In: Clinical gynecologic endocrinology and infertility. 4th ed. Baltimore: Williams and Wilkins, 1989:265-82.

Luteal phase defect

DAYA S. Efficacy of progesterone support for pregnancy in women with recurrent miscarriage. A meta-analysis of controlled trials. Brit J Obstet Gynaecol 1989;96:275-80.

GOLDSTEIN P, BERRIER J, ROSEN S, SACKS HS, CHALMERS TC. A meta-analysis of randomized control trials of progestational agents in pregnancy. Brit J Obstet Gynaecol 1989;96:265-74.

JONES GS. The luteal phase defect. Fertil Steril 1976;27:351-6.

JORDAN J, CRAIG K, CLIFTON DK, SOULES MR. Luteal phase defect: the sensitivity and specificity of diagnostic methods in common clinical use. Fertil Steril 1994;62:54-62.

SPEROFF L, GLASS RH, KASE NG (eds). Dysfunctional uterine bleeding. In: Clinical gynecologic endocrinology and infertility. 4th ed. Baltimore: Williams and Wilkins, 1989:536-8.

Female infertility

Michael G.R. Hull †

■ KEY POINTS ■

- Infertility affects a couple, and both partners should be investigated and treated together.
- Sperm disorders are the commonest cause of infertility but the female partner is usually directly involved in investigations (e.g., cervical mucus penetration) and treatments (e.g., donor insemination or assisted conception methods). In vitro fertilisation (IVF) employing intracytoplasmic sperm injection is the most effective treatment.
- Oligomenorrhea and amenorrhea are the only clear indications of anovulation. Except when due to ovarian failure, treatment possibilities are excellent, leading to virtually normal chances of conception.
- Tubal/pelvic infective damage is most commonly due to *Chlamydia trachomatis*, but the infection was often asymptomatic and *Chlamydia* serology is a useful screening test for likely damage requiring early diagnostic laparoscopy. Surgery offers limited benefit, mainly in a selective minority of cases, and IVF is often needed.
- Endometriosis is often asymptomatic and diagnosis requires laparoscopy. Surgery is the only treatment offering benefit for natural conception but IVF may be needed.
- Cervical mucus defects are an uncommon cause of infertility and difficult to define reliably.
- Uterine fibroids are a rare cause of infertility, only relevant when distorting the uterine cavity.
- Couples with unexplained infertility (normal menstrual cycles, laparoscopy, semen analysis, postcoital test and coital frequency) of less than 3 years duration are essentially normal and have simply been unlucky. They have no need for active treatment, but require basic advice.
- Couples with more prolonged unexplained infertility have poor prognosis for natural conception. They can benefit from intrauterine insemination and/or mild ovarian stimulation, abut IVF and related methods are the only treatments offering a normal chance of conception.
- The only treatment methods that can achieve normal rates of conception each cycle are the ovulation induction methods for oligomenorrhea or amenorrhea, and IVF and related methods of assisted conception. Reversal of sterilisation is almost equally effective, and achieves the highest cumulative rates in time, because tubal function had not been damaged by infection.
- Incidental factors strongly affecting fertility prognosis are the age of the woman, raised follicle-stimulating hormone level in the menstrual phase of the cycle, duration of infertility, and cigarette smoking. Extreme obesity or weight loss are only important when associated with oligomenorrhea of amenorrhea. Even when pregnancy occurs there is increased risk of miscarriage associated with age of the woman and polycystic ovarian disease.

This chapter is primarily concerned with female infertility. However, it is good clinical practice to deal with both partners as a couple; there is important physiological interaction between the male and female, and treatment of male infertility commonly involves the woman in artificial insemination or in vitro fertilization (IVF). Therefore, the organization of care as discussed in this chapter will apply to the couple, and basic screening tests of male as well as female fertility will be covered. Specialist practice will be covered only in so far as it will enable the general physician to advise patients what might be done for them.

Basic applied physiology

Infertility can be the result of several distinct functional elements of conception that fail, all of which must be considered in practice: ovulation, tubal transport of the oocyte, timed coital delivery of sperm, cervical mucus receptivity, sperm production and motility, fertilization, and uterine/endometrial receptivity for implantation. Some functions such as cervical mucus receptivity are cyclical and linked to follicular development and ovulation; others, such as sperm production or function, are independently controlled or can be damaged in isolation. The most frequently defined causes are described later in the chapter (Tab. 48.1). Best understood are the control of ovulation and the causes and treatment of ovulation failure, which are discussed in Chapter 46. Detailed analyses of the physiology and pathophysiology of the causes of infertility are beyond the scope of this chapter, but some of the key points of practical relevance are summarized below.

Ovulation (oocyte release and follicular maturation)

While follicular growth and rupture can be observed by serial ultrasonography, follicle size correlates only weakly with functional maturity, which is best reflected by hormone production. The functional capacity of the corpus luteum reflects preovulatory follicular maturation, and midluteal serum progesterone measurement is an accurate index of ovulation with potential for conception. Variation between cycles, however, requires repeated measurement. Assessment of multiple ovulation induced by stimulation therapy must take into account the progesterone contribution of the several mature and subsidiary follicles.

Oocyte quality Follicular maturation determines not only ovulation but also oocyte maturation and fertilizing ability (see below). Independent of those functions, however, is oocyte quality, which cannot be recognized clinically but determines embryo quality and ultimate viability. Declining oocyte quality is the main cause for declining fecundability as women age, and it is associated with declining follicle numbers in the ovaries. Thus, diminishing inhibin levels, and consequently rising follicle-stimulating hormone (FSH) levels during the early follicular phase, are clinically important indices of potential fertility.

Tubal transport of the oocyte

Oocyte uptake and transport along the tube depends on healthy, unrestricted fimbriae and ciliary action of the endotubal mucosa. Assessment of the fimbriae and mucosa is essential in clinical practice, as well as of mere patency and restrictive adhesions.

Timed coital delivery of sperm

Optimal timing of coitus to achieve conception is 1 to 2 days before ovulation, that is, the day of or day before the onset of the luteinizing hormone (LH) surge. That is linked to peak receptivity of cervical mucus; it appears that spermatozoa should be present and available to the oocyte as soon as ovulation occurs. Spermatozoa are stored in the female tract and normally retain fertilizing ability for at least 48 hours, effectively bridging intervals of 2 days between coitus. More frequent intercourse is more effective (not less as sometime believed), whereas infrequent intercourse reduces sperm quality.

Cervical mucus secretion and receptivity

Cervical mucus is a tissue, not a fluid, containing a mesh-like mucoprotein matrix that acts as a challenging selector of sperm that have favorable motility. Full development and receptivity peaks with the peak estradiol level, normally lasts 2 to 3 days, and is quickly interrupted by the antiestrogen effects of progesterone secreted in response to the LH surge even before ovulation.

Sperm production and motility

Spermatozoa are normally produced in vastly excessive numbers; what matters is functional ability. Sperm motility must be forwardly progressive with a fast tail beat and only slight lateral head movement to enable rapid progression through cervical mucus and onward to reach the oocyte. The pattern then changes dramatically to slow lashing of the tail and marked lateral head movement ("activated motility", a feature of "capacitation") to enable penetration of the outer coverings of the oocyte (granulosa cumulus cells and zona pellucida). Sperm motility in semen correlates only weakly, even when precisely quantitated using computerized imaging, with mucus penetration, fertilization, and the chance of natural conception.

Fertilization

To achieve fertilization the oocyte must have matured in response to the LH surge by resuming meiosis to reach metaphase II (extrusion of the first polar body), and the spermatozoa must have developed activated motility and undergone the acrosome reaction (shedding of the acrosomal cap) to release the proteolytic enzymes required to assist penetration of the zona pellucida and attachment to the oocyte membrane (vitelline). Entry of the oocyte by the (haploid) spermatozoon induces the second meiotic division of the oocyte (reducing it from diploid to haploid) and expulsion of the second polar body. Fertilization is defined by formation of the pronuclei of the oocyte and spermatozoon. Syngamy soon follows, and the first cleavage division of the embryo occurs about 24 hours after the meeting of oocyte and spermatozoa.

Uterine/endometrial receptivity for implantation

Endometrial proliferation in response to estrogen, and subsequent secretory differentiation in response to progesterone, generally occur normally when given appropriately timed hormone signals. Full secretory differentiation, that is, decidualization, is induced locally by paracrine signals from the blastocyst. There is virtually no clinical value to be gained from endometrial histology. Implantation success or failure is largely determined by embryo quality, which in turn reflects original gamete quality. For example, the age-related decline in female fecundability is primarily due to a decline in oocyte quality reducing implanting ability (without affecting ovulation and fertilization).

Measures of fertility: practice oriented to outcome

The logical development of a system of diagnosis and treatment of infertility depends on knowledge of some basic statistics: the relative frequency of causes to indicate the likelihood of finding a particular cause in practice; and outcome measures in terms of pregnancy and preferably birth rates, which can be related to each diagnostic investigation in order to determine its discriminant value, and to each treatment in order to determine its effectiveness. It is essential that the choice of any diagnostic or therapeutic method used is oriented to define the chance of achieving pregnancy and the birth of a child.

Outcome related to diagnostic and therapeutic procedures is best described by pregnancy or preferably birth rates related to specific time frames. Most results have been reported as pregnancy rates, though IVF results are more commonly presented as birth rates (by requirement). The difference is particularly important in women with a high risk of miscarriage, such as due to age or polycystic ovarian (PCO) disease.

The cumulative chance of success for a couple depends on the duration of the exposure to the chance of natural conception or to the number of cycles of active treatment. Rates given per cycle may be misleading if limited to the first cycle or two of treatment, because the rate tends to fall in subsequent cycles. For these reasons, cumulative time-specific or cycle-specific rates will be presented in this chapter whenever possible.

Cumulative rates are calculated using the life-table method, which takes into account those couples who are not followed-up or actively treated as long as others. Biases can occur that would lead to calculations of exaggerated success rates, due to selective reporting by successful patients or selective discontinuation of cyclical treatment. Therefore, all patients should be actively followed-up, and the life-table method must be applied to specifically defined groups of patients categorized by diagnosis, age, and duration of infertility, who would be treated consistently. Patients selectively withdrawn from treatment must remain in the life-table calculation as continuing failures. The calculation should be based upon the original intention to treat.

What patients want to know

If done in a valid way, the life-table method provides the only means of properly answering the question for each couple according to their specific conditions (categorized by diagnosis, age, and duration of infertility): "What is our chance of conceiving in a cycle of treatment, or if we keep going with treatment, what is our chance after two, or three, or more cycles?"; alternatively, "...after 6 months or a year or 2 years following an operation?"

Time-specific prognosis is of key practical importance to patients. Their expectations need to be measured in terms of months or at the most 1 to 2 years. A chance of success amounting to 10%, 20%, or 30% in the course of the next two years offers no realistic hope to a couple who have been trying to conceive for some years already. Even a greater chance may seem hopeless to a woman who is already in her late 30s.

Measuring effectiveness of treatments

Most "infertile" couples are really subfertile and have a chance of conceiving naturally without treatment. Therefore, controlled prospective studies are needed to assess the true benefits of many treatments. When tested in this way, some treatments that were in common use have been found to be of no benefit for fertility, such as hormonal suppression of endometriosis. In some cases, randomized studies are inappropriate because the condition is severe and treatments are obviously effective, such as ovulation induction methods in women with amenorrhea. However, in such cases, results can be compared with a common standard, namely normal rates of natural conception.

Normal fertility rates

In populations of proven fertility, the peak conception rate per cycle is about 33% in the first month of trying, but it falls quickly, settling to about 5%. The average is 20 to 25% per cycle, and expectations of any fertility treatment must be judged against that; however, less effective treatments may be acceptable if simple and inexpensive. Cumulative normal pregnancy rates amount to 90% after 1 year and 95% after 2 years (as illustrated for comparison in many of the following figures describing cumulative pregnancy rates in different causes of infertility). In other words, 5 to 10% of normal fertile couples take more than a year or two to conceive, and some may therefore present with a complaint of infertility, though investigations would show that they require no treatment. Because 90% of normal couples conceive within 1 year, a delay of more than 1 year is the usual criterion employed to define infertility, or strictly, subfertility.

Choosing treatment: a balance of factors

In couples with subfertility, the choice of treatment depends on a balance of known factors: the chance of pregnancy without treatment; or the chance with simple but only modestly effective treatment; or with more successful but more complex and costly treatment; and other factors having an important effect on prognosis must be taken into account, such as the duration of infertility and the woman's age.

There is only sufficient space to consider the more common causes of infertility in graphic detail. Cumulative pregnancy rates presented graphically are easy to interpret and useful to show patients, who understand them very well (see following figures).

Causes and treatments of infertility

The causes of infertility and their relative frequencies are listed in Table 48.1. They add up to more than 100% because some couples have more than one cause. In primary infertility, endometriosis and sperm disorders are relatively more frequent (because they are usually present from the start), whereas in secondary infertility tubal infective damage is more frequent (because that is acquired, sometimes due to complications of childbirth, miscarriage, or termination of pregnancy).

Spurious causes Other "causes" are often cited that are spurious, that is, apparent abnormalities that controlled studies have shown do not reduce fertility or have shown that corrective treatments do not improve it. These include: intermittent "luteal deficiency", hyperprolactinemia in ovulating women, endometrial polyps, minor endometrial adhesions (common after normal pregnancy), endotubal (cornual) polyps, and fibroids (at least in most cases).

OVULATION FAILURE

Ovulatory disorders in women with normal menstrual cycles rarely occur persistently enough to cause prolonged infertility. Any changes in circulating steroid patterns that can be linked to differences in outcome are too subtle for routine investigation and offer no specific effective treatment.

Amenorrhea and oligomenorrhea are the only clear indications of ovulatory failure and, after excluding primary ovarian failure, the patients are very successfully treated, as illustrated in Figure 48.1. Women with amenorrhea can be promised a chance of conception that is as good as normal, though they may require several cycles of treatment to achieve success. The results in women with oligomenorrhea are slightly below normal, which seems to be primarily because of the greater subtlety of disorder associated with polycystic ovarian (PCO) disease. PCO disease accounts for most cases of oligomenorrhea, and about one-third of those with amenorrhea, often without other features of the classical PCO syndrome.

The causes, diagnosis, and treatment of ovulation failure are discussed elsewhere in this book. All that needs to be emphasized here is that the chance of conception in each cycle of treatment is about 20%, ranging from 15 to 25% depending on the efficiency of each treatment, and on the degree of stimulation (multiple ovulation) if gonadotropins are used. Although those rates are equivalent to normal, treatment may have to be repeated for many cycles in order to build up a high cumulative chance for some patients.

To have the confidence to encourage such persistence requires confidence in the accuracy of diagnosis and choice of treatment, and in the reliability of the criteria used for ovulation in response to treatment. It also requires attention to other fertility factors that may adversely affect the chance of conception despite successful induction of ovulation.

Table 48.1 Causes of infertility and their approximate frequencies (from several sources)

Main causes

Sperm defects or dysfunction	30%
including spermatogenic failure	1-2%
seminal antisperm antibodies	5%
varicocele	1-2%
Ovulation failure (amenorrhea or oligomenorrhea)	25%
including primary ovarian failure	1-2%
Tubal infective damage	20%
Unexplained infertility	25%

Other causes

Endometriosis (causing damage)	5%
Coital failure or infrequency	5%
Cervical mucus defects or dysfunction	3%
Uterine abnormalities (e.g., fibroids), rare as a true cause	
Genital tuberculosis, rare in developed countries	
General debilitating illnesses, rare	

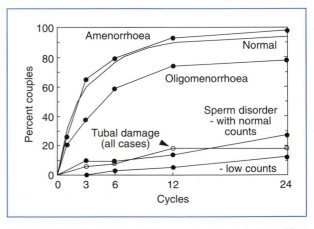

Figure 48.1 Overall cumulative conception rates resulting from treatment of the main causes of infertility, compared with normal rates, excluding the use of donor insemination, assisted conception methods, or reversal of sterilization. (Redrawn with permission from Hull et al. Br Med J 1985;291:1697.)

If ovulation is successfully induced and there is inexplicable failure to conceive after several cycles of treatment, assisted conception methods such as in vitro fertilization (IVF) or gamete intra-fallopian transfer (GIFT) can reasonably be considered. If there is an additional cause of infertility, IVF or intracytoplasmic sperm injection would of course be required. IVF will be used more often to enable control of the number of oocytes or embryos transferred in women who have been very difficult to control against multiple ovulation.

By contrast, IVF with donated oocytes is needed to treat women with primary ovarian failure, and the chance of success is as good as normal.

TUBAL/PELVIC INFECTIVE DAMAGE

Once the fallopian tubes have been damaged by infection, particularly the mucosa, they can never be restored to normal function. The prognosis for pregnancy is generally poor, even after surgery, as the results shown in Figure 48.1 illustrate. These findings are common to all studies of *complete* populations of women with tubal infertility; however, selected sub-groups can do better (as described below).

The most common problem is distal tubal occlusion with hydrosalpinx. Patency is easily restored by surgically opening the distal end and turning it back to form a cuff to maintain patency, but the chance of successful pregnancy is mostly poor. The problem does not usually lie with the limitations of surgery but with irreversible functional damage to the tubal mucosa and fimbriae. Other important prognostic factors are the extent and density of tubal-ovarian adhesions and fibrosis in the tubal wall.

When these various features are taken into combined account, tubal/pelvic infective damage can be graded into several degrees of severity, which provide useful predictive discrimination for the chance of pregnancy, with or without surgery. The results shown in Figure 48.2, in women who have *not* undergone surgery, highlight the marked impairment of fertility even in cases of minor damage, such as flimsy adhesions but otherwise apparently normal tubes.

The results of surgery illustrated in Figure 48.3 demonstrate that substantial benefit is gained from surgery, even in those patients with minor damage. However, it is also clear that surgery can never restore normal function; cumulative pregnancy rates amount to at best 50 to 60% after 2 years. In addition, the cases suitable to benefit from surgery are in the minority. The majority of cases have severe damage and gain little or no benefit from surgery. On the other hand, women with complete bilateral tubal occlusion may see a 10% chance of pregnancy from surgery as a worthwhile benefit, particularly if the alternative of IVF treatment is unaffordable, or they may prefer tubal surgery for psychological reasons as it offers a continuing chance of conceiving naturally and without risk of multiple pregnancy. The main risk is of tubal ectopic pregnancy (10 to 15% of pregnancies), though that is not entirely avoidable by IVF treatment despite direct transfer of embryos to the uterus (5 to 7%).

Clinical findings

It is generally agreed that laparoscopy is the definitive investigation of tubal/pelvic infective damage. It allows for testing of tubal patency as well as assessment of peritubal and periovarian adhesions. It can also conveniently be combined with hysteroscopy to detect intrauterine abnormalities though they are rarely true causes of infertility. The mucosa of the tubal ampulla can also be examined using an additional endoscope at laparoscopy, though not easily.

By contrast, endotubal examination can be simply done by X-ray hysterosalpingography with good prognostic discrimination. Hysterosalpingography is sometimes chosen to provide specific information on the endotubal state only after laparoscopic indication of tubal damage, but it is preferred by others as a preliminary routine assessment of tubal patency at a relatively early stage of investigations, being an out-patient procedure.

Hysterosalpingography can be further refined by transuterine catheterization (through the cervix) of the tubal

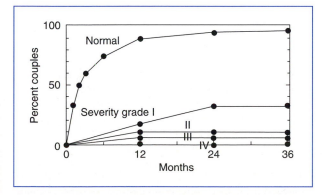

Figure 48.2 Cumulative conception rates with untreated tubal/pelvic infective disease related to disease grading, compared with normal rates. (Redrawn from Wu and Gocial. Int J Fert 1988;33:341, and reprinted with permission from Hull, Hum Reprod 1992; 7:985-96.)

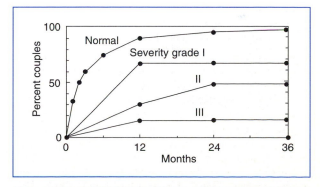

Figure 48.3 Results after surgery for tubal/pelvic infective disease related to grading as in Figure 48.2. The most severe cases (grade IV) were not treated surgically.

openings to check patency of each tube ("selective salpin-gography") when standard testing has suggested proximal tubal occlusion. That finding is often due to technical fail-ure, or to inflammatory plugs that can be dislodged by locally directed fluid pressure or a guided wire.

Other methods of tubal assessment that are advocated but are still being appraised include: ultrasound assess-ment of tubal patency by passage of reflective fluid medi-um endoscopy using a flexible fiberoptic system through the cervix (falloposcopy), or a rigid endoscope passed into the tubal ampulla (tuboscopy) at the time of laparoscopy.

Screening investigations Simple screening methods for likely tubal disease, applicable in primary care at an early stage of infertility, include: (1) *history* of sexually trans-mitted infections or acute pelvic peritonitis ("pelvic inflammatory disease"), complications of pregnancy, abdominal or pelvic surgery (often for appendicitis), and pelvic pain; (2) *examination* findings of pelvic tenderness or masses; and (3) *serology* indicative of past chlamydial infection. Even in the absence of any other clinical fea-tures, a raised chlamydia titre indicates at least a 50% likelihood of finding significant tubal damage, and early referral for specialist investigation is required.

Treatment

Surgery

The methods of surgery now employed are predominantly *laparoscopic*, because severe disease requiring open surgery usually has a poor prognosis. The main indication for *open* surgery is tubal anastomosis using microsurgical techniques to bypass *proximal* tubal occlusion, and similarly for the reversal of sterilization. However, open surgery also remains more successful for *distal* salpingostomy because it is possible to turn back the tube to form a better "cuff".

Proximal occlusion can sometimes be *canalized radi-ographically* by passing a wire and distending catheters under image control, which is used as a therapeutic step after attempting diagnostic selective salpingography.

Reversal of sterilization

Sterilization is not considered a cause of infertility in the usual sense. It is mentioned here only to emphasize the critical importance of infective damage limiting the suc-cess of tubal surgery for infertility. After sterilization, when only a short segment of the tube has been damaged as by a clip method, surgical anastomosis should lead to at least an 80% chance of pregnancy in women under 40 years old. Of course, many women requiring reversal of sterilization are older, but pregnancy rates of about 50% can be expected in women aged 40 to 42. Those rates approach normal rates of conception (qualified by age) and are far greater than can be expected from any tubal surgery undertaken for infective damage.

In vitro fertilization treatment

In the majority of cases of infective tubal damage, IVF and embryo transfer treatment will be needed to achieve pregnancy. Pregnancy rates of 20 to 25% each cycle can be expected, which is similar to the total cumulative chance of natural conception after tubal surgery in severe cases. With IVF treatment, cumulative pregnancy rates of at least 50% can be achieved after 3 to 4 cycles, though these may be spread out for practical and financial rea-sons over 1 or 2 years or more. Much higher rates can be achieved by women who are prepared to persist with treatment, though few are able to do so.

Preliminary tubal surgery?
The risk of tubal ectopic pregnancy is not completely avoided by embryo transfer to the uterine cavity; the rate is 5 to 7% of pregnancies. It seems that embryos can drift into the tubes because of functional damage to the tubal mucosa, which would nor-mally maintain embryo movement towards the uterus by ciliary action. For that reason, salpingectomy or proximal clipping of damaged tubes is sometimes considered prior to IVF treatment, but not usually unless ectopic pregnan-cy has previously occurred.

A greater reason for considering prior salpingectomy or proximal tubal clipping is the marked interference of a hydrosalpinx with the chance of implantation. Pregnancy rates when a hydrosalpinx is present are nearly halved. It seems that intermittent drainage of hydrosalpinx fluid into the uterus, or possibly loss of embryos by drift back into the tube, prevents successful implantation. However, salp-ingectomy is emotionally difficult for a young woman to accept, even though benefit is likely (it is yet to be for-mally proven). Salpingectomy or tubal clipping seems more readily acceptable in women around the age of 40 years because they need to optimize their chance of con-ceiving by IVF as quickly as possible.

ENDOMETRIOSIS

Endometriosis arises mainly by retrograde menstruation along the fallopian tubes, leading to implantation of endometrial tissue on the ovaries and pelvic peritoneum. Endometriosis can induce intense local fibrosis, presum-ably due to cyclical bleeding, leading to dense adhesions and blood-filled cysts, particularly involving the ovaries. Tubal function may be affected by restrictive adhesions, but the tubal mucosa usually remains unaffected and func-tionally favorable. Ovulation also continues normally. The main problem for conception is interference with oocyte release and access to the tubal fimbriae.

In most cases, however, endometriosis remains superfi-cial and causes no structural damage, apart perhaps from subperitoneal fibrosis. Nevertheless, fertility is moderate-ly impaired through several evident mechanisms, includ-ing subtle functional impairments of the granulosa cells and oocyte, and local peritoneal prostaglandin release and immune reactions, which possibly affect oocyte passage and pick-up and sperm function.

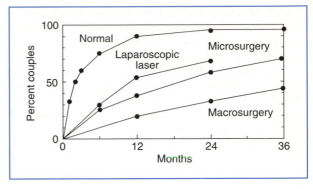

Endometriosis has been classified in complicated ways, but the critical distinguishing prognostic features are adhesions and cysts, particularly if the ovaries are involved even to an apparently slight extent. When endometriosis is classified on that simple basis, the prospects for natural conception without treatment are clearly distinguished, as shown in Figure 48.4. Severe endometriosis obviously demands treatment for infertility without delay.

Clinical findings

Severity of the disease does not correlate well with symptoms, typically pain, and tubal occlusion that might be easily detected radiographically is seldom a feature. Therefore, laparoscopy is needed even in the absence of suggestive symptoms after more than 2 years of failure to conceive.

Treatment

When there is structural damage – adhesions and cysts – surgical correction is the definitive method of treatment if technically possible. Hormonal treatment that suppresses endometriotic activity is only sometimes useful to facilitate surgery. If surgery is feasible, moderately successful results are possible (Fig. 48.5), particularly using modern methods of open microsurgery or laparoscopy. Pregnancy rates remain well below normal but amount to 50 to 60% after 2 years, and they appear to continue to accumulate presumably because of the healthy state of the tubal mucosa. However, after a year, or if corrective surgery was not possible, assisted conception methods must be considered.

In cases of superficial ("minor") endometriosis, the choice of treatment is not so clear as there is a modest chance of conceiving naturally without treatment (Fig. 48.4). Hormonal suppression, the old standard, now has no place. It has been clearly shown to lead to no improvement

Figure 48.5 Cumulative conception rates in severe endometriosis, related to the type of surgery when possible, collated and presented as in Figure 48.4, from the same review source.

in conception rates after stopping treatment, and it carries the disadvantages of unpleasant side effects and of preventing any chance of pregnancy during treatment. In effect, it reduces the chance of success. By contrast, there is now some evidence that destruction of superficial endometriosis, which can be done simply at the time of diagnostic laparoscopy, may improve the chance of conception, though only slightly. Benefit is presumably gained from prevention of the local release by active endometriosis of interfering factors (so-called "peritoneal factors").

If surgical treatment of either minor or severe endometriosis fails to achieve pregnancy within 1 to 2 years, it is then appropriate to consider assisted conception methods of treatment, which offer at least a 25% chance of conception each cycle. In vitro fertilization and embryo transfer are appropriate, but if tubal access is favorable and the mucosa is healthy, as is usual, GIFT is an alternative that seems to offer a better chance of pregnancy than IVF, but it requires laparoscopy.

CERVICAL MUCUS DEFECTS AND DISORDERS

Cervical mucus defects and functional disorders are infrequent causes of infertility (3%) and can be difficult to diagnosis with certainty. Defects are most obvious when they are the result of cervical surgery, particularly conization; this can almost completely remove the mucus-secreting epithelium, including the deep crypts of the lower cervical canal. Otherwise, deficient secretion, acidity, antisperm antibodies, and other, undefined features affecting sperm penetration are often misdiagnosed due to imperfect timing of sample collection before ovulation, coupled with the brief duration of the receptive phase in some individuals or the variation between cycles. To confirm inherent, persistent disorders of mucus function, detailed monitoring of ovulation and the LH surge is usually required in repeated cycles; together with postcoital test-

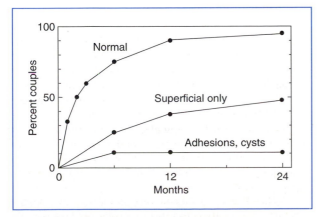

Figure 48.4 Cumulative conception rates with untreated endometriosis related to simplified disease grading, compared with normal rates. (Data collated from several sources and redrawn with permission from Hull, Hum Reprod 1992;7:785-96.)

ing of sperm uptake in vivo, and definitive testing of sperm-mucus penetration in vitro using normal donor mucus and semen samples as controls.

Antisperm antibodies detected in cervical mucus often do not interfere with sperm motility in mucus, and their origin and functional significance then remain obscure. Nor do cervical or vaginal infections seem to interfere with mucus receptivity to sperm, nor does antibiotic treatment seem to offer any benefit.

Deficient secretion due to cervical damage needs to be bypassed by treatments like intrauterine insemination, with or without the added benefit of superovulation, and if necessary by IVF or GIFT. If deficient secretion by an undamaged cervix can be shown to respond to increased stimulation using exogenous estrogen, leading to demonstrable receptivity to sperm, gonadotropin therapy can then be used in order to induce not only multiple ovulation but associated increased estrogen secretion to stimulate the mucus. Results of the treatments described are too few to have proven benefit since cervical mucus defects are uncommon, but they appear to be moderately successful.

Mucus acidity is also an uncommon problem, but it can often be corrected simply by douching with bicarbonate solution, and there is some evidence of benefit for conception. The diagnosis is less simple, however, because cervical mucus is often acidic if mistimed. Acidity (pH <5.5) must be demonstrated in several cycles when the mucus is fully developed. For treatment, the woman douches herself an hour or more before intercourse using a 50 mmolar bicarbonate solution, which she can prepare by dissolving domestic $NaHCO_3$ 1g (a level teaspoonful) in 250 ml warm tap water.

SPERM DISORDERS

The diagnosis and treatment of sperm disorders are discussed in detail elsewhere in this book (Chap. 41). They are discussed in the present context of female infertility, partly because standard semen microscopy is of such limited prognostic value in contrast to tests of function, and because testing functional ability by penetration of cervical mucus usually employs the partner's mucus in the first place. Testing cervical mucus penetration may be done in vitro or in vivo (postcoital testing).

Figure 48.1 shows cumulative pregnancy rates in men with sperm dysfunction detected by negative postcoital test results, according to whether seminal sperm counts were normal or subnormal. The prognosis for natural conception is almost equally poor, and it is clear that treatment is needed at an early stage when a diagnosis of sperm disorder has been definitely made. The most successful method of treatment is by IVF, employing intracytoplasmic sperm injection to achieve fertilization; this method involves the woman in the procedures of ovarian stimulation and monitoring, surgical oocyte collection, and embryo transfer. A much simpler alternative for the woman is donor insemination, but this involves great emotional and ethical issues for the couple.

Sperm-cervical mucus testing

Sperm-mucus interaction provides a biological and clinical interface between male and female infertility. The various methods employed have all been shown to provide valuable prognostic discrimination for either natural conception or in vitro fertilization. However, there is considerable overlap between tests of sperm-mucus interaction and independent tests of sperm function, leaving much room for different choices in practice.

Disorders of sperm function are the most common cause of impaired sperm-mucus interaction. Therefore, some specialists prefer to ignore the relatively small likelihood of a diagnosis of mucus dysfunction and instead concentrate assessment on the sperm independently. This is a legitimate and logical preference, however there also exists remarkable polarization of views about sperm-mucus testing, particularly the postcoital test. There are some who believe it has no prognostic value and is an unnecessary and stressful intrusion, or that it is difficult to time properly and requires a daily service. Others find it easy in practice, and there are sound data demonstrating strong prognostic discrimination, furthermore overriding the prognostic value of standard semen microscopy. The application and value of sperm-mucus testing needs to be clarified.

Types of tests, in vivo (postcoital testing) and in vitro In vivo testing by postcoital testing is only a screening test for several possible disorders: coital and ejaculatory competence, vaginal factors such as acidity, cervical mucus receptivity, and disorders of sperm function that are the commonest causes of failure.

In vitro testing offers the advantage of a definitive distinction between sperm and mucus dysfunction by inclusion of normal donor samples as controls ("crossed penetration testing"). Methods include measurement of distance penetrated by sperm into mucus within capillary columns or on a microscope slide; and qualitative assessments of behavior at the semen mucus interface that can reliably distinguish inherent sperm dysfunction from the effect of seminal antisperm antibodies, irrespective of seminal sperm "counts".

To be valid, mucus must be appropriately timed just before ovulation (which can be simply done when the woman recognizes her own mucus surge), and an appropriate criterion of sperm measurement must be used. The original World Health Organization criterion for the postcoital test of ten progressively motile sperm per high power microscopy field was arbitrary and based on no outcome analysis. It is now clear that the critical requirement is only one progressive sperm/hpf. There are several prospective studies demonstrating the prognostic discriminant power of sperm-mucus tests both in vitro and by the postcoital test.

If all adverse fertility factors including the woman's age are specifically controlled by exclusion, however, the predictive power of the postcoital test can be critically affected by the duration of infertility (Fig. 48.6). The negative postcoital test group primarily represents sperm dysfunction, and in couples with such a distinct cause of

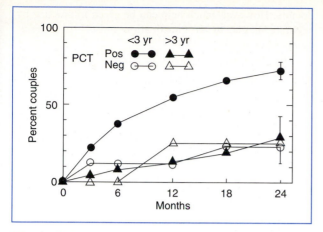

Figure 48.6 Cumulative conception rates in untreated infertile couples with normal ovulation, tubal state, and semen microscopy, related to their postcoital test (PCT) result and duration of infertility. Those with a positive PCT (closed symbols) have fully defined unexplained infertility. Those with negative PCTs (open symbols) are mostly due to sperm dysfunction. The prognosis in unexplained infertility is strongly affected by duration, unlike defined causes such as sperm dysfunction. (Data collated from Hull et al. Br Med J 1985;291:1697; Glazener et al. Hum Reprod 1987;2:665-71.)

infertility, duration of infertility has no importance. By contrast, the positive postcoital test group represents unexplained infertility, as all other factors were also favorable, and couples with a duration of less than 3 years had a much improved chance of natural conception; those with prolonged, unexplained infertility of more than 3 years duration had no better chance of natural conception than the couples with sperm dysfunction.

Thus the postcoital test is of prognostic discriminant value for natural conception only in couples with a relatively short duration of infertility. Those of long duration, whether with normal or defective sperm function, must all consider assisted conception treatment. However, the success and choice of IVF or GIFT on the one hand, or intracytoplasmic sperm injection on the other, is critically dependent on the assessment of sperm function. Therefore, the postcoital test or other sperm-mucus testing is of prognostic value for in vitro fertilization though not for natural conception in couples with prolonged infertility. The as yet undefined causes of failure to conceive naturally in couples with prolonged unexplained infertility are clearly not related to sperm-mucus interaction.

UTERINE ABNORMALITIES

There remains no clear evidence that non-occlusive uterine abnormalities of any sort cause infertility, nor that surgical treatment improves the chance of conception.

Congenital uterine abnormalities, including the effects of fetal exposure to maternal diethylstilbestrol, are of doubtful relevance for conception (except for rare occlusive types) or miscarriage, though some may be associated with later obstetric problems. Surgical correction is mostly of unproven benefit even if possible. Hysteroscopic resection of a septum is often done because it seems to be safe, but its value in the treatment of infertility remains speculative and should not be allowed to divert attention from more likely causes.

Small endometrial polyps, tubocornual polyps, and minor endometrial adhesions appear to be of no importance. Severe endometrial adhesions, however, obliterating the cavity and causing amenorrhea or hypomenorrhea (*Asherman's syndrome*) are probably significant and can be treated relatively simply by hysteroscopic dissection.

Myomata (fibroids) are the most common abnormality, but the only evidence that they can interfere with conception comes from IVF studies that demonstrate reduced chances of implantation when fibroids distort the uterine cavity. There is no sound evidence that they interfere with the continuation of pregnancy. Claims of benefit for the chance of natural conception from myomectomy have usually involved additional surgery for incidental conditions, particularly pelvic adhesions. Indeed, myomectomy often *leads* to adhesion formation, and it may therefore cause more harm than benefit to fertility. Myomectomy should therefore be reserved for fibroids that are impinging on the uterine cavity, particularly if they cause significant menorrhagia and anemia.

INFECTIONS

Upper genital tract infection causes infertility in women or men by structural damage, and in men it may induce autoantibodies to sperm. There is no other evidence of past infection or of present organisms detectable in the lower genital tract causing functional interference with conception or risk of miscarriage.

Ascending infection in women, due to sexual transmission or postabortal or puerperal sepsis, is particularly damaging due to the destruction of the tubal mucosa and fimbriae. Tuberculosis can cause the most severe damage but is rare in developed countries; it is most likely found in immigrants from countries where tuberculosis is common. By contrast, intra-abdominal infections due to appendicitis or following surgery cause mainly peritubal and periovarian adhesions with relative sparing of the tubal mucosa, which offers better prognosis for fertility, though the fimbriae may be destroyed.

In developed countries, *Chlamydia trachomatis* accounts for more than half of the cases of infective tubal/pelvic damage, often indicated only by serological evidence without any obvious episode of pelvic sepsis. An episode of acute pelvic infection leads to infertility in 10 to 15% of cases, and every additional episode doubles the risk. Among those who conceive, the risk of ectopic pregnancy is increased five- to tenfold. Early diagnosis and antibiotic treatment, appropriately selected to act effectively against both chlamydial and gonococcal infections, can reduce the risks of infertility and ectopic pregnancy by two-thirds.

Women with asymptomatic *C. trachomatis* in their lower genital tract have a risk of developing acute pelvic sepsis in up to 30% of cases. Screening for the organism in both the women (in a cervical swab and first-fraction early-morning urine sample) and their partners (in urine), and eradication by treatment, can halve the incidence of acute pelvic sepsis during the next year.

Thus primary care physicians as well as hospital-based specialists have a valuable role in the prevention of tubal infertility by early diagnosis and treatment of pelvic sepsis and appendicitis in young women and girls, and possibly in population screening for *C. trachomatis*.

IMMUNOLOGICAL DISORDERS

There are only two autoimmune disorders that can be clearly defined as causes of infertility: autoimmune ovarian failure and antisperm antibodies secreted into seminal plasma.

In *autoimmune ovarian failure*, antibodies bound to the follicle cells block the effect of gonadotropins. Follicles are not depleted, but the condition presents with the classic indices of ovarian failure – amenorrhea and postmenopausal levels of FSH – along with serological evidence of the antibodies, sometimes linked to polyglandular autoimmune failures.

Antisperm antibodies in blood correlate poorly with the locally secreted antibodies which cause dysfunction; testing for them on blood is of no clinical value. Antisperm antibodies in cervical mucus are seldom significant. By contrast, antisperm antibodies in semen are much more likely to by important. Nevertheless, they vary in type and site of attachment (e.g., sperm head or tail tip), and their functional relevance must be demonstrated: by sperm agglutination in semen, or attachment to the cervical mucus protein mesh preventing penetration. These disturbances are associated with impaired fertilizing ability that is demonstrable in vitro (see Chapter 41).

While antiovarian and antisperm antibody levels in the circulation can be suppressed by glucocorticoids, there is little or no benefit for fertility, presumably due to continuing high affinity of remaining antibody at the binding sites.

In conclusion, autoantibody screening in the investigation of infertility offers no defined diagnostic or prognostic value, or any therapeutic potential. There is an indication for specific testing only in women with ovarian failure or men with evident sperm dysfunction. A case can be made for routine testing for antisperm antibodies in seminal plasma, though in this author's view, the functional relevance of an abnormal result still needs to be tested by cervical mucus penetration.

UNEXPLAINED INFERTILITY

The elusive problem of unexplained infertility can cause extreme anguish to patients and extreme frustration to doctors. However, much help can be given in practice by accurate diagnostic prognostication and effective treatments when needed.

A diagnosis of unexplained infertility implies that critical investigations of all the key functions required for conception are normal. The definitive criteria have been discussed in the section on applied physiology. However, the diagnostic methods and criteria used in practice vary. They usually include midluteal serum progesterone in several cycles to assess ovulation, laparoscopy to detect tubal/pelvic infective damage or endometriosis, and semen microscopy to determine sperm concentration and the proportions that appear to be normal and motile (the traditional "sperm counts"). To this should be added the history of coital frequency (at least twice per week is required).

More importantly in this author's view, there should be assessment of sperm function (which is not adequately indicated simply by the numbers and proportion motile in semen), and preferably of sperm-cervical mucus interaction. Figure 48.6 shows that the prognosis for natural conception is poor if the postcoital test is negative, even if seminal sperm counts are normal. Figure 48.6 also shows that with a negative postcoital test, the prognosis remains poor, even if the duration of infertility is relatively short. By contrast, if the postcoital test is positive, irrespective of seminal sperm counts, the prognosis is favorable, at least in couples with a relatively short duration of infertility. However, in couples with prolonged infertility, the postcoital test remains prognostically useful for in vitro fertilization, indicating IVF and GIFT would be valuable therapeutic options.

By contrast, it has been shown that in the absence of any test of sperm function in couples with otherwise unexplained infertility of prolonged duration, fertilizing ability is seriously impaired in one-third.

No other investigations or apparent abnormalities (see the list of spurious causes after Table 48.1) have been shown to be of any prognostic significance and can therefore be ignored in the definition of unexplained infertility.

Duration less than three years

Figure 48.6 illustrates that couples with relatively short duration of unexplained infertility are essentially normal. They have simply been unlucky so far and are very likely to conceive without therapeutic intervention. There are no effective treatments to improve the chance of natural conception, and there is no need for methods of assisted conception. What is needed is careful explanation to the couple of the functional meaning of the findings and their chance of conceiving, and encouragement to keep trying.

Duration greater than three years

There is of course a progressive decline in the cumulative chance of natural conception with increasing duration of unexplained infertility, but the most important reduction in practice is seen after 3 years. The results shown in Figure 48.6 have therefore been divided at that point for simplicity and clarity. After 3 years, the chance of natural conception falls to unhopeful levels, equivalent to 1 to 2% each month, and treatment is needed.

The best explanation that can be offered for severe subfertility as a couple, despite all tests of function being within the normal range, is probably a compounding effect of suboptimal fecundability affecting both partners. The normal chance of conception each cycle has a wide range, with a lower limit of 5%. One partner with high fecundability could overcome low-normal fecundability in the other, but if *both* are of low-normal fecundability, it seems likely there would be a combined effect reducing their fecundability as a couple to the level of only 1 to 2% that is observed.

The potentially good news, however, is that the key elements required to achieve conception – oocyte and sperm production, fertilizing ability, and implanting ability – are usually favorable and can be employed effectively to assist conception if necessary.

Treatment

In the treatment of prolonged unexplained infertility, controlled trials of clomiphene to boost ovulation have shown only a slight benefit (cycle pregnancy rates of 4 to 5%). More powerful superovulation using gonadotropins, or treatment by IUI (intra-uterine insemination of specially prepared sperm), each achieve pregnancy rates of up to 10% each cycle. However, a combination of superovulation using gonadotropins with intrauterine insemination can achieve pregnancy rates of 10 to 25% each cycle. The large variation is apparently due to the degree to which the ovaries are stimulated. The higher rates appear to be achievable only with incautious overstimulation, which risks high-order multiple pregnancy. When intrauterine insemination is combined with cautious ovarian stimulation, success rates are usually around 15% per cycle. By contrast, IVF or GIFT treatment offers pregnancy rates of at least 25% each cycle, even when the number of embryos or oocytes transferred is limited to a maximum of three.

INCIDENTAL FACTORS AFFECTING FERTILITY

While specific causes of infertility may be defined, and effective treatments, either specific or empirical, are available, it needs to be recognized that the prognosis for conception and birth is often greatly affected by incidental factors, which are often uncorrectable: age of the woman (and of the man to a much smaller degree), ovarian aging (raised basal FSH), fatness of the woman (and fat distribution), cigarette smoking (and probably passive smoking) and other social drugs, duration of infertility (independent of age), previous pregnancy (secondary versus primary infertility), and increased risk of pregnancy failure.

Age of the woman

Fertility declines slowly after 30 years of age, with the fall accelerating around 37 to 38 years and sharply after 40 years. Only two-thirds of women aged 35 to 39 years will have a baby, and only one-third of those first trying to conceive at 40 to 44 years. The overriding importance of the woman's age was first demonstrated by results of donor insemination treatment, which controls for any effects of the man's age and coital frequency. All fertility treatments are affected in the same way.

Fertility, of course, depends on the duration of exposure and fecundability (per cycle). The age-related decline in fecundability is due to declining oocyte quality affecting implanting ability and the risk of miscarriage, and therefore it affects the potential success of fertility treatments, as it does the chance of natural conception. The decline is well-represented by the pregnancy and birth rates achieved per cycle of IVF treatment (Fig. 48.7). There is a greater decline in birth rates than pregnancy rates with age due to the marked rise in miscarriage rates. Compared with women under 30 years old, the chance of having a baby per cycle of treatment is reduced soon after 40 years by more than half, and at 44 to 45 years by 90%.

Thus it is clear that women who are infertile after the age of 35 years have no time to lose. They deserve relatively early investigations and treatment. After the age of 40 years, their first choice of treatment should be the most effective method, usually IVF or GIFT, though specific favorable choices are reversal of sterilization and ovulation induction in cases of oligo-amenorrhea not due to ovarian failure. There is no time to be wasted on less effective, speculative methods. However, alternatives are not necessarily mutually exclusive. Combinations may be appropriate: for example, tubal surgery followed very soon and as often as possible by IVF could offer a chance, though small, of natural conception between cycles of IVF.

Ovarian aging

As previously discussed, the basal serum FSH level is an index of ovarian follicular capacity (or "reserve") and

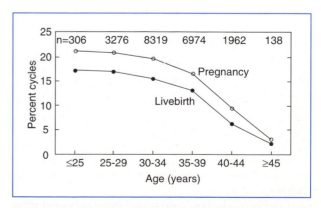

Figure 48.7 Clinical pregnancy and livebirth rates by IVF treatment per started cycle related to the woman's age. Complete United Kingdom national data for 1993, maximum of three embryos transferred by law. (From 4th Annual Report by HFEA, London E1 7LS, UK, 1995.)

indirectly of associated oocyte quality. Young women with a raised FSH level, though still ovulating, have reduced implanting ability of their fertilized oocytes comparable to women over 40 years old. Their prognosis for natural conception, as by IVF, is equally poor. FSH measurement is therefore a valuable routine investigation.

The basal serum FSH level (measured between days 1 and 5 of a cycle) is normally constant between cycles, but it becomes increasingly variable as levels rise. Therefore FSH needs to be measured in two or preferably three cycles, and it is the highest level that is prognostic. Attempts have been made to refine the diagnostic accuracy of FSH measurement by dynamic tests, but in this author's view, simple measurement of the basal level in several cycles is the best choice at present.

Fatness of the woman

Population studies show that only extremes of weight loss or obesity affect a woman's fertility, and then usually by obvious interference with menstrual cyclicity. Between those extremes, the distribution of fatness may also be relevant, with women with central obesity ("apple shaped") being at a disadvantage compared to women who accumulate fat around their hips ("pear shaped"); however, the difference is small. Fatness should not affect the management of infertility except in the specific treatment of associated ovulation failure.

Cigarette smoking and other social drug usage

Population studies show that fecundability (per cycle) is reduced in smokers, but in general their cumulative rates of pregnancy catch up with nonsmokers, though taking longer. In the treatment of infertility it is more relevant to take into account cycle fecundability. In the general population, the chance of natural conception per cycle is reduced by about 30% (proportionately), and this reduction is matched in fertility treatments such as IVF.

The effect is mainly due to smoking by the woman. Smoking products reach the oocyte via follicular fluid and appear to reduce fertilization, cleavage and implantation, and increase the risk of miscarriage. Smoking by the man has no clearly defined effect, but there is growing evidence of indirect effect via the woman due to passive smoking, including exposure in the workplace. Therefore in treating infertility, both partners should be strongly advised to stop smoking and the woman to minimize exposure to others smoking at work, if possible. Furthermore, the advice should be extended into pregnancy to minimize the risk of loss at that stage (see below).

Effects of alcohol, caffeinated beverages, and other recreational drugs are unclear. Population studies tend to suggest adverse effects of "excessive" usage, therefore infertile couples are usually advised on moderation.

Duration of infertility

In general the duration of infertility significantly affects the chance of natural conception, but its effect is critical on the prognosis for natural conception in cases of unexplained infertility or minor endometriosis (in which the mechanisms of infertility are largely unexplained), as discussed earlier. It is therefore a key determinant of the choice of treatment in those conditions. It also has an effect on treatment success rates, but to a much smaller extent and does not discourage treatment.

Previous pregnancy

Secondary infertility is more likely to be due to tubal/pelvic infective damage, and primary infertility to endometriosis or sperm disorders, but both primary and secondary infertility share all possible causes. A history of a previous pregnancy therefore does not help in reaching a diagnosis. It does indicate a significantly better prognosis for conception, both naturally and by treatment, but the differences are only slight. Thus, a history of previous pregnancy should be included in any audit for strictly comparative purposes but does not affect the choice of treatment.

Increased risk of pregnancy failure

The real goal for an infertile couple is to have a baby, indeed a healthy baby, not merely to conceive. In the treatment of infertility there is a tendency to not think beyond the achievement of pregnancy as the index of success. Yet a major contribution to failure, and an especially cruel blow to a couple after trying so long, is miscarriage of pregnancy or loss of their baby at a later stage. Furthermore, multiple pregnancy resulting from some fertility treatments involves increased risks of permanent cerebral damage in surviving premature babies.

In previously infertile women, the risk of miscarriage, even after conceiving naturally, is approximately doubled (from about 12% to 20-25%). This may be due mainly to the contribution of cases of subclinical as well as overt polycystic ovarian disease, associated with hypersecretion of LH or androgens, amongst whom the miscarriage rate is about 40%. In such cases, the risk might be reduced when gonadotropin therapy is required by combination with preliminary pituitary desensitization to suppress LH levels.

The woman's age is another major factor; by the time women reach IVF treatment, about half are over 35 years old. The risk of miscarriage increases exponentially, most notably from about 37 to 38 years. After 40 years the risk is increased threefold and seems to be higher in those women treated for infertility (33 to 50%). There is nothing that can be done about that of course, except to minimize the risk by avoiding earlier delays in infertility treatment. It is also increasingly important to give the prognosis of fertility treatment in terms of the chances of a baby, not merely conception. Obstetric risks later in pregnancy are increased but remain low and do not affect treatment decisions in older women, though they need to be discussed as they normally would be, including the genetic/chromosomal risks for the baby.

Risks of late fetal loss or damaged survival are mainly due to multiple pregnancy that results from uncontrolled gonadotropin therapy to induce ovulation or from unlimited transfer of embryos after IVF (or oocytes by GIFT). The risks, and the costs of care, double with each additional baby. Though selective reduction of multiple pregnancies can be done by destroying individual fetuses, most societies would prefer to avoid high-order multiple pregnancies (triplet or greater) in the first place. However, the choice of number of embryos to transfer after IVF depends on a difficult balance of probabilities, particularly in older women.

ORGANIZATION OF INFERTILITY PRACTICE IN PRIMARY CARE

While technical advances in diagnosis and treatment of infertility have become more complex, advancing knowl-

edge and evaluation of clinical methods has helped to clarify, reduce, and simplify the choices to be made in practice. Following the discussions of basic physiology and clinical findings in the first two parts of this chapter, it is now possible to develop a rational scheme of care in a summarized manner (Tab. 48.2). In addition, there need to be clear objectives in practice at each level of care: primary, secondary, and tertiary. In the present context, only primary care and the indications for referral to specialist care will be described.

Primary treatment

The only effective treatment suitable in primary care is clomiphene therapy to induce ovulation in women with oligo-amenorrhea. Likely responders are those with a presumptive diagnosis of polycystic ovarian disease (with or without obesity or hirsutism), indicated by normal FSH and prolactin levels and evidence of estrogenization (indicating ovarian activity, though disordered, and pituitary drive), which is demonstrated by a normal menstrual response after a short course of progestogen (e.g., oral medroxyprogesterone acetate 5 or 10 mg daily for 5 days) (see Chapter 46).

Following an interval of 7 days after the course of progestogen, clomiphene is given 50 to 100 mg daily for 5 days, and the response is checked by basal temperature charting and serum progesterone measurement during the temperature high-phase. If there is no response, clomiphene treatment should be repeated after 6 weeks

---

Table 48.2 Rational scheme of primary care of infertility

Clinical objectives

To assist couples with relatively short-term infertility (6-12 months) by:
Screening, using simple methods, for a likely cause; to indicate a need for early specialist referral
Information, through illustrated literature and practical advice (see below); to help the couple feel in control, autonomous
Promotion of pre-pregnancy health through Rubella immunity and advice on diet and for both partners to stop smoking

Investigations

Preliminary	Rubella serology
Ovulation	Menstrual cycle (normal or oligo-amenorrhea)
Tubal/pelvic disease	History of abdomino-pelvic infection, surgery, pain, intrauterine contraceptive device complications, abortion or obstetric complications, and menstrual excess or pain
	Examination finding of pelvic tenderness or tumor
	Chlamydia serology
Coital	History: penetration, ejaculation, as well as frequency; and if infrequent, what method of timing if any, and could it be wrong (see advice below)?
Semen assessment	Microscopy: sperm concentration, motility, morphology
	Antisperm antibody test

Primary advice

Chance nature of conception and normal rates
Timing of coitus: *before* ovulation, *don't* "save it up", *don't* use temperature charting, *do* use the mucus surge
Preovulatory cervical mucus surge recognition: copious, slippery, stretchy, for about 2 days
Stop smoking, both partners
Pre-pregnancy health: rubella immunization, diet, folate supplementation

---

Table 48.3 Indications for specialist referral

General

Duration of infertility more than 1-2 yr
Woman's age more than 35-40 yr: duration infertility more than 6-12 months

Oligo-amenorrhea

Raised FSH or prolactin
Failure to respond to or conceive by clomiphene treatment (see text)

Tubal/pelvic disease likely

History or pelvic examination abnormal
Chlamydia serology abnormal

Coital failure (rare)

Impotence
Ejaculatory failure

Semen defects

Severe (azoospermia or severe oligospermia, i.e., <5 million/ml)
Moderate oligospermia: refer, or arrange definitive sperm function testing if service available in specialist laboratory
Antisperm antibodies: refer, or arrange definitive testing of sperm-cervical mucus penetration if service available in specialist laboratory

for at least three attempts before concluding complete lack of responsiveness. If responsive, clomiphene can be repeated for six cycles before considering the need for specialist investigation of other fertility factors or other treatment (Tab. 48.3).

Collaborative care

Coordination of care by effective collaboration between primary care and specialist centers is an important practical aim. Specialists should be best able to provide guidelines for primary care that are up to date and coordinated with their own practice, and they should be able to offer access to the same laboratory services to ensure reliability of findings. Patients are deeply resentful of the duplication of investigations that should be avoidable when referred for specialist care, or from a secondary to a tertiary care center. Seminology services in particular can be highly variable and should only be provided by laboratories associated with specialist infertility centers, preferably tertiary centers.

Suggested readings

HILLIER SG, KITCHENER HC, NEILSON JP (eds). Scientific essentials of reproductive medicine. London: WB Saunders, 1996.

HULL MGR. Managed care of infertility. Current Opinion Obstet Gynecol, 1996;8:305-13.

HULL MGR. Fertility treatment options in women over 40 years old. In: RA Lobo (ed). Perimenopause. New York: Springer, 1997;287-307.

HULL MGR, FLEMING CF. Tubal surgery versus assisted reproduction: assessing their role in infertility therapy. Current Opinion Obstet Gynecol 1995;7:160-7.

SNICK HKA, SNICK TS, EVERS JLH, COLLINS JA. The spontaneous pregnancy prognosis in untreated subfertile couples: the Walcheren primary care study. Hum Reprod 1997;12:1582-8.

Complaints and diseases of the climacteric and postmenopausal period

Peter Kenemans

▰ KEY POINTS ▰

- Menopause is the point in time of a woman's last menstrual period.
- The climacteric is the period of transition around menopause characterized by a change in menstrual cycle pattern and typical complaints such as hot flushes, night sweats, and symptoms of urogenital atrophy.
- Osteoporosis and cardiovascular disease are, and Alzheimer's disease may be, menopause-related diseases.
- Estrogen replacement therapy has a beneficial effect on climacteric symptoms as well as on menopause-related diseases and should be prescribed continuously. It must be combined with progesterone or a progestogen unless the uterus has been removed.
- The daily progestogen dosage should be as low as possible but sufficiently high to prevent endometrial pathology. A nonandrogenic progestogen is preferred.
- Hormone replacement therapy should be started with the combined estrogen/progestogen-phase to avoid unexpected bleeding at the start of treatment, unless an ultrasound scan has shown the endometrium to be thinner than 5 mm (double-layer thickness).

Menopause is the point in time of a woman's last menstrual period. The median age at menopause is 51 years. The term menopause is also used in reference to the whole period of life after the point of menopause.

The climacteric is the period of transition around the menopause that begins with a time period in which marked menstrual cycle irregularity occurs, often accompanied by hot flashes and night sweats, which can still be present years after amenorrhea has occurred. During this time, signs and symptoms of urogenital atrophy and other more atypical complaints become apparent. A feeling of lack of well-being can also be present, in addition to depressive mood changes, joint and muscle pains, and signs of epithelial atrophy of the skin, mouth, and eyes.

Postmenopause is that period of a woman's life that follows the last menstruation. This part of her life will extend, for most women in Western society, for more than three decades. In the first decade of postmenopause, symptoms are climacteric in nature and related to the vasomotor and urogenital systems. There may also be conditions that are more psychosocially determined. After 60, many women will experience a variety of health problems and diseases that are related to the process of aging. Some of these diseases and conditions can also be linked to menopause. Osteoporosis and cardiovascular disease are prominent among these diseases. Early menopause has been shown to be a risk factor for both diseases. On the other hand, postmenopausal supplementation with estrogens has been shown to decrease the risk for both osteoporotic fractures and myocardial infarction. Therefore, these diseases will be discussed in this chapter as menopause-related diseases. Other diseases that have been shown to have a possible relation to the postmenopausal status of relative estrogen deficiency as well as estrogen supplementation will also be discussed, which include dementia due to Alzheimer's disease and cancer of the breast, endometrium, and colon.

Hormone replacement therapy (HRT) can be defined as perimenopausal and postmenopausal medication with estrogens or a combination of estrogens and progestogens (or any other sex steroid-like substance) for the treatment of climacteric symptoms and for the prevention of menopause-related diseases such as osteoporosis and cardiovascular disease. Indications for symptomatic HRT are vasomotor instability, urogenital atrophy, and perimenopausal cycle disorders. Preventive HRT should be considered seriously in women with a premature menopause (as a result of surgery, chemotherapy, radiation therapy, or premature ovarian failure) and in women who have an established increased risk of cardiovascular disease or osteoporosis.

Despite the well-documented advantages of HRT in women with an indication for preventive HRT, patient compliance is poor, with discontinuation of use frequently occurring long before the long-term benefits of HRT could be expected to manifest. For many women an important factor in compliance is the advice given by the general practitioner and the gynecologist; the counseling provided during the initial period of HRT is especially important. Therefore, general practitioners and specialists involved in counseling and monitoring women before and while following HRT should know about the basic rules that apply for HRT in hysterectomized and nonhysterectomized women. Women's general fear related to an increased cancer risk through the use of HRT should be discussed in depth with women contemplating HRT and placed in the overall perspective of potential risks and benefits of HRT.

Clinical findings

The climacteric years are the years in which definite changes take place in a woman's body, linked to the aging process of the ovaries. The first manifestation of this period is usually a change in cycle regularity. Concurrently, the first vasomotor symptoms often occur as well. These physical changes are often accompanied by changes in the family and the social environment, which may have a profound influence on a woman's psychosocial functioning during mid-life.

Perimenopausal cycle disorders

Changes in the menstrual cycle will often first be noticed by many women when they are in their forties. Many will also be confronted by troublesome vaginal bleeding episodes. The principal cause for this lies in the aging process of the ovary, which results in a progressive decline in the number of follicles. During the decade preceding the onset of the menstrual irregularity, a progressive increase in follicle-stimulating hormone (FSH) levels (at cycle day 3) can be observed, which can be interpreted as an early signal that stimulation of follicular growth is becoming more difficult. Menstrual cycles get longer due to inadequate folliculogenesis, resulting in impaired corpus luteum function and inadequate progesterone secretion. Perimenopausal cycle disorders are a common reason for consultation and referral.

At the start of the menopausal transition, about 60% of the cycles are still ovulatory, whereas in the last 6 months preceding menopause, ovulatory progesterone levels are found in only about 5% of cycles. Gradually more and more cycles are characterized by a follicular estradiol secretion that is insufficient to induce a mid-cycle luteinizing hormone (LH) surge, though it is sufficient to stimulate endometrial growth. The endometrium that builds up in this situation lacks the modifying effect of the normal luteal progesterone and disintegrates easily, resulting in vaginal bleeding that can vary from spotting to episodes of very heavy bleeding. Menopause marks the end of menstrual cycle disturbances. When menstruation is defined as endometrial bleeding following ovulation, for many women the last real menstrual period precedes menopause by many months or even years. Although distinct hormonal changes during the menopausal transition are recognized, hormonal markers are unreliable for diagnosis because of large intra-individual variations and also because of their fluctuating nature.

It is important during the perimenopausal period to rule out organic pathological causes for vaginal bleeding, especially those that relate to endometrial hyperplasia or trophoblastic disease. The peak incidence of endometrial hyperplasia is seen in the age group of 40 to 50 years and for endometrial cancer in the age group of 50 to 60 years. After having ruled out organic causes for abnormal vaginal bleeding, the clinician is left with a group of patients with a bleeding pattern that is often called dysfunctional. The management of women with perimenopausal dysfunctional bleeding should be directed at stopping the current bleeding episode and at taking measures aimed at the prevention of recurrence. The choice of treatment is primarily determined by the type of bleeding disorder (anovulatory or ovulatory), the need for contraception, and the presence of other climacteric complaints such as flushes and vaginal dryness.

Vasomotor instability

Sudden spells of sweating during the night may be the first sign of vasomotor instability. The hot flush (also known as hot flash) is the characteristic symptom of the climacteric syndrome. Sometimes an unpleasant sensation, originating in the abdomen or breast, precedes the visible flush. The flush presents as a sudden reddening of the skin on the head, neck, and chest; it is experienced as an explosion of heat lasting 3 to 4 minutes followed by profuse sweating. The heat-loss mechanism appears to be activated despite an apparently normal core body temperature, resulting in peripheral vasodilatation, tachycardia, and a decreased skin resistance.

Incidence, frequency, and severity of climacteric flushing varies widely in and between various cultures worldwide. Some women suffer severe flushes for many years, while others experience none, or only brief mild ones. Flushing starts in most women years before natural menopause, in others years after. After bilateral ovariectomy, flushing is normal and starts within days or weeks after surgery. An earlier onset of flushing is seen in hysterectomized women and in women who smoke cigarettes.

Vasomotor symptoms, usually mild, already occur in four out of ten women aged 40 years and over who have regular menstrual cycles. During the period of irregular menstrual cycles and oligomenorrhea, vasomotor symptoms become more severe and frequent. In a large Dutch study, 85% of women experienced hot flushes at the time of menopause, and 30% described them as severe. Even 10 years after menopause, many women (about 50%) still experienced hot flushes. In industrialized countries, a substantial portion of women will suffer from flushes that persist for 3 years or much longer.

In general, the most severe flushes occur between the moment of the last menstrual bleeding and 3 years thereafter. There are indications that women with severe vasomotor symptoms, that is five or more flushes daily, show the following characteristics: they have several other typical climacteric complaints (such as sexual dryness), they have more severe atypical complaints (such as irritability), and a greater feeling of a lack of well-being, and they may also have accelerated bone loss when compared to women without vasomotor symptoms.

At the present time, there is no theory that explains all aspects of the flush. The flush cannot be related to one specific hormone or the changes therein. Caused by the waning oocyte quality, an increasing hypothalamic gonadotropin-releasing hormone (GnRH) neuron activity could affect the activity of the adjacent neurons in the thermo-regulatory center via altered norepinephrine activity.

Urogenital symptoms and complaints

Being of a common embryological origin, both the female lower genital tract and the lower urinary tract are sensitive to the reduction in circulating estrogen levels during the climacteric and postmenopause. The prevalence of urogenital atrophy and related symptoms is high in postmenopausal women, and the true magnitude is probably underestimated. Symptoms related to the atrophic changes in the vagina include irritation, vaginal and sexual dryness, vaginal discharge and infection, vulvovaginal pruritus, dyspareunia, postcoital bleeding, and signs and symptoms of prolapse. Estrogen deficiency leads to atrophic changes in the urethral epithelium and the highly vascularized submucosal layer. This may give rise to inade-

quate urethral closure and an abnormal urine flow pattern. Related symptoms are frequency, nocturia, urgency, dysuria, and recurrent urinary tract infection. It is likely that postmenopause plays a contributing but minor role in the onset of symptoms of urinary incontinence.

Other climacteric symptoms and complaints

For many women, midlife as such, but not specifically the climacteric transition, is associated with a variety of symptoms that may influence their well-being. In general, the so-called menopausal syndrome is restricted to symptoms such as menstrual cycle disorders, bouts of excessive sweating, hot flushes, and sexual dryness. Sometimes atypical symptoms such as tiredness, palpitations, headache, dizziness, irritability, and sleeplessness are associated with severe vasomotor symptoms. These atypical symptoms can then be considered as menopause-related as these complaints will disappear together with vasomotor complaints – either spontaneously or with HRT. Most experts regard climacteric depressive mood changes as an atypical complaint that is linked to vasomotor symptoms. However, depressive illness as such is certainly not related to the climacteric.

Around the point of menopause, many women experience permanent or periodic episodes of pain in and around the small joints. On the whole, with this type of arthralgia, the joints usually show no abnormalities on physical examination or with X-rays. Due to their prevalence in the climacteric and their response to estrogen-containing replacement therapy in about half of these women, these complaints can sometimes be considered as menopause-related complaints.

The same is true for certain oral complaints (such as dry mouth, a burning sensation on the tongue, a sensation of altered taste) and complaints of dry eyes. However, controlled studies have not been performed in all of these conditions.

Complications

The cessation of the production of estradiol by the ovaries has profound effects on various organs in the female body. Urogenital atrophy is an early manifestation of estrogen deficiency, but the condition will extend throughout the entire postmenopausal period. In many women, the climacteric is a period of accelerated bone loss, leading to manifest osteoporosis and osteoporotic fractures only later in postmenopause. The impact of the lack of estrogens on cardiovascular disease in women, and especially on fatal myocardial infarction, is now well-documented. More recently, the importance of estrogens for the central nervous system has attracted attention.

Cardiovascular disease

Cardiovascular disease is the leading cause of death in American and European women. Epidemiological data show that there is a clear relation between menopause and mortality from cardiovascular disease. There is a strong increase in the risk of cardiovascular disease in women after the onset of menopause. Premenopausal women who undergo a bilateral oophorectomy are at a significantly higher risk of developing cardiovascular disease, while postmenopausal estrogen use leads to a substantial reduction of the relative risk of coronary heart disease. The cardioprotective effect of the ovarian hormone 17β-estradiol is not simply limited to changes in lipid and lipoprotein metabolism. Cardiac function, endothelium-dependent and endothelium-independent vasomotion, coagulation, and fibrinolysis, as well as homocysteine metabolism, have all been shown to be directly influenced by estrogens and the lack thereof.

Menopause-induced changes resulting in a more atherogenic lipid and lipoprotein profile have been known for a long time. Postmenopausal women have higher serum levels of total cholesterol and of low-density lipoprotein cholesterol (LDL-C) and lower serum levels of high density cholesterol (HDL-C) than premenopausal women. An elevated postmenopausal plasma level of lipoprotein (a) [Lp(a)] is a separate, independent cardiovascular risk factor, as it has been linked to premature atherosclerosis, coronary artery disease, and myocardial infarction in a variety of case control studies.

Osteopenia, osteoporosis and osteoporotic fractures

Bone loss with aging is a universal phenomenon. It is estimated that during the course of a woman's life, she will lose half of the bone from her spine and about 30% of her cortical bone, which is considerably more than a man will lose. The result of this bone loss is a low skeletal mass and loss of bone architecture, leading to an increase in fracture risk. A white woman at the age of 50 has a lifetime risk of suffering a hip fracture or a wrist fracture of 15% each and a 32% risk of a vertebral fracture, which results in an overall lifetime risk of any fracture of around 50%.

In healthy women, during the perimenopausal years, bone loss increases and often becomes significant. It has been estimated that within the perimenopause and the first three menopausal years, in total between 10 and 20% of bone mineral is lost from the lumbar spine. This accelerated bone loss in climacteric women results from an imbalance between bone resorption and bone formation. Many factors, such as hormones, cytokines, and immune cells, are involved in the interaction between osteoblasts and osteoclasts. Estradiol is thought to decrease the osteoclast formation and activity. However, estrogen acts not only directly on bone cells but also affects parathyroid function by resetting (lowering) the set-point of parathyroid hormone, and it also regulates calcium absorption by its intestinal receptors.

There is a large inter- and intra-individual variability in bone loss. Early postmenopausal women can probably be divided into fast and slow bone losers. Five years after menopause, 50% of all women will continue to lose bone at the same rate, while others will either show an increased rate or a decreased rate of bone loss.

The risk of osteoporotic fractures is not only influenced by peri- and postmenopausal bone loss and risk factors for falls. Bone mass in the postmenopausal women is also a function of the original peak bone mass, which is, in turn, regulated by genetic factors, calcium intake, and physical activity. Clinical risk factors are unreliable for identifying women at risk. A reliable indicator of fracture risk is bone mineral density. Indications for determining mineral bone mass can be the following: a history of oligo- or amenorrhea, a low Quetelet index, a suspect family history, hyperthyroidism during perimenopause, hyperparathyroidism, and long-term corticosteroid use.

Alzheimer's disease

Dementia due to Alzheimer's disease is a common disorder with an enormous impact on a person's quality of life. It has been shown that after menopause, cerebral blood flow in women decreases significantly, as does cognitive ability. While dementia related to vascular disease affects men more than women, the incidence of dementia due to Alzheimer's disease is greater in women. Alzheimer's disease is related to a disturbance in the cholinergic neurotransmission system, which is very important for memory and cognitive function. Estrogens are definitely involved in the process of acetylcholine synthesis, and they also have an influence on neuronal architecture and organization. With the decrease of estrogens after menopause, the total number of synaptic connections diminishes, making neurons prone to cell degeneration and death. In men, this process develops much more slowly, as testosterone can be aromatized to estrogen in the brain.

Treatment

Changes in endogenous estrogen levels during the climacteric and postmenopause have been related to symptoms, complaints, and diseases described earlier in this chapter. Reversal of many of these effects of menopause have been shown to occur after the administration of exogenous estrogen either alone or in combination with progestogens. Proof that restoration to a premenstrual situation is possible with hormone replacement therapy (HRT) comes not only from in vitro studies, animal studies, and experimental studies in humans, but also from various types of epidemiological studies. Hormone replacement therapy is highly effective for the symptomatic treatment of climacteric symptoms and can be used for the primary and secondary prevention of menopause-related diseases such as osteoporosis and cardiovascular disease. Thus, indications for HRT are either symptomatic or preventive in nature (Tab. 49.1). Generally, HRT for symptomatic treatment is short-term in nature (less than 5 years).

Preventive HRT is long-term in nature (5 years or more) and is intended to be lifelong in certain instances. Indications for long-term preventive treatment can be either established disease, such as osteoporotic fractures

Table 49.1 Indications for hormonal replacement therapy

Indications for symptomatic, short-term treatment

Hot flushes and sweating
Urogenital atrophy
Perimenopausal cycle disorders
Other climacteric complaints and symptoms

Indications for preventive, long-term treatment

Adolescents with ovarian dysfunction and
  amenorrhea (e.g., Turner's syndrome, anorexia
  nervosa, athletes)
Women with premature menopause (as a result of
  surgery, chemotherapy, radiation therapy, or
  premature ovarian failure)
Women with a bone mass value more than 1 SD below
  the age-adjusted mean
Women with a history of osteoporotic fractures
Women with existing CVD (myocardial infarction)
Women with risk factors for CVD, such as
  hyperlipidemia, high Lp(a), hyperhomocystinemia,
  especially when in combination with one of the
  following conditions:
    smoking
    hypertension
    diabetes mellitus
    familial CHD (in the first degree and <60 yr old)
    familial hyperlipidemia

(From Kenemans P, Barentsen R, van de Weijer PHM. Practical HRT. 2nd ed. Zeist: Medical Forum International, 1996.)

and severe coronary artery stenosis (tertiary prevention), or the presence of strong risk factors for the disease (e.g., low bone mineral content or hyperhomocystinemia, which is secondary prevention).

Hormonal treatment options for HRT consist of estrogens, progestogens, and androgens and/or a combination thereof, while other substances such as Tibolone, Tamoxifen, and Raloxifene can also be considered. The oral route is the most common way of administration, both for estrogens as well as for progestogens, however the transdermal route is becoming more popular. Transdermal application of estrogens results in a stable serum estrogen level since the first-pass effect on the liver is circumvented. The effect on the lipid profile is less pronounced, at least at the beginning of the treatment. Progestogens are also available in patches. Subcutaneous implantation of estradiol pellets has been used for many decades. Renewed implantation can lead to high serum estradiol levels. In some countries, particularly in the United Kingdom, estrogen implants are combined with testosterone.

The vaginal route is preferred for the treatment of vaginal epithelial atrophy and urogenital complaints. Various estrogens are available for vaginal application, such as estriol, 17β-estradiol, and conjugated equine estrogens in various formulations (creams, tablets, vaginal rings). Estrogens can also be administered intramuscularly (estradiol), percutaneously (estradiol cream), intranasally (estradiol spray), and sublingually (estradiol tablets). Progestogens can be administrated orally, trans-

dermally, or directly to the endometrium using a progestogen-releasing intrauterine device (IUD).

Estrogens Micronized estradiol, estradiol valerate, and conjugated equine estrogens are all widely used estrogens. Their effects are highly similar to those of 17β-estradiol, the natural estrogen. After oral administration, micronized 17β-estradiol is metabolized to estrone and estrone sulfate. Estradiol valerate has the same active metabolites. Conjugated equine estrogens, derived from the urine of pregnant mares, are mixtures of estrogens and estrogen sulfates, with some metabolites having a very long half-life.

Estriol and estriol succinate are weak estrogens and are mainly used for the treatment of urogenital symptoms. In the dosages commonly used, they affect neither the endometrium nor lipid metabolism.

Progestogens Steroid hormones that have an affinity for the progesterone receptor are called progestogens, progestins, or gestagens. Some may also show some affinity for other steroid receptors, including the androgen receptor. The synthetic testosterone-derived C-19 progestogens often have distinct androgenic effects, which sometimes are reflected in clinical signs such as acne, fluid retention, disturbed glucose metabolism, liver dysfunction, and changes in blood clotting. They might decrease HDL-C and cause LDL-C to rise, thus counteracting the protective cardiovascular effect of natural estrogens. With the dosages normally used in HRT, these effects are only minor or absent. This is especially true with the newer C-19 steroids, such as desogestrel and gestoden. The synthetic progesterone-derived C-21 steroids, and especially medroxyprogesterone acetate, are among the most widely used progestogens in combined HRT. Other C-21 progestogens are dydrogesterone, cyproterone acetate, and promegestone. Recently, the natural micronized progesterone has become available for use in HRT regimens. Micronized progesterone exerts no androgenic effects and does not influence the lipid or lipid protein metabolism.

Other drugs Androgens are sometimes added to therapy for the stimulation of libido and bone remodeling. For oral administration, the synthetic androgenic hormone methyltestosterone is available in combination with estrogen. One alternative is formed by the injectable esters of testosterone.

Tibolone is a synthetic C-19 steroid, of which metabolites have estrogenic and progestogenic as well as androgenic actions. As a result, it can be used as a monotherapy. Other drugs that are sometimes used for the postmenopausal replacement of estrogen are tamoxifen and raloxifene. These drugs have tissue-specific estrogenic and anti-estrogenic effects. Through its estrogenic action, tamoxifen influences bone mineral density and plasma lipid profile in a favorable way. It is also associated with thrombotic events and endometrial hyperplasia, polyps, and cancer. Tamoxifen is at the present time often used for adjuvant breast cancer therapy because of its anti-estrogenicity. In tamoxifen users, the anti-estrogenic action of tamoxifen is sometimes encountered as an increased frequency of flushes. Raloxifene belongs to the next generation of so-called SERMs (selective estrogen receptor modifiers). It is said to give fewer flushes and to not stimulate the endometrium.

HORMONE REPLACEMENT THERAPY REGIMENS

Basically, there are two HRT regimens, each with modifications. The two basic regimens are unopposed estrogen therapy (ERT) (or estrogen-only therapy) and estrogen combined with progestogen (combined HRT, cHRT).

Estrogen therapy used to be the preferred method, but it is now only recommended for hysterectomized women. In nonhysterectomized women, unopposed estrogen increases the risk of endometrial cancer. Estrogen therapy should be administered continuously, that is, daily without interruption, in an adequate dosage. The old regimen was a cyclic, that is, discontinuous, administration of estrogen, with a medication-free week. As climacteric symptoms are liable to reappear in the medication-free week, this regimen is generally not used anymore.

There are two different forms of combined HRT, namely sequentially combined HRT (scHRT) and continuously combined HRT (ccHRT). Continuous estrogen with sequential (or cyclic) addition of progestogen is a regimen in which the progestogen is administered sequentially for 10 to 14 days each artificial cycle, which is usually 28 days, in order to avoid endometrial neoplasia. Currently, a monthly regimen is recommended as a matter of choice for nonhysterectomized women. The so-called long cycle, a 3-monthly regimen with 12 to 14 days addition of progestogens has yet to be proven safe for the endometrium. Continuously combined HRT – continuous estrogen and continuous progestogen – is a method developed to produce amenorrhea while still achieving sufficiently high serum estrogen levels to generate the beneficial effects of estrogen replacement therapy. In the early postmenopause and in the initial phase of therapy, this regimen often causes breakthrough bleeding and spotting, leading to a reduced patient compliance. Continuous combinations should therefore only be used after an amenorrhea of at least 2 years duration. Tibolone is an agreeable alternative for this regimen, and raloxifene could be in the near future.

Indications for symptomatic hormone replacement therapy

Perimenopausal cycle disorders Menstrual irregularities and changes in bleeding pattern must lead to a careful evaluation, primarily directed to the detection of pathology, with dysfunctional bleeding usually considered a diagnosis of exclusion. Oral progestogens can be used for luteal supplementation (cycle day 16-25), and in addition for the suppression of endometrial proliferation (cycle day 5-25). The use of oral contraceptives can be considered, especially in women requiring contraception. Generally the use of oral contraceptives results in a regular cycle pattern, a significant reduction of vaginal blood loss (up to 50%), and adequate contraception. Therefore, oral contraceptives are considered to be the first choice in perimenopausal cycle disorders. Even the lowest estradiol regimen (20 µg EE) sustains adequate serum estrogen levels to prevent the short- and long-term sequela of estrogen deficiency, however, long-term oral contraceptives may be contraindicated in women in their forties with other risk factors for cardiovascular disease (such as smoking, diabetes mellitus, or hypertension), or in whom the use of sex steroids may be associated with an increased risk of thrombosis. Progestogen-releasing IUDs provide an alternative for the long-term use of oral contraceptives for perimenopausal cycle disorders.

Prostaglandin synthetase inhibitors and tranexamic acid could be considered as nonhormonal treatment options. In extreme cases, the use of GnRH analogues with the addition of a low-dose estrogen (the so-called add back therapy) could be helpful.

Hot flushes and night sweats Estradiol and conjugated estrogens are highly effective in the treatment of vasomotor symptoms. For premenopausal women, and especially for those in need of cycle control or contraception or both, again low-dose oral contraceptives are the first choice. Progestogens, when used daily in adequate doses (e.g., medroxyprogesterone acetate 10 mg; dydrogesterone 10 mg), have also been shown to be effective. Tibolone, 2.5 mg daily given continuously, reduces vasomotor symptoms. Tamoxifen and raloxifene are not effective at all, and tamoxifen is known to cause flushes. Hormonal treatment for vasomotor complaints must be continued for 1 to 2 years. If the complaints return after the discontinuation of medication, one more HRT treatment course should be considered.

Nonhormonal treatment options include: α2-adrenergic agonists such as clonidine. Clonidine 0.05 mg, taken twice daily, will in some patients reduce the number of hot flushes, but it may have side effects such as light sedation and a dry mouth. In an experimental setting, a combination of progressive muscle relaxation and slow deep breathing was shown to reduce the incidence of subjective hot flushes by approximately half. In addition to this so-called paced respiration training, daily outdoor exercises have been advocated.

Urogenital symptoms and other climacteric complaints The vaginal route is the route of choice of estrogen application for women with complaints of vaginal epithelial atrophy and for those women who need local estrogen therapy prior to lower genital tract surgery. For some women, the oral route is a better option. In this case, the first choice is estriol in tablets of 1 or 2 mg. Under normal circumstances this dosage will neither influence the endometrium nor the lipid metabolism. When standard systemic HRT is given for other indications, this is generally also sufficient for the treatment of urogenital complaints. However, in a small number of women on systemic HRT, there are still persistent symptoms of urogenital atrophy. In these women, additional vaginal applications of estrogen will help. Within 2 weeks of starting HRT, considerable improvement can be observed in vaginal cytology and vaginal blood flow, but it may sometimes take up to 6 to 12 months of therapy before complaints of vaginal dryness and dyspareunia disappear.

For the prevention of recurrent urinary tract infections, as a consequence of urogenital atrophy, medication should be continued for the rest of a woman's life. The scientific basis for the actual efficacy of estrogen therapy in urinary incontinence remains controversial. An overall small but significant subjective improvement for all types of incontinence with estrogen therapy compared to placebo, has been demonstrated. If atypical climacteric complaints are associated with vasomotor complaints, they will usually disappear with adequate treatment of the flushes. Without vasomotor symptoms, effective treatment is less certain. A trial treatment with HRT of 3 months duration may be considered, and should be continued only if a marked improvement is recorded. Oral complaints, such as dry mouth, burning tongue, altered or dirty taste can be treated with a trial treatment of 3 months of HRT. Therapy can be continued after proven improvement. The same is true for eye complaints like dry eyes and lack of lacrimal fluid.

Indications for preventive hormone replacement therapy

Hormone replacement therapy (HRT) in postmenopausal women substantially reduces both the risk of cardiovascular disease and of osteoporotic fractures. A reduction of the risk of stroke incidents and a reduction in the risk of stroke mortality have also been reported, but other important studies have not confirmed this. Estrogens have been shown to influence cognitive functioning in women, and some studies report that estrogen use also seems to benefit the cognitive functioning of patients with existing Alzheimer's disease. Reports on a possible relationship between estrogen use and the development of Alzheimer's disease are conflicting. Recently, a prospective cohort study demonstrated that estrogen use may delay the onset of, and also may decrease the risk of, Alzheimer's disease. Properly designed investigations are needed to clarify this relationship further. In this section, the use of HRT for the prevention of cardiovascular disease and for the prevention of osteoporotic fractures will be discussed in more detail.

Cardiovascular disease
Epidemiological evidence consistently supports the view that HRT provides substantial protection against cardiovascular disease in postmenopausal women.

Taken together, the data currently available with regard to combined HRT suggest that the addition of progesterone will not eliminate the benefits of estrogen on the cardiovascular system, but it could be that some types of progestogen will attenuate that benefit.

This cardioprotective effect of estrogens is probably largely mediated by increased HDL-C levels. HDL-C transports cholesterol from the periphery to the liver and may mobilize cholesterol already deposited in the arterial walls. In the liver, hepatic lipase is involved in the metabolism of HDL-C. Hepatic lipase is inactivated by estrogen, which may partly explain the increase in HDL-C during postmenopausal estrogen use. The reduction of LDL by estrogens is brought about through induction of LDL receptors in the liver. It should be noted that the production of triglycerides is increased by estrogens, which could be interpreted as an adverse effect.

The positive effect of estrogens on lipid profile is initiated within weeks of starting oral therapy and does not persist after termination of therapy. This could explain the consistent finding of a strong effect among users as compared to never and past users.

The decision to use HRT for reducing the risk of cardiovascular disease should be made on an individual basis. The American Heart Association advises HRT as a cardio-protective therapy, especially in women with pre-existing cardiovascular disease or in women with a high cardiovascular risk. Both sequentially combined and continuously combined HRT are effective in reducing elevated LDL cholesterol levels in hypercholesterolemic postmenopausal women and should be considered in their treatment. Hormone replacement therapy in healthy postmenopausal women to prevent their generally lower cardiovascular disease risk is still controversial. Large randomized clinical trials are needed before issuing any valid recommendation for primary prevention.

Concern about an adverse effect still exists with regard to the addition of progestogen. Some synthetic progestogens display an unfavorable effect on serum lipoprotein levels, while others do not show this at all. Natural progesterone may have the least impact on metabolic parameters.

Osteoporosis and osteoporotic fractures
By starting HRT soon after bilateral oophorectomy, bone loss can be prevented. When this treatment is extended for more than 10 years, lumbar spine bone mass is 30% higher and that of the femur 10% higher compared to those in untreated women.

In premature natural menopause, estrogen replacement has the same bone-sparing effect. When used for at least 5 years, HRT decreases the incidence of osteoporosis-related fractures by about half. Progestogens probably add to the beneficial effect and certainly do not counteract the effects of estrogens on the skeleton.

In established osteoporosis, estrogen therapy seems a realistic alternative to other therapies, such as diphosphonates, fluoride, and anabolic steroids. The minimum dosage or the minimum value of serum estradiol to prevent postmenopausal bone loss has not yet been determined. It should be realized that there is a large individual variation in estradiol plasma levels with a given dose of estrogen.

The best option for preventing fractures is to start HRT at menopause, or as soon as there is an indication for

HRT, and continue HRT lifelong. The decision to use HRT can be based on the results of bone mass measurement using the T-score (the number of standard deviations above or below the mean peak bone mass).

HRT is advised in the case of a low bone mass (T score < −1), as it will reduce the fracture rate by 50%. Some clinicians advise waiting until the age of 65 before starting HRT, based on the ability of estrogens to raise bone mass in older women with osteoporosis. This advice is based on the knowledge that hip fractures occur mostly after the age of 70. It should be realized, however, that although an increase in bone mass can be reached in older women, the structural integrity of the trabecular architecture is generally disrupted with early bone loss, and this will not necessarily be restored with estrogens taken at a later age.

Contraindications

There are only a few conditions in which HRT seems contraindicated (Tab. 49.2), and the contraindications are not absolute. Hormone replacement therapy is generally considered to be contraindicated in patients who have been treated for primary breast cancer, especially in cancers in which estrogen and progestogen receptors have been demonstrated to be present. In patients still left with hormone-sensitive micrometastasis, estrogen treatment may activate dormant cells or accelerate tumor recurrence. Therefore, it is only in those situations where there are important, well-defined reasons for prescribing estrogens that estrogen-containing HRT could be prescribed. At this time the issue is rather controversial.

Tamoxifen is an alternative medication as far as the indications of osteoporosis and an increased risk for cardiovascular disease are concerned. Tamoxifen has a beneficial effect on bone mass and on lipid profile. On the other hand, when using Tamoxifen, one should bear in mind the higher incidence of hot flushes, an increased risk of venous thrombosis, and also of endometrial abnormalities, including endometrial cancer. The new generation anti-estrogen Raloxifene has been reported to have a better profile: fewer hot flushes and no endometrial stimulation. Tibolone could also be a good option as it has been claimed to not stimulate the breast epithelium and to have a beneficial effect on hot flushes.

A history of endometrial carcinoma is also traditionally looked upon as an absolute contraindication for estrogen therapy. Given the assumption that micrometastasis still left in place may be stimulated by estrogens, a small number of nonrandomized retrospective studies do not substantiate this fear. In low-stage, low-grade disease, the risk of recurrence is extremely low even with postmenopausal HRT. If there are strong preventive indications, estrogen replacement may be given in these cases on the precondition that continuous progestogen is added to estrogen, also following hysterectomy. Preferably estrogen-containing HRT should not be started within 2 years after diagnosis, and for higher stages of endometrial cancer, HRT should be considered an absolute contraindication during the first 5 years.

Severe liver dysfunction is also considered to be a contraindication for HRT. Women with a severe liver dysfunction should not receive any substance that is specifically metabolized in the liver. Therefore, oral estrogens and progestogens should not be prescribed in cases of severe liver dysfunction, as they might influence liver metabolism.

Porphyria is a group of disorders caused by the shortage of one of the enzymes used in the synthesis of the heme group of hemoglobin. Estrogens have been shown to affect this enzyme activity adversely, especially in oral contraceptive users. This effect is probably mediated by the liver. The influence of non-oral HRT is unknown.

At this time there are no specific contra-indications for progestogens. Meningiomas have been shown to have a higher percentage of receptors for progesterone and are clinically arrested in their growth by anti-progestogens. Therefore, progestogens might be considered to be contraindicated for use in meningioma patients. There is no contraindication for estrogen-only HRT.

There are many conditions that have been considered to be a contraindication for HRT for a long time. However, HRT is not contraindicated in conditions such as prolactinoma, malignant melanoma, liver adenoma,

---

Table 49.2 Contraindications for hormonal replacement therapy, special conditions, and conditions in which HRT is not contraindicated

Contraindications (relative, not absolute)

Contraindications for estrogens
  A history of breast cancer
  A history of endometrial cancer
  Severe liver dysfunction
  Porphyria
Contraindications for progestogens
  Meningioma

Special conditions (requiring a special HRT approach)

Myoma uteri
Endometriosis
Mastopathy
Migraine
Venous thrombosis and embolism
Familial hypertriglyceridemia
Gallstones
Epilepsy
Increased breast cancer risk

Conditions in which HRT is not contraindicated

Prolactinoma
Malignant melanoma
Liver adenoma
Varices
Diabetes mellitus
Otosclerosis
Hyperthyroidism
Sickle cell anemia
Endometrial hyperplasia

(From Kenemans P, Barentsen R, van de Weijer PHM. Practical HRT. 2nd ed. Zeist: Medical Forum International, 1996.)

varices, diabetes mellitus, otosclerosis, hyperthyroidism, sickle cell anemia, endometrial hyperplasia, hypertension, and myocardial infarction. On the contrary, endometrial hyperplasia, as well as myocardial infarction, can be considered to be indications for HRT applied in an adequate way. The protective effects of HRT on cardiovascular risk may in fact be augmentative in diabetes mellitus. Women with uterine fibroids and those with endometriosis are among those who need special attention. On rare occasions, growth of these lesions occurs under HRT, in which case treatment should be stopped. In the case of endometriosis, a continuous combined regimen is often considered to be better.

Mastopathy or severe breast tenderness is mostly transient and will resolve in most cases within 6 months. Dose reduction, or in some cases a few days' interruption, of estrogen intake may be required. In women with migraines, blood level fluctuations should be avoided as much as possible by using transdermal estrogen and the lowest possible progesterone dose. In women with familial hypertriglyceridemia and in women with gallstones, non-oral estrogens might be preferred. In women with epilepsy, which reacts adversely to unopposed estrogens, a continuous combined estrogen-progestogen therapy should be used in slightly higher dosages. Caution is advised in women with an increased risk for breast cancer. Women with a positive family history for breast cancer, with BRCA-1 or -2 gene mutations, women with premalignant breast lesions, and those women who used DES during pregnancy are all reported to have an increased breast cancer risk. It is not known whether HRT increases this breast cancer risk further.

Practical remarks

When beginning HRT, a number of points should be given careful attention. Among these are the purpose of HRT for the specific client and the duration of medication, the expected bleeding pattern, the possible side effects (fluid retention and mastopathy and presumed changes in body weight), and the breast cancer risk. A basic examination should include a pelvic examination, blood pressure recording, and possibly mammography. The first evaluation should be done after 3 months, at which time side effects and bleeding pattern should be discussed. For motivation and therapy compliance, check-ups can be planned every 6 to 12 months thereafter. Mammography should be performed every other year. Endometrial monitoring should be carried out in the case of unscheduled vaginal bleeding events. It should be remembered that endometrial hyperplasia is more prevalent in postmenopausal breast cancer patients receiving tamoxifen, in diabetes mellitus patients, and in women on long-term unopposed estrogen replacement. Women with unscheduled bleeding should undergo vaginal ultrasonography. If endometrial thickness is greater than 4 mm (double endometrial layer), an outpatient endometrial sampling procedure should be carried out. In women with persistent unscheduled bleeding, a repeat endometrial sampling should then be performed either by Vabra-curette or D & C, or alternatively, a hysteroscopic evaluation of the uter-

ine cavity with endometrial sampling should be performed. It should be remembered that with adequate progestogen treatment, hyperplasia can be reversed to normal endometrial histology in nearly all cases.

Bone mass measurement is only helpful in women with a very low bone mass at the start of HRT, and permits the detection of the small group of women in whom bone loss is continuous in spite of the usual hormone dosages.

In general, for practical HRT, a few basic rules should be followed (Tab. 49.3).

Despite the well-documented advantages of HRT, patient compliance is generally poor, which means that HRT use is discontinued within the time treatment was originally intended to last. In many countries, the duration of therapy is only between 6 and 12 months, while one-third of the women never fill their prescription for HRT. Reasons for poor compliance are, in particular, the occurrence of withdrawal bleedings, weight increase, breast tenderness, and fear of cancer. To achieve optimal compliance, both physician and patient must accept the therapy and understand why hormone therapy is prescribed in her particular case. Counseling about the risks and benefits of long-term hormonal treatment may begin during the period when a woman is being treated for climacteric symptoms. A woman should understand the probable risks and benefits of hormone therapy and should decide, together with her physician, whether or not to take preventive hormone therapy. Among the risks to be discussed are those for thromboembolism and can-

---

Table 49.3 The seven basic rules of practical hormone replacement therapy

1. Estrogen replacement therapy (ERT) should be prescribed continuously

2. ERT must be combined with progesterone or a progestogen (P) unless the uterus has been removed

3. In any combined (E + P) HRT regimen, progestogen should be prescribed for at least 10 days, and preferably for 12-14 days

4. A monthly sequentially combined regimen (continuous E plus sequential P) is the standard method of choice

5. The daily progestogen dosage should be as low as possible, but sufficiently high to prevent endometrial pathology

6. A nonandrogenic progestogen is recommended

7. HRT should be started with the combined E/P-phase to avoid unexpected bleeding at the start of treatment, unless an ultrasound scan has shown the endometrium to be thinner than 5 mm (double-layer thickness)

(From Kenemans P, Barentsen R, van de Weijer PHM. Practical HRT. 2nd ed. Zeist: Medical Forum International, 1996.)

cer. Although the incidence of thromboembolism is very low under HRT, the risk is probably increased. The risk for cancer with HRT is not very clear. With adequately administered HRT, the risk for cancer in general is not increased. Uncertainty surrounds the risk for endometrial carcinoma and breast cancer in women consistently taking HRT for more than 5 years. With HRT, the risk for colorectal cancer is probably decreased. There are indications that the overall mortality, as well as the mortality from cancer in general, is decreased in HRT users compared to nonusers.

Suggested readings

GRADY D, RUBIN SM, PETITTI DB, et al. Hormone therapy to prevent disease and prolong life in postmenopausal women. Ann Intern Med 1992;117:1016-37.

KENEMANS P, BARENTSEN R, VAN DE WEIJER PHM. Practical HRT. 2nd ed. Zeist: Medical Forum International, 1996.

OLDENHAVE A, JASZMANN LJB, HASPELS AA, EVERAERD WThAM. Impact of climacteric on well-being: a survey based on 5213 women 39 to 60 years old. Am J Obstet Gynecol 1993;168:772-80.

Assisted reproduction

Grigoris Grimbizis, Paul P. Devroey

In vitro fertilization (IVF), initially developed in 1978 for women suffering from mechanical infertility, revolutionized the treatment of infertility. However, IVF and other techniques introduced since then have had extremely limited success in patients with severe impairment of spermatogenesis. In 1992, the establishment of the first pregnancies after intracytoplasmic sperm injection (ICSI) offered a new effective tool in the treatment of severe male infertility where the number of spermatozoa in the ejaculate is very low or even zero.

Infertility is a condition that affects the couple. It is usually defined as the inability to achieve a pregnancy within 12 months of unprotected intercourse. However, European Society of Human Reproduction and Embriology (ESHRE) has recently proposed changing the time of regular coital exposure from 12 to 24 months before characterizing a couple as infertile. In the industrially developed countries, approximately 8 to 15% of married couples are infertile. The overall incidence of

infertility seems to have been steady over recent years, but there has been a dramatic increase in visits to physicians for treatment.

Assisted reproduction techniques rely on two common elements: ovarian stimulation in order to bring multiple follicles to maturity, and mechanisms for bringing oocytes and spermatozoa into proximity in order to enhance fertilization. Enhancement of in vivo fertilization is attempted on the basis of intrauterine insemination with prepared spermatozoa, or with the transfer of retrieved oocytes into the tube together with the sperm. Where in vivo fertilization of the oocytes is not feasible, fertilization can be achieved by in vitro culture of the gametes, followed by the subsequent transfer either of the embryos into the uterus or of the zygotes/early embryos into the fallopian tube. Where fertilization of the oocytes cannot be achieved even by means of in vitro culture of the gametes because of severe male infertility, intracytoplasmic sperm injection should be used (Tab. 50.1).

Table 50.1 Assisted reproduction techniques according to the type of fertilization

Fertilization	Technique			Description
In vivo	Intrauterine insemination		IUI	Transfer of prepared spermatozoa into the uterine cavity
	Gamete intrafallopian transfer		GIFT	Transfer of oocytes together with spermatozoa into the tube
In vitro	In vitro fertilization and embryo transfer		IVF/ET	Transfer of embryos into the uterine cavity after fertilization in vitro
	Zygote intrafallopian transfer		ZIFT	Transfer of zygotes into the tube after fertilization in vitro
	Tubal embryo transfer		TET	Transfer of embryos into the tube after fertilization in vitro
Micro-insemination	Intracytoplasmic sperm injection		ICSI	Direct indroduction of a spermatozoon into the ooplasm
	After	Micro-epididymal sperm aspiration	MESA	Sperm recovery from the caput of epididymis by microsurgery
		Fine needle aspiration	FNA	Isolation of spermatozoa from the aspirate of testicular tissue
		Testicular exploration with sperm extraction	TESE	Isolation of spermatozoa from testicular biopsy tissue

Although IVF offers a successful solution for most infertile couples, those with no oocytes, no uterus or a serious uterine deformity, and those with no spermatozoa even in multiple testicular biopsies cannot be helped. Providing that the couple without gametes accepts gamete donation, and the couple without a uterus accepts use of a surrogate one, the physician is still able to offer a method of forming a family exclusive of adoption.

INDICATIONS

Male factor

Impaired sperm production, function, or transport is one of the leading causes of infertility. It is estimated that in approximately 30% of infertile couples an important abnormality is identified only in the man and in another 20% there is a contributing male factor in addition to a female one. Male-factor infertility is usually characterized by a profound decrease in the fertilizing potential of the sperm or by the absence of sperm in cases of azoospermia.

The introduction of these new techniques has shifted interest from the causes of male infertility to the semen and its characteristics, since the new treatments are primarily symptomatic. Nevertheless, it is essential that apart from the sperm characteristics the male partner be thoroughly investigated in order to clarify the possible etiology of his infertility. This is important not only because in some cases the patient may benefit from a cause-specific treatment (e.g., hypogonadotropic hypogonadism), but also for the genetic counseling of the couple. However, in more than 50% of the subfertile males, no etiological factor can be identified. The effectiveness of other therapeutic options in this group is extremely poor, while in other categories (such as varicocele) the effectiveness of therapy is controversial and the various assisted reproduction techniques seem to be the only efficient treatment alternative.

The normal semen parameters determined by the World Health Organization (WHO) are the threshold values under which the probability of natural conception is significantly reduced. With decreasing total sperm count and/or progressive sperm motility and/or sperm morphology, the results of IVF become doubtful and inconsistent. In cases of oligo-astheno-teratospermia, no universal standards have emerged for the selection of patients for either IVF or intracytoplasmic sperm injection. In general, intracytoplasmic sperm injection should be used after fertilization failure or very low fertilization rates in previous IVF cycles and when sperm parameters are extremely poor (<500 000 progressively motile spermatozoa in the whole ejaculate, <4% normal forms by Kruger's strict criteria) (Fig. 50.1). Repetition of an unsuccessful IVF treatment cycle may not be in the best interests of the patients and may be unethical, since aggressive stimulation is usually needed. It has therefore been proposed to use both standard IVF and intracytoplasmic sperm injection simultaneously in cases with marginal sperm characteristics, dividing the oocytes into two groups at the first attempt (Fig. 50.1).

The development of intracytoplasmic sperm injection also appears to offer an effective solution in the treatment of men with obstructive or non-obstructive azoospermia (Fig. 50.1). Obstructive azoospermia as a result of congenital absence of the vas deferens, failed reconstructive surgery, and other irreparable congenital or postinflammatory obstructions can now be dealt with by intracytoplasmic sperm injection, using spermatozoa obtained by microsurgical epididymal sperm aspiration (MESA), fine needle aspiration (FNA), or testicular exploration with sperm extraction (TESE). Nonobstructive azoospermia includes cases with Sertoli cell-only syndrome, maturation arrest, postcryptorchidism tubular atrophy, mumps, or Klinefelter's syndrome. These patients may have occasional foci of normal seminiferous tubules with spermatogenesis. Thus, a combination of testicular exploration with sperm extraction and intracytoplasmic sperm injection provides a solution for some cases previously regarded as hopeless.

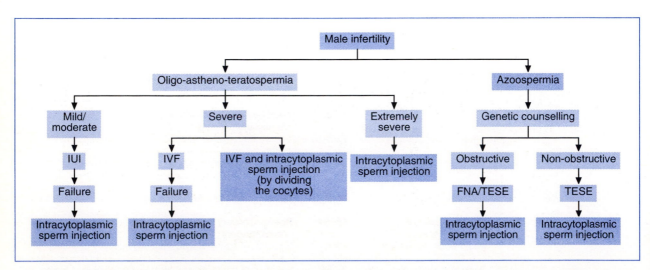

Figure 50.1 Treatment of male-related infertility. (IUI = intrauterine insemination; IVF = in vitro fertilization; TESE = testicular exploration with sperm extraction; FNA = fine needle aspiration.)

The use of intracytoplasmic sperm injection has given rise to fears that genetic abnormalities may be transmitted to the offspring because all of the physiological mechanisms of fertilization are bypassed. Although the technique in itself does not seem to increase the risk of genetic defects, certain categories of infertile males should have evaluation and counseling. Patients with congenital absence of the vas deferens are associated with a high incidence of mutations in the cystic fibrosis gene, and both partners should therefore be examined in order to avoid the risk of a child with cystic fibrosis. In cases of Klinefelter's syndrome, prenatal diagnosis is always necessary if chromosomal abnormalities are to be excluded. Finally, it is likely that some forms of severe male infertility could be genetically transmitted through deletions on the Y chromosome, and although there have been completely normal intracytoplasmic sperm injection offspring, the parents should be informed that a male child may have a problem with spermatogenesis.

Tubal factor

Abnormalities of the fallopian tubes comprise one of the largest diagnostic groups in most infertility centers. Pelvic inflammatory disease due to sexually transmitted microorganisms such as gonococci, chlamydia, and other pathogens is the main cause of tubal infertility. Tubal damage may also result from septic abortion, puerperal infection, suppurative appendicitis, peritonitis from other causes, previous abdominal pelvic surgery, and congenital malformations.

The majority of patients initially subjected to IVF for tubal infertility have already undergone at least one attempt at surgical reconstruction. However, technological advances and new laboratory techniques have significantly improved the efficiency of IVF and have caused doubts about the necessity of tubal reconstructive surgery. On the other hand, in a parallel trend, the field of reconstructive surgery has seen tremendous advances. Laparoscopic

management of infertile women now allows for a more objective estimation of the tubal status and repair of the damage that is as effective as with microsurgery, at a low cost, and with rapid recovery.

The choice between surgery and IVF depends essentially on the definite diagnosis of tubal pelvic damage and the prognosis for surgical treatment, but the coexistence of other factors (age of the woman; other types of infertility, such as in the male) may play a crucial role as well. Laparoscopy is always necessary in order to estimate tubal pelvic damage. Patients with adhesions, especially filmy adhesions, and partial distal tubal occlusion (phimosis) have a favorable prognosis, with pregnancy rates approximating 50% within 12 to 18 months postoperatively. Thus, adhesiolysis or fimbrioplasty (preferably laparoscopic) should initially be attempted, and IVF should be reserved for those who fail to conceive 12 to 18 months after surgery, given that monthly fecundity rates fall dramatically thereafter (Fig. 50.2). This treatment option offers the chance of natural conception and, if successful, the possibility of having more than one pregnancy. In cases of sterilization, re-anastomosis by microsurgery prior to IVF should always be used, with the exception of women with extremely damaged tubes (Fig. 50.2). The results in terms of pregnancy rates approximate 50%, depending of course on the type of re-anastomosis and the extent of damage.

In cases of total distal tubal occlusion (hydrosalpinx), the decision depends on the extent of tubal damage. Patients with mild damage to tubal mucosa, assessed by laparoscopy and if possible by salpingoscopy, have pregnancy rates of about 30 to 35% within 18 to 24 months postoperatively and should therefore be treated initially by salpingostomy (Fig. 50.2). The use of IVF should be delayed for at least 18 to 24 months, given that the tubes regain their function more slowly than in the other types of tubal pathology.

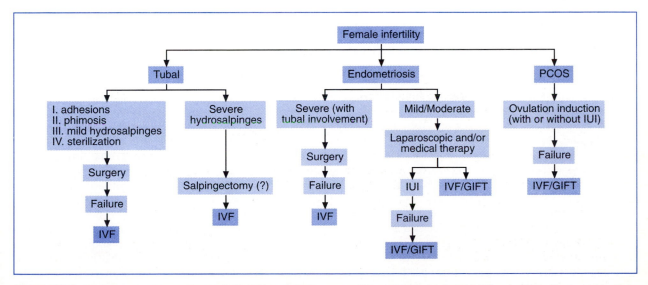

Figure 50.2 Treatment of female-related infertility. (PCOS = polycystic ovarian syndrome; IUI = intrauterine insemination; IVF = in vitro fertilization; GIFT = gamete intrafallopian transfer.)

Patients with hydrosalpinges and severe tubal damage should be oriented from the beginning toward IVF, although there is evidence hydrosalpinx is associated with a reduced conception rate. This is thought to be caused by the flow of toxic agents, microorganic debris, and lymphocytes as a result of chronic inflammation, or by a direct mechanical effect from fluid leaking from the hydrosalpinges to the uterine cavity. In this case, both receptivity of the endometrium and embryo viability are impaired. Preventive salpingectomy prior to IVF treatment is proposed as an alternative, but its results remain to be confirmed by prospective studies (Fig. 50.2). This practice may offer additional protection against ectopic implantation.

The occurrence of additional adverse factors is likely to be the overriding determinant in the choice of treatment. Women of advanced age should preferably be treated by IVF from the beginning because the possible delay in conception following surgery may be too long. Another alternative for women over 35 is to start with surgery if it seems favorable, but to fit in a cycle of IVF treatment two or three times each year as well. The coexistence of male subfertility is an indication for treatment with IVF combined with intracytoplasmic sperm injection from the beginning.

Endometriosis

Subfertility is one of the most frequent complaints in patients with endometriosis. It has been suggested that the pelvic peritoneal fluid environment is detrimental to sperm function. Production of prostaglandins by endometriotic implants is thought to affect tubal motility, folliculogenesis, or corpus luteum function, while activation of macrophages and elevated cytokines may also indicate immunological alterations interfering with fertility. Disordered follicular growth, ovulatory dysfunction, and impaired embryo development have also been suggested as possible causes of endometriosis-associated infertility.

There is no therapeutic approach directed at the etiology of the disease. The treatment remains empirical and its effectiveness unproven. Surgical therapy is indicated in cases of tubal obstruction, ovarian endometriomas, extensive adhesions, and cul-de-sac obliteration (Fig. 50.2). Laparoscopic ablation is probably effective in cases of endometriotic implants. Medical treatment in cases of mild or moderate disease includes suppression of ovulation with progestogens, oral contraceptives, danazol, or gonadotropin-releasing hormone agonists, but their usefulness is still under clinical investigation.

Assisted reproduction techniques are usually recommended 1 to 2 years after prior unsuccessful medical or surgical therapy (Fig. 50.2). The use of superovulation with intrauterine insemination (IUI) in cases of endometriotic patients with patent tubes has been reported to increase fecundity rates. Failure to achieve a pregnancy is an indication for IVF. In patients without tubal involvement, gamete intrafallopian transfer (GIFT) appears to be another effective alternative. The decision whether to utilize IVF must also take into account the couple's age, the existence of other infertility factors, the duration of infertility, and the patients' wishes. There are some reports that severe endometriosis may affect the IVF results because of an impaired response to ovarian stimulation, poor oocyte/embryo quality with defective implantation capacity, and a lower number of embryos transferred.

Polycystic ovarian syndrome

Infertility in patients with polycystic ovarian syndrome (PCOS) is primarily associated with anovulation. Ovulation induction with clomiphene citrate and/or gonadotropins, either for natural conception or for intrauterine insemination, is accompanied by high ovulation and pregnancy rates. In cases of long-standing infertility that is resistant to other in vivo treatments, IVF provides an alternative mode of therapy. IVF also gives an opportunity to assess the fertilizing potential of the gametes, bypassing factors that can interfere in the in vivo fertilizing process, such as lack of follicle rupture, oocyte entrapment within ruptured follicles, mechanical difficulties of the fimbriae in reaching all surfaces of the enlarged ovaries, and abnormalities in sperm or embryo transport. Patients are referred to IVF after four to six unsuccessful cycles of ovulation induction.

Immunological infertility

The exposure of spermatozoal antigens to the mucosal and the systemic immune systems results in the development of immunity to multiple spermatozoal epitopes. The presence of antisperm antibodies has a fertility-reducing effect.

Antisperm antibodies can be present locally, in semen, and in the female genital tract (cervical mucus), or in the systemic circulation. Both IgA and IgG isotypes have been described. Antisperm antibodies directed against the head of the spermatozoon can interfere with gamete interaction by inhibiting sperm from binding to the oocyte, while tail-directed antisperm antibodies tend to impair sperm motility. Thus, in vivo and even in vitro fertilization are reduced.

Therapy for antisperm-antibody-associated infertility is empiric and largely unproven. Short-time condom use does not improve conception rates. The administration of corticosteroids was abandoned after a few years of doubtful results and potentially dangerous side-effects. Intrauterine insemination was proposed as a method to overcome infertility associated with cervical mucous antisperm antibodies. Separation of antibody-free from antibody-bound spermatozoa by various techniques, as well as the treatment of spermatozoa with pentoxifylline, was also tried by several investigators in combination with IVF. The general experience shows that in severe cases none of these techniques is able to provide acceptable results. Only intracytoplasmic sperm injection can offer an effective alternative in such cases.

Unexplained infertility

The term unexplained infertility is applied to an infertile couple that fails to conceive after 2 years of unprotected intercourse and whose routine infertility work-up yields normal values. The standard infertility investigations should include history, physical examination of both partners, semen analysis, hormonal profile, hysterosalpingography, and/or laparoscopy and immunological tests. A more extensive evaluation is currently proposed, including bacteriological studies, a post-coital test, a sperm penetration test, and an estimation of the major histocompatibility complex and serial ultrasound monitoring (for luteinized unruptured follicle), but it has not been established that all of these additional investigations contribute to effective diagnosis.

Since the infertility is unexplained, only empirical strategies have been proposed for its therapy. A more rational use of assisted reproduction techniques can now be offered to such couples, based on the provision of data concerning the effectiveness of the various treatments. It is estimated that without treatment 40 to 80% of these couples will become pregnant in 3 years. The duration of infertility (>3 years), the age of the female partner (>30 years), the history of a previous pregnancy, and the frequency of coitus can affect the results. Ovarian stimulation with gonadotropins and intrauterine insemination each double the likelihood of conception independently of each other, while their simultaneous application increases pregnancy rates fourfold. Treatment with clomiphene citrate also increases conception rates, but to a lesser extent, and only in women with >3 years of infertility.

In cases of unexplained infertility, ovarian stimulation, usually combined with intrauterine insemination, should be initially advised for at least four cycles. The next step for those who fail to conceive and who wish to pursue treatment is IVF or gamete intrafallopian transfer (Fig. 50.3). However, this decision may be influenced by the age of the female partner, the duration of infertility, and the patients' wishes.

OVARIAN STIMULATION

Basic concepts

The first IVF pregnancy was established in a natural cycle, but this natural-cycle IVF was abandoned in the early 1980s and replaced by controlled ovarian hyperstimulation in order to obtain a large number of fertilizable eggs. Many different protocols have emerged for this purpose, using clomiphene citrate and/or gonadotropins with or without gonadotropin-releasing hormone (GnRH)-analogues for follicular rescue and development.

In the physiologic ovulatory cycle, the recruitment of the oocytes available in each cycle occurs about 3 months before ovulation and is gonadotropin-independent. A slight but significant rise in follicle-stimulating hormone (FSH) over a certain threshold level during the preceding late luteal phase and early follicular phase is responsible for the rescue of a follicular cohort. One of the rescued follicles then usually matures earlier, a process known as

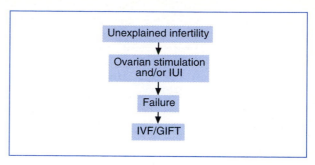

Figure 50.3 Treatment of couples with unexplained infertility. (IUI = intrauterine insemination; IVF = in vitro fertilization; GIFT = gamete intrafallopian transfer.)

selection of the dominant follicle. After this, the dominant follicle's hormonal activity modulates pituitary secretion of gonadotropins and restricts the growth of the other rescued follicles by reducing FSH levels.

Gonadotropins and/or antiestrogens can be used to restore the ovulation process in cases of hypothalamic-pituitary failure or dysfunction, such as anovulatory patients with PCOS, a process known as ovulation induction. On the other hand, ovarian stimulation in assisted reproduction technique programs is usually applied in cases of normal ovulatory women in order to increase the cohort of follicles achieving maturation. Although the general principles of treatment are similar, the intensity of stimulation, the course of treatment, and the hormonal patterns differ between these two groups. The aim of ovulation induction therapy is to provide gonadotropin levels that mimic the pattern of natural cycles and thus allow for the selection and maturation of a limited number of the rescued follicles. In controlled ovarian hyperstimulation, the FSH concentration is increased and sustained throughout the treatment above the threshold level. This leads to the rescue of more follicles from atresia and their development up to full or partial maturation.

Agents and stimulation protocols

Clomiphene citrate and gonadotropins

The antiestrogenic effect of clomiphene citrate on the central nervous system increases FSH and luteinizing hormone (LH) pulse frequency, providing a moderate gonadotropin stimulus to the ovary and thus increasing the cohort of follicles reaching ovulation. It is usually administered from cycle day 3 or 5 for 5 days at a dose of 50 to 100 mg (Fig. 50.4).

Ovarian stimulation for assisted reproduction techniques is based primarily on the use of gonadotropins. Gonadotropins induce multifollicular development by directly increasing FSH levels above the threshold values and consequently stimulating follicular growth. Initially, human pituitary gonadotropins (hPG) were used, but their use was abandoned because of the scarcity of human pitu-

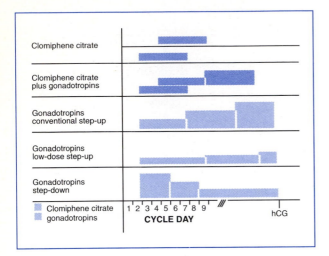

Figure 50.4 Ovarian stimulation with clomiphene citrate and/or gonadotropins: treatment protocols.

itaries and the occurrences of Creutzfeldt-Jacob disease. Since the late 1970s, predominantly human menopausal gonadotropins (hMG) have been used in ovarian stimulation, and several preparations are currently available for clinical use (Tab. 50.2). Recombinant FSH (recFSH) is now being prepared on an industrial scale and will probably soon be joined with recLH and rechCG. RecFSH preparations have high purity, high specific activity, no biological contamination, and no LH activity, and their use for ovarian stimulation compares favorably with urinary gonadotropins. The design and production of therapeutically active gonadotropin agonists and antagonists by recombinant DNA technology is a challenge for the future.

Several treatment schemes for gonadotropin therapy have been proposed over the years. The fixed-dose initial regimes, including the administration of certain doses of hMG on predetermined cycle days, were gradually aban-

doned for the more effective and flexible individually adjusted schemes. In the present day, the step-up protocols are widely used (Fig. 50.4). The conventional regime includes the administration of 150 IU hMG and/or FSH from cycle day 3, while the dose is adjusted after 5 days (from cycle day 8) according to each patient's response. More recently the low-dose step-up and the step-down protocols were proposed as alternatives to the conventional step-up regime in order to induce oligofollicular development (Fig. 50.4). The low-dose step-up regimen is characterized by low initial doses (37.5-75 IU), a slower increase (7 to 14 days), and smaller gonadotropin increments (37.5 IU). The step-down protocol involves the administration of a high initial dose (150-225 IU), followed by a decrease (to 112.5 IU), with the appearance of the dominant follicle (diameter >10 mm) and a further reduction (to 75 IU) 3 days later. These schemes of gonadotropin administration seem to be useful in cases of PCOS patients stimulated for natural conception or intrauterine insemination. A combination of gonadotropins and clomiphene citrate has also been proposed (Fig. 50.4) in order to reduce the amount of hMG required and to induce a more intense ovarian response with better synchronization, but it does not seem to be more efficient than the conventional hMG-regime.

GnRH analogues (agonists and antagonists)

In about 15% of the cycles stimulated with gonadotropins and/or clomiphene citrate, the exaggerated estradiol levels – due to the multifollicular response – provoke high LH concentrations during the follicular phase or untimely spontaneous LH surge. This leads to impaired oocyte quality or, more often, to cycle cancellation. For this reason, a combined therapy of gonadotropins and gonadotropin-releasing hormone (GnRH) analogues have been gradually introduced in order to avoid interference from endogenous gonadotropin secretion. The GnRH analogues are a group of synthetic compounds synthesized from natural GnRH by changing its amino acid sequence. They are divided into the agonists and the antagonists according to their mode of action. The GnRH agonists

Table 50.2 Gonadotropin preparations and their characteristics

Name		Origin	FSH/LH activity	Purity	Production method
Human menopausal gonadotropins	hMG	Urine	1:1	3-5%	Kaolin extracts of women's menopausal urine
Human menopausal gonadotropins	hMG FD	Urine	3:1	3-5%	Partial separation of LH from other urinary proteins
Pure FSH	pFSH	Urine	FSH ≈ 99%	<5%	Separation of LH from other urinary proteins
Highly purified FSH	FSH HP	Urine	FSH ≈ 99.9%	=95%	Selective separation of FSH from urine
Recombinant FSH	recFSH	Cell cultures	FSH ≈ 100%	=100%	Recombinant technology applied in cell lines of Chinese hamster ovary

suppress pituitary function by down-regulating the GnRH receptors and inhibiting the post-receptor mechanisms, after an initial flare-up effect. Their use is safe and their action transient. The GnRH antagonists cause immediate and sustained suppression of pituitary secretion by competitive inhibition of GnRH action without an initial flare-up effect. The more recent third-generation GnRH antagonists should allow for freedom from allergic reactions, and their action is transient.

The GnRH agonists are usually administered according to two different protocols, the short and the long protocols (Fig. 50.5), which are designed to achieve pituitary desensitization and suppression of the endogenous gonadotropin production. In the short protocol, the GnRH agonists are given from cycle day 1, while the gonadotropins are usually started on cycle day 3, making use of the initial stimulatory effect of the GnRH agonists on gonadotropin secretion before pituitary suppression in the late follicular phase. In the long protocol, the GnRH agonists are administered from mid-luteal or early follicular phase until hCG injection, while gonadotropins are administered after pituitary desensitization. Its use is based on the complete suppression of the pituitary ovarian axis before gonadotropin initiation. Alternatively, the ultrashort protocol is designed to enhance follicular development by making use of the initial flare-up effect (Fig. 50.5). In this case, the GnRH agonists are administered only on cycle days 2 to 4, while stimulation with gonadotropins is started from cycle day 3.

Although the GnRH antagonists are still not available for clinical use, the basic concepts and design of their administration for ovarian superovulation are different due to the immediate suppression of pituitary action. Thus, stimulation with gonadotropins begins from cycle day 3 and the GnRH antagonist is added later, usually from cycle day 5 or 7 (Fig. 50.5).

Monitoring of treatment

Proper monitoring of the patient during gonadotropin therapy is essential in order to obtain enough good quality oocytes, to avoid the risk of ovarian hyperstimulation syndrome, and, in cases of ovulation induction for intrauterine insemination, to reduce the incidence of high-order multiple pregnancy. Patient monitoring is based mainly on hormonal and ultrasound examinations.

An ultrasound assessment is necessary before the initiation of treatment in order to exclude the presence of ovarian cystic masses. During the initial latent phase, the gonadotropin dose is adjusted according to the plasma estradiol levels since the ovaries are usually silent. An increase shows an effective dose, while low estradiol levels for more than 5 to 7 days indicate the need for a dose increase. On the other hand, in the "active" phase of treatment, the number and size of the developing follicles have to be estimated by ultrasound examination and by their hormonal activity by plasma estradiol measurements in order to regulate the gonadotropin dose and to determine the timing of the ovulatory hCG dose. Ultrasound examinations can also provide useful information on endometrial thickness and pattern.

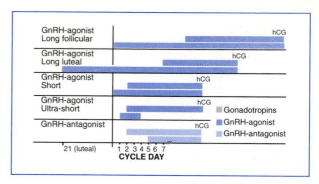

Figure 50.5 Ovarian stimulation with gonadotropin-releasing hormone (GnRH) analogues and gonadotropins: treatment protocols.

Induction of follicular maturation and ovulation

Induction of follicular maturation and subsequent ovulation can be achieved by administering hCG. This is usually the practice in cycles stimulated with clomiphene citrate and/or gonadotropins so as to avoid the need for accurate detection of LH surge onset and ovulation. However, the administration of hCG for follicular maturation and ovulation is necessary in cycles stimulated with GnRH analogues plus gonadotropins, due to the absence here of an endogenous LH surge.

In cycles stimulated without GnRH analogues, hCG is usually given when at least one follicle with a diameter of >17 mm is observed and estradiol levels of about 0.92 to 1.10 nmol/l per follicle >15 mm are reached. In cycles stimulated with GnRH analogues, hCG is administered when two or more follicles with a diameter of approximately 20 mm are identified and estradiol also increases to 0.92 to 1.10 nmol/l per follicle >15 mm. The hCG dose is usually 10 000 IU, although in cases of imminent ovarian hyperstimulation syndrome it can be reduced to 5 000 IU.

IN VITRO FERTILIZATION

Oocyte pick-up and isolation

Pick-up

Oocyte retrieval is performed 36 hours after hCG injection (Fig. 50.6). It was initially carried out by the use of laparoscopy, but this practice has been gradually abandoned and is now used only in exceptional cases. In the present day, transvaginal ultrasound-guided follicular aspiration is primarily used.

The laparoscopic ovum pick-up is usually performed under general anesthesia. The follicles are punctured under direct view of the ovaries with a needle that is passed through a second puncture trocar. The follicles can be flushed and washed with culture media to ensure the recovery of the oocytes. The transvaginal ultrasound-guided oocyte retrieval is performed with an aspiration

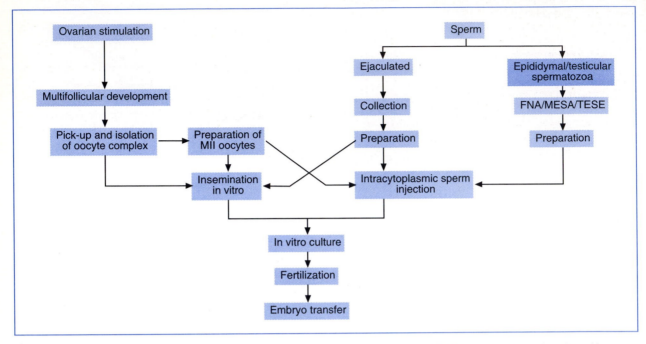

Figure 50.6 In vitro fertilization and intracytoplasmic sperm injection: main steps. (TESE = testicular exploration with sperm extraction; MESA = microsurgical epididymal sperm aspiration; FNA = fine needle aspiration.)

needle connected to the vaginal transducer with a guide under general or local anesthesia. The follicles are aspirated through the vaginal wall during direct viewing of the ultrasound screen. If necessary, the follicles can also be flashed.

Isolation and classification

The recovered oocytes are searched for under a microscope, removed from the follicular fluid, washed, and transferred into culture media. Oocyte maturity is evaluated during this procedure. The classification of the oocytes is based on cumulus-cell density, the appearance of the corona radiata around the oocytes, and the presence of the first polar body (Fig. 50.7).

Sperm preparation

Sperm must always be prepared before in vitro insemination of the oocytes (Fig. 50.6). Several techniques have been devised to remove the seminal plasma, which is thought to prevent capacitation and fertilization of the oocytes. The cellular detritus must be removed as well as to increase the concentration of progressively motile sperm. Centrifugation and washing were initially used in preparing the IVF semen samples, which still remains a useful technique. The swim-up technique is based on the ability of progressively motile spermatozoa to migrate actively and is widely used for IVF samples. The Percoll method usually makes use of a medium with discontinu-

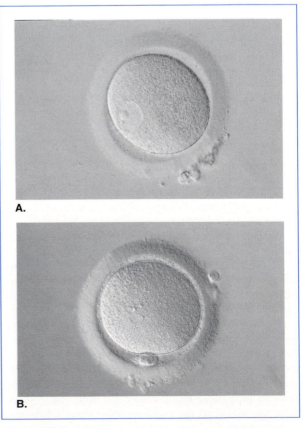

A.

B.

Figure 50.7 (**A**) An immature oocyte and (**B**) a mature metaphase II oocyte.

ous density gradients for centrifugation of the sperm in order to achieve higher concentrations of motile sperm and increased purity because of the fewer abnormal forms, cells, and debris.

Insemination in vitro

The oocytes are inseminated 1 to 4 hours after follicular aspiration. In cases with normal sperm characteristics, 20 000 to 100 000 motile spermatozoa are usually delivered to each oocyte. The number may be raised to 500 000 in cases with poor semen samples. The inseminated oocytes are then cultured for 16 to 20 hours. Open Petri dishes or even tubes can be used for culture in an incubator containing 5% CO_2. Their use, however, is accompanied by fluctuations in the pH and osmotic pressure during the manipulations, by risk of contamination, and the need for a larger amount of medium. The culture of inseminated oocytes in microdrops of medium under paraffin oil in Petri dishes is thought to offer a better and more stable environment and is now used with increasing frequency.

Intracytoplasmic sperm injection

Preparation of the oocytes

The removal of the cumulus and the corona cells from the cumulus-corona-oocyte complexes is a prerequisite for the application of intracytoplasmic sperm injection (Fig. 50.6). This is achieved by a combination of enzymatic and mechanical procedures. Oocytes are then rinsed several times in droplets of medium and inspected for an assessment of their status under an inverted microscope. Only metaphase II (Fig. 50.7b) oocytes are used for intracytoplasmic sperm injection.

Preparation of the spermatozoa

Three types of spermatozoa can be used for intracytoplasmic sperm injection: ejaculated, epididymal, and testicular (Fig. 50.6). The ejaculated sperm, after mixture with medium, are initially centrifuged at high speeds. Then the pellet is passed through a Percoll gradient and submitted to a final centrifugation just before microinjection. The epididymal sperm is recovered from the caput of the epididymis by microsurgery and then treated in the same way as ejaculated sperm. Testicular spermatozoa are isolated from testicular biopsy tissue. The specimens are initially shredded into small pieces in Petri dishes with medium. The medium is then centrifuged after removal of the tissue pieces and the pellet is used for intracytoplasmic sperm injection.

Procedure

Two types of pipettes are prepared carefully for the injection procedure: (1) the injection pipette, and (2) the holding pipette. The pipettes are fixed into the tool-holder of an inverted microscope, connected to a micrometer-type microinjector, and moved by a hydraulic remote-control manipulator. A single, living, immobilized spermatozoon is aspirated, tail first, into the tip of the injection pipette. The oocyte is fixed on the holding pipette with its polar body at 6 o'clock. The injection pipette is pushed into the cytoplasm at the 3 o'clock position, the cytoplasm is aspirated to ensure the penetration of the zona pellucida and the spermatozoon is delivered carefully with a small amount of medium (Fig. 50.8). The injected oocytes are washed and cultured in micro-drops of medium under paraffin oil in a CO_2 incubator.

Embryo transfer

Assessment of fertilization

The oocytes are usually evaluated for fertilization 16 to 18 hours after insemination or micro-injection. Normally fertilized oocytes have two intact or fragmented polar bodies and, more significantly, two distinct pronuclei (Fig. 50.9). This is an important step in the assessment of normal fertilization, since oocytes with one or more than two pronuclei can also cleave. However, such abnormally fertilized but cleaved oocytes should not be transferred.

The embryo cleavage of the two-pronuclei oocytes as well as the evaluation of embryo quality are assessed after a further 24 hours of culture, shortly before transfer. The embryos are graded according to fragmentation, to the number of blastomeres (cleavage rate), and to their equality (Fig. 50.10). Embryos without anucleate fragments are considered to be of excellent quality, while the presence of fragments decreases their quality accordingly.

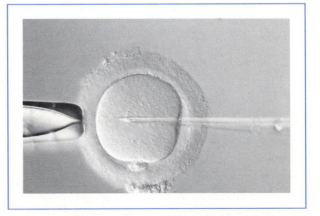

Figure 50.8 Intracytoplasmic sperm injection procedure: The oocyte is fixed on the holding pipette with its polar body at 6 o'clock. The injection pipette is pushed into the cytoplasm at the 3 o'clock position, the cytoplasm is aspirated to ensure the penetration of the zona pellucida and the spermatozoon is delivered carefully with a small amount of medium.

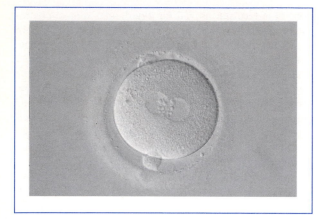

Figure 50.9 A normally fertilized oocyte characterized by the presence of two distinct pronuclei.

Procedure

The transfer of the embryos back into the uterine cavity is usually carried out 2 days after the pick-up and occasionally 3 days after, as in cases of delayed fertilization. The embryos are aspirated with a small amount of culture medium into a polyfluorethylene catheter connected to an insulin syringe. A second, guide catheter is introduced into the uterus through the cervical canal. The transfer catheter is then advanced through the guide catheter close to the fundus, and the embryos are injected carefully and slowly into the uterine cavity.

Luteal phase

The implantation of the transferred embryos is a significant step in the setting up of a successful pregnancy. Maturation of the endometrium during the luteal phase is necessary to make it receptive to the invading embryos. Hormonal supplementation with hCG or progesterone is used routinely for the support of the luteal phase. This is thought to be especially necessary in cycles stimulated with GnRH agonists plus gonadotropins. The use of hCG improves pregnancy rates significantly, but it is also associated with the development of ovarian hyperstimulation syndrome in high-risk patients. On the other hand, the use of progesterone, especially the natural one in the form of vaginal suppositories, is as effective as hCG, and it is not linked with the appearance of ovarian hyperstimulation syndrome.

Results

The fertilization rates of the oocytes inseminated in vitro are usually ~60%. The application of intracytoplasmic sperm injection is associated with an incidence of oocytes damaged by the procedure of 7 to 10% and a fertilization rate of ~60%. The achievement of pregnancy depends on the number and the quality of the embryos transferred as well as on the age of the patient. The pregnancy rates are 20 to 30% for both regular IVF and intracytoplasmic

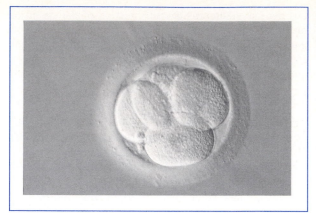

Figure 50.10 A four-cell stage embryo.

sperm injection, while abortion rates are ~15 to 20%. Ectopic pregnancy rates are ~4% for regular IVF and ~1.5% for intracytoplasmic sperm injection. Tubal damage is the main factor associated with ectopic implantation. Approximately 20% of the pregnancies achieved are multifetal.

INTRAUTERINE INSEMINATION

Intrauterine insemination using husband or donor sperm has been performed since the late 1800s. Today, intrauterine insemination is always carried out with prepared spermatozoa. The removal of the seminal plasma by sperm processing methods is thought to enhance capacitation and thus the fertilizing potential of the semen, while a higher concentration of progressively motile and morphologically normal spermatozoa is achieved. The introduction of the prepared sperm into the uterine cavity increases the concentration of the vital spermatozoa in the ampulla by avoiding the filtration effect of the cervix, while the elimination of the distance to be traveled by the spermatozoa is thought also to increase the probability of gamete interaction. Tubal patency, as well as the absence of peritoneal factors impeding ovum release and pick-up, are prerequisites for the use of intrauterine insemination.

The concentration and the total number of the motile spermatozoa inseminated seem to be the most crucial parameters in determining the chances of conception. Normal morphology also seems to be significant in establishing pregnancy. Sperm preparation can be carried out with the same methods as for IVF. Swim-up is commonly used with relatively normal semen samples since it is associated with an excellent isolation of the motile and morphologically normal spermatozoa, but the sperm loss is often high. In the presence of sperm disorders, Percoll methods seem to be better since they are associated with higher sperm recovery rates and greater selection of progressively motile spermatozoa. However, there are no absolute rules.

Intrauterine insemination can be performed in both spontaneous and stimulated cycles. Its use in spontaneous cycles is not associated with increased conception rates.

Ovarian stimulation can be carried out by several regimes, including the use of clomiphene citrate and the use of gonadotropins. The use of gonadotropins is usually more effective, but the development of more than four oocytes must be avoided since the risk of high-order multiple pregnancy is then higher. A low-dose step-up protocol is usually indicated. Accurate estimation of spontaneous ovulation or of ovulation induced by hCG is important. This is achieved with appropriate ultrasound and hormonal monitoring (estradiol and LH levels). The procedure takes place shortly before ovulation. A catheter is passed through the cervix, and 0.3 to 0.5 ml of prepared spermatozoa are usually introduced.

The use of clomiphene citrate for intrauterine insemination is associated with an ~8 to 10% pregnancy rate per cycle and a ~10 to 15% multifetal pregnancy rate, usually twins. The administration of clomiphene citrate and/or gonadotropins increases the pregnancy rate to ~15% per cycle, with a concomitant increase in the incidence of multiple pregnancies to ~20%. The addition of GnRH agonists in the stimulation protocols further increases the pregnancy rate to ~20% per cycle, but it is also accompanied with a multiple pregnancy rate of ~25%. Nowadays, most of the higher order multifetal pregnancies are the direct result of ovarian stimulation with gonadotropins and/or intrauterine insemination.

INTRAFALLOPIAN TRANSFERS

Gamete intrafallopian transfer

Gamete intrafallopian transfer is the replacement of freshly collected oocytes together with prepared spermatozoa in the oviduct. The presence of intact oviducts is an absolute prerequisite for the use of any tubal transfer. The rationale for its use is that the gametes would benefit from the optimal intrafallopian environment, while a better synchronization between embryonal and endometrial development may enhance implantation of the resulting embryos. An additional advantage of laparoscopic tubal transfers is thought to be the absence of endometrial damage.

After proper ovarian stimulation, oocyte retrieval is usually performed transvaginally by ultrasound guidance as for IVF. However, the laparoscopic route can also be used, since access to the fallopian tubes is needed, shortly thereafter, for the replacement of the gametes. Sperm is prepared before the pick-up with the standard IVF preparation techniques. Usually four mature oocytes are replaced, two on each side. The oocytes and the spermatozoa of one side are aspirated separately or mixed into the replacement catheter, and they are then expelled carefully into the tube through a cannula inserted into the ampulla. The same is repeated for the other side.

Zygote intrafallopian transfer

Zygote intrafallopian transfer (ZIFT) was devised as an alternative to gamete intrafallopian transfer in order to bypass the latter's main disadvantage: the lack of any control of fertilization. During zygote intrafallopian transfer, pronuclear-stage embryos are transferred into the tubes; for this reason it also referred to as pronuclear-stage transfer (PROST). Another variant is the tubal embryo transfer (TET), which includes the replacement of day 2 embryos. The application of these techniques is thought to combine the advantages of gamete intrafallopian transfer with those of IVF, that is, the proof of normal fertilization and the exclusion from transfer of polyploid embryos.

Oocytes are aspirated transvaginally by ultrasound guidance. The sperm is prepared with one of the several available techniques. The oocytes are then inseminated and cultured as already described. Fertilization is assessed 16 to 18 hours later and usually up to three normally fertilized oocytes are replaced by the same laparoscopic technique as in gamete intrafallopian transfer. Day 2 embryos can also be transferred, while the transcervical route by retrograde tubal catheterization can be used.

Comments

The application of tubal transfers gave way to serious criticism as to their relative effectiveness. Intrafallopian transfers offer no advantage in terms of implantation and pregnancy rates in systems with optimal in vitro culture conditions. However, in IVF laboratories with suboptimal culture conditions, the patients may benefit from tubal transfers. Also, in cases with difficult or impossible transcervical embryo transfer, a tubal transfer can be called for.

The combination of gamete intrafallopian transfer with diagnostic and/or therapeutic laparoscopy has also been proposed as possibly yielding good results. In these cases, ovarian stimulation has to be moderate (e.g., with clomiphene citrate) in order to avoid problems with visualization, since the existence of stimulated ovaries is thought to be a contraindication for their accurate clinical assessment during laparoscopy. Tubal transfers may also be useful in cases where embryos are of poor quality and reduced implantation capacity, such as frozen-thawed embryos and embryos of women over 40 years old. Tubal transfers may be an alternative to co-culture systems in patients with poor embryonic development in vitro. The validity of these special indications has to be proven by prospective studies.

COMPLICATIONS

Ovarian hyperstimulation syndrome

The ovarian stimulation used in assisted conception cycles is associated with a non-physiological ovarian response and may occasionally lead to the development of ovarian hyperstimulation syndrome. This condition is characterized by a broad spectrum of clinical and laboratory manifestations, and in extreme cases it can be accompanied by serious and potentially life-threatening complications. The pathophysiological change responsible for ovarian hyperstimulation syndrome presentation is an acute increase in vascular permeability, leading to third space shifting (abdominal, pleural, and pericardial cavities as well as anasarca). This also results in a rapid depletion of intravascular plasma volume and, consequently, in hypovolemia, hypotension, and hemoconcentration. The severity of ascites and the rising hematocrit are usually used as parameters in the management of ovarian hyperstimulation syndrome.

The hallmark in ovarian hyperstimulation syndrome establishment is either the exogenous hCG given for follicular maturation/ovulation or the endogenous hCG produced by an ongoing pregnancy. Several strategies have been proposed for the prevention of ovarian hyperstimulation syndrome. In patients with PCOS, the low-dose step-up and the step-down protocols should be used for ovulation induction. In cases of imminent ovarian hyperstimulation syndrome, discontinuation of ovarian stimulation and either cancellation of pre-ovulatory hCG injection or administration of hCG after a pause of several days can prevent the occurrence of ovarian hyperstimulation syndrome. The use of GnRHa for follicular maturation/ovulation has also been proposed as preventive manipulation. Another alternative is to cancel embryo transfer and cryopreserve the resulting embryos to avoid endogenous hCG production from a pregnancy. The luteal phase should be supported with progesterone since hCG could induce ovarian hyperstimulation syndrome presentation.

Mild cases of ovarian hyperstimulation syndrome can be managed on an outpatient basis with careful clinical and laboratory assessment of the affected women. Moderate and severe cases need hospitalization, and the existence of life-threatening complications necessitates intensive care management. Balanced and careful restoration of intravascular volume depletion with crystalloids and/or colloids is essential. Abdominal paracentesis should be considered in cases of tense ascites, impairment of renal function, and hemoconcentration unresponsive to medical therapy. Severe complications (hypovolemic shock, renal failure, thromboembolic phenomena, and adult respiratory distress syndrome) need additional treatment measures. Surgery should be avoided except for in the events of the rupture of ovarian cysts, torsion of the ovaries, or ectopic pregnancy.

Multiple pregnancies

Multiple pregnancies should be considered as a complication because they are accompanied by serious problems at the level of gestational management and fetal outcome. Sociological and economic problems, even of secondary value, are quite serious as well. In order to avoid the occurrence of multifetal pregnancies after assisted reproduction techniques, there is a need for innovations that can balance between seemingly contradictory purposes: maintaining the effectiveness of these techniques in terms of pregnancy rates and at the same time reducing the risk of multiple births.

In cases of ovulation induction, with or without intrauterine insemination, the number of preovulatory follicles ≥ 14 mm is the most significant parameter affecting multiple implantation. Oligofollicular development is essential in the prevention of multiple pregnancies and should be based on the more judicious use of stimulatory agents and/or the choice of the appropriate protocols such as the low-dose step-up or the step-down protocols. In cases of multifollicular development, discontinuation of ovarian stimulation and either cycle cancellation or administration of hCG after a pause of several days could be used as preventive measures. Conversion of an intrauterine insemination to an IVF cycle (with limitation of the transferred embryos) and elective oocyte retrieval before intrauterine insemination (in order to leave only a limited number of oocytes) are other effective alternatives.

In IVF and gamete intrafallopian transfer, the incidence of multiple pregnancies can be controlled by reducing the number of the embryos/oocytes transferred into the uterus/tubes. In young women until three embryos should be transferred. However, the elective transfer of two good quality embryos is another alternative that can prevent triplets without decreasing pregnancy rates. On the other hand, in older patients, a more aggressive embryo transfer policy is allowed due to the lower implantation capacity of the embryos that result.

Once a multiple pregnancy is achieved, selective embryo reduction to twins seems to be an effective treatment alternative. Due to the serious ethical problems associated with its application, preventive measures should always be applied very strictly.

Suggested readings

ANDERSEN AN, LINDHARD A, LOFT A, ZIEBE S, ANDERSEN CY. The infertile patient with hydrosalpinges - IVF with or without salpingectomy? Hum Reprod 1996;11:2081-4.

DE KRETSER DM. Male infertility. Lancet 1997;349:787-90.

DEVROEY P, NAGY P, TOURNAYE H, LIU J, SILBER S, VAN STEIRTEGHEM A. Outcome of intracytoplasmic sperm injection with testicular spermatozoa in obstructive and non-obstructive azoospermia. Hum Reprod 1996;11:1015-8.

FAUSER B, VAN HEUSDEN A. Manipulation of human ovarian function: physiological concepts and clinical consequences.

Endocr Rev 1997;18:71-106.

HULL MGR, FLEMING CF. Tubal surgery versus assisted reproduction: assessing their role in infertility therapy. Curr Opin Obstet Gynecol 1995;7:160-7.

JONES HW, TONER JP. The infertile couple. N Engl J Med 1993;329:1710-5.

MARSHBURN PB, KUTTEH WH. The role of antisperm antibodies in infertility. Fertil Steril 1994;61:799-811.

PELLICER A, OLIVEIRA N, RUIZ A, REMOHI J, SIMÓN C. Exploring the mechanism(s) of endometriosis-related infertility: an analysis of embryo development and implantation in assisted reproduction. Hum Reprod 1995;10 (Suppl. 2):91-7.

Reissmann T, Felderbaum R, Diedrich K, Engel J, Comary-Schally AM, Schally AV. Development and applications of luteinizing hormone antagonists in the treatment of infertility: an overview. Hum Reprod 1995;10:1974-81.

Smitz J, Ron-El R, Tarlatzis BC. The use of gonadotrophin releasing hormone agonists for in vitro fertilization and other assisted procreation techniques: Experience from three centres. Hum Reprod 1992;7 (Suppl 1):49-66.

Soliman S, Daya S, Collins J, Hughes E. The role of luteal phase support in infertility treatment: a meta-analysis of randomized trials. Fertil Steril 1994;61:1068-76.

The ESHRE Capri Workshop. Infertility revisited: The state of the art today and tomorrow. Hum Reprod 1996;11:1779-807.

Tournaye H, Camus M, Ubaldi F, Clasen K, Van Steirteghem A, Devroey P. Tubal transfer: a forgotten ART? Is there still an important role for tubal transfer procedures? Hum Reprod 1996;11:1815-22.

Van Steirteghem AC, Liu J, Joris H, et al. Higher success rate by intracytoplasmic sperm injection than by subzonal insemination. Report of a second series of 300 consecutive treatment cycles. Hum Reprod 1993;8:1055-60.

Van Steirteghem AC, Nagy Z, Joris H, et al. High fertilization and implantation rates after intracytoplasmic sperm injection. Hum Reprod 1993;8:1061-6.

Endocrinology of pregnancy

Felice Petraglia

ENDOCRINOLOGY OF THE PLACENTA

Placental hormonal substances include two major groups: (1) protein and peptides (including cytokines and growth factors), and (2) steroid hormones. Hormones are localized in the cytotrophoblast and syncytiotrophoblast layers of the placenta. They act on placental growth and differentiation through autocrine/paracrine mechanisms, and they modulate a variety of placental functions, such as hormonogenesis, blood flow, and immune function. Several of these products are released into the maternal circulation. Other than the trophoblast, the maternal decidua and fetal membranes (amnion and chorion) produce several of the hormones typically expressed from placental cells. These hormones may be secreted in amniotic fluid and/or maternal circulation and locally act in the placental fetal-maternal interface. Some of these placental hormones exert their effects on the fetus as well as on the mother, participating in fetal and maternal homeostasis during pregnancy.

Protein and peptide hormones

Human chorionic gonadotropin To rescue the corpus luteum and to maintain progesterone secretion for the maintenance of pregnancy, the placental cytotrophoblast secretes a luteinizing hormone (LH)-like hormone, human chorionic gonadotropin (hCG), which prevents the lysis of the corpus luteum, resulting in a persistent secretion of progesterone that maintains the endometrium for implantation and development of the blastocyst.

Human chorionic gonadotropin is a glycoprotein hormone with biological and immunological characteristics similar to pituitary LH. It is composed of two noncovalently linked subunits: α (which is common to LH, follicle-stimulating hormone [FSH], and thyroid-stimulating hormone [TSH]) and β (which confers specificity). Human chorionic gonadotropin is secreted from trophoblastic tissues and is primarily released into the maternal circulation, with only 1% released into the fetal compartment. The concentration in maternal circulation peaks during the first 12 weeks of gestation (60-100 IU/ml), decreasing at about 18 to 20 weeks to a plateau that remains stable throughout gestation. The kidneys are the major route for metabolizing plasma hCG. The placental production of hCG is not subjected to the negative feedback action of sex steroids. Human chorionic gonadotropin receptors have been located in fetal testis, ovary, adrenal gland, kidney and thymus. Human chorionic gonadotropin may play an important role either in preventing the maternal rejection of the fetus, because it causes a specific and noncytotoxic inhibition of lymphocytes, or in stimulating fetal thyroid cell function. Human chorionic gonadotropin levels are measured in urine or maternal plasma for the diagnosis of pregnancy, in cases of miscarriage and therapeutic abortion, ectopic pregnancy, and molar pregnancy.

Human placental lactogen Human placental lactogen (hPL) is composed of a single-chain polypeptide (191 amino acids) with 85% homology to pituitary growth hormone (GH) and prolactin. Human placental lactogen has effects on lipid and glucose metabolism, as well as on body weight gain, similar to those of GH. Maternal serum or urine human placental lactogen levels increase steadily throughout pregnancy. This hormone is produced by the syncytiotrophoblast and exerts its major metabolic effect on the mother, ensuring increased nutritional demands of the fetus. A major effect of human placental lactogen is on insulin and glucose metabolism, as well as on lipolysis, an action that involves insulin-like growth factor I (IGF-I). Indeed, human placental lactogen also stimulates IGF-1 production and substrate availability, contributing to the growth of the fetus.

In multiple gestation and in diabetic pregnancies, when the placentas are larger, higher maternal human placental lactogen levels are observed. Low human placental lactogen levels in maternal serum have been found in intrauterine growth retardation, prolonged gestation, hypertension, and preeclampsia.

Adrenocorticotropic hormone and pro-opiomelanocortin related peptides Adrenocorticotropic hormone (ACTH) is secreted by the syncytiotrophoblast from a precursor molecule, pro-opiomelanocortin (POMC). Other important peptides derived from the same glycoprotein precursor are *β-endorphin (β-END), β-lipotropin (β-LPH)*, and *β-MSH*. Production and release of ACTH and *β-END* from the placenta is increased by corticotropin-releasing factor (CRF), suggesting a regulating pathway similar to the hypothalamus-pituitary-adrenal axis. Plasma ACTH levels rise during the third trimester of gestation, reaching high concentrations during labor and delivery. Furthermore, maternal levels of β-END are correlated with the degree of pain perception during labor and delivery. Conditions such as hypoxia and acidosis result in an increase of ACTH and β-END levels.

Neurohormones

Gonadotropin-releasing hormone (GnRH) and its precursor are produced by cytotrophoblast cells. GnRH is immunologically and chemically identical to hypothalamic GnRH; its production of placental GnRH is stimulated by estrogen, activin, prostaglandins, and adrenaline, and production is inhibited by progesterone, inhibin, and endogenous opioid peptides. Placental GnRH regulates local hCG and steroid hormone release, and it stimulates the release of prostaglandins. It is secreted in maternal plasma. The concentration varies in a pulsatile fashion. A correlation between plasma GnRH and hCG concentrations exists; for example, the highest circulating levels of both hormones occur during the first trimester of gestation.

Corticotropin-releasing factor is secreted by the trophoblast, fetal membranes, and the decidua; and it is identical to hypothalamic CRF, a neurohormone that stimulates ACTH and POMC-derived peptide release from pituitary cells. Placental CRF regulates ACTH and β-END release from cultured trophoblast cells. Placental CRF release is stimulated by glucocorticoids, prostaglandins, noradrenaline, acetylcholine, interleukin 1, arginine-vasopressin, angiotensin II, oxytocin, and neuropeptide Y, while it is inhibited by nitric oxide and progesterone. Glucocorticoids stimulate its production by fetal membranes. Maternal plasma CRF levels increase during pregnancy and reach peak values at term. The major role of placental CRF is to stimulate the maternal and fetal pituitary-adrenal axes. Other local functions of CRF include the stimulation of prostaglandin secretion from the placenta and fetal membranes, the vasodilatation of utero-placental vessels, and the myometrial contractility is increased.

CRF-binding protein, a protein that binds CRF and reduces its biological action, is produced by the syncytiotrophoblast, the decidua, and fetal membranes. Its circulating levels in pregnant women are not higher than those of nonpregnant women or men. Maternal CRF-binding protein levels decrease two- to threefold during the last 4 weeks of pregnancy. These changes induce an increase of free CRF, which may exert local actions on the intrauterine tissues approaching parturition.

Somatostatin is secreted by cytotrophoblast cells during the first trimester of pregnancy. It is secreted in maternal circulation and its levels decrease with advancing gestational age. Its possible function is to inhibit the release of human placental lactogen.

Neuropeptide Y is produced by cytotrophoblast cells. Maternal levels of neuropeptide Y reach peak values at parturition and fall rapidly after delivery. Neuropeptide Y plays a role in modulating placental hormone secretion and probably in local vasculature tone.

Oxytocin stimulates uterine contractions by acting both directly on the myometrium and indirectly on decidual prostaglandin production. The origin of oxytocin is the posterior pituitary lobe, although recent data also indicate the expression of a placental oxytocin. Oxytocin metabolism apparently does not change during pregnancy. The increase in the sensitivity of the uterus to this hormone with advancing gestational age is mediated by a specific increase in the density of oxytocin receptors. Oxytocin also plays a major role in milk ejection during lactation; it binds to receptors on myoepithelial cells of the mammary gland, producing contraction of the mammary smooth muscle.

Relaxin is a double chain protein hormone secreted in pregnancy mainly by the corpus luteum, and also by the placenta, decidua, and chorion. This hormone may influence prostaglandin secretion in the membranes. During the first trimester, maternal serum relaxin levels increase, suggesting a role in maintaining early pregnancy, possibly in synergy with progesterone. It is also involved in the softening and ripening of the pregnant cervix, in advancing the Bishop Score, in relaxation of the pubic symphysis, and in inhibition of uterine contractility. During the second trimester, relaxin concentration in the maternal serum declines.

Growth factors

Growth factors synthesized by the trophoblast include *epidermal growth factor* (EGF), *platelet-derived growth factor* (PDGF), *nerve growth factor* (NGF), *fibroblast growth factor* (FGF), and *transforming growth factor* (TGF). They are involved in placental differentiation, proliferation, and growth during pregnancy, acting on specific receptors. The production of these factors is mainly localized in cytotrophoblast cells. They are poorly secreted in maternal circulation.

Recently a new family of growth factors has been characterized in human placenta called the inhibin-related proteins. Placental inhibin, activin, and follistatin are produced by trophoblast cells and have different roles in gestational physiology. It has been suggested that these inhibin-related proteins take part in regulating hCG and progesterone secretion, in modulating immune function, in embryogenesis, and in prostaglandin release. Maternal serum and amniotic fluid levels of inhibin, activin, and follistatin increase throughout pregnancy. Activin levels reach their peak value at the onset of spontaneous labor, and they are higher in women with preeclampsia and preterm labor.

Maternal insulin-like growth factor I (IGF-I) levels increase approximately threefold throughout gestation, whereas IGF-II concentration does not change. These two growth factors may be involved either in prenatal fetal growth or in placental growth. In the circulation, they are primarily complexed to IGF-binding proteins to reduce their clearance from the blood. During normal gestation serum IGF-binding protein 1 levels increase, while in healthy pregnant women serum levels of IGF-binding protein 2 and IGF-binding protein 3 decrease. Newborn birth weight is directly correlated with maternal levels of IGF-I and inversely with IGF-binding protein 1. The increase of IGF-I levels during the third trimester of pregnancy may result from placental GH stimulation of IGF-I and IGF-binding protein 3 secretion, which may reduce the metabolic clearance rate of IGF-I.

Cytokines

Cytokines secreted from the trophoblast and the decidua include: *interleukins* (ILs), *tumor necrosis factor-alpha* (TNF-α), and *interferons* (IFNs). In the human placenta the two major forms of interleukins are IL-1 (IL-1α, IL-1β,) and IL-6. Interferon alpha is the form more diffuse in the feto-placental unit, being present in the various intrauterine tissues, including placenta, fetal membranes, and maternal decidua; however, it is not detectable in maternal blood. Women with preterm labor and intra-amniotic infection have significantly higher amniotic fluid IL-1β and IL-6 levels. Amniotic fluid IL-6 levels correlate with histological chorioamnionitis and amniotic fluid cultures in women in premature labor with intact membranes, suggesting that elevated amniotic fluid IL-6 is predictive of preterm delivery even in the absence of a positive amniotic culture of chorioamnionitis.

Steroid hormones

Progestogens

Progesterone prepares and maintains the endometrium to allow for implantation, probably suppressing the maternal immunological response to fetal antigens and preventing maternal rejection of the trophoblast. Progesterone is largely produced by the corpus luteum until about 10 weeks of pregnancy, and thereafter, the placenta is the major source. Precursors are derived from the maternal bloodstream, while the fetal contribution is negligible. Serum progesterone levels increase throughout pregnancy

Some progesterone metabolites, such as 21-hydroxylated derivatives, may be biologically active and responsible for the drowsiness and behavioral effects associated with pregnancy. For this reason, and also because they are synthesized by neuronal/glial cells, they have been named neuroactive steroids or neurosteroids. The decidua and fetal membranes also synthesize and metabolize progesterone, using pregnenolone sulfate as a precursor. This local steroidogenesis may play a role at parturition. The fetus may die in utero without a change in progesterone levels; progesterone is not affected in cases of anencephaly or placental sulfatase deficiency.

Androgens

Dehydroepiandrosterone sulfate (DHEAS) from both the mother and the fetus provides the substrate for estrogen production by the placenta. DHEAS is actively metabolized by the placenta by an active sulfatase that converts DHEAS to free DHEA. Free DHEA can diffuse into the syncytiotrophoblasts, where it is actively metabolized to estrogen. The metabolic clearance rate of DHEAS increases throughout pregnancy.

Another important change in the metabolism of DHEAS during pregnancy is an estrogen-induced increase in maternal hepatic 16-hydroxylation of DHEAS. Because the conversion of DHEAS to estrogen occurs via its irreversible placental metabolism, this is a better marker of placental activity than the total metabolic clearance rate of DHEAS. The conversion of DHEAS to estrogen increases from about 5% in the first trimester to 5 to 25% in the second trimester, to 25 to 40% in the third trimester. The placental conversion of *androstenedione* to estrogen also increases with advancing gestation. The levels of sex hormone-binding globulin (SHBG) increase early in pregnancy, while the metabolic clearance rate of both *testosterone* and *5-dihydrotestosterone* is significantly decreased compared with those of nonpregnant women.

Estrogens

Placental estrogen production during pregnancy largely results from the conversion of maternal and fetal adrenal precursors. The basic precursors of estrogens are 19-carbon androgens (androstenedione and DHEA). Estrogen concentrations in the maternal circulation increase steadily throughout pregnancy. In the first trimester of gestation, *estrone (E_1)* and *estradiol (E_2)* predominate. The ovary is a major source of estrogens, while the maternal adrenal cortex remains the major source of androgen precursors for placental estrogen formation. In the second and third trimesters, *estriol (E_3)* becomes the most important estrogen. Because human placenta lacks a 16-hydroxylation activity, fetal liver provides the androgen precursor 16-OH-DHEAS (derived from fetal adrenal DHEAS) for placental estriol production. Estrogen, in turn, feeds back to the fetal adrenal to direct steroidogenesis along the pathway to provide even more of its precursor, DHEAS. With birth and loss of exposure to estrogen, neonatal 16-hydroxylation activity rapidly disappears. Therefore, fetal endocrine function is characterized by rapid and extensive conjugation of steroids with sulfate for protection from the biologic effects of the steroids present in such great quantities.

Estriol is formed from a nonfunctional or dysfunctional fetal adrenal. Anencephaly is associated with relative absence of the fetal zone of the adrenal cortex. Decreased levels of fetal adrenal androgen precursors lead to a greatly decreased estriol output from the placenta. When fetal low density lipoprotein-cholesterol precursors are decreased, as in hypobetalipoproteinemia and placental sulfatase deficiency, the lack of lipoprotein for androgen production and enzyme for sulfate cleavage lead to a decrease in estriol production. Hydatiform molar pregnancies are also associated with low estriol output.

MATERNAL ENDOCRINE CHANGES DURING PREGNANCY

Pituitary gland

The volume of the pituitary gland increases by 136% from early to term pregnancy. The number, structure, and function of thyrotrope, gonadotrope, corticotrope, soma-totrope, and lactotrope cells change significantly during pregnancy. The greatest gestation-related changes occur in the lactotropes. In fact, in the third trimester they represent 60% of the pituitary cells. By one month postpartum, the number of lactotropes decrease in nonlactating women. The number of gonadotropes and ACTH-secreting cells markedly decrease during pregnancy, as well as the number or somatotropes. Thyrotrope cells show little changes.

Growth hormone During pregnancy, the secretion of growth hormone by the maternal pituitary is markedly suppressed. Human placenta produces a variant of GH (GH-V) that is encoded by its own gene and differs by 13 amino acids from pituitary GH. This variant of GH is secreted in a nonpulsatile manner, with minimal diurnal variation, and is biologically active. Near term, only 3% of circulating GH bioactivity is derived from maternal pituitary secretion, while 85% is derived from placental secretion of GH-V, and 12% is derived from the actions of chorionic somatomammotropin. This circulating GH-V probably stimulates IGF-1 secretion, which results in a negative feedback suppression of maternal GH secretion. At the third trimester of pregnancy, the elevated GH-V and IGF-1 concentrations and the decreased IGF-BP concentrations create an "acromegalic-like" state.

Thyroid-stimulating hormone Maternal concentrations of TSH are within the normal range, and the TSH response to thyrotropin-releasing hormone (TRH) is normal throughout pregnancy. A small change in maternal circulating TSH levels is observed between 9 and 13 weeks of gestation, at the same time as the peak placental production of hCG. This decrease may be due to the weak thyrotropic properties of hCG.

Luteinizing hormone and follicular-stimulating hormone The markedly elevated concentrations of estradiol and progesterone during pregnancy suppress maternal LH and FSH. The increased inhibin secretion by the placenta and corpus luteum may act synergistically with estradiol to suppress FSH secretion. Maternal serum LH and FSH levels are decreased by 6 to 7 weeks of pregnancy and are near or below the detection limits of most assays in the second and third trimester. After delivery, maternal concentrations of estradiol, progesterone, and inhibin decrease rapidly, and circulating LH and FSH levels slowly return to normal.

Prolactin During pregnancy *prolactin* is produced by the maternal and fetal pituitary glands, and particularly by the maternal decidua. The decidual secretion of prolactin is the source of the amniotic prolactin, while prolactin detected both in the fetal and maternal circulation is secreted from the pituitary gland. Amniotic fluid levels of prolactin are similar to those found in the maternal serum until 10 weeks of pregnancy, then rise markedly until the 20th week, and finally decrease. Maternal serum prolactin levels progressively increase throughout pregnancy. Amniotic prolactin reduces the permeability of the human amnion in the fetal to maternal direction, and it may be important (as well as renin) in the regulation of water and electrolytes in amniotic fluid. In the maternal compartment, prolactin prepares the mammary glands for future lactation.

Following delivery, in non-nursing mothers, prolactin concentration decreases to nonpregnant levels within 3 months. In nursing women, baseline serum prolactin concentration slowly decreases to nonpregnant levels, and intermittent episodic pulses of prolactin secretion in conjunction with nursing are observed.

Adrenal cortex

Adrenal morphology does not change substantially during pregnancy, even though the most complex and fascinating endocrine changes in pregnancy are those involving the maternal adrenal cortex. The increase in adrenal steroid biosynthesis in pregnancy modulates metabolic, fluid, and electrolyte changes that occur in pregnancy. Although adrenal androgen synthesis is increased, DHEA levels are lower during pregnancy because of increased placental uptake and metabolism.

In nonpregnant individuals, *cortisol* secretion is under control of the central nervous system. In fact, CRF secreted from the hypothalamus directly stimulates the release of ACTH, which is the major secretagogue for cortisol. During pregnancy, the human placenta secretes large amounts of CRF into the maternal and fetal circulation. This probably explains the increase in maternal cortisol levels during the second and third trimesters. The levels of the cortisol-binding globulin also increase two- to three-fold, though both bound and unbound cortisol increase. During pregnancy there is an increase in the overall conversion of cortisol to cortisone, modulated by cytotrophoblastic 11-OH-dehydrogenase. Human placental cortisol-cortisone interconversion decreases with gestational age.

The elevated free cortisol in pregnancy probably contributes to insulin resistance, in particular in the third trimester, when both free cortisol and insulin resistance are maximal. Hypercortisolism may also contribute to abnormal striae during pregnancy, but most full-blown signs of Cushing's syndrome do not appear. The high progesterone levels may act as a glucocorticoid antagonist and prevent some cortisol effects during pregnancy.

Maternal serum concentrations of *11-deoxycorticosterone* are much higher in the third trimester of pregnancy than in nonpregnant women. The source of these elevated 11-deoxycorticosterone levels is the peripheral 21-hydroxylation of progesterone, such as in the kidney.

Maternal plasma *aldosterone* levels steadily increase throughout pregnancy, reaching a peak in midpregnancy; these levels are maintained until delivery, when they rapidly fall. The augmented aldosterone secretion in pregnancy is due to increased zona glomerulosa stimulation by angiotensin II, ACTH, and extracellular potassium. Aldosterone during pregnancy is secreted predominantly in the urine as tetrahydro-aldosterone, 18-monoglucuronide aldosterone, and free aldosterone. The main role of aldosterone in pregnancy is to stimulate transepithelial sodium transport across the kidneys, sweat glands, salivary glands, and the gastrointestinal tract.

Thyroid gland

Total concentrations of both *3,5,3'-triiodothyronine (T$_3$) and thyroxine (T$_4$)* are significantly increased. Plasma T$_4$ levels rise before T$_3$ levels. Thyroxine is present in the circulation bound to thyroxine-binding globulin, albumin, and prealbumin, whereas only a small percentage is present as free T$_4$. During the first half of gestation the levels of thyroxine-binding globulin increase from two- to three-fold, and they remain constant thereafter. Human placenta is able to deiodinate T$_4$ to T$_3$ and convert these active hormones to inactive derivatives, in particular early in pregnancy. This metabolization steadily decreases with the progression of gestation because of a rapid decline in the activity of this enzyme, and it may account for the apparent maintenance of a low placental extraction of T$_3$ and T$_4$. Furthermore, during normal pregnancy, the increase in thyroxine-binding globulin may cause a transient decrease in the free T$_4$ and T$_3$ levels, which may account for the increase in TSH levels and in thyroid size (from 10 to 30%).

Human placenta contains TRH-like immunoreactivity, but it is not known whether this placental TRH-like material has physiological significance. Human chorionic gonadotropin plays an important role as a thyrotropic hormone because of its structural resemblance to TSH; it can bind to the TSH receptor and have intrinsic thyrotropic activity. In addition, hCG accounts for a substantial minority of the total serum thyrotropic activity in early pregnancy and contributes to the increase in maternal thyroid size.

Parathyroid glands

Parathyroid hormone (PTH) is the main regulator of the serum calcium concentration in pregnancy. In fact, normal fetal skeletal mineralization requires that 30 g of calcium be supplied to the fetus by the pregnant woman. PTH and vitamin D interact in modulating the calcium uptake from the fetus (Fig. 51.1). During pregnancy, serum intact PTH levels fall by an average of about 50%, probably in response to increased vitamin D levels and intestinal calcium absorption. Calcitriol, on the other hand, stimulates intestinal calcium absorption. Calcitriol is normally produced from precursors by the kidney, and by human placenta increasing the serum calcitriol concentration to double.

Pancreas

Normal pregnancy is characterized by a reduction in the ability of insulin to stimulate glucose uptake and by an enhancement of β cell insulin secretion (Fig. 51.2). From conception to delivery, the ability of insulin to stimulate glucose utilization declines from 50 to 70%, and insulin secretory responses to nutrients such as glucose increase from two- to threefold. Early pregnancy is characterized

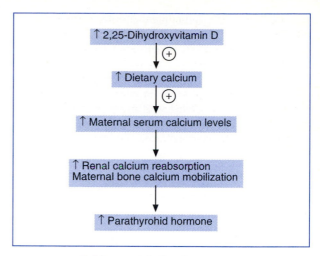

Figure 51.1 Calcium metabolism in pregnancy.

by increased insulin secretion from the maternal pancreas, and a decrease in maternal glucose levels; at term, an increased insulin resistance results in stimulating gluconeogenesis and increased maternal glucose levels. In nondiabetic women during the third trimester of pregnancy, insulin resistance and hyperinsulinemia are both increased in response to glucose, but the metabolic clearance rate of insulin is not altered. In fact, the increased insulin resistance that occurs in pregnancy is primarily due to the action of other hormones (human placental lactogen, cortisol, and GH).

In pregnant women during the fed state, the disposal of glucose is impaired, which produces somewhat higher maternal blood levels. Diabetic pregnant women have high glucose levels, and the flow of nutritional substrates is directed from maternal circulation to the fetus. The subsequent fetal hyperinsulinemia represents a strong stimulus for growth, whereas human placental lactogen directly affects fetal tissue metabolism, including synergistic

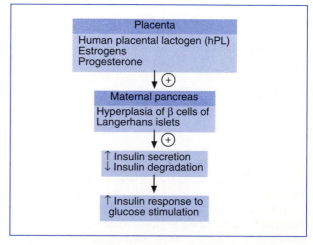

Figure 51.2 Placental hormones and glucose metabolism.

actions with insulin and in particular liver gluconeogenesis. Later in gestation, human placental lactogen enhances lipolysis and ketogenesis, which are metabolic sources for the fetus.

Insulin also directly inhibits pulmonary surfactant protein secretion, leading to the increase in respiratory distress syndrome associated with hyperglycemia in pregnancy. Thus, the effective control of maternal diabetes reduces the risk of neonatal respiratory distress syndrome.

Cardiovascular hormones

The kidneys and decidua secrete *renin* during pregnancy, which plays an important role in regulating water and electrolytes in amniotic fluid.

Posterior pituitary *vasopressin* is involved in the control of osmolarity, acting by inhibiting water loss in the kidney. Plasma osmolarity starts to decrease in early gestation and ends up at significantly lower than nonpregnant levels by the fifth week of gestation. It reaches a nadir at about the tenth week, and this level is then maintained until term. After the first trimester, the degradative enzyme vasopressinase, secreted by the syncytiotrophoblast, is detected in the circulation and increases to maximum levels at 36 weeks of gestation. This is probably an important factor for the increase in the metabolic clearance rate of vasopressin during pregnancy. The metabolic clearance rate of vasopressin increases in the second half of gestation, and it decreases after delivery. During pregnancy, increased renal blood flow does not significantly contribute to the increase in metabolic clearance rate. The two major stimuli for vasopressin secretion are osmolarity and blood volume, but also nausea, hypoglycemia, angiotensin, and stress.

Human atrial tissue produces a hormone called *atrial natriuretic peptide*, which causes a potent natriuretic effect and smooth muscle relaxation. This peptide has been found both in maternal and fetal circulation, and its plasma concentrations rise during labor.

ENDOCRINOLOGY OF PARTURITION

During the last weeks of normal pregnancy, two major processes occur: increased uterine contractions, and a softening and thinning of the lower uterine segment and cervix. Labor is the final event of gestation, and its onset is usually fairly abrupt with the establishment of regular contractions every 2 to 5 minutes. At this time, several factors and mechanisms allow for the beginning of the myometrial contractions and dilatation of the cervix, and the fetus is subsequently expelled in less than 24 hours.

Estrogens play an important role in the activation of myometrial contractions. They rise in concentration throughout pregnancy, reaching their peak value at term. They act by stimulating oxytocin secretion, by increasing the uterine sensibility to oxytocin, and by stimulating prostaglandin secretion and cervical maturation.

Because *progesterone* is essential for the maintenance of early pregnancy, it has been suggested that its withdrawal leads to termination of pregnancy. Progesterone has an inhibitory role on myometrial contractions. Furthermore, progesterone decreases adrenergic receptors, inhibits estrogen and oxytocin receptor synthesis, and promotes the storage of prostaglandin precursors in the decidua and fetal membranes. At the end of the gestational period, the estrogen/progesterone ratio increases, probably due to (1) an inhibitory feedback of estrogens on the progesterone secretion, (2) placental maturation, or (3) a signal from the fetus.

Prostaglandins have a major role at parturition. During pregnancy amniotic fluid prostaglandin concentrations remain unchanged until labor, upon which they rise subsequent to the rupture of membranes and dilatation of the lower uterine segment. The major sources of prostaglandins are the placenta, decidua, and fetal membranes. Some endocrine/paracrine factors stimulate the production of prostaglandins: oxytocin, CRF, ACTH, interleukins, activin A, TGFβ, and EGF. Interestingly, the concentration of these factors increases at term. The two major enzymes responsible for prostaglandin levels are prostaglandin synthetase and hydroxyprostaglandin dehydrogenase. The clinical use of prostaglandins for the induction of labor is quite common, and the local intracervical application of prostaglandins is useful for cervical ripening. Their major function is to stimulate the myometrial contractility. Prostaglandins are almost certainly involved in the maintenance of labor once it is established.

Catecholamines exert their effects on myometrial contractility: in fact, β-adrenergic activity stimulates contractions, whereas β-adrenergic activity inhibits labor. Progesterone increases the receptor/receptor ratio at the myometrial level, thus favoring continued pregnancy. There is no evidence that changes in catecholamine levels or their receptor density initiate labor, but it is likely that such changes occur when labor is established. The β-adrenergic drug ritodrine has proved to be a valuable agent in the management of premature labor.

At parturition, plasma levels of *oxytocin* are fivefold more elevated than plasma levels of neurohypophyseal oxytocin. Both maternal and fetal oxytocin levels reach their peak value in correspondence with the expulsive time of parturition, but neither has been convincingly shown to increase prior to labor. This hormone is perhaps the main stimulating factor of myometrial contractility at delivery, and it is suggested that its role in the initiation of labor is due to an increased sensitivity of the uterus to it rather than increased plasma concentrations of the hormone. Another mechanistic action of oxytocin is the stimulation of prostaglandin $F_{2\alpha}$ ($PGF_{2\alpha}$) secretion by the decidua and fetal membranes. The clinical use of oxytocin for the induction of labor is a classic approach.

Another important factor at delivery is the increase of free *CRF* and the decline of CRF-binding protein levels. This represents a response to the stress of parturition through the increased secretion of *ACTH* and *cortisol*. In addition, CRF has paracrine control on uterine contractility by increasing the secretion of prostaglandins.

Relaxin represents an autocrine/paracrine factor that inhibits uterine contractions and activates cervical maturation. Maternal plasma concentrations are elevated throughout pregnancy and decrease at labor, allowing delivery.

ENDOCRINE CHANGES DURING THE PUERPERIUM

After delivery, hormonal levels return to normal values. Plasma steroid levels decline rapidly. As a consequence of continued low-level production by the corpus luteum, *progesterone* does not reach basal prenatal levels as rapidly as does estradiol; it falls to luteal-phase levels within 24 hours after delivery, but it reaches follicular-phase levels only after several days. *Estradiol* falls to early follicular-phase levels within 1 to 3 days after delivery. The levels of hCG and human placental lactogen decline progressively within a week, and the decrease of other placental protein levels (inhibin, activin A, CRF) occurs as a function of their half-life.

The pituitary gland does not reduce in size until lactation ends. During the early weeks of puerperium, the secretion of *FSH* and *LH* continue to be suppressed, and responsiveness to GnRH is subnormal. Only by the third or fourth postpartum week are most women presenting follicular-phase levels of LH and FSH, and also responsiveness to GnRH returns to normal. At the onset of labor, a fall in *prolactin* serum levels occurs, which is followed by a surge in concentrations at delivery. Prolactin then exhibits variable patterns of secretion depending upon whether breast feeding occurs. In nonlactating women, delivery is followed by a rapid fall in serum prolactin concentrations over 1 to 2 weeks, whereas the return of normal cyclic function and ovulation may be expected in the second postpartum month. In lactating women, serum prolactin concentrations remain elevated, inhibiting GnRH secretion, and causing a persistence of anovulation. Thus, the average time for ovulation in women who lactate is about 4 to 6 months.

LACTATION

Throughout pregnancy, development of the breast alveolar lobules occurs: this requires the concerted participation of *prolactin, human placental lactogen, estrogen, progesterone, GH,* and *glucocorticoids*. In the puerperium, milk secretion is associated with further enlargement of the lobules and requires *prolactin, insulin,* and *adrenal steroids*. Prolactin, in particular, is essential for lactation. However, it does not occur until unconjugated estrogens fall to nonpregnant levels at about 36 to 48 hours postpartum.

Milk production requires the additional stimulus of surges of *oxytocin*, which acts on the smooth muscle of the gland ductules and causes contractile responses. The release of this hormone is occasioned by stimuli of a visual, psychologic, or physical nature that prepare the mother for suckling. The continued maintenance of established

milk secretion requires the establishment of periodic suckling, as well as periodic removal of the breast milk.

The use of dopamine receptor agonists (bromocriptine, cabergoline) can be clinically applied to inhibit lactation. Some reports have demonstrated efficacy of dopamine receptor antagonists (domperidone, metoclopramide) in stimulating lactation.

FETAL ENDOCRINOLOGY

Much of our information about fetal endocrinology is indirect from knowledge of the adult endocrine system. Study of the fetal endocrine system is further complicated by the multiplicity of sources of the various hormones: In fact, the fetus is exposed to maternal and placental hormones besides its own amniotic fluid, which also contains a variety of fetal and maternal hormones.

Fetal hypothalamus

In the fetus, the hypothalamic hormones (*CRF, TRH, GnRH, GH-RH,* and *somatostatin*) are detectable by 8 to 10 weeks of gestation, whereas all of the hormones of the adult anterior pituitary are extractable from the fetal adenohypophysis by 12 weeks. The direct circulatory connection between the hypothalamus and the pituitary gland develops at about 16 weeks of age.

Fetal adenohypophysis

During the first trimester, the fetal pituitary gland exerts a negligible role in organogenesis of target organs. GH does not play any role in fetal growth, as its total absence is consistent with normal development at birth. Similarly, the development of the gonads and adrenal gland during the first trimester appears to be directed by hCG rather than fetal tropic hormones, whereas the development of the thyroid gland occurs independently of TSH production by the fetus.

During the second trimester, the secretion of anterior pituitary hormones (*GH, TSH, gonadotropins, ACTH,* and *prolactin*) occurs, coincidentally with maturation of the hypophyseal portal system. LH has been detected in the fetal pituitary gland by 10 weeks with a sexual dimorphism; pituitary LH content is higher in the female than in the male fetuses. Luteinizing hormone in pituitary glands in both male and female fetuses rises sharply between 10 and 27 weeks, with little change thereafter. This sexual dimorphism is likely to be related in part to the higher concentrations of plasma testosterone in the male fetuses. FSH, detected in the fetal pituitary as early as 10 weeks of gestation, shows a sexual dimorphism that is similar to that of LH. The FSH/LH ratio is higher in female fetuses, but in both sexes there is a rise in FSH content between 10 and 25 weeks, after which FSH remains constant. The concentration of FSH falls in both sexes in late pregnancy.

Luteinizing hormone is present in fetal plasma as early as it is detectable in the fetal pituitary gland. Higher concentrations are found in midgestation, with lower levels toward term. In cord blood the levels of LH are low, and plasma FSH levels follow the same pattern as LH. No significant sex difference exists in cord FSH levels, which are very low, but in older neonates, FSH values in plasma are higher in the female.

Even though sex differentiation in the human fetus does not depend on pituitary gonadotropins, LH and FSH are essential for the normal development of the differentiated testis and ovary and the external genitalia in the male.

The fetal ovary does not have a critical function in female sexual differentiation. Primordial and primary follicles develop in the fetal ovary between 20 and 25 weeks, which is when peak concentrations of FSH and LH are observed. The growth, development, and maintenance of the fetal ovary are influenced by gonadotropins.

Fetal gonadotropins do not influence the events of organogenesis, but they are essential for normal development of the differentiated gonads and external genitalia. Indeed, female fetuses have higher FSH levels than male.

Fetal neurohypophysis

Vasopressin and *oxytocin* are detected in the fetal pituitary gland by 12 to 18 weeks, when their sites of production, the supraoptic and paraventricular nuclei, develop. The pituitary content of these hormones increase to term, with no evidence of feedback control.

Fetal thyroid gland

During the early first trimester, the thyroid gland develops at the same time as pituitary gland development, independent of a TSH stimulus. By 12 weeks, the thyroid is capable of iodine-concentrating activity and thyroid hormone synthesis. During the second trimester, the secretion of TRH, TSH, and *free T_4* is increased. The maturation of the feedback mechanisms is suggested by the plateau of TSH levels at about 20 fetal weeks.

During the third trimester, *free T_3* and *reverse T_3 (r T_3)*, the inactive metabolite of T_4, also start to be secreted. Thyroxine is the thyroid hormone produced in the largest amounts throughout fetal life, and at birth the conversion of T_4 to T_3 becomes demonstrable.

The development of thyroid hormones occurs independently from maternal systems, and very little placental transfer of these hormones occurs in physiologic concentrations. This also prevents maternal hypersecretion of thyroid hormone due to the influence of the fetal compartment. However, placental transfer prevents maternal supplementation from being effective therapy for fetal hypothyroidism. Conversely, goitrogenic agents are transferred across the placenta and may induce fetal hypothyroidism and goiter.

Fetal parathyroid glands

At the end of the first trimester, fetal parathyroid glands are capable of synthesizing *parathyroid hormone*, even if the placenta actively transports calcium into the fetal compartment, with a subsequent relative fetal hypercalcemia. This contributes to a suppression of fetal parathyroid hormone secretion, whose serum levels remain low or undetectable, whereas fetal serum calcitonin levels increase.

Fetal adrenal cortex

By 4 weeks of age, the cortex becomes identifiable, and steroid hormone production is detectable in the inner zone layer by 7 weeks. Early in pregnancy, the adrenal gland grows remarkably and has a size similar to that of the fetus's kidney. Most of the adrenal cortex is composed of a thick inner (fetal) zone, which subsequently regresses or is transformed into the outer (adult or definitive) zone during the early neonatal period. This inner fetal zone is the source of most fetal steroids. Before 20 weeks, it can function without ACTH, perhaps in response to hCG, whereas after this time fetal ACTH is required. The adrenal gland slowly decreases in size until 34 to 35 weeks, when a second spurt in its growth occurs under ACTH control.

The main function of the fetal adrenal gland is to provide *DHEAS* as the basic precursor for placental estrogen production. Estrogens at high concentrations, in turn, inhibit 3-hydroxysteroid dehydrogenase-isomerase activity and pregnenolone sulfate transformation to cortisol in the adrenal gland, leading to increased enhancement of the pituitary ACTH secretion. The high ACTH levels, due to the relatively low cortisol levels, are responsible for the hyperplasia of the fetal adrenal gland and the increase of DHEAS secretion. With birth and loss of exposure to estrogen, the fetal adrenal gland quickly changes to the adult type of gland.

Fetal gonads

The testes become detectable by about 6 weeks when they start to synthesize *testosterone*. The maximum production of testosterone coincides with the peak levels of circulating hCG. Fetal testes also produce *dihydrotestosterone*, the reduced testosterone metabolite, which is responsible for the development of the male external genitalia. It is also responsible for the *müllerian* duct inhibitory factor, which suppresses the further development of the müllerian ducts into its derivates: the fallopian tubes, the uterus and the upper part of the vagina.

The ovaries become evident by about 8 weeks; however, the significance of the steroids produced by fetal ovaries remains unclear.

ENDOCRINE DISEASES OF EARLY PREGNANCY: RECURRENT EARLY PREGNANCY LOSSES

Abortion or early pregnancy loss can be defined as the spontaneous termination of gestation before 20 weeks of gestational age or below a fetal weight of 500 g. If pregnancy losses that go unrecognized are also considered, the rate of spontaneous abortion is close to 50% of all pregnancies. About 80% of abortions occur in the first 12 weeks of pregnancy. The occurrence of 3 or more consecutive abortions is defined as "habitual early pregnancy loss," and the probability to start a successful pregnancy decreases after every subsequent abortion. Recurrent early pregnancy loss in about 70% of cases is due to gene abnormalities, in accordance with the observation that the incidence of spontaneous abortions rises dramatically in women over age 40.

Even if the causes of the majority of early spontaneous abortions remain unknown, quite often the determination of the karyotype of the parents can reveal some defects, such as balanced chromosomal rearrangement, mosaicism, chromosome inversions, or ring chromosomes. Parental karyotyping is not necessarily definitive, however, since there are many genetic defects that can cause recurrent early pregnancy losses, such as gene expression defects that are not detectable by karyotyping. Sometimes the karyotypes of the parents are normal but fetal chromosomal defects can be detected: the most common defects are the trisomies of chromosomes 13, 16, 18, 21, and 22. Several environmental factors are also associated with spontaneous abortion, in particular smoking and alcohol abuse. There is no hard evidence that infectious agents can cause pregnancy loss, although a significantly higher incidence of anti-*Chlamydia* antibodies was reported in women with habitual abortion. Many anatomical uterine abnormalities may result in recurrent abortion, the most frequent being a septate uterus.

It is very unlikely that a mild subclinical endocrine disease may cause recurrent pregnancy loss. The endocrine abnormality that may cause this event is an inadequate luteal phase, in particular the deficiency of progesterone and its metabolites. Nevertheless, the treatment with exogenous progesterone in such cases is most often useless. A different approach has been to diagnose an inadequate luteal phase during the nonpregnant period and to treat patients with progesterone a few days after ovulation, but there is no evidence that this progestational treatment makes any difference either.

Early recurrent pregnancy loss may also be caused by immunologic problems. In several autoimmune diseases, such as LES, serum autoantibodies can block the production of prostacyclin with an unbalanced thromboxane activity; this results in vasoconstriction and thrombosis that can lead to pregnancy complications, such as abortion, intrauterine growth retardation, and preterm delivery.

There is also the possibility of an abnormal maternal immune response to antigens on the placental or fetal tissues, deriving from the lack of formation of blocking factors (antigen-antibody complexes) that modulate the maternal immune response at the beginning of a normal pregnancy.

ENDOCRINE DISEASES DURING PREGNANCY

Endocrine aspects of (pre) eclampsia

In pregnancy, the association of gestational edema and proteinuria with hypertensive disorders has been termed preeclampsia or eclampsia, depending on whether the patient has seizures. The incidence of gestational hypertension is about 7%, and about half of the women with progestational hypertension develop exacerbations of hypertension in the third trimester of pregnancy. Clinically, preeclampsia usually appears after 32 weeks of gestation, or, most frequently, around term. However, in severe cases (and in particular in cases of chronic hypertension), it may appear as early as 26 weeks. Signs of this disease are edema, proteinuria (1 to 10 g daily), and a rise in diastolic blood pressure by 15 mmHg or more over first trimester values.

In preeclamptic pregnancies, the activity of all of the components of the *renin-angiotensin-aldosterone* system is reduced, reflecting an appropriate feedback response. The most important finding in women with hypertension in pregnancy is an increased arteriolar constriction in response to angiotensin.

Amniotic fluid concentrations of *prolactin* are lower in pregnancy complicated by hypertension or polyhydramnios than in normal pregnancy. The secretion of several placental hormones is augmented in preeclamptic patients such as hCG, estriol, activin A, and inhibin A, as well as maternal CRF, possibly due to hyperplasia of the cytotrophoblast. Interestingly, in these patients, plasma CRF-binding protein levels are lower than in normal pregnant women, thus the amount of circulating free CRF levels is increased, which may subsequently act on the various target functions.

Maternal diabetes

Diabetes complicates pregnancy in two situations: in women with diabetes who become pregnant with metabolic abnormalities from the time of conception onward (*progestational diabetes*); and in women who are first found to have abnormalities of glucose tolerance during routine testing in pregnancy (*gestational diabetes mellitus* [GDM]). In GDM women, hyperglycemia is usually too mild to cause overt diabetic symptoms in the mother, but it is sufficient to alter fetal growth and development during the second and third trimesters. In addition, these women have a high risk for developing diabetes in subsequent years.

Progestational diabetes

Pregnancy has a significant metabolic impact on type I (insulin-dependent diabetes mellitus [IDDM]) and type II diabetes (non-insulin-dependent diabetes mellitus [NIDDM]), greatly increasing insulin resistance. In the second half of pregnancy, there is a progressive increase in the amount of insulin required to maintain euglycemia. As a result of the progressive insulin resistance, patients must be checked at frequent intervals during the second and third trimesters for blood glucose level monitoring and adjustments of insulin doses. Placental uptake of glucose, which is not dependent on maternal insulin, may cause hypoglycemia in pregnant type I patients who have not recently consumed food. In addition, because insulin is the major hormone suppressing lipolysis and ketogenesis, pregnant women with type I diabetes are at an increased risk for accelerated ketone production and ketoacidosis whenever they omit their insulin therapy or experience an intercurrent illness. The ketoacidosis may occur rapidly and at lower plasma glucose concentrations than typical ketoacidosis in nonpregnant women. Because of the tendency of ketosis during caloric deprivation in pregnancy, diets providing less than approximately 25 kcal/kg actual body weight should not be prescribed to avoid exposure of the fetus to elevated maternal ketone levels. The insulin resistance of pregnancy rapidly decreases after delivery, and several patients need very little insulin during the first few days postpartum.

Gestational diabetes mellitus

Glucose screening for gestational diabetes mellitus should be carried out between 24 and 28 weeks of gestation, when insulin requirements are maximal. If the fasting and 1-hour or 2-hour screening plasma glucose levels are abnormal, a glucose tolerance test may not be required. For borderline screening tests, a 3-hour glucose tolerance test should be performed, preceded by a special diet containing about 300 g of carbohydrates for 3 days. Any patient with one or more of the risk factors (obesity, family history of diabetes mellitus, previous infant weighing greater than 4000 g, previous stillborn infant, previous congenitally deformed infant, previous polyhydramnios, history of recurrent abortions) should be screened at the first visit if the first visit is prior to 24 weeks. In patients who prove positive, a diet of 1800 calories should be prescribed: 50 to 60% of the caloric requirements are given as carbohydrate, 18 to 22% as protein, and the remainder (about 25%) as fat. Less than 10% of the fat is saturated, up to 10% polyunsaturated fatty acids, and the remainder is nonsaturated.

Oral hypoglycemic agents are not recommended during pregnancy because they cross the placental barrier and may induce fetal and neonatal hypoglycemia. Short-acting, intermediate-acting, and long-acting insulin may be used in combination with dosage schedules designed to maintain maternal euglycemia. For diabetic control during pregnancy, long-acting insulins are seldom used, but a combination of short-acting and intermediate-acting insulins are given as a split morning and evening dose (insulin units administered should be equal to the body weight in kilograms x 0.6 in the first trimester, x 0.7 in the second trimester, and x 0.8 in the third trimester). A mean daily serum glucose level of less than 120 mg/dl is encouraged, with fasting levels 60 to 90 mg/dl, preprandial blood glucose levels between 60 and 105 mg/dl, postprandial levels less than 120 mg/dl, and levels greater than 60 mg/dl between 2 and 6 AM.

Hyper- and hypothyroidism

Hyperthyroidism is common in pregnancy, occurring in about 1 to 2 per 1000 pregnancies. It is associated with increased cardiac output and peripheral vasodilatation. Maternal hyperthyroidism is associated with an increased risk of maternal heart failure, premature delivery, and a modestly increased risk for early abortion. The most common form of hyperthyroidism during pregnancy is Graves' disease; because TSH-receptor antibody may cross the placenta, maternal disease may cause fetal goiter and transient neonatal hyperthyroidism. The minimum findings needed to establish the diagnosis are clearly elevated values of serum free T_3 and free T_4, combined with a suppressed TSH.

The treatment of maternal hyperthyroidism is complex in pregnancy because antithyroid drugs cross the placenta and may cause fetal hypothyroidism and goiter or cretinism in the newborn. The choices include antithyroid drugs, β-adrenergic blocking drugs, and thyroid surgery. [131]I treatment is contraindicated during pregnancy. Further supportive measures include an adequate dietary caloric intake and multiple vitamins, because both pregnancy and hyperthyroidism increase caloric needs, and vitamin deficiency may accompany hyperthyroidism. The antithyroid drugs are the thioamides, which block the synthesis of thyroid hormone. It usually takes about 1 week for the amelioration of symptoms and 4 to 6 weeks for full control. Propylthiouracil and methimazole have both been used. The patient should be started on 100 to 150 mg of propylthiouracil every 8 hours. After a reduction of symptoms and a decrease of serum T_4, the dose of propylthiouracil should gradually be lowered to about 100 mg/day and maintained for the duration of the pregnancy. Since propylthiouracil crosses the placental barrier, a major concern during maternal treatment is the development of fetal goiter and hypothyroidism. Children exposed to thioamides in utero attain full physical and intellectual development and have normal thyroid function studies. β-adrenergic receptor blockers have been used in conjunction with propylthiouracil (propranolol at the dose of 40 mg every 6 hours). However, some reports have indicated propranolol as an etiologic agent in intrauterine growth retardation, fetal demise, impaired fetal response to hypoxic stress, and postnatal hypoglycemia and bradycardia. Surgical treatment of hyperthyroidism is recommended only if medical treatment fails.

The major risk for pregnant patients with thyrotoxicosis is the development of a thyroid storm. Precipitating factors include infection, labor, cesarean section, or noncompliance with medication. Hyperthermia, marked tachycardia, perspiration, and severe dehydration are blocked with propranolol (20 to 80 mg every 6 hours); sodium iodide (which blocks thyroid hormone, 1 g iv); propylthiouracil (1200 to 1800 mg given in divided doses); replacing fluid losses with at least 5 liters of fluid; and rapidly lowering the temperature with hypothermic techniques.

Hypothyroidism is uncommon in pregnancy since most women with the untreated disorder are oligomenorrheic. The most important laboratory findings to confirm the diagnosis are elevated TSH and low T_4 levels. Maternal hypothyroidism may be hazardous to the developing fetus, as thyroid hormones are important particularly in the development of neural and skeletal systems. Thus, fetal hypothyroidism leads to cretinism, with mental retardation and dwarfism. The correlation between the maternal and fetal thyroid states is poor, and most hypothyroid mothers deliver euthyroid newborns. The fetus is dependent upon hormones synthesized by its own thyroid gland, generally from about 11 weeks of gestation. Women taking thyroid medication at the time of conception may need an adjustment of the dose during pregnancy.

Hyper- and hypoparathyroidism

Hyperparathyroidism is caused by a single parathyroid adenoma (80 to 90%), multiglandular disease (10 to 20%), or carcinoma (1%). The most common symptoms are fatigue, muscle weakness, renal stones, emotional changes, headache, gastrointestinal symptoms, and bone disease (see Chapter 18). Hyperparathyroidism causes additional problems during pregnancy. About 6% of reported patients with hyperparathyroidism have pancreatitis. Spontaneous abortion or fetal death occurs in about 15% and neonatal hypocalcemic tetany in about 30%. The diagnosis of hyperparathyroidism is established by demonstrating elevated serum PTH levels and hypercalcemia. The standard treatment of hyperparathyroidism during pregnancy is surgery, which reduces the risk of complications.

Hypoparathyroidism is an uncommon disease that results in low PTH and total and ionized calcium concentrations from permanent parathyroid damage or removal of all parathyroid tissue. Spontaneous hypoparathyroidism is rare. Hypocalcemia causes neuromuscular irritability, paraesthesias, carpopedal spasm, and in the most severe cases, laryngospasm and seizures. During pregnancy, untreated maternal hypoparathyroidism causes fetal hypocalcemia and, in response, fetal parathyroid hyperplasia. Therapy for hypoparathyroidism consists of oral calcium and vitamin D.

Hormonal therapy in maturing fetal lung during pregnancy

Preterm labor (between 28 and 36 weeks of pregnancy) is associated with a distress syndrome. In these cases, a short-term treatment with glucocorticoids enhances fetal lung maturation. When fetal lungs mature (about 35 weeks of pregnancy), type II pneumocytes produce a surfactant that decreases alveolar surface tension, thus facilitating lung expansion and preventing atelectasia. The synergistic action between cortisol and other hormones (such as prolactin, thyroxine, estrogens, prostaglandins, and so on) is the main requisite for surfactant production.

It has been shown that lung maturation correlates more closely with cortisol levels than with fetal age. Indeed, glucocorticoids stimulate lung surfactant protein synthesis. Studies have clearly demonstrated that glucocorticoid administration to the mother or directly to the fetus accelerates fetal lung maturation. Intrafetal administration, however, is complicated by the fact that the injection per se is associated with some maturational responses. Thus, the administration via the maternal compartment provides a more clear-cut demonstration of the effect. Maternal cortisol is effective in large doses. Synthetic glucocorticoids, such as betamethasone or dexamethasone, are effective in lower concentrations as in other glucocorticoid target tissues. Glucocorticoid administration to the mother is effective prior to weeks gestation. The benefits derived seem to depend on a number of factors, including fetal sex (female infants benefit more than male) and ethnic group (black infants benefit more than white). The most used glucocorticoid is betamethasone (12 mg im every 12 hours for three times).

In addition to glucocorticoids, thyroid hormones have been advocated to enhance pulmonary maturation, but because thyroid hormone does not effectively cross the placenta, TRH has been the most active agent used. Studies have shown poor results.

TUMORS ASSOCIATED WITH PREGNANCY

Luteoma of pregnancy

Due to a prolonged hCG stimulation during pregnancy, a transient luteoma of pregnancy or a very rare extensive luteinization of ovarian theca cells may occur. It is correlated with multiple pregnancy or hydramnios, and secretes androgens, responsible for maternal hirsutism, as well as abnormal genitalia in the female fetus. Regression of the luteoma takes place postpartum.

Prolactinomas

Pregnancy may be induced in patients with a microprolactinoma treated with bromocriptine or cabergoline. In the absence of any symptoms, when pregnancy occurs, the treatment with dopamine receptor agonists is discontinued. For the patients with a macroprolactinoma, mild neurosurgical complications frequently occur. In general, these can be treated by the restitution of dopaminergic drugs throughout pregnancy.

Gestational trophoblastic neoplasia

Gestational trophoblastic neoplasia include hydatidiform mole (the benign form) and choriocarcinoma (the malignant and metastasizing form). In Europe their incidence is about 1/1500 pregnancies, but it varies in relation to the geographical zone, race, and age. Furthermore, the risk of developing a second molar pregnancy is about 40 times greater than that of developing the first. A sensitive tumor marker is represented by elevated serum levels of hCG (from 3 to 100 times higher than in normal pregnancy), frequently by 3 weeks and usually by 6 weeks of pregnancy. A diagnosis of trophoblastic disease is possible when the hCG level rises over a 2-week period, or when values remain higher after 16 weeks. Rarely, trophoblastic diseases are associated with hyperthyroidism, due to the thyrotropic activity of hCG.

Benign form: hydatidiform mole Patients with a hydatiform mole generally present with irregular or heavy vaginal bleeding during the first or early second trimester of pregnancy. The bleeding is usually painless, although it can be associated with uterine contractions, and patients may expel molar "vesicles" from the vagina. They also occasionally develop excessive nausea and even "hyperemesis gravidarum." Irritability, dizziness, and photophobia may occur, since some patients develop preeclampsia. Patients may occasionally exhibit symptoms related to hyperthyroidism, such as nervousness, anorexia, and tremors. Trophoblastic tissue may occasionally embolize to the lungs. A definitive diagnosis of hydatidiform mole is made by ultrasonography. Hydatidiform mole may be complete or incomplete, and it is characterized by elevated urinary concentrations of hCG that return to normal values at about 60 to 90 days after uterine evacuation. At this time, the persistence of normal values for at least 3 weeks may be considered a sign for a good prognosis. Undetectable levels should be reached within 12 to 16 weeks. If the hCG titers plateau or rise at any time, chemotherapy should be initiated.

The standard treatment of hydatidiform mole is suction evacuation, followed by sharp curettage of the uterus. Following the evacuation of a hydatiform mole, the patients must be monitored with weekly serum assays of hCG.

Malignant forms: invasive mole and choriocarcinoma
Invasive moles, also named chorioadenoma destruens, are usually locally invasive tumors that may penetrate the entire myometrium. They are associated, although rarely, with metastasis, particularly to the vagina or lung; brain metastases have also been demonstrated. It represents the majority of molar pregnancies. Human chorionic gonadotropin titers are persistent 90 days after uterine evacuation.

Choriocarcinoma is a malignant trophoblastic disease that may occur in pregnant women (from a malignant degeneration of a hydatidiform mole, and also from an abortion or an extrauterine pregnancy), as well as in nonpregnant women. Vaginal bleeding is a common symptom of uterine choriocarcinoma or vaginal metastases. Because of the gonadotropin excretion, amenorrhea may develop, simulating early pregnancy. Hemoptysis, cough, or dyspnea may occur as a result of lung metastases. In the presence of central nervous system metastases, the patient may complain of headaches, dizzy spells, "blacking out", or other symptoms referable to a space-occupying lesion in the brain. Rectal bleeding or "dark stools" could be a presentation of disease that has metastasized to the gastrointestinal tract. Choriocarcinoma in the prepubertal child causes precocious puberty, presenting with the appearance of pubic hair, the development of mammary glands, and vaginal bleeding. This tumor is always characterized by very high levels of hCG (greater than 500 000-1 000 000 mIU/ml or more in 24 hours in urine). These levels are related to the extension of the tumor and to the presence of metastases, and often a further increase 3 weeks after uterine evacuation is observed.

In this case, chemotherapy is usually initiated without histologic confirmation of disease. Before initiating chemotherapy, a full metastatic work-up must be done to determine whether metastatic disease is present.

Suggested readings

JAFFE RB. Protein hormones in human placental, decidual, and fetal membranes. In: Yen SSC, Jaffe RB (eds). Reproductive endocrinology. Philadelphia: WB Saunders Company, 1991; 920-35.

PETRAGLIA F, VOLPE A, GENAZZANI AR, RIVIER J, SAWCHENKO PE, VALE W. Neuroendocrinology of the human placenta. Frontiers Neuroendo 1990;11:6-37

PETRAGLIA F, CALZÀ L, GARUTI GC, DERAMUNDO BM, ANGIONI S. New aspects of placental endocrinology. J Endocrinol Inv 1990;13:353-71

PETRAGLIA F, FLORIO, P, NAPPI C, GENAZZANI AR. Peptide signalling in human placenta and membranes: autocrine, paracrine, and endocrine mechanisms. Endocrine Rev 1996; 17:156-86.

TULCHINSKY D, LITTLE A.B. Maternal-fetal endocrinology. Philadelphia: WB Saunders Company. 2nd ed. 1994.

52

Contraception

Douwe J. Hemrika

Fertility regulation is an important issue because it limits the rapid growth of the world population and prevents the occurrence of unintended pregnancy. The prevention of sexually transmitted diseases (STDs) is an issue closely related to contraception. The long-term sequelae of sexually transmitted diseases, such as tubal factor infertility, ectopic pregnancy, and infection with the human immunodeficiency virus (HIV), pose serious health problems to individual patients and are a burden on health economics. The choice of a contraceptive method is governed by a number of factors:

- *Contraceptive efficacy* Failure of contraception can be due to "method-failure" or "user-failure". Rates of failure are usually higher due to incorrect or inconsistent use by the average user than from a correctly used contraception product or method that failed (Tab. 52.1).
- *Acceptability* To ensure maximum patient compliance, the method should not, or only minimally, interfere with the act of sexual intercourse and must be easy to use.
- *Side effects* Ideally, the method should be devoid of serious side effects. In this respect, patient selection is important. While side effects of contraceptives usually receive ample public attention and often cause general concern, physicians should be able to balance the risks of a particular contraceptive method against the risk of unintended pregnancy and the sequelae of induced abortion, also taking into account possible health benefits of contraception.
- *Reversibility* Except for male and female sterilization, any contraceptive method should be easily reversible and allow for the prompt return of normal fertility upon discontinuation.

BARRIER METHODS

Vaginal contraceptives aimed at preventing the entry of spermatozoa into the upper female genital tract include the condom, the diaphragm, the cervical cap, and spermicides. Adequate instruction to the proper use and a high level of motivation are essential to ensure adequate contraceptive efficacy. Nonetheless, barrier methods are of limited contraceptive reliability compared to other methods (Tab. 52.1), but they have the advantage of protecting against sexually transmitted diseases.

Condoms

Modern condoms are made of thin latex (±0.5 mm thick) that is not only impermeable to spermatozoa, but also to bacteria that cause sexually transmitted diseases and to viruses such as HIV and the human papilloma virus (HPV). Consequently, condoms provide protection against both pregnancy and sexually transmitted diseases.

Many condom failures are the result of inappropriate application. The condom should be placed on the erect penis before vaginal penetration, and immediately after ejaculation the penis should be withdrawn, holding the condom in place to avoid spill of semen.

The addition of spermicidal agents is controversial. With proper use spermicides are unnecessary, while it is unsafe to rely on a spermicidal agent when inadvertent spill of sperm has occurred.

Some vaginal lubricants and vaginal medication (such as the anti-fungal agent ketoconazole) can weaken the latex and compromise contraceptive reliability.

Table 52.1 Efficacy of various contraceptive methods

Method	Annual failure rates (%)	
	Perfect use	Average use
Combined oral contraceptives	0.1	3
Progestin-only pill	0.5	5
Progestin implants	0.2	0.3
IUD	0.2	0.4
Condoms	2	12
Diaphragm and spermicides	6	18
Cervical cap	6	30
Spermicides	3	21
Periodic abstinence	5	20
Withdrawal	4	19
Male sterilization	0.1	0.04
Female sterilization	0.2	0.2

(Hatcher RA, Trussell J, Stewart F. Contraceptive technology. 16th revised ed. New York: Irvington Publishers, 1994.)

The female condom consists of a sheath of 15 cm length made of polyurethane inserted into the vagina. Although the female condom offers protection against sexually transmitted diseases and should be as reliable as a male condom, acceptability remains a problem.

The diaphragm

A diaphragm consists of a latex dome fixed to a flat coil spring 50 to 100 mm in diameter. The anterior rim is placed behind the symphysis pubis and the posterior rim rests in the posterior vaginal fornix, thereby completely covering the portio vaginalis of the cervix. Contraceptive reliability of the diaphragm depends on proper use by the woman, but also on proper fitting by the doctor. A set of fitting rings is necessary to determine the largest ring that can easily be brought in the right position without discomfort to the woman.

A diaphragm will never completely seal off the cervix form the distal vagina, so the addition of spermicides is essential to ensure efficacy of 10 to 20 times higher. Spermicide jelly should be applied to both sides of the dome and around the brim. The diaphragm can be inserted maximally 6 hours before coitus, and it should be left in place for at least 6 to 8 hours after intercourse to assure that no viable spermatozoa are present in the vagina upon removal. After removal, the diaphragm can be cleaned with warm water and checked for leaks.

The cervical cap

The cervical cap is a smaller device than the diaphragm that is designed to snugly fit over the portio vaginalis of the cervix and is kept in place by the surface tension created by cervical and vaginal secretions. The use of a spermicide is advisable. The cap should be inserted at least 30 minutes before intercourse, and, like the diaphragm, should not be removed until at least 6 to 8 hours after coitus. The cap can be left in place for longer than 24 hours (up to 3 days) without adverse outcome. Proper placement of the cap over the cervix must be checked by the woman herself after insertion and before every new episode of intercourse.

Spermicides

Spermicidal agents come in the form of creams, jellies, suppositories, and vaginal sponges. They usually contain nonoxynol-9, which acts by damaging the cell membrane of spermatozoa. Spermicides are applied to the vagina no longer than 10 to 20 minutes before coitus and remain active for a limited time span (less than 1 hour). Their use should be advocated only in conjunction with other (barrier) methods of contraception. Allergic reactions resulting in vaginal irritation and discharge are the most commonly observed side-effects. Spermicides offer no protection against sexually transmitted diseases.

INTRA-UTERINE DEVICE

Modern intra-uterine devices (IUDs) have a polyurethane, T-shaped frame with a copper thread fitted on the vertical arm, while some have additional copper sleeves on the horizontal arms. The initial addition of copper to the older inert IUDs and the subsequent increase of the copper surface from 200 mm^2 to 380 mm^2 greatly increased contraceptive reliability, which approaches that of surgical sterilization.

In addition to copper IUDs, systems for intra-uterine hormone release (designated as intra-uterine systems, IUS) have been developed. Drawbacks of the older systems, which released 0.065 mg of progesterone per 24 hours, such as a life-span of only 1 year and a high ectopic pregnancy rate, are alleviated by newer systems. An example of such a system is the levonorgestrel-IUS (LNG-IUS), which releases 0.020 mg of levonorgestrel per 24 hours and can be left in situ for 5 years; it gives excellent protection to both intra- and extra-uterine pregnancy. The added advantage of the LNG-IUS is a considerable reduction in menstrual flow.

Intra-uterine devices induce a sterile inflammatory reaction in the endometrium, which impairs implantation. Copper has a profound toxic effect on spermatozoa and prevents fertilization. The progesterone-medicated IUDs induce decidualization of the endometrium with atrophy of the glands, making implantation unlikely to occur. The cervical mucus plug is made thick and viscous, inhibiting sperm penetration. In addition, progesterone affects the motility of spermatozoa, inhibits the acrosome reaction, and alters tubal motility. Due to these effects, fertilization virtually does not occur, although ovarian function is unaffected in 80% of LNG-IUS users.

The effects of IUDs on the endometrium are rapidly reversible, since fertility is completely restored immediately after removal of an IUD.

The high incidence of pelvic inflammatory disease occurring during the use of the Dalkon Shield brand of IUD has given IUDs a bad name and continues to raise concern in both women and health professionals. Since it was recognized that the multifilament thread of the Dalkon Shield was responsible for this phenomenon, the new IUDs were fitted with a monofilamentous string. It has now convincingly been shown that sexual behavior (that is, the risk of acquiring a sexually transmitted disease) is the only risk factor for the occurrence of pelvic inflammatory disease in users of contemporary IUDs. An increased risk for ascending infection only exists during the first 20 days after insertion of the IUD.

The new copper- and levonorgestrel-medicated IUDs prevent fertilization and protect against ectopic pregnancy as compared to women who do not use contraception. When a patient is pregnant with an IUD in situ, 2 to 3% of these pregnancies will prove to be ectopic.

Patient selection Most healthy women are eligible for IUD use. Nulliparity is no contraindication, although nulliparous women are somewhat more likely to experience side effects like heavy menstrual periods or dysmenorrhea. A stable, monogamous relationship is an important prerequisite for IUD use, in view of the risk of STD (Tab. 52.2). Women with menorrhagia or frank dysmenorrhea are obviously not good candidates for standard IUDs, but a LNG-IUS can be an attractive alternative in these cases.

IUD insertion Although an IUD can be inserted at any time, insertion during or shortly after a normal menstrual period is preferred, since it rules out pregnancy. IUDs can be inserted at any time after an abortion or delivery, although immediate post partum insertion carries a higher risk of expulsion. When the prevalence of sexually transmitted diseases in the population under care is high, routine cervical swabs before insertion or prophylactic antibiotics (such as doxycycline 200 mg orally 1 hour before insertion) are recommended. Care should be taken to position the IUD high in the uterine cavity in the fundal area. Since expulsion of an IUD often occurs during the first subsequent menstrual period, 6 weeks after insertion is a good time to check the presence of the IUD. Routine check-up visits are not needed thereafter. The copper IUDs can be left in situ for at least 8 years, and the progestogen reservoir of the LNG-IUS has a life span of 5 years.

Common problems with IUDs Copper IUDs are expected to increase menstrual flow by 50%. Antifibrinolytic drugs may be useful when excessive bleeding occurs. In case of severe dysmenorrhea, nonsteroidal anti-inflammatory drugs may be prescribed. Approximately 10 percent of IUDs are removed in the first year because of bleeding and pain. The LNG-IUS significantly reduces menstrual blood loss. However, intermenstrual spotting or complete amenorrhea (in 20% of cases) can be reasons for discontinuation.

The expulsion rate of IUDs is approximately 5% in the first year (most frequently in the first month after insertion) and 1 to 2% per year after the first year.

If the intra-uterine device perforates the intrauterine wall, it almost always occurs during insertion (1 in 1000 insertions) and is related to the skill and experience of the clinician performing the procedure.

Table 52.2 Contraindications to use of intra-uterine devices

Absolute
Confirmed or suspected pregnancy
Known or suspected pelvic infection
At-risk for sexually transmitted disease
Undiagnosed vaginal bleeding
Known or suspected pelvic malignancy
Allergy to copper or Wilson's disease (copper IUDs only)

Relative
Uterine size <6 cm or >9 cm
Submucous myoma
Uterus didelphis, bicornis, or septus
Valvular heart disease, chronic corticosteroid therapy, immune suppression
History of pelvic inflammatory disease
Undiagnosed abnormal PAP smear

When a patient becomes pregnant with an intra-uterine device in situ, ultrasonography should be used to document an intra-uterine pregnancy, exclude an ectopic pregnancy, and verify the presence of the intra-uterine device in the uterine cavity. If the string of the intra-uterine device is still visible in the cervical canal, the intra-uterine device should be removed. The risk of miscarriage is not increased by this procedure. If, due to the growth of the uterus, the string of the intra-uterine device is no longer visible, and the woman wants to carry the pregnancy to term, the intra-uterine device can be left in situ, but there is an increased risk of miscarriage (with the possibility of infectious complications) and immature delivery. If during delivery the intra-uterine device is not expelled spontaneously together with the placenta, it has to be removed manually immediately post partum. When the string of the intra-uterine device is no longer visibly protruding from the cervix and ultrasound shows the intra-uterine device in its proper intrauterine position, no action needs to be undertaken. If the intra-uterine device cannot be located inside the uterus, an abdominal X-ray should be obtained to detect a perforated, intra-abdominally located intra-uterine device. In this situation, removal by laparoscopy/laparotomy is mandatory because of the risk of migration and occasional bowel perforation. In cases where the intra-uterine device cannot be removed by applying simple traction on the string, (partial) embedment into the myometrium is the usual cause. Removal under direct hysteroscopic inspection is preferred to blind procedures because it is less traumatic.

ORAL CONTRACEPTIVES

Since the introduction of oral contraceptives in the early sixties, there has been a continuous effort to reduce the dosage of the steroids in the pill without compromising contraceptive reliability and cycle control. Dose reduction of the estrogenic component from 0.08 mg of ethinylestradiol in the first oral contraceptives to 0.020 to 0.030 mg in contemporary oral contraceptives has led to a dramatic decline of thromboembolic complications. Almost all modern oral contraceptives use ethinylestradiol as their estrogen source. The progestogens in the older oral contraceptives were norethisterone and its derivatives, while in modern preparations levonorgestrel (second generation oral contraceptives) or desogestrel/gestodene (third generation oral contraceptives) are used, with less impact on carbohydrate and lipid metabolism.

Modern oral contraceptives are safe, carrying only minimal risks in healthy women and providing considerable health benefits, while keeping an excellent contraceptive record. Although almost all pregnancies that occur during oral contraceptive use are due to poor patient compliance or mistakes in pill intake, gastrointestinal disorders and drug interactions can sometimes be the cause of oral contraceptives failure.

Oral contraceptives suppress ovarian folliculogenesis and ovulation by inhibition of the production of follicle-stimulating hormone and luteinizing hormone. The suppression of gonadotrophins is effected within a few days (<7 days) of pill ingestion and is rapidly reversed after 7 day's discontinuation. Although inhibition of ovulation is the prime mechanism of action of oral contraceptives, progestogens exert additional contraceptive effects on the endometrium (pseudodecidualization and atrophy inhibiting implantation) and the cervix (viscous cervical mucus impeding sperm transport).

Oral contraceptives are generally administered in a 21-day cycle with a 7-day pill-free interval. Sequential dose regimens, where the first seven pills contain estrogens only, have largely been replaced by combined-dose regimens. In monophasic combined formulations, every pill contains the same amount of the estrogenic and gestagenic component, while in bi- or triphasic preparations the gestagenic component is increased in one or two incremental steps during the pill cycle. Standard oral contraceptives contain 0.050 mg of ethinylestradiol, and modern oral contraceptives have 0.030 to 0.020 mg of ethinylestradiol ("sub-fifty preparations") (Tab. 52.3).

Risk factors, complications, and contraindications The risk factors, complications, and contraindications of oral contraceptive use are outlined in Tables 52.4 and 52.5. The risk of venous thromboembolism is increased by estrogens in a dose-dependent manner. The absolute incidence of venous thromboembolism in oral contraceptive users of preparations containing more than 0.050, 0.050, and less than 0.050 mg of ethinylestradiol is estimated at 8, 4, and 3 per 10 000 women years, respectively. For comparison, in normal pregnancy the risk for venous thromboembolism is 8 per 10 000 women years, while non-users have a risk of 1 per 10 000. There is at present no reason to assume that oral contraceptives with third generation progestogens carry a higher risk for venous thromboembolism. Patient selection is important, and a history of venous thromboembolism, pre-existent coagulation disorders, a family history positive for venous thromboembolism, obesity, and advanced age are separate risk factors to be taken into account before prescribing oral contraceptives.

Modern oral contraceptives, containing non-androgenic second and third generation progestogens, have no impact on lipid metabolism, do not increase the risk of cardiovascular disease, and can safely be prescribed to non-smoking women up to the age of menopause.

Hypertension induced by oral contraceptives is rare, but it does occur even with low-dose preparations. Recent data seem to indicate a marginally increased risk for breast cancer in oral contraceptive users. In patients who develop breast cancer before the age of 35 and in those who started oral contraceptives at a young age (<20 years), a relative risk of 1.4 for long-term users has been found. The incidence of benign lesions of the breast is not increased by oral contraceptives, and women diagnosed with these lesions can safely use oral contraceptives.

Table 52.3 Composition of frequently used oral contraceptives

Sequential formulations with 0.050 mg EE
EE 7 x 0.050 mg/d + lynestrenol/EE 15 x 2.50/0.050 mg/d
EE 7 x 0.050 mg/d + lynestrenol/EE 15 x 1.00/0.050 mg/d
EE 7 x 0.050 mg/d + desogestrel/EE 15 x 0.125/0.050 mg/d

Combined formulations with 0.050 mg EE
Monophasic
  Etynodiolacetate/EE 21 x 1.00/0.050 mg/d
  Lynestrenol/EE 22 x 2.50/0.050 mg/d
  Lynestrol/EE 22 x 1.00/0.050 mg/d
  Lynestrol/EE 22 x 1.00/0.050 mg/d + 6 x placebo
  Norethisterone/mestranol 21 x 1.00/0.050 mg/d
  Levonorgestrel/EE 21 x 0.250/0.050 mg/d
  Levonorgestrel/EE 21 x 0.125/0.050 mg/d

Biphasic
  Levonorgestrel/EE 11 x 0.05/0.050 + 10 x 0.125/0.050 mg/d

Combined formulations with less than 0.050 mg EE
Monophasic
  Lynestrenol/EE 22 x 0.75/0.0375 mg/d
  Lynestrenol/EE 22 x 0.75/0.0375 mg/d + 6 x placebo
  Norethisterone/EE 21 x 1.00/0.035 mg/d
  Norethisterone/EE 21 x 0.50/0.035 mg/d
  Levonorgestrel/EE 21 x 0.150/0.030 mg/d
  Desogestrel/EE 21 x 0.150/0.030 mg/d
  Gestodene/EE 21 x 0.075/0.030 mg/d
  Norgestimate/EE 21 x 0.250/0.035 mg/d

Biphasic
  Desogestrel/EE 7 x 0.025/0.040 + 15 x 0.125/0.030 mg/d

Triphasic
  Levonorgestrel/EE 6 x 0.050/0.030 + 5 x 0.075/0.040 + 10 x 0.125/0.030 mg/d
  Norethisterone/EE 7 x 0.500/0.035 + 7 x 0.750/0.035 + 7 x 1.000/0.035 mg/d
  Gestodene/EE 6 x 0.050/0.030 + 5 x 0.070/0.040 + 10 x 0.100/0.030 mg/d
  Gestodene/EE 6 x 0.050/0.030 + 5 x 0.070/0.040 + 10 x 0.100/0.030 mg/d
  Norgestimate/EE 7 x 0.180/0.035 + 7 x 0.215/0.035 + 7 x 0.250/0.035 mg/d

Combined formulations with less than 0.030 mg EE

Desogestrel/EE 21 x 0.150/0.020 mg/d
Gestodene/EE 21 x 0.075/0.020 mg/d

Progestogen-only formulations

Lynestrenol 0.500 mg
Ethynodiol diacetate 0.500 mg
Norethindrone 0.350 mg
Levonorgestrel 0.030 mg
Levonorgestrel 0.075 mg

(EE = ethinylestradiol.)

Beneficial effects of oral contraceptives Oral contraceptives reduce the incidence and discomfort of menstrual disturbances, both in adolescents suffering from irregular, anovulatory bleeding, and in women in the fourth decade who experience menorrhagia with resulting anemia

Table 52.4 Contraindications to oral contraceptive use

Absolute

Thrombophlebitis or thromboembolic disorders
A past history of deep venous thrombosis
or thromboembolic disorders
Cerebrovascular or coronary artery disease
Known or suspected carcinoma of the breast
Known or suspected estrogen-dependent neoplasia
Undiagnosed, abnormal vaginal bleeding
Cholestatic jaundice (during pregnancy or with prior pill use)
Hepatic adenomas or carcinomas
Congenital hyperlipidemia

Relative

Significant (uncontrolled) hypertension
Severe impairment of liver or renal function
Smokers (>15 cigarettes/d) who are over 35 years of age

Table 52.5 Contraindications and risk factors associated with oral contraceptive use

Complication	Risk with oral contraceptive use	Additional risk factors
Venous thromboembolism		History of VTE, coagulation disorders, obesity, age, hypertension
Cardiovascular disease	=	Smoking, hypertension, obesity, diabetes
Breast cancer	Slightly	Family history, age <20 yrs at OC start, late age at first pregnancy
Diabetes mellitus	=	No impact of low-dose OCs on carbohydrate metabolism; risk of VTE increased in diabetics over 35 who smoke
Liver adenomas	?	Anecdotal evidence with older OCs; clinically not relevant
Cervical cancer	=	
Epilepsy	=	Possible effect of anti-epileptic drugs on OC efficacy observed
Migraine	?	Increase in attacks in patients with vascular migraine; for non-vascular migraine, often relief of symptoms
Sickle cell disease	?	Probably no effect on sickling, observed risk of VTE

(VTE = venous thromboembolism; OC = oral contraceptives.)

caused by fibroids, adenomyosis, and the like. The risk of ever acquiring endometrial cancer is reduced in OC users by 50%. The risk of ovarian cancer is reduced by at least 40% in ever-users, and by 80% in long-term users. The risk of pelvic inflammatory disease is reduced by 50% due to the thick, viscous cervical mucus plug.

Patient management When starting with an oral contraceptive, a low-dose preparation (≤ 0.030 mg of ethinylestradiol) should initially be chosen. Monophasic formulations are preferable because of their simplicity.

If oral contraceptives are started on the first day of the menstrual period, contraceptive reliability is immediately guaranteed, but breakthrough bleeding may occur during the first cycle. If the pill is started on the fifth day of the cycle, cycle control is better, but additional contraception is advisable during the first week. Oral contraceptives can be started immediately post-abortion. Post partum oral contraceptives can be reinitiated after 3 weeks, and they should probably be started within 2 weeks in women who receive medical suppression of lactation. Women who breastfeed should be informed that milk production can decrease, even with low-dose oral contraceptives. They should be advised to use alternative methods of contraception from 6 weeks post partum onwards.

When switching to another formulation, the new preparation can be started after the usual 7-day pill-free interval. Contraceptive efficacy is not affected, even when switching to a lower-dose preparation.

Monitoring recommended during oral contraceptive use consists of annual blood pressure measurements and a breast examination. A cervical PAP smear can be taken at the usual intervals. Routine laboratory tests are not warranted except in high-risk patients.

Drugs that cause liver-enzyme induction (such as anti-epileptic drugs and rifampicin) can increase the metabolism of steroids and consequently lead to a reduction of contraceptive reliability and to an increased incidence of breakthrough bleeding. Patients using anti-epileptic drugs should use an oral contraceptive with 0.050 mg of ethinylestradiol. There are no firm data to incriminate antibiotics in reducing the contraceptive performance of oral contraceptives.

Common problems with oral contraceptives Breakthrough bleeding occurring after many months or years of oral contraceptive use is caused by atrophy of the endometrium due to continuous exposure to progestogens. A 7-day course of estrogens (1.25 mg of conjugated estrogens or 2 mg ethinylestradiol) during any part of the pill cycle or during the pill-free interval will usually solve the problem.

Absence of withdrawal bleeding occurs in approximately 5% of women on low-dose oral contraceptives. Although benign in nature (the low estrogen dose induces insufficient endometrial proliferation), many women are anxious about the possibility of pregnancy or will not accept amenorrhea. An oral contraceptive with less progestational dominance (not necessarily with a higher dose of ethinylestradiol) can sometimes relieve this problem.

Reduced libido can be caused by suppression of ovarian androgen production in combination with a non-androgenic progestogen in the oral contraceptive, especially in third generation oral contraceptives. Switching to a second or even first generation oral contraceptive may solve the problem.

Nausea usually is a transient feature in the woman first starting oral contraceptives and is related to the estrogenic component of the pill. Taking the pill during a meal or at bedtime can reduce discomfort. When vomiting occurs within 1 hour after ingestion of the pill, the patient should take an additional pill or temporarily revert to another form of contraception.

Breast tenderness (mastodynia) is related to the estrogenic component of the oral contraceptive. Switching to a more progestogen-dominant preparation and avoiding excessive xanthines in the diet (coffee, tea, chocolate) may be helpful.

What to do about missed pills? The omission of one or more pills from a pack occurs frequently: approximately 25% of oral contraceptive users forget to take the pill regularly. When the omission is corrected within 36 hours, contraceptive reliability is not impaired. When more than 36 hours have elapsed since the last pill, the action to be taken depends on the part of the pill cycle in which the omission occurred:

- first week: complete the pill cycle and use additional contraception for 7 days. If intercourse occurred within 48 hours before or after the omitted pill, morning-after contraception is advisable;
- second week: complete the pill cycle as usual. Additional contraception is unnecessary;
- third week: complete the pill cycle, and continue with a new pillstrip without the usual 7-day pill-free interval.

In general, contraceptive failure is most likely to occur when pills are omitted at the end of a pill cycle or at the beginning of a new cycle, since in these cases the 7-day pill-free interval is likely to be prolonged. When withdrawal bleeding does not occur after a defective pill cycle, a urinary pregnancy test is mandatory.

PROGESTINS ALONE

Progestin-only contraception can be achieved by continuous administration of a progestogen, either orally (the minipill), or as long-acting injectables or subdermal implants. The mechanism of action depends on progesta-

tional effects on the cervix and the endometrium, since ovulation is not uniformly suppressed.

All progestin-only methods share the same side-effects and problems, in particular irregular bleeding: up to 40 to 60% of users will experience irregular cycles, and a minority a patients have continuous spotting or amenorrhea. Other side-effects include acne, mood swings, headaches, and hair loss. However, bleeding problems are by far the main reason for discontinuation of progestin-only contraception.

Progestin-only pills

Women who do not tolerate estrogens or in whom estrogens are contra-indicated may be eligible for progestin-only pills. The pill is started on the first day of a menstrual period and taken continuously without a pill-free interval. Users of progestin-only pills should be highly motivated, since taking the minipill daily at the same time of the day is imperative to assure reliable contraception. Whenever a pill is omitted or taken more than 3 hours too late, additional contraceptive measures should be used for 48 hours.

Injectables

Available preparations of injectable contraceptives are medroxyprogesterone 150 mg administered once every 3 months, and norethindrone enanthate 200 mg, given every other month. The start of treatment is during the first 5 days of the cycle to assure immediate contraceptive reliability. The high dose of medroxyprogesterone suppresses ovulation and induces complete amenorrhea. Breakthrough bleeding is common and can be treated by a 7-day course of oral estrogens. A major drawback of this method is reversibility of fertility upon discontinuation, as it may take 3 to 12 months for regular menstrual periods to return.

Long-acting implants

The most-used long-acting implant system consists of six silastic capsules releasing small amounts of levonorgestrel. Newer systems are those with two rods with levonorgestrel and those with a single rod containing 3-ketodesogestrel. Subdermal implantation at the medial aspect of the upper arm, as well as removal of the device, requires a small surgical procedure under local anesthesia by trained personnel. Due to the slow-release mechanism of these devices, they provide adequate contraception for at least 5 years. Although progestational effects on cervical mucus and endometrium are the prime mechanisms of contraceptive action, almost 60% of cycles in long-term users are characterized by anovulation. Irregular bleeding (60% in the first year declining to 35% in subsequent years) is the main reason for discontinuation. Adequate, pre-insertion counseling with regard to cycle disruption is essential in assuring adequate patient compliance. After removal of the device, normal regular cycles promptly return, resulting in excellent and immediate reversibility.

HEMRIKA DJ, SCHOEMAKER J. The oral contraceptive. In: Grossman A (ed). Clinical endocrinology. 2nd ed. Oxford: Blackwell Science, 1997;717-30.

NEWTON JR. New hormonal methods of contraception. In: Glasier A (ed). Contraception. Baillière's Clinical Obstetrics and Gynecology. Vol. 10. Philadelphia: WB Saunders, 1996;87-101.

ODLIND V. Modern intra-uterine devices. In: Glasier A (ed). Contraception. Baillière's Clinical Obstetrics and Gynecology. Vol. 10. Philadelphia: WB Saunders, 1996;55-67.

SPEROFF L, GLASS RH, KASE NG. Clinical gynecologic endocrinology and infertility. 5th ed. Baltimore: Williams & Wilkins, 1994.

Hirsutism

Hirsutism

Johannes Schoemaker

■ **KEY POINTS** ■

- Hirsutism is defined as excessive hair growth in women in the areas of the male sexual hair pattern.
- Hirsutism is caused either by elevated plasma concentrations of androgens or by increased sensitivity of the hair follicle to androgens.
- Hyperandrogenism is caused either by intake of exogenous androgens or by an increased production of androgens by the adrenal glands or the ovaries.
- Adrenal causes include stress, pituitary or adrenal tumors, and enzyme deficiencies.
- Ovarian causes include ovarian tumors, polycystic ovarian disease, and hyperthecosis.
- Step 1 in the diagnosis is to determine whether hyperandrogenism exists. Step 2 is to detect the source of hyperandrogenism – either adrenal or ovarian – by suppressing either of the two organs. Step 3 is to make the final diagnosis.
- Therapy is first and foremost in the hands of the beautician.
- Medical therapy is realized by either suppression of the adrenals, suppression of the ovaries, or anti-androgenic drugs.

Hirsutism is defined as excessive hair growth on women in the areas of the male sexual hair pattern. It should be distinguished from hypertrichosis, which is excessive hair growth all over the body, which can occur in males as well as in females. Although patients who complain of hirsutism find it annoying, the condition is rarely the symptom of a serious illness. Particularly in the western hemisphere, the complaint has its roots in culture rather than in medicine. The ideal female body image of today requires that sexual hair only grows in the armpits and the lower triangle of the pubic area. Even the slightest sign of a moustache, perimammillary hair, or hair in the abdominal midline is undesirable or even unacceptable, as is hair on the extremities. In the multicultural societies of today, this beauty idol is worshipped without taking the ethnic differences into account. This culture of the practically hairless female body leads to many complaints that are not based on real pathology, and therefore often the beautician rather than the doctor should be consulted. On the other hand, having a body hair pattern that does not comply with the current concept of beauty may lead to depres-

sion, social isolation, and so on, and as such may lead to real pathology, albeit psychosocial rather than somatic. Moreover, occasionally excessive sexual hair may be the symptom of an underlying disease. The complaint should therefore always be taken seriously. The patient is helped better with an understanding approach than with a denial of her complaint.

Physiology of hair growth

Hair growth takes place in hair follicles, epithelial downgrowths from the surface of the skin, which are usually associated with an apocrine sebaceous gland, also of epithelial origin (Fig. 53.1). The growth of each individual hair consists of three phases: anagen, catagen, and telogen. Anagen is the phase of active growth, which may vary in length from some 3 weeks to as long as 3 years, depending on the area of the body where the hair is located. Telogen is the resting phase, which may last from 3 to 5 months. Catagen is the transitional phase from anagen to telogen and usually lasts for only a few days. At the

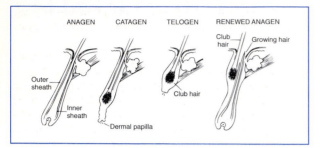

Figure 53.1 Hair and hair follicle in the different stages of development. (Reproduced with permission of the editor from Adashi EY, Rock JA, Rosenwaks Z [eds]. Reproductive endocrinology, surgery, and technology. In: Hyperandrogenic disorders, Vol. 2. Philadelphia-New York: Lippincott-Raven Publishers, 1998;1489-634.

end of telogen, the hair is shed and a new hair is formed, growing from the same follicle. The number of hair follicles is determined while the fetus is still in utero. No new follicles arise during life. Hair distribution is obviously dependent on the distribution of hair follicles over the body surface and as such is genetically determined.

Three different types of hair are distinguished. Lanugo hair is the thin, downy hair of babies and is shed in the first few months of life. Vellus hair is the soft hair that is distributed all over the body, also fine in texture. Terminal hair is more course and usually pigmented. It should be realized, however, that the line between vellus and terminal hair is not sharp, and intermediate types of hair are often seen. Hair can also be distinguished on the basis of its body distribution. Hence, we distinguish general body hair as being comprised of the hair of the scalp, eyebrows, eyelashes, and the vellus hair distributed all over the body. During puberty the hair pattern that develops first is the ambosexual hair, which grows under the armpits, on the external genitalia, and in the lower triangle of the pubic area. In women in general this comprises the full sexual hair pattern, although, depending on ethnic background, a considerable proportion of women also overlap into the third pattern: the male sexual hair. This grows on the upper lip, the cheeks and the chin, on the breast, often starting in the periareolar area, on the lower abdomen and upwards, and also on the back.

Hair growth is regulated by growth hormone (GH) as well as by androgens. General hair growth is, amongst others, GH-dependent; thyroid hormone, and particularly the lack of it, may lead to hypertrichosis. Examples of the effect of GH, or its placental equivalent human placental lactogen (HPL), are found in the increased vellus hair during pregnancy and in anorexia nervosa. The major determinants of hair growth, however, are the androgens. Increased androgen production, first of the adrenals and later on of the testes and the ovaries, is responsible for the initiation of the growth of ambosexual hair and then of male sexual hair during puberty. The amount of hair growing is determined by the level of androgens, the

duration of exposure to these androgens, and the sensitivity of the end organ, determined among other things by the number of androgen receptors in the hair follicle. The most important androgen to stimulate the hair follicle is testosterone. Hair follicles, however, do not have receptors for testosterone, only for 5-dihydrotestosterone (5-DHT). Inside the cells of the hair follicle, testosterone is converted into 5-DHT by the enzyme 5α-reductase and subsequently binds to the receptor. Other androgens such as androstenedione and dehydroepiandrosterone (DHEA) are in fact precursors of testosterone. Either in peripheral tissue such as fat, or inside the cells of the hair follicle, these precursors are further metabolized into testosterone and subsequently into 5-DHT.

Pathophysiology

Hirsutism is brought about either by high levels of androgens or by an increased sensitivity of the hair follicle to androgens. Increased sensitivity of the hair follicles cannot be diagnosed as such and is therefore diagnosed by exclusion of hyperandrogenism. Such hirsutism is usually called idiopathic. Hyperandrogenism is either caused by an increased production of androgens from the adrenals or the ovaries or by a decreased metabolic clearance rate for androgens, or by exogenous intake of (often synthetic) androgens. The decreased metabolic clearance rate is a rare condition and usually does not require specific diagnostic attention.

Adrenal causes for hyperandrogenism include functional disturbances, such as when the patient is under stress, has tumors – either adrenocorticotropic hormone (ACTH)-producing in the anterior pituitary (Cushing's disease) or cortisol-producing in the adrenal itself (Cushing's syndrome) – or enzyme deficiencies in the pathway of cortisol and sex steroid synthesis (Fig. 53.2).

Ovarian causes for hyperandrogenism include androgen-producing tumors, such as androblastomas and adrenal rest tumors, as well as functional disturbances of unknown etiology, such as polycystic ovarian disease and hyperthecosis (Fig. 53.2).

Examples of drugs that have androgenic (side) effects are, in addition to androgens themselves, testosterone for mastodynia and the anabolic steroids. DHEA is a popular drug because many believe it slows down the aging process. Minoxidil, cyclosporin, and diazoxide may cause hypertrichosis.

Clinical findings

Intake of exogenous hormones should be revealed by the patient's history.

Clinically, hirsutism is evaluated by inspection. The severity of the symptom is classically scored on the Ferriman and Gallway scale. This score assesses hair growth at eleven different areas of the body and rates these areas on a scale of 1 to 4. For daily practice the scale is not of much importance, because the interindividual variation of the assessment is quite large. A simple description usually suffices.

The first step in making a diagnosis is assessing hyperandrogenism. The effect of androgens on the end organ is mainly determined by the plasma concentration of androgens. However, testosterone is bound to sex hormone-binding globulin (SHBG), as well as to albumin, and the major part of DHEA is present in plasma in its sulfated form (DHEA-S). Assaying free testosterone is difficult and expensive. For this reason several substitutes for free testosterone have been developed, such as the free androgen index: This index is calculated as T (testosterone) x 100/SHBG. DHEA and androstenedione circulate freely in plasma and can therefore be assessed directly. Hence, to determine hyperandrogenism, ideally testosterone, DHEA, androstenedione, the free androgen index, and SHBG are all determined. The first three, however, for practical reasons, usually suffice. If no hyperandrogenism is present, the diagnosis of exclusion is idiopathic hirsutism.

If hyperandrogenism is present, the next step is to determine whether the excessive androgen secretion is coming from the adrenal glands or from the ovaries. This can be done by suppressing androgen secretion from either of the two sources. The ovaries can be suppressed by a GnRH agonist. For obtaining full suppression, the agonist should be applied for at least 2 weeks at the normally prescribed dose. More commonly, the adrenal is suppressed by dexamethasone. For obtaining full suppression of the adrenal, dexamethasone should be given for at least 7 days in a dose of at least 2.5 mg for every 20 kg of body weight. If at the time of maximal suppression androgen secretion is still excessive, the source is in the other organ or secretion is not under normal control, such as in the case of a tumor. The latter can be excluded by also suppressing the other source.

It is usually not necessary to go to the full extent of performing these tests. A number of rules of thumb can be very helpful, which are: (1) If androstenedione is the predominantly elevated androgen, hyperandrogenism is usually of ovarian origin, particularly if luteinizing hormone (LH) is also elevated; (2) if DHEA(-S) is the predominantly elevated androgen, hyperandrogenism is usually of adrenal origin; (3) if hirsutism is accompanied by disturbances of the menstrual cycle, hyperandrogenism is usu-

ally of ovarian or mixed origin; and (4) if testosterone does not surpass 6 nmol/l, an androgen producing tumor is unlikely.

If hyperandrogenism is of adrenal origin and not likely to be caused by a tumor, enzyme deficiencies of the cortisol pathway must be diagnosed, particularly because enzyme deficiencies require corticosteroid therapy rather than anti-androgenic therapy. Mild deficiencies in particular, such as in pubertal-onset or heterozygous forms of 21-hydroxylase and 11β-hydroxylase deficiencies, are commonly diagnosed. A corticotropin stimulation test, with special attention to be paid to the increase in 17-hydroxyprogesterone, may be helpful in distinguishing enzyme deficiencies from functional hyperandrogenism. A 17-hydroxyprogesterone level higher than 15 ng/ml 1 hour after the IV injection of 250 mg of synthetic corticotropin is diagnostic for late-onset (pubertal-onset) 21-hydroxylase deficiency.

Treatment

The most important therapy for hirsutism generally lies in the hands of the beautician. Electrocoagulation of hair follicles is the only definitive treatment for this condition. Waxing, depilatory creams, and tweezers are also part of a beautician's practice.

Medical treatment for hirsutism rests on three pillars: (1) suppression of the adrenals, (2) suppression of the ovaries, and (3) anti-androgen therapy.

Suppression of the adrenals can be done by corticosteroids, preferably dexamethasone. In general, a relatively low dose is used. The best indication is obviously adrenal hyperandrogenism. The therapy is monitored by measuring the elevated androgens. Full suppression of the adrenals is not the aim. Although relatively low doses are used, the patient should be warned of the well-known side effects of corticosteroids such as osteoporosis, stomach ulcer, disturbances of glucose metabolism, and hypertension. Moreover, the patient should be warned that under

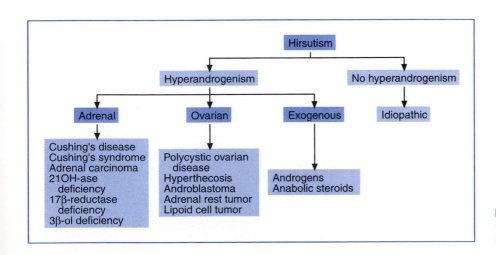

Figure 53.2 Causes of hirsutism (3β-ol = 3β-hydroxysteroid dehydrogenase.)

acute stress, such as surgery, major accidents, or a severe infectious disease, the dose should be increased five- to eightfold for a short period of time.

Suppression of the ovaries can be done either by steroids or by gonadotropin-releasing hormone agonists (GnRH-a). For steroids, oral contraceptives are a good choice, provided that older generation pills are used. Modern low-dose oral contraceptives generally have only a relatively small suppressive effect on the gonadotrophs and thus on the ovaries. Luteinizing hormone in particular continues to be secreted under those pills. Oral contraceptives have the additional advantage that they increase SHBG, which reduces the free circulating testosterone. GnRH agonists cannot be given for longer periods of time because of their total suppression of estrogens, which in turn would lead to a substantial loss of bone minerals. Add-back therapy, with small amounts of estrogens or a combination of estrogens and progesterone, would compensate for that, though giving oral contraceptives would be much easier.

Anti-androgens often exert their action through different pathways. Some of these pathways are suppressing gonadotropins, stimulating SHBG synthesis, suppressing 5α-reductase and thereby reducing the conversion from testosterone into 5-DHT, and, finally, binding to and thereby inactivating the androgen receptor. Often the effect of one anti-androgen is exerted through a combination of those actions.

Spironolactone is an aldosterone antagonist and also an anti-androgen by binding to the androgen receptor and by its 5α-reductase suppressing activity. It is the weakest of the anti-androgens currently available. Cyproterone-acetate is the oldest of the anti-androgens. Being a very strong progestogen in addition to its anti-androgenic activity, it suppresses gonadotropins but also has a receptor effect. Flutamide is a relatively pure receptor antagonist, and finasteride is a 5α-reductase inhibitor. Particularly the latter three are potent drugs. It should be realized, however, that anti-androgenic therapy takes a long time. Its effect cannot accurately be estimated before 6 to 9 months of treatment. The major effect is demonstrated by the reduction in the number of tweezing or depilatory sessions. The most important side effect of all anti-androgens is their feminizing effect on a male fetus during pregnancy. Anti-androgens should thus always be combined with a 100% safe method of contraception.

Suggested readings

ADASHI EY, ROCK JA, ROSENWAKS Z (eds). Reproductive endocrinology, surgery, and technology. In: Hyperandrogenic disorders. Vol. 2, Section 17. Philadelphia-New York: Lippincott-Raven Publishers, 1996;1489-634.

Endocrinology
of aging

Endocrinology of aging

Clark T. Sawin

We are now reasonably fortunate in that life expectancy has significantly lengthened in the last century, such that in modern times many survive to age 80 years and beyond. Moreover, it is noticeable that older persons are not merely dry husks of past selves, but they can have active and productive lives. Nevertheless, changes with age still exist. In this chapter we will explore the possibility that some of these changes are due to parallel changes in the endocrine system, and whether these changes might be reversed or slowed by endocrine therapy.

The major distinction to be made is between an age-related change, that is, an endocrine shift that occurs as persons become older, and a disease-related change, that is, a disorder that is more common in older persons. The distinction is simple in concept but is not simple in practice. There may be endocrine changes with age that occur in most persons, but the changes might occur with such a large variation that in some persons the changes are never evident. Even centenarians may have perfectly normal endocrine function. As a practical approach, most endocrine changes that occur in the majority of older persons can be considered as due to age. The major example is the hypogonadism that occurs in all older women; arguments continue as to whether or not it should be called a disease. While there are many other generalized endocrine changes with age, most are subtle and have only a few apparent clinical consequences. However, when a change occurs in only some older persons, it can be considered disease-related, particularly when there are identifiable clinical consequences. The primary diseases of concern are those related to dysfunction of the thyroid gland and pancreatic beta-cells.

Galen (129-199 A.D.), the ancient physician, believed that as years passed the body simply dried out. This to him explained all the features of aging, such as wrinkles and sagging skin. A more recent 19th century endocrine view was that aging was due to failure of the thyroid gland, because the changes myxedema caused looked so much like those caused by aging per se. In the first few decades of the 20th century, this concept broadened, and some physicians thought that there was benefit in giving older persons a wide range of glandular preparations; the results, such as they were, were in retrospect largely due to a placebo effect.

Viewpoints then shifted to the idea that we should use our new investigative tools to determine if in fact there were endocrine changes with advancing age and, as a separate question, to determine whether the consequences of any such changes might be ameliorated by specific endocrine therapy. This initiative has been the focus of ideas, symposia, and reviews during the past 70 years. Three general themes emerge: (1) there is no general "running down" of all hormonal secretions with increasing age; (2) the secretion of certain specific hormones does in fact decrease, due to either disease or age itself; and (3) the action of certain hormones, or at least the sensitivity of the body's tissues to these hormones, can decrease because of age (increased hormonal secretion may or may not make up for this lower tissue response). Age is not associated with generally raised endocrine activity, except in response to lower tissue response, nor is hyperfunctioning endocrine disease related to age.

HYPOTHALAMIC-PINEAL-PITUITARY CHANGES IN AGING

There are shifts in the timing of the circadian rhythms of cortisol, thyrotropin (thyroid-stimulating hormone, or TSH), and melatonin with age, as well as reduced levels of TSH, melatonin, growth hormone (GH) and prolactin, either during the day or the night, in older persons. Older persons may also have a somewhat higher level of vasopressin. Most of these changes are slight and have no clear pathological significance. For example, these hormones, as well as parathyroid and thyroid hormones, are essentially normal even in centenarians. Nevertheless, there may be some clinical significance to the lower levels of melatonin and GH and the raised level of vasopressin.

Melatonin

There is no evidence that melatonin administration delays aging in man. However, it is true that melatonin levels are lower in older persons, particularly during sleep, the usual time of maximal melatonin secretion. Some investigators believe that the lower level of melatonin found in older persons is a cause of poor sleep, which is supported by data that show improved sleep in older persons when they take small doses of melatonin (1-2 mg) before retiring. The evidence is limited, however, and more studies are needed before one can make a general recommendation to give melatonin to older persons with insomnia.

Growth hormone

It is clear that there is a fall in GH levels with age, along with a parallel decrease in insulin-like growth factor I (IGF-I), a GH-dependent hormone, and that some of the decrease in lean and adipose body mass and in bone density can be reversed with injections of GH. However, there is controversy over whether or not there is lasting benefit from the administration of GH or IGF-I (or even the hypothalamic hormone, GH-releasing hormone) to older persons who have low levels of GH or IGF-I but do not have hypothalamic or pituitary disease. For example, the effects of GH on muscle mass and strength add little to the effects of exercise alone, and the effect on bone is slight. Furthermore, current data represent only 1 to 2 years of therapy; whether the short-term benefits and high costs outweigh the side-effects and the possibility of inducing mild acromegaly over many years is unknown. A reasonable position would be to encourage further studies, await more data that show a clear benefit at low risk, and defer treating patients at the present time.

There are no data to show that older persons are more susceptible to acromegaly, though this would be difficult to demonstrate because of the rarity of the disease.

Vasopressin and water balance

Older persons may have a somewhat higher level of vasopressin, which appears to be in response to a lower sensitivity of the kidney to vasopressin. Thus, the raised serum levels are compensatory to the decreased renal response. There is also a parallel decrease in thirst in some older persons that, with the fall in renal sensitivity to vasopressin, can lead to older persons becoming more easily dehydrated. There can be some concurrent difficulty in excreting salt and water in older persons, perhaps exacerbated by a higher level of atrial natriuretic peptide; more likely, the raised levels of atrial natriuretic peptide are compensatory to a reduced renal sensitivity to the hormone. Clinically, whether or not these changes have major effects on salt and water balance, it is important to be cautious in administering fluids in older persons and to pay particular attention to avoiding dehydration.

Diabetes insipidus appears to be no more common in older persons than in younger ones.

ADRENAL CHANGES

Cortisol

The level of serum cortisol is well-maintained into oldest age, along with the regulation of the adrenocorticotropic hormone (ACTH)-cortisol feedback system. Nevertheless, the control of cortisol may be somewhat affected by age, as some data suggest that there is a more prolonged cortisol response to stress and a slower inhibition of ACTH by cortisol in older persons. No data, however, have indicated that these changes have led to an untoward outcome. The main disorders of ACTH-cortisol function, Addison's and Cushing's diseases, are uncommon and seem not to occur more frequently in older persons than in younger persons.

Aldosterone

The secretion of aldosterone clearly falls with age due to a parallel fall in renin secretion. By approximately 70 years of age the decrease can be as much as 50%. This decrease, when marked, can occasionally contribute to salt loss in older persons and in a few, particularly when there is mild renal failure, can lead to the syndrome of isolated aldosterone deficiency (i.e., aldosterone deficiency without a lack of cortisol). The treatment is replacement therapy with small doses of mineralocorticoid (e.g., fludrocortisone, 0.05-0.15 mg/day) with due caution for the side effects of overtreatment: hypertension, salt retention, or exacerbation of congestive heart failure.

The relative lack of aldosterone in older persons may also contribute to the development of orthostatic hypotension, a disorder that is usually of multifactorial origin. Even if orthostatic hypotension is not caused by a deficiency of aldosterone, in some patients the administration of fludrocortisone may help, although the doses needed (sometimes up to 0.2-0.3 mg/day) are often higher than the replacement doses used in isolated aldosterone deficiency.

Aldosterone excess does not occur more often in older persons.

Dehydroepiandrosterone

Dehydroepiandrosterone (DHEA) and its sulfate are major secretions of the adrenal cortex yet have no certain function except as minor precursors of active androgens. Because the secretion and serum levels of both markedly decrease with age, there is a common thought among the public that "replacement" with oral DHEA will slow the aging process and have a number of other beneficial effects, such as the prevention of cardiovascular disease, osteoporosis, cancer, and cognitive decay. There is no solid evidence for any of these effects in man.

In the United States DHEA can be sold over the counter as a food supplement and so can be, and is, taken by hundreds of thousands of persons, many of them of older age. While there are no data for long-term benefit, the question remains whether short-term benefit is possible. All that can be said to date, however, is that there are no evident problems associated with the lower level of DHEA and its sulfate in older persons, and there are probably no outright harmful effects from taking it by mouth. From a clinical viewpoint, there is as yet no clear indication for the supplemental use of DHEA.

Catecholamines

Serum levels of both the catecholamines epinephrine and norepinephrine are higher in older persons than in younger adults. While this may represent a higher level of sympathetic nervous system activity, it is more likely that the raised levels are compensatory to the decreased responsiveness of tissues to epinephrine and norepinephrine. For example, both alpha-adrenergic (vascular) and beta-adrenergic (vascular and lymphocytic) responses to adrenergic stimuli are diminished in older persons. Thus, the changes in serum levels can be considered physiologic.

There are no data to indicate that pheochromocytoma is more common in older persons.

THYROID CHANGES

Thyroid hormone metabolism

As Victor Horsley noted over 100 years ago, both hypothyroid monkeys and persons look older than they are; consequently, older persons look as though they might be hypothyroid. When this hypothesis was finally studied using modern analytic techniques, it was apparent that the level of serum thyroxine (T_4) was no different in older persons than in their younger counterparts. It turned out, however, that this is due to a parallel decrease in both metabolism and secretion of T_4; the decrease in metabolic breakdown of T_4, which might be expected to raise the serum T_4 level, is balanced by a slight and barely perceptible fall in the activity of the TSH-thyroid axis. The serum level of T_4 is thus maintained on an even keel even to age 100 years and more.

Whether or not there is an age-related fall in the serum level of triiodothyronine (T_3) is somewhat controversial. The initial reports of a fall in serum T_3 with age were countered by data that suggested that any fall was due to concomitant non-thyroid disease and not to a change in the thyroid gland. The likely answer is that there is a modest fall in serum T_3 levels with age that can be exacerbated by other illness; the slight decrease in serum T_3 with age has no known adverse effects. Thus, measurement of serum T_4 in older persons is clinically useful, while measurement of serum T_3 is less so.

Thyrotropin

There have been many investigations studying changes in the serum level of TSH with age, however, the results are confusing. Some data show a slight fall in mean serum TSH, generally within the range for younger adults, and some show a rise. A slight fall would be expected, based on the known shift in T_4 metabolism; when this result is found, the persons studied are usually selected to be normal older persons. When a slight rise is found, this is usually the result of including among the persons studied a modest fraction of patients with unsuspected thyroid failure, which would be expected to raise the mean level of serum TSH. Overall serum TSH may show a slight fall with age, but the value remains in the normal range for younger persons. Hence, with some qualification (see below under Hyperthyroidism), measurement of serum TSH remains a useful and practical guide to the diagnosis of thyroid dysfunction.

Hypothyroidism

Almost all (>99%) thyroid failure in adults is due to primary hypothyroidism unless there is known pituitary or hypothalamic disease. Primary thyroid failure, characterized by a raised serum TSH, is conspicuously more common in older persons, and more so in women than in men. When the concurrently measured serum level of T_4 is within the reference range, the condition is called "subclinical hypothyroidism," a convention that does not always take into account that some of these patients do have symptoms when questioned closely. When the T_4 level is below the reference range, it is called "clinical" or "overt" hypothyroidism, again an arbitrary convention as some of these patients have no symptoms and may feel quite well. The prevalence of thyroid failure depends somewhat on the cut-off used to define a raised serum TSH level. When limited to a significantly raised serum TSH, that is, ≥10 mU/l, the prevalence in persons over 60 years of age is about 4 to 7% in iodine-replete areas of the world and about 1% in iodine-deficient areas. As expected, the prevalence is higher in women than in men, but even in men the prevalence is 2 to 3%, which is a minor percentage but a substantial number of affected persons.

The rise in hypothyroidism with age is most likely due to a parallel partial failure of immune regulation with age. Most patients have an abnormally high level of antibodies to thyroid peroxidase (anti-TPO). Still, it is not clear why only some become hypothyroid if the immune shift is a general one due to age itself, nor is it clear why many with abnormal anti-TPO antibodies never become hypothyroid.

The prevalence of raised serum TSH levels is high enough in older persons to make screening for thyroid failure a reasonably cost-effective maneuver. In women over age 60 years, it is actually cost-saving; screening can even be fairly cost-effective in women as young as 35 years old. Our current recommendation is to measure the serum TSH concentration in everyone over age 60 years and to consider the measurement in those between 35 and 59 years.

Treatment of thyroid deficiency is straightforward: one gives oral T_4, beginning with small doses, such as 25 μg/day, in doses that are increased every 2 months or so by 25 μg/day until the serum TSH level has fallen to the reference range. The dose of T_4 is generally lower than in younger persons because, as indicated by the physiology of T_4 in older persons, less T_4 is needed to provide a given biologic effect. Treatment will remove any symptoms that are related to the lack of thyroid hormone but will not, of course, cure the many other complaints often found in older persons. Treatment will also probably lower the serum level of cholesterol enough to affect the cardiovascular outcome beneficially.

The main difficulty in treating older persons with oral T_4 is poor compliance with therapy. This problem needs to be assessed not only by interviewing the patient but by periodic measurement of the serum TSH value. Serum TSH should be measured from 1 to 4 times a year, depending on the physician's assessment of the individual patient's ability to take oral T_4 reliably.

Hyperthyroidism

Hyperthyroidism is much less common in older persons than is hypothyroidism. Although some have suggested that hyperthyroidism is more common in older persons than in younger persons, this is probably not the case except in areas of the world where there is (or was) iodine deficiency. When hyperthyroidism occurs, the signs and symptoms are far from typical compared to younger persons with the disease. Actively hyperthyroid older persons may show only weight loss as the presenting symptom and often do not have a goiter; they can be apathetic instead of nervous and irritable and may not have a rapid pulse, as in younger persons. It is easy to misdiagnose. One should check for hyperthyroidism in any older patient with unexplained weight loss, atrial fibrillation, or depression.

The test for hyperthyroidism is the same as for hypothyroidism: measurement of serum TSH. Most who are tested will not have the disease because it is far less common than hypothyroidism (the prevalence of proven hyperthyroidism is about 0.2 to 0.3%). The serum TSH concentration should be less than 0.1 mU/l. The diagnosis is quite rare when the serum TSH value is only slightly low, such as between 0.1 and 0.4 mU/l. To achieve the required sensitivity and specificity of diagnosis, however, the assay used must have an appropriate functional sensitivity, that is an interassay coefficient of variation <20% at the desired cut-off of 0.1 mU/l.

Note that when one screens older persons for hypothyroidism, one will always be screening for the rarer hyperthyroidism. When one finds a truly low serum TSH value by this route, rather than as a result of a clinical suspicion of hyperthyroidism, there is a new problem created: a small fraction of older persons (<1%) have a spontaneously low serum TSH (i.e., <0.1 mU/l) and yet do not have hyperthyroidism even when followed up for several years. Sometimes the serum T_4 in these patients is in the high end of the reference range and sometimes it is normal. While most of these patients are not hyperthyroid when further studied, they are at risk both for later hyperthyroidism and for atrial fibrillation; they should be monitored periodically for these conditions by checking the pulse and measuring the serum levels of both TSH and T_4.

When hyperthyroidism is diagnosed in an older person, the treatment is no different than in a younger person. Depending on the geographic location, the treatment may be more likely to be radioiodine, but in some areas of the world antithyroid drugs are the preferred therapy.

Thyroid nodules and cancer

Thyroid nodules are common, but their prevalence depends heavily on the means of diagnosis. Ultrasound detects many more than does palpation. The likelihood of finding a thyroid nodule as an incidental finding after a carotid ultrasound study is high whether or not there is iodine deficiency in the area. With either means, it is difficult to show a distinct rise in prevalence with increasing age unless the patient has had prolonged iodine deficiency in the past. There is little question, however, that thyroid cancer, when it occurs in older persons, has a poorer outcome than in younger ones.

As the vast majority of these thyroid "incidentalomas" are benign, it is not always clear what to do about them. Many clinicians are inclined to do fine-needle aspiration cytology of any nodule, perhaps because of concern over thyroid cancer or liability. A reasonable balance might be to follow the patient by palpation and perform fine-needle aspiration only if an incidentaloma becomes palpable, or if a palpable nodule grows in size. Surgery might then be done if the cytopathology result suggested a need for it. Another approach, over 100 years old, is the use of thyroid hormone. Though currently controversial due to several controlled trials that have suggested that therapy with oral T_4 is of limited value, it does seem effective in some circumstances. Until there are better data, clinical judgment should prevail as to whether or not to use thyroid hormone as primary therapy for a thyroid nodule or after its resection.

GONADAL CHANGES

Women

All older women undergo menopause and become hypogonadal. Estrogen therapy, often combined with a progestin, benefits the cardiovascular system (there is less coronary heart disease and stroke), the bones (there is less osteoporosis), sexual function, and a number of other bodily systems. The biologic cost is a probable, though not certain, increase in the incidence of breast cancer, which has only a small effect on the overall lower mortality provided by the hormone therapy. Many women do not want to continue to have periodic bleeding after menopause, which also must be considered. Overall, most recommend the use of estrogen and/or progestin therapy after menopause unless there is a clear contraindication, such as a previous history of breast cancer. A regimen can usually be found that obviates periodic bleeding, such as continuous administration of the hormone(s).

Men

There is no "male menopause". Though men do not have menses and hence cannot have cessation of menses, some men, but by no means all, do have a decrease in gonadal function as they become older. Primary hypogonadism, characterized by a low normal or low serum level of testosterone and a significantly raised serum level of luteinizing hormone (LH), occurs in 5 to 25% of men about the age of 60 years. The percentage is higher as age increases. In addition, another uncertain but minor fraction of men over age 60 years has a lower than expected serum level of testosterone without a clear rise in the serum concentration of LH. These men may have a type of hypothalamic hypogonadism, because LH function appears intact, or they may be simply normal variants.

While there are improvements in various functions when testosterone replacement is given to older men with spontaneously lower than expected serum levels of testosterone, there is no agreement on how widespread such therapy should be. Treatment does increase muscle strength and bone mass but has no certain effect on future fractures. Treatment may improve cognitive function and can improve sexual function, even though sexual dysfunction is related to hypogonadism in only a few older men. Some clinicians would reserve testosterone therapy only to those with clear symptoms of hypogonadism; they point to the possible worsening of prostate and cardiovascular disease as adverse outcomes of such therapy. Others think that therapy might be offered to anyone with a low testosterone level. Primarily, data is lacking in assessing the benefits and risks over the long-term, as most available data analyze effects over only a year or two. Ongoing studies will provide some answers. In the meantime, a reasonable recommendation is to treat only those men with proven hypogonadism (distinctly low serum testosterone level or a low testosterone level with a significantly raised serum LH level) and to focus on clinical symptoms rather than on presumed long-term benefits.

CHANGES IN CALCIUM REGULATION

Parathyroid hormone and vitamin D

Parathyroid hormone (PTH) levels are somewhat higher in older persons than in younger persons, although the values are mainly within the reference range for younger adults. Hence, the assay remains useful without adjustment of the reference range. The slight rise in serum PTH concentration with age may be age-related, but there is probably a real contribution to the rise from a modest degree of concomitant vitamin D deficiency. The mild lack of vitamin D leads to less absorption of gut calcium, which in turn leads to a slight lowering of the serum calcium concentration. The result is a small rise in PTH in compensation. The fact that modest doses of vitamin D reverse the slightly raised level of PTH support this idea. There is also a probable contribution to this overall effect on PTH by a sluggish conversion of the inactive 25-hydroxy-vitamin D to the active 1,25-dihydroxy-vitamin D by the kidney, and perhaps a parallel contribution by a lesser ability of the gut to respond to active vitamin D. Overall, older persons are slightly behind younger persons in their calcium absorption. A reasonable recommendation, at least in areas of the world with poor sunlight in the winter, is to give older persons approximately 800 U/day of vitamin D as a supplement.

Hyperparathyroidism

Hyperparathyroidism is more common in older women than in younger women, and it may also be somewhat more common in older men than younger men. In part the increased prevalence in older women is related to estrogen deficiency, as estrogen replacement often lowers the raised serum level of calcium to or toward the reference range. If this maneuver does not work or cannot be done, the treatment of clear-cut hyperparathyroidism with a distinctly raised serum calcium (i.e., >12.0 mg/dl) is the same as for younger persons, which is surgery. However, it remains unresolved whether or not milder degrees of hyperparathyroidism need to be treated with surgery. Expectant, watchful waiting may make sense for a number of these patients. Again, clinical judgment should prevail: completely asymptomatic patients can be followed and the serum calcium monitored every few months, while those with end-organ changes, such as renal stones or worsening osteoporosis, can be treated by surgery.

Osteoporosis/osteopenia

Clearly, the prevalence of both osteopenia and the more severe osteoporosis is higher in older persons (see Chap. 25, Osteoporosis). Whether these changes in bone mineral density, which increase the risk for future fractures, are inherent in the bone itself or whether there is a significant effect of the raised PTH to diminish bone density is not clear. There is no doubt, however, that vitamin D deficiency can cause a lower bone mineral density, which is one reason why prophylaxis makes sense. It is also well-known that estrogen therapy prevents bone loss and decreases fractures in women; again, prophylaxis is sensible.

CHANGES IN CARBOHYDRATE BALANCE AND DIABETES

Insulin and glucose metabolism

Older persons develop a slight degree of insulin resistance as evidenced by a modest decrease in glucose tolerance, although there is a minor contribution of slight beta-cell dysfunction to the glucose intolerance. The appearance of insulin resistance in older persons appears to be related to a decrease in the muscle content of the glucose carrier protein, GLUT 4. A contrary view is that there is no significant increase in insulin resistance with age and that any such observation can be explained by taking into account the increase in body mass index that usually accompanies increased age. Some support for this view is seen in the reversal of insulin resistance, at least in part, by raising the level of physical activity.

Diabetes mellitus

Diabetes mellitus in older persons is almost always of the type 2 variant. Defining the line between normal levels of serum glucose in older persons and diabetes continues to be problematic, despite new recommendations that the diagnosis of diabetes mellitus be redefined as a fasting serum glucose of ≥ 126 mg/dl. It is possible, for example, that the definition is too strict to apply universally to older persons, as evidenced by the slight rise in HbA1c that appears to occur with aging. The fact remains that, by whatever definition, diabetes mellitus type 2 is clearly more common in older persons: the prevalence in the United States is approximately 10 to 11% and will probably be higher when the new criteria are applied.

The approach to patients with diabetes mellitus type 2 has not been changed by the new criteria for diagnosis. In general, treatment is no different for older persons with type 2 diabetes mellitus than for younger persons. The difficulty, however, is determining whether or not there is benefit in these older, often obese, patients in treating them intensively so as to normalize the serum glucose.

This approach, which was successful in reducing complications in younger, thinner patients with type 1 diabetes mellitus, may or may not apply to these older patients with the type 2 variant. The issue remains unresolved, although a recent short-term study of type 2 diabetes suggested that there may be no net benefit and perhaps potential harm in tightly controlling the serum glucose. At the present time a reasonable recommendation is to treat patients with type 2 diabetes mellitus sufficiently to remove symptoms. This should result in a HbA1c of approximately 8.5 to 9.0%. Further control of the serum glucose and HbA1c would be sought if the patient were expected to live for many years (so that any presumed benefits would have time to appear); the goal would then be a HbA1c between 7.0 and 8.0%. Attempts to "tighten" control of the HbA1c make sense only if benefit is likely and the patient is highly cooperative; otherwise, the resources needed would be wasted. Further data are badly needed to aid clinicians in deciding whether more intensive therapy to lower the serum glucose is justified in older patients with type 2 diabetes mellitus.

Suggested readings

CHEN M, BERGMAN RN, PACINI G, PORTE D JR. Pathogenesis of age-related glucose intolerance in man: insulin resistance and decreased beta-cell function. J Clin Endocrinol Metab 1985;60:13-20.

GARFINKEL D, LAUDON M, NOF D, ZISAPEL N. Improvement of sleep quality in elderly people by controlled-release melatonin. Lancet 1995;346:541-4.

HOLLOWAY L, BUTTERFIELD G, HINTZ RL, GESUNDHEIT N, MARCUS R. Effects of recombinant human growth hormone on metabolic indices, body composition, and bone turnover in healthy elderly women. J Clin Endocrinol Metab 1994;79:470-9.

LIPS P, WIERSINGA A, VAN GINKEL FC, et al. The effect of vitamin D supplementation on vitamin D status and parathyroid function in elderly subjects. J Clin Endocrinol Metab 1988;67:644-50.

MICCOLI P, ANTONELLI A, IACCONI P, ALBERTI B, GAMBUZZA C, BASCHIE RL. Prospective, randomized, double-blind study about effectiveness of levothyroxine suppressive therapy in prevention of recurrence after operation: result at the third year of follow-up. Surgery 1993;114:1097-101.

ROSS DS. Thyroid hormone suppressive therapy of sporadic nontoxic goiter. Thyroid 1992;2:263-9.

SAWIN CT. Thyroid disease in older persons. In: Braverman LE (ed). Contemporary endocrinology: diseases of the thyroid, Totowa, NJ, Humana Press, 1997;103-124.

SEEMAN TE, ROBBINS RJ. Aging and hypothalamic-pituitary-adrenal response to challenge in humans. Endocr Rev 1994;15:233-60.

TENOVER JL. Testosterone and the aging male. J Androl 18:103, 1997.

VAN COEVORDEN A, MOCKEL J, LAURENT E, et al. Neuroendocrine rhythms and sleep in aging men. Amer J Physiol 1991;260:651-61.

VELDHUIS JD, URBAN RJ, LIZARRALDE G, JOHNSON ML, IRAN-MANESH A. Attenuation of luteinizing hormone secretory burst amplitude as a proximate basis for the hypoandrogenism of healthy aging in men. J Clin Endocrinol Metab 1992;75:52-8.

YARASHESKI KE, ZACHWIEJA JJ, CAMPBELL JA, BIER DM. Effect of growth hormone and resistance exercise on muscle growth and strength in older men. Amer J Physiol 1995;268:268-76.

Diabetes mellitus and metabolic disorders

Diabetes mellitus: diagnosis, classification, epidemiology and metabolic disturbances

Leif Groop

Diabetes mellitus represents a group of metabolic disorders characterized by chronic hyperglycemia with or without typical symptoms. These symptoms include thirst, polyuria, fatigue, and sometimes weight loss and blurred vision. The Greek term "diabetes" means "to pass through" and was already A.D. used to indicate an increased urine output. Although ancient Indian medicine had previously recognized that urine of certain polyuric patients tasted of honey, it was not until the 18th century that the word "mellitus" (from Greek and Latin meaning honey) was added to distinguish polyuria associated with glycosuria from other causes of polyuria.

The chronic hyperglycemia of diabetes results from defects in insulin secretion, insulin action, or both. It is associated with long-term organ damage, particularly in the eyes, kidneys, nerves, heart, and blood vessels. More specifically, these long-term complications of diabetes include retinopathy, which can lead to loss of vision; nephropathy leading to renal failure; nephropathy with an increased risk of foot ulcers, amputations, and foot deformations; and autonomic neuropathy causing cardiovascular, gastrointestinal, genitourinary, and sexual dysfunction. Patients with diabetes also have an increased risk of atherosclerotic cardiovascular, peripheral vascular, and cerebrovascular disease; in addition to an increased incidence of obesity, particularly abdominal obesity, hypertension, and lipid disorders. The clustering of abdominal obesity, hypertension, lipid disorders with diabetes (especially type 2 diabetes) and cardiovascular disease is often called a "metabolic syndrome" or insulin resistance syndrome, to indicate that insulin resistance could be a common denominator for the syndrome. The burden of life-threatening chronic disease may have a serious emotional and social impact on the patients and their families.

Epidemiology

Aging and Westernization of developing countries have lead to a dramatic increase in the worldwide prevalence of diabetes, growing from 100 million in 1994 to an estimated 165 million in 2000 and 230 million in 2010. This increase is primarily due to an increase in type 2 diabetes, particularly in developing countries. There are marked differences in the prevalences of type 1 and type 2 diabetes across different populations. In Europe, about 10 to 15% of all patients with diabetes have type 1 diabetes. In the age group of 0 to 15 years, the highest incidence of type 1 diabetes is seen in Finland (40/100 000 per year) and Sweden (30/100 000 per year), while the lowest is seen in Japan (1/100 000 per year). Although there are no definite explanations for these gross differences, a reciprocal relationship is seen with type 2 diabetes, which is common in countries where type 1 diabetes is rare, such as Japan.

A combination of environmental factors and genetic susceptibility is thought to explain most of these differences. In developing countries, the epidemic of type 2 diabetes is ascribed to the accumulation of so-called "thrifty genes." Genes predisposing a person to abdominal fat accumulation, energy preservation, and insulin resistance may have been beneficial during periods of famine. These "thrifty genes" would thus have increased the probability of survival in a harsh environment. With the increase in energy intake and decrease in energy expenditure (exercise), they are no longer survival genes; instead, in the wrong environment, they are associated with shorter survival. In general, mortality is increased more than twofold in patients with type 2 diabetes, and cardiovascular mortality is usually increased even more.

At the present time, the total prevalence of diabetes varies between 0.8% in Africa to 3.6% in Europe and 5.3% in North America. There are, however, populations with a very high prevalence of diabetes. In India, the prevalence is about 13% in the age group 30 to 64 years, in Micronesians on the Island of Nauru it is about 40% in the same age-group, while it approaches 50% in the Pima Indians from Arizona (Fig. 55.1). The prevalence of impaired glucose tolerance follows a somewhat different geographical pattern: it is about 7% in Europe, 15% in Native Americans and Pima Indians, and the highest prevalence is about 20% in Micronesians.

Etiopathogenesis

Normal energy metabolism

The ultimate goal of substrate metabolism is to ensure adequate energy supply to the body. About two-thirds of total energy expenditure is made up by resting energy expenditure, while thermogenesis (loss of ingested energy as heat) and exercise account for the remaining third. Energy is derived from the oxidation of fat (9 kcal/g), carbohydrates (4 kcal/g), and, to a very small extent, protein (4 kcal/g). In the body energy is stored either as glycogen in skeletal muscle (about 1500-2000 kcal) or as triglycerides in fat tissue (about 100 000-200 000 kcal). During starvation, body proteins can be broken down to amino acids, which are converted into glucose (gluconeogenesis) to meet the energy demands of the brain.

Carbohydrate metabolism In man, plasma glucose levels are maintained within narrow limits of 3.6-5.8 mmol/l or 65-105 mg/dl. Glucose is transported across plasma membranes into tissues (and back) by a family of specific glucose transporters. Of them, the glucose transporter 1 (Glut1) is considered the major glucose transporter in the postabsorptive state, whereas the insulin-sensitive Glut4 transports glucose into the cell after a meal. In the postabsorptive (fasting) state, the majority of glucose disposal occurs in insulin-independent tissues, such as brain (50%) and splanchnic tissues (25%), while the remaining 25% occurs in insulin-dependent tissues such as muscle. Basal glucose uptake, which averages about 2 mg/kg per minute, is precisely matched by the release of glucose from the liver, and to a smaller extent from the kidneys. Hepatic glucose production is made up of two compo-

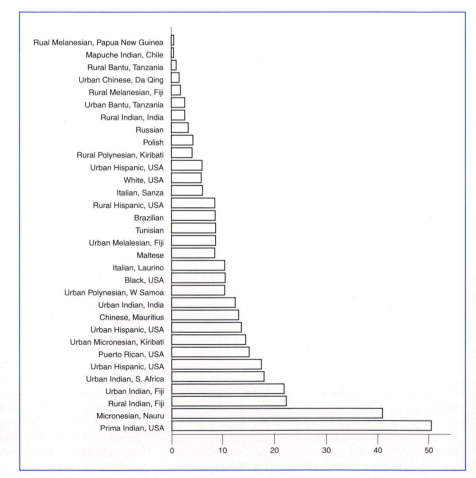

Figure 55.1 Prevalence of diabetes in persons aged 35-65 years in relation to income. (From King H, et al. Global estimates for prevalence of diabetes mellitus and impaired glucose tolerance in adults. Diabetes Care 1993;16:157-77.)

nents, gluconeogenesis (about 25% from the formation of new glucose from lactate, pyruvate, glycerol, and gluconeogenic amino acids such as alanine) and glycogenolysis (about 75% from glycogen breakdown). Glucagon and catecholamines stimulate hepatic glucose production, whereas insulin suppresses it. After a meal, insulin concentrations rise from 5-10 to about 50-70 mU/l, which results in the suppression of hepatic glucose production and the replenishment of liver glycogen stores.

A major part of insulin-stimulated glucose uptake occurs in muscle, while glucose uptake into adipose tissue is small. After entering the cell by facilitative transport (Glut4), glucose is phosphorylated to glucose-6-phosphate. Thereafter, it can either enter the glycolytic pathway and the Krebs cycle – yielding ATP, carbon dioxide, and water – or be stored as glycogen in skeletal muscle (Fig. 55.2).

Notably, hepatic glucose production is about 3 times more sensitive to the inhibitory action of insulin than peripheral tissues are sensitive to the stimulatory action of insulin (Fig. 55.3). To exert its effect on insulin-sensitive tissues, insulin first binds to a specific receptor and stimulates its receptor tyrosine kinase. This in turn results in tyrosine phosphorylation of the receptor and intracellular substrates, including the insulin receptor substrate 1 (IRS1) and phosphatidylinositol 3-kinase (PI-3K). They link the tyrosine phosphorylated insulin receptor to the downstream part of the insulin signaling pathway and the biological effectors, including the glucose transporters and enzymes of glycogen synthesis.

Fat metabolism In fat cells and in the liver, insulin stimulates the synthesis of triglycerides from free fatty acids and glycerol. During starvation, triglycerides are mobilized by the process of lipolysis, which liberates free fatty acids and glycerol. Lipolysis is stimulated by catecholamines, which after binding to specific G-protein-coupled β-receptors, stimulate the hormone-sensitive lipase. This enzyme is very sensitive to inhibition by insulin. Free fatty acids can be oxidized by many tissues – including fat, muscle, and liver – and fat oxidation is usually proportional to the availability of free fatty acids. In the postabsorptive state, free fatty acid levels vary between 0.4-1.0 mmol/l and decrease to 0.1-0.4 mmol/l

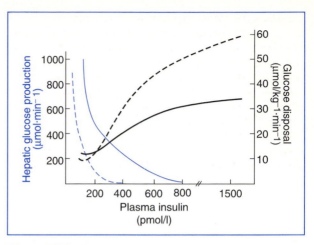

Figure 55.3 Dose-response curve for the stimulation of glucose uptake and suppression of hepatic glucose production by insulin in healthy control subjects (broken line) and in patients with type 2 diabetes (solid lines). (Adapted from Groop L. et al. Glucose and free fatty acid metabolism in non-insulin dependent diabetes mellitus: evidence for multiple sites of insulin resistance. J Clin Invest 1989;84:205-13.)

after a meal. In order to be oxidized, free fatty acids have to be transported into the mitochondrion by the enzyme carnitine palmitoyl transferase. In the mitochondrion, protons are generated by oxidative phosphorylation and transported out to the cytosol, where they convert ADP to ATP (Fig. 55.4). On the mitochondrial membrane are also located so-called uncoupling proteins (ucp), which serve as a short circuit transporting protons back into the mitochondrion and thereby yielding heat rather than ATP. This is the reason for the process called thermogenesis, that is, the ability to expend energy as heat after a meal. Several uncoupling proteins have been described: ucp1, which is primarily expressed in brown adipose tissue (and thereby rare in humans); ucp2, found in most tissues; and ucp3, expressed in muscle and fat.

Ketone bodies, acetoacetate, 3-hydroxybutyrate, and acetone are generated by partial fat oxidation in the liver, generally when there is a lack of insulin. Beta-oxidation of free fatty acids produces acetyl-coenzyme A (CoA), which can either condense with oxaloacetate in the Krebs cycle to form citrate, or in the lack of insulin condense with another acetyl-CoA molecule in ketogenesis to form acetoacetate (Fig. 55.5). Acetoacetate can either be converted to 3-hydroxybutyrate (this process is dependent upon the redox state of the cell) or decarboxylated to acetone. Following an overnight fast, ketone bodies in the plasma average 0.1-0.4 mmol/l; after prolonged fasting for 5 days, the levels can rise to 7-10 mmol/l. Ketone bodies represent an important energy fuel for the brain when glucose is lacking. However, it takes a few days until the brain adapts to the use of ketone bodies as fuels. After an overnight fast, ketone bodies supply only 2 to 5% of total energy expenditure.

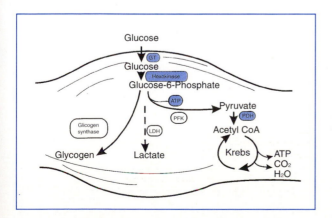

Figure 55.2 Pathways of intracellular glucose metabolism.

Protein metabolism In the fed state, oxidation of proteins do not contribute much to total body energy expenditure, whereas the situation markedly changes during long periods of starvation. Protein metabolism is the sum of two ongoing simultaneous processes, protein degradation (proteolysis) and protein synthesis. The daily turnover of proteins is much larger than the daily intake of proteins (200-300 g/day compared with 80-120 g/day), suggesting that degraded amino acids are used for the synthesis of new proteins. Protein degradation is stimulated by glucagon and insulin deficiency. Nitrogen from protein breakdown is excreted as urea or ammonium. Insulin inhibits proteolysis and stimulates protein synthesis. Protein synthesis is also stimulated by amino acids, such as leucine.

Metabolic disturbances in diabetes mellitus

Hyperglycemia develops when insulin secretion is inadequate for the degree of insulin resistance. At the onset of type 1 diabetes and maturity-onset of diabetes in the young (MODY), insulin sensitivity is usually normal, which means that patients usually display severe impairment in insulin secretion. Patients who develop type 2 diabetes are usually obese and insulin-resistant at the onset of the disease. They may be able to compensate this situation for several years by increasing their insulin secretion two- to threefold. Ultimately they reach a stage when this is no longer possible and hyperglycemia develops.

Type 1 diabetes Autoimmune destruction of the β-cells leading to more or less absolute insulin deficiency characterizes type 1 diabetes. This is usually seen when the β-cell mass is reduced <10% of normal. Insulin is a hormone with strong anabolic effects. Insuline suppresses

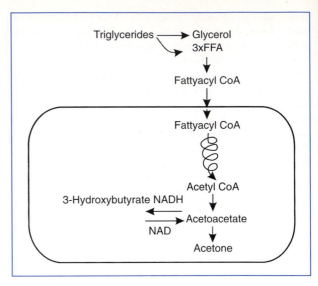

Figure 55.5 Oxidation of free fatty acids and ketogenesis.

hepatic glucose production, lipolysis, ketogenesis, and protein breakdown; whereas it stimulates peripheral glucose uptake, lipogenesis, and protein synthesis. Lack of insulin therefore has profound metabolic effects on all of these pathways. Fasting hyperglycemia results from increased hepatic glucose production, particularly increased gluconeogenesis. Postprandial hyperglycemia is usually the consequence of unstrained hepatic glucose production and impaired glucose uptake in peripheral tissues. Part of the excess glucose is lost in urine, which means a loss of energy; each gram of glucose excreted means a loss of 4 kcal. Severe glycosuria is the most important reason for the weight loss seen in uncontrolled type 1 diabetes. Lipolysis is grossly increased, providing an abundance of free fatty acids for oxidation. Increased

Figure 55.4 Lipolysis and oxidation of free fatty acids in the mitochondria. Catecholamines bind to G-protein-coupled β-receptors and activate adenylate cyclase, which hydrolyzes ATP to cAMP. This in turn stimulates the hormone-sensitive lipase (HSL), which catalyzes the breakdown of triglycerides to glycerol and free fatty acids. Free fatty acids are transported into the mitochondrion by carnitine palmityl transferase and oxidized to acyl-CoA, which can enter the Krebs cycle and undergo oxidative phosphorylation to generate ATP and protons. The latter are transported out to the cytosol, but they can also be transported back into the mitochondrion in a short circuit by the uncoupling proteins (ucp). This reaction yields heat rather than ATP.

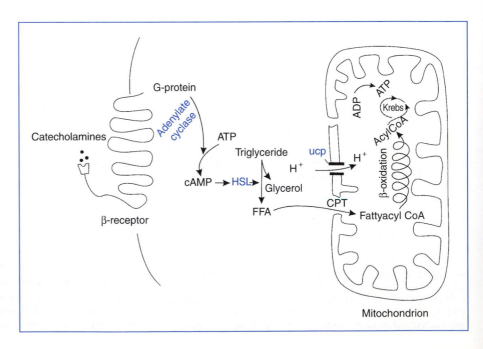

β-oxidation of free fatty acids results in an increase in acetyl-CoA, which will further stimulate hepatic glucose production by stimulating the key enzyme of gluconeogenesis, pyruvate carboxylase (Fig. 55.6). The increased rate of free fatty acid oxidation also provides energy needed to drive gluconeogenesis, which is a very energy-demanding process. A high rate of gluconeogenesis further aggravates the severe loss of energy seen in type 1 diabetes. In the lack of insulin, the Krebs cycle is inhibited, and this inhibition is further emphasized by an increase in the NADH/NAD ratio. Acetyl-CoA is now preferentially used for synthesis of acetoacetate. The plasma ketone body levels can rise to 10-20 mmol/l. Ketone bodies are strong organic acids, and the ensuing metabolic acidosis results in a special form of hyperventilation (Kussmaul). Both glucose and ketone bodies induce osmotic diuresis and dehydration, resulting in polyuria and thirst. Ketone bodies can also induce vomiting, resulting in electrolyte disturbances, and particularly high plasma potassium levels in the face of intracellular potassium depletion. This is further aggravated by a lack of insulin, as insulin normally stimulates the transport of potassium inside the cell. An increased rate of free fatty acid oxidation can lead to further impairment in peripheral glucose uptake by substrate competition (Randle cycle), that is, an increased rate of free fatty acid oxidation inhibits the oxidation of glucose. Finally, a lack of insulin leads to unstrained proteolysis, that is, increased protein catabolism, negative nitrogen balance, and muscle wasting. In children this can be manifested as growth retardation.

Patients with long-standing, poorly controlled type 1 diabetes often develop a secondary form of insulin resistance called *glucose toxicity*. This is manifested as impaired insulin-stimulated glucose transport. It has been proposed that an increased activity of the glucosamine pathway could contribute to down-regulation of the glucose transport system. This quantitatively minor pathway of glucose metabolism involves conversion of fructose-6-phosphate and glutamine to glucosamine-6-phosphate via the enzyme glutamine:fructose-6-phosphate aminotransferase (GFAT).

Type 2 diabetes Although both peripheral (skeletal muscle) and hepatic insulin resistance and impaired β-cell function contribute to hyperglycemia in a patient with manifest type 2 diabetes, hyperglycemia per se can further impair insulin sensitivity and β-cell function. A vicious cycle ensues that maintains hyperglycemia, a situation also referred to as glucose toxicity. Since subjects with manifest hyperglycemia usually display all defects of diabetes, it is not possible from studying type 2 diabetic patients to discern what is inherited and what is acquired in type 2 diabetes. To circumvent this problem, we have studied persons at an increased risk of type 2 diabetes, that is, first-degree relatives of patients with type 2 diabetes. We quantitated insulin sensitivity and β-cell function in these individuals using the euglycemic and hyperglycemic clamp techniques. Nondiabetic individuals with normal glucose tolerance showed a 30% reduction in their rate of insulin-stimulated glucose metabolism. Glucose oxidation was normal at this stage; therefore the defect in glucose uptake was completely accounted for by the defect in glucose storage as glycogen. The defect in glucose storage was associated with impaired activation of glycogen synthase by insulin, that is, the key enzyme of the glucose storage pathway in muscle. This does not a priori localize the defect to the glycogen synthase step, as more proximal defects in the insulin signaling pathway could also result in impaired activity of the glycogen synthase by insulin.

Impaired suppression of hepatic glucose production by insulin is a hallmark of manifest type 2 diabetes. In type 2 diabetes hepatic glucose overproduction is primarily due to enhanced gluconeogenesis, whereas glycogenolysis seems to play a smaller role. Hepatic glucose production and its suppression by insulin is normal in glucose-tolerant first-degree relatives of patients with type 2 diabetes. In contrast, suppression of hepatic glucose production may be impaired after a meal in individuals with impaired glucose tolerance, and it could contribute to the postprandial rise in blood glucose. Diabetes develops when the β-cells cannot compensate the insulin resistance. The transition from normal to impaired glucose tolerance and type 2 diabetes is mainly dependent upon a deterioration of β-cell function. Importantly, type 2 diabetes usually begins years, and possibly decades, before diagnosis. At diagnosis, about 50% of the patients already have hypertension or are showing signs of macroangiopathy.

Classification of diabetes

The proposed new WHO classification of diabetes encompasses both clinical stages and etiologic types of diabetes and other categories of hyperglycemia. The clinical staging takes into consideration the fact that many diabetic subgroups progress through several clinical stages during their natural history. All subjects with diabetes mellitus can be categorized according to clinical stage from normoglycemia to manifest hyperglycemia; this should be achievable worldwide regardless of the availability of sophisticated diagnostic tools. The etiologic

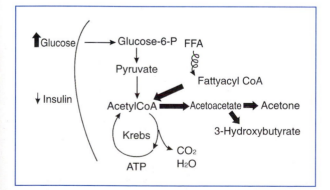

Figure 55.6 Intracellular metabolism in the diabetic state. Lack of insulin leads to an inhibition of glucose uptake, glycolysis, and glucose oxidation (*thin arrows*), while lipolysis and free fatty acid oxidation are increased (*thick arrows*), generating acetyl-CoA, which condenses to acetoacetate.

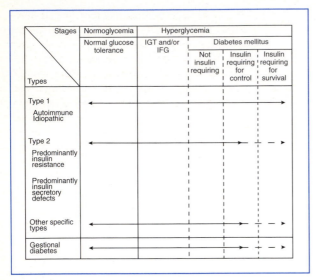

Figure 55.7 World Health Organization classification of disorders of hyperglycemia (1998).

classification is based upon the identification of the underlying disease process (Fig. 55.7).

The clinical staging goes from normoglycemia (fasting venous plasma glucose <6.1 mmol/l or 110 mg/dl) to gross hyperglycemia or diabetes. *Impaired glucose tolerance* is defined as a 2-hour glucose concentration during an oral glucose tolerance test of 7.8 -11.0 mmol/l or 140-200 mg/dl. In addition, a new stage called *impaired fasting glucose or nondiabetic fasting hyperglycemia* is based upon fasting glucose concentrations of 5.6-6.0 mmol/l or 100-110 mg/dl (Tab. 55.1). Diabetes mellitus, regardless of the underlying cause, is subdivided into (1) *non-insulin requiring*, that is, those patients who may be satisfactorily controlled with diet and/or oral antidiabetic agents (formerly non-insulin-dependent diabetes mellitus, NIDDM), (2) *insulin-requiring for control* (a new form corresponding to type 2 diabetic patients requiring insulin therapy for metabolic control rather than for survival), and (3) *insulin-requiring for survival* (corresponding to the former class of insulin-requiring diabetes, IDDM).

The etiologic types designate disease processes that result in diabetes mellitus (Tab. 55.2). The etiologic classification may be possible only if appropriate measurements of autoimmune or genetic markers are available.

Type 1 diabetes indicates processes of β-cell destruction that may ultimately lead to diabetes mellitus requiring insulin for survival or prevention of ketoacidosis, coma, and death. Type 1 diabetes can be subclassified into an autoimmune and an idiopathic form. The autoimmune form is identified by the presence of islet cell (ICA), glutamic acid decarboxylase (GAD), insulin autoantibodies (IAA) or other antibodies directed against β-cell antigens. In a small proportion of patients with type 1 diabetes, no autoantibodies can be demonstrated; this form of type 1

diabetes is called "*idiopathic*". Although this form is relatively rare in Europe (<10%), it may be more common in non-Europeans. Autoimmune diabetes is further subdivided into a rapidly progressive form that is commonly observed in children younger than 15 years, but it may also occur in adults, and a slowly progressive form that mostly occurs in adults. The latter is also referred to as latent autoimmune diabetes in adults (LADA) and defined as glutamic acid decarboxylase antibody-positive diabetes when the onset is after the age of 35. These patients are usually misclassified as type 2 diabetic patients; in fact, about 10% of type 2 diabetic patients have latent autoimmune diabetes in adults.

Type 2 diabetes encompasses the group of patients previously called non-insulin-dependent diabetes mellitus (NIDDM). People with type 2 diabetes usually have two metabolic defects, impaired insulin action and insufficient insulin secretion to compensate for the degree of insulin resistance. At least initially these patients do not usually need insulin to survive. The disease often remains undiagnosed for many years. The patients are at increased risk of both macrovascular and microvascular disease. The etiology is not known, but there are most likely several different causes of type 2 diabetes. A majority of the patients display features of the *metabolic syndrome* (insulin resistance syndrome or syndrome X); these patients are at particular risk of developing macrovascular disease. Evidence is accumulating that insulin resistance may be the common etiologic factor for the individual components of the metabolic syndrome. The metabolic syndrome is defined as glucose intolerance, impaired glucose tolerance or diabetes

Table 55.1 Glucose concentrations (mmol/l) for the diagnosis of diabetes mellitus and other categories of hyperglycemia

	Venous whole blood	Capillary whole blood	Venous plasma	Capillary plasma
Diabete mellitus				
Fasting or	≥6.1 (110)	≥6.1 (110)	≥7.0 (126)	≥7.0 (126)
2-h of OGTT	≥10.0 (180)	≥11.1 (200)	≥11.1 (200)	≥12.2 (220)
IGT				
Fasting and				
2-h of OGTT	<6.1 (110)	<6.1 (110)	<7.0 (126)	<7.0 (126)
	6.7-9.9	7.8-11.0	7.8-11.0	8.9-12.1
	(120-179)	(140-199)	(140-199)	(140-199)
IFG				
Fasting	5.6-6.0	5.6 -6.0	6.1-6.9	6.1-6.9
2-h	(100-109)	(100-109)	(110-125)	(110-125)
(if measured)	<6.7 (120)	<7.8 (140)	<7.8 (140)	<8.9 (160)

Values are given as mg/dl within brackets. To convert blood glucose to plasma glucose, multiply by 1.13; to convert mg/dl to mmol/l, divide by 18.

For epidemiological or population screening purposes, the fasting or 2-hour value after 75 g oral glucose load may be used alone.

(IGT = impaired glucose tolerance; IFG = impaired fasting glucose; OGTT = 75 g oral glucose tolerance test.)

Table 55.2 Etiological classification of disorders of glycemia

Type 1 (β-cell destruction, usually leading to absolute insulin deficiency)

Autoimmune
  Clinically rapidly progressing (classical juvenile-onset type 1 diabetes)
  Clinically slowly progressing (LADA)

Idiopathic

Type 2 (may range from predominantly insulin resistance with relative insulin deficiency to a predominantly secretory defect with or without insulin resistance)

Other specific types

Genetic defects of β-cell function
  HNF-1α (formerly MODY3)
  Glucokinase (MODY2)
  HNF-4α (MODY1)
  IPF-1 (MODY4)
  HNF-1β (MODY5)?
  Mitochondrial diabetes with deafness (MIDD)
  Others

Genetic defects in insulin action
  Type A insulin resistance
  Leprechaunism
  Rabson-Mendelhall syndrome
  Lipoatrophic diabetes
  Others

Diseases of the exocrine pancreas
  Fibrocalculous pancreatopathy
  Pancreatitis
  Trauma/pancreatectomy
  Neoplasia
  Cystic fibrosis
  Hemochromatosis
  Others

Endocrinopathies
  Cushing's syndrome
  Acromegaly
  Pheochromocytoma
  Glucagonoma
  Hyperthyroidism
  Somatostatinoma
  Others

Drug- or chemical-induced diabetes
  Nicotinic acid
  Glucocorticoids
  Thyroid hormone
  Alpha-adrenergic agonists
  Beta-adrenergic agonists
  Thiazides
  Dilantin
  Pentamidine
  Vacor
  Interferonalpha
  Others

Uncommon forms of immune-mediated diabetes
  Insulin autoimmune syndrome (antibodies to insulin)
  Anti-insulin receptor antibodies
  Stiff man syndrome
  Others

Other genetic syndromes sometimes associated with diabetes
  Down's syndrome
  Friedreich's ataxia
  Huntington's chorea
  Klinefelter syndrome
  Lawrence-Moon-Biedel syndrome
  Myotonic dystrophy
  Porphyria
  Prader-Willi syndrome
  Turner's syndrome
  Wolframís syndrome
  Others

mellitus, and/or insulin resistance, together with two or more of the components listed in Figure 55.8.

The metabolic syndrome with normal glucose tolerance identifies a group of subjects at a high risk of future diabetes. Alone, each component of the metabolic syndrome conveys an increased risk of cardiovascular disease, but together they increase the risk manifold. Thus, it follows that the management of persons with hyperglycemia should focus not only on glucose control but also include strategies for reducing their cardiovascular risk. Insulin resistance is defined as the lowest quartile of a normal population applying their own method for measuring insulin sensitivity. If one uses the gold standard method – the euglycemic insulin clamp and an insulin infusion rate of 40 mU/kg per minute or 287 pmol/kg per minute – this refers to values of < 4.5 mg/kg per minute.

Other specific types Genetic defects of β-cell function. Several monogenic forms of diabetes with impaired β-cell function have been described in past years. These include the different forms of MODY (maturity-onset diabetes of the young) (Tab. 55.3), mitochondrial diabetes with deafness (MIDD), and other types. Maturity-onset diabetes of the young is inherited in an autosomal dominant fashion and usually becomes manifested at less than 25 years of age. MODY1 is rare and is due to mutations in a liver transcription factor, HNF-4α on chromosome 20. MODY2 is due to several mutations in the glucokinase gene on chromosome 7. The disease is characterized by mild elevations in blood glucose, and complications are rare or absent. MODY3 is the most common form of MODY and due to mutations in another hepatocyte nuclear factor, HNF-1α on chromosome 12. Patients with MODY1 and MODY3 are susceptible to microangiopathic but not to macroangiopathic complications. One reason could be that they display almost normal insulin sensitivity. A fourth form of MODY was recently described. It is caused by heterozygous mutations in the insulin transcription factor IPF-1. In its homozygous form, the mutation causes complete agenesis of the pancreas. MODY5 is thought to be due to mutations in the HNF-1β

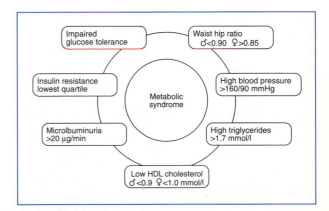

Figure 55.8 Definition of the metabolic syndrome. (World Health Organization, 1998.)

Table 55.3 Monogenic forms of diabetes with a predominant β-cell defect

Diabetes type	Chromosome	Gene	Complications
MODY1	20	HNF-4α	Retinopathy common
MODY2	7	Glucokinase	Rare or absent
MODY3	12	HNF-1α	Microangiopathy common
MODY4	13	IPF-1	?
MODY5		HNF-1β	Cystic kidney disease
MIDD	Mitochondrial DNA	3243 tRNA leucine	Deafness

Table 55.4 The spectrum of diabetes in Scandinavia

Type 2 diabetes with metabolic syndrome	60%
Mixed type 1 and type 2 diabetes (MIN)	10%
Type 1 diabetes	15%
Latent autoimmune diabetes in adults (LADA)	10%
Maturity-onset of diabetes in the young (MODY)	<5%
Mitochondrial diabetes with deafness (MIDD)	1%
Insulin receptor defects	<1%

gene, the heterodimer of HNF-1α. These patients usually display severe kidney disease with cystic deformations.

Mutations in mitochondrial DNA have been found in diabetic patients with deafness (MIDD). As mitochondrial DNA is only inherited from the mother, the disease has a maternal transmission. The most common mutation occurs at position 3243 in the transferRNA leucine gene. The same mutation can cause a number of neurological disorders such as the "mitochondrial myopathy, encephalopathy, lactic acidosis, and stroke-like" syndrome (the MELAS syndrome). Other specific subtypes are listed in Table 55.2.

Diseases of the exocrine pancreas. Diabetes can be the consequence of any process destroying the pancreas, such as pancreatitis, carcinoma, trauma, infection, cystic fibrosis, hemochromatosis, and pancreatectomy. Damage to the pancreas must be rather extensive to cause diabetes. Malnutrition-related diabetes is due to fibrocalculous pancreatopathy in most circumstances, and it is accompanied by pancreatic fibrosis and calcium stones in the exocrine ducts.

Heterogeneity of diabetes. It has become clear that diabetes is a heterogeneous spectrum of disorders, including classical type 1 diabetes, latent autoimmune diabetes in adults, monogenic forms with β-cell dysfunction and impaired insulin action, as well as classical type 2 diabetes with the metabolic syndrome. In Europe about 25% of diabetes patients would belong to the group of autoimmune diabetes. If we apply the criteria for the metabolic syndrome, about 60% of type 2 diabetic patients in Europe will have the metabolic syndrome (Tab. 55.4). This figure will obviously change over the next few years, when hopefully our knowledge about the etiology of diabetic subtypes increases.

Clinical findings

The diagnosis of diabetes requires the establishment of the presence of chronic hyperglycemia. Therefore, under most circumstances, one elevated blood glucose or plasma glucose measurement is not enough: it must be confirmed by another measurement on another day. The definition of chronic hyperglycemia has varied over the years. The current criteria were established by the National Diabetes Data Group (NDDG) by the United States National Institutes of Health in 1979 and subsequently endorsed by the World Health Organization (WHO) Expert Committee on Diabetes in 1980. The criteria were revised in 1985.

The current definition of chronic hyperglycemia is based upon a 2-hour venous plasma glucose value during an oral glucose tolerance test (OGTT) that exceeds 11.1 mmol/l or 220 mg/dl (equivalent to a venous blood glucose value of 10.0 mmol/l or 180 mg/dl). The rationale for choosing this cut-off level is that it indicates an increased risk of diabetic retinopathy. This was considered to be reflected by a fasting plasma glucose of ≥7.8 mmol/l or 140 mg/dl (blood glucose of 6.7 mmol/l or 120 mg/dl). However, the OGTT is cumbersome for diagnostic purposes, and therefore the majority of diagnoses are based upon the fasting value, which shows less variation than the 2-hour value during the OGTT (6.4% compared with 16.7%). It has also become evident that the fasting plasma glucose cut-off level of 7.8 mmol/l or 140 mg/dl underestimates the prevalence of diabetes compared with the 2-hour value during the OGTT. To obtain the same prevalence of diabetes by using only a fasting plasma glucose value as the 2-hour glucose value, the cut-off level for fasting plasma glucose must be lowered to 7.0 mmol/l or 127 mg/dl (blood glucose 6.7 mmol/l or 120 mg/dl). Another argument for this change is that the risk for cardiovascular disease is already increased at fasting blood glucose concentrations in this range.

The use of these lower fasting plasma glucose values for the diagnosis of diabetes would not increase the prevalence of diabetes if the disease was previously diagnosed by a 2-hour value. In contrast, it would decrease the prevalence by about 14%. In practice, diabetes was in most cases diagnosed based upon the higher fasting plasma glucose value of 7.8 mmol/l or 140 mg/dl. It can therefore be anticipated that the decrease of this cut-off level to 7.0 mmol/l or 127 mg/dl would increase the number of diabetic patients by 5 to 10% (Tab. 55.1). These new diagnostic criteria for diabetes have been endorsed by both the American Diabetes Association and WHO.

It is preferable to use plasma glucose instead of blood glucose measurements, as the latter is influenced by the hematocrit value. Furthermore, plasma glucose gives a better estimate of the glucose concentration seen by the tissues than the blood glucose concentration. Although the plasma glucose concentration is roughly 1.13 times higher than the blood glucose concentration, this relationship is not linear through the entire range of glucose concentrations.

It is also preferable to use venous instead of capillary (fingerprick) samples, because the variation coefficient of the latter is much higher than those of venous samples. At the present time, the use of hemoglobin A_{1c} cannot be recommended for diagnostic purposes.

Impaired glucose tolerance and impaired glucose metabolism

In accordance with the 1985 WHO criteria, impaired glucose tolerance was defined as a 2-hour plasma glucose value during an OGTT of 7.8-11.0 mmol/l or 140-220 mg/dl (blood glucose 6.7-10.0 mmol/l). This is still valid, but it is impracticable if no OGGT's are used for diagnosis. To circumvent this problem, a fasting plasma glucose concentration of 6.1-6.9 mmol/l or 110-125 mg/dl (blood glucose 5.5 -6.0 mmol/l or 100-110 mg/dl) was proposed to identify a risk group with impaired glucose metabolism. The long-term risks of this new risk group need to be established.

Normal glucose tolerance is thus defined as a fasting plasma glucose concentration <5.5 mmol/l 100 mg/dl or a 2-hour glucose concentration of <7.8 mmol/l or 140 mg/dl.

Gestational diabetes

Gestational diabetes is used to define a condition of chronic hyperglycemia (including both impaired glucose tolerance and diabetes mellitus) with the onset or first recognition occurring during pregnancy. It does not exclude the possibility that the glucose intolerance may antedate pregnancy but was previously unrecognized. Glucose levels are usually lower during the first trimester; elevated plasma glucose levels in the first part of pregnancy may therefore indicate previously undiagnosed diabetes.

It seems to be difficult to achieve worldwide acceptance for uniform diagnostic criteria for gestational diabetes. World Health Organization recommends screening for gestational diabetes at pregnancy weeks 26 to 28 with a 75 g OGTT. A 2-hour plasma glucose value ≥7.8 mmol/l or 140 mg/dl indicates gestational diabetes according to WHO, which now also includes gestational impaired glucose tolerance. After the pregnancy, the woman should be re-classified as having either diabetes mellitus, impaired glucose tolerance, or normal glucose tolerance based upon an OGTT performed later than 6 weeks after delivery.

Suggested readings

ALBERTI KGMM, ZIMMET PZ FOR THE WHO CONSULTATION GROUP. Definition, diagnosis and classification of diabetes mellitus and its complications. Part 1: Diagnosis and classification of diabetes mellitus. Diabetic Medicine, in press.

BECK-NIELSEN H, GROOP L. Metabolic and genetic characterization of prediabetic states. Sequence of events leading to non-insulin-dependent diabetes mellitus. J Clin Invest 1994;94: 1714-21.

FERRANNINI E, GROOP L. Hepatic glucose production in insulin-resistant states. Diabetes/Metabolism Reviews 1989;8:711-26.

FROGUEL P, ZOUALI P, VIONNET N, et al. Familial hyperglycemia due to mutations in glucokinase: definition of a subtype of diabetes mellitus. New Engl J Med 1993;328:697-702.

GROOP LC, BONADONNA RC, DELPRATO S, et al. Glucose and free fatty acid metabolism in non-insulin dependent diabetes mellitus: evidence for multiple sites of insulin resistance. J Clin Invest 1989;84:205-13.

GROOP L, FERRANNINI E. Insulin action and substrate competition. In: Ferrannini E (ed). Insulin resistance and disease. Baillière's Clinical Endocrinology and Metabolism 1994;7:1007-32.

GROOP L, WIDÉN E, FERRANNINI E. Insulin deficiency or insulin resistance in the pathogenesis of IDDM. Error of metabolism or methods? Diabetologia 1993;36:1326-31.

KING H, REWERS M, WHO AD HOC DIABETES REPORTING GROUP. Global estimates for prevalence of diabetes mellitus and impaired glucose tolerance in adults. Diabetes Care 1993;16:157-77.

NATIONAL DIABETES DATA GROUP. Classification and diagnosis of diabetes mellitus and other categories of glucose intolerance. Diabetes 1979;28:1039-57.

REAVEN GM. Role of insulin resistance in human disease. Diabetes 1988;37:1595-1607.

THE EXPERT COMMITTEE ON THE DIAGNOSIS AND CLASSIFICATION OF DIABETES MELLITUS. Report of the expert committee on the diagnosis and classification of diabetes mellitus. Diabetes Care 1997;20:1183-97.

WORLD HEALTH ORGANIZATION. Diabetes mellitus: Report of a WHO study group. Geneva, WHO 1985. Technical Report Series 727.

YAMAGATA K, ODA N, KAISAKI PJ, et al. Mutations in the hepatocyte nuclear factor-1α gene in maturity-onset diabetes of the young (MODY3). Nature 1997;384:455-8.

Type 1 diabetes

████ KEY POINTS ████

- A complex picture emerges in the etiopathogenesis of type 1 diabetes, where not one but several genes provide a necessary but insufficient genetic susceptibility to type 1 diabetes. Epidemiological research strategies have identified a number of risk determinants that may be causally related to the development of type 1 diabetes.
- Genes located within the HLA region are the most important in conferring susceptibility, but several other susceptibility regions have been identified. The influence of the environment on the etiopathogenesis of type 1 diabetes is also evident, such as in the differences in disease incidence among genetically homogeneous countries and between monozygotic and dizygotic twins.
- It is now possible to screen thousands of sera for autoantibodies assigning risk for type 1 diabetes in simple assays based upon well-characterized recombinant autoantigens.
- The general goals for treatment of patients with type 1 diabetes are to maintain a degree of metabolic control that prevents both hypoglycemic and hyperglycemic symptoms, and that prevents short-term and long-term diabetic complications with as little restriction as possible of their eating habits, leisure-time activities, and personal and professional lives.
- The care for patients with type 1 diabetes is best provided by a diabetes team with a diabetes physician, a diabetes nurse, a dietitian, and an orthoptist.

ETIOPATHOGENESIS

Flemming Pociot, Allan E. Karlsen,
Thomas Mandrup-Poulsen

Diabetes mellitus represents a heterogeneous group of disorders. Some distinct diabetic phenotypes can be characterized in terms of specific etiology and/or pathogenesis, but in most cases overlapping phenotypes make etiological and pathogenetical classification difficult.

Type 1 diabetes (formerly called insulin-dependent diabetes mellitus (or IDDM) is characterized by absolute insulin deficiency, abrupt onset of symptoms, proneness to ketosis, and dependency on exogenous insulin to sustain life. It is the most common form of diabetes among children and young adults in populations of Caucasoid origin.

Type 1 diabetes is the result of pancreatic beta-cell destruction. The development of type 1 diabetes requires a genetic predisposition to the disease and putative environmental triggers that activate pathogenetic mechanisms, leading to a progressive loss of pancreatic islet beta-cells. Although these beta-cell destructive processes are associated with a variety of immune phenomena, the immunological mechanisms directly involved in beta-cell killing have not yet been clearly defined in man.

Epidemiology

The prevalence of type 1 diabetes in most Caucasoid populations is approximately 0.4%. Type 1 diabetes is traditionally regarded as a disease of the childhood and adolescent periods. The age-specific incidence pattern is similar worldwide within this age group, although the worldwide incidence differs markedly for the age group of up to 15 years (Fig. 56.1). The disease is extremely rare before 6 months of age, but the incidence increases up to puberty,

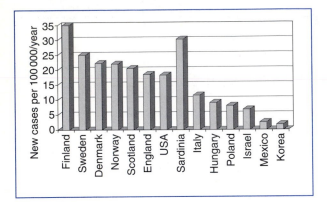

Figure 56.1 Incidence of type 1 diabetes in children aged under 15 years from fourteen selected countries. There is a 20- to 60-fold difference between the countries with the highest incidence rate and those with the lowest. Recent studies have not only identified new high-risk areas for type 1 diabetes, such as Sardinia, but also suggested an increasing incidence of type 1 diabetes, particularly in Europe. (Numbers are adapted from the WHO Technical Report Series 844: Prevention of Diabetes Mellitus, 1994.)

and it declines thereafter. An increasing incidence of type 1 diabetes for individuals <15 years of age has been observed in many countries. It has been estimated that in 1994 there were 11.5 million individuals with type 1 diabetes; in year 2000 the number will reach 18.1 million; and by year 2010 it will be 23.7 million. Recent studies have suggested that more than 50% of all type 1 diabetes cases develop after the age of 21 years, and that the cumulative incidence (up to age 80 years) may reach approximately 1%.

Migration studies and twin studies have provided evidence that nongenetically determined factors are important in causing type 1 diabetes. Such studies have demonstrated abrupt changes in diabetes incidence within one generation upon migration. The strongest evidence for nongenetic factors comes from studies of identical twins. All diabetic twin studies to date indicate a higher concordance rate for type 1 diabetes in monozygotic (MZ) than in dizygotic (DZ) twins. Most studies of MZ twins have shown that the majority of co-twins of type 1 diabetes patients are not diabetic, although recent data suggest a cumulative proband risk of 70% from birth to age 35.

Genetics of type 1 diabetes

Type 1 diabetes is a multifactorial disorder with a polygenic basis. Type 1 diabetes does not follow a clear Mendelian pattern of inheritance. Nevertheless, it is clear that genetic factors play an important role. Hence, type 1 diabetes has been classified as a polygenic or multifactorial disease, although it is not precisely known how many genetic loci are involved or how they interact with environmental factors. Though diabetes was already clinically recognized in ancient Egypt, the use of family data to evaluate the genetic component of diabetes was not feasible until the

introduction of insulin therapy 75 years ago. Difficulties in interpreting these original family data arose because the two major forms of diabetes, type 1 diabetes and non-insulin dependent (type 2) diabetes, were not recognized as separate disease entities until 25 years ago. Nonetheless, evidence of a familial component to diabetes was strongly indicated, as well as a role for environmental factors.

In the 1970s, association and affected-sib pair linkage studies established the role of human leukocyte antigen (HLA) genes in type 1 diabetes predisposition (the HLA contribution of disease is now referred to as *IDDM1*). HLA also revealed the heterogeneity of type 1 diabetes and type 2 diabetes, since type 2 diabetes generally does not show an association with HLA, although certain subsets may demonstrate some association. The comparison of rates of type 1 diabetes disease concordance in siblings who share two identical and zero parental HLA chromosomes with the concordance rate in monozygotic twins, the risk in relatives, and the population prevalence (Tab. 56.1) implicates additional non-HLA genetic factors.

The increased type 1 diabetes risk in siblings over the population prevalence (λ_s) is t15 (lifetime sib risk 6%/population frequency = 0.4%). This λ_s value is comparable to that of other autoimmune polygenic diseases such as multiple sclerosis and systemic lupus erythematosus. However, it is much lower than for monogenetic disorders caused by rare, highly penetrant mutations. In general, the lower the λ_s, the more difficult it wil be to identify, that is, clone, the genes involved. It will also be difficult to prove which of the many polymorphisms in a type 1 diabetes-associated region is of etiological importance. In addition, it is possible that the clustering of type 1 diabetes in families is due to shared environmental factors, such as viral infections, cow's milk protein, and certain other nutritional factors. However, environmental factors are notoriously difficult to identify, so genetics studies offer a more realistic option to address the question of how much of the familial clustering can be accounted for by genetic predisposition. Over the last 3 years extensive efforts have been invested to genetically map chromosomal regions that would demonstrate evidence of linkage to type 1 diabetes. This has been done by typing microsatellites (abundant loci with high rates of polymorphism) in large collections of type 1 diabetes multiplex families, that is, families with two affected offspring. This has led to the identification of at least 16 non-HLA loci demonstrating some evidence of linkage to type 1 diabetes (Tab. 56.2).

Table 56.1 Empirical risks of type 1 diabetes

	% (concordance rate for relatives)
General population	0.4
Average risk for siblings	6
HLA-identical siblings	12-15
One parent with type 1 diabetes	2-5
Both parents with type 1 diabetes	5-20
Monozygotic twins	30-70

Table 56.2 IDDM susceptibility loci and their chromosomal localization

Susceptibility locus	Chromosomal localization
IDDM1	6p21
IDDM2	11p15.5
IDDM3	15q26
IDDM4	11q13
IDDM5	6q25
IDDM6	18q21
IDDM7	2q31
IDDM8	6q25-q27
IDDM10	11p11.2-q11.2
IDDM11	14q24.3-q31
IDDM12	2q33
IDDM13	2q34
IDDM15	6q21
GCK	7p
DXS1068	Xq

(Loci demonstrating some evidence of linkage to IDDM and their chromosomal localization. No details are been published on *IDDM9* and *IDDM14*.)

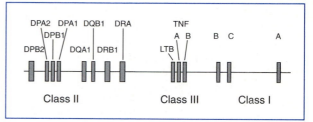

Figure 56.2 Schematic map of the human MHC, spanning a continuous region of about 4 Mb on the short arm of chromosome 6. Class I genes include HLA-A, -B, and -C, as well as the class I-like genes E, F, G, and H. Class II genes are divided into the main subregions DR, DQ, DN/DO, and DP. Other genes in this region include the large multifunctional protease (LMP) and transporter associated with antigen processing (TAP) genes. The class III region comprises a great number of genes encoding products with a variety of functions, such as complement components, tumor necrosis factor α (TNFα) and β, and heat shock protein (HSP) 70. (LTB = lymphotoxin beta.)

For all of these loci, including the HLA (*IDDM1*), the etiological mutation(s) *in sensu strictu* has not been identified. For the HLA region, several genes are probably involved (see below).

IDDM2 corresponds to the insulin gene (*INS*) region on chromosome 11p15.5. Most of the other regions are 5 to 20 centimorgans (cM) in size and may contain several hundred genes. In addition, heterogeneity within and between racial groups exists for the different type 1 diabetes loci listed in Table 56.2. Whether this reflects true heterogeneity in type 1 diabetes susceptibility between populations or whether this is due to differences in study design is at not entirely clear at the present time.

The genes

HLA-encoded susceptibility of type 1 diabetes

The best evidence for a genetic component of the susceptibility to type 1 diabetes comes from studies of the II.A region. The HLA region is a cluster of genes located within the major histocompatibility complex (MHC) on chromosome 6p21. According to structural and functional characteristics, the many genes in this region have been classified into three families, classes I, II, and III (Fig. 56.2).

The strongest genetic association with type 1 diabetes is conferred by class II genes. One of these, *DQB1*0302*, represents the predominant, but not the only, class II allele associated with type 1 diabetes in Caucasoid populations. Although numerous studies have emphasized the primary role of DQ in predisposition to type 1 diabetes, the involvement of DR is likely in some cases. Thus, analysis of the linkage between DQ and DR alleles on haplotypes that carry *DQB1*0302* genes demonstrated that only certain DR4-associated DRB1 alleles are prevalent among type 1 diabetes patients. The strong linkage disequilibri-

um of the HLA region makes it difficult to determine whether the DQ or the DR genes, or indeed other, non-class II genes, are the principal IDDM-associated loci on certain haplotypes. The frequencies of HLA gene alleles as well as their combinations differ greatly among various ethnic groups. This is due to evolutionary recombination events that have re-sorted specific HLA alleles among different human lineages and resulted in different type 1 diabetes associated genotypes by breaking up the linkage disequilibrium among class II genes present in a single ethnic group. Table 56.3 lists the various haplotypes that have been implicated in contributing to type 1 diabetes susceptibility.

Interestingly, a strong negative association with type 1 diabetes of certain haplotypes is observed (Tab. 56.3). DR2 haplotypes are negatively associated with type 1 diabetes in most populations, and they are protective of type 1 diabetes even in heterozygotes who carry a disease-susceptibility haplotype such as *DRB1*04-DQB1*0302*. There are several different DR2 positive haplotypes, and only the *DRB1*1501-DQB1*0602* combination is negatively associated with type 1 diabetes. Other haplotypes, including DR5 and DR6 haplotypes, may be associated with reduced susceptibility.

The correlation of specific amino acid residues with HLA-DQ/DR encoded susceptibility to type 1 diabetes

The fact that multiple different class II alleles and combinations of alleles are associated with type 1 diabetes can be reconciled by the hypothesis that these alleles share something in common that is central to disease susceptibility, such as specific amino acid substitutions. Indeed, certain amino acids in the DQ and DRβ chains correlate with disease susceptibility/resistance, and these amino acids are known to be critical for the function of the class II molecule in peptide binding and T cell recognition. For example, aspartic acid (Asp) at position 57 of the DQβ chain is encoded by DQ8 protective alleles; while an alanine, valine or serine residue at the same position is present in predisposing alleles. Although it has been shown that Asp 57 does in fact have a pronounced role in the function of class II molecules with respect to peptide binding, it cannot account for all of the complexity of HLA and type 1 diabetes associations. To evaluate the role of specific residues of the DRβ chain, an informative approach has been to compare the *DRB1*04* subtype alleles (Tab. 56.4). Clearly, no single residue explains the type 1 diabetes associations of the respective alleles. Rather, a combination of polymorphic residues in the DQα and DQB chains and the DRβ chain may be influencing the conformation of the antigen-binding groove of the DQ/DR molecules and hence conferring the risk determination.

Non-HLA encoded susceptibility to type 1 diabetes. Which are the genes?

Which are the genes responsible for conferring the non-HLA-encoded susceptibility to type 1 diabetes? As discussed above, very little is known. In broad terms, such genes/loci/regions have been identified and/or analyzed either by a candidate gene approach or by whole or partial genome screenings. For the loci listed in Table 56.2, candidate genes have been identified and properly analyzed in only two cases in order to qualify as the susceptibility gene of the region.

IDDM2 – The insulin gene (INS) region

The immune-mediated process leading to type 1 diabetes is highly specifically directed at the insulin-producing pancreatic beta-cells. The insulin gene is, therefore, a plausible candidate for the susceptibility locus since insulin or insulin precursors may act as autoantigens. Alternatively, insulin levels could modulate the interaction between the immune system and the beta-cells.

A unique minisatellite (variable number of tandem repeats, VNTR) that arises from tandem repetition of 14-15 bp oligonucleotide sequences is located in the 5' regulatory region of the human insulin gene (*INS*) on chromosome 11p15.5. Repeat numbers vary from about 26 to over 200, and VNTR alleles occur in three discrete size classes: class I (26-63 repeats), class II (mean of 80 repeats), and class III (141-209 repeats). Class II alleles are extremely rare in Caucasoid populations, whereas the frequencies of class I and class III alleles are 0.71 and 0.29, respectively. The class I/I homozygous genotype is associated with a two- to fivefold increase in the risk of developing type 1 diabetes.

This susceptibility locus, *IDDM2*, has been mapped and identified as corresponding to an *INS* VNTR allelic variation. Data indicate that the VNTR modulates INS transcription in the pancreas and thymus. Class III alleles, as compared to class I alleles, correlate with low INS

Table 56.4 Critical polymorphic residues of the HLA-DRB1*04 beta chain associated with predisposition to type 1 diabetes

DRB1*04 allele	Polymorphic residues					Disease predisposition
	37	57	71	74	86	
0401	Tyr	Asp	Lys	Ala	Gly	++
0402	Tyr	Asp	Glu	Ala	Val	+/−
0403	Tyr	Asp	Arg	Glu	Val	−
0404	Tyr	Asp	Arg	Ala	Val	+/−
0405	Tyr	Ser	Arg	Ala	Gly	+++
0406	Ser	Asp	Arg	Glu	Val	− − −

Table 56.3 Class II molecules and haplotypes associated with type 1 diabetes

DQ Molecules	DR-haplotypes	Population	RR
POSITIVE ASSOCIATIONS			
A1*0301-B1*0302	DRB1*04	Multiple	2.5-9.5
A1*0501-B1*0201	DRB1*301	Multiple	2.5-5.0
A1*0501-B1*0302	DRB1*301/DRB1*04	Multiple	12.0-32.0
A1*0301-B1*0201	DRB1*301/DRB1*04	Multiple	
A1*0301-B1*0402	DRB1*04/DRB1*801	Caucasians	4.0-15.0
A1*0301-B1*0201	DRB1*701	Blacks	8.0-13.0
A1*0301-B1*0201	DRB1*901	Blacks	5.5
A1*0301-B1*0401	DRB1*04	Japanese	3.5-4.5
A1*0301-B1*0303	DRB1*901	Japanese	2.0-4.5
NEGATIVE ASSOCIATIONS			
A1*0102-B1*0602	DRB1*1501	Multiple	0.03-0.2
A1*0103-B1*0603	DRB1*1301	Multiple	0.05-0.25
A1*0301-B1*0301	DRB1*04	Multiple	0.2-0.5
A1*0501-B1*0301	DRB1*1101	Multiple	0.05-0.5

mRNA levels in the pancreas but with higher levels in the thymus. Greater INS expression in the thymus may explain the dominant protective effect of class III VNTR alleles reported in type 1 diabetes by enhancing tolerance to the preproinsulin protein.

IDDM12 – The CTLA4 gene

The role of the cytotoxic T-lymphocyte-associated-4 (CTLA4) gene on chromosome 2q33 has been examined in various autoimmune diseases. CTLA-4 has been shown to mediate antigen-specific T-cell apoptosis, and biochemical abnormalities related to apoptosis are associated with autoimmune disease in patients and animal models (see below). An association between type 1 diabetes and CTLA4 polymorphisms has been demonstrated in several populations. Even though CTLA4 is the most likely gene candidate for IDDM12, the etiological mutation has not been identified, and detailed physical and genetic mapping of the region will be required.

Other non-HLA genes

Even less evidence exists for specific candidate genes of the other regions demonstrating evidence of linkage to type 1 diabetes, IDDM3, IDDM4, and so on. The identification of such genes awaits further mapping of these regions. Support for the different regions may come from different sources: (1) identification of candidate genes in such regions; (2) identification of syntenic regions, such as regions demonstrating correspondence in gene order between the chromosomes of different species, conferring susceptibility to diabetes in the spontaneous animal models, such as the NOD mouse and the BB rat; (3) overlapping with regions identified through genome scans in other autoimmune or inflammatory diseases such as rheumatoid arthritis and celiac disease.

In summary, molecular genetics and epidemiological research over the last decade has increased our knowledge of the etiopathogenesis tremendously. A complex picture emerges where not one but several genes provide a necessary but insufficient genetic susceptibility to type 1 diabetes. Epidemiological research strategies have identified a number of risk determinants that may be causally related to the development of type 1 diabetes.

Genes located within the HLA region are the most important in conferring susceptibility, but several other susceptibility regions have been identified. Fine mapping of all susceptibility regions should facilitate genetic population screening for individuals at high risk and ultimately lead to the identification of the pathophysiologically relevant mutations of the individual genes.

Etiology

As evident from the sections above, genetics are indeed involved in the etiopathogenesis of type 1 diabetes. However, the influence of the environment on the etiopathogenesis of type 1 diabetes is also evident, such as in the differences in disease incidence among genetically homogeneous populations, and between monozygotic and dizygotic twins described above. Diet, viral infections, and other environmental exposures are potential etiologic factors. One example of diet as an etiological agent in type 1 diabetes is the early exposure to bovine albumin in cow's milk. Others are nitrite and nitrates from food and drinking water. Although a single major component in the diet has still not been demonstrated in type 1 diabetes, studies of the increasing incidence rate in low-risk populations migrating to high-risk areas strongly suggest environmental component(s) in the etiology of this disease. This may also include infections, and indeed several viruses including Enterovirus, Coxsackievirus, cytomegalovirus, ECHO virus, Epstein-Barr virus, rubella, mumps and rotaviruses have all been implicated in human type 1 diabetes. This may either be directly due to infection of the beta-cells or through molecular mimicry with beta-cell proteins/antigens, resulting in a cross-reactive autoimmune reaction against beta-cell antigens. Whereas this aspect still remains controversial, an example of amino acid sequence homology between Coxsackie B virus and an immunogenic epitope on a putative beta-cell autoantigen glutamic acid decarboxylase (GAD) has been demonstrated.

In conclusion, though autoimmunity is most certainly involved in the pathogenesis of type 1 diabetes (see below), questions remain to be answered regarding the etiology of the disease, some of the most important of which are: (1) what triggers the disease? and, (2) is the fact that beta-cell destruction eventually results in type 1 diabetes the result of a primary autoimmune disorder directed specifically against the beta-cells or, rather, is the autoimmunity associated with type 1 diabetes the result and perpetuator of a non-immune mediated initial beta-cell destruction? In other words, what comes first, the chicken or the egg?

Autoimmunity in type 1 diabetes

The specific loss of the beta-cells in the pathology of type 1 diabetes is generally accepted to be primarily of autoimmune origin. This notion is initially based upon the finding of islet infiltrating mononuclear cells and specific beta-cell destruction (insulitis) in most patients who died in the pre-insulin treatment era. Although this infiltration could be a secondary immune response to a primary non-immune destruction of the pancreatic beta-cells, several lines of evidence support the involvement of autoimmunity in type 1 diabetes pathogenesis. Due to the inherent difficulties of studying the disease process in humans, the use of animal models to study type 1 diabetes has provided additional valuable information to the observations made in human type 1 diabetes. The two most well-characterized and frequently used animal models of spontaneous autoimmune type 1 diabetes are the non-obese diabetic (NOD) mice and the Bio-Breeding (BB) rats. These inbred animal models demonstrate several similarities to the development of type 1 diabetes in humans.

Nevertheless, it is important to keep in mind that each of these models at best represents the counterpart of one individual human being in multiple copies, that is, one genetic set-up. Thus, despite the polygenic nature of type 1 diabetes in both human and NOD mice, the complexity of human type 1 diabetes is much larger due to different etiology/pathogenesis among individuals.

In addition to insulitis and an association with certain HLA tissue-types (see above), the presence of several islet cell autoantibodies and autoreactive T lymphocytes in prediabetic and recent-onset diabetic humans and animals supports an autoimmune involvement. Furthermore, a vast number of experiments in the animal type 1 diabetes models with transfer of T-lymphocyte subsets from diabetic to nondiabetic recipients have demonstrated that both CD4+ T helper cells, as well as the CD8+ cytotoxic T cells, may indeed transfer the disease, either directly or as accelerators of other beta-cell destructive processes.

Autoantigens in type 1 diabetes

Autoantigens in type 1 diabetes can be identified and characterized by islet reactivity with autoantibodies and/or T-cell receptors.

Autoantibodies in type 1 diabetes

The existence of islet cell cytoplasmic autoantibodies (ICA) in sera from newly diagnosed diabetic patients was first described in 1974 by indirect immunofluorescence analysis on human pancreatic tissue. This technique is restricted by the availability of human pancreata, and the reproducibility is rather poor between laboratories. However, in standardized analyses approximately 60 to 80% of recent-onset type 1 diabetes patients display ICA in their serum versus less than 2 to 3% of the healthy control individuals. It should, however, be kept in mind that 2 to 3% of the healthy population is much more than the incidence of type 1 diabetes in the population (0.1 to 0.5%), demonstrating that ICA positivity per se is not a sufficient marker for disease development in general population screenings. Nevertheless, ICA is a useful marker for disease development in first-degree relatives of diabetic patients and in population screenings.

In 1982, insulin was the first islet autoantigen to be positively identified. However, insulin constituted only a minor part of islet cell cytoplasmic autoantibody binding, since insulin autoantibodies were only detected in approximately 40% of recent-onset type 1 diabetes patients. Shortly thereafter, another islet autoantigen, named the 64K autoantigen based upon its molecular weight, was immunoprecipitated from isolated rat islets with sera from diabetic individuals. Antibody reactivity against this antigen was later demonstrated to be present in approximately 70 to 80% of recent-onset type 1 diabetes patents, in contrast to less than 5% in healthy individuals. Furthermore, both ICA and the 64K autoantibodies could be identified up to 10 years before the clinical onset of type 1 diabetes.

This suggested that they may be both predictive of and involved in ongoing beta-cell destruction preceding the acute onset of type 1 diabetes.

In 1990, glutamic acid decarboxylase (GAD) was finally demonstrated as one of the major proteins in the immunoprecipitated 64K gel band. GAD is an enzyme that before this identification was primarily known within the area of neuroscience research due to its catalytic activity in the synthesis of the neurotransmitter gamma-amino butyric acid (GABA). However, the role of this amino acid in pancreatic beta-cells still remains to be clarified. GAD has been cloned from both rat and human islets, and the existence of two distinct GAD isoforms (named GAD65 and GAD67 according to their molecular weight) encoded by different genes were found. Whereas both isoforms were found in rat islets, only the GAD65 isoform was expressed in human islets; it was demonstrated that this GAD65 isoform represents the major autoantigen included in the original diabetes associated 64K immunoprecipitate. Preabsorption of ICA-positive sera with GAD65 did not remove all antibody reactivity within pancreatic islets, which suggested that other autoantigens were involved in type 1 diabetes. Indeed, trypsin treatment of islet proteins resulted in immunoprecipitation with diabetic sera of additional antigens with molecular weight following SDS gel separation of 37 kD, 40 kD, and 50 kD. In early studies it was demonstrated that the prevalence of 50 kD autoantibodies correlated with GAD autoantibody reactivity, whereas 37 kD and 40 kD autoantibodies were suggested as better predictors of type 1 diabetes-development in prediabetic individuals than GAD autoantibodies. The proteins behind these diabetes-associated immunoprecipitates have recently been identified, and the corresponding cDNAs were cloned. The 40 kD tryptic fragment, being identical to the recently cloned IA-2 antigen, is a member of the membrane-bound protein tyrosine phosphatase (PTP) family.

Another autoantigen, named ICA512, is considered to represent a fragment of IA-2. The 37 kD tryptic fragment appears to originate from phogrin (also referred to as IA-2-beta), a new member of the protein tyrosine phosphatase family, showing high degree of sequence homology with IA-2.

The autoantigenic epitopes are located in the intracellular domains of both of these transmembrane protein tyrosine phosphatases. Following post-translational processing, phogrin is cleaved into proteins of 60 to 64 kD. Thus, the originally immunoprecipitated 64K autoantigen may include both GAD and phogrin. Finally, the 50kD fragment is described as a trypsinization product of GAD. It is of interest that both GAD and the protein tyrosine phosphatases are primarily expressed in neuronal (brain) and islet tissue.

Over the last decade, a long list of islet cell and non-islet cell-related autoantibodies with varying type 1 diabetes association and specificity have been demonstrated. An increasing number of the corresponding autoantigens are being identified, some of which are listed in Table 56.5. The hitherto-identified major autoantigens in type 1 diabetes are mostly intracellular or secreted components of the beta-cells, making their direct involvement in beta-

Table 56.5 Identified autoantigens in autoimmune type 1 diabetes

Insulin
Glutamic acid decarboxylase (GAD65)
GM2-1 ganglioside
GT3 ganglioside
Sulfatide
Protein tyrosine phosphatase (IA-2)
Phogrin (IA-2β)
Hsp65
Peripherin
Carboxypeptidase H
Glucose transporter 2 (GLUT2)

cell killing by cytolysis unlikely. Furthermore, high-titer autoantibodies to GAD are frequently found in another autoimmune disease, the Stiff-man syndrome, but only a small proportion of those patients develops type 1 diabetes, and vice versa, Stiff-man syndrome is extremely rare in diabetic patients. In addition, newborns with a high ICA titer due to transplacental transfer from their type 1 diabetic mothers do not show any aberrations of insulin production or develop type 1 diabetes as a result of these antibodies. Nevertheless, autoantibodies to islet-cell surface antigens (ICSA), such as gangliosides that directly influence beta-cell function, have been described in a few studies of animal models of type 1 diabetes.

Prediction of type 1 diabetes, autoantibody screening

Whereas the direct pathogenetic involvement of autoantibodies in type 1 diabetes sems unlikely, their presence in sera from diabetic – and in particular prediabetic – patients have made them valuable tools as markers for disease progression. Until recently the time- and resource-consuming method for ICA screening described above was the preferred method for screening sera, such as in the large ongoing international intervention studies with nicotinamide or oral insulin-treatment in first-degree relatives of type 1 diabetes patients. The complexity of the method is, however, reflected by the low reproducibility of data between laboratories, which makes it necessary to select core laboratories for screening in such intervention trials.

Following the cloning of cDNA encoding the GAD65 autoantigen, it was possible for the first time to develop reproducible, fast, and cost-efficient assays based on a defined recombinant autoantigen. The first assays based on radioimmuno-detection of immunoprecipitated ^{35}S-methionine-labeled *in vitro* transcribed and translated GAD yielded the same high recognition of GAD-autoantibodies in diabetic sera as described above. After the identification of another of the major autoantigens, the IA-2/ICA512 (see above), similar semiautomated assays for this antigen were developed, and the combination of GAD- and IA-2, and in some cases insulin autoantibodies, has been associated with a near 100% risk of type 1 diabetes onset within 5 years in first-degree relatives. These screening systems have also proven useful in the early detection of patients diagnosed

as type 2 diabetes patients, who later become insulin-requiring (LADA, late-onset autoimmune diabetes in the adult).

In summary, it is now possible to screen thousands of sera in easy assays based upon well-characterized recombinant autoantigens, allowing for the evaluation of the predictive value of these assays (perhaps combined with, for example, HLA typing) for later development of type 1 diabetes in screening the general population. Combined with intravenous glucose tolerance tests of individuals in risk groups, this may be a feasible screening method once safe and effective interventions are available for the prevention of type 1 diabetes.

T-cell reactivity in type 1 diabetes

Whereas autoantibodies and their autoantigens in human type 1 diabetes are rather well-characterized, the demonstration of autoreactive T-cell clones in human type 1 diabetes has been lagging behind. Despite this, type 1 diabetes is generally regarded as a T-cell mediated autoimmune disease primarily based upon observations in animal models of type 1 diabetes. Indeed, several CD4+ and CD8+ T-cell clones have been isolated from these models that may induce type 1 diabetes when transferred to non-diabetic recipients. Thus, although both helper, suppressor, and cytotoxic T cells are involved in and may even be necessary for beta-cell destruction to progress to overt type 1 diabetes in animal models, the precise role and interaction of those cells remain to be established.

Experiments in NOD mice have demonstrated that a hierarchy of T-cell autoreactivity exists, some of which are primarily associated with the development of disease and some of which are secondary to the appearance of autoantigens liberated after beta-cell destruction. Thus, it has been demonstrated that neonatal tolerization with GAD peptides – in contrast to other T-cell autoantigens in the NOD mice – may prevent the onset of type 1 diabetes depending on timing, concentration, and the route of administration of the tolerizing antigen.

In recent years another aspect of T-cell involvement and regulation of immune-reactions has become evident in the animal models of type 1 diabetes. The CD4+ T cells may differentiate into or switch between two subsets or phenotypes, the Th1 and Th2 phenotypes, characterized by their cytokine secretion profile and function. Th1 cells – which primarily secrete IL-2, interferon gamma, and tumor necrosis factor β – are involved in cell-mediated immune responses, whereas Th2 cells secreting IL-4 and IL-10 stimulate antibody producing B-lymphocytes. Furthermore, the Th2 cytokine profile may inhibit the effect of the Th1 cells and vice versa. The existence of such an inhibitory Th2 cell system may in part explain the controversy regarding the existence and function of suppressor T cells. In NOD mice, a shift of islet reactive Th2-lymphocytes toward a Th1 profile has been suggested to be associated with the development of type 1 diabetes, and in animal studies of so-called oral tolerance, where early feeding with insulin prevents or reduces the incidence of type 1 diabetes, the mechanism has been proposed to be migration of Th2-positive cells to the islets, thus inhibiting the Th1 help necessary for the autoimmune beta-cell destruction.

Effector mechanisms in type 1 diabetes

Insulitis: an inflammatory reaction

In inflammatory lesions, including those observed in the target organs in autoimmune disorders, persistent synthesis and secretion of soluble mediators of inflammation (such as cytokines, proteases, complement and coagulation factors, and free radicals) take place, leading to high local tissue concentrations of these mediators. Cytokines are released by macrophages. T cells and B cells mediate leukocyte chemotaxis, proliferation and differentiation, endothelial cell activation, and many other local and systemic biological activities important for the immune response. Some cytokines – such as interleukin 1 (IL-1), tumor necrosis factor (TNF) α, and interferon gamma – also have cytostatic or cytotoxic actions, primarily contributing to host defense against tumor cells and microorganisms, but also to destruction of some normal cells.

Cytokines as effector molecules in type 1 diabetes

There is increasing evidence to support the role of cytokines as effector molecules leading to beta-cell destruction and type 1 diabetes:

1. *In vitro* IL-1, either alone or in synergy with TNFα and/or interferon gamma causes selective beta-cell destruction in isolated islets and the perfused pancreas by inhibiting mitochondrial glucose oxidation causing DNA damage and inducting apoptosis. These effects are associated with induction of cytokine-inducible nitric oxide synthase (iNOS) and nitric oxide (NO) synthesis specifically in the beta-cells (Fig. 56.3).

2. *Ex vivo* the function of islets isolated from IL-1-pretreated normal rats or of syngeneic islet explants exposed *in vivo* to cytokines during the rejection process in mixed islet syn- and xenografts is irreversibly inhibited.

3. *In vivo*
   - daily IL-1 injections for 5 days cause a transient insulinopenic diabetes in normal rats, associated with induction of islet iNOS expression;
   - expression of IL-1, IL-2, TNFα, interferon gamma, IL-6, and IL-12 has been demonstrated early in the insulitis lesion in animal models of type 1 diabetes; and IL-1 and interferon gamma mRNA expression correlates with beta-cell and macropage iNOS expression;
   - anti-IL1 treatment with soluble IL-1 receptors or the naturally occurring IL-1 receptor antagonist (IL-1Ra) reduces type 1 diabetes incidence in animal models, in the first approach without affecting T-cell function;
   - transgenic expression of interferon gamma in beta-cells under the control of the insulin promotor causes insulitis and IDDM, probably by recruiting and activating macrophages to produce IL-1, TNFα, and other mediators;
   - interferon gamma gene knock-out delays type 1 diabetes in the NOD mouse, but does not prevent type 1 diabetes, underlining the importance of the synergistic interaction of several proinflammatory cytokines.

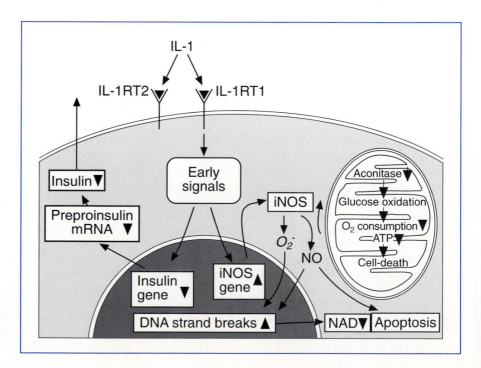

Figure 56.3 A schematic representation of intracellular second messengers of IL-1 in beta-cells.

4. In man several cytokines are expressed in the insulitis lesion at diagnosis, the combinations of IL-1, TNFα, and interferon gamma or TNFα and interferon gamma damage human beta-cells, and polymorphisms of several cytokine genes have been implied as type 1 diabetes susceptibility loci in association studies.

Cytokine signaling in beta-cells

IL-1, TNFα, and interferon gamma have pleiotropic and overlapping effects. Cells of different types and stages of activation and differentiation may utilize distinct cytokine signaling pathways, lending hope for development of tissue and disease-specific intervention strategies based upon tissue-specific cytokine action. Most of the work on cytokine signaling in beta-cells has been performed using IL-1.

IL-1 signaling. IL-1 exerts its action by binding to the IL-1 type 1 receptor (IL-1RT1)-associated peptide (IL-1RT1AcP) complex. Ligand binding causes rapid association and phosphorylation of IL-1RT1-associated tyrosine kinase (IRAK), which is essential for the activation of NFkB, a nuclear transcription factor binding to responsive gene sequences thereby regulating gene transcription.

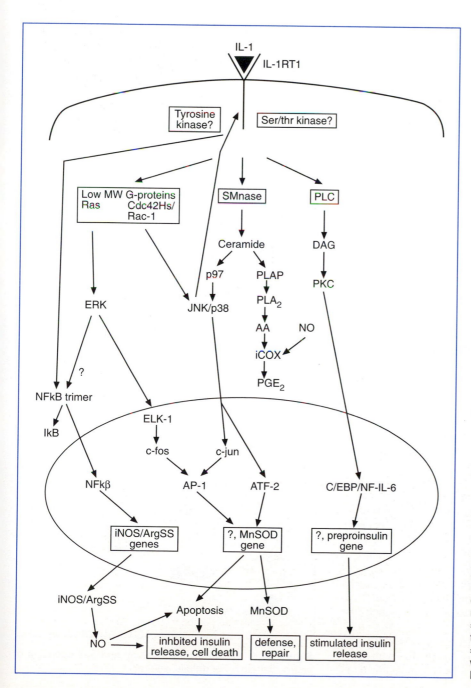

Figure 56.4 A model for IL-1-signaling in beta-cells. (IL-1 = interleukin-1; IL-1RTI = IL-1 type 1 receptor; ser/thr = serine/threonine; MW = molecular weight; SMnase = sphingomyelinase; PLC = phospholipase C; DAG = diacylglycerol; PLAP = phospholipase A$_2$ activating protein; PLA$_2$ = phospholipase A$_2$; AA = arachidonic acid; iCOX = inducible cyclooxygenase; PGE$_2$ = prostaglandin E$_2$; NO = nitric oxide; PKC = protein kinase C; iNOS = cytokine-inducible nitric oxide synthase; ArgSS = argininosuccinate synthetase; MnSOD = manganese superoxide dismutase; X, Y = unknown genes; NF = nuclear factor.) (Reproduced with kind permission from Diabetologia.)

IL-1 postreceptor signaling events involve TNF receptor-associated factor (TRAF) 6, guanidin tris phosphate (GTP)-binding proteins, adenyl cyclase activation, phospholipid hydrolysis by nonphosphatidylinositol phospholipase Cs (PLC), release of arachidonic acid from phospholipids by phospholipase A_2 (PLA$_2$), and perhaps release of ceramide from sphingomyelin catalyzed by membrane sphingomyelinase. These early events lead to the activation of a cascade of protein kinases, including the p38 mitogen-activated protein kinase (MAPK) and INK MAPK. This results in the activation of nuclear transcription factors NFkB, NF-IL-6, c-fos, AP-1 (activating protein 1), and the expression of IL-1-regulated genes. Based on extrapolation of the available studies on IL-1 signaling in non-beta-cells and data on IL-1 signaling in beta-cells, a model for IL-1 signal transduction in beta-cells is shown in Figure 56.4.

Second messengers of cytokine effects in beta-cells

As mentioned above, nitric oxide may be an important second messenger for cytokine signaling that leads to beta-cell destruction. There are, however, observations to suggest that nitric oxide production may neither be a necessary nor sufficient precondition for cytokine-induced beta-cell destruction. Hence, additional mediators of cytokine-induced beta-cell death may be necessary, such as free oxygen radical generation or the facilitation of other apoptosis-inducing pathways (e.g., JNK mitogen-activated protein kinase cascade or the Fas/FasL system). Furthermore, available data suggest that pathways may exist that depend on cytokine profile, concentration, exposure time, islet species, and/or metabolic state.

Fas/Fas ligand

In addition to their role in beta-cell cytotoxic cytokine production, direct T-cell-mediated cytotoxicity may be exerted via two major complementary pathways, which are based upon exocytosis of perforin-containing granules or engagement of the apoptosis-inducing Fas/Fas-ligand (FasL) system. Recently a possible involvement of this Fas/FasL system in type 1 diabetes, which may depend on cytokines, has become evident. The Fas/FasL system is normally believed to be involved in controlling tissue homeostasis, such as regulation of the T-cell pool. Both Fas and FasL are expressed by activated T lymphocytes, which results in apoptosis when a Fas-expressing activated T cell encounters a FasL-expressing T cell (or other cell-type). This is mediated through an apoptosis-transducing signal from the "death-domain" in the cytoplasmic region of the receptor for FasL, Fas, following cross-linking. By a similar mechanism, expression of FasL on cells in immune-privileged sites such as the eye or testis have been associated with protection against the immune system characteristic of these sites.

It was recently reported that beta-cells may also be induced to express Fas following stimulation with IL-1. Furthermore, this has been shown to be coupled to IL-1-induced nitric oxide production. Finally, NOD Fas gene knock-out mice did not develop diabetes.

Interleukin-1 converting enzyme (ICE) is a cysteine protease shown to be one of the accelerating mechanisms involved in apoptosis induced by various stimuli, including Fas-mediated apoptosis. Inhibition of ICE or one of the ICE family proteases has been shown to block Fas-induced death signaling in mouse lymphoma cell systems. It has recently been demonstrated that interferon gamma upregulates ICE in beta-cells. In human islets, 6 to 9 days of cytokine exposure has been shown to induce apoptosis in a nitric oxide-independent way. It has been suggested that upregulated expression of ICE may be an important component of this scenario.

Beta-cell destruction in type 1 diabetes, as well as following cytokine exposure, however, seems to be a complex interaction of several pathways that may result in a mixture of necrosis and apoptosis. It seems plausible that a competition between protective and deleterious pathways/mechanisms may be induced in the beta-cell, and that the outcome depends upon the type and magnitude of the stimuli as well as the metabolic state of the beta-cell itself. Future studies will clarify the potential involvement of the Fas/FasL systems and other mechanisms in human diabetes, with the possibility in the future of developing novel and rational intervention strategies for IDDM.

A model for the etiology and pathogenesis of type 1 diabetes

One model for the etiology and pathogenesis of type 1 diabetes (Fig. 56.5) predicts that anything from the external or internal environment that can destroy a beta-cell (nutrients? virus? chemical? IL-1?) will lead to the release of beta-cell proteins. These proteins will be taken up by residing antigen-presenting cells (APCs) in the islets, will be processed to antigenic peptides, and as such will be presented by MHC class II molecules on the cell surface. This activates the APC to produce and secrete monokines (IL-1, TNFα) and co-stimulatory signal(s) which – if T helper lymphocytes with receptors that specifically recognize the antigenic peptide are present in the islet – induce the transcription of a series of lymphokine genes. One of

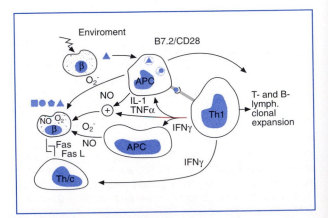

Figure 56.5 Model for the etiology and pathogenesis of type 1 diabetes. For details, see text.

these, interferon (IFN), will stimulate via feedback the APC to increase expression of MHC class II molecules and IL-1 and TNFα. In addition, other cells of the APC lineage present in the islets are also induced to secrete monokines. IL-1, potentiated by TNF and interferon, is cytotoxic to beta-cells through the induction of free radical (e.g., NO, O_2) formation in the islet. These cytokines also upregulate the Fas receptor, making the beta-cell susceptible to killing by activated T-cells by binding of the ligand for Fas, FasL.

The model described above has the following implications:

1. There is no need to suggest a ubiquitous environmental trigger.
2. There is no specific type 1 diabetes genes, rather
   - type 1 diabetes is a polygenic disorder;
   - susceptibility is conferred by common alleles of normal genes occurring in unfavorable combinations; and
   - each of these genes are involved in quantitative control of a specific element of the pathogenetic process.
3. There is no one single autoantigen, but rather polyclonal immune activation directed toward the multitude of modified beta-cell proteins.
4. Specificity in antigen recognition by T-helper cells directs the immune response toward the islets, but the earliest beta-cell destruction effector pathway is dependent upon an antigen-nonspecific inflammatory process.
5. As part of the inflammatory process, high concentrations of combinations of cytokines as well as other exogenous mediators lead to beta-cell destruction.
6. Beta-cell destruction is primarily the result of cytokine-mediated induction of beta-cell apoptosis and perhaps also specific expression of inducible nitric oxide synthase (iNOS).
7. Nitric oxide (NO) is beta-cell cytotoxic due to the inhibition of mitochondrial ATP-generation, induction of DNA damage, and activation of the apoptotic program.
8. Cytokines (IL-1) cause Fas expression on the beta-cells, making beta-cells more susceptible to antigen-specific killing by activated T helper or T cytotoxic lymphocytes expressing FasL, which implies there is a secondary role for T-cell-mediated effector mechanisms.

MANAGEMENT OF TYPE 1 DIABETES

Carl-David Agardh, Kristian F. Hanssen

Type 1 diabetes is an inherited autoimmune disease characterized by a progressive destruction of the insulin-producing beta-cells of the islets of Langerhans in the pancreas, which leads to an absolute insulin deficiency and results in a patient requiring insulin treatment for survival. The disease is not directly inherited, since only about 50% of identical twins are concordant for diabetes. The increased life-time risk for a child of a mother with type 1 diabetes to develop the same type of diabetes is 1 to 2%

and about three times higher if the father has the disease. The disease is associated with certain HLA types, and at the time of diagnosis several autoantibodies, such as islet cell antibodies (ICA), glutamic acid decarboxylase (GAD) antibodies, and insulin antibodies are present in the blood. The clinical symptoms of diabetes occur when the beta-cell mass has decreased to about 20% and can be related to the lack of insulin and hyperglycemia. The cause of diabetes is mostly unknown, but it is thought to be a combination of environmental factors and genetic susceptibility.

The prevalence of type 1 diabetes is different in different populations. In Europe, about 10 to 15% of all diabetic patients have type 1 diabetes; the highest incidence is seen in Finland and Sweden, and the lowest is seen in Japan. The disease usually appears before the age of 35 years, but it can occur at all ages, with the most frequent age at onset between 12 and 14 years. A related form of type 1 diabetes is late-onset autoimmune diabetes in adults (LADA), which is characterized by a presence of GAD antibodies, an age at onset of over 35 years, and a need for insulin treatment, usually within 1 to 2 years after clinical onset of the disease.

Clinical findings

The clinical symptoms that occur that lead to a diagnosis of diabetes or during periods of poor metabolic control in type 1 diabetic patients are an effect of absolute or relative insulin deficiency. Lack of insulin leads to increased lipolysis, protein breakdown, increased glucose production and hyperglycemia, and decreased uptake of glucose in peripheral tissues. Increased lipolysis leads to an excess of free fatty acids for oxidation, which leads to ketone body production in the liver and metabolic acidosis, and protein breakdown leads to muscle wasting. The increased glucose production and decreased uptake of glucose in peripheral tissues lead to hyperglycemia, glucosuria, and osmotic diuresis.

At clinical onset of diabetes, most symptoms can be explained by a lack of the effects of insulin. The increased osmotic diuresis causes polyuria and dehydration, and the loss of body water causes polydipsia. The loss of glucose in urine and the breakdown of fat and muscle tissues lead to weight-loss despite polyphagia. Hyperglycemia and osmotic changes result in refractive errors and blurred vision. Glucosuria is often associated with monilial overgrowth and pruritus vulvae and balanitis. If untreated, an increased production of ketone bodies ensues and leads to metabolic acidosis. The patient is then dehydrated, with hyperventilation, abdominal pain, and vomiting. A substantial urinary loss of electrolytes such as sodium, potassium, magnesium, bicarbonate, and chloride takes place. Eventually, signs of central nervous dysfunction appear, though coma only occurs in about 10% of the patients. If not diagnosed and treated with fluids, insulin, and potassium, diabetic ketoacidosis is a life-threatening condition.

The onset of symptoms is more rapid and severe in children than in adults. The symptoms usually develop over some weeks to a few months, but they may occur after only a few days in small children.

The same symptoms can appear in a patient with known type 1 diabetes during periods of poor metabolic control due to a relative insulin deficiency or an increased need of insulin during concurrent illnesses such as infection and increased stress due to trauma.

Diagnosis

Clinical symptoms together with chronic hyperglycemia establish the diabetes diagnosis. It is important to keep the diagnosis of diabetes in mind, especially in small children who often present with ketoacidosis, which is sometimes misdiagnosed as gastroenteritis. If possible, one should aim at an etiological diagnosis to exclude other specific types of diabetes, such as genetic defects causing different forms of maturity-onset diabetes of the young (MODY). Repeated fasting plasma glucose values ≥ 7.0 mmol/l, a presence of GAD-antibodies, and low plasma levels of C-peptide strongly suggest that the patient has type 1 diabetes.

Treatment

Treatment goals

The general goals for treatment of patients with type 1 diabetes are to prevent short-term and long-term diabetic complications; promote independence, equity, and self-sufficiency; and to remove hindrances so that they may have the fullest possible integration into society. The goal is to achieve and to maintain a degree of metabolic control that prevents both hypoglycemic and hyperglycemic symptoms, and prevents long-term diabetic complications with as little restriction as possible of their eating habits, leisure-time activities, and personal and professional lives.

To achieve this, there is a need for an intensified insulin treatment strategy that includes self-monitoring and self-management skills based upon a structured educational program provided by a diabetes team that consists of a diabetologist, a diabetes nurse, a dietitian, and a podiatrist.

Insulin treatment

Most type 1 diabetic patients are treated with a four times-daily insulin regimen. The total daily dose usually varies between 0.5 to 0.8 U/kg. The doses must be individualized depending on the patient's daily activities, but as a rule of thumb, 25% of the daily dose is given before breakfast, 15% before lunch, 25% before dinner as short-acting insulin, and 35 to 40% as medium-acting insulin at bedtime. Two alternatives of short-acting insulins are presently available for use before meals.

Rapid-acting insulin analogues are given immediately before each main meal. Since the duration of action is short (3 to 4 hours), medium-acting insulin often has to be given at lunchtime and always at bedtime. The advantages with the insulin analogues are that they are given in connection with the meal, the absorption is fast and not dependent upon the injection site, they give a lower postprandial rise in blood glucose, and there is no need for snacks between meals. The disadvantage is the shorter duration of action, which often makes supplementary injections of medium-acting insulin a requirement if the between-meal interval is to be longer than 5 hours.

Short-acting soluble insulins are given 30 to 40 minutes before each meal and medium-acting insulin at bedtime. The duration of action is dependent upon the insulin dose: the higher the dose, the longer the action. To obtain a faster absorption, it is recommended that the short-acting insulin be injected in the abdomen. The disadvantage with this insulin preparation is its relatively slow-onset of action, which leads to higher postprandial blood glucose levels. Due to its longer duration of action, snacks between meals are often necessary to avoid hypoglycemic symptoms before the next main meal.

An alternative to the four times-daily insulin regimen is a *three-times daily insulin regimen*. A mixture of short-acting and medium-acting insulin is given before breakfast, short-acting insulin before the evening meal, and medium-acting insulin before bedtime.

Insulin pump treatment Subcutaneous insulin infusion therapy using an electronic insulin pump is an alternative insulin regimen for selected, highly motivated patients. The insulin pump contains a vial of short-acting insulin and is connected to the patient through a catheter and a needle inserted in the abdominal subcutaneous tissue. The pump delivers a continuous amount of insulin per hour, and short-acting insulin is given before meals by the patient activating the pump. In many patients, this treatment mode leads to very good metabolic control. Due to the small amount of insulin given per hour, however, there is an increased risk for ketoacidosis if the delivery of insulin is interrupted for technical or other reasons.

Self-monitoring of blood glucose

All type 1 diabetic patients should self-monitor their blood glucose as an integrated part of insulin treatment. Reagent strips with or without meters can be used. A blood glucose profile is recommended at least two to three times per week, with blood glucose measurements before breakfast, lunch, dinner, and bedtime. In addition, further measurements can be performed when needed, such as to check for hypoglycemia and during concurrent illnesses. The results must be recorded by the patient to provide a cumulative record as a basis for day-to-day insulin dose self-adjustment; education on the effects of lifestyle on blood glucose; and for coping with illness and new situations, hypoglycemia management, and avoidance. At each out-patient visit, the records should be evaluated and discussed with the patient, and the skill to perform self-monitoring and interpret the results should be assessed. HbA_{1c} levels reflect the mean glucose level during the past 30 days and should be measured 3 to 4 times per year. The result only gives a measure of the mean metabolic control, and in patients with values normal or close to normal, the occurrence of hypoglycemia must be evaluated.

Healthy eating

The dietary recommendations for people with type 1 diabetes are not different from the population in general. The most important issue is to provide the patient with knowledge about how different types of food influence the blood glucose response. In general, the proposed contribution to energy intake should be:

- fat: saturated fat <10%. Replace excess saturated fat with monounsaturants, or polyunsaturates (up to 10%), or carbohydrates;
- carbohydrates: around 50 to 55%. Use foods containing soluble fiber in a carbohydrate-rich diet. Simple sugars need not be rigorously excluded from the diet, but they often need to be limited;
- protein: approximately 15% or less (0.8 g/kg).

Alcohol intake should be moderate due to its content of calories and due to the increased risk for hypoglycemia in connection with alcohol intake.

Physical exercise

Physical exercise can be recommended since it benefits insulin sensitivity, hypertension, and blood lipid control. It is recommended that the physical activity take place on a regular basis in order to facilitate insulin reduction and increase food intake in order to avoid hypoglycemia. The patient should use self-monitoring to learn about the exercise response, and how insulin and dietary changes affect this. The patient must be informed about the resultant delayed hypoglycemia, especially with more prolonged, severe, or unusual exercise, and a possible need for less insulin overnight and the next day. He or she should also be instructed to avoid exercise during insulin deficiency, which will raise the blood glucose and ketone levels.

SPECIAL SITUATIONS

Pregnancy

To avoid the increased risk for fetal malformation, pre-

pregnancy management is essential in order to optimize glucose control before conception. If the patient is on statins or ACE-inhibitors, these drugs should be withdrawn; if there is a need for antihypertensive treatment, labetalol or nifedipine should be prescribed. The patient should be urged to stop smoking. During pregnancy, care should be provided jointly by a diabetologist, an obstetrician, a midwife, a dietitian, and a neonatologist. During pregnancy, there is often a reduced need for insulin during the first trimester, with an increased risk for hypoglycemia. Thereafter, there is a gradual increased need for insulin, often 60 to 80% of prepregnancy doses. It is essential to gradually increase the doses to achieve a near-normal blood glucose level while avoiding hypoglycemia in order to achieve normal fetal development. After delivery, the insulin doses can be restored to normal.

Surgery

During major surgery, insulin should be given by continuous intravenous infusion, supplemented with dextrose and potassium (GIK). The infusion should begin in the morning and continue until the patient eats normally after surgery. Blood glucose should be measured before, during, and after (1-4 times hourly) surgery. One should aim for blood glucose levels of 6.0 to 10.0 mmol/l. Normal insulin injections should start as soon as practicable, but one must continue the GIK infusion until 30 to 60 minutes after the first subcutaneous injection.

Organization of care

The care for patients with type 1 diabetes is best provided by a diabetes team with a diabetes physician, a diabetes nurse, a dietitian, and an orthoptist. This team should provide the patient with a structured educational program to form the basis for self-management of the disease and be available to the patient in case of acute problems. The team also should perform screening procedures in order to detect and treat signs of late diabetic complications, such as regular screening for retinopathy, microalbuminuria, hypertension, and foot problems. The team should provide a system for shared care between general practitioners and hospital specialists.

Suggested readings

A Desktop Guide to Type 1 (Insulin-Dependent) Diabetes Mellitus. European Diabetes Policy Group 1998. ISBN 0 7017 00807.

Bach JF. Insulin-dependent diabetes mellitus as an autoimmune disease. Endocrine Rev 1994;15:516-42.

Christie MR. Aetiology of type 1 diabetes: immunological aspects. In: Ashcroft FM, Ashcroft SJH (eds.) Insulin, molecular biology to pathology. Oxford: IRL Press, 1992.

Corbett JA, McDaniel ML. Does nitric oxide mediate autoimmune destruction of β-cells? Diabetes 1992; 41:897-903.

Dahcquis G. Environmental risk factors in human type 1 diabetes – an epidemiological perspective. Diabetes/Metabol Rev 1995;11:37-46.

House DV, Winter WE. Autoimmune diabetes: the role of autoantibody markers in the prediction and prevention of insulin-dependent diabetes mellitus. Clin Lab Med 1997;17:499-545.

EIZIRIK C, FLOSTRÖM M, KARLSEN AE, WELSH N.The harmony of the spheres: inducible nitric oxide synthase and related genes in pancreatic beta-cells. Diabetologica 1996;39:875-90.

LERNMARK A, BÄRMEIER H, DUBE S, HAGOPIAN W, KARLSEN A. Autoimmunity of diabetes. In: Daughaday WH (ed). Endocrinology and Metabolism Clinics of North America 1991;20: 589-617.

KARLSEN AF, DYRBERG T. Molecular mimicry between non-self, modified self and self in autoimmunity. Immunology 1998;10:25-34.

MANDRUP-POULSEN T. The role of interleukin-1 in the pathogenesis of IDDM. Diabetologica 1996;39:1005-29.

POCIOT T. Insulin-dependent diabetes mellitus – a polygenic disorder? Dan Med Bull 1996;43:216-48.

TODD JA. Genetic analysis of type 1 diabetes using whole genome approaches. Proc Natl Acad Sc USA 1995;92:8560-5.

Type 2 diabetes mellitus: pathogenesis and treatment

Leif Groop

Epidemiology

About 3% of the population, or 100 million people, suffer from type 2 diabetes mellitus in the world. It has been predicted that this number will double within 10 years. Therefore, type 2 diabetes (non-insulin-dependent diabetes mellitus) is one of the most common, non-communicable diseases in the world. It is associated with devastating complications that severely influence the quality of life. In addition, or because of this, type 2 diabetes imposes an enormous burden on health care systems all over the world.

There are large ethnic and geographic variations in the prevalence of type 2 diabetes. In Scandinavia, where type 1 diabetes is common, type 2 diabetes accounts for about 85% of all cases with diabetes. In Asia and Japan, where type 1 diabetes is rare, type 2 diabetes represents almost 99% of the cases of diabetes. In certain ethnic populations, such as the Pima Indians and the Nauruans, the prevalence of type 2 diabetes approaches 40%. However, the distinction between type 1 and type 2 diabetes may not be as clear as hitherto believed.

Etiopathogenesis

Inheritance of type 2 diabetes

The concordance rate of type 2 diabetes in monozygotic twins has been found to be around 70 to 80% compared with 10 to 20% in dizygotic twins. Type 2 diabetes and impaired glucose tolerance cluster in families. The lifetime risk of developing type 2 diabetes is about 40% in offspring of diabetic parents. If both parents have type 2 diabetes, the risk in the offspring has been estimated to be as high as 70%. Type 2 diabetes seems to have a predominant maternal mode of transmission in Caucasians, with a relatively low prevalence of the disease. After adjustment for age and age at onset (mothers live longer than fathers),

patients with type 2 diabetes in Scandinavia show a 1.5- to 2-times higher prevalence of type 2 diabetes in mothers than in fathers.

What is inherited in type 2 diabetes?

In general, both insulin resistance and impaired insulin secretion are required to manifest type 2 diabetes. Insulin resistance by itself cannot cause diabetes, with the exception of some rare conditions with insulin receptor mutations. As long as the β-cell can compensate for the degree of insulin resistance, glucose tolerance remains normal. Therefore, impaired β-cell function is always involved in the pathogenesis of type 2 diabetes.

One can thus assume that at least two genetic defects must be involved: one causing insulin resistance, and one causing impaired β-cell function. Insulin resistance is manifested as impaired insulin-stimulated glucose uptake by skeletal muscle. Insulin resistance can be triggered by many conditions, such as obesity, pregnancy, aging, and infections. The question thus arises whether skeletal muscle insulin resistance represents a primary inherited defect or whether it develops as a consequence of stimulus such as obesity.

Insulin resistance

Insulin resistance can be defined as the condition in which insulin is no longer able to exert a normal biological effect on its target tissues. These can be skeletal muscle, adipose tissue, and liver. Insulin resistance can involve the metabolism of three major substrates: glucose, free fatty acids, and protein. In most situations we limit the definition of insulin resistance to the glycoregulatory effect of insulin. Adipose tissue is metabolically less active and considered to take up less than 5% of the glucose metabolized in the body.

The metabolic syndrome

Skeletal muscle insulin resistance is not unique to type 2 diabetes, as it is also observed in association with hypertension, hypertriglyceridemia, abdominal obesity, microalbuminuria, and hyperuricemia. These conditions tend to cluster together. This syndrome has been referred to as syndrome X or the metabolic or insulin resistance syndrome, as it is believed that insulin resistance is the common denominator of the different conditions. The sequence of events by which insulin resistance would cause these abnormalities is not clear. Nevertheless, the simultaneous occurrence of these conditions is associated with a markedly increased risk for cardiovascular disease, and they may be used as markers for a subgroup of type 2 diabetes characterized by severe insulin resistance and a high risk of cardiovascular disease.

Obesity

Obesity is a well-recognized risk factor for type 2 diabetes: about 60 to 80% of type 2 diabetic patients are obese. It is not known, however, whether obesity actually predisposes a person to type 2 diabetes or whether it is a consequence of the inherited metabolic milieu of type 2 diabetes. A low metabolic rate predisposes Pima Indians to weight gain. Nondiabetic first degree relatives of patients with type 2 diabetes are characterized by abdominal obesity and a decreased metabolic rate compared with spouses without a family history of type 2 diabetes. Further, there is a strong correlation between the amount of intra-abdominal fat measured by CT scan and insulin sensitivity.

Thrifty genotype

Why does insulin resistance develop, and why is non-insulin-dependent diabetes mellitus (NIDDM) increasing in individuals switching from a rural to an urban lifestyle? The "thrifty gene hypothesis" was put forward in 1962 by Neel, who proposed that individuals living in a harsh environment with an unstable food supply would maximize their probability of survival if they could maximize the storage of surplus energy. Genetic selection would thus favor energy-conserving genotypes in such environments. Storage of energy as fat, especially as intra-abdominal fat, is a more efficient way of storing energy than storing energy as glycogen in skeletal muscle. The theory goes that when this energy-storing genotype is exposed to the abundance of food typical of Western society, it becomes detrimental and causes insulin resistance and type 2 diabetes.

Insulin secretion

It has long been debated whether insulin resistance or insulin deficiency is the primary defect in the pathogenesis of type 2 diabetes. Both defects can be inherited, although the presence of the former is required to manifest the lat-

ter. If one uses the first phase (the first 10 minutes) of insulin release from an intravenous glucose tolerance test (IVGTT) as a measure of β-cell function, insulin secretion first increases with increasing blood glucose concentrations. When the 2-hour blood glucose value during an oral glucose tolerance test (OGTT) exceeds 9 mmol/l, insulin secretion begins to become impaired (Fig. 57.1). In the transition from impaired glucose tolerance to type 2 diabetes, only a moderate deterioration of insulin sensitivity takes place, while there is a clear impairment in insulin secretion. Of note, type 2 diabetes typically begins years, and possibly decades, before diagnosis. Macroangiopathy is the secret killer of type 2 diabetic patients. At diagnosis, about 50% of the patients already show hypertension or signs of macroangiopathy (Fig. 57.2).

Search for the type 2 diabetes genes

Two major approaches are being used in the search for the type 2 diabetes genes. The candidate gene approach aims at identifying of the type 2 diabetes genes based upon information of their function. While this approach has been successful in a number of monogenic disorders with

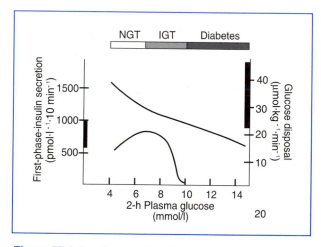

Figure 57.1 Insulin secretion and insulin sensitivity in relation to glucose tolerance. When 2-hour blood glucose during the oral glucose tolerance test exceeds 9 mmol/l, insulin secretion becomes impaired. (From Groop L, Widén E, Ferrannini E. Insulin deficiency or insulin resistance in the pathogenesis of IDDM. Error of metabolism or methods? Diabetologia 1993;36:1326-31.)

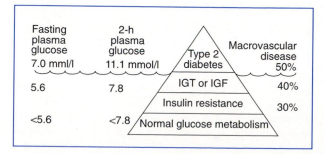

Figure 57.2 Phases in the development of type 2 diabetes.

known biochemical defects (e.g., phenylketonuria), our knowledge about the underlying defects in type 2 diabetes is limited. It is therefore not surprising that the candidate gene approach has not been very successful for the identification of type 2 diabetes genes.

The random gene search, also referred to as positional cloning, assumes no knowledge of the underlying defects. Instead, positional cloning aims at localizing the disease gene on the basis of its position in the genome. If a chromosomal region has been linked to the disease, the next step could be the search for attractive candidate genes in this region. This approach has been successful in a number of monogenic disorders (e.g., dystrophic dysplasia) where the relationship between genotype and penetrance of the phenotype is more straightforward than for type 2 diabetes. The situation for type 2 diabetes is most likely more complicated, however, where we can assume that a number of genes will increase susceptibility to the disease and that these genes will act in concert with a number of environmental factors.

Candidate genes for insulin resistance and the metabolic syndrome

The first step in insulin action is the binding of insulin to its receptor. A reduced ability of insulin to stimulate autophosphorylation of tyrosine residues on the β-subunit of the receptor has been demonstrated in patients with type 2 diabetes. This may, however, represent a secondary phenomenon, since tyrosine kinase activity is restored in fat cells after weight reduction. Mutations in the tyrosine kinase domain of the insulin receptor result in the phenotype of type A insulin resistance and acanthosis nigricans. Other rare mutations in the insulin receptor give rise to the severe clinical syndromes of leprechaunism and Rabson-Mendelhal syndrome. Mutations in the insulin receptor are rare and cannot explain inherited insulin resistance in type 2 diabetes.

IRS-1 and IRS-2: the docking protein IRS1 links the tyrosine-phosphorylated insulin receptor to the downstream part of the insulin signaling pathway. IRS1 is phosphorylated on multiple tyrosine residues, and it could be a candidate for genetic insulin resistance. The frequency of an aminoacid polymorphism (codon 972), which is located close to the tyrosine phosphorylation site, is increased in type 2 diabetic patients with the metabolic syndrome. Targeted disruption of IRS-1 in the mouse does not lead to diabetes, however the heterozygous knock-out mouse with disruption of both IRS-1 and the insulin receptor tyrosine kinase develops diabetes. This suggests that multiple defects are required to manifest the disease. More recently another insulin receptor substrate 2 (IRS-2) has been identified. Interestingly, disruption of this gene causes diabetes not only due to insulin resistance, but also due to a marked β-cell defect.

Glycogen synthase: impaired stimulation of glycogen synthesis by insulin is a hallmark of type 2 diabetes and impaired glucose tolerance. The key enzyme of this pathway, glycogen synthase, could therefore be an important candidate for a genetic defect causing insulin resistance. Polymorphism of the glycogen synthase gene has been

associated with type 2 diabetes in some populations, particularly with type 2 diabetes associated with the metabolic syndrome. Of sib pairs discordant for the polymorphism, carriers of the rare (disease-associated allele) showed more features of the metabolic syndrome than carriers of the common allele.

Obesity genes The thrifty gene hypothesis proposes that efficient storage of energy could have been associated with a survival advantage during human evolution. Efficient storage of energy must include storage of fat and weight gain. Therefore, obesity genes could predispose one to insulin resistance and type 2 diabetes. Despite large fluctuations in food intake and energy expenditure, body fat is tightly regulated in humans. A powerful feedback system (also referred to as the *lipostat hypothesis*) between fat and a satiety/energy expenditure center in the hypothalamus has been postulated, since damage to this region causes morbid obesity.

This field of research has moved into a new, exciting era with the discovery of the ob-gene, which codes for a novel protein called *leptin* that is expressed in fat. A mutation in the leptin gene results in the complete absence of the protein in the ob/ob mouse. Treatment of the ob/ob mouse with leptin resulted in marked weight loss. However, man is not mouse, and when obese humans were studied, they had elevated rather than decreased levels of leptin. In fact, the leptin levels showed a strong positive correlation with the total fat mass. In this regard, humans resembled the db/db mouse. A putative defective leptin receptor gene was postulated. The db mutation is due to an abnormally spliced leptin receptor in the hypothalamus. Some rare cases of mutations in the leptin and leptin receptor gene have been described in humans. In addition to morbid obesity, these individuals also displayed pituitary dysfunction.

The *β₃-adrenergic receptor* is expressed in brown adipose tissue of rodents and considered responsible for thermogenesis. The β₃-adrenergic receptor thereby became a candidate gene for human obesity. A low β₃-adrenergic receptor activity could promote obesity by decreased thermogenesis and by slow lipolysis with retention of lipids in fat cells. A mutation in the first intracellular loop of the receptor changes a tryptophan in position 64 to arginine. Individuals with the mutation have a decreased metabolic rate and a tendency toward weight gain. We observed that nondiabetic individuals heterozygous for the Trp64Arg mutation had a higher waist-hip-ratio, higher insulin values, higher blood pressure, and were more insulin-resistant than individuals homozygous for the wild type Trp64Arg.

Candidate genes for impaired insulin secretion

A subgroup of about 10% of patients with type 2 diabetes present with GAD antibodies and slowly develop insulin deficiency. They are called LADA (latent autoimmune diabetes in adults), or slowly progressing type 1 diabetes.

It is important to identify them, since they are usually misdiagnosed as having type 2 diabetes. In Europe, approximately 20% of diabetic families have both type 1 and type 2 patients. In these families, the patients with type 2 diabetes usually present with some degree of insulin deficiency.

Several monogenic forms of diabetes with impaired β-cell function have been described in the past years. They include the different forms of MODY (maturity onset diabetes of the young), mitochondrial diabetes with deafness (MIDD), and other types.

Treatment

Regardless of whether insulin resistance or insulin deficiency predominates in the pathogenesis of diabetes, hyperglycemia can itself impair both β-cell function and insulin action. The optimal treatment for type 2 diabetes should therefore not only improve β-cell function and insulin action but also break the vicious cycle through which hyperglycemia impairs these functions.

Treatment should also aim to relieve symptoms, improve quality of life, and prevent acute metabolic problems of hyperosmolar non-ketotic coma and the chronic micro- and macrovascular complications. There is strong evidence for an association between chronic hyperglycemia and the development of microangiopathic complications, whereas the link between blood glucose control and macrovascular disease is less clear. The target glucose concentrations advocated by the European NIDDM Policy Group are thought to prevent microvascular complications (Tab. 57.1), but there is no proof that lowering blood glucose below these values will prevent macrovascular disease. Treatment that aims at the prevention of cardiovascular disease should not only influence glucose concentrations, but it should also have beneficial effects on plasma lipids and blood pressure. Few therapeutic agents fulfill these criteria.

Medical treatment

Type 2 diabetes may be treated by oral hypoglycemic agents, insulin, or a combination of both. The oral agents have traditionally included the sulfonylureas and metformin. The α-glycosides inhibitor acarbose and agents belonging to the group of thiazolidinediones, such as troglitazone, have more recently been introduced for the treatment of type 2 diabetes.

Oral agents

Sulfonylureas Sulfonylureas have represented the backbone of type 2 diabetes therapy for 40 years, yet there is still much controversy about their mode of action. The main effect of sulfonylureas is the stimulation of insulin secretion. Sulfonylureas exert this effect by closing ATP-sensitive potassium channels in the β cells, which results in depolarization of the cell membrane. This in turn promotes an influx of calcium, which stimulates insulin secretion. Sulfonylureas bind to receptor-like structures (sulfonylurea receptor or ATP-sensitive potassium channel) on the β-cell. The binding capacity of different sulfonylureas for these receptors closely parallels their ability to stimulate insulin secretion.

Many earlier studies came to the conclusion that sulfonylureas enhanced insulin sensitivity. These studies did not take into account the fact that hyperglycemia itself can induce insulin resistance and that this will improve as blood glucose levels fall.

Sulfonylureas are weak acids that are extensively protein-bound (over 90%), metabolized in the liver, and excreted in the feces or through the kidney. There are clear differences in absorption, metabolism, and elimination between various sulfonylureas. In addition, several factors influence the absorption and bioavailability. Probably the most important of them is hyperglycemia, which slows absorption by slowing gastric emptying. Most sulfonylureas have traditionally been given twice daily 30 minutes before meals. This may not be necessary, since even short-acting sulfonylureas like glipizide seem to exert a much longer biological effect than predicted from its half-life (Tab. 57.2).

The average plasma glucose-lowering effect of sulfonylureas during chronic treatment is about 3 mmol/l. If the treatment goal is not achieved, the drug dose is usually increased to the recommended maximum. This practice assumes that there is a linear relationship between the drug dose and its biological effect. Such a relationship does not exist; instead, maximum effects are achieved with relatively low doses, such as for glibenclamide at 10 mg/day, or for glipizide at 15 mg/day. Therefore, increasing the drug dose is a poor substitute for starting insulin therapy in a patient who no longer satisfactorily responds to the drug.

Table 57.1 Treatment targets for patients with type 2 diabetes

	Good	Acceptable	Poor
Blood glucose (mmol/l)			
Fasting	4-4 -6.7	<7.8	<7.8
Postprandial peak	4.4 -8.9	<10.0	>10.0
HbA₁c*	<2	<4	>4
Cholesterol (mmol/l)	<5.2	<6.5	>6.5
HDL-cholesterol (mmol/l)	>1.1	>0.9	>0.9
Triglycerides (mmol/l)	<1.7	<2.2	>2.2
BMI (kg/m²)			
Men	<25	<27	>27
Women	<24	<<26	>26
Blood pressure (mmHg)	<140/90	<160/95	>160/95

* 1 SD above the non-diabetic mean.

Table 57.2 Pharmacokinetic properties of some sulfonyl-ureas and sulfonylurea-like compounds

Drug	Circulating half-life (h)[1]	Effect duration (h)	Daily dose (mg)	Doses/day
Acetohexamide	0.8 -2.4	12-18	250-1500	2
Chlorpropamide	24-48	24-72	100-500	1
Gliclazide	6-15	10-15	40-320	1-2
Glibenclamide[2]	2-4	20-24	2.5-20	1-2
Glipizide	1-5	12-14	2.5-20	1(-2)
Tolbutamide	3-28	6-10	500-3000	2-3
Tolazamide	4-7	16-24	100-1000	1-2
Glimepiride	5-8	24	1-4	1

[1] Elimination half-life of the active metabolite is about 4-6 h.
[2] Using more sensitive assays for glibenclamide determination, the half-life has been considerably longer.

Choice of sulfonylurea There is little evidence to suggest that one sulfonylurea is more effective than another, and there is particularly little documentation to suggest that the new sulfonylurea-like drugs (glimepiride and repaglinide) are more efficient than older sulfonylureas. There may, however, be some differences in timing of the effect. Glibenclamide lowers fasting plasma glucose better than glipizide, probably through a better suppression of hepatic glucose production. In contrast, glipizide results in greater postprandial insulin release and lower postprandial glucose excursions. Long-acting agents such as chlorpropamide and glibenclamide should be avoided in the elderly because of the high risk of adverse effects.

Adverse effects Sulfonylureas are usually well-tolerated, and adverse effects are rare. The main problem is hypoglycemia. It can be very prolonged and in elderly subjects lead to neurological damage and death. In the elderly, hypoglycemia can easily be misdiagnosed as a cerebrovascular event. About 20% of patients treated with sulfonylureas in the United Kingdom reported at least one episode of symptomatic hypoglycemia during the preceding 6 months. Data from the Swedish and Swiss registries of adverse reaction report only 0.22 episodes per 1000 patient-years, which should be compared with the rate of 100 episodes per 1000 patient-years during insulin therapy. Glibenclamide carries a greater risk of hypoglycemia than other agents, probably because of its profound effect on the liver. Of note, almost all cases of severe hypoglycemia have occurred in patients over the age of 75 years who had other risk factors such as poor nutrition and renal disease. It is important to identify the persons at risk to avoid long-acting sulfonylureas in such individuals.

Biguanides Extracts of goat's rue (*Galega officinalis*), which contains guanidine, were already used for the treatment of diabetes in medieval times. Synthetic biguanides

(metformin and phenformin) were introduced in the late 1950s for the treatment of NIDDM. Phenformin was withdrawn in most countries in the late 1970s because of its high risk of lactic acidosis. However, the use of metformin has been increasing in most countries, particularly for the treatment of the obese insulin-resistant NIDDM patients.

Metformin reduces the plasma glucose concentration by about 2-3 mmol/l, but it does not seem to lower blood glucose concentration below normal. Therefore, metformin treatment is not associated with any increased risk of hypoglycemia. A dose-response relationship has been reported between 500 and 3000 mg. One of the advantages of metformin is that its use is not associated with weight gain; if anything, there may be a slight reduction in body weight. Metformin has also been shown to reduce elevated triglyceride concentrations and blood pressure in some studies. In addition, metformin seems to have beneficial effects on fibrinolysis and platelet aggregation.

Given these considerations, the obese, insulin-resistant patient is the best candidate for metformin monotherapy. A daily dosage of 1.5-3.0 g is frequently required. A combination with sulfonylurea is beneficial in patients with fasting plasma glucose concentrations >10 mmol/l. It is important, however, to evaluate the success of this combination therapy at regular intervals, since further deterioration of β-cell function usually requires insulin therapy.

Various mechanisms have been proposed to explain the antihyperglycemic effect of metformin. It is likely that the drug has small effects on multiple metabolic pathways with the net result of lowering blood glucose. In patients with manifest diabetes, it undoubtedly decreases hepatic glucose production, primarily by inhibiting gluconeogenesis. In addition, it has a modest effect on insulin-stimulated glucose uptake, averaging about 20%. This effect is also seen in patients with impaired glucose tolerance, which makes metformin a potential candidate for preventing impaired glucose tolerance from progressing to manifest NIDDM.

Adverse effects The major concern with the biguanides has been the risk of lactic acidosis. This risk is much lower with metformin than with phenformin, as it is about 3 cases per 100 000 patient-years for metformin compared with 60 cases per 100 000 patient-years with phenformin. Phenformin binds strongly to mitochondrial membranes, where it acts to uncouple oxidative phosphorylation and inhibit the oxidation of lactate, hence allowing it to accumulate. Metformin binds poorly to mitochondrial membranes but may have an effect on lactate uptake into the cells. However, it inhibits lactate oxidation only if the drug accumulates in plasma, such as it does in renal failure. Lactic acidosis can also develop in patients with severe shock or hypoxia (both of which increase the production of lactate) or hepatic failure. Avoiding the high-risk categories of alcohol abuse and renal, hepatic, respiratory, and cardiac failure will greatly reduce the risk of this life-threatening complication.

Alpha-glucosidase inhibitors Alpha-glucosidase inhibitors (acarbose) delay carbohydrate absorption in the gut by selectively inhibiting disaccharidases in the intestinal brush border. In high doses the drugs can cause malabsorption. Acarbose is taken in dosages of 50-100 mg with each meal. The drug preferentially lowers postprandial blood glucose by 1-2 mmol/l and is most effective in patients with a high carbohydrate intake. Acarbose thus has an Antabuse-like effect. A high carbohydrate intake frequently results in carbohydrate malabsorption with side-effects such as flatulence, abdominal bloating, and diarrhea; to reduce the side effects, many patients learn to reduce their carbohydrate intake, which leads to improvement of glycemic control. The drug can be combined with sulfonylureas, metformin, or insulin.

Thiazolidinediones (glitazones) As most patients with type 2 diabetes are characterized by severe insulin resistance, drugs that increase insulin sensitivity have long been on the wish-list for the treatment of type 2 diabetes. A new group of drugs, the thizolidinediones (glitazones), are mainly insulin-sensitizers, that is, they improve insulin sensitivity. The first member of the group, troglitazone, has been launched in a number of countries, including the United States. This drug lowers blood glucose concentrations primarily by improving insulin sensitivity. It also seems to have beneficial effects on triglyceride and free fatty acid levels and blood pressure. Treatment is often associated with a slight weight gain. The thiazolidinediones function as ligands for a nuclear receptor, the peroxisome proliferator activated receptors (PPARγ), which are important regulators of free fatty acid metabolism in the fat cell. The drug has no effect on hepatic glucose production, and treatment with glitazones is consequently not associated with any increased risk of hypoglycemia. Unfortunately, troglitazone has in so me cases caused severe liver damage, which is most likely due to the extensive liver metabolism of the drug. Several other drugs from the same group, including rosiglitazone and pioglitazone, are under development. Preclinical studies indicate that these new glitazones would have less effects on the liver, but their use has so far been limited.

Failure of oral agents Oral hypoglycemic agents may fail to control hyperglycemia or diabetic symptoms, either from the onset (primary failure) or after a period of therapeutic success (secondary failure). Primary failure is usually due to the incorrect use of oral agents in patients with type 2 diabetes, while the causes of secondary drug failure are less clear. The frequency of secondary failure increases with the duration of the disease. In most studies there is an increase in blood glucose of about 0.25 mmol/l per year (Fig. 57.3). This would inevitably lead to a 100% rate of secondary drug failure after 10 to 15 years.

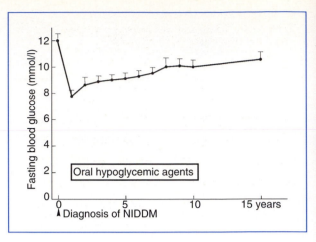

Figure 57.3 Mean annual fasting blood glucose concentrations in 156 type 2 diabetic patients treated with diet and/or oral antidiabetic agents. The annual increase in fasting blood glucose was 0.25 mmol/l. (From Groop L. Sulfonylureas in NIDDM. Diabetes Care 1992;15:737-54.)

Although poor compliance with diet is thought to be an important reason for poor response to treatment, disease-related factors seem to be the major determinants of secondary drug failure. A progressive decline in β-cell function may be part of the natural history of type 2 diabetes. Patients with an autoimmune form of diabetes (LADA) also develop secondary failure with increased frequency.

Insulin

There is no general agreement about how to treat patients with secondary failure to oral agents, but insulin therapy is obviously needed in most circumstances. The main options include: (1) premixed short- and intermediate-acting insulin twice daily before breakfast and dinner, and (2) a combination of NPH insulin at bedtime (or in the morning) with oral agents (Fig. 57.4).

A single daily dose of NPH insulin given in the evening or in the morning is rarely sufficient to achieve the treatment goals. Multiple insulin injections result in unacceptable weight gain and are not as well-tolerated in the elderly. The insulin treatment of choice for patients with type 2 diabetes is probably two doses of premixed insulin (e.g., 30% of short-acting plus 70% of NPH insulin) before breakfast and dinner. Insulin is best given by an insulin pen, which makes the adjustment of the doses easy. Pens with other mixtures, such as 50%/50% are also available and are preferred when there is a tendency toward large postprandial rises in blood glucose. In general, 60% of the total dose is given in the morning and 40% before dinner, but this should be adjusted to the individual needs of the patient. In some circumstances, if the treatment goals are not achieved or the daily insulin dose exceeds 60 U/day, this insulin regimen can also be combined with oral agents. In the obese, insulin-resistant patient, the combination of insulin with metformin has

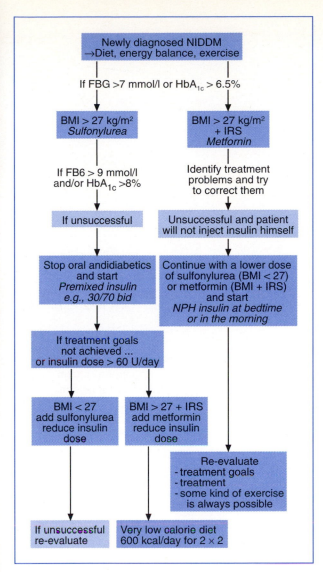

Figure 57.4 Treatment schedule for type 2 diabetes.

proven quite effective. A beneficial effect is usually seen within a few days in the form of reduced glycemia and lower insulin dosage (about 30-40% lower).

Home-monitoring of blood glucose is a prerequisite for any insulin therapy. A reliable representation of overall glycemic control can be obtained from measurements of blood glucose before breakfast, lunch, and dinner and at bedtime twice a week.

General measures

Treatment of type 2 diabetes should start by correcting the imbalance between energy intake and energy requirements. A diet rich in fat can induce insulin resistance before it induces weight gain. A low-fat diet rich in complex carbohydrates is prescribed to fit an individual's needs with the following aims: (1) to adjust energy intake to match energy requirements, (2) to reduce the risk for macrovascular disease, and (3) to correct the metabolic factors leading to hyperglycemia. Unfortunately, diet alone is only able to normalize blood glucose concentrations in about 20 to 30% of the patients. Other means are therefore required to overcome insulin resistance in type 2 diabetes.

Exercise represents the most powerful tool for improving insulin sensitivity, and a 100% improvement in insulin sensitivity is not uncommon. In practical terms, an extra 30 minutes walk each day may enhance insulin sensitivity more than doubling the dose of oral antidiabetic agents or increasing the insulin dose by 20 U. In the Malmö study, a program of moderate exercise twice weekly plus diet modification over a 6-year period was able to prevent progression from impaired glucose tolerance to manifest type 2 diabetes. More importantly, this intervention program also significantly reduced mortality.

Suggested readings

BECK-NIELSEN H, GROOP LC. Metabolic and genetic characterization of prediabetic states. Sequence of events leading to non-insulin-dependent diabetes mellitus. J Clin Invest 1994;94:1714-21.

ERIKSSON J, FRANSSILA-KALLUNKI A, EKSTRAND A, et al. Early metabolic defects in persons at increased risk for non-insulin dependent diabetes mellitus. New Engl J Med 1989;321:337-43.

GROOP L, WIDÉN E, FRANSSILA-KALLUNKI A, et al. Different effects of insulin and oral antidiabetic agents on glucose and energy metabolism in type 2 (non-insulin-dependent) diabetes mellitus. Diabetologia 1989;32:599-605.

GROOP L. Sulfonylureas in NIDDM. Diabetes Care 1992;15:737-54.

GROOP L, WIDÉN E, FERRANNINI E. Insulin deficiency or insulin resistance in the pathogenesis of IDDM. Error of metabolism or methods? Diabetologia 1993;36:1326-31.

GROOP L, KANKURI M, SCHALIN-JÄNTTI C, et al. Association between polymorphism of the skeletal muscle glycogen synthase gene and non-insulin dependent diabetes mellitus. New Engl J Med 1993;328:11-4.

GROOP LC. The etiology of non-insulin-dependent diabetes mellitus. In molecular pathogenesis of diabetes mellitus. In: Leslie RDG (ed). Front Horm Res 22;131-56, Basel: Karger, 1997.

INZUCCHI SE, MAGGS DG, SPOLETT GR, et al. Efficacy and metabolic effects of metformin and troglitazone in type II diabetes mellitus. New Engl J Med 1998;338:867-72.

KAHN R. Insulin action, diabetogenes and the cause of type II diabetes. Diabetes 1994;43:1066-84.

WIDÉN E, GROOP L. Biguanides: metabolic effects and potential use in the in the treatment of the insulin resistance syndrome. Diabetes Ann 1994;8:227-41.

WIDÉN E, LEHTO M, KANNINEN T, WALSTON J, SHULDINER A, GROOP L. Association between a polymorphism of the (3-adrenergic receptor gene and insulin resistance in Finnish nondiabetic subjects. New Engl J Med 1995;333:348-51.

YKI-JÄRVINEN H, KAUPPILA M, KUJANASUU E, et al. Comparison of insulin regimens in patients with non-insulin-dependent diabetes mellitus. New Engl J Med 1992;327:1426-33.

Acute metabolic complications in diabetes mellitus

Kristian F. Hanssen

▌ KEY POINTS ▌

- Diabetic ketoacidosis results from absolute or relative insulin deficiency.
- Diabetic ketoacidosis is defined as severe and uncontrolled diabetes requiring emergency treatment with insulin and intravenous fluids, and a blood ketone body (acetoacetate and 3-hydroxybutyrate) concentration of greater than 5 mmol/l. It can be identified by a strong positive Ketostix test of urine and blood glucose >15-30 mmol/l.
- Increasing polyuria and thirst with associated nausea, vomiting, anorexia, dehydration, and occasionally abdominal pain are the main clinical findings.
- The treatment consists of the replacement of fluids, electrolytes, and insulin; the diagnosis and treatment of precipitating factors; and high quality general medical care and close surveillance.
- Almost all cases of diabetic ketoacidosis are preventable, making the education of patients vitally important.
- Diabetic nonketotic hyperosmolar syndrome is characterized by marked hyperglycemia (>30 mmol/l) and severe dehydration. It most often occurs in elderly patients.

DIABETIC KETOACIDOSIS

Diabetic ketoacidosis is still a major cause of morbidity and mortality in insulin-dependent diabetes mellitus (type I diabetes), though it is preventable in most instances. Its major biochemical features are hyperglycemia, hyperketonemia, and metabolic acidosis. It is often defined as severe uncontrolled diabetes requiring emergency treatment with insulin and intravenous fluid, and a blood ketone body (acetoacetate and 3-hydroxybutyrate) concentration greater than 5 mmol/l. For practical purposes, a strong positive Ketostix test (urine Ketostix test ++ or plasma Ketostix test + or more) and plasma bicarbonate <15 mmol/l are considered together with hyperglycemia (blood glucose >15-20 mmol/l) to identify diabetic ketoacidosis.

The annual incidence rates of ketoacidosis vary between 1 to 5 episodes/100 type 1 diabetes patients per year in Europe and the United States. This variation is due to the social environment, including the cost and availability of insulin, and the availability and quality of health care.

Pathophysiology

In type I diabetes, plasma ketone levels rise because of their overproduction by the liver. Insulin inhibits lipolysis via an insulin-sensitive lipase. In the insulin-deficient state, particularly if there is an increased secretion of catecholamines, excessive amounts of free fatty acids are released from the adipose tissue and transported to the liver. In the liver, the free fatty acids can either be re-esterified or enter the mitochondria and be oxidized to ketones. In patients with hypoinsulinemia and hyperglucagonemia, fatty acids preferentially enter the mitochondria at an accelerated rate, which results in an increased production of ketones. Acidosis then results from the accumulation of the keto acids beta-hydroxybutyrate and acetoacetate, which causes low serum bicarbonate levels and an increased anion gap. Insulin deficiency and elevated levels of glucagon and catecholamines result in increased rates of hepatic glycogenolysis and gluconeogenesis, leading to hyperglycemia. Glucose disposal by muscle and adipose tissue is reduced by insulin deficiency, while raised plasma levels of catabolic hormones and fatty acids induce tissue insulin resistance. Blood glucose levels may therefore fall relatively slowly during treatment in patients with higher levels of catabolic hormones, such as in infection. This may be readily overcome by increasing the infusion rate of insulin.

Hyperglycemia causes an osmotic diuresis when the renal threshold for glucose is exceeded, leading to dehydration and secondary losses of electrolytes. Urinary sodium losses are exacerbated by the deficiency of insulin. Hyperventilation, fever, and sweating may further worsen fluid and electrolyte depletion. Contraction of extracellular fluid volume causes a reduction in renal blood flow, which impairs the ability of the kidneys to clear glucose and ketone bodies. Correction of dehydration is therefore crucial.

Although total body potassium is considerably depleted, plasma potassium levels at presentation are usually normal or high. Hypokalemia at presentation normally signifies a marked deficiency of body potassium.

Clinical findings

Symptoms and signs

Diabetic ketoacidosis occurs in both young and old patients and may be the presenting manifestation of diabetes. After several days of polyuria and polydipsia, patients experiencing diabetic ketoacidosis usually present with associated nausea, vomiting, anorexia, and occasionally abdominal pain (Tab. 58.1). Abdominal pain can sometimes mimic an acute abdominal condition. Infections, trauma, cardiovascular events, emotional stress, and omission or inadequate doses of insulin are common precipitating causes. The failure to increase insulin doses during infections, or the tendency to reduce insulin dosage when the patient eats less because of intercurrent illness, may lead to relative or absolute insulin deficiency. Patients with ketoacidosis have tachypnea (Kussmaul respiration), tachycardia, dehydration, and an odor of acetone (though many persons cannot smell acetone), and in later stages, an altered mental status ranging from disorientation to coma. Acidosis causes peripheral vasodilatation and may lead to hypothermia, which may mask signs of infection. Leucocytosis is common and does not necessarily indicate infection.

Table 58.1 Data to collect in case of diabetic ketoacidosis

History
    Precipitating cause ?
    Current treatment ?
    Treatment failure ?
 	
Physical examination
    Dehydration
    Ketosis (smell ?)
    Acidosis (deep breathing, Kussmaul respiration ?)
    Precipitating causes: pneumonia ?, myocardial
       infarction ?, urinary tract infection ?
    Diabetic complications, especially at cardiovascular
       and/or renal level
    Hypothermia
    Gastric stasis
 	
Laboratory investigations
    Glucose
    Na^+, K^+, Cl^-
    Urea, creatinine
    Acid-base status including pO_2 and pCO_2
    Osmolality
    Ketone bodies (e.g., Ketostix)
    Lactate (if high lactate is suspected)

Diabetic ketoacidosis is a medical emergency requiring prompt diagnosis and treatment. Hyperglycemia may be rapidly confirmed by a blood glucose stix before the results from the laboratory are available. A strong positive Ketostix measurement in urine and plasma confirms ketoacidosis. Metabolic acidosis is present when there are reduced serum bicarbonate levels and an increased anionic gap. Table 58.1 lists the principal biochemical parameters to monitor.

Treatment

High quality general care, often in an intensive care unit, is needed in diabetic ketoacidosis. The condition leads to gastric paresis, and the stomach may contain 1 to 2 liters of fluid. A nasogastric tube is therefore often indicated, and control of urinary output is mandatory. Furthermore, in patients suspected of having cardiovascular disease, central venous pressure measurements are helpful.

There are three important treatment principles: (1) replacement of fluids and electrolytes and insulin treatment must be administered; (2) precipitating diseases must be diagnosed and treated, and (3) high quality general medical care must be given and the patient must be kept under close surveillance.

Rehydration is very important and should be started immediately with isotonic NaCl 0.9% containing appropriate potassium supplements (see below), at a rate of 1 liter per hour for the first 3 hours (Tab. 58.2). In patients with cardiovascular or renal disease, a slower rate of administration may be necessary, and monitoring of central venous pressure is helpful. After 3 hours, the infusion rate is adjusted to the clinical situation. A rising serum sodium >150 mmol/l may necessitate the temporary intro-

Table 58.2 Initial treatment of diabetic ketoacidosis in adults

NaCl 0.9 %(1 l/h first 3 h, usually 4-6 l/24 h)

Insulin: continuous iv infusion 5-10 U/h (average 6 U/h)

When blood glucose has fallen to 15 mmol/l, 5%, glucose 1 liter with 20-28 U regular insulin infused for 4-6 h instead of NaCl infusion. If the patient is still dehydrated, give both NaCl and glucose

Potassium: no potassium 1 h unless plasma K⁺ <3.5 mmol/l. Thereafter to each liter of fluid: give 20 mmol KCl (in case of plasma K⁺ 3.5-5.5 mmol/l); give 40 mmol KCl (in case of plasma K⁺ < 3.5 mmol/l); do not give KCl (in case of plasma K⁺ > 5.5).

Sodium bicarbonate 100 mmol (700 ml of 1.3%) if pH <7.0

duction of hypotonic NaCl (0.45%) or 5% glucose (with appropriate insulin). The total amount of fluid is approximately 5 to 6 liters in the first 24 hours.

Insulin treatment and rising pH stimulate the uptake of potassium into the cells, which can result in extracellular hypokalemia. Hypokalemia can bring about cardiac arrhythmias and weakness of the respiratory muscles. Twenty mmol of potassium are needed on average for each liter of fluid replacement after the start of insulin treatment. Special care should be taken if renal failure occurs and if urine output is less than 40 ml/hour. Many medical centers postpone the start of potassium supplement until satisfactory urine output is achieved and serum potassium is below 5 mmol/l. When hypokalemia is present, the potassium supplement should be doubled to 40 mmol/hour.

In adult patients, insulin is best given intravenously, but intramuscular injections every hour is an option, particularly in children. Regular (soluble) insulin at a rate of 5 to 10 U per hour (average 6 U/hour) is given intravenously. Insulin is diluted to a convenient concentration in a syringe pump or added to a 500 ml bag of isotonic saline before infusion. This regimen should produce a steady fall in plasma glucose concentration of about 4-6 mmol/h; if not, the insulin infusion rate should be increased by 2 U per hour. It is important to note that a common reason for failure is mechanical problems with the pump or the infusion line.

In diabetic ketoacidosis, there is a variable degree of insulin resistance: when blood glucose levels are decreased, the insulin resistance diminishes, leading to lower insulin requirements. It is therefore necessary to monitor blood glucose levels, acid-base levels, and electrolytes every hour for the first few hours. When blood glucose levels are about 15 mmol/l, the insulin infusion should be stopped and changed to glucose (5.5%) 1000 ml with regular insulin (20-28 U) in the glucose bag and an infusion rate of 200 ml/h. The goal is to maintain blood glucose levels at 5-12 mmol/l. If significant acidosis is still present, the insulin dose should be slightly increased. Hypoglycemia after diabetic ketoacidosis should be

avoided by changing to glucose/insulin infusion early. When the patient is able to eat, subcutaneous insulin should be initiated instead. The injection dose of subcutaneous insulin should include some regular insulin and be given before terminating the intravenous infusion of insulin. It is particularly important to remember that the half-life of iv insulin is only 5 minutes, so subcutaneous insulin must be given at once when stopping the intravenous insulin.

Bicarbonate treatment is controversial. However, small doses of bicarbonate are beneficial if there is severe acidosis (pH <7.0) or if cardiorespiratory failure seems imminent. Bicarbonate (approximately 100 mmol) should be infused as 700 ml of 1.26%.

Raising arterial pH to 7.10-7.20 should be tried, though fully normalizing acid-base status should not be attempted, as concomitant insulin treatment will lessen the acidosis by reducing ketone body production. Administration of bicarbonate can lead to hypokalemia, and extra potassium (20 mmol per 100 mmol bicarbonate) must be administrated.

Complications

Cerebral edema is a rare, but serious complication of diabetic ketoacidosis, especially in children. It presents with a decline in the level of consciousness, often with respiratory arrest within a few hours. The process generally starts some hours after the start of treatment for diabetic ketoacidosis. After an initial satisfactory response to treatment, some patients deteriorate without warning. The diagnosis should be confirmed by a computed tomography or a magnetic resonance scanning of the brain. The poor prognosis of fully developed cerebral edema may in part be due to delays in diagnosis and treatment. Reasonable measures to treat include slowing intravenous fluids and slowing insulin infusion, and administering Mannitol (0.2 g/kg iv over 30 minutes, repeated if necessary). Dexamethasone 4 mg four times per day may be tried, but the prognosis is poor.

Thromboembolism Thromboembolic complications are significant causes of death in diabetic ketoacidosis, as both dehydration, increased blood viscosity, and increased coagulability may be present. Routine prophylactic anticoagulation is indicated in high-risk patients.

Kidney failure Some patients with diabetic ketoacidosis may have pre-existing kidney disease, particularly diabetic nephropathy. In this situation, careful monitoring of urine flow and electrolyte and fluid balance, including central venous pressure monitoring, is necessary. Some patients may otherwise have irreversible kidney failure.

Lactic acidosis Some patients with diabetic ketoacidosis also have lactic acidosis, especially with concomitant severe infection. In very rare cases, oral biguanide therapy with metformin can lead to lactic acidosis.

Other complications   Adult respiratory distress syndrome, rhinocerebral mucormycosis (fungal infection), and rhabdomyolysis are rare complications of diabetic ketoacidosis.

Prevention

Almost all cases of diabetic ketoacidosis are preventable. Educating the patient to monitor blood glucose levels closely, check urine for ketone bodies by Ketostix in case of intercurrent illness, and increase insulin dosage and take extra regular insulin when blood glucose values are over 15 mmol/l are all very important. Furthermore, it must be taught that insulin dosage often should be increased during intercurrent illness, even if food intake is reduced due to the illness. Patients must also be aware that vomiting and abdominal pain may be the first signs of diabetic ketosis; they must know that their blood glucose levels and urine Ketostix should be monitored intensively in such situations and that regular insulin in extra doses should be given if appropriate. Patients with type I diabetes using insulin pumps have an increased risk of diabetic ketoacidosis if mechanical failure of the pump or block in the fittings develop.

DIABETIC NON-KETOTIC HYPEROSMOLAR SYNDROME

Clinical findings

Patients with diabetic non-ketotic hyperosmolar syndrome have marked hyperglycemia (>30 mmol/l) without significant ketonemia and acidosis. They have marked hyperosmolarity (>340 mOsmol/l), Ketostix in serum is < ++, and plasma bicarbonate is >18 mmol/l. They are usually profoundly dehydrated and often have depressed consciousness. Most people with the syndrome are middle aged or elderly, and it is often precipitated by thiazide diuretics. The patients mostly have non-insulin-dependent diabetes mellitus (type 2 diabetes), which in many patients is undiagnosed, and they often have coexisting diseases and therefore a high mortality (approximately 30%). Characteristic symptoms are polyuria, thirst, and declining consciousness. Severe dehydration and hypotension are common. The degree of dehydration is generally larger than in diabetic ketoacidosis and averages approximately 9 liters of body fluid lost. Although total body sodium is depleted through renal losses, plasma sodium may be low, normal, or high, depending on the degree of water deficit. Symptoms generally develop over several days and may be mistaken for stroke or dementia. Vomiting is not common, and Kussmaul respiration is not a feature because significant acidosis is absent.

Treatment

The treatment principles are similar to diabetic ketoacidosis, including rehydration, electrolyte substitution, insulin administration, a search for precipitating factors, and excellent medical care. In general, the insulin doses needed to reduce blood glucose levels are lower (2-4 U/h), and the fluid deficit is larger than in diabetic ketoacidosis. Because many patients are elderly and have co-existing cardiovascular disease, it is wise to normalize both the glucose levels and fluid deficit gradually. Whether to use 0.9% or 0.45% NaCl in rehydration is controversial. This author recommends NaCl 0.9% in general, but one may try 0.45% if a patientís serum sodium concentration is above 150 mmol/l. Thromboembolic episodes are common; hence thrombosis prophylaxis may be indicated.

Suggested readings

ALBERTI KGMM, MARSCHALL SM. Hyperglycemic emergencies: a further look. In: Albert KGMM, Krall LP (eds). The diabetes annual. Vol 6. 1991.

PICKUP J, WILLIAMS G. Textbook of diabetes. 2nd ed. Oxford: Blackwell Science, 1997.

Late diabetic complications

DIABETIC RETINOPATHY

Elisabet Agardh

Diabetic retinopathy is the leading cause of blindness among people under 65 years of age in the Western world. The fundus changes vary from occasional hemorrhages and microaneurysms to multiple hemorrhages, severe exudation along the blood vessels as well as in the central part of the macula, fibrovascular proliferations accompanied by preretinal or vitreous hemorrhages, and retinal detachment. Visual loss can be prevented by laser treatment provided it is performed before irreversible damage of the retina has occurred. It is therefore of utmost importance to screen for diabetic retinopathy regularly; 1- to 2-year intervals are generally recommended.

Epidemiology

Diabetic retinopathy occurs in both type 1 and type 2 diabetic patients. The rate of both mild and severe retinopathy is correlated to the duration of the diabetes: the longer the duration, the higher the risk (Figs. 59.1-59.3). Type 1 diabetic patients do not have any retinopathy at the diagnosis of diabetes. In type 2 diabetic patients, however, diabetic retinopathy is present in about 25% at diagnosis, which probably reflects the fact that many of these patients have had diabetes for several years before diagnosis. Potentially sight-threatening retinopathy, such as leakage in the most central parts of the retina (macular edema) and neovascularizations (proliferative retinopathy) occur in both type 1 and type 2 diabetic patients, but they are more common in type 1 and insulin-treated type 2 diabetic patients than in noninsulin-treated diabetic patients.

Pathophysiology

The retinal vessel wall is composed of three structures: endothelial cells, pericytes, and a basal membrane. The

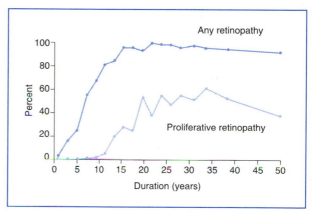

Figure 59.1 Frequency of retinopathy or proliferative retinopathy by duration of diabetes (years) in persons taking insulin who had diagnosis of diabetes before 30 years of age. Wisconsin Epidemiologic Study of Diabetic Retinopathy. (From Arch Ophthalmol 1984;102:520-26, reproduced by permission.)

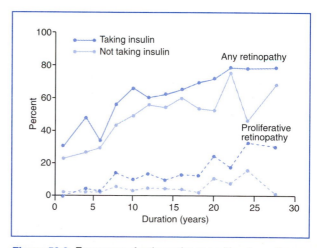

Figure 59.2 Frequency of retinopathy or proliferative retinopathy by duration of diabetes (years) in persons receiving or not receiving insulin who had a diagnosis of diabetes at or after 30 years of age. Wisconsin Epidemiologic Study of Diabetic Retinopathy. (From Arch Ophthalmol 1984;102:527-32, reproduced by permission.)

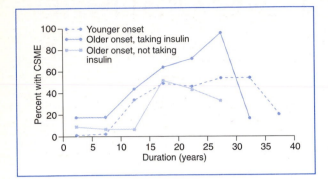

Figure 59.3 The frequency of macular edema by duration of diabetes. Wisconsin Epidemiologic Study of Diabetic Retinopathy. (From Int Ophthalmol Clin 1987;27:230-38, reproduced by permission.)

endothelial cells are located nearest the vessel lumen, forming tight junctions with components of the basement membrane. These structures are important for the maintenance of the blood-retinal barrier, as they allow only small molecules to pass through. The exact function of the pericytes is not known, but they probably serve as contractile elements that maintain the vascular tone. In addition, they seem to inhibit endothelial cell proliferation.

One of the earliest signs of diabetic retinopathy is basal membrane thickening and pericyte loss. Occlusion of small vessels may also be associated with endothelial cell loss, and in areas of nonperfusion some capillaries may appear as cylinders of thickened basal membrane or as acellular strands. In other capillaries, however, the loss of pericytes may induce endothelial cell proliferation and microaneurysm formation.

Course

Vascular occlusion Vascular occlusion creates areas of nonperfusion. Microaneurysm formation is an early sign of vascular closure. Rupture of microaneurysms, capillaries, or venules result in intraretinal hemorrhages. As the process of vascular occlusion proceeds, small infarcts occur in the nerve fiber layer and fluffy white spots ("cotton wool spots") appear as a result of axoplasmic swelling. Other signs of nonperfusion are venous dilation and formation of loops, as well as focal narrowing, making the venules appear as strings of beads. New vascular channels between arterioles and venules are created in the damaged capillary bed, appearing as fine blood-filled vessels within the retinal tissue: that is, intraretinal microvascular abnormalities (IRMA). Later in the course, new blood vessels arise from the retina and optic disc. Initially they proliferate along the surface of the retina, but as they make contact with the adjacent vitreous, they adhere to its posterior membrane. Posterior vitreous detachment will cause bleeding from the new delicate vessels, resulting in trapped blood between the retina and vitreous or in intravitreous hemorrhage, often with a deterioration of vision as

a result. The new vessels are accompanied by fibrous tissue, which creates fibrovascular complexes that extend from the retinal vessels into the vitreous. If the fibrovascular tissue undergoes contraction, retinal detachment may occur and result in severe visual impairment.

Neovascularization may also occur in the iris and angle inhibiting absorption of fluid through the trabecular meshwork and secondary elevated intraocular pressure, that is, neovascular glaucoma.

Increased vascular permeability Microaneurysms, dilated capillaries and venules, and IRMA all impair the blood retinal barrier. The increased vascular permeability results in an extracellular accumulation of serum lipids, lipoproteins, and other plasma constituents, which are visible as a thickening of the retina and/or yellow dots, that is, hard exudates, sometimes in circinate or stellate patterns. Leakage from microaneurysms is usually focal, whereas leakage from dilated capillaries is diffuse. Visual impairment depends upon the location, severity, and extension of leakage.

Classification

Nonproliferative retinopathy Nonproliferative retinopathy is characterized by varying numbers of microaneurysms, hemorrhages, cotton wool spots, hard exudates (Fig. 59.4, see Color Atlas), IRMA, and/or venous abnormalities. Depending upon the amount of changes, it can be classified as mild, moderate, or severe.

Proliferative retinopathy Proliferative retinopathy is characterized by neovascularization on the disc or elsewhere (Fig. 59.5, see Color Atlas). In addition, all changes characteristic for nonproliferative retinopathy may be present.

Macular edema Macular edema is characterized by thickening of the retina, with or without hard exudates, within one optic disc diameter from the retina (Fig. 59.6, see Color Atlas). Macular edema can be present in nonproliferative as well as in proliferative retinopathy.

Putative pathogenetic mechanisms

There is a strong correlation between the development and progression of diabetic retinopathy and the degree of metabolic control. The exact mechanisms, however, are not yet fully understood. Several hypotheses have been proposed and tested in animal studies, but the results are not yet applicable to man.

Sorbitol Glucose is metabolized to sorbitol by the enzyme aldose reductase. Sorbitol is osmotically active and binds water. Elevated blood glucose levels result in increased sorbitol concentrations. Since this substance cannot pass through cell membranes, it accumulates intracellularly and causes an increased retention of fluid. In addition, it creates a redox imbalance that may cause an increased production of reactive oxygen species, which will have a further negative impact on cellular function.

Clinical trials, however, have not shown that aldose reductase inhibitors prevent the development or progression of diabetic retinopathy.

Glycosylation products Elevated blood glucose levels result in the formation of advanced glycosylation end products (AGE). Glucose rapidly attaches to amino groups of proteins. Initially, these products are short-lived and reversible, but glycosylated proteins may undergo auto-oxidation, thereby generating reactive oxygen species that may contribute to protein cross-linking, degradation and tissue damage in diabetic blood vessels. Aminoguanidine inhibits AGE formation, but there are so far no reports on clinical trials of this drug.

Growth factors Several growth factors have been proposed to be involved in ischemia-induced diabetic retinopathy. Of those proposed, vascular endothelial growth factor (VEGF) seems to fulfill most criteria for a major mediator of neovascularization. It promotes stimulation of endothelial cell growth in culture. High-affinity tyrosine-autophosphorylating VEGF receptors have been demonstrated on endothelial cells, pericytes, and retinal pigment epithelia. Hypoxia increases the VEGF production in cells in the vessel walls as well as in some retinal cells. Furthermore, increased levels of VEGF have been demonstrated in the vitreous of patients with proliferative diabetic retinopathy. Recent studies also suggest that VEGF can induce vascular permeability. The mode of action is likely an induction of an intracellular signal transduction cascade that leads to an activation and translocation of protein kinase C (PKC) through several steps. Growth and vasopermeability effects seem to be induced by one of its isoforms, PKC beta. A clinical trial on the effect of a PKC beta inhibitor (LY 333 351) is underway.

Treatment

Severe forms of diabetic retinopathy should be treated with photocoagulation. The argon green wavelength is most commonly used. Laser treatment should be performed in eyes with proliferative retinopathy provided the proliferative vessels have caused preretinal or vitreous hemorrhage, or reached a certain size (1/3 of the optic disc close to or on the optic disc, or 1/2 of the optic disc elsewhere), and in eyes with macular edema provided it is located close enough to the center of the macula (within 500 μ) or is located slightly more peripherally (within one optic disc diameter from the center of the macula) and has reached a certain size (at least one optic disc). In these cases – that is, high-risk proliferative retinopathy and clinically significant macular edema – laser treatment reduces the risk of visual impairment and blindness by at least 50%.

Techniques Before considering treatment for macular edema, a fluorescein angiogram is usually obtained in order to visualize the type and extension of leakage as well as the obstruction of vessels (Fig. 59.7). The passage of intravenously injected fluorescein is documented through the retinal circulation by a series of photographs.

The fluorescein angiogram gives useful information, particularly regarding the type and localization of macular edema, information that is important when choosing a mode of treatment. Focal leakage, which can be localized to microaneurysms, is treated by direct coagulation of the individual aneurysms. Diffuse leakage is covered by weak burns in a grid pattern. The laser burns probably cause a closure of the leaking microaneurysms and/or promotes a reestablishment of the blood-retinal barrier and, when successfully performed, results in the absorption of edema and hard exudates (Fig. 59.8, see Color Atlas).

Proliferative retinopathy is treated by panretinal photocoagulation (Fig. 59.9, see Color Atlas). The posterior half of the retina, with the exception of the area between the branches of the temporal vessels, is covered with laser burns at approximately one burn width apart. By this laser treatment, the demand for oxygen may be reduced by destruction of the outer retina, thereby permitting an increased supply of oxygen to the inner retina and reducing one stimulus for neovascularization. The destruction may also inhibit the release of ischemia-induced growth factors.

Removal of the vitreous is considered when vitreous, or severe preretinal hemorrhage in tight apposition to the macula, do not clear up; when fibrovascular complexes exert traction on the macula; or when there is a tractional retinal detachment in combination with a retinal hole. The vitreous can be replaced by sodium chloride, gas, or silicon oil.

Side effects The most common side effects of photocoagulation are visual impairment due to progressive scar formation after central treatment and impaired dark adaptation after panretinal photocoagulation.

Risk factors

Early age at the onset of diabetes, diabetes duration, and poor metabolic control are all prominent risk factors for both the development and progression of diabetic

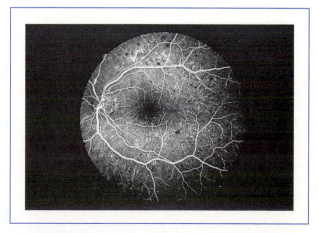

Figure 59.7 Fluorescein angiogram demonstrating multiple microaneurysms.

retinopathy. Good metabolic control from early on reduces the risk in both type 1 and type 2 diabetes. In addition, it has been shown that improved metabolic control is also beneficial later in the course of diabetes. Clinical studies have shown that intensified treatment reduces the risk for development and progression of retinopathy in type 1 diabetes by 50% and in type 2 diabetes by 25%. Retinopathy that is already established is not affected and may even worsen if the blood glucose levels are reduced too quickly, such as during pregnancy. Diabetic women should therefore have extra eye examinations during pregnancy.

Other risk factors are hypertension and nephropathy. Smoking has not yet been established as a major risk factor.

Cataract

Before 30 years of age, cataract occurs more frequently in type 1 diabetes than in a nondiabetic population. After 30 years of age, the occurrence of cataract is similar in these two groups, whereas it is higher in type 2 diabetes. Surgical techniques used for cataract removal and lens implantation are the same as for nondiabetic patients. Since progression of existing diabetic retinopathy after cataract extraction has been reported, a preoperative retinal examination should be performed and, in patients with diabetic retinopathy, a postoperative one as well.

DIABETIC RENAL DISEASE

Allan Kofoed-Enevoldsen

The spectrum of renal disease associated with diabetes includes *diabetic nephropathy, renal papillary necrosis, urinary tract infection, and neurogenic bladder dysfunction.*

Of these, diabetic nephropathy is by far the most prevalent and the only one specifically found in diabetes. Diabetic nephropathy is responsible for a large portion (25-35%) of all patients treated for end-stage chronic renal failure. In addition, through its association to the development of generalized cardiovascular disease, diabetic nephropathy is the main cause of the excess mortality in diabetes.

DIABETIC NEPHROPATHY

Diabetic nephropathy is a gradually progressing disease characterized by the development of proteinuria, hypertension with subsequent loss of glomerular function, and uremia. It carries a high risk of death from uremia and cardiovascular disease, and it causes excess morbidity due to severe diabetic retinopathy. During the past decade, well-documented therapeutic strategies for primary and secondary prevention have been established, thus making routine screening procedures for identifying at-risk subjects highly successful.

Diagnosis

The clinical diagnosis diabetic nephropathy refers to the development of persistent proteinuria ("macroproteinuria," i.e., above 0.5 g total urinary protein or 300 mg urinary albumin per 24 hours in at least two of three samples obtained with one month interval) in a diabetic patient free from other renal or urinary tract diseases and cardiac insufficiency.

Urinary albumin excretion in the otherwise healthy diabetic patient normally does not exceed 30 mg per 24 hours. It follows that any patient developing diabetic nephropathy will necessarily have to pass through a phase of elevated urinary albumin excretion (30-300 mg per 24 hours) in which the criterion for clinical diabetic nephropathy is not yet fulfilled. Urinary albumin excretion in this range is termed *microalbuminuria*.

Urine for the measurement of albumin excretion may be sampled as a timed (24-hour or overnight) urine sample. An early morning urine may be sufficient, given both albumin and creatinine concentrations are determined to calculate the albumin/creatinine excretion ratio (reference values in Table 59.1). Obviously longer sampling periods will serve to neutralize the impact of naturally occurring variability in albumin excretion. However, even the day-to-day coefficient of variation in diurnal albumin excretion measured during 24-hour sampling periods is 30 to 50%. Samples for the measurement of urinary albumin excretion may be stored at +5°C for one week. Physical activity tends to increase urinary albumin excretion, and urinary tract infection should be ruled out, although the effect on urinary albumin excretion will usually be ignorable unless pyuria is present.

The diagnosis of diabetic nephropathy may be confirmed by renal biopsy, which should be considered only in cases of unexpected presentation of albuminuria. Such situations include the development of albuminuria before 5 years of IDDM duration, albuminuria in an NIDDM patient without evidence of diabetic retinopathy, or suspected nondiabetic renal disease where specific therapy may be indicated. Hematuria and even red cell casts may be seen in diabetic nephropathy, but they require consideration of the differential diagnoses.

Epidemiology

The incidence of diabetic nephropathy relates to the quality of blood glucose control and other therapeutic interven-

---

Table 59.1 Urinary albumin excretion reference values

	Albumin (mg/24 h)	Albumin (µg/min)	Alb /creatinine (mg/g)	Alb /creatinine (mg/mmol)
Normal	<30	<20	<30	<2.5
Microalbuminuria	30-300	20-200	30-300	2.5-25
"Macroalbuminuria"	>300	>200	>300	>25

tions (see below). Among the cohorts of insulin-treated diabetic patients with diabetes diagnosed from 1930 to 1950, as many as 50% developed diabetic nephropathy. Through the sixties the incidence was reduced to 30 to 40%, but it remained stable thereafter. It is likely that further improvements in blood glucose and blood pressure control during the past decade has lead to further reduction the cumulative incidence of diabetic nephropathy. The cumulative incidence of diabetic nephropathy in patients with NIDDM (10 to 15%) is generally lower than in IDDM. In IDDM, diabetic nephropathy generally does not develop before 10 years of diabetes duration, whereas even newly diagnosed NIDDM patients may present with diabetic nephropathy.

The annual incidence curve follows a bell-shaped pattern, with its maximum reached after 15 to 20 years of diabetes duration (IDDM) (Fig. 59.10). Thereafter the incidence declines, indicating that the remaining population is protected against the development of diabetic nephropathy. Thus the risk of developing diabetic nephropathy in a normoalbuminuric IDDM patient with more than 25 years of diabetes duration is very low.

This pattern does not simply reflect differences in the quality of blood glucose control, but it indicates that certain, possibly genetically related factors are responsible for differences in the individual susceptibility for the development of diabetic nephropathy. Another indicator of genetic involvement is the finding of an accumulation of cases of diabetic nephropathy within families, as evidenced from several sibling studies. A number of susceptibility genes have been identified, typically conferring a two- to fourfold increase in risk, but genetic screening is so far not considered to be of clinical relevance.

The quality of blood glucose control has a major influence on the incidence of diabetic nephropathy. The risk of developing diabetic nephropathy seems to increase progressively when average blood glucose values exceed 8 to 9 mmol/l. Conversely, keeping long-term blood glucose tightly regulated (corresponding to glycosylated hemoglobin-A_{1c} below 7.0 to 7.5%) would be a highly effective preventive strategy. However, this is not easily achieved in the daily clinical setting.

Pathogenesis

Diabetic nephropathy is a slowly progressing disease with a time span of up to 30 years from the onset of microalbuminuria until the final stage of chronic end-stage renal failure is reached. In this process several stages may be identified. A suggested classification of five stages is shown in Table 59.2. The staging is principally based upon two renal physiologic parameters: *glomerular filtration* and *glomerular macromolecular permeability*. It is also possible to allocate certain characteristic findings related to glomerular morphology and biochemistry to this suggested staging.

Morphology

Since Kimmelstiel and Wilson in 1936 reported that broadening of the glomerular intercapillary connective tissue was a characteristic finding in diabetic patients presenting with renal failure, the focus in unraveling the pathogenesis of diabetic nephropathy has been on the glomerulus. In addition, the extracellular matrix has remained a *locus in quo*.

The key morphological abnormalities include glomerular basement membrane thickening, increased mesangial matrix volume fraction, glomerular sclerosis resulting in glomerular closure, and loss of functioning nephrons (Fig. 59.11).

Glomerular basement membrane thickening is not specifically related to diabetic nephropathy, but it may be found in diabetic patients with normal urinary albumin

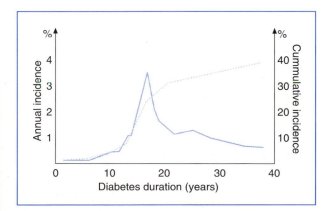

Figure 59.10 The annual (———) and cumulative (..........) incidence of diabetic nephropathy in type 1 diabetes patients with diabetes diagnosed between 1933 and 1972. (Redrawn with permission from Kofoed-Enevoldsen et al. Diabetes 1987; 36:5-9.)

Table 59.2 Stages in the development of diabetic nephropathy

I **Glomerular hyperfunction and hypertrophy**
UAE normal or eventually slightly raised.
Glomerular filtration rate elevated

II **Silent stage**
UAE normal. Structural lesions are building up.
May not progress

III **Microalbuminuria (*incipient diabetic nephropathy*)**
UAE elevated (30-300 mg/24 h). Structural lesions present. High risk of progressing to overt diabetic nephropathy if no intervention is undertaken

IV **Overt diabetic nephropathy**
Persistent macroalbuminuria (above 300 mg/24 h).
Glomerular filtration is declining

V **End-stage renal failure**

(UAE = urinary albumin excretion.)
(Adapted from Mogensen CE,ed. The kidney and hypertension in diabetes mellitus. Dordrecht: Kluwer Academic Pub, 1996.)

excretion as well. However, the glomerular basement membrane width increases with the development of microalbuminuria until, in overt diabetic nephropathy, glomerular basement membrane width is doubled compared to healthy nondiabetic controls.

Mesangial matrix volume fraction remains within the normal range (10% of total glomerular volume) in patients with normal urinary albumin excretion. It then significantly increases in patients with microalbuminuria until in overt diabetic nephropathy the mesangial matrix may occupy 25% of the total glomerular volume.

The distribution of advanced glomerular lesions is even within the juxtamedullary and cortical zones.

Physiology

Increased glomerular macromolecular permeability underlies the development of albuminuria, which is the diagnostic criterion for diabetic nephropathy.

The glomerular filtration barrier consists of the endothelial cell lining the glomerular capillary luminal surface, the glomerular basement membrane, and the glomerular epithelial cell (Fig. 59.11). The integrated function of these three layers is necessary to maintain intact glomerular filtration. The restriction of trans glomerular passage of macromolecules is governed by two characteristics of the filtration process: size and charge selectivity *Size selectivity* leads to progressive restriction of the passage of large molecules, such that those larger than 60 Å display a fractional clearance of less than 0005. *Charge selectivity* restricts the passage of negatively charged macromolecules. It is due to this charge selectivity that the anionic albumin molecules are effectively retained in spite of their relatively small size (36 Å). Both loss of glomeru-

lar size and charge selectivity are found in diabetic nephropathy. It seems that the initial event, explaining the onset of microalbuminuria, is a loss of charge selectivity.

Glomerular filtration rate is often elevated in newly onset diabetes (IDDM). Hyperglycemia, ketosis, and elevated glucagon and growth hormone levels may explain the elevated glomerular filtration rate, which is also linked to an increase in renal plasma flow and possibly to an increase in glomerular capillary pressure. Elevated glomerular filtration rate may be a risk marker for later development of diabetic nephropathy. At the onset of microalbuminuria, glomerular filtration rate is, however, not increased, and it will remain unchanged until microalbuminuria progresses to overt diabetic nephropathy. A steady decrease in glomerular filtration rate follows at the onset of overt diabetic nephropathy. Although great individual variability is found, a fall rate of 1 ml/min per month is to be expected when no therapeutic intervention is undertaken.

Biochemistry

Defining the molecular pathobiology of diabetic nephropathy remains an area of active research, with the obvious ultimate goal of introducing novel therapeutic strategies.

Subtle changes in the composition of the glomerular extracellular matrix may play a central role in the pathogenesis of diabetic nephropathy. Major macromolecular constituents of the extracellular matrices are collagen (type IV), laminin, and heparan sulfate proteoglycan. Diabetes-induced increased synthesis of collagen IV and laminin, in combination with a relative or absolute decrease in the synthesis of heparan sulfate proteoglycan, results in a selective decrease in the glomerular basement membrane content of heparan sulfate proteoglycan. This, in turn, may explain the loss of the charge selectivity of the glomerular filtration barrier and the appearance of albuminuria.

Multiple mechanisms through which diabetes may exert the abnormalities in the extracellular matrix metabolism have been demonstrated. Among those directly linking the level of blood glucose to a possible pathogenetic mechanism are the activation of the *polyol pathway* and the consequences of *nonenzymatic glycation*. Activation of protein kinase C and increased expression of transforming growth factor β also appear to characterize the disease process.

Drugs specifically designed to interfere with either of these pathogenetic pathways have been designed and may offer novel therapeutic possibilities in the near future.

As stated above, there are major differences in the individual susceptibility of the development of diabetic nephropathy. The familiar accumulation of cases of diabetic nephropathy has lead to an exploration of several proposed candidate genes. Particularly, the genetics of the renin-angiotensin system have been extensively investigated. Neither the DD genotype of the angiotensin converting enzyme "Insertion/Deletion" polymorphism nor polymorphisms in the angiotensinogen gene and the

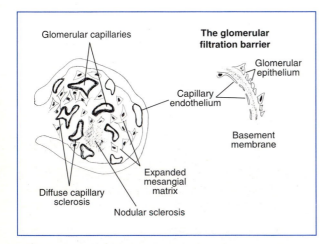

Figure 59.11 *(Left)* An illustration of key morphological features of diabetic glomerulosclerosis. The expanded mesangial matrix together with diffuse capillary sclerosis leads to glomerular capillary closure and loss of functioning glomeruli. *(Right)* Insert illustrating the principal components of the glomerular filtration barrier. The filtration barrier loses its charge - and size - selectivity during the development of diabetic nephropathy.

angiotensin-II type 1 receptor have stood confirmatory test in secondary populations, however.

Ongoing family studies using a whole genome screening approach may identify clinically meaningful genetic risk markers.

Diabetic nephropathy and "malignant angiopathy"

It is important to recognize that diabetic nephropathy should be considered merely an organ-specific manifestation of a generalized *malignant angiopathy*, rather than an isolated diabetes-induced renal complication. The term "malignant angiopathy" has been coined to embrace the concurrent appearance of sight-threatening retinal vessel disease, increased morbidity and mortality from atherosclerotic cardiovascular disease, and progressive glomerulosclerotic nephropathy.

Atherosclerotic cardiovascular disease Cardiovascular mortality is two to ten times higher in IDDM and NIDDM patients with diabetic nephropathy compared to patients with normal urinary albumin excretion. This is at least partly explained by the presence of known cardiovascular risk factors.

Arterial hypertension is present in 40% of patients at the onset of diabetic nephropathy. An increase in blood pressure accompanies the progression of microalbuminuria to diabetic nephropathy, and hypertension is generally not present at the onset of microalbuminuria. Hypertension itself, through a vicious circle, increases the progression rate of diabetic nephropathy. The mechanism responsible for the rise in blood pressure remains to be resolved, but it is known that it includes sodium (and water) retention, which accelerates through the impaired capability of compensatory increasing the glomerular filtration rate in patients with diabetic nephropathy.

An atherogenic plasma lipid profile with elevated LDL cholesterol and triglyceride is often found, and the plasma fibrinogen concentration is elevated in patients with diabetic nephropathy. The specific association of these risk factors with elevated urinary albumin excretion is strongest in IDDM as normoalbuminuric IDDM patients (in contrast to NIDDM) in good metabolic control display no abnormalities in their blood lipid profile. As with hypertension, hyperlipidemia may also increase the rate of the progression of nephropathy.

Retinopathy The annual incidence of severe, sight-threatening proliferative retinopathy is increased tenfold in patients with diabetic nephropathy (Fig. 59.12), and virtually all patients with end-stage renal failure will have developed proliferative retinopathy.

Simple background retinopathy should be demonstrable in all patients when urinary albumin excretion exceeds 300 mg per 24 hours.

An absence of retinopathy is not an uncommon finding in NIDDM patients presenting with proteinuria. In that case, the likelihood of a nondiabetic cause of the proteinuria increases above 50%, and renal biopsy should be considered before the diagnosis of diabetic nephropathy is decided.

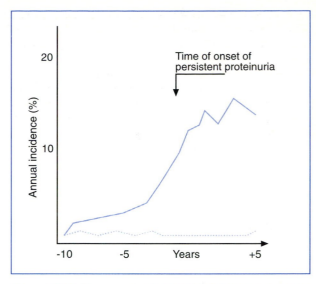

Figure 59.12 The annual incidence of proliferative retinopathy in type 1 diabetes patients with (———) and without (..........) diabetic nephropathy. The two groups are matched for diabetes duration, and the incidence of retinopathy is shown during the 15-year period from 10 years before the onset of overt diabetic nephropathy until 5 years after. (Redrawn with permission from Kofoed-Enevoldsen et al. J Diab Compl 1987;1:96-9.)

The pathogenetic background for the combined appearance of diabetic renal and retinal disease is not known. The development of both complications may, however, be retarded by strict blood glucose control.

Treatment

Monitoring glomerular function

Urinary albumin excretion Urinary albumin excretion should be followed regularly in diabetic patients from the onset of diabetes. Guidelines for urine sampling and evaluation of measurements are given above (see "Diagnosis"). Yearly measurements are advocated until the eventual occurrence of elevated levels appear (rarely before 5 years of diabetes duration in IDDM, frequently earlier in NIDDM). In order to confirm the presence of persistently elevated urinary albumin excretion, repeated samples should then be scheduled at each visit. When persistently elevated urinary albumin excretion is confirmed, samples may be requested, such as twice yearly, to monitor further progression.

Glomerular filtration rate Routine measurement of the glomerular filtration rate in newly onset diabetic patients is generally not indicated. However in patients with overt diabetic nephropathy, monitoring of the glomerular filtration rate is of major importance. The most simple approach is to measure serum creatinine; it has long been known that in terms of the natural history of the disease, a plain plot of repeated reciprocal serum creatinine values (when above 200 µmol/l) against time will predict the time until development of end-stage renal failure with remarkable certainty. However, serum creatinine is dependent upon other factors, such as dietary protein intake and extra renal creatinine losses, and is not a sufficient method for monitoring glomerular filtration rate.

Measuring creatinine clearance offers a more specific assessment of glomerular filtration rate, although it leads to systematic overestimation by 10 to 40% and is less reliable in monitoring the course of advanced renal disease.

The traditional insulin constant infusion technique remains a gold standard. The less elaborate single shot techniques measuring ^{51}CrEDTA clearance, for example, also produces state-of-the-art individual follow up data.

A steady decrease in glomerular filtration rate follows the onset of overt diabetic nephropathy. Although great individual variability is found, a fall rate of 1 ml/min per month is to be expected when no therapeutic intervention is undertaken. With long-term antihypertensive treatment, this fall rate may be reduced by as much as 90%.

Renal biopsy Renal biopsy, although rarely needed, can provide conclusive evidence for establishing the diagnosis of diabetic nephropathy. Factors that should alert the clinician to consider a renal biopsy include development of albuminuria before 5 years IDDM duration, albuminuria in an NIDDM patient without evidence of diabetic retinopathy, or suspected nondiabetic renal disease where specific therapy may be indicated.

Sequential biopsies have been performed to document the effect of intervention, such as improved metabolic control. With an interval of 2 years between biopsies, it is possible to document retarded progression of morphological disease markers such as basement membrane thickness and matrix/glomerular volume fraction, even with only moderate improvement in blood glucose control (i.e., a reduction in hemoglobin A_{1c} from 9.9 to 8.7%).

Electromicroscopic examination is required to calculate the delicate extracellular matrix morphometric data, but it is generally of no use in the differential diagnosis of diabetic nephropathy.

Primary prevention

Primary prevention is preventing or retarding the onset of microalbuminuria in a previously normoalbuminuric diabetic patient. Preventing the onset of microalbuminuria obviously blocks the track toward developing progressive renal disease. Among IDDM patients with more than 5 years of diabetes duration, the incidence of microalbuminuria will be 1 to 3% per year unless strict metabolic control is achieved. However, this adds to a cumulative incidence of around 50% after 25 years of diabetes duration. The potential benefit of an effective preventive strategy is therefore considerable.

Improved blood glucose control The cornerstone in primary prevention of diabetic nephropathy is strict blood glucose control. If possible, blood glucose should be kept within 4 to 10 mmol/l and with a hemoglobulin A_{1c} level below 7.5%. To obtain this degree of blood glucose control, it is often necessary to replace conventional insulin therapy with a multiple dose regimen, or continuous subcutaneous insulin infusion. Under these circumstances, the ideal goal of glucose control may not be achievable in many patients. It is important to realize, however, that all improvements in glucose control – even if the optimal level cannot be achieved – seem to have significant beneficial effects, such that any improvement can be considered worthwhile.

Experience from the American DCCT trial suggests that improving average hemoglobin A_{1c} in an IDDM population from 9 to 7% results in a 40% reduction in the risk of developing microalbuminuria.

The increase of hypoglycemic episodes and increased risk of ketoacidosis (with continuous subcutaneous insulin infusion) must of course be considered in deciding individual therapeutic goals.

Improved blood glucose control retards or prevents both the onset of microalbuminuria and (most likely) also glomerular morphological changes associated with the development of microalbuminuria. Some of the presumed renal risk markers for development of microalbuminuria may be reverted as well, such as glomerular hyperfiltration and renal enlargement.

Antihypertensive therapy Hypertension in *normoalbuminuric* diabetic patients should be treated using the indications that are also used in the nondiabetic population, recognizing that diabetes *per se* constitutes an additional cardiovascular risk factor.

The drugs of choice would be diuretics, ACE inhibitors, or calcium antagonists (possibly not nifedipine), favored for their efficacy in the *secondary prevention* and *treatment* of diabetic nephropathy (see below). Beta-blocking agents may be as effective, but they warrant specific attention to the risk of aggravating hypoglycemic episodes and exacerbation of insulin resistance.

The availability of ambulatory 24-hour blood pressure measurements may widen the indications for antihypertensive therapy.

Normotensive normoalbuminuric diabetic patients should not receive "antihypertensive" therapy with the aim of primary prevention of microalbuminuria.

Secondary prevention

Secondary prevention consists of preventing or retarding progression from the stage of microalbuminuria to overt diabetic nephropathy. Success in secondary prevention would then be to keep urinary albumin excretion below 300 mg per 24 hours. In addition, although not a formal criterion for the diagnosis of diabetic nephropathy, an additional goal of secondary prevention would be to keep the glomerular filtration rate within or slightly above the normal range.

More than half of the patients with microalbuminuria in the range of 100 to 300 mg per 24 hours will progress to overt diabetic nephropathy within 5 years. This number can be markedly reduced by early effective antihypertensive treatment, the use of ACE inhibitors even in normotensive patients, and possibly by strict metabolic control.

Routine clinical screening for the presence of microalbuminuria is mandatory in order to identify cases to enter the secondary prevention program.

Improved blood glucose control   Strict blood glucose control according to the criteria described under "primary prevention" reduces the rate of progression of microalbuminuria to diabetic nephropathy, including the associated development of arterial hypertension. Strict blood glucose control may also prevent the slight reduction in glomerular filtration rate appearing in some patients already at the stage of microalbuminuria. In addition, the development and progression of diabetic retinopathy is retarded in spite of the tendency to initial worsening of the retinopathy with sudden tightening of the metabolic control.

Again, the increased risk of hypoglycemic episodes and increased risk of ketoacidosis (with continuous subcutaneous insulin infusion) must be considered in deciding individual therapeutic goals.

It is estimated that the development of diabetic nephropathy can be prevented or retarded in two out of three microalbuminuria IDDM patients with successful improvement of blood glucose control. The clinical trials with improved blood glucose control have generally not included patients on regular antihypertensive treatment.

Antihypertensive therapy   "Antihypertensive" therapy retards or prevents the progression of microalbuminuria to overt diabetic nephropathy, notwithstanding the presence or absence of arterial hypertension. Both progression of albuminuria and decline in glomerular filtration rate are affected.

With ACE inhibitors, the beneficial effect is already seen at doses that do not reduce the systemic blood pressure. This reflects a specific effect of ACE inhibitors on intraglomerular pressure, which is being reduced through preferential dilatation of the glomerular efferent arteriole. Over 2 years, administration of an ACE inhibitor may prevent progression from microalbuminuria to overt diabetic nephropathy in two of three normotensive patients. The efficacy has been demonstrated both in IDDM and NIDDM patients.

With diuretics, beta-blockers, or calcium-antagonists, a decrease in albuminuria is seen only with lowering of the systemic blood pressure.

The short-acting calcium-antagonist nifedipine has not been very effective in preventing the development of diabetic nephropathy. The reason for its failure may be specific sympathetic and renin-angiotensin system-activating properties of nifedipine.

It follows that all diabetic patients with microalbuminuria should be considered for treatment with an ACE inhibitor, whether or not arterial hypertension is present.

Treatment of overt diabetic nephropathy

Improved blood glucose control   Unlike in primary or secondary prevention, strict blood glucose control has

only minor if any effects on the progression of diabetic nephropathy once persistent proteinuria above 300 mg per 24 hour is reached. This statement should not lead to ignoring the quality of blood glucose control, as other organ systems – such as the retina and the myocardium – may benefit from improved metabolic control. As noted above, the incidence of severe retinopathy and coronary heart disease is markedly elevated in patients with diabetic nephropathy.

Antihypertensive therapy   Antihypertensive therapy is the cornerstone of retarding the progression of established diabetic nephropathy. The treatment retards the progression of albuminuria and preserves kidney function so that the time until end-stage renal failure is markedly prolonged.

Unlike in microalbuminuric type 1 diabetes patients, the majority of patients with diabetic nephropathy will have arterial hypertension. As with microalbuminuria, however, the prescription of an antihypertensive drug must be considered in normotensive patients. The choice of treatment follows the considerations mentioned above (see "Secondary prevention"). Thus an ACE inhibition deserves specific attention in the treatment of diabetic nephropathy.

Effective antihypertensive therapy usually leads to an initial drop in glomerular filtration rate. The decline of the glomerular filtration rate is hereafter slowed down to 1/10 of the pre-treatment fall rate, so that the preventive effect of the treatment soon becomes apparent. Whereas the median survival time of patients was previously only 7 years from the onset of diabetic nephropathy, 10-year survival of more than 80% has been reported following administration of effective antihypertensive therapy.

Protein restriction has only a limited role in the treatment of diabetic nephropathy. A low protein diet (0.6-0.8 g/kg per day), however, can prevent or retard the progression of glomerulosclerosis, most likely by reducing glomerular hemodynamic stress. The readily measurable consequences of a shift to a low protein diet (and preferably with vegetable protein) is a reduction in urinary albumin excretion and in glomerular filtration rate, an effect similar to that obtained with antihypertensive treatment. An additive effect of protein restriction to ongoing antihypertensive treatment has not been demonstrated in diabetes.

A second major problem in protein restriction is poor patient compliance, hence long-term observance to a low protein diet is rather unlikely.

The recommendation is thus to generally avoid the *high* protein diet (above 1.0 g/kg per day) that is otherwise often prescribed to diabetic patients, and to consider a low protein diet only in the situation where massive proteinuria and declining glomerular filtration rate progresses, despite ongoing antihypertensive therapy.

Renal replacement therapy   Renal replacement therapy (dialysis and transplantation) must be considered in patients with diabetic nephropathy at an earlier time point than in nondiabetic patients with chronic renal insufficiency. This is because of the relatively poor general condition of the uremic diabetic patient due to the concurrent presence of generalized vascular disease.

When the glomerular filtration rate approaches 25 ml per minute measured with a valid technique (e.g., ^{51}CrEDTA clearance), the time has come for referral to a nephrologist. Dependent upon muscle mass and dietary protein consumption, this may correspond to a serum creatinine level as low as 150 µmol/l.

The choice between dialysis (CAPD or hemodialysis) or transplantation depends upon individual preference and the availability of a suitable donor. Diabetics generally experience only a slightly poorer prognosis on renal replacement therapy than nondiabetics.

Blood glucose control is complicated by fluctuating insulin requirements. In addition, measurement of hemoglobin-A_{1c} may not give a valid estimate of long-term metabolic control in the uremic patient. When peritoneal dialysis is preferred, addition of insulin to the dialysis solution will often lead to a marked improvement of blood glucose control.

To prevent malnutrition, diabetic patients on renal replacement therapy should receive a high protein content diet.

An extensive work-up to disclose the presence of associated coronary heart disease, which is often silent, must be considered.

Successful combined renal and pancreas transplantation obviously creates optimal metabolic control. The initial enthusiasm with the procedure has declined, however, due to the associated technical problems.

Handling of associated angiopathy The increased prevalence of associated vascular disease demands specific attention in all patients with diabetic nephropathy.

Coronary heart disease – often silent – should be pursued and treated with persistence.

Plasma lipid status should be obtained, and elevated LDL and triglyceride levels should be treated vigorously. The use of beta-blocking agents in patients with established coronary heart disease should generally not be withheld unless the patients are faced with unwieldy problems with hypoglycemic events or other contraindications.

Annual ophthalmological examinations should be performed, even in the rare patient with no initial evidence of diabetic retinopathy.

Prognosis

The potential prognostic impact of the preventive and therapeutic regimens are described above. Early aggressive antihypertensive treatment in patients with established diabetic nephropathy has been implemented for more than a decade. The current data suggests that the 10-year mortality rate in IDDM patients following onset of diabetic nephropathy is now reduced to 10 to 20%. The

major causes of death are end-stage renal disease (2/3) and cardiovascular disease (1/4). The ultimate prospect for future prevention and treatment of diabetic nephropathy will be to reduce the mortality to match normoalbuminuric diabetic patients, that is, a relative mortality of 2 to 4 compared to the nondiabetic population.

The prognosis of diabetic nephropathy in older Caucasian NIDDM patients differs from that described above in the IDDM patients. Whereas the 10-year incidence of end-stage renal disease is 50% in IDDM, it is only 5 to 10% in NIDDM; and whereas the mortality in IDDM patients with diabetic nephropathy is up to 40-fold higher than in normoalbuminuric IDDM patients, the excess mortality in the older Caucasian NIDDM patients with diabetic nephropathy is around twofold. The differences are mainly due to the increased prevalence of competing causes of mortality in the aged NIDDM patient. Selected populations of young NIDDM patients show prognostic features much like that of IDDM patients.

It is still discussed whether late onset microalbuminuria (e.g., onset after 20 years of diabetes duration) may carry a better prognosis than early onset microalbuminuria. If this is the case, a less strenuous therapeutic attitude may be justified. This is often reflected in recommendations to initiate treatment "especially in young diabetic patients". However, there is only very little evidence to suggest that the differences in time of onset reflects essentially different diseases.

SELECTED TOPICS

Diabetic nephropathy in IDDM versus NIDDM

The Pima Indians, who have a high risk of developing NIDDM at young age, develop a diabetic nephropathy that functionally, morphologically, and with regard to prognosis for survival and development of end-stage renal failure, is virtually identical to that of IDDM patients. Otherwise, the occurrence of diabetic nephropathy in, for example, older Caucasian NIDDM patients, is influenced by their much more prevalent competing causes of morbidity and mortality. Current knowledge gives no reason to doubt that similar central mechanisms are operating in the pathogenesis of diabetic nephropathy in NIDDM and IDDM, however.

Among the preventive and therapeutic regimes discussed above, the efficacy of antihypertensive treatment – including the use of ACE inhibitors in normotensive microalbuminuria patients – is also documented in NIDDM. Reduced insulin sensitivity following beta-blocker or thiazide prescription may promote hyperglycemia in the NIDDM patient.

The efficacy of strict blood glucose control in the primary and secondary prevention of diabetic nephropathy in NIDDM has not been evaluated as yet.

Diabetic nephropathy and pregnancy

Pregnancy in diabetic nephropathy remains a challenge due to an increased risk of pregnancy complications. The complications are primarily preeclampsia and anemia, occurring in as many as every second case. Malformations and perinatal death have been reported in 8 and 5%, respectively. The number of complications increases and maternal postpartum life expectancy decreases with decreasing renal function. The decision to counsel against pregnancy must be individualized.

When glomerular filtration rate has declined below 40 to 50 ml per minute, pregnancy should probably be considered contraindicated.

As in all diabetic women, pregnancy must be carefully planned and preceded by strict blood glucose control. Ongoing antihypertensive treatment should be adjusted, recalling that *ACE inhibitors are contraindicated* in pregnancy and that several calcium-antagonists are best avoided during the first trimester.

Pregnancy may induce transient progression of diabetic nephropathy, especially an increase in urinary albumin excretion, but it is not generally associated with a worsening of the prognosis. Retinopathy may progress, and a sudden onset of proliferative lesions can require prompt treatment.

OTHER RENAL AND URINARY TRACT DISEASES ASSOCIATED WITH DIABETES

Renal papillary necrosis

Renal papillary necrosis (RPN) has been found in 4 to 8% of diabetic patients at autopsy. On the other hand, diabetes represents the single most common disease associated with RPN (50 to 60% of cases in the United States), exceeded by analgesics abuse in countries with more liberal access to these drugs. The course of the disease is often silent, except for a moderate increase in urinary protein excretion and sometimes gross hematuria, but RPN can ultimately lead to renal failure.

The main causes of RPN in diabetes are ischemia and pyelonephritis. Analgesics that inhibit cyclooxygenase (i.e., NSAIDs) may provoke ischemic papillary lesions.

Prompt treatment of urinary tract infections and discouraging the use of NSAIDs in diabetic patients is therefore recommended.

Urinary tract infection

Diabetic patients are more susceptible to the development of urinary tract infections, both bacterial and fungal, and they are more likely to cause complications in diabetic patients. Ascending infection with renal involvement should be suspected in the diabetic patient who does not respond to relevant antibiotic therapy in 3 to 4 days.

The diagnosis of fungal infections demands characterization to exclude simple colonization. More than 10 000 colonies per ml indicates a need for antifungal treatment.

Neurogenic bladder dysfunction

Neurogenic bladder dysfunction with a decreased sensation of fullness, bladder enlargement, and abnormal contractions resulting in significant residual urine is very common in diabetes. Therapy includes scheduled repetitive voiding, cholinergic drugs (bethanechol), alpha-adrenergic blocking agents, intermittent self-catheterization, and surgical release of the internal bladder sphincter.

Measurement of postvoidal residual urine assures therapeutic efficacy.

DIABETIC NEUROPATHY

Göran Sundkvist

Three main types of diabetic neuropathies are distinguishable: (1) peripheral neuropathy, (2) autonomic neuropathy, and (3) mononeuropathies.

PERIPHERAL NEUROPATHY

Epidemiology

Diabetic peripheral neuropathy is a frequent complication of diabetes, particularly if quantitative objective neurophysiological nerve function tests are included. Depending on the definition of neuropathy, the frequency of peripheral neuropathy varies between 25 to 35%, and it is over 40% in elderly diabetic patients. If peripheral neuropathy is defined as absent ankle reflexes and/or an abnormal vibration sense, 50% of patients have peripheral neuropathy after 25 years of diabetes. There are no major differences between type 1 and type 2 diabetes with regard to peripheral neuropathy.

Pathogenesis

Peripheral neuropathy is associated with hyperglycemia. Hyperglycemia favors deterioration in nerve function and normalization of glycemic control improvement. The mechanism behind this association is not completely clear; several different factors are thought to be involved. Hyperglycemia favors accumulation of sorbitol, advanced glycosylation end products, and free radicals in nerve tissue. In the experimental situation, all of these biochemical factors contribute to impairments in peripheral nerve function. Vascular factors, however, also contribute to nerve damage; occlusions and functional disturbances in the nutritive vessels of the peripheral nerves are found in diabetic patients.

Clinical findings

Peripheral neuropathy is defined as the presence of symptoms and/or signs of peripheral nerve dysfunction in people with diabetes when other causes of neuropathy have been excluded. The main symptoms of peripheral neuropathy are described in Table 59.3 and shown in Figure 59.13.

Symptoms and signs

Absent ankle tendon reflexes

Testing ankle reflexes is a simple but surprisingly reliable test of peripheral nerve function. Indeed, if examination of the ankle reflexes is compared with a complete neurological examination, this simple test seems to be as efficient to detect peripheral neuropathy as a complete neurological examination conducted by a neurologist.

Abnormal vibration sense

Using a 128 Hz tuning fork, a lack or a clearly deficient vibration sense on the toe or the ankle is abnormal. Determination of vibration thresholds with a biothesiometer give quantitative values easy to follow prospectively. A biothesiometer vibration threshold value >25 V predicts future foot complications.

Pressure (protective) perception

Absence of sensation in the foot to a 5.07 (10 g bending force) disposable nylon-monofilament is abnormal. The plantar aspects of the distal phalanx of the great toe and the first, third, and fifth metatarsal heads are tested. If the filament is not felt on any of the test sites, there is a clear loss of pressure perception, thus increasing the risk for foot ulcers.

Pin prick Use a disposable pin and ask the patient whether it is painful. Do not ask if it is felt!

Light touch Use a cotton wisp and ask the patient whether it is felt or not.

Most of these signs will be detected by a simple clinical examination that should be conducted at least once a year in all diabetic patients. Only unclear cases need further investigation at a neurophysiological laboratory.

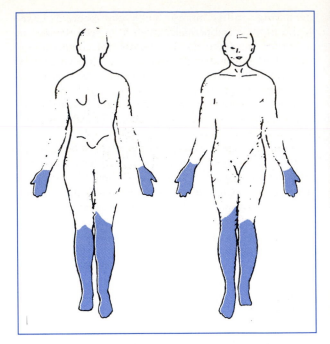

Figure 59.13 In diabetic peripheral neuropathy, sensory loss is most severe in distal (shadowed in blue) parts of the extremities. In the legs, sensory loss is mostly associated with absent ankle reflexes. Sensory loss may be perceived as a "dead feeling" or "emptiness" but is often not noticed by the patient. Diabetic peripheral neuropathy is sometimes accompanied by different types of pain: unusual tenderness (allodynia), "prickling" or "tingling", "jabbing" needle-like or pulses, burning, or aching.

Diagnosis

If a patient has both symptoms and signs of peripheral neuropathy, there is no doubt about the diagnosis of clinical peripheral neuropathy. The most frequent form of peripheral neuropathy is, however, asymptomatic (no symptoms but positive signs of peripheral neuropathy). On the other hand, it is not always clear that a patient with symptoms but without signs is affected by peripheral neuropathy. After the start of insulin treatment, however, recently diagnosed patients with poorly controlled diabetes sometimes develop an acute painful neuropathy without showing signs of peripheral neuropathy.

There are disorders associated with diabetes that may result in peripheral neuropathy. Hence, in diabetic patients with peripheral neuropathy, always consider: (1) vitamin B_{12} deficiency, (2) hypothyroidism, (3) gluten intolerance, (4) high consumption of alcohol, and (5) hepatological problems.

Actions to be taken after diagnosis of peripheral neuropathy

Acute/chronic painful peripheral neuropathy

- Improve and stabilize glycemic control (normalization of HbA_{1c}).
- Simple analgesics.

Table 59.3 Symptoms of peripheral neuropathy

Pain (burning, shooting, stabbing); often increased at night

Pins and needles (paresthesia)

Increased skin sensitivity (allodynia)

Foot lesions (pes cavus, toe deformities, callus formation on foot plant, ulcers below metatarsal heads)

Charcot joints (swelling of foot and ankle; pseudoinflammation, pseudofractures)

Negative symptoms (inability to perceive due to sensory loss)

- Tricyclic antidepressive drugs such as amitriptyline, nortriptyline ("old antidepressives"; blockers of noradrenaline uptake should be used) are effective. Start with 25 mg at bedtime and increase to 50 mg after 2 weeks; if needed increase to 75 to 100 mg. Inform the patient that it will take 2 to 3 weeks until there is an effect. Clarify that the drug has an effect on peripheral nerves and not on the mood. Serotonin reuptake inhibitors and mianserin do not work.
- In patients not responding to tricyclic antidepressive drugs gabapentin (300 mg × 3 increasing to 1800 mg/day orally) may be worth a trial.
- In patients with lancinating (electric shock-like) pain, carbamazepine (100 mg once or twice a day; if needed gradually increasing to a maximal dosage of 800 to 1000 mg) may be of value. If carbamazepine does not work, phenytoin (100-400 mg per day) or valproate (100-500 mg per day) may be tried.
- Lignocaine iv and/or mexiletine orally are the third choice but must be considered as drugs for the specialist to prescribe (refer the patient).
- Trials with local treatment with capsaicin have suggested some effect against burning pain, but the results are not very convincing. In some countries the analgesic drug tramadol has been suggested when simple analgesics such as aspirin or acetaminophen are unsatisfactory for pain control in patients with diabetic neuropathy. Tramadol should not be combined with tricyclic medication, however.
- No improvement of pain: refer to a diabetologist/neurologist.

Painless peripheral neuropathy (loss of sensation neuropathy)

- Educating the patient on good foot care is very important.
- Improve glycemic control.
- Follow the patient carefully.

Based on the presumed pathogenesis, many clinical control trials of aldose reductase inhibitors, antioxidants, and vasodilators have been conducted. Unfortunately, although these compounds have been most successful in experimental diabetes, all clinical trials with these compounds have been without effect on human diabetic neuropathy. In addition, no controlled clinical trials supports the use of vitamin B (thiamine) as a remedy for diabetic neuropathy. Certainly there is a need for new and effective drugs to prevent and treat peripheral neuropathy in diabetic patients.

AUTONOMIC NEUROPATHY

Epidemiology

Signs of autonomic neuropathy, based on cardiovascular tests, are frequent (16 to 40%) in clinical reports, but large population-based studies are missing. The frequency of symptoms of autonomic neuropathy in diabetic patients is unknown.

Pathogenesis

Similar pathogenic mechanisms of peripheral neuropathy are considered for autonomic neuropathy. There are differences between autonomic neuropathy and peripheral neuropathy, however; hypoinsulinemia predicts peripheral neuropathy whereas hyperinsulinemia is associated with autonomic neuropathy, and autoimmunity against nerve structures may have a role in the development of autonomic neuropathy. Nevertheless, hyperglycemia seems to be deleterious for the autonomic nervous system; improvement in glycemic control is associated with improved autonomic nerve function both in type 1 and type 2 diabetes.

Clinical findings

Ideally, the presence of symptoms (Tab. 59.4) in combination with objective signs of autonomic neuropathy is the definition of autonomic neuropathy. In clinical practice, however, the definition is not that simple. A variety of symptoms have been attributed to autonomic neuropathy. Accordingly, the concept that autonomic neuropathy should be considered as a patchy disorder has been coined; that is, in the individual patient, autonomic neuropathy may affect one, several, or all innervated organs. However, the autonomic nervous system has two main components: the parasympathetic and the sympathetic systems. Hence, from a holistic point of view, autonomic neuropathy is a generalized disorder of parasympathetic and/or sympathetic damage involving parasympathetic and/or parasympathetic target organs. Thus a patchy engagement may simply reflect the difficulties in assessment. More sensitive meth-

---

Table 59.4 Important symptoms of autonomic neurophathy

Cardiovascular symptoms
  General
    Disturbed circadian blood pressure, sudden death
  Dizziness (unsteady when standing)
  Edema

Genital and urological symptoms
  Male sexual dysfunction
    Insufficient erection
    Disturbed ejaculation
    Retrograde ejaculation
  Female sexual dsyfunction
    Reduced lubrication
  Bladder dysfunction

Gastrointestinal symptoms
  Vomiting
  Diarrhea

Sweating disturbances
  Gustatory sweating
  Deficient sweating

ods than those currently available should enable a more extensive autonomic neuropathy to be revealed.

A large variation of symptoms has been associated with autonomic neuropathy. In many patients symptoms are vague and difficult to distinguish from those of other possible disorders. Although the recent development of quantitative tests of autonomic nerve function has facilitated the diagnosis of autonomic neuropathy, most tests are cardiovascular, and autonomic neuropathy is not only a cardiovascular disorder. Some tests are complicated and not available for clinical use. Accordingly, in clinical practice an evaluation of symptoms reported by the patient, a simple test of autonomic function such as the heart rate reaction during deep breathing (see below), and the general impression (other complications, etc.) of the diabetic patient are the basis for the clinical diagnosis of autonomic neuropathy. Quantitative tests may show abnormalities, however – that is, signs of autonomic neuropathy – although no symptoms are usually reported.

In clinical practice, the physician must resolve the patient's complaints. Specific diagnostic methods and treatments are symptom-oriented. Before discussing the handling of various symptoms, a simple quantitative test of autonomic neuropathy will be described below.

Deep breathing test

The deep breathing test is still the simplest and most reliable test of autonomic nerve function and can be carried out at any doctor's office. In this test, the patient breathes deeply during one minute of continuous ECG recording. The longest RR intervals of the ECG (during Expiration) and the shortest (during Inspiration) are selected (Fig. 59.14), and the E/I ratio is then calculated (E/I ratio = mean longest RR interval/mean shortest RR interval).

The E/I ratio measures parasympathetic nerve function, that is, a low value indicates parasympathetic nerve dysfunction. A value of the E/I ratio <1.21 is clearly abnormal in individuals below 40 years of age, <1.15 in those between 40 to 50 years of age, and <1.10 is clearly abnormal in those

>50 years of age. The interpretation is simple. If a patient with symptoms of autonomic neuropathy (AN) shows a normal E/I ratio then the diagnosis of AN is unlikely; whereas if the test is positive, the diagnosis of AN is confirmed.

Cardiovascular manifestations

General (including "sudden death")

Sudden death is a symptom of autonomic neuropathy. It has been suggested that disturbed respiratory reflexes rather than disturbed cardiac reflexes are involved. Recently, however, autonomic neuropathy has been associated with ventricular extra-systoles, disturbed cardiac function, and silent myocardial ischemia. The 24-hour circadian blood pressure profile is disturbed in diabetic patients with autonomic neuropathy; the normal dip in blood pressure during the night is lost. The abnormality is associated with increased cardiac muscle wall thickness and may also contribute to kidney dysfunction; autonomic neuropathy predicts future falls in glomerular filtration rate. In diabetic patients, beta-blockers are particularly life saving after myocardial infarction. Beta-blockers increase parasympathetic nerve tone via the central nervous system; normalization of parasympathetic nerve tone may explain the favorable effect of beta-blockers on survival after myocardial infarction in diabetic patients.

Dizziness

Postural symptoms are often vague and anemia, epilepsy, and cardiovascular diseases must always be excluded.

Diagnosis A systolic blood pressure drop of ≥ 30 mmHg indicates an abnormal systolic blood pressure fall. The normal postural diastolic blood pressure reaction is an increase in diastolic blood pressure; a lack of rise or fall in diastolic blood pressure is therefore a sign of autonomic neuropathy.

Treatment Physical training and the compression of legs and/or lower body (corset) may be tried. Circulatory stimulating pharmacological agents in general have been used

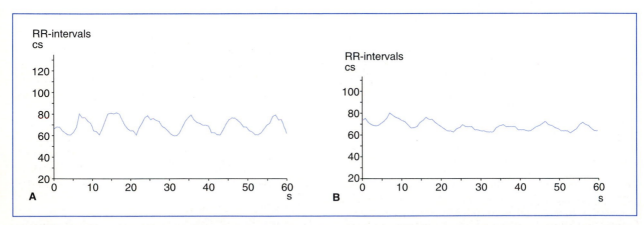

Figure 59.14 **(A)** A patient demonstrating a normal E/I ratio (1.33 in a 43-year-old woman). **(B)** A patient demonstrating an abnormal E/I ratio (1.13 in a 38-year-old woman.)

without success. Recently the peripherally alpha agonist midodrine has been registered in some countries for use in orthostatic hypotension. In severe cases, mineralocorticoids (fludrocortisone) may be used.

Edema

Edema, unrelated to renal or cardiac dysfunction, has been described in patients with a long duration of diabetes. Increased arterio-venous shunting has been assumed to explain this condition. Treatment with ephedrine orally may reduce this type of edema; the mechanism is believed to be closure of the shunts.

Genital and urological symptoms

Erectile dysfunction is defined as an inability to achieve or maintain an erection sufficient for coitus. In diabetic men a mixture of psychogenic, arterial, and nervous factors contribute. In principle, there is a gradual loss of erectile function when organic causes are involved. Total impotency may develop in as many as 50% of diabetic men. The nerve component of erectile dysfunction is parasympathetic neuropathy. Diabetic men may also suffer from ejaculative failure, a sympathetic neuropathy manifestation, that could lead to retrograde ejaculation and fertility problems.

Diagnosis A progressive erectile disturbance in a patient with at lest 15 to 20 years of diabetes is consistent with a diabetes-related disturbance. The clinical examination should include penile inspection and palpation, testicular palpation, palpation of the prosthetic gland, examination of secondary sexual characteristics, pulse palpation of leg and inguinal vessels, and a neurological examination with regard to peripheral neuropathy.

Treatment If erectile dysfunction is suspected, it might also be appropriate for the primary caring physician to give an iv injection of vasoactive drugs, most often prostaglandin E1 (alprostadil) or a combination of papaverine and phentolamine (15-60 mg/0.5-2 mg). If a sustained erection is achieved, venous incompetence and sinusoidal disorder can be ruled out and the patient can be directly offered autoinjection treatment with the appropriate drug; urethral suppository of alprostadil is available in some countries, or vacuum devices. If the physician is unfamiliar with intracavernous injections or if the case is untypical, the patient should be referred to a urologist. Patients with ejaculation disturbances with a wish to conceive should always be referred to a urologist.

Recently sildenafil has been introduced for oral treatment of erectile dysfunction. Sildenafil inhibits phosphodiesterase type 5 leading to elevation in cGMP thereby increasing smooth muscle relaxation and erection. Sildanafil has to be taken one hour before planned sexual activity; 50 mg as a start dose is recommended. In diabetic men 100 mg is often needed. Sildenafil should not be used together with nitroglycerine or in patients with recent myocardial infarction.

Female sexual dysfunction

Compared with men, women with diabetes have previously been thought to be spared from sexual dysfunction,

however, recent studies have shown that this is not true. Women with diabetes often have a reduced sexual desire, which not only could be due to difficulties to coping with the disease and hypoglycemia but also to reduced lubrication, reported in higher frequency among women with diabetes than in other women. Although this reduction could be related to hyperglycemia, nerve dysfunction is a plausible explanation. Reduced lubrication reduces sexual pleasure and treatment with lubricants or estrogen creams are appropriate.

Bladder dysfunction

Bladder problems are an uncommon clinical problem. A large, nonsensitive bladder is not infrequent in long-term diabetic patients, however, and it is sometimes a problem in kidney transplanted patients.

Gastrointestinal symptoms

Vomiting

Gastric atonia may explain vomiting. Autonomic neuropathy may slow gastric emptying; however, hyperglycemia may also lead to a functional slowing of gastric motility, reversible when normoglycemia is achieved. Anorectic behavior in young women with diabetes must always also be considered. Although esophageal motility disturbances have been connected with autonomic neuropathy, this is associated with difficulties in swallowing rather than vomiting.

Diagnosis A normal E/I ratio in the deep breathing test makes it unlikely that autonomic neuropathy causes vomiting. If hyperglycemia and anorectic behavior are unlikely, further investigation is needed (manometry, scintigraphy, electrogastrography) at special laboratories.

Treatment Normalization of hyperglycemia. If a motility disturbance has been proven, motility stimulating drugs – that is, oral cisapride or oral erythromycin (the latter works on the motilin receptor) – may be tried.

Diarrhea

Nocturnal diarrhea is a rare symptom of autonomic neuropathy. The background is obscure and could be bacterial overgrowth in, by autonomic neuropathy, primarily obstipated bowels. Anal sphincter insufficiency is sometimes also present.

Diagnosis Other causes of diarrhea to be considered are gluten intolerance and exocrine pancreatic failure. Rectal palpation may reveal a loose anal sphincter. Some favor a test of bacterial overgrowth (hydrogen breathing test) before treatment.

Treatment A trial with oral tetracycline for 2 to 4 weeks is the first option. Temporary codeine may be necessary.

Antibiotics of other types may also be tried if tetracycline does not inhibit the diarrhea. In most cases the diarrhea disappears but may later return; in such cases, repeat the previous treatment.

Sweating disturbances

Gustatory sweating

Profuse sweating appears in the face and on the neck when eating spicy food. The background is thought to be a degeneration of sympathetic nerves leading to a regeneration of parasympathetic nerves growing into the cervical ganglion.

Diagnosis Provocation confirms the clinical suspicion. Almost all patients demonstrate abnormal deep breathing tests.

Treatment Topical glycopyrrolate was recently shown to be the specific treatment for diabetic gustatory sweating.

Deficient sweating

Sympathetic denervation leads to a lack of sweating on the leg. Patients may therefore have compensatory increased sweating on other parts of the body, sometimes by mistake considered as hypoglycemic sweating. Lack of sweating on the lower leg makes the skin dry and thereby increases the risk for skin lesions and ulcers.

Diagnosis Dry skin at clinical examination.

Treatment Moisture creams.

MONONEUROPATHIES

Epidemiology

The prevalence of mononeuropathies is rare: 2 to 3 cases per 1000 patients per year. It is more frequent in type 2 than in type 1 diabetic patients.

Pathogenesis

Pathogenesis is unclear, but vascular occlusion and secondary infarctions are suspected. There is no clear relationship to high blood glucose values.

Clinical findings

Cranial nerves (N.III) leading to ptosis and lateral deviation of the eye or (N.VI) paralysis of the abducent nerve. The paralysis is often preceded by pain. Paralysis of the facial nerve may be another manifestation.

Diagnosis

Most patients need to be referred to an ophthalmologist and/or otologist for diagnosis and local treatment.

Treatment

Paralysis mostly improves during a month or two, and persistent problems are rare. Glycemic control in most patients is satisfactory. Insulin treatment in type 2 diabetes patients will not improve the neuropathy.

Truncal neuropathy

Patients with long-term diabetes suddenly develop intensive local pain on the chest or on the abdomen. The pain is often radiating and most intense during the night. Weight loss may be a feature.

Diagnosis In the region of pain, there is sensory loss and a flaccid muscle; the muscle is bulging. Electromyography shows denervation phenomenon.

Treatment Treatment involves symptomatic analgesics and careful explanation to the patient about the nature of the disorder. Symptomatic truncal neuropathy mostly disappears within 2 to 3 months.

Compression neuropathies

Median nerve entrapment in the carpal tunnel is 2 to 3 times more frequent in diabetic patients compared with others. Ulnar nerve entrapment at the elbow is also more frequent in diabetic than other subjects.

Pathogenesis Diabetic nerves are vulnerable to pressure (ischemia?).

Diagnosis Pain in the hand in the morning combined with difficulties in using the fingers are symptoms suggestive of median nerve entrapment. Muscle atrophy of the thenar eminence of the palm, loss of palmar sensation of the first, second, third, and lateral half of the fourth fingers and of the major portion of the palm confirms the diagnosis. Ulnar nerve entrapment is suggested from pain in the elbow region in combination with loss of sensation from the medial part of the hand, the fifth finger, and the medial side of the fourth finger, and atrophy of the intrinsic muscle in the space between the thumb and the index finger at the first dorsal interosseous muscle (defective thumb adduction).

Treatment Treatment is surgical decompression.

Diabetic amyotrophy (proximal motor neuropathy)

Diabetic amyotrophy (proximal motor neuropathy) is a rare but serious complication that usually affects elderly diabetic patients.

Pathogenesis Unknown.

Symptoms A sudden weakness in the tight muscle unilaterally, sometimes bilaterally, develops. The patient has clear difficulties walking. The patellar reflex deficiency corresponds to the muscle weakness.

Diagnosis The patient should be referred to a specialist/diabetologist. Electrophysiology is always indicated.

Treatment Insulin treatment motivated in orally treated type 2 diabetic patients. Physical treatment and rehabilitation are essential. Most patients improve within 2 years.

THE DIABETIC FOOT

Jan M. Apelqvist

Epidemiology

The diabetic foot can be defined as a condition that includes infection, ulceration, and destruction of deep tissues associated with neurological abnormalities and peripheral vascular disease in the lower limbs. In the Western world, diabetic foot lesions are the most common reason for hospital admission in patients with diabetes. Treatment of diabetic foot lesions are associated with high cost, especially in cases of amputation due to in-hospitalization, rehabilitation, and an increased need for home care and social services. Forty to 60% of all lower leg amputations are related to diabetes mellitus. In some areas, proportions of up to 70 to 90% have been reported. More than 70% of all diabetes-related amputations are preceded by a foot ulcer. The most common reason for an amputation is a foot ulcer deteriorating due to deep infection or ischemia. The prevalence of foot ulcers has been estimated to be 4 to 10% in patients with NIDDM, with a majority of patients over 60 years of age. The incidence of foot ulcers in diabetic persons has been reported to range from 2.4 to 5.7%.

Factors associated with foot ulcer

The major factors that increase the risk of ulcers and amputations are peripheral neuropathy, altered biomechanics, peripheral vascular disease, and skin pathology, including a history of foot ulcers (Tab. 59.5). Signs of sensomotor-neuropathy has been established in 70 to 100% of diabetic subjects with a foot ulcer. The progress of loss of protective sensation is slowly (usually not initially) recognized by the patient, which makes regular foot inspection mandatory (monofilament, vibratory sensation, tendon reflexes) for signs of muscle wasting and/or atrophy. In 4 out of 5 cases of foot ulcer, a precipitating extrinsic or intrinsic trauma can be verified. The most common extrinsic factors are the use of poor footwear, walking barefoot, and other trauma caused by loss of protective sensations, including pain, pressure, and temperature. The motor-neuropathy results in atrophy of

Table 59.5 Factors associated with foot ulcer
Age

Socioeconomic status
     Low social position
     Access to health care
     Compliance/neglect
     Education

Neuropathy
     Sensomotor dysfunction
     Autonomic neuropathy

Peripheral vascular disease
Metabolic control

Extrinsic factors
     Poor footwear
     Walking barefoot
     Fall/accidents
     Objects inside shoes

Intrinsic factors
     Limited joint mobility
     Bony prominences
     Foot deformity/osteoarthropathy
     Callus

intrinsic muscles that result in foot deformities (prominent metatarsal heads, claw-toes).

In the presence of sensory neuropathy that leads to an elevated plant of pressure and shear stress to specific regions of the plantar area of the foot during walking. This pressure causes initial tissue damage such as blister, hemorrhage, minor skin injury, and later as callus formation. If this condition continues without proper protection, an intrinsic ulcer (stress ulcer, mal perforance) develops, with a high probability for developing foot infection. A strong relation has been established between abnormal foot pressure and incidence of these plantar ulcerations. The autonomic neuropathy creates changes in skin-blood flow, impaired sweating (cracked/dry skin), arterial-venous shunting and edema. Diabetes has also been shown to be associated with restrictions in range of motion of the joints and tendons, which causes the ligaments to be stiff, creating what is often called the "stiff foot syndrome." The mechanism has been related to a disturbed metabolism of collagen and nonenzymatic glycosylation. Neuropathy is further considered to be one of the fundamental factors leading to diabetic osteoarthropathy.

Stiff foot syndrome is one of the most devastating foot complications of diabetes. Initial symptoms usually included hot, erythematous edema in a foot with or without pain and initially no radiographic changes. There is often a rapid progression on X-ray of bone destruction, fractures, and destruction of joints. Collapse of the medial longitudinal arch of the foot leads to deformities under which large ulcers typically develop. Precipitating trauma is often reported by the patient. Treatment in the acute face is immediate nonweight bearing, usually with total contact casting. Weight-bearing should not be started until inflammatory signs have diminished. In cases of severe foot deformities, orthopedic reconstruction of inactive osteoarthropathic feet can be performed. The etiology of this process is unknown, but it is clearly related to neuropathy and believed to be caused from a combination of sensomotor dysfunction and arterio-venous shunting, causing hyperperfusion, bone-demineralization and increased mechanical stress. Suspected neuro-osteoarthropathy should always be referred to a specialist of the diabetic foot. Vibrate threshold tests for vibration and light touch provide the best tools in the clinical setting for identifying persons with a loss of protective sensation. The most commonly recommended tools are the Semmes-Weinstein monofilament (5.07; 10 g) or tuning fork (128 Hz) (Tab. 59.6).

Prevalence of neuropathy increases with age, duration of diabetes, microangiopathy, and poor glycemic control (IDDM).

Peripheral vascular disease in diabetic subjects usually affects the femoral and iliac arteries in similar rates as nondiabetics, but it is more likely to distally involve the vessels below the knee and usually spares the foot. The most common symptoms of peripheral vascular disease are claudication and rest pain. These symptoms are strongly related to the probability of amputation, but a substantial number of diabetic patients with foot ulcerations do not have them despite the presence of severe peripheral vascular disease. Only 50% of patients with diabetes and gangrene have been shown to have rest pain.

Absence of palpable pedal pulses is a sign of peripheral vascular disease. However, palpation is greatly effected by a room temperature, biological variation, and skill of the practitioner, and it is considered to have poor reproducibility. As a consequence, noninvasive vascular testing is usually recommended in cases of the diabetic foot and foot ulcer. Noninvasive vascular evaluation, such as systolic toe or ankle blood pressure, are important to identify ischemia in the diabetic foot.

The risk of foot ulcers and amputation increases with both age and duration of diabetes. Male-sex has been associated with an increased risk of ulcers and amputation in most studies of patients with NIDDM. However, the findings are inconsistent, and short-term outcome studies of foot ulcers found no relation with regard to sex. Increased probability for foot ulcer and amputation has also been related to socioeconomic status such as low social position, lack of access to health care, and lack of patient education. The condition of willful self-neglect has also been described. The influence of race is controversial. Nonwhite race has been associated with increased risk of foot ulcer or amputation in some reports. In most cases, however, they have not been corrected for socioeconomic status. Poor glycemic control increases a risk for microangiopathy and neuropathy and has been related to amputation. The risk of diabetic foot disease is associated with co-morbid conditions including microangiopathy, especially albuminuria and macrovascular disease (stroke, congestive heart failure, and ischemic heart disease).

Prevention

The feet should be examined regularly at every routine visit (Tab. 59.6). Socks and shoes should be removed and the patient should be encouraged to examine their own feet. The patient should be educated regarding self-care practices of foot care (Tab. 59.12).

Shoes and particularly insoles should be frequently inspected and replaced when necessary. Patients with high risk feet should have access to podiatric care. Programs including regular foot inspection, education, podiatric care, and the use of adequate protective shoes and education have shown to substantially decrease the number of foot lesions.

Table 59.6 Physical examination of the foot

Neuropathy
  Muscle wasting/atropathy
  Sensory/vibratory threshold
  Tuning fork (128 Hz)
  Monofilament (5.07/10 g)
  Biothesiometer (>25)

Vascular
  Palpable pulses
  Rubor on dependency
  Capillary filling time

Skin
  Skin temperature
  Ingrown nails
  Callosities ulcer
  Edema

Bone
  Foot deformities
  Joint deformities
  Bony prominences
  Limited joint mobility
  Previous amputation

Table 59.7 Factors associated with outcome for foot ulceration

Age, sex, race
Duration and type of diabetes
Peripheral vascular disease
Infection
Microangiopathy
Type, site, cause of ulcer
Limited joint mobility, foot deformity
Edema
Multiple cardiovascular disease
Smoking
Metabolic factors

Diabetic foot: outcome and management

There is a complexity of factors related to outcome of foot ulcer in diabetic subjects, and the importance of evaluating these factors is well recognized (Tabs. 59.7-59.9).

Type, sight, and cause of ulcer

Most ulcers can be classified as either neuropathic, ischemic, or neuroischemic. Only a minority of ulcers are purely ischemic. The majority of ulcers are caused by a combination of neuropathy and varying degrees of peripheral vascular disease. An ulcer caused by extrinsic trauma such as ill-fitting shoes or acute mechanical trauma are usually localized to digits or dorsum of the foot. An intrinsic ulcer is usually localized to metatarsal heads and decubital ulcers, mostly to the heel (see Fig. 59.15, see Color Atlas). Ischemic ulcers are more common on the tips of the toes or the lateral border of the foot. Foot ulcers located to the heel and multiple ulcers are strongly related to amputation or death because of more severe peripheral vascular disease and multiple cardiovascular disease. Ulcers on the metatarsal heads have a high probability for primary healing but also have a high recurrence rate. The healing rate of the lesion is also related to the exposure of tissue such as muscle, bone, or continuous necrosis of skin and underlying tissue (gangrene). A systematic assessment of foot and corresponding ulcer is mandatory for management of the patient (Tab. 59.8). It can be concluded that type, site, and cause of ulcer are related to outcome and must be considered when treatment strategies are chosen.

Peripheral vascular disease

Peripheral vascular disease is the most important factor related to the outcome of foot ulcer and to the probability

Table 59.9 Management of diabetic foot ulcer

Improve circulation
  Noninvasive vascular testing
  PTA
  Vascular surgery

Treat edema

Treat infection
  Antibiotics
  Oral
  Parenteral
  Culture, biopsy
  X-ray, CT, bone scan, MRI

Treat pain

Non-weight-bearing
  Protective/therapeutic shoes
  Insoles/orthoses
  Contact casting
  Crutches
  Wheelchair

Topical treatment
  Debridement
  Dressings
  Topical agents
  Skin grafting

Improve metabolic control

Foot surgery
  Incision/drainage
  Corrective surgery
  Amputation

General condition
  Cardiovascular treatment
  Microangiopathy
  Malnutrition
  Smoking

Setting
  Patient/staff education
  Compliance
  Support follow-up
  Multidisciplinary

Table 59.8 Assessment of foot ulcer

Cause	Neuropathy, ischemia, extrinsic/intrinsic trauma
Site, size, type	Plantar, dorsal, interdigital, depth, size, tissue involved (bone, muscle, tendon)
Ulcer condition	Necrosis dry/wet, granulation, exudation
Skin margin	Maceration, hyperkeratosis, dry/cracked skin induration
Periwound area	Cellulitis, edema, erythema, fibrosis, fluctuation
Limb characteristics	Edema, pulses, capillary filling time, rubor on dependency
Weight bearing	Walking capacity, motility, need for immobilization, bony prominences/foot deformity
Pain	Location, type, cause, duration

of amputation. It is important to establish the extent of peripheral vascular disease and consider the benefit of angioplasty and reconstructive vascular surgery. A systolic toe blood pressure <30 to 45 mmHg or ankle pressure <50 to 80 mmHg have been suggested as critical levels for primary healing or healing with minor amputation in cases of foot ulcer. Transcutaneous oxygen measurement (<20 mmHg), laser doppler, and capillary microscopy has also been suggested to be of value. No patient with diabetes should undergo amputation without vascular evaluation regarding the possibility for angioplasty or vascular surgery. Different vasoactive drugs have been suggested to be of benefit in cases of peripheral vascular disease, but sufficient data are lacking for a general conclusion. A microangiopathy characterized by thickening of basement membranes of the small vessels and capillaries have been demonstrated in patients with foot lesions, but this has not been confirmed by others. There is also some evidence for increased capillary leakage and functional microvascular lesions, which might be of importance for the outcome of foot ulcers. A relationship between these functional disturbances and histological findings has not been established; the implications of these findings must be further evaluated.

Edema and pain

Edema is related to outcome of foot ulcer and is often of multifactorial origin, of which congestive heart failure, neuropathy, venous insufficiency, and neuropathic/hydrostatic edema are of most importance. Treatment of edema must be focused on its predisposing cause.

Pain, when present, is strongly related to the probability of amputation. Aggressive treatment of pain irrespective of cause is mandatory to avoid amputation in case of an ulcer. Factors that need to be considered are ischemia, neuralgia, pressure, local wound pain, and anxiety. Treatment must be focused on the most important factor in each case.

Infection

Infection in the diabetic foot is a limb-threatening condition and has been claimed to be the immediate cause for amputation in 25 to 50% of diabetic patients. It has been suggested that the more severe courses of foot infection in diabetes are consequences of defect inflammatory response, metabolic abnormalities, neuropathy, edema, and vascular disease. A superficial infection is considered to be present where signs of cellulitis are present with and without bacteriological confirmation. A deep infection is considered to be present when signs of infections are combined with evidence of involvement of deep tissue structures such as bone, tendon, and muscle. A superficial microbiological colonization of foot ulcer is virtually universal. A culture of fluid from a lesion, aspiration from deep tissues, or biopsy specimens might in cases of deep infection provide more reliable data. A superficial infection is typically due to aerobic gram positive cocci, like in particular *Staphylococcus aureus* and/or streptococcus. A deep infection, or an infection with ischemia or necrosis, is usually polymicrobial due to Gram-positive cocci, strict anaerobes, and gram-negative bacilli. It is likely that bacterial species, which are usually not pathogenic, can cause a true infection in the diabetic foot when part of a mixed flora. A substantial number of patients with deep foot infection do not have severe symptoms and signs indicating the presence of deep infection such as increased body temperature, increased CRP or sedimentating rate, or a substantially increased white serum blood count. However, when abnormal laboratory parameters are present, they usually indicate substantial tissue damage and the presence of an abscess. Bone X-ray is an essential part of the evaluation of the infected foot. A normal bone X-ray cannot exclude the possibility of a deep infection, and in many cases a bone X-ray cannot distinguish between osteomyelitis or neuro-osteoarthropathy. Under these conditions investigations such as bone scan, CT or MRI (magnetic resonance imaging) can be helpful for the diagnosis of bone infection in the diabetic foot. However, there is no golden standard, and judgments are still based upon clinical symptoms and signs. The general approach to superficial infection is to debride devitalized tissue, including surrounding callus. Antibiotic treatment chosen is empiric and should be active against the above-mentioned specimens. Antibiotics are given until clinical signs of inflammations have disappeared. Hospitalization for surgical intervention and broad spectrum antibiotics are usually essential in the management of deep foot infection. A surgical approach is often necessary, particularly in the case of acute deep soft tissue infection. For limb-threatening infection, intravenous antibiotics that have activity both against aerobic and anaerobic cultures are usually necessary. Intravenous antibiotics should be maintained until clinical signs of inflammatory reactions have diminished, and overlaid antibiotics must be used for another 3 to 6 months unless all infected tissue has been removed. The diagnosis and management of chronic osteomyelitis is an area of major controversy. It is crucial to establish differentiation versus osteoarthropathy. Standard treatment for osteomyelitis includes surgical removal of infected bone and prolonged antibiotic treatment.

Protective, therapeutic footwear

Relief of mechanical stress caused by bony prominences, foot deformities, and limited joint mobility are important factors in the treatment of foot ulcers, especially for intrinsic ulcers. Relief of mechanical stress by therapeutic shoes and in-soles is mandatory for ulcers to heal in those cases. There is sufficient data recommending the use of total contact casting or other similar devices, particularly in cases of plantar ulcers in short-term treatment of foot ulcers when shoes are not sufficient. However, this technique must be used with caution and by experienced staff due to the risk of new ulceration, especially in the presence of edema. Protective shoes are essential in the treatment and prevention of extrinsic ulcers. It is also important to recognize the need for pressure relief in pressure ulcers, both when sitting and in bed. Patients usually must be equipped with adequate footwear both for in- and outdoor use. Compliance is often a problem. It is important to encourage patients to wear the footwear at all times. The patient must understand that even a few steps of load-bearing on an ulcerated foot may prevent healing.

Treatment

Topical treatment

Topical treatment is a part of the total management of foot ulcers. The choice of topical strategy (agents or dressing) are in most cases empiric. The choice of topical treatment should be based on the general condition of the ulcer (Tab. 59.8). Assessment of foot ulcer and the use of different approaches are probably of benefit in different phases of healing. Promising studies regarding different strategies have been presented regarding topical growth factors, fibroblasts, different topical agents, and hyperbaric oxygen treatment, but further studies are needed before a consensus can be reached. Skin- or punch-grafting has been used with success in the cases with adequate perfusion and control of infection.

Improvement of glycemic control has been related to a reduction in microangiopathy and neuropathy in IDDM. There is no evidence at the moment that improved glycemic control will reduce the development of peripheral vascular disease. HbA_{1c} and random blood glucose levels have been considered risk factors for amputation in some studies but not by all. Short-term metabolic control has been related to wound healing in case reports and experimental studies of wound healing. Glycemic control has been suggested to be related to decreased levels of growth factors, changes in collagen metabolism, nonenzymatic glucosylation, defective host defense and hemorrhagic disturbances. It is generally believed that improved metabolic control is mandatory to improve the healing velocity of foot ulcers.

Foot surgery

Incision and draining is mandatory in cases of deep infection, as debridement of calluses and necrotic tissue. In cases of foot surgery it is usually not recommended unless a vascular procedure to improve circulation has been achieved. Selective correction of structural deformity – such as bony prominences, hammertoes, hallux valgus, or osteoartropathy deformity – has been used in selected cases. Great care must be taken to intervene at an optimal time and only when arterial insufficiency is not present or has been previously corrected. Amputation should only be performed at the lowest possible level according to tissue damage, ischemia, and infection. Indication for amputation is a toxic condition not responding to treatment, progressive gangrene, and intractable pain not responding to treatment. Nonhealing ulcers should not be considered as an indication for amputation.

Comorbidity

The presence of congestive heart failure, ischemic heart disease, and cerebrovascular disease have been related to the outcome of foot ulcers. The major risk factors associated with development of atherosclerosis in nondiabetic subjects are smoking, hyperlipoproteinemia, and high blood pressure. These factors have all been assumed to be similarly atherogenic in diabetic populations and must be treated aggressively; all patients should stop smoking. Diabetic nephropathy, defined as albuminuria, has been identified both as a risk factor for the outcome of foot ulcers and for lower extremity amputation. Proteinuria is considered to be a widespread vascular disease marker in diabetic patients.

The basic principle for the management of foot ulcers is to recognize that the lesion is a sign of a multiorgan disease. Improved nutrition has been related to the outcome of foot ulcers, especially in cases of foot infection, ischemia, and amputation. It is of importance to consider socioeconomic factors and compliance in the outcome and choice of strategy in the treatment of foot ulcers.

Prognosis

Management of the diabetic foot is complex and limited by multiple factors and necessitates a multifactorial approach (Tab. 59.10). The healing rate of foot ulcers are known, with the exception of centers of excellence where it is claimed to be between 80 to 90%. However, diabetic patients with previous foot ulcers have a high risk of developing new ulcers, and a high probability for future amputations and increased mortality.

These findings stress the need for lifelong observation of the diabetic foot at risk and the necessity of preventive foot care, especially among diabetic patients with previous foot ulcers or amputations. A multidisciplinary approach that includes prevention, patient education, and multifactorial treatment of foot ulcers has been reported to reduce amputation rates by 49 to 85% (Tabs. 59.11-59.12).

DIABETIC MACROANGIOPATHY

Markku Laakso

All manifestations of macroangiopathy, coronary heart disease (CHD), cerebrovascular disease, and peripheral vascular disease (PVD) are substantially more common in patients with diabetes mellitus than in nondiabetic subjects. The most important of these manifestations is CHD; over 50% of all diabetic patients die of this complication.

Insulin-dependent diabetes mellitus and noninsulin-dependent diabetes mellitus (NIDDM) are the two main sub-

---

Table 59.10 Diabetic foot ulcer: basic principles of management

Team approach
    Diabetologist
    Orthopedic surgeon
    Diabetes nurse
    Podiatrist
    Orthotist
    Close contact with vascular surgeon
Early comprehensive evaluation of risk factor
Early and coordinated intervention
Confirmed close follow-up until final result
Strict criteria for amputation
Continuity, accessibility

Table 59.11 Essential of the management of the diabetic foot

Regular inspection of foot and footwear at patient's regular visits

Preventive foot and shoe care in high-risk feet (podiatry, shoe care, education)

A multifactorial and multidisciplinary approach in the case of an established foot lesion

Early diagnoses of peripheral vascular disease and invasive angiological intervention

Continuous follow-up of patients with previous foot ulcers

Registration of amputation and foot ulcer

Table 59.12 Advice to patients regarding footcare

Inspect your feet daily and always check between the toes

If you cannot inspect your feet yourself, ask someone to do it for you

Wash your feet regularly. Dry them carefully, especially between the toes

Do not put your feet in hot water; the temperature should always be <37 °C

Do not walk barefoot in- or outdoors and never wear shoes without socks

Do not use chemical agents or plasters to remove corn and calluses

Inspect and feel with your hands the insides of your shoes daily

For dry feet, use lubricating oils or creams, but not between the toes

Change stockings daily

Cut nails straight across, and do not cut corns and calluses

Notify your physician at once if you develop a blister, cut, scratch, or sore

types of diabetes. This review concentrates only on NIDDM because >85% of all diabetic patients have NIDDM, and because data on risk factors for macroangiopathy in patients with insulin-dependent diabetes are limited.

In order to understand risk factors for macroangiopathy in NIDDM, it is crucial to realize that NIDDM is preceded by a prediabetic state, a phase of asymptomatic hyperglycemia of variable duration. This prediabetic state has to be important for the risk of macroangiopathy because the duration of NIDDM does not have a strong effect on the risk of CHD. Even this mild abnormality in glucose tolerance increases the risk for CHD. Impaired glucose tolerance, a category between normal glucose tolerance and NIDDM, is characterized by several adverse changes in cardiovascular risk factors. Subjects with impaired glucose tolerance often have hypertension, obesity, central obesity, hyperinsulinemia, and serum lipid and lipoprotein abnormalities (elevated serum total triglycerides and low high-density lipoprotein [HDL] cholesterol). These abnormalities become more severe when the subjects develop frank diabetes. Although patients with NIDDM often have a clustering of adverse changes in cardiovascular risk factors, a significant proportion of the risk for macroangiopathy among these patients remains unexplained. Therefore, macroangiopathy must be partly caused by the diabetic state itself or by yet unidentified risk factors.

Different manifestations of macroangiopathy in patients with NIDDM

Coronary heart disease

All manifestations of CHD, myocardial infarction (MI), sudden death, and angina pectoris are more common in patients with NIDDM than in corresponding control subjects. The prognosis after an acute MI is poor in diabetic patients. These patients have a two- to threefold higher mortality than nondiabetic subjects, primarily due to higher in-hospital mortality. Among women with NIDDM, the risk for fatal and nonfatal CHD is relatively higher than among men with NIDDM.

We have recently completed a study that included a population-based sample of 1059 patients (581 men, 478 women) with NIDDM, aged 45 to 64 years at baseline. These patients were followed up to 7 years with respect to CHD events. Altogether 16.7% of male and 12.8% of female NIDDM patients died of CHD, and 26.8% male and 20.9% female patients had a serious CHD event (death from CHD or nonfatal myocardial infarction). Diabetic men had a three- to fourfold higher risk and diabetic women an eight- to elevenfold higher risk for CHD than corresponding nondiabetic subjects. The high risk for CHD in patients with NIDDM seems to be largely independent of age, because in our study on elderly NIDDM patients, aged 65 to 74 years, 3.4% of nondiabetic and 14.8% of NIDDM subjects died from CHD or had a nonfatal MI during the 3.5-year follow-up.

Cerebrovascular disease

Population-based studies have indicated higher mortality after stroke in diabetic patients than in nondiabetic individuals. In our study on 1059 patients with NIDDM, diabetic men had a two- to threefold and diabetic women a fivefold higher risk for stroke during the 7-year follow-up than corresponding nondiabetic subjects. Ischemic stroke was the most common cause for a cerebrovascular event in NIDDM patients. Similarly, elderly patients with NIDDM had a considerably increased risk for fatal and nonfatal stroke compared to nondiabetic subjects (6.1 versus 3.4%) during the 3.5-year follow-up. The incidence of stroke was particularly high among diabetic women.

Peripheral vascular disease

All manifestations of PVD ranging from absent peripheral leg and foot pulses to amputation are more common in patients with diabetes than in nondiabetic subjects. Several studies have indicated that patients with NIDDM have a 10- to 15-fold higher risk for lower extremity amputation compared to that in nondiabetic subjects. In our study on 1059 middle-aged patients with NIDDM, the incidence of amputation during the 7-year follow-up was similar in both genders (5.6% in men and 5.3% in women). Ischemic amputation was practically nonexistent among nondiabetic subjects. Of the 58 first amputations performed during the study period, 31 (53.5%) were amputations of toes, 17 (29.3%) amputations were performed below the knee, and 10 (17.2%) above the knee.

Intimal calcification is not the only atherosclerotic complication in peripheral arteries among diabetic subjects. Medial artery calcification (known also as Mönckeberg's arteriosclerosis) is a condition that leads to stiffening of the elastic layer of the arterial wall, but it does not obstruct the arterial lumen, in contrast to intimal artery calcification. Medial artery calcification is frequent among patients with NIDDM and is associated with the risk of all-cause mortality and macroangiopathic complications. According to our results on 1059 middle-aged patients with NIDDM, those who had medial artery calcification had significantly higher total mortality (38.0 versus 22.3%), CHD mortality (20.3 versus 11.1%) and stroke mortality (4.6 versus 2.3%) than patients without medial artery calcification during the 7-year follow-up.

Abnormalities in cardiovascular risk factors and their predictive value for macroangiopathy in subjects with NIDDM

Subjects with NIDDM have multiple abnormalities in cardiovascular risk factors, including dyslipidemia, elevation of blood pressure, obesity, hemostatic factors, hyperinsulinemia, and hyperglycemia.

Serum lipids and lipoproteins

In patients with NIDDM, the most common dyslipidemia is hypertriglyceridemia due to an increase in the number of very-low-density lipoprotein (VLDL) and intermediate-density lipoprotein particles. In contrast, the results concerning serum total and low-density lipoprotein cholesterol (LDL) levels in patients with NIDDM have been conflicting. However, in the majority of studies, the levels of total and LDL cholesterol have been reported to be normal. Although LDL concentration is normal, compositional changes in LDL particles occur in NIDDM. The most important of these is the predominance of small, dense LDL particles, which may increase the risk for CHD in

patients with NIDDM. A decrease in serum HDL cholesterol, and particularly in the HDL_2 subfraction, is typical for patients with NIDDM.

Several studies, among them the Multiple Risk Factor Intervention Trial, the Whitehall Study, and the Framingham Study, have indicated that total (and LDL) cholesterol are similar risk factors for CHD in patients with NIDDM as in nondiabetic subjects. Total and LDL also predicted CHD events in our study including 1059 middle-aged patients with NIDDM. Contradictory results have been reported on the importance of high total cholesterol as a risk factor for stroke in patients with NIDDM. Hypercholesterolemia has been shown to be related to an increased occurrence of PVD. Several studies indicate an inverse relationship between HDL cholesterol and the risk of CHD, stroke, and PVD in patients with NIDDM. Total triglycerides were first shown to be associated with the risk of cardiovascular death in the Paris Prospective Study. Most, but not all, recent studies have confirmed this finding.

Blood pressure

The prevalence of essential hypertension in patients with NIDDM is substantially greater than in the general population. According to several studies, more than 50% of patients with NIDDM have elevated blood pressure. The cause for higher risk of hypertension in patients with NIDDM remains unknown, but it is associated with insulin resistance and hyperinsulinemia. Elevated levels of blood pressure increase the risk for cardiovascular disease morbidity and mortality similarly in diabetic patients as they do in nondiabetic subjects. The World Health Organization Multinational Study on diabetes demonstrated that the presence of proteinuria in hypertensive patients with NIDDM increased mortality by fivefold among men and by eightfold among women compared with those without hypertension and proteinuria. Hypertension is the single most important risk factor for stroke in nondiabetic subjects as well as in diabetic patients. High blood pressure level is also a significant risk factor for PVD in NIDDM, and it has been linked with the progression of PVD as well as with the risk of amputation.

Obesity

Patients with NIDDM are often obese. Obesity and its central distribution are associated particularly with dyslipidemia among these patients as well as elevated blood pressure and hyperinsulinemia. The importance of obesity as an independent risk factor for CHD and stroke remains controversial in patients with NIDDM. Central obesity has predicted CHD in prospective studies independent of overall obesity in diabetic patients.

Hemostatic factors

Hemostatic abnormalities are common in patients with NIDDM. Increased levels of fibrinogen, PAI-1, Factor

VII, and von Willebrand factor levels have been reported in patients with NIDDM. Although hemostatic factors have been shown to predict CHD in several large prospective studies in nondiabetic subjects, no studies are available on their impact on the risk of CHD, stroke, or PVD in diabetic patients.

Microalbuminuria

NIDDM patients with an increased urinary albumin and protein excretion rate are at increased risk of cardiovascular mortality, independent of classic cardiovascular risk factors. The mechanisms behind this association are poorly understood, but increased urinary albumin excretion rate is often associated with adverse changes in cardiovascular risk factors. The association between stroke and proteinuria or albuminuria is controversial.

Hyperglycemia

By definition patients with NIDDM are hyperglycemic. Several recent prospective studies have indicated that poor metabolic control increases the risk for cardiovascular disease. In a 10-year prospective study on newly-detected patients with NIDDM aged 45 to 64 years in Kuopio, in eastern Finland, high fasting blood glucose significantly predicted cardiovascular mortality independent of other risk factors. Furthermore, cardiovascular mortality was increased by threefold in NIDDM patients included into the highest blood glucose tertile compared to the lowest blood glucose tertile, irrespective of the mode of treatment. Quite similar results were obtained from Sweden from a study aiming to investigate the influence of long-term glycemic control on cardiovascular mortality in a cohort of about 400 newly-detected NIDDM patients. In our study on elderly patients with NIDDM, hyperglycemia was significantly associated with the risk of CHD. In that study there was a significant dose-response relationship between glycated hemoglobin A_{1c} (GHbA$_{1c}$) and the risk of CHD death. A long duration of diabetes without concomitant high GHbA$_{1c}$ increased the CHD event rate considerably less than did high GHbA1c with a short duration of diabetes. In our study on middle-aged patients with NIDDM, high fasting glucose also independently predicted CHD events.

Hyperglycemia predicts poor prognosis after stroke and worsens the ischemic brain damage from a stroke in diabetic patients. In our studies of middle-aged and elderly patients with NIDDM, poor glycemic control was a significant and independent predictor of stroke. Similarly, in the Wisconsin Epidemiological Study of Diabetic Retinopathy, high HbA$_{1c}$ levels were significantly associated with stroke mortality in diabetic patients.

Poor glycemic control and a long duration of diabetes are strong predictors for PVD according to studies from different populations, including Pima Indians, Oklahoma Indians, and Caucasians. Our study is consistent with these studies showing that high fasting glucose and a long

duration of diabetes were associated with a high risk of PVD in middle-aged patients with NIDDM. High GhbA and high fasting glucose were associated with a twofold risk for amputation.

Hyperinsulinemia and insulin resistance

Three prospective population studies, published originally over 15 years ago – the Helsinki Policemen Study, the Paris Prospective Study, and the Busselton Study – have demonstrated that high plasma insulin is associated with an increased risk for CHD independent of other risk factors in nondiabetic subjects. Thus far about twenty different studies have been published on that issue, and there is still controversy whether or not hyperinsulinemia predicts cardiovascular events in nondiabetic subjects. The majority of patients with NIDDM are hyperinsulinemic, but only a few studies have been published on high plasma insulin as a predictor of CHD in patients with NIDDM. No studies are available on the association between hyperinsulinemia and the risk for stroke or PVD in patients with NIDDM.

Table 59.13 presents a summary of risk factors for macroangiopathy in patients with NIDDM. NIDDM is characterized by normal (or elevated) levels of total (and LDL) cholesterol, low levels of HDL cholesterol, high levels of total triglycerides, obesity, hyperglycemia, and hyperinsulinemia. Several population-based studies indicate that classic risk factors, total cholesterol, elevated blood pressure, and smoking are similar risk factors for CHD among patients with NIDDM, as they are among nondiabetic subjects. In addition, low HDL cholesterol concentration and high levels of total triglycerides are likely to be more important risk factors for macroangiopathy in patients with NIDDM than they are in nondiabetic subjects. The role of obesity as an independent risk factor

Table 59.13 Summary of risk factors for macroangiopathy in patients with NIDDM

Risk factor	Abnormality	Proven risk factor	Positive treatment effect
Total cholesterol	±	Yes	Yes
HDL cholesterol	↓	Yes	NA
Total triglycerides	↑	Yes	NA
Blood pressure	↑	Yes	Yes
Smoking	±	Yes	NA
Obesity	↑	No	NA
Hyperglycemia	↑	Yes	NA
Hyperinsulinemia	↑	?	NA

(NA = data not available; ± = no change; ↓ = decrease; ↑ = increase.)

for macroangiopathy in NIDDM has remained controversial. However, obesity and its central distribution have several adverse effects on cardiovascular risk factors. Several recent studies indicate that poor glycemic control predicts macrovascular complications, but the role of hyperinsulinemia remains to be clarified in future studies.

Because several modifiable risk factors predict macroangiopathy, there is a great potential to reduce the burden of atherothrombotic complications among patients with NIDDM. Treatment of classic risk factors should considerably reduce the risk for macroangiopathy in NIDDM patients. Unfortunately, the data are limited to support this notion since only a few clinical trials are available, and all of these are subgroup analyses of trials including mainly nondiabetic subjects. However, the Scandinavian Simvastatin Survival Study and the Cholesterol And Recurrent Events (CARE) trial have shown that the reduction of total and LDL cholesterol by simvastatin or pravastatin significantly reduces the incidence of cardiovascular events in diabetic patients, most of them having NIDDM. Similarly, a subgroup analysis of the Systolic Hypertension in the Elderly Program (SHEP) indicates that the treatment of isolated systolic hypertension in elderly subjects with thiazide diuretics also reduced cardiovascular events in diabetic patients. Unfortunately, we do not have any evidence to substantiate the notion that the treatment of low HDL cholesterol and high triglycerides would be beneficial. Although poor glycemic control is an independent risk factor for macroangiopathy, we do not have trial evidence to indicate that the normalization of glucose control could result in the lowering of the risk of atherothrombotic events. The UK Prospective Study may reduce uncertainty in this respect.

Even though we have been successful in treating all abnormal cardiovascular events, it is not likely that we could prevent macrovascular complications in patients with NIDDM because macroangiopathy is often already present at the diagnosis of diabetes. Abnormal cardiovascular risk factors in the prediabetic state must be primarily responsible for an excess risk for macroangiopathy in NIDDM. Therefore, we should identify persons at high risk of developing diabetes and prevent the progression to NIDDM. Prevention of NIDDM by diet, weight loss, exercise, or drug treatment is highly relevant, as well as for all efforts to prevent macroangiopathy in subjects with abnormal glucose tolerance.

Acknowledgements

The research projects referred to in the part of the review by Markku Laasko have been financially supported by grants from the Academy of Finland.

Suggested readings

APELQVIST J. The wound healing in diabetes. outcome and costs. In: Harkless L, Armstrong G (eds). Healing the diabetic foot wound. Clin Podiatr Med Surg. 1998;15:21-39.

BRENNER MB (ed). The kidney. 5th ed. Philadelphia: WB Saunders Company, 1996.

DIABETES CONTROL AND COMPLICATIONS TRIAL RESEARCH GROUP. The effect of intensive treatment of diabetes on the development and progression of long-term complications in insulin-dependent diabetes mellitus. New Engl J Med 1993;329:977-86.

KING GL, BROWNLEE M. The cellular and molecular mechanisms of diabetic complications. Endocrinol Metab Clin N America 1996;25:255-70.

KLEIN R. Hyperglycemia and microvascular and macrovascular disease in diabetes. Diabetes Care 1995;18:258-68.

LAAKSO M. Insulin resistance and coronary heart disease. Curr Opin Lipidol 1996;7:217-26.

LAAKSO M, LEHTO S. Epidemiology of macrovascular disease in diabetes. Diabetes Rev 1997;5:294-9.

LARSSON J, APELQVIST J. Towards less amputations in diabetic patients: incidence, causes, cost, treatment and prevention - A review. Acta Ortop Scand 1995;66:181-92.

MOGENSEN CE (ed). The kidney and hypertension in diabetes mellitus. 3rd ed. London: Kluwer Academic Publishers, 1996.

PORTE D, SHERWIN RS (eds). Diabetes mellitus. 5th ed. East Norwalk: Appleton & Lange, 1996.

REIBER G.E. The epidemiology of diabetic foot problems. Diabet Med 1996;13S:6.

UK PROSPECTIVE DIABETES STUDY (UKPDS) GROUP. Intensive blood-glucose control with suphonylureas or insulin compared with conventional treatment and risk of complications in patients with type 2 diabetes (UKPDS 33). Lancet 1998;352:837-53.

WARD JD, TESFAYE XX. Pathogenesis of diabetic neuropathy. In: Pickup JC, Williams G (eds). Textbook of diabetes. 2nd ed. Oxford: Blackwell Science, 1997.

WATKINS PJ, EDMONDS ME. Clinical features of diabetic neuropathy. In: Pickup JC, Williams G (eds). Textbook of diabetes. 2nd ed. Oxford: Blackwell Science, 1997.

YOUNG RJ. The management of diabetic neuropathy. In: Pickup JC, Williams G (eds). Textbook of diabetes. 2nd ed. Oxford: Blackwell Science, 1997.

Diabetes and pregnancy

Kerstin E. Berntorp, Anders H. Frid

◼ KEY POINTS

- The outcome of diabetic pregnancies has improved considerably in many countries during recent years, in large part due to improvements in diabetic care and metabolic control.
- Normal pregnancy induces insulin resistance through the diabetogenic effect of placental hormones and progesterone. Postprandial blood glucose levels rise with a compensatory hyperinsulinemia, reaching a peak at 28 to 32 gestational weeks. This condition favors nutrient transfer to the fetus.
- Maternal diabetes may cause fetal malformations, which are related to the severity of hyperglycemia. Increased transport of glucose from the mother to the fetus induces fetal hyperinsulinemia and causes accelerated and inappropriate fetal growth (large-for-gestational-age fetus and macrosomia).
- There is some controversy regarding the influence of gestational diabetes on the morbidity and mortality of the fetus and newborn. There is also controversy over which screening and diagnostic procedure to use during pregnancy. There is, however, no controversy regarding the high future risk of the mother developing non-insulin-dependent diabetes mellitus (type 2 diabetes).
- In light of the recent trend toward screening for and early intervention of type 2 diabetes, it seems justifiable to have screening programs for gestational diabetes in order to find and follow a high-risk group of women, with the added advantage of a high probability of a beneficial effect on the well-being of the fetus.

Maternal diabetes in pregnancy can be classified as either pregestational diabetes or gestational diabetes. The term pregestational diabetes includes both type 1 diabetes (insulin-dependent diabetes mellitus, or IDDM) and type 2 diabetes (non-insulin-dependent diabetes mellitus, or NIDDM). Gestational diabetes is defined as abnormal glucose tolerance first recognized during pregnancy regardless of whether the condition persists after pregnancy. The best known classification of diabetes in pregnancy was published by Priscilla White from Boston, USA, in 1949 and subsequently modified by her (Hare and White, 1980). This was an attempt to predict the outcome of pregnancy based on the duration and age of onset of dia-

betes or the presence of vascular disease. The prognosis is graded from A (best) to T (worst) (Tab. 60.1).

METABOLIC ADAPTATION IN NORMAL PREGNANCY

In normal pregnancy, fasting blood glucose concentrations tend to decrease with gestation, while postprandial glucose levels tend to rise; fasting insulin concentrations progressively increase, as does glucose-stimulated insulin secretion, reaching a peak at 28 to 32 gestational weeks. Hormonal changes, including an increase in growth hor-

Table 60.1 White classification of pregestational diabetes. All classes below class A require insulin therapy. Classes R, F, RF, H, and T have no onset/duration criteria but usually occur in long-term diabetes. The development of a complication moves the patient to the lower class

Class A	Diet alone, any duration or onset age
Class B	Onset age 20 yr or older and duration less than 10 yr
Class C	Onset age 10-19 yr or duration over 10-19 yr
Class D	Onset age under 10 yr, duration over 20 yr, background retinopathy, or hypertension (not preeclampsia)
Class R	Proliferative retinopathy or vitreous hemorrhage
Class F	Nephropathy with over 500 mg/day proteinuria
Class RF	Criteria for both classes R and F coexist
Class H	Arteriosclerotic heart disease clinically evident
Class T	Prior renal transplantation

(From Hare JW, White P. Gestational diabetes and the White Classification. Diabetes Care 1980;3:394.)

mone of placental origin, are held responsible for this marked increase in insulin resistance. Glucose is a major metabolic substrate for the infant and traverses the placenta by facilitated diffusion. The blood glucose level in pregnancy is normally regulated within a narrow interval, which is between 3.5 and 6.5 mmol/l, and there is a very close relationship between maternal and fetal glucose concentrations.

PREGESTATIONAL DIABETES

Effect of diabetes on the fetus

There is a strong association between elevated glycated hemoglobin (HbA_{1c}) in early pregnancy and the occurrence of fetal malformations. Furthermore, maternal hyperglycemia leads to fetal hyperglycemia, which, in turn, stimulates B cells to increase insulin production. Several neonatal complications seen in diabetic pregnancies may be directly or indirectly associated with fetal hyperinsulinemia. The classical diabetes fetopathy is characterized by the large-for-gestational-age fetus or the macrosomic infant. Fetal growth acceleration is usually seen in association with poor metabolic control, particularly in mothers with a short duration of diabetes without major manifestations of microangiopathy. The opposite, that is, fetal growth retardation, is often associated with severe diabetic microangiopathy in the mother.

Preconceptional planning

All potential diabetic mothers should be given contraceptive and pregnancy advice in the routine diabetic clinic. They should be informed about the importance of strict glycemic control from the time of conception and throughout pregnancy. Once a women expresses an interest in becoming pregnant, she should have access to the diabetic clinic for more specific preconceptional advice in order to optimize glycemic control and to screen for diabetic complications. She also needs information about what a diabetic pregnancy requires, including frequent home blood glucose monitoring and frequent antenatal visits. Appropriate advice should be given by a dietitian. Oral hypoglycemic drugs should be withdrawn, since these drugs cross the placenta and are potentially teratogenic. Sulfonylureas also stimulate B cells directly, aggravating fetal hyperinsulinemia and macrosomia.

Most diabetic women are concerned about the risk of diabetes in their children. The lifetime risk for diabetes is small, at about 3% of children with mothers with IDDM and about 9% of children who have fathers with IDDM, which should be viewed against a background prevalence of approximately 0.15% in the general population. When both parents have IDDM the risk is greater and may reach 30%. The discrepancy of maternal and paternal transmission is not fully understood. The risk of an infant of a NIDDM mother or father is much higher, at about 15%, and it may reach 75% if both parents are diabetic.

Nephropathy and hypertension

If the patient has persistent proteinuria in the absence of urinary tract infection, with concomitant systemic hypertension, diabetic nephropathy should be suspected. Proteinuria usually increases during pregnancy, but there is no evidence that pregnancy accelerates progression of renal disease. Patients with nephropathy are at great risk of developing hypertension, and during the last trimester worsening of nephropathy may be clinically difficult to distinguish from pre-eclampsia. Hypertension should be controlled with drugs considered safe in pregnancy.

Retinopathy

Whenever possible, optimal regulation of the diabetic state should take place before conception. Retinopathy may deteriorate rapidly when glycemic control is tightened over a short period. Women with poor glycemic control and severe baseline retinopathy are at the greatest risk for progression. An acute decrease in retinal perfusion with an impaired supply of oxygen and glucose may be responsible. An ophthalmological examination should preferably take place before pregnancy, but otherwise in the beginning, and thereafter in case of background retinopathy in each trimester. Patients with proliferative retinopathy and those who are prone to develop systemic hypertension should be examined more frequently. Laser photocoagulation may be safely used during pregnancy, but ideally patients with proliferative retinopathy should be adequately treated before pregnancy.

Glucose control and insulin treatment during pregnancy

Early in pregnancy most diabetic women need to be seen at weekly intervals. Thereafter they should be encouraged to attend outpatient visits every 1 to 2 weeks. Self-monitoring of blood glucose should be applied throughout pregnancy. Monitoring should be performed at least four times per day, that is, preprandial, and preferably 1 hour postprandial as well. The main objective is to attain normoglycemia, which ideally means fasting glucose concentrations less than 5 mmol/l and postprandial glucose concentrations less than 7 mmol/l. HbA_{1c} levels should be determined at monthly intervals and should be normalized during the second and third trimester. To achieve normoglycemia, virtually all IDDM women will require short-acting insulin before meals and intermediate-acting insulin at bedtime. In women with NIDDM, a combination of short-acting and medium-acting insulin twice daily is often enough to attain near-normoglycemia. For many women, insulin requirement does not begin to increase until the second trimester, and some women need to reduce their dose during the first 3 months. By the end of the second trimester, the insulin requirements will often have doubled. Generally the insulin requirement continues to increase until around 36 gestational weeks, when it often plateaus or even declines slightly, probably due to the increased transfer of glucose to the fetus in late pregnancy.

Obstetric care and labor

Ideally the pregnant woman should have access to a combined diabetic and obstetric clinic or team comprised of a diabetologist, an obstetrician, a diabetes specialist nurse, a midwife, and a dietitian. A detailed ultrasound scan should be performed at gestational weeks 17 to 19 for confirmation of gestational age and for detection of major fetal malformation. Frequent ultrasound scans should be performed during the last trimester to assess fetal growth as well as frequent registrations of the fetal heart rate to detect fetal hypoxia. Measurement of umbilical and placental blood flow velocity waveforms might also be valuable.

The management of diabetes during labor and the postpartum period should be well-planned and discussed with the patient. According to modern policy, delivery is not induced until term or after at least 39 completed weeks of pregnancy if maternal blood glucose is well-regulated. If pregnancy complications occur, or if there is coexisting severe diabetic angiopathy, the mode and time of delivery must be individualized. During labor it is essential to attain normoglycemia (blood glucose around 5-6 mmol/l). Blood glucose should therefore be monitored on an hourly basis. Continuous intravenous infusion of glucose together with multiple subcutaneous injections of insulin (or as continuous infusion) should be adjusted according to blood glucose levels. In the immediate postpartum period insulin requirements normally decrease rapidly to prepregnancy levels or lower. It is important that the first hours of contact between mother and child are not disturbed by hypoglycemia.

GESTATIONAL DIABETES

The most simple definition of gestational diabetes (GDM) is glucose intolerance that presents in pregnancy. GDM may develop at any time during pregnancy but most commonly appears in the beginning of the third trimester. There is a lack of consensus regarding how and when to test for GDM and which patients should be tested, beginning with the pioneering studies of O'Sullivan in the 1960s. Part of the problem lies in the fact that two considerations have to be made: the risk for the fetus of the present pregnancy, and the risk of the mother to develop diabetes in the future.

Epidemiology _____

According to the National Diabetes Data Group criteria, 2 to 4% of pregnant women are reported as having GDM. When using the World Health Organization (WHO) criteria for "impaired glucose tolerance during pregnancy," as many as 5 to 10% of the women will be diagnosed. In southern Sweden, where all pregnant women undergo a 75 g oral glucose tolerance test (OGTT) in the 28th week of gestation, 1.5 % are diagnosed as having GDM using the European Association for the Study of Diabetes (EASD) criteria, and 5% of the women have impaired glucose tolerance during pregnancy according to the WHO criteria. Treatment is, however, considered only when the 2-hour value is 9.0 mmol/l (162 mg/dl) or more. The major OGTT criteria are summarized in Table 60.2. In addition, all high-risk women should be screened at presentation (Tab. 60.3).

Diagnosis _____

The National Diabetes Data Group and the American Diabetes Association recommend a 3-hour 100 g OGTT for diagnosis. Screening is performed in the 24th to 28th week of gestation using a non-fasting 1-hour 50 g OGTT. In women exceeding a 1-hour value of 7.8 mmol/l (140 mg/dl), a 3-hour 100 g OGTT is performed. The WHO proposes the fasting 2-hour 75 g OGTT for diagnosis. A 2-hour blood glucose value between 7.8 mmol/l (140 mg/dl) and 11.0 (198 mg/dl) is called impaired glucose tolerance during pregnancy, and a 2-hour value 11.1 (200 mg/dl) and higher is called gestational diabetes. However, in many countries the diagnosis of GDM is made when pregnant women have 2-hour values exceeding 7.8 mmol/l (140 mg/dl), which is in accordance with the new criteria recently proposed by the WHO Consultation Group (1998). A study group of the EASD has proposed the 2-hour 75 g OGTT with the cut-off limit of 9.0 mmol/l (162 mg/dl) for the diagnosis of "gestational impaired glucose tolerance (IGT)." These criteria have gained acceptance in the Scandinavian countries and also elsewhere.

Prognosis for the fetus

In gestational diabetes, hyperglycemia during pregnancy may cause diabetic fetopathy with macrosomia and disturbed fetal maturation. There is, however, no prospective study in women with GDM comparing treatment with no treatment. Screening for GDM was instituted in Sweden in 1987. In a nationwide study, earlier-born siblings to children of mothers diagnosed as having GDM in 1987-1992 (3958 cases) were compared to a control group (7916 cases), assuming that a large part of the mothers had undiagnosed GDM in the preceding pregnancy. A significantly higher rate (odds ratio 1.56) of stillborn infants in the GDM group was found compared to controls.

Treatment

Ideally, all women at risk for GDM should be treated at clinics with a special interest in GDM, where they should be given dietary advice and instructions in glucose self-monitoring. Dietary advice should be focused on carbohydrates with low glycemic index. Frequent measurements of blood glucose is necessary in order to detect those who deteriorate. Glycemic targets should be similar to those in women with pregestational diabetes. Fasting blood glucose <5 mmol/l and postprandial blood glucose < 8 mmol/l can be considered as therapeutic goals. If this is not achieved with dietary changes alone, insulin therapy should be initiated. Normoglycemia can usually be

Table 60.3 High-risk women for gestional diabetes

Previous gestational diabetes
Previously large-for-gestational-age fetus
First order relative with diabetes mellitus
Obesity
Excessive weight gain during pregnancy
Fetal macrosomia

attained using a combination of short-acting and medium-acting insulin twice daily.

Obstetric care and labor

Women with GDM who require insulin therapy should be followed according to the guidelines outlined previously in this chapter for women with pregestational diabetes, although in most cases insulin requirement ceases at the onset of labor. If blood glucose is carefully controlled on diet alone, there is usually no need to initiate fetal surveillance, and the same routines as for normal pregnancies could be followed. In most cases, immediately postpartum, or rather during labor, blood glucose concentrations return to prepregnancy levels.

Prognosis for the mother

All studies show that women who have had gestational diabetes run an increased risk of developing diabetes later in life; thus, a follow-up program should be instituted. Since insulin sensitivity is high during lactation, glucose measurements may be misleading. It is feasible to check fasting or random blood glucose 6 to 8 weeks after birth to detect persisting diabetes in women. An OGTT should be performed after lactation, 6 to 12 months after birth.

Table 60.2 The major screening and diagnostic OGTT criteria used (values refers to venous plasma)

OGTT	Fasting	1 h	2 h	3 h	Comment
50 g non-fasting		≥7.8 mmol/l ≥140 mg/dl			Followed by 100 g OGTT
100 g fasting (O'Sullivan)	5.8 mmol/l 105 mg/dl	10.6 mmol/l 190 mg/dl	9.2 mmol/l 165 mg/dl	8.1 mmol/l 145 mg/dl	Two or more met or exceeded
75 g fasting (EASD)			>8.9 mmol/l >161 mg/dl		Gestational IGT or GDM
75 g fasting (WHO, 1985)			7.8-11.0 mmol/l 140-198 mg/dl >11.0 mmol/l >198 mg/dl		IGT during pregnancy GDM
75 g fasting (WHO, 1998)			≥7.8 mmol/l ≥140 mg/dl		GDM

(OGTT = oral glucose tolerance test; EASD = European Association for the Study of Diabetes; IGT = impaired glucose tolerance; GDM = gestational diabetes.)

As many as 10% of the women may have diabetes 12 months after birth. After several years, a wide range of incidence rates have been reported, some as high as 60%. The variability is most likely due to different screening and diagnostic procedures.

Suggested readings

ÅBERG A, RYDHSTRÖM H, KÄLLÉN B, KÄLLÉN K. Impaired glucose tolerance during pregnancy is associated with increased fetal mortality in preceding sibs. Acta Obstet Gynecol Scand 1997;76:212-7.

BUCHANAN TA, METZGER BE, FREINKEL N, BERGMAN RN. Insulin sensitivity and β-cell responsiveness to glucose during late pregnancy in lean and moderately obese women with normal glucose tolerance or mild gestational diabetes. Am J Obstet Gynecol 1990;162:1008-14.

CHEW EY, MILLS JL, METZGER BE, et al. Metabolic control and progression of retinopathy. Diabetes Care 1995;18:631-7.

ERIKSSON L, FRANKENNE F, EDÉN S, HENNEN G, VON SCHOULTZ B. Growth hormone 24-h serum profiles during pregnancy - lack of pulsatility for the secretion of the placental variant. Br J Obstet Gynaecol 1989;96:949-53.

GIRLING JC, DORNHORST A. Pregnancy and diabetes mellitus. In: Pickup and Williams (ed). Textbook of diabetes. 2nd ed. Oxford: Blackwell Science, 1997.

HANSSON U, PERSSON B. Relationship between haemoglobin A_{1C} in early type 1 (insulin dependent) diabetic pregnancy and the occurrence of spontaneous abortion and fetal malformation in Sweden. Diabetologia 1990;33:100-4.

LESLIE D. Genetic counselling and diabetes mellitus. In: Pickup and Williams (eds). Textbook of diabetes. 2nd ed. Oxford: Blackwell Science, 1997.

LIND T, PHILLIPS PR. Influence of pregnancy on the 75-g OGTT, a prospective muticenter study. The Diabetic Pregnancy Study Group of the EASD. Diabetes 1991;40 (suppl 2):8-13.

O'SULLIVAN JB. Diabetes mellitus after GDM. Diabetes 1991;40 (suppl 2):131-5.

O'SULLIVAN JB, MAHAN CM. Criteria for the oral glucose tolerance test in pregnancy. Diabetes 1964;13:278-85.

REECE EA, COUSTAN DR, HAYSLETT JP, et al. Diabetic nephropathy: pregnancy performance and fetomaternal outcome. Am J Obstet Gynecol 1988;159:56-66.

STANGENBERG M, PERSSON B, NORDLANDER E. Random capillary blood glucose and conventional selection criteria for glucose tolerance testing during pregnancy. Diabetes Res 1985; 2:29-33.

THE SECOND INTERNATIONAL WORKSHOP CONFERENCE ON GESTATIONAL DIABETES MELLITUS. Diabetes 1985;34:(suppl 2).

Organization of diabetes care

Carl-David Agardh

███ KEY POINTS ███

- In the future there will be an increasing number of people who have diabetes and who will develop late diabetic complications.
- Goals for improved diabetes care were defined by the World Health Organization and the International Diabetes Federation in St. Vincent, Italy, in 1989 ("the St.Vincent Declaration").
- Implementing the goals of the St.Vincent Declaration can form the basis for organizing diabetes care, irrespective of the health care system in any individual country, but it requires a planned strategy.
- Management of diabetes requires comprehensive knowledge and time of the doctor and the diabetes health care team (e.g., time for patient visits, education, treatment), and a two-way collaboration with the diabetic person.
- A continuous system for quality development must be instituted to evaluate structure, process, and outcome of care.

Diabetes mellitus is a significant, growing health problem, affecting at least 10 million European citizens and approximately 100 million people worldwide. Diabetes is more prevalent in the elderly, with 50 to 55% of the patients aged 65 years or older, and 10% aged less than 35 years. The prevalence seems to be increasing worldwide, due either to an increase in incidence or to other factors, such as earlier detection and longer survival. It has been estimated that the prevalence of diabetes will reach 216 million people by the year 2010. Regardless of the reason for the increased prevalence, an increasing number of people with the disease and those who will develop late diabetic complications will have to be cared for in the future.

Diabetes causes substantial morbidity and mortality, primarily through cardiovascular, eye and kidney disease, and limb amputation. Compared with nondiabetic individuals, people with diabetes have a fourfold higher risk of dying from heart disease or developing peripheral arterial disease, and a twofold higher risk of having a stroke. Specific diabetes complications are responsible for approximately 12000 cases of legal blindness each year in the United States, making it a leading cause of new cases of blindness in adults aged 25 to 74 years. Moreover, 32% of new cases of end-stage renal disease are attributable to diabetes.

In the United States the total direct costs are estimated to be $ 45.2 billion, and the total indirect costs, including short- and long-term morbidity and mortality, are estimated to be $ 46.6 billion. The total cost of diabetes mellitus has also been calculated in the County Council of Malmöhus in southern Sweden for 1993-1994. The total population of the county was 568 709, or approximately 6.5% that of Sweden, and the age distribution corresponds well to the national average. The prevalence of diabetes was 2.6%. People with diabetes accounted for 6.3% of all out-patient visits and 9.5% of all in-patient episodes. The total cost of health care consumption was SEK 27 885 per patient per year, which corresponds to 8% of the total cost of health care in the region.

When taking into account the increasing demand for health services for these patients, it is important for society to organize the care of diabetic patients in a cost-effective way in order to be able to provide good quality diabetes care in the future. This increasing demand also shows the need for a systematic and continuous quality improvement of diabetes care, and it demonstrates the importance of standards and recommendations of medical procedures. It also demonstrates the need for organizing the health care system through flexible integration of primary health care, specialist teams, and patient groups on a local basis.

THE GOALS OF DIABETES TREATMENT

In order to reduce the burden of diabetes, representatives of government health departments and patient organizations from all European countries met with diabetes experts under the aegis of the Regional Offices of the World Health Organization (WHO) and the International Diabetes Federation in St. Vincent, Italy, in 1989. At the meeting, they unanimously agreed upon some recommendations to form the basis of improved diabetes care in Europe, and they urged that they be presented in all countries throughout Europe for implementation. In the St. Vincent Declaration, general goals and five-year targets were set (Tab. 61.1) and can be achieved by the organized activities of the medical services in active partnership with people with diabetes and their families, friends, workmates, and organizations.

Implementing the goals of the St. Vincent Declaration can form the basis for organizing diabetes care, irrespective of the health care system in any individual country, but it requires a planned strategy together with structured information for monitoring and evaluation, both of which are essential for progressive improvement in the quality of diabetes care. The starting point for such a systematic and continuous process is to evaluate the structure, process, and outcome of care in order to define the basis for future improvement. These points are described below.

The structure of care

In most countries, and as stated in the WHO program "Health for All", the focus of the health care system is on primary health care to meet the basic needs of each community through services provided as close as possible to where people live and work, and to be readily acceptable to all.

To fulfill the goals of the St. Vincent Declaration, the organization of diabetes care in general practice must include some key elements (Tab. 61.2).

Table 61.1 General goals and five-year targets for children and adults with diabetes

General goals

Sustained improvement in health experience and a life approaching normal expectation in quality and quantity
Prevention and cure of diabetes and of its complications by intensifying research effort

Five-year targets

Elaborate, initiate, and evaluate comprehensive programs for detection and control of diabetes and of its complications with self-care and community support as major components
Raise awareness in the population and among health care professionals of the present opportunities and the future needs for prevention of the complications of diabetes and of diabetes itself
Organize training in diabetes management and care for people of all ages with diabetes, for their families, friends and working associates and for the health care team
Ensure that care for children with diabetes is provided by individuals and teams specialized both in the management of diabetes and of children, and that families with a diabetic child get the necessary social, economic, and emotional support
Reinforce existing centers of excellence in diabetes care, education, and research. Create new centers where the need and potential exist
Promote independence, equity, and self-sufficiency for all people with diabetes - children, adolescents, those in the working years of life, and in the elderly
Remove hindrances to the diabetic citizen into society, which is fully possible
Implement effective measures for the prevention of costly complications
Establish monitoring and control systems using state of the art information technology for quality assurance of diabetes health care provisions and for laboratory and technical procedures in diabetes diagnosis, treatment, and self-management

The process of care

Management of diabetes requires – of the doctor and the diabetes health care team – comprehensive knowledge and time (e.g. time for patient visits, education, treatment), and a two-way collaboration with the diabetic person. In 1991, a subcommittee of the European Region of the International Diabetes Federation and the St. Vincent Declaration Steering Committee of WHO Europe formulated The European Patients' Charter since it was felt that many people with diabetes were receiving suboptimal care, and that they have the right to know what care they should expect to receive. By providing this information to patients it was felt that they could stimulate appropriate improvement in care with clear benefit for their own health. Equally, it was felt that the diabetic person also has responsibilities in self-care, and these points are also included in the Charter.

In the Charter it is stated that the health care team should provide the following:
• *A treatment plan and self targets*. This should include plans on eating and physical activity, advice on how to

Table 61.2 Key elements for diabetes care in general practice

A well-trained general practitioner
Access to a diabetes nurse taking care of patient education
Access to a dietician to give nutrition advice
Access to a podiatrist and orthotist for preventive foot care and for treatment
A close collaboration with hospital diabetes clinics for shared care, when necessary
Access to a screening program for diabetic retinopathy
A close collaboration with a biochemistry laboratory, including quality control of laboratory procedures used in general practice

change doses and timing of tablets or insulin based on the self-monitoring of blood glucose, and individual target values for blood glucose, blood lipids, blood pressure, and body weight (Tab. 61.3).
- *Regular check-ups*. At the regular visits, the individual targets should be discussed, and the self-monitoring results and current treatment reviewed. On a regular basis, two to four times per year, the degree of long-term metabolic control should be checked as assessed by HbA1c, body weight, blood pressure, and blood lipids, and the feet should be inspected. At least once a year, or more often according to individual needs, the eyes and kidney function should be checked, as well as self-monitoring and injection techniques and eating habits. Each visit should also include a period of continued education about diabetes and its treatment.
- *Continuing education*. Continuous education includes, among several things, teaching why and how to control blood glucose levels, how to monitor blood and urine tests and how to react on the results, knowledge about signs of low and high blood glucose levels including ketosis, how to treat these conditions and how to prevent them, knowledge about long-term complications,

and how to deal with life-style variations such as exercise and alcohol.
- *Special situations*. Information must be provided to the patient regarding how to act in special situations as such planning to become pregnant, in emergencies, and when having problems with long-term complications.

The Patients' Charter not only describes what should be available to the patient from the health care providers to achieve the treatment goals, but also stresses that the diabetic person also has responsibilities in self-care, and these responsibilities are also delineated.

QUALITY DEVELOPMENT

The recognition of quality as the focal point of health care in diabetes, and the excess cost of the disease for society, have prompted several lines of activity in Sweden. They are aimed at identifying, elaborating, and diffusing adequate methods and instruments for the development of quality and cost-effectiveness of diabetes care and at making it possible to implement the St. Vincent Declaration goals.

From 1991 to 1994, several regional surveys were performed by professionals under the supervision of the Swedish National Board of Health and Welfare. These surveys demonstrated regional differences in care provided and in some outcome measures and showed the need for a systematic and continuous improvement in quality of diabetes care. They also demonstrated the importance of standards and recommendations for medical procedures and tools in outcome measures.

In 1993, under the supervision of the Swedish National Board of Health and Welfare, together with professional organizations, a database (Medical Access and Result System, or MARS) was created, consisting of state-of-the-art articles describing the current knowledge and development within the field of diabetes. The content is continuously updated, and the system is distributed to health care providers on CD-ROM, the Internet, or as paper copies.

Based on the knowledge described in the Medical Access and Result System, the National Consensus Guidelines for the Management of Diabetes were presented in 1996 to assist health officials, health planners, health service administrators, and diabetes professionals in the development of local policies and programs, and to help provide adequate patient information. The guidelines cover all aspects of diabetes care, irrespective of age, cultural, and behavioral differences. Similar European guidelines have been published for type 1 and type 2 diabetes mellitus.

With the purpose of creating a tool for systematic, continuous quality assessment, the Swedish National Diabetes Register was launched in 1996 (Tab. 61.4). Each diabetes health care provider will report outcome indicators on an annual basis. Complete anonymity of the patient, the center, and the individual doctor who provides the information is assured. In the first version of the register, true outcome indicators will be registered on visual impairment, leg amputation, end stage renal disease,

Table 61.3 Targets for diabetes control

	Good	Acceptable	Poor
Blood glucose (mmol/l)			
Fasting	4.4-6.1	<7.8	>7.8
Postprandial	4.4-8.0	<10.0	>10.0
HbA$_{1c}$ (%)	<6.5	<7.5	>7.5
Total cholesterol (mmol/l)	<5.2	<6.5	>6.5
HDL cholesterol (mmol/l)	>1.1	>0.9	<0.9
Fasting triglycerides (mmol/l)	<1.7	<2.2	>2.2
Body mass index (kg/m^2)			
Males	20-25	≤27	>27
Females	19-24	≤26	>26
Blood pressure (mmHg)	≤140/90	≤160/95	>160/95

These targets are ideal and may have to be modified. Therefore, individual targets should be established for each patient. E.g., the goals may be too strict in the elderly, while the blood pressure goals in patients with signs of nephropathy need to be even stricter. (HDL = high density lipoprotein.)

Table 61.4 The Swedish National Diabetes Register

Date for registration	....
Patient identity	....
Calendar year for diagnosis of diabetes	....
Diabetes treatment	□ insulin □ oral agents □ diet
HbA$_{1c}$ (%)	....
Body weight (kg)	....
Height (m)	....
Blood pressure (mmHg)	....
Antihypertensive treatment	□ yes □ no
Lipid-lowering treatment	□ yes □ no
Nephropathy (U-albumin >200 μg/min or >300 mg/l)	□ yes □ no
Dialysis/kidney transplantation	□ yes □ no
Visual impairment (<0.3 on the best eye)	□ yes □ no
Myocardial infarction	□ yes □ no
Stroke	□ yes □ no
Amputation above the ankle	□ yes □ no
Smoker (>1 cigarette/day)	□ yes □ no

(Events occurring during each individual calendar year are registered.)

myocardial infarction, and stroke occurring during the past calendar year. Some intermediate outcome indicators, such as degree of metabolic control (HbA$_{1c}$), type of diabetes treatment, presence of antihypertensive, and lipid-lowering treatment will also be registered. In addition, patient-oriented indicators, such as body mass index and smoking habits, will be included. Feedback information will be given annually to each center, together with data representing the whole country and different regions, for comparison. Data will also be stratified according to age and type of diabetes treatment in relation to the degree of metabolic control in order to avoid the influence of case-mix between different health care providers.

Suggested readings

ALBERTI KGMM, APFEL J, GRIES FA, et al. The European Patients' Charter. Diabetic Med 1991;8:782.

ALBERTI KGMM, GRIES FA, JERVELL J, KRANS HMJ FOR THE EUROPEAN IDDM POLICY GROUP. A desktop guide for the management of non-insulin-dependent diabetes (NIDDM). An update. Diabetic Med 1994;11:899.

BERNE C, AGARDH C-D. Diabetes mellitus - current Swedish national guidelines Nord Med 1997;112:151.

DIABETES 1993. Vital statistics. American Diabetes Association, Alexandria, VA, 1993.

DIRECT AND INDIRECT COSTS OF DIABETES IN THE UNITED STATES IN 1992. American Diabetes Association, Alexandria, VA, 1993.

EUROPEAN IDDM POLICY GROUP. Consensus guidelines for the management of insulin-dependent (type 1) diabetes. Diabetic Med 1993;10:990.

HEALTH FOR ALL - TARGETS YEAR 2000. The health policy in Europe. In: Anonymous, (ed). European Health for All - Series 4. Copenhagen: WHO Regional Office for Europe, 1991.

WORKSHOP REPORT. Diabetes care and research in Europe: the Saint Vincent Declaration. Diabetic Med 1990;7:360.

ZIMMET P, MCCARTY D. The NIDDM epidemic: global estimates and projections - a look into the crystal ball. IDF Bulletin 1995;40:8.

Hypoglycemia in type 1 diabetes mellitus

Geremia B. Bolli

KEY POINTS

- The prevention of hypoglycemia is essential for survival because the brain uses only glucose for its metabolism.
- Several mechanisms have evolved in the physiology of glucose counter-regulation to protect brain function against hypoglycemia. These mechanisms are named counter-regulatory mechanisms and involve the secretion of hormones, changes in substrate concentrations, and neural mechanisms that cooperate in a complex fashion to prevent hypoglycemia.
- In type 1 diabetes mellitus, hypoglycemia is frequent because of therapeutic (iatrogenic) hypoglycemia, and also because counter-regulatory defenses are impaired. The reduced responses of glucagon and adrenaline are the most important alterations in this regard.
- While the reasons of reduced responses of glucagon at times of hypoglycemia are not known, much is known about reduced responses of adrenaline. Recent antecedent hypoglycemia is responsible largely for, if not fully, the loss of responses of adrenaline to hypoglycemia in type 1 diabetes mellitus.
- Because optimal insulin treatment should be directed at improving long-term blood glucose control without increasing the number and severity of hypoglycemic episodes, it is essential that the insulin plan is based on a rational strategy to minimize the frequency of hypoglycemia. Otherwise, it is possible that a vicious circle of "hypoglycemia-reduced responses of adrenaline-more hypoglycemia could be created".

Hypoglycemia is a fact of life for people with type 1 diabetes mellitus (T1DM). Mild, asymptomatic episodes occur once or twice a week in insulin-treated diabetic subjects. Nocturnal, asymptomatic hypoglycemia occurs in about 25% of diabetic subjects treated with either "conventional" or "intensive" insulin therapy. Mild hypoglycemia, if recurrent, induces unawareness of hypoglycemia and impairs glucose counterregulation, which in turn predisposes to severe hypoglycemia. In the Diabetes Control and Complications Trial (DCCT), the frequency of severe hypoglycemia, i.e. coma or hypoglycemia severe enough to require assistance from a third party,

increased ~3 fold in diabetic subjects treated with intensive insulin therapy as compared to subjects on "conventional" therapy (from ~0.2 to ~0.6 episodes/patient-year). Notably, also in type 1 diabetic patients, including children and adolescents on "conventional" therapy, the frequency of severe hypoglycemia reported is as high as ~0.20 episodes/patient-year.

Even brief hypoglycemia can cause profound dysfunction of the brain. Prolonged, severe hypoglycemia can cause permanent neurological sequelae. In addition, it is possible that hypoglycemia may accelerate the vascular complications of diabetes by increasing platelet aggregation and/or fibrinogen formation. Finally, hypoglycemia may be fatal. Pooling the data of literature, at least 4% of deaths of nearly one thousand patients with type 1 diabetes mellitus are considered to be the result of hypoglycemia. However, because of lack of good epidemiological data, it is likely that this figure is underestimated. Clearly, better knowledge of the causes and mechanisms of insulin-induced hypoglycemia, is highly desirable to reduce the frequency and the consequences of recurrent hypoglycemia, hypoglycemia unawareness, and severe hypoglycemia among insulin-treated diabetic patients.

The importance of glucose for brain metabolism

Tissues such as muscle and liver may easily switch from oxidation of glucose to other non-glucose fuels such as non-esterified free fatty acids, ketones and lactate. In contrast, the brain is a fragile organ regarding its metabolism because from a practical point of view, it utilises only glucose as source of energy. In fact, although in theory the brain can oxidise ketones and lactate, this occurs in humans only under experimental conditions where supraphysiological concentrations of these substrates are produced in plasma by means of exogenous infusion. During insulin-induced hypoglycemia closely mimicking the spontaneous condition of insulin-treated IDDM, plasma ketone concentration decreases, and lactate concentration does not increase substantially. In a late phase of hypoglycemia, plasma ketones increase, but this does not help the brain probably because it is already neuroglycopenic. Because it cannot operate gluconeogenesis, neither store considerable amounts of glucose under the form of glycogen, the brain is strictly dependent on continuous glucose delivery from the circulation for its metabolism and function.

Physiology of responses to hypoglycemia in humans

Because maintenance of plasma glucose concentration above a given threshold is crucial for brain function and thus survival of whole body, it is no surprise that multiple mechanisms cooperate to prevent hypoglycemia in mammals. These counterregulatory mechanisms become especially important under adverse conditions, such as prolonged fasting, failure of vital organs (kidney, heart, liver), or after administration of glucose lowering drugs. The homeostatic mechanisms include, first, suppression of endogenous insulin secretion; second, release of counterregulatory hormones; and, third, generation of specific symptoms. The latter include the autonomic (anxiety, palpitations, hunger, sweating, irritability, tremor), and neuroglycopenic (dizziness, tingling, blurred vision, difficulty in thinking, faintness) symptoms.

When a low dose of insulin is infused in normal, non-diabetic subjects, suppression of endogenous insulin secretion which limits portal hyperinsulinemia is the first observable event against progression into severe hypoglycemia. If blood glucose continues to fall, then the

counterregulatory hormones are released and increase in plasma. Taken together, these mecanhisms result in an increase in hepatic glucose production by the liver and kidney, as well as in a suppression of peripheral glucose utilization in the muscle. These are the key mechanisms which limit the decrease of glucose in plasma aiming at priviledging is use by the brain.

All counterregulatory hormones are important in defense against hypoglycemia, but they play a different role in different phases of hypoglycemia. Both glucagon and adrenaline increase hepatic glucose production acutely and in the long-term. In contrast to glucagon, which does not possess extra-hepatic effects, adrenaline increases also glucose production by the kidney, reduces the uptake of glucose in the muscle, and stimulates lipolysis. The latter effect increases plasma free fatty acid concentration, which in turn contributes to sustained gluconeogenesis in the liver and suppresses oxidation and utilization of glucose in the muscle (Randle's cycle). Growth hormone and cortisol are named "slow" counterregulatory hormones because it takes two to three hours after they are released to observe an insulin-antagonistic effect. Both growth hormone and cortisol increase glucose production from the liver (most likely by accelerating gluconeogenesis), and suppress glucose utilization in the muscle. In addition, they stimulate lipolysis.

If for any reason a single counterregulatory factor, namely a hormone, or a substrate, or the liver *per se* (autoregulation), fails to respond to prolonged hypoglycemia, counterregulation becomes less efficient, and more severe hypoglycemia eventually develops despite larger increases in the remaining counterregulatory hormones (Fig. 62.1). For example, in the early phase of insulin-induced hypoglycemia, the responses of *both* glucagon and adrenaline are similarly important in preventing more severe hypoglycemia. In fact, if glucagon or adrenaline fails to increase, severe hypoglycemia develops despite compensatory increase in the other hormone (Fig. 62.1). Similarly, in the late phase of hypoglycemia, failure of growth hormone or cortisol to increase, is followed by a more severe hypoglycemia despite larger increases in other counterregulatory hormones (Fig. 62.1). Nevertheless, the responses of the "rapid" hormones glucagon and adrenaline to hypoglycemia are more important than those of the "slow" hormones growth hormone and cortisol simply because they exert their counterregulatory effects in an earlier phase before hypoglycemia progresses from mild into severe. The summary of physiology of glucose counterregulation is given in Table 62.1.

An important concept which has evolved during the last few years, is that the brain responses to hypoglycemia are hierarchic. During progressive decrements in plasma glucose, the release of counterregulatory hormones begins *before* the symptoms of hypoglycemia are generated. Several studies have concordantly indicated that all counterregulatory hormones (glucagon, adrenaline, cortisol, growth hormone) are released at a (arterial) plasma glucose threshold of ~65 mg/dl (~3.5 mmol/l); that symptoms (both autonomic and neuroglycopenic) appear when plasma glucose decreases to below ~55 mg/dl (~3.0

Table 62.1 Mechanisms of glucose counterregulation during prolonged, insulin-induced hypoglycemia in normal humans

Factor	Phase	Mechanism(s)
Suppression of insulin secretion by the pancreatic β-cell	Early & late	Limits portal hyperinsulinemia
Secretion of counter-regulatory hormones (glucagon, adrenaline, growth hormone, cortisol)	Early & late	Increase hepatic (and renal?) glucose production Suppress peripheral glucose utilization
Increase of substrates (free fatty acids)	Late	Increase hepatic glucose production Suppress peripheral glucose utilization
Hepatic autoregulation	Late	Increases hepatic glucose production (only in severe hypoglycemia)

(From Bolli GB. From physiology of glucose counter-regulation to prevention of hypoglycemia in type 1 diabetes mellitus. Diab Nutr Metab 1990;4:333-49.)

mmol/l); and that cognitive function deteriorates when plasma glucose decreases to below 50 mg/dl (~2.7 mmol/l).

Definition of hypoglycemia

In classic textbooks of the recent past, hypoglycemia is usually defined as plasma glucose concentration below 50

mg/dl (~2.7 mmol). However, normally the release of counterregulatory hormones to hypoglycemia is already evident for modest decreases in plasma glucose below normal, post-absorptive values. It takes a decrease of only ~10 mg/dl (~0.5 mmol/l) plasma glucose to elicit the counterregulatory response of pancreatic beta-cell, and ~20 mg/dl (~1 mmol/l) decrease in plasma glucose to observe the response of counterregulatory hormones. Thus, a more conservative, physiological definition of hypoglycemia is any decrease in plasma glucose concentration to below ~70 mg/dl (~4.0 mmol/l). This concept is important not only in physiology, but also to define safe glycemic targets of intensive therapy of type 1 and type 2 diabetes mellitus.

Pathophysiology of hypoglycemia in IDDM

Inappropriate therapeutic hyperinsulinemia, either absolute or relative, is the initiating cause of hypoglycemia in diabetes mellitus. Unfortunately, hyperinsulinemia is the rule in diabetes mellitus both T1 and T2 (T2DM), because of the therapeutic delivery of insulin into the peripheral rather than portal circulation, and because of the empirical algorithms used to administer insulin. However, when IDDM patients and non-diabetic subjects are experimentally exposed to similar hyperinsulinemia, hypoglycemia is more severe and prolonged in the former. Clearly, the mechanisms of defense against hypoglycemia are impaired in T1DM. The most common and nearly universal defect is loss of glucagon response to hypoglycemia. Under these conditions, it is the response of the remaining rapid counterregulatory hormone adrena-

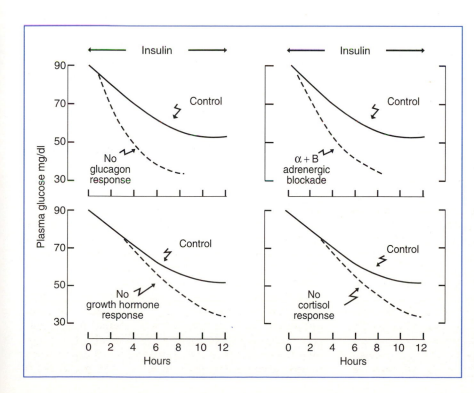

Figure 62.1 Summary of the roles of counterregulatory hormones in defense against prolonged insulin-induced hypoglycemia in normal humans. Lack of increase in a single counterregulatory hormone (broken line) is followed by a more severe hypoglycemia as compared to control studies (solid line) in an early phase of hypoglycemia for glucagon and adrenaline (*rapid* hormones), and in a late phase for growth hormone and cortisol (*late* hormones), despite greater responses of the other remaining counterregulatory hormones. (From Diabetes 1988;37:1608-1617, with permission.)

line, which is critical for counterregulation. Unfortunately, however, many T1DM patients also suffer from reduced responses of adrenaline, especially after recurrent hypoglycemia, and/or in the presence of duration of T1DM greater than 15-20 years. Clearly, it is especially T1DM patients with combined defects of glucagon and adrenaline who are at high risk for severe hypoglycemia during therapeutic administration of insulin which aims at near-normoglycemia.

Glycemic control and glucose thresholds of brain responses to hypoglycemia

One of the most important findings over the last few years has been the observation that the glycemic thresholds of physiological responses to hypoglycemia, i.e. release of counterregulatory hormoens, generation of specific symptoms and impairment in cognitive function, are not fixed, but may shift up- or downwards depending on antecedent glycemic control. For example, chronic hypoglycemia in insulinoma patients and recurrent hypoglycemia in T1DM patients is associated with high thresholds of responses of counterregulatory hormones and symptoms to hypoglycemia (i.e. responses occur at lower than normal plasma glucose). On the other hand, chronic hyperglycemia in diabetes mellitus is associated with low thresholds (i.e., responses occur at higher than normal plasma glucose). The importance of such an observation relies on the fact that a given IDDM patient may, or may not experience symptoms of hypoglycemia depending on his/her recent, antecedent blood glucose control. For example, in case he/she had had recurrent (i.e., daily) episodes of hypoglycemia, it is likely that he/she would not be able to recognise hypoglycemia at all, or possibly become aware of it at lower than normal plasma glucose concentration. However, if hypoglycemia is prevented, the patient may quickly recover symptoms and recognise hypoglycemia at a physiological plasma glucose threshold (see below).

Hypoglycemia and cognitive function

The physiological hierarchy of responses indicates that brain function becomes impaired when plasma glucose concentration decreases to below 50 mg/dl (2.7 mmol/l). However, in patients with history of chronic or recurrent hypoglycemia, brain function is "protected", i.e. onset of cognitive dysfunction occurs at lower than normal plasma glucose concentration. Unfortunately, however, the protection is limited to quite a narrow range of plasma glucose. In fact, if plasma glucose drops below 2.2 mmol/l, then brain function becomes impaired *at the same time*, or even slightly *before* the warning symptoms of hypoglycemia appear. Thus, under these circumstances, the patient becomes severely neuroglycopenic before he/she can take measures to correct neuroglycemia (by eating food). In the absence of immediate external help, this condition may ultimately progress into unconsciousness (coma).

Effect of rate of fall on responses to hypoglycemia

Contrary to common wisdom, a fast fall of blood glucose in patients with type 1 diabetes mellitus, does not elicit greater counterregulatory hormone responses as compared to a slow fall. However, a fast fall of blood glucose results in greater impairment in cognitive function as compared to slow fall. Notably, this effect is less evident in diabetic patients with hypoglycemia unawareness, in keeping with the concept of brain protection by antecedent, recurrent hypoglycemia.

Treatment of hypoglycemia

Minor episodes The standard advice is to rest and take 10-20 g of carbohydrate. In practice patients often overtreat hypoglycemia. It is important to stress the need for both short-acting and longer-acting carbohydrates, e.g. the regimen might be half a glass of orange juice and two biscuits. When circumstances permit, symptoms suggestive of hypoglycemia should be checked by measuring a blood glucose level. This helps patients to correctly interpret their subjective feelings and avoids unnecessary treatment.

Hypoglycemic coma or severe hypoglycemia Some episodes of coma may recover spontaneously (if the patient is alone or asleep) or with the help of glucose forced into the mouth by friends or relatives. As the teeth are often clenched, this may not be easy, and glucose tablets are of little use because the mouth is too dry to dissolve them. Glucose solutions or gels delivered into the cheek space are effective. Failing this, the helpers can give an injection of glucagon. Glucagon is supplied as a powder which must be dissolved before injection.

Medical treatment is either by injection of glucagon 1 mg i.m. or glucose 25 g iv. Although glucose is conventionally given as a bolus dose of 50% glucose (50 ml), lower-strength glucose infusions are preferable and less likely to produce thrombophlebitis. Glucagon is claimed to be of comparable speed and efficacy to glucose, and is simpler and less traumatic to administer.

Antecedent hypoglycemia as primary cause of hypoglycemia unawareness in diabetes mellitus

Evidence has accumulated over the last few years that loss of symptoms of hypoglycemia in IDDM patients is largely, if not fully the result of antecedent, frequent hypoglycemia. The observation in insulinoma patients that cure of hypoglycemia after surgical resection of the tumor, is followed by full recovery of appropriate responses of counterregulatory hormones, symptoms, as well as onset of cognitive dysfunction, has prompted similar observations in T1DM patients. Fanelli et al. have been the first to report that meticulous prevention of hypoglycemia in T1DM patients previously experiencing nearly one episode of hypoglycemia/day, is followed by rapid recovery of symptoms (both autonomic and neuroglycopenic) and counterregulatory responses (Figs. 62.2 and 62.3). In that study, symptoms normalized both in terms of plasma glucose thresholds as well as magnitude. The release of counterregulatory hormones improved, particularly for adrenaline (Fig. 62.3). In normal human volunteers, two episodes of mild and brief insulin-induced hypoglycemia (~50 mg/dl, ~2.7 mmol/l for ~90 minutes, one episode in the morning, the other in the afternoon), or a single episode of nocturnal hypoglycemia, blunt the hormonal and symptom responses to hypoglycemia induced on the following day. Similar observations have been made in IDDM patients. This pattern of responses mimics closely the spontaneous responses of IDDM patients unaware of hypoglycemia.

Thus, frequent iatrogenic hypoglycemia in type 1 diabetes mellitus, rapidly induces loss of symptoms and blunt the release of counterregulatory hormones in response to hypoglycemia. The good news for patients and the important information for diabetologists, is that prevention of hypoglycemia largely, if not fully reverses unawareness of, and improves counterregulation to, hypoglycemia.

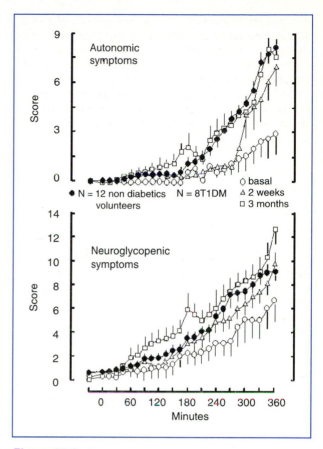

Figure 62.3 Score of autonomic and neuroglycopenic symptoms in responses to the experimental hypoglycemia of Figure 62.2, before, and two weeks and three months after meticulous prevention of hypoglycemia in a group of T1DM patients (From Fanelli C, Epifano L, Rambotti AM, et al. Meticulous prevention of hypoglycemia (near-)normalizes magnitude and glycemic threshold of neuroendocrine responses. Diabetes 1993;42:1683-89.)

Hypoglycemia unawareness and impaired glucose counterregulation

T1DM patients unaware of hypoglycemia suffer from greater impairment of the glucose counterregulatory system, primarily because of more suppressed release of adrenaline. Meticulous prevention of hypoglycemia which recovers symptoms, improves the responses of glucagon, although slightly, at least in short-term T1DM. Prevention of hypoglycemia also normalises the responses of adrenaline to hypoglycemia. However, the effect of prevention of hypoglycemia on responses of adrenaline is more evident in T1DM of short, as compared to T1DM of long duration, and in T1DM without, as compared to those with, clinically overt autonomic neuropathy.

Taken together, these observations point it out that prevention of hypoglycemia reverses most of the suppressed adrenaline responses to hypoglycemia in T1DM. Sometimes, the responses of adrenaline to hypoglycemia

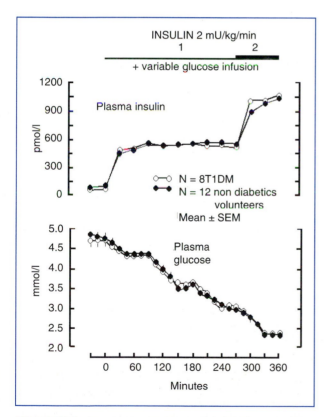

Figure 62.2 Plasma insulin and glucose concentrations during experimental step-wise decreases in plasma glucose (hyperinsulinemic-hypoglycemic glucose clamp) in a group of T1DM patients and non-diabetic subjects. Responses of counterregulatory hormones, symptoms and cognitive function were measured at each plateau plasma glucose concentration (From Fanelli C, Epifano L, Rambotti AM, et al. Meticulous prevention of hypoglycemia (near-) normalizes magnitude and glycemic threshold of neuroendocrine responses. Diabetes 1993;42:1683-89.)

are apparently irreversibly lost in long-term diabetes mellitus despite meticulous prevention of hypoglycemia and absence of autonomic neuropathy. This cannot be easily explained at the present time. However, these data indicate that loss of adrenaline responses to hypoglycemia are not necessarily the result of autonomic neuropathy, although clinically overt autonomic neuropathy importantly contributes to this. In addition, these data indicate that it is especially long-term IDDM which requires a careful approach with insulin treatment to prevent hypoglycemia, because it is long-term diabetes which is associated with loss of glucagon responses and most of adrenaline responses, to hypoglycemia.

Mechanisms of hypoglycemia unawareness

In rats, chronic hypoglycemia increases, whereas chronic hyperglycemia decreases, glucose transport to the brain. In humans, prolonged hypoglycemia increases fractional extraction of glucose from blood. In T1DM with low values of glycosylated hemoglobin (HbA$_{1c}$) due to

antecedent, frequent hypoglycemia, fractional extraction of glucose does not decrease during hypoglycemia in contrast to T1DM patients with elevated HbA$_{1c}$ and nondiabetic subjects. Taken together, these observations support the view that brain glucose transport is influenced by antecedent prevailing plasma glucose concentration. Hypoglycemia accelerates delivery of glucose to the brain. Thus, during subsequent hypoglycemia, the brain is not, or at least is less, neuroglycopenic than normal, and does not need to generate the counterregulatory responses and the autonomic symptoms to defend and alert the subject about pending hypoglycemia. More recently, Davis et al. have provided evidence for an additional mechanism of hypoglycemia unawareness, i.e. that the responses of cortisol to antecedent hypoglycemia blunt the autonomic hormone responses to subsequent hypoglycemia. Although in theory both mechanisms may be involved, at present time their relative contribution to hypoglycemia unawareness in diabetes mellitus is not known.

The vicious circle "recurrent hypoglycemia-unawareness"

Intensive insulin therapy aims at (near-)normoglycemia. Because subcutaneous insulin replacement is so imperfect, mild hypoglycemia is inevitably induced from time to time. In turn, if hypoglycemia is frequent (e.g. one episode/day), glucose transport to the brain accelerates and/or cortisol is released. If the former mechanism were operating, it would result in the the paradoxical situation of low glucose concentration in blood (hypoglycemia), but normal or near-normal glucose in the brain (absence of neuroglycopenia). This would explain the suppression of brain responses to hypoglycemia, i.e. less generation of the autonomic responses and blunted release of adrenaline. This also explains the preservation of cognitive function below the plasma glucose threshold of onset of cognitive dysfunction. However, as any compensatory mechanism, if glucose concentration falls below a given threshold in plasma, glucose transport suddenly decreases despite the above mentioned greater activity of glucose transporters at the level of the blood brain barrier, and severe neuroglycopenia suddenly develops.

Prevention of hypoglycemia is an important part of the modern intensive therapy. In theory, if one were able to prevent hypoglycemia since the very first clinical onset of T1DM and to keep preventing hypoglycemia during the following years, hypoglycemia unawareness should not appear in the natural history of diabetes mellitus. In fact, meticulous prevention of hypoglycemia in T1DM patients previously suffering from recurrent hypoglycemia, fully reverses the syndrome of hypoglycemia unawareness and impaired release of adrenaline in short-term T1DM. In addition, if intensive therapy is conducted in a way that prevents the decrease in HbA$_{1c}$ below 6.0%, the frequency of hypoglycemia is minimised, secretion of adrenaline and generation of symptoms in response to hypoglycemia appear to be appropriate.

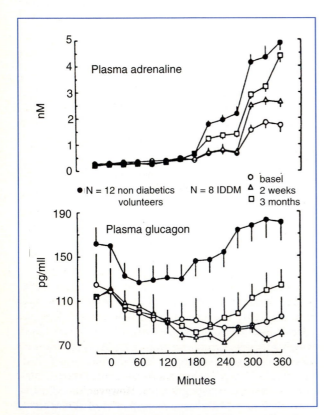

Figure 62.4 Plasma adrenaline and glucagon responses to the experimental hypoglycemia of Figure 62.2, before, and two weeks and three months after meticulous prevention of hypoglycemia in a group of T1DM patients (from Fanelli C, Epifano L, Rambotti AM, et al. Meticulous prevention of hypoglycemia (near-)normalizes magnitude and glycemic thresholds of neuroendocrine responses... Diabetes 1993;42:1683-89.)

Need of combining intensive therapy which aims at (near)-normoglycemia with prevention of hypoglycemia to prevent hypoglycemia unawareness

The DCCT study has indicated that intensive insulin therapy which decreases HbA_{1c} <7.0% strongly protects against onset/progression of long-term microvascular complications. However, the DCCT has also reported an increase in the risk for severe hypoglycemia by ~3 times. The key "post-DCCT" question is if it is possible to reconcile the goal of long-term near-normoglycemia with that of prevention of recurrent hypoglycemia, to prevent hypoglycemia unawareness and loss of adrenaline responses to hypoglycemia (impaired counterregulation).

The answer is YES. Interestingly, a therapeutic program which prevents hypoglycemia is compatible with long-term near-normoglycemia and HbA_{1c} <7.0%. This programme is based on good knowledge of insulin pharmacokinetics and pharmacodynamics. In short, it is primarily based on a rational scheme of insulin delivery, good education of the patient, and close contact between patient and the treating team to choose an appropriate insulin dose.

In the prevention of diurnal hypoglycemia, the model of insulin therapy is the first pre-requisite for success. It should be based on multiple daily doses of insulin. Because both the short-acting insulin analogue lispro and the long-acting insulin analogue glargine prevent hypoglycemia better than human insulin, short-acting insulin analogues at meal-time and glargine insulin at dinner-time should be given. If NPH insulin is still used, in totally C-peptide negative T1DM patients, a second intermediate-acting insulin dose at lunch (~30% of the total lunch dose) is often useful to improve blood glucose concentration at dinner time. However, intermediate-acting insulin should not be given at breakfast, because it increases the risk for hypoglycemia before, or immediately after lunch. The only exception is small kids who need a midmorning snack. In this case a small dose of intermediate-acting insulin (~30% of the total dose) should be given at breakfast.

In the prevention of nocturnal hypoglycemia, it is *essential* to split the evening insulin dose into regular insulin at dinner, and a fourth injection of NPH insulin at 23:00-24:00 hours. In fact, NPH insulin has a peak of action between 4-6 hours after s.c. injection and, if injected at dinner with the aim of improving fasting blood glucose, it increases the risk for nocturnal hypoglycemia despite the bed-time snack.

To prevent hypoglycemia, self-monitoring of blood glucose and close contact with the diabetologist (cellular phone may be essential) are of course key factors for the success. The glycemic target should be 130-140 mg/dl (7-8 mmol/l) in the fasting state, prior to each meal and at bed-time. If this goal is successfully achieved, the percentage of HbA_{1c} should range between 6.0-7.0%, i.e in an interval of good protection against onset/progression of microvascular complications. If the short-acting insulin analogue lispro is used with NPH, glycemic control improves long-term without increasing the risk for hypo-

glycemia. However, this can be achieved solely if NPH insulin is added to the meal doses of lispro according to a new strategy of replacement of basal insulin.

In summary, the challenge of the modern treatment of T1DM, especially young, new-onset patients, is to achieve long-term near-normoglycemia while minimising the frequency of hypoglycemia. This is nowdays possible and feasible. It is expected to be even easier with increasing experience in combining short-acting and long-acting insulin analogues.

HYPOGLYCEMIA IN TYPE 2 DIABETES MELLITUS

Hypoglycemia in T2DM is less frequent than in T1DM because of insulin resistance, and intact counterregulation, at least in patients with short duration of diabetes. As diabetes duration increases and beta-cell function deteriorates substantially (plasma C-peptide <0.1 nmol/l), glucagon responses to hypoglycemia may become as abnormal as in T1DM. Nevertheless, hypoglycemia may occur in T2DM, especially if treatment is directed at achieving the goals of intensive therapy. Hypoglycemia may occur as consequence of both insulin and/or sulphonylurea treatment.

Sulphonylurea-induced hypoglycemia

Sulphonylurea-induced hypoglycemia may be severe and protracted, especially during treatment with long-acting sulphonylureas such as chlorpropamide and glibenclamide. It is recommended that short-acting sulphonylureas (e.g. tolbutamide) or short-acting insulin secretagogues (e.g. replaglinide, nateglinide) are used at meals to minimise the risk for inappropriate hyperinsulinemia after prolonged stimulation of pancreatic beta-cells. Sulphonylureas should not be used in the presence of failure of a vital organ (liver, heart, kidney, lung). Old age is a relative, but important contra-indication because of the erratic nutrition of the elderly and because of the decline in glomerul filtration rate at advanced age. Under these circumstances, meal-time administration of short-acting insulin is preferable to sulphonylureas because insulin can be more easily adapted to the individual nutritional plan of every day. An interesting alternative is the administration of the long-acting insulin analogue glargine in the evening.

One important aspect of the risk for hypoglycemia with sulphonylureas in T2DM, is the greater insulin sensitivity in the afternoon as compared to the morning hours. It means that the limiting blood glucose during sulphonylurea administration in the morning or at lunchtime, is the pre-dinner, not the pre-breakfast value, because if the dose is titrated on the pre-breakfast value, the risk for late afternoon hypoglycemia increases.

Hypoglycemia following sulphonylurea treatment should be regarded to as an emergency, especially in the elderly who may suffer at the same time of concomitant diseases such as hypertension, and cerebral and/or cardiac artery disease. Intravenous glucose (10-20% solution) at the rate of 200-300 mg/min should be initiated preferably in the hospital, and maintained for several hours, sometimes for more than 24 hours, at the rate to be decided based on blood glucose determination every 30 minutes), because of the long plasma half-life of sulphonylureas and/or its metabolites.

Because of the above considerations, sulphylureas are not the ideal pharmacological candidate for intensive treatment of T2DM nowdays required after the conclusion of the UKPDS. Sulphonylureas should be cautiously used at low doses, keeping it in mind the seriousness of hypoglycemia they can induce which is complicated by 10-20% mortality. It will be interesting in the future to assess whether the new short-acting insulin secretagogues (repaglanide, nateglinide) will decrease the risk for hypoglycemia in intensive treatment of T2DM.

Acknowledgements

The friendly support from the BBC & B Co., Inc., is gratefully acknowledged.

Suggested readings

BOLLI GB. From physiology of glucose counterregulation to prevention of hypoglycemia in Type 1 diabetes mellitus. Diab Nutr Metab 1990;4:333-49.

BOLLI GB, DI MARCHI RD, PARK GD, PRAMMING S, KOIVISTO VA. Insulin analogues and their potential in the management of diabetes mellitus. Diabetologia 1999;42:1151-67.

BOYLE P, KEMPERS S, O'CONNOR AM, NAGY RJ. Brain glucose uptake and hypoglycemia unawareness in patients with insulin-dependent diabetes mellitus. N Engl J Med 1995;333:1726-31.

CRYER PE. Iatrogenic hypoglycemia as a cause of hypoglycemia-associated autonomic failure in IDDM: a vicious circle. Diabetes 1992;41:255-60.

DAVIS SN, SHAVERS C, COSTA F, MOSQUEDA-GARCIA R. Role of cortisol in the pathogenesis of deficient counterregulation after antecedent hypoglycemia in normal humans. J Clin Invest 1996;98:680-91.

FANELLI C, DI VINCENZO A, MODARELLI F, et al. Post-hypoglycemic hyperketonemia does not contribute to brain metabolism during insulin-induced neuroglycopenia in humans. Diabetologia 1993;36:1191-97.

FANELLI C, EPIFANO L, RAMBOTTI AM, et al. Meticulous prevention of hypoglycemia (near-)normalizes magnitude and glycemic thresholds of neuroendocrine responses to, symptoms of, and cognitive function during hypoglycemia in intensively treated patients with IDDM of short duration. Diabetes 1993;42:1683-89.

FANELLI C, PAMPANELLI S, LALLI C, et al. Long-term intensive therapy of IDDM diabetic patients with clinically overt autonomic neuropathy: effects on awareness of, and counterregulation to hypoglycemia. Diabetes 1997;46:1172-81.

FANELLI C, PAMPANELLI S, LEPORE M, et al. Prevention of nocturnal hypoglycemia in intensive therapy of IDDM. Diabetes 1998;47 (Suppl 1):A109.

FANELLI C, PAMPANELLI S, PORCELLATI F, et al. Effect of rate of blood glucose fall on responses to hypoglycemia in T1 DM. Diabetes 2000;49 (Suppl 1):A133.

FANELLI CG, PAMPANELLI S, PORCELLATI F, BOLLI GB. Shift of glycemic thresholds for cognitive function in hypoglycemia unawareness in humans. Diabetologia 1998; 41:720-23.

GERICH J, MOKAN M, VENEMAN T, KORYTKOWSKI M, MITRAKOU A. Hypoglycemia unawareness. Endo Rev 1991;12:356-71.

PAMPANELLI S, FANELLI C, LALLI C, et al. Long-term intensive insulin therapy: effects of HbA1c, risk for severe and mild hypoglycemia, status of counterregulation and unawareness of hypoglycemia. Diabetologia 1996;39:677-86.

PERRIELLO G, PIMENTA W, PAMPANELLI S, et al. Demonstration of a day-night variations in systemic glucose production, but not in systemic and muscle glucose uptake in Type 2 diabetes mellitus. Diabetes 1998;47 (Suppl 1):A41.

RATTNER R, HIRSCH IB, NEIFING JL, GARG SK, MECCA TE, WILSON CA, for the USA Study group of Insulin Glargine in Type 1 diabetes: Less hypoglycemia with insulin glargine in intensive treatment for Type 1 diabetes. Diabetes Care 2000;23:639-43.

THE DIABETES CONTROL AND COMPLICATIONS TRIAL RESEARCH GROUP. The effect of intensive treatment of diabetes on the development and progression of long-term complications in insulin-dependent diabetes mellitus. N Engl J Med 1993;329:977-86.

UK PROSPECTIVE DIABETES STUDY (UKPDS) GROUP. Intensive blood-glucose control with sulphonylureas or insulin compared with conventional treatment and risk of complications in patients with type 2 diabetes (UKPDS 33). Lancet 1998;352:837-53.

YKI-JÄRVINEN H, DRESSLER A, ZIEMEN M, HOE 901/3002 Study Group: Less nocturnal hypoglycemia and better post-dinner glucose control with bedtime insulin glargine compared with bedtime NPH insulin during insulin combination therapy in type 2 diabetes. Diabetes Care 2000; 23:1130-36.

63

Obesity and metabolic syndrome

Peter Arner

Obesity is defined as an excess of body fat in relation to other body compartments. Non-obese women have a higher percentage of body fat than non-obese men. There is no consensus on how much excess fat is needed for a subject to be diagnosed as being obese, however, >25% body fat in men and >30% in women are common cut-off points for the diagnosis of obesity. Fat distribution is an additional aspect of obesity. Men and women of normal weight have gender differences in fat distribution: it is evenly distributed in men and peripherally distributed (around the gluteofemoral region and lower abdominal area) in women. In obesity, the gender differences are often further pronounced. Most men develop an upper-body type of obesity with excess fat being localized in the abdominal subcutaneous and visceral fatty regions. Obese women, on the other hand, usually deposit excess fat in the peripheral regions. This difference in body fat distribution is of clinical importance (see below). However, there are women with upper-body obesity and men with peripheral obesity. When obesity is marked (i.e., body fat >40 to 50%), the fat is distributed in a uniform fashion in all depots.

Body fat and body fat distribution can be measured in a number of ways (Tab. 63.1). Weight-to-height ratios are useful measures of body fat since they are simple and inexpensive. The most commonly used index is the body mass index (BMI = weight/height^2). Obesity is often defined as BMI >27 to 28 kg/m^2, since mortality risk starts to increase above this BMI range. Other frequently used measures of body fat are skin-folds (reflecting subcutaneous fat) and bioelectric impedance (all fat stores). Body fat distribution can be measured indirectly by circumferences. The most commonly used one is waist-to-hip-ratio. Upper-body fat distribution is usually defined as waist-hip ratio of >1.00 in men and >0.90 in women. Direct (but expensive) measures of body fat distribution are computed tomography and magnetic resonance imaging.

The prevalence of obesity is steadily increasing in most countries. In particular, the increase is apparent in the parts of the Pacific Ocean region where there has been a recent change from a traditional to a Westernized life-

Table 63.1 Some methods to measure body fat (BF) and body fat distribution (BFD)

Method	Remarks
Under water weighing	Complicated but exact measure of BF
Isotope techniques	Expensive but exact measure of BF
Skin-folds	Very easy but measures only subcutaneous BF
Impedance	Easy but less accurate measure of BF
Weight-to-height ratio	Very easy but less accurate indirect measurement of BF
DEXA	Expensive; can measure BF and BFD
Computed tomography	Very expensive measure of BFD; exposure to radioactivity
Nuclear magnetic resonance	Very expensive measure of BFD
Ultrasound	Easy measure of subcutaneous BFD
Circumferences	Very easy and indirect but less accurate measure of BFD
Sagittal measure	Easy and indirect but less accurate measure of visceral BFD

style. For example, obesity (defined as BMI >30 kg/m^2) was almost unknown in Micronesian and Polynesian populations 20 to 30 years ago, but it is now present in 60 to 70% of the adults. There are comprehensive data in Europe on the prevalence of obesity; approximately 15% of adult men and 22% of adult women are obese (BMI >30 kg/m^2).

Etiology

In the majority of cases, obesity is primarily caused by *high energy intake* in combination with a *low level of physical activity*. The epidemiological evidence for this assumption is evident. The change in lifestyle among populations in the Pacific Ocean region and among minority populations in North America (such as Pima Indians) from their traditional lifestyle (low calorie density food and high physical activity) to a Westernized one (high calorie density nutrients and sedentary living) occurred in parallel with a dramatic increase in obesity prevalence, as discussed above. However, other factors may contribute to the development of obesity (Tab. 63.2). Eating disorders are relatively common, affecting 1 to 3% of the general population. *Bulimia* nervosa is characterized by frequent episodes of excessive eating, accompanied by emotional distress and compensatory behavior to avoid weight gain. *Binge eating* is characterized by frequent excess food intake accompanied by emotional distress, but without compensatory behavior to avoid weight increase. Both conditions are associated with the development of obesity. *Affective psychiatric disorders* are sometimes accompanied by binge eating, and the pharmacotherapy of several affective disorders has increased appetite as a side effect. In many countries obesity is more common among the poor than among the rich, perhaps due to the differences in *socioeconomic status*. *Cultural differences* may also play a role. There are different trends in body imaging between ethnic groups. For example, dissatisfaction with being overweight is less frequently observed among African-American women than among Caucasian women.

Genetic factors are most likely of importance for the development of obesity. Results of family studies suggest that up to 40% of the variance in body fat between individuals is hereditary. Body fat distribution is also at least partly determined by genetic factors. Regarding the mode of inheritance, the vast majority of obesity cases do not segregate in families with a clear Mendelian pattern, indicating a complex heritability. In rare cases such as Prader-Willi syndrome and Pardent-Beedle syndrome, obesity might be attributed to a single gene defect. However, in most cases it is likely that obesity is due to the interaction between a number of environmental and genetic factors.

In spite of intensive research during the last years, the genes causing human obesity are unknown. This is in contrast to animal models of obesity. Thus, the genes causing obesity in rodents have all been characterized recently. Except for some rare examples, the "animal obesity genes" do not, however, seem to be of importance for

Table 63.2 Etiology of obesity
High caloric intake in combination with low physical activity
Psychosocial factors
Eating disorders
Affective disorders
Socioeconomic background
Ethnic factors
Genetic factors
Altered function of adipose tissue
Decreased lipolysis
Increased lipid synthesis
Endocrine (i.e., leptin) abnormalities
Increased development of white fat cells
Dysfunctional sympatho-adrenal activity
Decreased energy expenditure
Miscellaneous (appetite regulation, thyroid hormones, glucocorticosteroid)

human obesity. There has been much attention in genetic epidemiology studies of human obesity focused on so-called thrifty genes. It is postulated that a high ability to conserve energy, for example as fat, was a survival advantage in ancient living conditions when the availability of food was small and/or unpredictable. Such a "thrifty" genetic variance becomes a burden in modern society with an abundance of food available and less need of physically demanding activities. Indeed, the best examples of common human obesity genes are the recently described polymorphisms in several of the beta-adrenoceptor genes. These genes could be considered thrifty because of their role in energy mobilization (glycogen breakdown in liver, triglyceride hydrolysis in fat tissue). Polymorphisms in codon 64 of the β_3-adrenoceptor gene and in codon 27 of the β_2-adrenoceptor gene are independently associated with obesity in humans.

An additional reason for becoming obese could be malfunctioning adipose tissue. Adipose tissue is the major site for lipid storage and mobilization (Fig. 63.1), which is regulated by two enzymes, lipoprotein lipase and hormone-sensitive lipase. The former enzyme is synthesized by fat cells and transported to the stroma-vascular part of adipose tissue, where it can hydrolyze circulating triglycerides produced by the liver or derived alimentary. This results in the liberation of free fatty acids, which are taken up by the fat cells to be esterified to triglycerides. The intracellular triglycerides in fat cells are hydrolyzed (lipolysis) by the

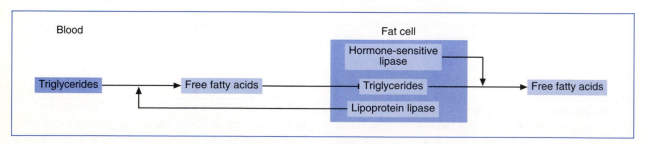

Figure 63.1 Regulation of triglyceride storage and mobilization in fat cells.

hormone-sensitive lipase, which is produced and exclusively localized inside the cell. The end products of lipolysis (glycerol and fatty acids) are liberated into the bloodstream to be utilized by other organs. Both the lipoprotein and the hormone-sensitive lipase enzymes are regulated by hormones, in particular insulin and catecholamines. Insulin stimulates lipoprotein lipase and inhibits hormone-sensitive lipase, whereas the opposite effect is obtained with catecholamines. Increased activity of lipoprotein lipase and decreased function of hormone-sensitive lipase have been repeatedly demonstrated in adipose tissue of obese humans, which can at least partly be ascribed to alterations in the function of insulin and catecholamines. These alterations may promote obesity since they favor net storage of fat in the fat cells. However, it remains to be established whether alterations in adipose tissue lipases are primary or secondary events in obesity.

It has recently become evident that adipose tissue, besides its metabolic function, also has an important endocrine role (Fig. 63.2). A number of proteins are produced in adipose tissue. They are either acting within the tissue in a para-endocrine fashion or transported to other organs, where they are active in a classical endocrine fashion. The most well-known adipose tissue hormone is *leptin*. Leptin is produced by adipose tissue (and the placenta) and is transported to the brain, where it inhibits appetite and stimulates thermogenesis. Results of animal studies suggest that leptin is the key protein in the so-called *lipostate mechanism*, by which the brain senses the amount of body fat in order to keep body weight constant in adult life. It is well-established that defects in leptin and/or in the leptin receptor cause obesity in animal models and that treatment of obese animals with leptin reduces body weight. However, the role of leptin in human obesity is not yet known, although a few obese patients with defective leptin protein have been reported. In most obese humans the circulating levels of leptin are increased. These leptin molecules seem to have a normal structure, and no major leptin receptor defects have been reported in man except for in a few families. In other words, it appears that obese humans, if anything, are resistant to leptin. This, of course, makes leptin a less likely candidate for anti-obesity drug therapy (see below).

Another adipose-specific hormone is *acylation-stimulating protein*. Its precursor, adipsin, is produced by fat cells and is converted to acylation-stimulating protein in the adipose tissue. This hormone stimulates lipid synthesis and inhibits lipolysis by adipose tissue through specific receptors. It has been suggested (but not proven) that altered action of acylation-stimulating protein in fat cells is of importance for the development of obesity.

In theory, obesity could develop through increased formation of new fat cells. In contrast to the development of brown adipose tissue, which takes place primarily before birth, the development of white adipose tissue, which predominates in humans, is a continuous process. The growth of new fat cells is a complex process that begins with the transformation of stem cells in the adipose tissue stroma differentiating into adipoplasts and pre-adipocytes; these cells then mature to adipocytes. So far there is no evidence that altered fat cell differentiation and development are of importance for the development of obesity.

Disturbances in the sympathetic nervous system have often been observed in obesity. Bearing in mind the important role of catecholamines in energy mobilization (lipolysis, glycogenolysis), energy expenditure (skeletal muscle work), and energy delivery (blood vessels), it is an attractive speculation that altered sympathetic activity could promote obesity. However, the role of the sympathetic system in obesity is controversial since both increased and decreased activity has been demonstrated. This inconsistency in findings might be due to methodological difficulties in measuring the sympathetic neuronal activity and adrenal production of catecholamines.

Decreased energy expenditure has sometimes been linked to obesity. However, the results have to be interpreted with caution because of difficulties in performing thorough comparative measurements in energy expenditure between obese and non-obese subjects. For example, basal metabolic rate, which is a major component of energy expenditure, is proportional to the lean body mass as well as to the fat mass.

Finally, a number of additional factors could be of importance for developing obesity such as defects in appetite regulation and hormonal abnormalities (thyroid, hormone, glucocorticosteroids). However, there is no evidence that such abnormalities are of importance for common cases of obesity.

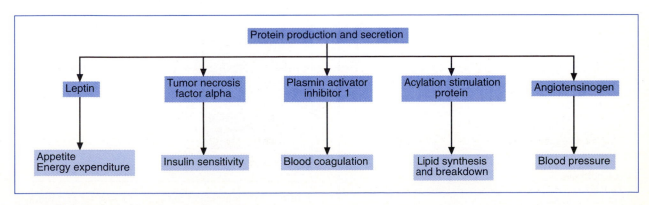

Figure 63.2 Endocrine function of adipose tissue.

Complications

One of the major health implications of obesity is its strong association with a number of medical disorders and decreased longevity (Tab. 63.3). Obesity usually coexists with several metabolic and cardiovascular abnormalities, in particular hyperglycemia, dyslipidemia, high blood pressure, and atherosclerotic cardiovascular disorders (i.e., stroke, coronary heart disease). This relation is most evident in upper-body obesity; peripheral obesity has little or no association with the mentioned clinical abnormalities. When several of these abnormalities occur together they form a so-called metabolic syndrome. Insulin resistance and hyperinsulinemia seem to be the key factors linking the different components in the metabolic syndrome together. Insulin resistance is due to a combination of decreased insulin cell surface receptor expression and a decrease in the less well-defined postreceptor intracellular signaling pathways. The insulin resistance and/or hyperinsulinemia could explain many of the metabolic and cardiovascular abnormalities of obese subjects. For example, hyperinsulinemia can increase the sympathetic nervous activity and alter the intracellular electrolyte balance that causes hypertension. Hyperinsulinemia can also alter lipoprotein synthesis by the liver and stimulate growth of arterial vessel wall (insulin is a growth factor), thereby causing dyslipidemia and atherosclerosis. When the insulin resistance is not adequately compensated by increased insulin production by the pancreatic beta cells, hyperglycemia is a result. Other abnormalities associated with the metabolic syndrome of obese subjects are hyperuricemia, coagulation abnormalities, and microalbuminuria.

There are additional pathophysiological mechanisms to consider in the metabolic syndrome of obese subjects. The circulating fatty acid level is increased in most obese subjects, which is at least in part due to a mass effect of the expanded fat tissue. High levels of fatty acids may inhibit insulin action, stimulate liver synthesis of triglycerides and glucose, as well as inhibit muscular uptake of glucose. Alterations of the endocrine function of adipose tissue could be involved as well (Fig. 63.1). For example, increased production and release of tumor necrosis factor alpha from adipose tissue of obese subjects may induce insulin resistance (because the cytokine modulates insulin action). Increased leptin production by adipose tissue could alter appetite regulation and change energy expenditure. Increased production of plasminogen activator inhibitor-1 by adipose tissue could impair blood coagulation. Increased angiotensinogen productions might cause hypertension. Another factor could be elevated sensitivity of the hypothalamopituitary-adrenal axis in the metabolic syndrome, which is followed by increased secretion of corticotropin-releasing hormone, adrenocorticotropin, cortisol and, in women, adrenal androgens. These alterations can, at least in part, explain several features of the metabolic syndrome such as upper-body fat distribution and insulin resistance. Finally, visceral fat must be considered (Fig. 63.3). Visceral fat mass is increased in most upper-body obese subjects, and there is a strong correlation between the amount of visceral fat and many features of metabolic syndrome. Visceral fat is, unlike other fat depots, directly drained by the liver through the portal vein. Visceral fat lipolysis is increased in upper-body obese subjects. This, in combination with a mass effect, may lead to a marked increase in the portal fatty acid concentration of upper body-obesity subjects that, in turn, can cause stimulation of gluconeogenesis and lipoprotein synthesis in the liver, as well as inhibition of insulin action and insulin breakdown by the liver.

The diabetes in obese subjects is usually type 2 (non-insulin-dependent). It is well-established that obesity complicates the management of diabetes; oral anti-diabetic drugs and/or insulin often do not normalize the hyperglycemia in the obese diabetic patient. However, weight-reduction often greatly improves the metabolic control, probably because it increases insulin sensitivity and improves beta-cell response to insulin secretory stimuli.

The *hypertension* in obese subjects is characterized by an elevation of both systolic and diastolic blood pressure.

Table 63.3 Important complications of obesity

Metabolic (insulin resistance) syndrome
Diabetes mellitus
Hypertension
Dyslipidemia
Gallstones
Cardiac disorders
  Coronary heart disease
  Heart failure
  Arrhythmias
  Sudden death
Pulmonary disorders
  Respiratory insufficiency
  Obstructive sleep apnea
  Pickwickian syndrome
Osteoarthritis
Infertility
Increased mortality

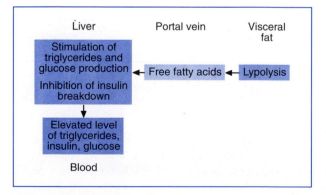

Figure 63.3 Interaction between visceral fat and the liver in upper body obesity.

Of practical importance when measuring blood pressure in obese subjects is the use of an appropriate-size compression cuff. A cuff which is too small will give falsely high pressure. Weight loss is the cornerstone of hypertension management in the obese patient, as even a moderate weight reduction can reduce blood pressure. When physical conditioning is incorporated with weight loss, there is an additive effect on blood pressure that is probably related to improved insulin sensitivity. When choosing an antihypertensive agent, it is important to remember that several of the drugs may worsen some of the metabolic and endocrine disturbances that accompany obesity. For example, thiazide diuretics may worsen insulin resistance and impair insulin secretion by the beta cells, and beta-adrenoceptor blockers may cause insulin resistance, glucose intolerance, and dyslipidemia. Calcium blockers and angiotensin-converting enzyme inhibitors are free of such side effects and may even improve insulin sensitivity and glucose tolerance.

There are a number of different dyslipidemia patterns that are associated with obesity. The most common are low levels of high density lipoprotein (HDL) and elevated levels of very low density lipoprotein resulting in low plasma HDL-cholesterol and high plasma triglycerides. There is no consensus if or how dyslipidemia of obese subjects should be treated. However, weight reduction, even a modest one, normalizes the dyslipidemia of obesity. The use of lipid-lowering drugs in obese subjects should depend on the severity of dyslipidemia and the coexistence of other atherogenetic factors such as diabetes and hypertension.

Obese subjects are predisposed to gall bladder disease, in particular gallstones. Increased biliary secretion of cholesterol and decreased gall bladder motility are important pathophysiological factors.

Obese subjects are also at high risk of developing a number of cardiovascular disorders. Atherosclerotic coronary heart disease is an end-point in the metabolic syndrome. Heart failure may develop as a result of altered loading from both the mechanical effect of increased fat mass and of the hypertension that is induced by obesity. Obesity is also associated with an increased risk of arrhythmia and cardiac arrest. The frequency of venous thrombosis is increased in obesity.

Obese subjects often suffer from dyspnea during moderate exercise or at rest. Obstructive sleep-apnea is also common in obesity and sometimes coexists with obesity-hyperventilation (Pickwickian syndrome). These pulmonary complications are partly mechanical and partly due to muscle dysfunction and the metabolic consequences of obesity.

Osteoarthritis in knees and/or hips is common in obese subjects. Both the metabolic changes and mechanical factors contribute to the association between obesity and joint disorders.

Obese women are often infertile and have gotten pregnant when losing weight. It has been speculated that increased leptin levels (which is observed in most obese subjects) inhibits ovary function. Furthermore, obesity often coexists with polycystic ovarian syndrome which, in itself, may cause infertility.

The impact of obesity on longevity must by considered. From data obtained by life insurance companies, we have known for more than 100 years that a high body weight is associated with excess mortality. However, a number of factors influence this relationship. Being moderately overweight (BMI <30 kg/m^2) is associated with no or only a slight increase in mortality. At high BMI levels, there is a dramatic increase in the risk. The fatty distribution is also of importance. Central fat distribution is associated with higher mortality risk than peripheral fat distribution at each BMI level. Finally, age is important. A relationship between body weight and mortality is present up to about retirement age; thereafter, obesity does not have an important impact on longevity.

Treatment

It is estimated that more than 30 billion dollars are spent each year in the United States on weight loss efforts. A lot of these resources are used to treat mild obesity or undesired fat distribution for cosmetic reasons. Nevertheless, medical treatment for an overweight subject should always be considered, bearing in mind the significant health consequences of excessive obesity and/or unfavorable fat distribution.

The indications for treatment are outlined in Table 63.4. While there is no firmly established consensus regarding indications, some guidelines can be provided. Subjects with BMI <30 kg/m^2 in combination with a peripheral fat distribution (usually women) have no or little medical risk and should be restricted from weight reduction programs unless they have overt medical complications to their obesity. Subjects with a BMI of 30 to 40 kg/m^2 have a moderate mortality risk and should be considered for treatment, in particular if they have upper-body fat distribution and/or medical complications and are not elderly (<65 years). Subjects with BMI >40 kg/m^2 are at high risk and should always be treated.

Treatment options for obese patients are outlined in Table 63.5. It is probably well-known that no long-term effective and safe cure exists for the moment. A conservative therapy should be the first choice. Today this constitutes a very-low-calorie diet (VLCD) in combination with exercise and some behavior modification. There are a

Table 63.4 Indications to treat obesity

Relative
  Body mass index 30-40 kg/m^2
  Fat distribution
  Obesity complications
  Age <65 years

Absolute
  Body mass index >40 kg/m^2

Table 63.5 Treatment of obesity
Conservative
Very-low-calorie diet (VLCD)
Exercise
Behavioral modifications
Pharmacological
Lipase inhibitors
Appetite suppressants
Thermogenic drugs
Surgical
Intestinal bypass
Gastric bypass
Vertical-stapled gastroplasty
Adjustable gastric banding

number of commercial VLCD formulas that contain all necessary nutrients with a daily energy intake of about 600 kcal. Very-low-calorie diet is often used for 2 to 3 months, but treatment for up to 6 months has been reported to be safe. Thereafter the patient must adapt to a balanced diet in combination with exercise. A minimum amount of recommended exercise is 30 minutes of strenuous walking 3 times per week or another equivalent exercise performance. The behavior modification should aim at improving the self esteem of the patient, change the sedentary type of lifestyle, and alter the eating behavior. In the best hands and with motivated patients, the conservative treatment can be successful; some large centers report up to a 50% long-term success rate. Usually, however, there is failure in 80 to 90% of the cases.

Since cure of obesity with conservative therapy often fails, a number of pharmacological treatments have been introduced. None, however, has been proven to be effective for a long time. In addition, many of the drugs used have been withdrawn because of dangerous or even lethal side effects. Perhaps because of the enormous potential market many drug companies have, there remain major ongoing anti-obesity drug discovery projects that will, hopefully, in the near future result in the introduction of drugs that are both effective and safe. Recently a lipase inhibitor (orlistat, tetrahydrolipstatin) has been introduced. It inhibits the breakdown of triglycerides in the food so that most of the lipids in a meal are lost in the stool. The drug is not very effective in reducing weight, but it may be effective in weight maintenance after VLCD. Due to the effects on the intestines, the use of this drug is associated with bowel problems and fatty diarrheas. The patient avoids eating food containing high amounts of fat because that induces the intestinal effects. The long-term effect of

the drug remains to be established. A serotonin uptake inhibitor (sibutramine) is near registration in many countries. It seems effective in combination with VLCD and does not appear to have the dangerous cardiac side effects that were caused by earlier serotonin uptake inhibitors; the latter drugs have been withdrawn from the market. Again, no long-term results are available. Finally, thermogenetic drugs have been tested. The most important ones are so-called β_3-adrenoceptor agonists. These agents stimulate the development of brown adipose tissue (which combusts fatty acids) and increase the breakdown of lipids to fatty acids in white fat tissue. The first-generation drugs were developed with the rat beta3-receptor as target and were very effective on obese animal models. Unfortunately, they were ineffective in obese human. New β_3-agonists are in current trials. They have been developed against the human β_3-receptor. In summary, there is no drug currently available that has a long-term and safe effect on obesity. At the present time, drug therapy should be reserved to physicians who are specialists in the field.

For many patients who have made many unsuccessful conservative attempts to reduce body weight, surgery could be an alternative. Simply removing adipose tissue (lipectomy, liposuction) cannot be considered as a method to treat obesity since it is not possible to remove more than about 10 kg of fat without causing dangerous side effects such as bleeding and fat embolism. Instead, bypass of the gastrointestinal tract is used. Various intestinal bypass operations have been used in the past that induce a decrease in energy uptake. These methods are effective in lowering body weight, but they are associated with long-term serious complications, in particular metabolic ones. Therefore, most surgeons today prefer to reduce the stomach volume so that the obese person can no longer eat large portions of food and thereby cause decreased energy intake. Several methods are used (gastric bypass, vertical-stapled gastroplasty, and placing adjustable bands around the upper part of the ventricle). All methods have advantages and disadvantages. They are all effective in reducing body weight, and many centers report good long-term results on body weight. On the other hand, several patients relapse in body weight because they adapt to the small stomach (for example, they eat liquid energy-rich nutrients), and/or the remaining "active" stomach dilutes so that they again can eat large amounts of foods. Alternatively, stapling of the stomach breaks or the adjustable band stops working. So far no long-term prospective and randomized studies have been performed on obesity surgery versus conservative therapy. However, a large Swedish one is ongoing (Swedish Obese Subjects); results will appear in about 5 years. Obesity surgery should above all be reserved for well-motivated and cooperating patients with BMI >40 kg/m² who have a documented failure to respond adequately to previous conservative therapies. A 2 to 4 kg/m² lower body mass index limit is sometimes used for men.

Suggested readings

ARNER P. Regulation of lipolysis in fat cells. Diabetes Reviews 1996;4:450-63.

BONADONNA RC, BONORA E. Glucose and free fatty acid metabolism in human obesity. Diabetes Reviews 1997;5:21-51.

BRAY GA, BOUCHARD C, JAMES WPT (eds). Handbook of obesity. New York: Marcel Dekker 1998.

DESPRÉS JP. Dyslipidemia and obesity. Ballièrés Clin Endocrinol Metab 1994;8:629-60.

HODGE AM, ZIMMET PZ. The epidemiology of obesity. Ballièrés Clin Endocrinol Metab 1994;8:577-99.

HSUEH WA, BUCHANAN TA. Obesity hypertension. Endocrinol Metab Clin North Am 1994;23:405-27.

KISSEBAH AH, KRAKOWER GR. Regional adiposity and morbidity. Physiol Rev 1994;74:761-811.

KOLANOWSKI J. Surgical treatment of morbid obesity. Br Med Bulletin 1997;53:433-44.

KOPELMAN PG, ALBON L. Obesity, non-insulin-dependent diabetes mellitus and the metabolic syndrome. Brit Med Bulletin 1997;53:322-40.

WEISER M, FRISHMAN WH, MICHAELSON MD, ABDEEN MA. The pharmacologic approach to treatment of obesity. J Clin Pharmacol 1997;37:453-73.

Lipid disorders

Lipid disorders in diabetes

Marja-Riitta Taskinen

KEY POINTS

- Cardiovascular diseases are the major complication of diabetes, and approximately 75% of diabetic patients die from them.
- In general, the lipoprotein pattern is anti-atherogenic in individuals with type 1 diabetes (insulin-dependent diabetes mellitus) who are insulin-treated and have optimal glycemic control.
- The major lipid abnormalities found in type 2 diabetic patients are elevated serum and VLDL triglycerides associated with a low concentration of HDL cholesterol.
- Because diabetic patients appear to have a greatly increased risk of coronary heart disease, they belong to the high-risk category as defined by the guidelines of American Diabetes Association (ADA) consensus conferences. This means that a borderline high LDL cholesterol in diabetic patients means a much higher LDL cholesterol in terms of risk. Consequently, the optimal LDL cholesterol for each diabetic patient is <2.6 mmol/l (<100 mg/dl). Raised concentrations of triglycerides and lowering of HDL cholesterol are also recognized as targets for treatment in diabetes.

Cardiovascular diseases are the major complication of diabetes and represent the greatest burden of diabetes at both individual and population levels. Today approximately 75% of diabetic patients die from cardiovascular diseases. The mortality rate of coronary artery disease is at least three times higher in type 2 diabetic (non-insulin-dependent diabetes mellitus) patients than persons without diabetes. The recognition of the magnitude of this problem has raised much concern regarding how to alleviate it. Reasons for excess cardiovascular diseases in diabetes are multifaceted, but it is most likely that dyslipidemia contributes to excess vascular risk. Since dyslipidemia is a preventable factor causing excess atherosclerosis, it represents a challenge for setting up treatment strategies. Management decisions should be based upon the recognition of the atherogenic lipid/lipoprotein components and on the understanding of the metabolic pathways to allow targeted treatment.

Function of lipoproteins

Lipoproteins are the vehicles in plasma that transport water-insoluble lipid molecules from sites of absorption (intestine) and synthesis (liver) to sites of storage and utilization. The primary lipid components are free and esterified cholesterol, triglycerides, and phospholipids. Lipoproteins are complex aggregates of lipids and specific apoproteins. In circulation, lipoproteins are exposed to the action of enzymes and lipid transfer proteins, and they interact with cellular receptors in liver and other tissues. In fact, apoproteins on the surface of lipoproteins have specific functions through their interactions with enzymes and receptors and thus regulate the fate of lipoprotein particles. These processes modify lipoprotein particles and also serve to regulate lipid and lipoprotein metabolism. The major classes of this lipid transport system are chylomicrons, very low density lipoproteins (VLDL), intermediate density lipoproteins (IDL), low density lipoproteins (LDL), and high density lipoproteins (HDL). Perturbation of any pathways that are involved with the lipid transport system results in abnormalities of serum lipids and lipoproteins.

Structure and composition of lipoproteins

The characteristics of the major lipoprotein classes differ with respect to chemical composition, size, density, physical structure, and metabolism (Fig. 64.1). The structure of lipoproteins is spherical and composed of apolar lipids (triglyceride, esterified cholesterol) containing a core that is surrounded by a hydrophobic surface containing apoproteins, phospholipids, and free unesterified cholesterol. The size of the lipoprotein varies according to the quantity of lipids in its core. The size of the particle and its lipid content affect its density and flotation rate in salt solutions. The outer shell stabilizes the lipoprotein particles. The different lipoprotein classes can be separated according to their density by using ultracentrifugation, according to immunoaffinity, or size using chromatography techniques. The recognition that there is heterogeneity within each major lipoprotein class depending on different lipid content, apoprotein content, and altered protein conformation has expanded the understanding of lipoprotein metabolism and pathophysiology of dyslipidemias and atherogenesis.

The cardinal task of chylomicrons and VLDL particles is to transport triglycerides; these particles are larger than LDL and HDL, which transport cholesterol in circulation. Chylomicrons and VLDL are primary particles, whereas IDL, LDL, and HDL are secondary particles derived from the metabolism of primary particles.

Exogenous and endogenous lipid transport system

Intravascular lipid metabolism involves the transport of exogenous (dietary) lipids and the transport of endogenous lipids derived from the liver (Fig. 64.2). The two transport pathways are closely intertwined. Chylomicrons transport dietary fat (triglyceride, cholesterol) that is absorbed and incorporated into chylomicrons in intestinal cells. Chylomicrons can be separated from other lipoproteins by the presence of specific apoprotein B48 synthesized in intestinal cells. Triglycerides make up 90% of the lipids in chylomicrons, which are the largest and lightest lipoprotein particles.

The nascent particles also contain some apoprotein (apo) A-I and A-II. During their circulation, chylomicrons acquire apoE and apoC molecules. Chylomicron metabolism consists of two steps: (1) delipidation of particles via action of lipoprotein lipase (LPL), which hydrolyzes triglycerides, and (2) uptake and degradation of remnant particles in the liver. The triglycerides in chylomicrons are rapidly lipolyzed by LPL; and the end-products are smaller, Tg-depleted but cholesterylester-rich remnant particles that still contain apoB48 and apoE. The released free fatty acids are taken up by tissues. An excess of circulating free fatty acids may dissociate LPL molecules from heparin-binding sites and result in cessation of lipolysis. Chylomicron remnant particles interact with receptors in the liver. This process is dependent upon the interaction of apo E with the LDL receptor-related protein (LRP) and the LDL receptor. Both hepatic lipase and LPL may contribute to this process by facilitating the interaction between remnants and receptors.

Endogenous lipid transport consists of two systems: (1) apoB-100 lipoprotein cascade (VLDL, IDL, LDL), and (2) the HDL cascade. Triglyceride-rich VLDL particles are secreted by the liver to provide an energy source for tissues in the fasting state. The formation of VLDL particles is initiated by the assembly of apoB100 and lipids in the liver. The maturation of nascent particles as they pass along the secretory pathway in hepatocytes and the conversion into mature VLDL particles is a complex process, and its regulation is not well-established. The assembly of lipids and apoB100 occurs in two steps (Fig. 64.3). The microsomal triglyceride transfer protein has a central role in the cotranslational formation of the pre-assembly pool of apoB100 and the initial assembly of lipids. This process is essential for the secretion of apoB100. In the

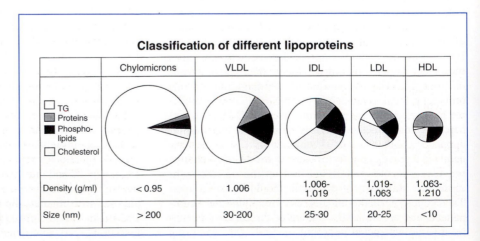

Figure 64.1 The composition, size and density of different lipoprotein classes.

Classification of different lipoproteins

	Chylomicrons	VLDL	IDL	LDL	HDL
TG / Proteins / Phospholipids / Cholesterol					
Density (g/ml)	< 0.95	1.006	1.006-1.019	1.019-1.063	1.063-1.210
Size (nm)	> 200	30-200	25-30	20-25	<10

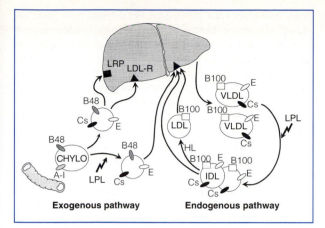

Figure 64.2 Schematic presentation of exogenous and endogenous lipoprotein pathways. Chylomicrons synthesized in intestinal cells contain apoB48 and A-I (and apoA-IV). Chylomicrons accumulate apoCs and apoE in circulation. Lipolysis by LPL produces remnant particles which are removed by uptake via "remnant" receptor (LRP)(n) or via LDL receptor (D). VLDL containing apoB100, apoE and apoCs (CI, CII, CIII) are lipolyzed by LPL into IDL particles which are removed directly by liver or further converted into LDL particles.

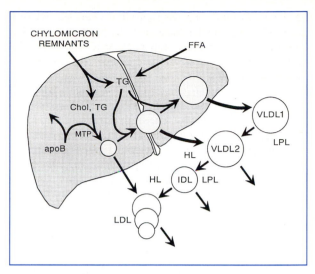

Figure 64.3 Schematic presentation of VLD assembly in the liver and maturation into large buoyant VLDL1 particles. The major secretory products are VLDL1 and VLDL2 particles whereas direct LDL output is much less. (MTP= microsomal transfer protein; HL=hepatic lipase, LPL=lipoprotein lipase; TG=triclycerides; Chol=cholesterol; FFA=free fatty acids.)

second step, addition of lipids converts the nascent particles into mature VLDL particles. The liver secretes VLDL particles that range in size and density, the two main products being VLDL1 (Sf 60-400) and VLDL2 (Sf 20-60). Importantly, the production of VLDL1 and VLDL2 seems to be regulated independently of one another. Plentiful availability of triglyceride for packaging into VLDL favors the production of large VLDL1 particles. The formation of large VLDL is also under hormonal control, being regulated by insulin and estrogen. It is also important to note that the VLDL1 production rate shows a positive correlation with plasma triglyceride levels. Kinetic data have revealed that the VLDL2 production rate and the fractional catabolic rate of LDL together explain 50% of the variation in plasma LDL concentration. Thus, the current concept is that VLDL1 overproduction causes elevation of plasma triglycerides and that VLDL2 overproduction results in raised LDL concentration. However, the factors that specifically determine VLDL2 secretion are not well-known.

Upon entering the circulation, apoB-containing particles are exposed to lipolysis by lipolytic enzymes lipoprotein lipase (LPL) and hepatic lipase (HL); and they are remodeled by cholesterol ester transfer protein (CETP), resulting in changes of coat and core apoproteins and lipids during the course of their intravascular metabolism. In the delipidation process, VLDL particles lose the triglyceride core, surface phospholipids, and apoproteins. At the same time, particles gain cholesterol esters from LDL and/or HDL via the lipid exchange process mediated by CETP. The triglyceride-rich particles are gradually converted through IDL into LDL. Thus, the VLDL-IDL-LDL cascade regulated by coordinated actions of LPL, HL, and CETP directs the metabolic channeling and remodeling of apoB100-containing

particles. During this cascade, VLDL particles can be directly removed from the circulation by receptor-mediated uptake in the liver. The ligand for the putative receptor is probably apoE on large VLDL particles. Recognizing that the subfraction distribution of LDL particles depends heavily on its pedigree is the key to understanding the generation of small dense LDL. The long residence time of large VLDL1 particles will favor an increased rate of transfer of core lipids. The rate of hydrolysis of triglyceride-rich LDL by hepatic lipase determines the formation of small dense LDL. The most important point is that different forms of VLDL particles give rise to varying LDL subclasses having different structural and metabolic properties. The LDL receptor described by Goldstein and Brown is responsible for the majority of LDL uptake in the liver. Importantly, the expression of LDL receptors is regulated by cholesterol content in liver cells. This feedback mechanism is critical in the regulation of plasma LDL cholesterol levels.

High density lipoproteins Nascent HDL particles are secreted as disc-shaped structures by the liver and intestine. Discoidal HDL particles become converted into spherical particles by the action of lecithin:cholesterol acyltransferase (LCAT) on free cholesterol derived from cells (Fig. 64.4). This reaction generates a hydrophobic core of increasing size due to accumulation of cholesterylesters. This initial step is critical in the reverse cholesterol transport process. In circulation, HDL particles are exposed to further modification by various enzymes and lipid transfer proteins (CETP and PLTP), which are responsible for the conversion of small dense HDL particles (HDL3) into large and light HDL particles (HDL2), and vice versa. As HDL particles enlarge, they can accommodate more apoproteins (apoC-II, apoC-III) and phospholipids on their surface. These components are derived from lipolysis of triglyceride-rich particles by LPL. The action of CETP is to transfer cholesterylesters out from HDL3 particles in exchange for triglycerides derived from triglyceride-rich particles. The triglyceride-enriched HDL particles are a good substrate for hepatic lipase, which promotes the formation of lipid-poor small HDL particles (HDL3). Thus, the size of HDL particles is in fact regulated in a fashion similar to that of LDL particles.

Mature HDL in plasma exits in two major density classes, HDL2 and HDL3, which can be further subdivided on the basis of apoA content. HDL particles contain at least two species of apoA-I-containing particles, namely particles containing only apoA-I (LpA-I) and particles containing both apoA-I and apoA-II (LpA-I/A-II). Strong evidence indicates that the metabolic fate of LpA-I and LpA-I/A-II particles is different. The majority of Lp-AI particles resides within HDL2 density range and LpA-I/A-II particles within HDL3 density range. Plasma apoA-I levels are primarily regulated by the catabolic rate of apoA-I. In fact, lipid composition of HDL particles seems to determine the catabolic rate of apoA-I. In contrast, plasma levels of apoA-II are primarily regulated by the production rate of apoA-II. The ambient concentrations of HDL2 and HDL3 in plasma are dependent on the coordinated action of LPL, HL, LCAT, CETP, and PLTP, in addition to the metabolism of apoA-I and A-II.

LIPID DISORDERS IN TYPE 1 DIABETES

In general, the lipoprotein pattern is anti-atherogenic in individuals with type 1 diabetes (insulin-dependent dia-

betes mellitus) who are insulin-treated and have optimal glycemic control. In the DCCT substudy, healthy type 1 diabetic patients men had normal lipid and lipoprotein values. Abnormal values, including elevated total and LDL cholesterol and decreased HDL cholesterol, were observed in younger female patients with higher HbA_{1C} levels. Nikkilä and Hormila were the first to report subnormal VLDL triglycerides and raised HDL cholesterol levels in type 1 diabetic patients with good glycemic control. The elevation of HDL cholesterol is primarily attributed to raised HDL2 cholesterol due to an elevation of LpA-I particles, particularly in women. LpA-I particles represent the antiatherogenic fraction of HDL and are proposed to have a key role in reverse cholesterol transport. In contrast, the concentration of HDL3 cholesterol and apo A-II seems to be within the normal range. Subnormal VLDL triglyceride and raised HDL2 cholesterol levels are attributed to a high lipolytic rate due to an increase in LPL activity caused by peripheral hyperinsulinemia. This is supported by the positive correlation found between LPL/HL ratio and the concentration of LpA-I particles. The current tenet is that a high lipolytic rate results in low VLDL triglyceride levels, and triglyceride-poor HDL consequently results in delayed catabolism of apoA-I. This is consistent with the observation that an inverse correlation exists between HDL2 cholesterol and the catabolism of LpA-I particles.

The lack of abnormalities of lipoprotein levels does not exclude the possibility that there are compositional changes that may be atherogenic. James and Pometta found that in poorly controlled type 1 diabetic patients, both VLDL and LDL subfractions showed multiple abnormalities. First, all three VLDL subclasses (VLDL1 Sf >100, VLDL2 Sf 60-100, and VLDL3 Sf 20-60) separated by gradient ultracentrifugation were increased and contained an excess of non-apoB apolipoproteins (apoCs and apoEs). Second, LDL subclass distribution demonstrated a shift to relative excess of small dense LDL. In addition, LDL particles were more triglyceride-rich but depleted in esterified cholesterol as compared to normal subjects. Of

Figure 64.4 Regulation of HDL subfraction distribution. Lipolysis of TRLs by LPL, HL and CETP and LCAT activities regulate the distribution of HDL subclasses. SR-B1 denotes scavenger receptor in the liver that mediates the selective uptake of cholesterol from HDL particles. The lipid exchange/lipolysis cascade regulates the size of HDL particles.

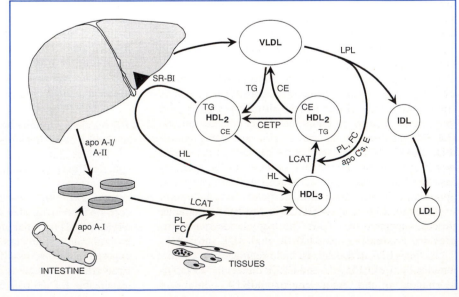

note, treatment with intensive insulin therapy was associated with a marked fall of VLDL particles and also corrected the distribution of LDL subclasses. We have reported that in normoalbuminuric type 1 diabetic patients, LDL particles are larger and less dense than in nondiabetic control subjects. LDL size correlated inversely with serum total and VLDL triglycerides and positively with HDL cholesterol. Caixas et al. found similar LDL phenotype distribution in type 1 diabetic subjects and in nondiabetic subjects. Rivellese et al. observed an increase of triglyceride-poor and cholesterol-rich small VLDL fractions in normolipidemic type 1 diabetic patients. This change was more marked in patients with unsatisfactory blood glucose control. Interestingly, the shift in VLDL subclass distribution seems to be related to low hepatic lipase activity in type 1 diabetic subjects treated with peripheral insulin injections. Of physiological relevance is that diabetic VLDL and LDL in vitro induces abnormal responses of cellular cholesterol metabolism in human macrophages.

In addition, lipoprotein particles in type 1 diabetic patients also show distinct abnormalities in the distribution of surface and core lipids. First, plasma and VLDL+LDL fractions had a higher free cholesterol-lecithin ratio, which is an index of coronary heart disease (CHD) risk. Second, there are subtle changes of phospholipid components in HDL that may impair the function of HDL in reverse cholesterol transport. Thus, high HDL cholesterol may not be as protective as in nondiabetic subjects. Paradoxically, these changes were not fully reversed after the achievement of optimal glycemic control. The clinical relevance of these compositional changes with respect to coronary heart disease risk can only be defined in prospective clinical studies.

Glycemic control in relation to lipoprotein pattern in type 1 diabetes

Glycemic control and the regimen of insulin therapy are factors that can markedly modify lipoprotein patterns in type 1 diabetes. Intensive insulin treatment that normalizes the glycemic control lowers VLDL and LDL but increases HDL. In the DCCT study (Diabetes Control and Complication Trial), favorable changes of serum lipids and lipoproteins were observed as a result of intensive insulin therapy. Optimization of glycemic control is particularly powerful in reducing VLDL concentration, but the response of HDL is less marked and slower. The effect is due to both reduction of the VLDL apoB synthetic rate and overstimulation of lipoprotein lipase by elevated peripheral insulin values. Consequently many type 1 patients have subnormal concentrations of VLDL and LDL. The overall effect of glycemic control on plasma triglyceride levels is estimated to average 0.08 mM (7.1 mg/dl, 8%) for each percentage-point fall of glycohemoglobin in a random type 1 diabetic cohort.

If metabolic control is poor, the major lipid abnormality is the elevation of the plasma triglyceride level, although elevation of serum total and LDL cholesterol also occurs.

In ketoacidosis due to insulin deficiency, plasma can be clearly lipemic due to a marked elevation of triglyceride-rich particles, and the concentration of HDL cholesterol is reduced. Insulin deficiency is followed by decreased clearance of triglyceride-rich particles because lipoprotein lipase activity is diminished. Optimization of insulin therapy rapidly restores LPL activity and corrects the abnormalities of VLDL metabolism.

The route of insulin delivery seems to have important consequences on lipid metabolism. Insulin delivery sc by conventional regimens results in peripheral hyperinsulinemia, whereas relative hypoinsulinemia supervenes in portal circulation. The exposure of the liver to subnormal insulin concentration is associated with reduced hepatic lipase activity that is reflected in changes of VLDL and LDL subclasses. Intraperitoneal insulin delivery is able to restore the hepatic lipase activity, which is reflected in a slight reduction of HDL levels. Unfortunately, the results on plasma and VLDL triglycerides have been partly inconsistent, probably due to the small number of patients in these studies. Much more work is required to establish if IP insulin delivery is more beneficial than conventional insulin regimens for lipoprotein metabolism.

Lipid disorders in diabetic renal disease

Type 1 diabetic patients with overt albuminuria and clinical nephropathy show a broad spectrum of lipid abnormalities characterized by elevations of serum total and LDL cholesterol, serum total and VLDL triglyceride, and apoB100. Substantial evidence shows that abnormalities of serum lipids and lipoproteins already occur in type 1 diabetic patients with microalbuminuria. We recently reported that type 1 diabetic patients with microalbuminuria have multiple abnormalities of apoB100 containing triglyceride-rich particles. The most significant change is the elevation of IDL concentration in patients with raised albumin excretion rate; this may contribute to the excess coronary heart disease risk in these patients. In addition, type 1 diabetic patients show mild hypertriglyceridemia and elevated LDL cholesterol. The mean diameter of LDL particles was smaller in type 1 patients with microalbuminuria or proteinuria than in normoalbuminuric patients. On the other hand, type 1 diabetic patients with microalbuminuria exhibit only trivial changes of HDL subclasses, and they are not of clinical relevance. Most studies have reported that Lp(a) levels are elevated in type 1 diabetic patients with microalbuminuria or proteinuria. However, conclusive evidence that elevation of Lp(a) may contribute to the excess coronary heart disease is still lacking in patients with renal disease.

Prevalence of dyslipidemia in type 1 diabetes

Surprisingly little data exists on the prevalence of lipid abnormalities in type 1 diabetic populations. The number of patients have been small in most studies, and consequently the data is partly inconsistent. Winocour et al. reported that in adults with type 1 diabetes, hypertriglyceridemia was found in 31% of cases and hypercholesterolemia in 27% of cases. In the WESDR (Wisconsin

Epidemiologic Study of Diabetic Retinopathy) cohort of type 1 diabetic subjects, the prevalence of moderate hypercholesterolemia (>6.2 mmol/l or >240 mg/dl) was 17% and only 29% of subject had borderline high cholesterol. The numbers are closely similar to nondiabetic agematched control subjects. Taking into consideration the impact of glycemic control, the numbers are probably much smaller in subjects with good glycemic control, as evidenced by DCCT data. In young adults with type 1 diabetes, the overall prevalence of lipid disorders is at the least less than in the nondiabetic population.

DIABETIC DYSLIPIDEMIA IN TYPE 2 DIABETES

The major lipid abnormalities found in type 2 diabetic patients are elevated serum and VLDL triglycerides associated with a low concentration of HDL cholesterol. The concentrations of serum and LDL cholesterol are similar or even lower than those in the general population. The elevation of serum triglycerides is usually mild or moderate, and the triglyceride values are 1.5 to 3.0-fold compared with those of nondiabetic cohorts matched for age, sex, and body mass index (BMI). In practice, the measurement of triglyceride values are between 1.5 and 3.0 mmol/l. The lack of striking abnormalities may give the clinician a false sense of security and lead to therapeutic negligence. Some type 2 diabetic patients with poor glycemic control may have severe hypertriglyceridemia and milky serum with extremely high plasma triglycerides (between 50 and 100 mmol/l). Such patients commonly have concomitant genetic hyperlipidemias or other secondary causes of dyslipidemias. Severe hypertriglyceridemia should prompt an examination of family members. Mutations in the LPL gene have recently been identified as a cause for severe hypertriglyceridemia in some diabetic patients.

HDL cholesterol is on average reduced in type 2 diabetic patients by 10 to 20%, and the actual values are close to or slightly below 0.9 mmol/l in men and 1.1 mmol/l in women. Importantly, the gender difference for HDL is less in type 2 diabetic patients than in nondiabetic cohorts. HDL has traditionally been subfractionated into HDL2 and HDL3 according to the flotation rate. The concentration of HDL2 cholesterol is reduced more than that of HDL3 in type 2 diabetic patients in most studies. In a cross-sectional study, we found that type 2 diabetic patients have low concentrations of LpA-I particles, particularly those of LpA-I/A-II particles and apoA-II.

New components of diabetic dyslipidemia

Changes of triglycerides and HDL cholesterol in type 2 diabetes are not isolated metabolic aberrations but commonly go hand in hand. The recognition that hypertriglyceridemia is associated with multiple alterations of other lipoproteins that are potentially atherogenic has expanded the picture of diabetic dyslipidemia.

Postprandial lipemia in type 2 diabetes The concept that atherosclerosis is a postprandial phenomenon was introduced by Zilversmit almost 20 years ago. Data from several cross-sectional studies indicate that increased postprandial lipemia is not only a risk factor for coronary heart disease, but that it also predicts the progression of angiographically defined coronary artery disease. This finding is important because the postprandial period after a fatty meal lasts for over 6 hours, indicating that man is feasting for more of the 24 hours than fasting. Since the magnitude of postprandial lipemia is known to be dependent upon the fasting serum triglyceride concentration, an obvious question becomes whether type 2 diabetic subjects are fat-intolerant. Our group and others have shown that the rise of triglyceride-rich lipoprotein concentration after a fat-containing meal is greater in type 2 diabetic patients than in people without diabetes. Available data suggest that type 2 diabetic subjects have prolonged residence time of triglyceride-rich lipoprotein remnants in circulation due to their defective removal, and fat intolerance seems to be an inherent feature of dyslipidemia in type 2 diabetes.

Postprandial lipemia comprises particles of both exogenous and endogenous origin. Chylomicrons and VLDL particles compete in the common lipolytic pathway at the level of lipoprotein lipase. Since chylomicrons are a superior substrate for LPL compared to VLDL particles, an accumulation of VLDL particles occur, which saturates the lipolytic capacity (Fig. 64.5). The corollary of this process is elevated triglyceride-rich lipoproteins and fat intolerance. These processes will be exaggerated in states where VLDL production is increased, as occurs in type 2 diabetes. Likewise, if VLDL production is not efficiently shut down in the postprandial phase due to impaired inhibitory action of insulin on VLDL production, or due to excess free fatty acid flux to the liver.

The metabolic capacity would be exceeded. In fact, both abnormalities seem to supervene in type 2 diabetes. Alternative mechanisms for impaired removal of triglyceride-rich lipoproteins may be suboptimal lipolysis due to reduced LPL activity and elevation of circulating free fatty acids, which may impede the binding of LPL to triglyceride-rich lipoproteins and endothelium-bound heparin sulphate. The remnant metabolism may also be delayed due to impaired interaction of remnants with hepatic receptors.

LDL subclasses in type 2 diabetes LDL is comprised of a heterogenous spectrum of particles that differ in density, size, chemical composition, and atherogenicity. Small dense LDL is defined as a particle with a mean diameter of less than 25.5 nm. Two distinct patterns of LDL patterns, A and B, can be separated based on the predominant particle size with nondenaturing gradient gel electrophoresis. Small dense LDL is the major component in pattern B, whereas pattern A consists of large buoyant particles with a mean diameter of greater than 25.5 nm. Small dense LDL is associated with the risk of myocardial infarction and CAD and is considered to be the most atherogenic LDL subclass. LDL size has been shown to be dependent on triglyceride levels in nondiabetic and diabetic cohorts. In addition, small dense LDL is associated with decreased HDL cholesterol levels, visceral obesity, and in some studies with insulin resistance and hyperinsulinemia. However, body mass index, visceral obesity, and hyperinsulinemia are not independent predictors of LDL size after adjusting for triglyceride and HDL cholesterol values or in multivariate models. Recently Austin et al. reported that small dense LDL is a risk factor for future development of diabetes independent of glucose intolerance, family history of diabetes, hypertension, and waist/hip ratio, but it is not independent of fasting triglyceride or insulin values. We have reported that first-degree relatives of type 2 diabetic subjects who have normal glucose tolerance but who are insulin-resistant have smaller LDL size than relatives who have no signs of insulin resistance. Thus, there seems to be a decrease of LDL size when subjects with normal glucose tolerance are compared to those with insulin resistance or impaired glucose tolerance through to type 2 diabetic subjects. Overall the LDL size seems to be a reflection of altered metabolic abnormalities of triglyceride-rich lipoproteins and HDL. Consequently, it is not unexpected that a number of studies has found a preponderance of small dense LDLs in type 2 diabetic patients. Emerging evidence indicate that there is a threshold of plasma triglyceride level for the preponderance of small dense LDLs somewhere between 1.5 to 1.7 mmol/l. Since the majority of type 2 diabetic patients have plasma triglycerides above 1.5 mmol/l, in practice small dense LDL is an integral feature of diabetic dyslipidemia. Interestingly, the association between small dense LDL and diabetes seems to be stronger in women than in men; this may partly explain the fatal lipid profile in diabetic women. Recently Caixas et al. reported that in type 2 diabetic patients, optimization of glycemic control by intensive insulin therapy caused a shift from the non-A to A phenotype of the LDL subclasses. Likewise, James et al. observed a decrease of LDL3 fraction representing small dense LDL after correction of glycemic control. The incidence of small dense LDL seems to be increased in type 2 diabetic patients with microalbuminuria and macroalbuminuria.

Lipoprotein (a) in type 2 diabetes The majority of studies indicate that type 2 diabetic patients do not have elevated Lp(a) levels, although some studies have shown increased values of Lp(a). However, the data are based on studies with a small number of subjects, and most studies have not included the apo(a) phenotype determinations. Likewise, the significance of Lp(a) as a coronary heart disease risk factor in type 2 diabetes is unclear due to a paucity of large clinical studies. However, some studies have provided positive evidence for the role of high Lp(a) as a risk factor for coronary artery disease in type 2 diabetes.

Prevalence of dyslipidemia in type 2 diabetes

The prevalence of dyslipidemia is common in type 2 diabetic populations, but it varies according to the used cutoff values. Hypertriglyceridemia varies between 20 and 60% in different studies, being two- to threefold higher than in nondiabetic populations of the same age. In the Procam Study, the prevalence of hypertriglyceridemia, defined as triglyceride levels above 2.3 mmol/l, averaged 39% in the diabetic population compared to 21% in the nondiabetic population. The respective prevalences of low HDL cholesterol (<0.9 mmol/l) were 27% and 17%. In the Framingham Study, the prevalence of hypertriglyceridemia (>2.7 mmol/l) was 19% and 9% in type 2 diabetic and nondiabetic men, and the respective numbers for women were 17% and 8%. Salomaa et al. recently reported that the prevalence of hypertriglyceridemia (TG >2.3 mmol/l) was 47.6% in men and 51.9% in women with type 2 diabetes in a Finnish cohort. In the San Antonio

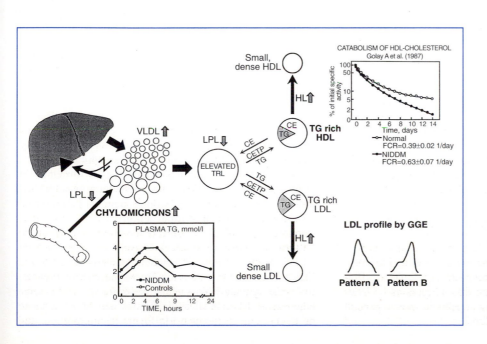

Figure 64.5 Schematic presentation of pertubations in the lipoprotein metabolism in type 2 diabetes. The key feature is increased production of VLDL in the liver that coincides with subnormal LPL activity and increased hepatic lipase activity. (From Syvänne M, Taskinen M-R. Lipids and lipoproteins as coronary risk factors in non-insulin-dependent diabetes mellitus. Lancet 1997;350:20-23.)

Heart Study population, 5% of diabetic women and 15% of diabetic men had triglyceride values above 4.5 mmol/l. The prevalence of hypercholesterolemia and high LDL cholesterol levels reflect those in the background population. The data from the National Health and Nutrition Examination Survey (NHANES) indicate that high or borderline total and LDL cholesterol values are found in 70% and 60% of adults with diagnosed diabetes. Rönnemaa et al. reported that in a Finnish cohort of type 2 diabetic subjects, the prevalence of hypercholesterolemia (serum cholesterol >6.5 mmol/l) was 54%, which was similar to the nondiabetic population.

A specific feature of diabetic dyslipidemia is that lipid abnormalities are frequently found at the time of diagnosis of diabetes, and they are present independently of the mode of treatment in cross-sectional studies. Similar abnormalities are also observed in glucose-tolerant first-degree relatives of type 2 diabetic patients. In the Botnia Study, we found that glucose-tolerant first-degree relatives of type 2 diabetic patients who were defined to be insulin-resistant on the basis of fasting insulin values (>10 μU/ml) have higher triglycerides and lower HDL cholesterol than insulin-sensitive relatives. Of note, these differences were observed despite the fact that both lipid values were within the normal range. The association between raised triglycerides and low HDL cholesterol with insulin resistance is well-documented in several studies before the onset of diabetes as well as in type 2 diabetic patients. Taken together, a long history of a proatherogenic lipid profile is likely to contribute to the excess coronary heart disease risk in type 2 diabetes.

Pathophysiology

The key feature of diabetic dyslipidemia is the elevation of plasma triglycerides and reduced HDL cholesterol. The current view is that these two abnormalities are not isolated metabolic aberrations but metabolically closely linked. The concept also includes the idea that disturbances of VLDL metabolism are associated with multiple alterations in the metabolic products IDL and LDL. Type 2 diabetic patients commonly have increased production of VLDL particles, and this defect is the principal cause for raised levels of plasma triglycerides. In addition, impaired clearance of triglyceride-rich particles contributes to the elevation of plasma triglycerides. This brings about the question of why the production rate of VLDL particles is increased in type 2 diabetes. The traditional belief has been that hyperinsulinemia, compensatory to insulin resistance, stimulates VLDL production in the liver in the presence of enhanced free fatty acid flux. This concept has been a topic of ongoing debate for the last decade. Data from in vitro studies using cell cultures and recently from kinetic studies in normal subjects indicate that insulin acutely suppresses both VLDL apoB and VLDL triglyceride production. Insulin appears to have a pivotal role in controlling the free fatty acid flux to the liver and

to have a direct effect on VLDL assembly and release processes. There is convincing evidence that the substrate flux of free fatty acids into liver is markedly increased in type 2 diabetes as well as in insulin resistance. The recognition that VLDL is secreted as a heterogenous spectrum of particles divided according to density into large buoyant VLDL1 particles and small dense VLDL2 particles has raised the question of whether insulin regulates the channeling of VLDL1 and VLDL2 particles. Recently Malmström et al. reported that in normal healthy men, acute hyperinsulinemia suppressed VLDL1 apoB production but had no effect on de novo VLDL2 apoB production. The suppression of VLDL apoB production averaged 50% in normal men. Thus, insulin seems to have a specific inhibitory action on the flux of large buoyant VLDL1 particles. This new concept envisages large VLDL1 particles as liver's chylomicrons, which should be released only in the fasting state but not in the postprandial phase when lipids from food are available. Thus one physiological action of insulin is to maintain the balance between intestinally derived and liver-derived triglyceride-rich lipoproteins and to respond to the shifts of energy needs during transition from the fasted to the fed state.

The recognition of this novel concept raises the question of whether this site of insulin action is dysregulated in insulin resistance. Recently Malmström et al. reported that type 2 diabetic subjects, in contrast to normal men, failed to suppress VLDL1 apoB production in response to acute hyperinsulinism. This failure of insulin to suppress VLDL1 particle release in type 2 diabetes results in inappropriate production of VLDL1 particles in the postprandial phase, and it most likely contributes to postprandial lipemia and is a major cause of the raised triglyceride levels.

Lipoprotein lipase (LPL) and hepatic lipase (HL) are key enzymes in the VLDL-IDL-LDL delipidation cascade and in HDL metabolism. LPL is an insulin-sensitive enzyme and hence is a candidate to be insulin-resistant. Type 2 diabetic patients with poor or moderate glycemic control have low or subnormal postheparin plasma LPL activity. The observations that low levels of postheparin plasma LPL activity and the LPL:HL lipase ratio cluster with insulin resistance, raised triglycerides, and low HDL cholesterol in healthy normoglycemic first-degree relatives of type 2 patients support the view that both lipases are modulated by insulin resistance. In type 2 diabetes the delipidation rate of triglyceride-rich particles is delayed for multiple reasons: paucity of LPL enzyme, saturation of binding sites due to overproduction of VLDL particles, and disassociation of LPL by excess free fatty acids.

A sequence of events leads to increased formation of small dense LDL in diabetic dyslipidemia. A principal key observation is that the metabolic properties of LDL particles are dependent upon the pedigree of the particles. Small dense LDL is postulated to be the product of VLDL1 delipidation, which is the principal component of VLDL subclasses in type 2 diabetic patients. The delayed passage of triglyceride-rich lipoproteins through the lipolytic cascade favors enhanced core lipid exchange between triglyceride-rich lipoproteins and LDL mediated by CETP. Large lipid-rich LDL particles are a good substrate for hepatic lipase and its action leads to formation of smaller dense LDL particles. Substantial evidence indicates that hepatic lipase activity is commonly increased in type 2 diabetes. The formation of small dense LDL depends upon the rate of transfer of triglycerides to LDL and the rate of their hydrolysis by hepatic lipase, both processes being enhanced in diabetic dyslipidemia.

There appears to be a symmetry of mechanism in the lowering of HDL cholesterol to the formation of small dense LDL. The long residence time of triglyceride-rich lipoproteins in circulation also results in an enhanced exchange of core lipids between triglyceride-rich lipoproteins and HDL particles. This process leads to a formation of triglyceride-rich HDL particles, which are good substrates for hepatic lipase. In this scenario, triglyceride-rich HDL particles have an enhanced catabolic rate, resulting in a reduced number and small size of circulating HDL particles. The end-result of this process is HDL3 particles that are the principal subclass of HDL particles in type 2 diabetes. Growing evidence indicates that indeed the catabolic rate of HDL particles and HDL apoA-I is increased in type 2 diabetic patients.

Lipid levels and coronary heart disease in diabetes

Type 1 diabetes   Type 1 diabetic patients have markedly higher coronary heart disease risk than nondiabetic populations despite normal levels of lipoproteins. On average the coronary heart disease risk has varied between 8 to 10% in both men and women in patients without proteinuria. It is well-established that the development of nephropathy accelerates the coronary heart disease risk up to 25-fold in patients with established diabetic nephropathy. Unfortunately, there is relatively little data on lipoproteins and coronary heart disease, and there are no clinical trials relating lipoproteins to coronary heart disease. The limited data that are available indicate that LDL cholesterol is a coronary heart disease risk factor in type 1 diabetes. Growing evidence suggests that the relative risk for coronary heart disease increases with elevation of serum triglycerides. In type 1 diabetic patients with coronary heart disease, serum HDL cholesterol levels are lower and serum triglyceride levels higher than in patients without coronary heart disease.

Type 2 diabetes   Determining the primary atherogenic lipid/or lipoprotein in type 2 diabetes is the key question for treatment strategies. Prospective epidemiological studies have established raised serum triglycerides to be a significant predictor of cardiovascular mortality and morbidity in type 2 diabetes. Data collected from six epidemiological studies, including a total of 4500 type 2 diabetic patients with a follow-up for periods of 7 to 13 years, lend evidence to the predictive power of triglycerides. In five of the six studies, hypertriglyceridemia was a predictor for future coronary heart disease events, and in three studies it predicted coronary heart disease mortality. Importantly, serum cholesterol was not a predictive factor in any of the six studies in multivariate analyses when adjusted for other risk factors. Unfortunately most of these studies have not included simultaneous measurements of HDL cholesterol and glycemic parameters together with lipid measures. High triglycerides/low HDL cholesterol was clearly a coronary heart disease risk factor in the recent study by Lehto et al., which included 1059 type 2 diabetic patients followed for up to 7 years. The presence of a total triglyceride level above 2.3 mmol/l, non-HDL cholesterol above 5.2 mmol/l, and HDL cholesterol <0.9 mmol/l increased the risk of coronary heart disease events twofold. Simultaneous presence of dyslipidemia and high fasting plasma glucose (>13.4 mmol/l) further increased the risk of coronary heart disease events up to threefold. There are several plausible mechanisms to explain how triglyceride-rich lipoproteins may promote atherogenesis. Smaller species of triglyceride-rich particles can have direct effects on the arterial wall to promote foam cell formation. Elevation of triglyceride-rich lipoproteins is associated with the formation of small dense LDL and excessive accumulation of remnants in the postprandial phase. However, which specific triglyceride-rich lipoprotein is the most atherogenic is still unknown. The fact, that the metabolism of triglyceride-rich lipoproteins is so intimately linked with that of HDL questions the inclusion of both parameters as separate variables in statistical analyses. In conclusion, strong evidence indicates that hypertriglyceridemia influences the risk of coronary heart disease in type 2 diabetic patients.

The power of cholesterol as a coronary heart disease risk factor was demonstrated in the Multiple Risk Factor Intervention Trial (MRFIT), where cardiovascular disease death rates over 12 years of follow-up rose more steeply with higher serum cholesterol in diabetic than in nondiabetic populations. In fact, at any given cholesterol level, the risk of cardiovascular mortality was higher in diabetic patients than in nondiabetic subjects. This observation raises the speculation as to whether any given amount of LDL cholesterol is more atherogenic in diabetic individuals. Several types of evidence support the tenet that "normal" LDL concentration may indeed be more atherogenic in type 2 diabetic patients than in nondiabetic individuals. First, the majority of LDL particles represent small dense LDL, which is more prone to oxidation and has a prolonged half-life due to poor affinity to LDL receptors. Small dense LDL also penetrates more readily into the arterial wall than large particles, and it has high binding affinity to proteoglycans, promoting its retention and consequent modification. Second, glycosylation of LDL impairs its removal via the LDL receptor pathway, which leads to its increased uptake by macrophages and promotes foam cell formation. Thus, glycation of LDL also enhances its atherogenic potential.

Treatment

Given the strong evidence that diabetic patients have a greatly increased risk of coronary heart disease, each diabetic patient belongs to the high-risk category as defined

Table 64.1 Target levels of lipids in diabetes	
Triglycerides	<2.3 mmol/l
and	
HDL-cholesterol	
women	>1.1 mmol/l
men	>0.9 mmol/l
LDL-cholesterol	<2.6 mmol/l
Cholesterol/HDL-cholesterol	<3.4 mmol/l

by the guidelines of American Diabetes Association (ADA) consensus conferences. In practice this means that a borderline high LDL cholesterol (between 3.4 to 4.1 mmol/l or 130 to 160 mg/dl) in diabetic patients means a much higher LDL cholesterol in terms of coronary heart disease risk. Consequently, the optimal LDL cholesterol for each diabetic patient is <2.6 mmol/l (<100 mg/dl) (Tab. 64.1). Raised concentrations of triglycerides and lowering of HDL cholesterol are also recognized as targets for treatment in diabetes. However, setting targets for triglyceride and cholesterol levels has been more difficult and guidelines are less consistent than for LDL cholesterol. Desirable triglyceride levels are <2.3 mmol/l (<200 mg/dl), but to avoid the deleterious metabolic consequences of raised triglycerides, the levels should be as low as possible. Optimal levels of HDL cholesterol should be above 1.1 mmol/l (>45 mg/dl), though it may be desirable to have even higher levels in women. The use of "non-HDL cholesterol" (serum cholesterol - HDL cholesterol) as a target has recently been widely emphasized. This measure includes cholesterol in VLDL and IDL in addition to that in LDL. This measure may thus be particularly important in disorders such as diabetic dyslipidemia in which the concentrations of VLDL and IDL are elevated. The optimal goal for non-HDL cholesterol is <3.4 mmol/l.

Since HMG-CoA (β-hydroxy-β-methyglutaryl-CoA) reductase inhibitors (statins) are highly effective in lowering LDL cholesterol, the primary target of therapy should be to lower LDL cholesterol. For diabetic patients with clinical coronary heart disease, the optimal goal of LDL cholesterol should be <2.6 mmol/l. Since diabetic patients with a first myocardial infarction have a poor short-term as well as long-term prognosis, aggressive lowering of LDL cholesterol should also be applied to diabetic patients who have not yet had a clinical event. Consequently, the targets of primary and secondary prevention are the same in diabetic patients (Tab. 64.1).

Second implications for treatment should be raised triglyceride and reduced HDL cholesterol levels. The fact that raised triglycerides act as a synergistic risk factor with other lipid risk factors justifies this approach. However, the lack of clinical trials that specifically target the correction of high triglyceride/low HDL cholesterol clustering hamper the active treatment in clinical practice, though future clinical trials may justify more aggressive approach. The concept of global risk factor management should be the basis for treatment strategies.

Treatment of dyslipidemia in diabetic patients consists of a stepwise approach with three major components. The first-line therapy is comprised of life-style changes aiming at weight loss, increased physical activity, smoking cessation, and moderation of alcohol intake. These actions aim to correct metabolic risk factors linked to insulin resistance. Effective use of lifestyle intervention is associated with clear benefits. Weight loss is generally associated with improvements in triglycerides and HDL cholesterol levels. Similar improvements are also seen with regular exercise programs aimed to improve physical fitness. Recommendations for physical activity should be individualized. Since smoking induces insulin-resistance and an unfavorable lipid profile, including fat intolerance, the cessation of smoking is extremely important.

If these therapies are insufficient to improve glycemic control to achieve targets, the second step is to intensify strategies to improve glycemic control. The more frequent use of combination therapy has facilitated the improvement of glycemic control in type 2 diabetic patients. Aggressive treatment of hyperglycemia improves triglyceride levels in particular but has less effect on HDL cholesterol. Drugs that are adversely influencing insulin resistance and lipid and lipoprotein metabolism should be avoided. It should be recognized that, unfortunately, optimization of glycemic control frequently fails to fully correct dyslipidemia in a sizable portion of type 2 diabetic patients. Consequently, if the specific target for lipid levels are not achieved, it becomes mandatory to institute therapies to correct specific components of dyslipidemia.

Treatment for LDL lowering

The drugs of first choice to reduce LDL cholesterol are statins, since they are highly effective, generally well-tolerated, safe, and do not have adverse effects on glycemic control. All statins inhibit HMG-CoA reductase activity and consequently decrease hepatic cholesterol content. The principal mechanism for lowering LDL cholesterol is enhanced expression of LDL receptors in the liver. Since VLDL remnants are also removed via binding to LDL receptors, statins also reduce cholesterol in VLDL and IDL particles and remnants. The potency of different statins to lower LDL cholesterol is dose-related. When the effects of various statins has been evaluated, the following potency (LDL response per mg dose) was discovered: fluvastatin < lovastatin = pravastatin < simvastatin < atorvastatin < cerivastatin. Recent data indicate that all statins are effective to lower triglycerides in hypertriglyceridemic subjects, but the effects are only trivial in normotriglyceridemic subjects. The efficacy to lower triglycerides seems to be comparable at equipotent doses for LDL cholesterol lowering. These new observations justify the use of statins in type 2 diabetic patients, representing the atherogenic lipid triad with high LDL cholesterol together with raised triglycerides and lowering of HDL cholesterol. In fact, many lipid experts consider statins to be the first-choice drug to treat diabetic dyslipidemia.

Hard evidence for the benefits of triglyceride lowering is so far lacking, but ongoing studies should yield further information. However, strong evidence from epidemiological and metabolic studies make a compelling argument that triglyceride-lowering in the global management of diabetic dyslipidemia would be beneficial. The situation shows parallels to the cholesterol controversy from some 10 years ago. Despite considerable evidence pointed to the causal connection between elevated cholesterol and CHD, it took several years and data from large-scale intervention studies to finally convince the skeptics.

Theoretically nicotinic acid is an ideal drug to treat diabetic dyslipidemia. Nicotinic acid is a powerful triglyceride-lowering agent, and it also markedly raises HDL cholesterol. Since nicotinic acid can worsen glycemic control, it should be avoided in the treatment of diabetic dyslipidemia. Consequently, drugs of the fibrate class are used as a first-line therapy to treat hypertriglyceridemia. Fibrates not only lower elevated triglyceride values but also effectively reduce postprandial lipemia, shift the distribution of LDL particles to less dense and more buoyant particles, and increase HDL cholesterol. Thus, fibrates have positive effects on all components of diabetic dyslipidemia. Fibrates exert multiple effects on lipoprotein metabolism as a result of their action on the peroxisome proliferator-activator receptors. Fibrates stimulate peroxisome proliferator-activator receptors in the liver and this action is followed by down-regulation of apoC-III gene and decrease of apoCIII synthesis. Fibrates also increase gene expression of apoA-I and A-II and consequently protein synthesis. The end-result is enhanced catabolism and reduced secretion of triglyceride-rich particles and increase of HDL particles. Whether the action of different fibrates on the peroxisome proliferator-activator receptor system is comparable is unknown, but the best studied compound is fenofibrate, and its effects are well-established.

In the present day, the most commonly used fibrates are bezafibrate, fenofibrate, and gemfibrozil. There are no studies on efficacy of different fibrates available, but extrapolation of the data from different studies indicates that fenofibrate may be more effective than other fibrates. In general, fibrates are well-tolerated and have no adverse effects on glycemic control.

What is the evidence for effectiveness of lipid lowering therapy in diabetes?

Although controlled clinical trials have conclusively shown a beneficial effect of cholesterol lowering in nondiabetic populations so far, no clinical trials have specifically studied the effects of lipid lowering in diabetic populations. However, the post hoc analyses of diabetic patients included in three clinical trials have given encouraging results (Tab. 64.2). The Scandinavian Simvastatin Survival Trial (4S) included 202 diabetic patients. The subgroup analysis demonstrated that simvastatin reduced lipids to a similar extent in diabetic and nondiabetic patients. This is the first study to show that lowering LDL cholesterol in type 2 diabetic patients decreases the risk of coronary heart disease events. The reduction of the coronary heart disease events was 55% in the diabetic cohort as compared to 32% in the nondiabetic cohort. The primary endpoint of total mortality was not significant because of low numbers. It should be kept in mind that in the 4S study, the diabetic patients had relatively high baseline cholesterol levels (5.5 to 8.0 mmol/l), and patients with triglycerides above 2.5 mmol/l were excluded. Hence, there is a caveat in extrapolating these data to the general diabetic population, because these lipid abnormalities are not typical of diabetic dyslipidemia. Likewise, CARE and TexCAP reported significant clinical benefits of lipid lowering in subgroups of diabetic patients. In these two studies, individuals with coronary heart disease had moderate cholesterol levels. In conclusion, the available data from these studies strongly suggests that LDL lowering will produce at least similar clinical benefits in type 2 diabetic patients as in nondiabetic subjects.

Although triglyceride levels are powerful predictors of CHD in diabetes, no clinical trial with the main focus on lowering triglyceride levels has been completed. The data from a subgroup analysis of diabetic subjects included in the Helsinki Heart Study indicated that the reduction of coronary heart disease risk by 60% in the gemfibrozil group, but the figure was not statistically significant due to low numbers of actual events. Two ongoing trials, Diabetes Atherosclerosis Trial (DAIS) and the FIELD

Table 64.2 Clinical trials of lipid therapy in diabetic subjects (subgroup analyses)

Study	Journal	n	LDL lowering	Baseline LDL	CHD reduction
Primary prevention					
Helsinki	Diabetes Care, 1992	135	-6.1%	191	-60% (NS)
AFCAPS/TexCAP	JAMA, 1998	264	-25%	150	-43%
Secondary prevention					
CARE	NEJM, 1996[1]	586	-28%	137	-25% (p=0.05)
4S	Diabetes Care, 1997	202	-37%	186	-55% (p=0.002)

[1] Not a full report on the diabetic group. LDL lowering refers to the overall group.
(AFCAPS/TexCAP= The Air Force/Texas Coronary Atherosclerosis Prevention Study; CARE= Cholesterol and Recurrent Events Trial; CHD=coronary heart disease; LDL= low density lipoproteins.)

Study are designed to evaluate the effects of fenofibrate on the coronary heart disease risk in type 2 diabetic populations. These trials aim to answer the question of whether the clinical benefits are mediated through changes in plasma triglycerides and/or HDL cholesterol. DAIS is a placebo-controlled double-blind multicenter study testing the efficacy of lipid lowering on coronary atherosclerosis, as determined by quantitative coronary angiography. The FIELD Study (Fenofibrate Intervention and Event Lowering in Diabetes) will recruit 6000 type 2 diabetic patients in the primary prevention arm, and 2000 type 2 diabetic patients in the secondary prevention arm. These trials, now in progress, will provide evidence to ascertain if the correction of diabetic dyslipidemia provides clinical benefits.

Suggested readings

CAIXÀS A, ORDÓNEZ-LLANOS J, DE LEIVA A, PAYÉS A, HOMS R, PÉREZ A. Optimization of glycemic control by insulin therapy decreases the proportion of small dense LDL particles in diabetic patients. Diabetes 1997;46:1207-13.

DCCT RESEARCH GROUP. Lipid and lipoproteins levels in patients with IDDM: Diabetes Control and Complications Trial Experience. Diabetes Care 1992;15:886-94.

DE MAN FHAF, CASTRO-CABEAZ M, VAN BARLINGEN HHJJ, et al. Triglyceride-rich lipoproteinsin non-insulin-dependent diabetes mellitus: post-prandial metabolism and relation to premature atherosclerosis. Eur J Clin Invest 1996;26:89-108.

GOLDEBERG RB, MELLIES MJ, SACKS FM, et al. for the CARE Investigators. Cardiovascular events and their reduction with pravastatin in diabetic and glucose-intolerant myocardial infarction survivors with average cholesterol levels: subgroup analyses in the cholesterol and recurrent events (CARE) trial. Circulation 1998;98:2513-9.

GROOP P-H, ELLIOTT T, EKSTRAND A, et al. Multiple lipoprotein abnormalities in type 1 diabetic patients with renal disease. Diabetes 1996;45:974-9.

HAFFNER SM. Lipoprotein(a) and diabetes. Diabetes Care 1993;16:835-40.

HAFFNER SM. Management of dyslipidemia in adults with diabetes. Diabetes Care 1998;21:160-78.

KOIVISTO VA, STEVENS LK, MATTOCK M, et al. and the EURODIAB IDDM Complications Study Group. Cardiovascular disease and its risk factors in IDDM in Europe. Diabetes Care 1996;19:689-97.

LEWIS GF. Fatty acid regulation of very low density lipoprotein production. Curr Opin Lipidol 1997;8:146-53.

LOPES-VIRELLA M, KLEIN RL, VIRELLA G. Modification of lipoproteins in diabetes. Diabetes/Metabolism Reviews 1996;12:69-90.

MALMSTRÖMJ, CASLAKE M, et al. Defective regulation of triglyceride metabolism by insulin in the liver in NIDDM. Diabetologia 1997;40:454-62.

PACKARD CJ, SHEPERD J. Lipoprotein heterogeneity and apolipoprotein B metabolism. Arterioscler Thromb Vasc Biol 1997;17:3542-56.

PYÖRÄLÄ K, PEDERSEN TR, KJEKSHUS J, FAERGEMAN O, OLSSON AG, THORGEIRSSON G, AND THE SCANDINAVIAN SIMVASTATIN SURVIVAL STUDY (4S) GROUP. Cholesterol lowering with simvastatin improves prognosis of diabetic patients with coronary heart disease. Diabetes Care 1997;20:614-20.

STAMLER J, VACCARO O, NEATON JD, WENTWORTH D for the Multiple Risk Factor Intervention Trial Research Group. Diabetes, other risk factors, and 12-yr cardiovascular mortality for men screened in the multiple risk factor intervention trial. Diabetes Care 1993;16:434-44.

STEINER G FOR THE DAIS PROJECT GROUP. The Diabetes Atherosclerosis Intervention Study (DAIS): a study conducted in cooperation with the World Health Organization. Diabetologia 1996;39:1655-61.

SYVÄNNE M, TASKINEN M-R. Lipids and lipoproteins as coronary risk factors in non-insulin-dependent diabetes mellitus. Lancet 1997;350:20-3.

TASKINEN M-R. Quantitative and qualitative lipoprotein abnormalities in diabetes mellitus. Diabetes 1992;41:12-7.

TASKINEN M-R, LAHDENPERÄ S, SYVÄNNE M. New insights into lipid metabolism in non-insulin-dependent diabetes mellitus. Ann Med 1996;28:335-40.

Diffuse hormone systems

65

Gastrointestinal hormones

Bo Ahrén

In 1902, Bayliss and Starling reported that extracts of the duodenal mucosa stimulated pancreatic exocrine secretion. It was therefore hypothesized that pancreatic secretion was regulated by a substance released from the duodenum. The substance was named secretin. Three years later, the word *hormone* (meaning "rouse to activity"), as first suggested by Hardy, was introduced by Starling as a name for substances such as secretin that are released into the bloodstream from one organ and act as chemical messengers on target cells in distantly located organs. Many gastrointestinal hormones of a peptide nature that meet the above criteria have been described. The gastrointestinal tract also produces other regulatory peptides that act locally in the tissue of production, or are neuropeptides that are produced in neural tissues and act as neurotransmitters. Altogether, gastrointestinal peptides regulate numerous physiological processes, such as gastrointestinal motility and secretion, endocrine and exocrine pancreatic secretion, and gallbladder contraction.

GASTROINTESTINAL ENDOCRINE CELLS

Numerous neuroendocrine cells exist in the gastrointestinal tract, and several regulatory peptides are produced by them (Tab. 65.1). These endocrine cells are characteristically located diffusely in the mucosa of the stomach or small and large intestines, among the mucosal cells (enterocytes) responsible for secretion and absorption. Each endocrine cell type is not randomly distributed throughout the gastrointestinal tract, but instead is concentrated in certain areas of the gastrointestinal tract. For example, the gastric inhibitory peptide (GIP)-producing K cells are distributed primarily in the duodenum, with a falling concentration of cells distally; whereas the glucagon-like peptide 1 (GLP-1)-producing L cells are most concentrated in the distal ileum, with falling concentrations proximal to this location. Since the main regulators of the release of the peptides from the endocrine cells are stimuli from the gastrointestinal lumen, this anatomical organization of endocrine cells allows stimuli to reach the cells at different time points after meal intake. Consequently, the regulatory peptides are released in a

defined manner in relation to food intake. For example, gastrin-producing G cells are located in the stomach and release gastrin immediately after food intake to stimulate gastric acid secretion; when nutrients at a somewhat later time point reach the duodenum, duodenal I and S cells release cholecystokinin (CCK) and secretin, respectively, and the gallbladder is contracted and the exocrine pancreatic secretion is stimulated, which are processes leading to neutralization of the gut content.

A given endocrine cell usually produces and secretes only one main regulatory peptide, although some cells produce more than one peptide (Tab. 65.1). In addition, a given endocrine cell expresses only a limited number of different receptors, allowing external regulation only by a limited number of influences. An endocrine cell regulates its function by adjusting the expression of regulatory peptides, and appropriate receptors, as well as enzymes responsible for the final synthesis of regulatory peptides and receptors. The regulation of such programming of each cell is at present poorly understood.

It was previously thought that gastrointestinal endocrine cells were derived from the neural crest and migrated into the primitive endoderm forming the gut. The rationale for this hypothesis was that the endocrine cells show a remarkable similarity to neuroendocrine cells in the central nervous system in terms of expression of regulatory peptides and enzymes. For example, the gastrointestinal cells are capable of taking up and decarboxylating amine precursors into the corresponding amine – as exemplified by dopa being converted to dopamine by a number of gastrointestinal endocrine cells – which is similar to a number of neuroendocrine cells in the brain. This ability has grouped the cells together under the name APUD cells (amine precursor uptake and decarboxylation cells). Another similarity is that some of the regulatory peptides produced in gastrointestinal endocrine cells are also neuropeptides in neurons in the central nervous system, as are cholecystokinin and glucagon-like peptide 1, for example. However, it was later demonstrated that the endocrine cells of the gastrointestinal tract originate in the endoderm and develop from pluripotent stem cells, which also give rise to the enterocytes. Antral G cells, for example, arise from immature precursor cells in the middle of the crypts and migrate downward to the base; the half-life of such a migration is 15 days. The regulation of development and maturation of these stem cells is not yet established, however.

Following their release from cells of production, the regulatory peptides may function as classical hormones by passing through the circulation and affecting distally located cells or organs (*endocrine* regulation). This is exemplified by secretin and cholecystokinin stimulating exocrine pancreatic secretion and glucagon-like peptide 1 stimulating insulin secretion. The regulatory peptides could also affect cells located nearby following passage through the intracellular space (*paracrine* or *autocrine* regulation), as exemplified by somatostatin, which is released from the stomach D cells and inhibits the closely located G cells from secreting gastrin. A third mode of influence by the gastrointestinal regulatory peptides is *neurocrine* regulation, which is when a neuropeptide is released from nerve endings and affects local gastrointestinal function. For example, galanin and neuropeptide

Y (NPY) are released from nerve endings and regulate gastrointestinal motility.

The organization of the peptide system in the gastrointestinal tract allows for a concerted action of various processes with high specificity. For example, the regulation of gastrointestinal function often requires a high local concentration of the messenger, which is permitted by the paracrine or neurocrine regulation of cells and nerves located in close apposition to the effector cells. The organization also precludes the released peptides from acting on other processes, since they degrade rapidly after acting, and it also precludes circulatory levels of the peptides in question to affect the processes since the circulating concentrations of such local regulatory peptides are low. Specificity is also permitted by the occurrence of specific peptide receptors on the target cells, precluding the regulatory peptides to act on other cells.

Action and degradation of the regulatory peptides

Following their extracellular release from the cells of production, the regulatory peptides reach their receptors

Table 65.1 Regulatory peptides of the gastrointestinal tract

Primary anatomical location	Cell type	Regulatory peptide	Abbreviation	No. of amino acids[1]
Stomach endocrine cells	G cells	Gastrin		17,34
		Peptide YY	PYY	36
		Pancreastatin		49
	D cells	Somatostatin		14,28
	A cells	Glucagon		29
	ECL cells	Not known		
Proximal intestinal endocrine cells	S cells	Secretin		27
	I cells	Cholecystokinin	CCK	8,33
	EC$_2$ cells	Motilin		22
	EC$_1$ cells	Substance P		11
		Neurokinin A		10
	K cells	Gastric inhibitory polypeptide	GIP	42
Distal intestinal endocrine cells	L cells	Glucagon-like peptide 1	GLP-1	30
		Oxyntomodulin		37
		Glucagon-like peptide 2	GLP-2	33
	PYY cells	Peptide YY	PYY	36
	N cells	Neurotensin		13
Stomach or intestinal nerve terminals	Vasoactive intestinal polypeptide		VIP	28
	Peptide histidine-isoleucin		PHI	27
	Galanin			29,30
	Gastrin releasing peptide		SRP	27
	Neuropeptide Y		NPY	36
	Calcitonin gene-related peptide		CGRP	37
	Substance P		SP	11
	Neuromedin U		NMU	26
	Pituitary adenylate cyclase-activating polypeptide		PACAP	27,38
	Neurokinin A		NKA	10
	Neurokinin B		NKB	10

[1] The number of amino acids is the human sequence thought to be of the most important physiological function.

located in the plasma membrane of their target cells. Most receptors of the gastrointestinal regulatory peptides are of the seven transmembrane spanning receptor type. Often a gastrointestinal regulatory peptide binds to several different receptors, as exemplified by cholecystokinin binding to CCK_A as well as CCK_B receptors, and, conversely, a given receptor might bind several regulatory peptides, as exemplified by CCK_B receptors binding cholecystokinin as well as gastrin. Following binding of the peptide to the receptor, a signal is transmitted to the interior of the cells, usually activating intramembranously located G proteins. G proteins consist of three subunits, called α-, β- and γ-units. Two main transduction pathways are activated by the Ga proteins: (1) the activation of adenylate cyclase to form cyclic adenosine monophosphate (AMP), which activates protein kinase A, and (2) the activation of phospholipase C, which through phosphoinositide hydrolysis yields the formation of diacyl glycerol and inositol-1,3,4-trisphosphate (IP_3), with the subsequent release of calcium from storage pools and activation of protein kinase C. Some regulatory peptides also activate ion channels in the plasma membranes.

Following activation of its receptor, the regulatory peptide itself is rapidly inactivated by peptidases located in tissues and in the circulation. Due to the rapid action of these enzymes, the half-life of a regulatory peptide is usually only a few minutes.

Gastrointestinal regulatory peptides as "classical" gastrointestinal hormones

Gastrin

Gastrin is produced in endocrine G cells along the mucosa of the gastric antrum. Its precursor is the 101-amino acid preprogastrin, which is processed through a 34-amino acid gastrin (G34, big gastrin) to the 17-amino acid sequence G17 (little gastrin). Both forms of gastrin are C-terminally amidated, and the C-terminal pentapeptide is identical to the corresponding sequence in CCK. Under fasting conditions, G34 (half-life 30 minutes) is the main circulatory form of gastrin, whereas after a meal, the main form is G17 (half-life 7 minutes). Gastrin exerts its action through the activation of CCK_B-receptors, which are G protein-coupled receptors of the seven transmembrane domain type, binding gastrin and cholecystokinin with equal affinity. The CCK_B-receptors are mainly coupled to the activation of phospholipase C.

Gastrin is released into the bloodstream after food intake. The primary stimulators of gastrin secretion are gastric distension, high pH, the cholinergic and peptidergic nerves by the neurotransmitters acetyl choline and gastrin-releasing peptide (GRP), and the luminal content of small peptides and amino acids. Gastrin secretion is also stimulated by coffee, wine, and beer, whereas fat and carbohydrates are poor secretagogues of the G cells. Conversely, gastrin secretion is inhibited by low pH in the stomach, by somatostatin produced in the proximally located D cells, and by adrenergic nerves, as well as by gut hormones released from the small intestine (mainly gastric inhibitory peptide and glucagon-like peptide 1).

The main function of gastrin is to stimulate acid secretion from the oxyntic mucosa, which is an effect executed directly on the parietal cells and indirectly through local release of histamine from ECL cells. Gastrin also increases gastric emptying and stimulates gastrointestinal motility. Hence, gastrin is important during the early postprandial period for the initiation of digestion and propulsion of food. Since its release is inhibited by low pH, that is, acid in the gastric lumen, and removal of food content from the stomach, its secretion vanishes in time after food intake. It has also been shown that gastrin stimulates hypertrophy and hyperplasia of the oxyntic mucosa, and that it stimulates proliferation of the ECL cells.

In addition to the G cells, gastrin is also expressed in duodenal mucosal cells. In these cells, however, the dominant gastrin form is G34. Gastrin is also expressed in the fetal pancreatic islets, and the gastrin gene has been found to be expressed in some colon cancer cells. In some neurons, primarily in the central nervous system, a small molecular form of gastrin, the C-terminal tetrapeptide of gastrin (G4; mini-gastrin), is expressed and apparently functions as a neurotransmitter. Gastrin may also be important during fetal development of the pancreas. In addition, gastrin may stimulate growth of colon cancers in an autocrine manner, though this latter hypothesis is less likely, since colon cancer cells do not usually posses gastrin receptors.

Circulating gastrin is markedly elevated in gastrin-producing endocrine tumors (gastrinoma, Zollinger-Ellison syndrome), which occur in the pancreas (80%) or duodenum (20%). The incidence of the disease is approximately 1 to 2 per million per year. Approximately 60% of the cases are malignant with metastases in the regional lymph nodes and/or in the liver, and 30% of the cases with gastrinoma are associated with multiple endocrine neoplasia (MEN-1). The dominating symptoms in gastrinoma are multiple and severe peptic ulceration and excessive secretory diarrhea, the latter being caused by enzyme inactivation and mucosal damage by the excessive production of acid. The diagnosis is usually made by the determination of grossly elevated circulating gastrin in the presence of increased basal acid output. In suspected cases, the gastrin response to iv provocation with secretin can be determined. Under normal conditions, secretin inhibits gastrin secretion, but in gastrinoma, secretin stimulates gastrin secretion. Treatment includes, in addition to surgical removal of the tumors, antisecretory treatment.

Circulating gastrin is usually elevated in peptic disorders associated with *Helicobacter pylori* infection, possibly due to the inhibition of somatostatin secretion. This may occur because of a selective loss of antral D cells, which in turn elevates gastrin secretion. It has also been shown that hypergastrinemia evolves in association with atrophic gastritis; this is the cause of the often concomitant occurrence of gastric carcinoid, that is, tumor development of the ECL cells due to the proliferative action of these cells exerted by gastrin. This condition may thus be treated with antrectomy and removal of the gastrin-producing cells. Finally, an important cause of hypergastrinemia is the long-term use of inhibitors of gastric acid secretion (H_2-receptor antagonists or proton pump inhibitors), since these drugs increase the gastric pH, which stimulates gastrin secretion. It is debated whether gastric carcinoid could also evolve in association with hypergastrinemia secondary to these drugs, but this risk seems to be minimal in humans.

Cholecystokinin

Cholecystokinin (CCK) is produced in the intestinal I cells, which are situated primarily along the mucosa of the duodenum and the proximal jejunum. The precursor of cholecystokinin is a 115-amino acid prepro-CCK, and the initial translational product is CCK83, which is further processed to several different forms of cholecystokinin that consist of the residues 58, 39, 33, 25, 22, 18, 12, 8, 7, and 5. The mechanisms of this processing and the functions of this number of intermediates or cholecystokinin forms are not yet established. CCK58, CCK39, CCK33, and CCK8 appear to be the main forms of cholecystokinin in the circulation. The circulating half-life of cholecystokinin is very short (for CCK8 only 1 minute), which is mostly due to rapid first passage degradation in the liver. Cholecystokinin is also produced in nerves, occurring as a neurotransmitter in intestinal nerves, in nerves in the pancreatic islets, and in the central nervous system. Studies on its processing in the nerves have revealed that the same CCK gene is expressed in nerves and in I cells, although the molecular form of CCK in the nerves is probably CCK4 rather than the longer forms.

Two different types of CCK receptors have been described, both of which are of the G protein seven transmembraneous domain type linked to activation of phospholipase C. One type is the CCK_A-receptors, which are expressed in the gallbladder smooth muscle cells, pancreatic acinar and islet cells, in gastrointestinal muscular cells, and in various parts of the brain. This receptor type shows almost a 1000-fold higher affinity for CCK than for gastrin. The other type is the CCK_B-receptors, which are expressed in the cerebral cortex and in other brain areas, in gastric parietal cells, in ECL cells, and in gastrointestinal muscular cells. This receptor type shows equal affinity for cholecystokinin and gastrin.

Cholecystokinin is released from the I cells into the circulation following a meal intake. The most efficient stimulators of cholecystokinin secretion are proteins, individual amino acids, and fat (triglycerides) in the intestinal lumen, whereas carbohydrates are only poor cholecystokinin secretagogues. The autonomic nervous system is also involved in cholecystokinin secretion since the parasympathetic nervous system and the neurotransmitter GRP stimulate cholecystokinin secretion. In addition, it has been hypothesized that a cholecystokinin-releasing peptide exists, presumably produced in the duodenum. This putative peptide would mediate the marked cholecystokinin secretion that occurs when the intraduodenal content of trypsin or chymotrypsin is reduced, implying a negative feedback between pancreatic enzyme secretion and cholecystokinin release. This hypothesis is supported by findings that pancreatic enzymes inhibit cholecystokinin release. The most potent inhibitor of cholecystokinin release is bile in the intestinal lumen, in addition to the negative feedback of pancreatic secretion, and somatostatin produced in D cells in close apposition to the I cells. Hence, cholecystokinin secretion seems to be precisely regulated by a variety of influences.

Cholecystokinin induces a variety of effects. Following the development of specific cholecystokinin receptor antagonists, the physiological significance of these effects was explored. It was demonstrated that the main physiological function of cholecystokinin is stimulation of gallbladder contraction, stimulation of pancreatic enzyme and bicarbonate secretion, inhibition of gastric emptying, stimulation of gastric somatostatin secretion, acceleration of intestinal transport, and prolongation of colonic transport. It should be emphasized that, in general, these actions are also regulated by other factors, such as the parasympathetic nervous system and other hormones. Thus, whereas cholecystokinin has been shown to be the single most important regulator of gallbladder contraction, stimulation of pancreatic enzyme secretion is also regulated by the cholinergic nerves, and pancreatic bicarbonate secretion is also regulated by secretin. Cholecystokinin, however, potentiates these responses and is therefore an important portion of the redundant regulation of these events.

In terms of physiology, cholecystokinin is thought to represent the key mediator of the responses to food entering the small intestine: it inhibits gastric acid and gastrin secretion through its stimulation of somatostatin secretion, as well as initiates digestive small intestine function (gallbladder contraction, pancreatic enzyme and bicarbonate secretion, acceleration of intestinal passing time). As a neurotransmitter, cholecystokinin may also be involved in other processes, such as the regulation of islet hormone secretion: cholecystokinin is an islet neurotransmitter and exerts powerful stimulatory action on insulin secretion. Finally, the ubiquitous distribution of cholecystokinin receptors in various parts of the brain has prompted studies on a potential central action of cholecystokinin, either as a hormone or as a central neurotransmitter. One interesting observation in this context is that cholecystokinin administered locally into the third cerebroventricular space in rats inhibits food intake, making cholecystokinin a candidate peptide involved in the regulation of food intake.

Overproduction of cholecystokinin is not a clinical entity, since no CCK-producing tumor has been described. Reduction of cholecystokinin release is, however, sometimes seen in subjects with celiac disease, although the clinical value of this is not known. A recent clinical interest in cholecystokinin has been stimulated by findings that CCK_A-receptor antagonists increase colonic passing time.

Secretin

Secretin is produced in the intestinal S cells, which are mostly located in the upper duodenum, with a falling degree of density distally. Secretin is a 27-amino acid peptide; it is processed from the 134-amino acid long pre-prosecretin. The major stimulus for secretin release is the presence of acid in the duodenum, although fatty acids, alcohol, and bile also stimulate secretin secretion. In the circulation, secretin has a short half-life of approximately 2 to 3 minutes because of rapid clearance in the kidney. The secretin receptor is a classical G protein-coupled seven transmembranous domain type, which occurs in two forms: one shows high affinity for secretin and is linked to adenylate cyclase, and another shows low affinity for secretin and is linked to phospholipase C.

The primary physiological function of secretin is to stimulate pancreatic water and bicarbonate secretion, which was the function first postulated to be a hormonal action in 1902 by Bayliss and Starling. The action to stimulate pancreatic secretion is potentiated by cholecystokinin and cholinergic nerves, although secretin appears to be the most important single regulator of this type of exocrine secretion. Pharmacologically, secretin also inhibits gastric acid secretion and stimulates bile and pancreatic enzyme secretion. However, only the stimulation of pancreatic water and bicarbonate secretion appear to be physiologically induced. Hence, the main function of secretin is to neutralize the acid content discharged into the duodenum, which provides the optimal environment in the intestinal lumen and thus promotes further digestion. As is cholecystokinin, secretin is reduced in the circulation in celiac disease, which may further compromise food digestion and pancreatic secretion in this disease.

Gastric inhibitory peptide

Gastric inhibitory peptide (GIP) is produced by the K cells located along the mucosa of the duodenum. Prepro-GIP is a 153-amino acid sequence that is processed to the final gastric inhibitory peptide, a 42-amino acid peptide. Gastric inhibitory peptide secretion from the K cells is stimulated after food ingestion; glucose, triglycerides, and amino acids are potent gastric inhibitory peptide secretagogues, as they activate the K cells from the luminal side. Furthermore, both sympathetic and parasympathetic nerves and neurotransmitters stimulate gastric inhibitory peptide secretion. The circulating half-life of gastric inhibitory peptide after its secretion into plasma is approximately 18 minutes.

Gastric inhibitory peptide activates specific, high-affinity G protein-coupled receptors that are of the seven transmembraneous domain type and coupled to adenylate cyclase. Gastric inhibitory peptide stimulates insulin secretion by an action dependent on the prevailing glucose concentration and exerted at dose levels circulating postprandially. It is therefore thought that gastric inhibitory peptide together with glucagon-like peptide 1 are the two main incretin hormones, which mediate the large insulin secretion seen postprandially. Gastric inhibitory peptide also inhibits gastric acid secretion, hence it has been suggested that gastric inhibitory peptide is a so-called enterogastrone factor, that is, a hormone that inhibits gastric function. However, whether gastric inhibitory peptide actually exerts the enterogastrone action under physiological conditions remains to be established.

No tumor oversecreting gastric inhibitory peptide has yet been described, but gastric inhibitory peptide may be of clinical interest as a pathogenetic factor in type 2 diabetes. The gastric inhibitory peptide response to oral glucose is inhibited in impaired glucose tolerance, which precedes type 2 diabetes, and, furthermore, the insulinotropic action of gastric inhibitory peptide is impaired in type 2 diabetes. In celiac disease, a low circulating level of gastric inhibitory peptide is usually seen.

Glucagon-like peptide 1 and other enteroglucagon hormones

In 1948 it was already demonstrated by Sutherland and deDuve that glucagon-like bioactivity existed in the gut, and in the early 1970s, so-called enteroglucagon cells were visualized in the distal small intestine in immunocytochemistry studies using antibodies directed against glucagon. We know today that the glucagon gene is expressed in the L cells located along the mucosa of the gut, with particular density in the distal small intestine and in the rectum. The same 180-amino acid preproglucagon is produced in these L cells as in the pancreatic A cells, but the post-translational processing of proglucagon is different in the two cells. In the L cells, at least five different peptide products of proglucagon are produced: glicentin (proglucagon$_{1-69}$), oxyntomodulin (proglucagon$_{33-69}$), intervening peptide 1 (IVP1, proglucagon$_{64-69}$), glucagon-like peptide 1 (proglucagon$_{78-107amide}$), and glucagon-like peptide 2 (proglucagon$_{126-159}$). The main and most important hormone secreted from these cells is glucagon-like peptide 1, which shows approximately 50% identity in its structure with glucagon. Glucagon-like peptide 1 is released following a meal intake and particularly by the action of carbohydrates and lipids. Furthermore, glucagon-like peptide 1 circulates as a hormone with a circulating half-life of 3 to 7 minutes and activates specific G protein-coupled seven transmembranous domain receptors coupled mainly to adenylate cyclase.

The most important function of glucagon-like peptide 1 is its glucose-dependent stimulation of insulin secretion. Glucagon-like peptide 1 also inhibits glucagon secretion and inhibits gastric acid secretion and gastric emptying. These latter effects are probably indirectly exerted by glucagon-like peptide 1 through the stimulation of somatostatin secretion. Available evidence suggests that both the insulinotropic action *and* the inhibitory action on gastric acid secretion and gastric emptying exerted by glucagon-like peptide 1 are physiological; hence, it is likely that glucagon-like peptide 1 is both an incretin and an enterogastrone factor.

During the 1990s, glucagon-like peptide 1 has gained considerable interest as a promising new therapeutic modality in the treatment of type 2 diabetes. This is because glucagon-like peptide 1 exerts a potent pattern of antidiabetogenic actions (stimulation of insulin secretion, inhibition of glucagon secretion, and reduction of gastric emptying), which is retained in subjects with diabetes. Several groups are now working with this possibility.

Although no true GLP-1oma has been documented, glucagon-like peptide 1 has been shown to be expressed in some neuroendocrine tumors of the pancreas and gut. However, elevated glucagon-like peptide 1 levels are rarely seen in these patients. Interestingly, subjects with tumors exhibiting glucagon-like peptide 1 immunoreactivity appear to exhibit a lower rate of distant metastases and a higher rate of curative resections than other abdominal endocrine tumors. Pathophysiologically, glucagon-like peptide 1 might also be involved in the dumping syndrome, in which high levels of glucagon-like peptide 1 are seen after food intake.

The other peptides processed from proglucagon in the intestinal L cells are also released postprandially. However, in comparison to the effects of glucagon-like peptide 1, very little is known about the physiological function of these other peptides. Oxyntomodulin has the capacity to inhibit gastric acid secretion and gastric emptying, and glucagon-like peptide 2 may be a trophic hormone stimulating regeneration and growth of the gut mucosa. Whether these actions are exerted physiologically is still unknown.

Peptide YY

Peptide YY (PYY) was first isolated in extracts of porcine duodenal mucosa, but later studies have shown that the peptide is mainly produced in the intestinal L cells; that is, in the same cells that produce glucagon-like peptide 1 and the other proglucagon-derived intestinal peptides. Peptide YY is therefore primarily produced in the distal portion of the small intestine and in the colon. Peptide YY is processed from a 98-amino acid prepro-peptide YY. The final form consists of a C-terminally amidated 36-amino acid sequence, although PYY_{3-36} is also produced, a 34-amino acid form. Peptide YY is released into the circulation following a meal intake in parallel to the increase in circulating glucagon-like peptide 1. Ingested fat and carbohydrates are particularly powerful stimulators of peptide YY secretion. In the circulation, the half-life of peptide YY is approximately 12 minutes.

Peptide YY shows a high structural similarity to neuropeptide Y and pancreatic polypeptide, and peptide YY and neuropeptide Y activate a number of different receptors with approximately the same affinity. At present, six different PYY/NPY receptors have been identified and cloned. These receptors have been identified in smooth muscle cells in the vascular bed, in the gastrointestinal tract, and in various parts of the brain. Several different effects are thought to be exerted by enteric peptide YY: induction of vasoconstriction, inhibition of pancreatic enzyme secretion, inhibition of gastric acid secretion, inhibition of gastric emptying, and inhibition of gut motility. Several of these actions seem to be indirectly mediated rather than exerted through action of the target cells.

For example, the inhibition of pancreatic enzyme secretion seems mediated by the inhibition of pancreatic blood flow, inhibition of cholecystokinin release, and inhibition of the activity of cholinergic nerves. Based on these actions and the release of peptide YY from the distal portion of the gut, it has been hypothesized that the main function of the peptide is to function as an enterogastrone and a pancreatone, that is, to inhibit stomach and pancreatic functions induced by the ingestion of food.

Motilin

Motilin is produced in endocrine cells (EC_2 cells) located in the upper portion of the small intestine, largely in the duodenum and proximal jejunum. Motilin is a peptide with 22 amino acids, and its circulating half-life is 5 minutes. Motilin seems to be cyclically released into the circulation irrespective of meal intake. The main effect of motilin is stimulation of smooth muscle contraction in the esophagus, stomach, duodenum, and proximal jejunum. Although not established, it is thought that the function of motilin is related to regulation of gastrointestinal motility during fasting, and in particular, it has been suggested that motilin initiates interdigestive motor activity. Motilin may therefore be the hormone responsible for clearance of the stomach and proximal small intestine from food content and bacteria in between meals. However, much remains to be studied on the regulation of synthesis and secretion of motilin, as well as on its physiological function. Circulating motilin is increased after partial intestinal resection, in acute diarrhea, and in ulcerative colitis. Erythromycin is a specific motilin receptor agonist, which may explain the adverse effect of diarrhea in the treatment with this antibiotic. Erythromycin has also been examined for its potential use in gastroparesis.

Neurotensin

Neurotensin is a non-amidated 13-amino acid peptide produced in the intestinal N cells, which are found along the mucosa primarily in the ileum, but also to some extent in the colon. Neurotensin is also expressed in a variety of neurons, both in the enteric nervous system and in the central nervous system. It is processed from a 170-amino acid preproneurotensin, which in its sequence also contains the peptide neuromedin N at its C-terminal end. Its receptor is a 424-amino acid peptide sequence that is coupled to the activation of guanylate cyclase, forming cyclic guanosin monophosphate in combination with the inhibition of cyclic adenosin monophosphate formation. Neurotensin is released into the circulation after a meal intake; fatty acids are particularly powerful neurotensin secretagogues. In addition, neurotensin secretion is stimulated by gastrin-releasing peptide, gastric inhibitory peptide, and cholecystokinin. The half-life of circulating neurotensin is under 6 minutes.

Neurotensin exerts a variety of effects, some of which are considered to be of physiological importance. These are the inhibition of gastric emptying and small intestinal motility, and the stimulation of colon contraction and defecation. Neurotensin may therefore be mediating the gastro-colic reflex, although this needs to be more firmly established. Neurotensin also stimulates pancreatic exocrine secretion and insulin secretion, though the physiological significance of these actions is not yet known.

Excessive expression of neurotensin is not unusual in gut endocrine tumors, and some tumors may consist mainly of neurotensin-producing cells. These patients have been shown to exhibit severe gastroesophageal reflux, which has been suggested to be due to increased intestinal contractions with enhanced enteric pressure.

Other regulatory peptides mainly produced by gastrointestinal endocrine cells

Somatostatin

Somatostatin is a ubiquitously distributed peptide expressed in endocrine cells and nerve terminals in a variety of organs. In the gastrointestinal tract, somatostatin is produced in the D cells, which occur along the mucosa in the stomach and small intestine. The D cells are usually equipped with long processes, making paracrine regulation by somatostatin on neighboring cells likely. Somatostatin is, however, also an enteric neuropeptide, and it occurs as such in nerve terminals primarily in the muscular layer of the small intestine. Somatostatin is processed from prosomatostatin, which consists of 92 amino acids, and it occurs as a cyclic 14-amino acid peptide (SS14) in the stomach D cells and as a 28-amino acid peptide (SS28) in enteric endocrine cells. Somatostatin is released into the circulation following a meal intake, and its circulating half-life is very short, only approximately 1 minute. Five different somatostatin receptors have so far been described (SSTR1 through 5). These are all G protein-coupled seven transmembranous domain receptors, and the different receptor types are expressed in different cells. The different types are also coupled to different signaling mechanisms. Somatostatin has in different target cells been shown to inhibit adenylate cyclase, phosphoinositide hydrolysis, calcium uptake, and protein phosphorylation.

Somatostatin exerts a variety of inhibitory influences on different gastrointestinal functions, most of which are probably mediated by paracrine or neurocrine actions. In the stomach, the somatostatin peptide inhibits gastrin secretion and gastric acid secretion, and it may be the final common path for a number of other hormones inhibiting acid secretion. For example, cholecystokinin stimulates somatostatin secretion, as does the neuropeptide calcitonin gene-related peptide (CGRP), implying that the inhibitory action of these peptides on gastric acid secretion could be mediated by somatostatin. Furthermore, somatostatin inhibits gastric emptying, and in the small intestine, somatostatin inhibits the release of other gut regulatory peptides (such as secretin, cholecystokinin, gastric inhibitory peptide, motilin, and glucagon-like peptide 1) and inhibits intestinal motility. Somatostatin may therefore be of great physiological importance in inhibit-

ing the stimulatory actions of other regulatory peptides after food intake. However, the exact physiological role of the peptide in relation to other regulatory peptides remains to be established.

Somatostatin is also expressed in the islet D cells and inhibits both insulin and glucagon secretion. A powerful inhibition of somatostatin is exerted on pancreatic exocrine secretion and gallbladder contraction as well.

Approximately 30 cases of somatostatinoma have been described in the literature, most of which are of pancreatic origin from the islet D cells. Most of the somatostatinomas are malignant. Interestingly, in spite of excessive circulating levels of this powerful inhibitory substance, few symptoms have been seen in these patients, the most common symptoms being dyspepsia, mild diabetes, cholelithiasis, diarrhea, hypochlorhydria, and goiter. Down-regulation of receptor activity is the likely reason for the lack of severe symptoms in these subjects.

Clinically, the main interest in somatostatin has evolved due to the development of powerful somatostatin analogues, such as octreotide, vapreotide, and lanreotide, which can be used in subjects with overproduction of regulatory peptides. The purpose of these analogues is to relieve symptoms associated with the overproduction of other peptides in the treatment of endocrine tumors, such as carcinoid tumors and acromegaly. Interestingly, somatostatin has also been shown to exert antiproliferative action, which may be explained by the inhibition of protein phosphorylation, which could add to the beneficial effect of somatostatin analogues in the treatment of endocrine tumors. Radiolabeled somatostatin analogues are also used for localization and treatment of endocrine tumors.

Pancreastatin

Pancreastatin is a 49-amino acid peptide that is processed from its precursor, chromogranin A. Chromogranin A and pancreastatin are processed in a number of different endocrine cells throughout the body, including G, D, and ECL cells in the stomach mucosa; the EC cells in the small intestine; in all types of islet endocrine cells; in the pituitary gland; and in the adrenals. Pancreastatin is released into the circulation after a meal intake and exerts a variety of effects, although no specific pancreastatin receptor has so far been described. The most important action of pancreastatin is the inhibition of pancreatic exocrine secretion, insulin secretion, and gastric acid secretion. Conversely, pancreastatin stimulates glucagon secretion and hepatic glucose production. However, the physiological importance of pancreastatin is yet to be established.

Pancreastatin and chromogranin A are excessively produced in carcinoid tumors and in other endocrine abdominal tumors, though the clinical significance of this in relation to symptomatology is not established. The presence of chromogranin A is often used histopathologically in the characterization of the tumors, and the determination of plasma levels of chromogranin A is often used both in the diagnostic work-up of the subjects and in the clinical follow-up of treated subjects.

Gastrointestinal neuropeptides

Vasoactive intestinal polypeptide and peptide histidine-isoleucin/histidine methionine

Under normal conditions vasoactive intestinal polypeptide (VIP) and peptide histidine-isoleucin (PHI)/peptide histidine methionine are expressed exclusively in nerves (and not in endocrine cells) and are processed from the same precursor. Vasoactive intestinal polypeptide is a 28-amino acid peptide with structural identity to the glucagon family, and PHI/peptide histidine methionine shows approximately 50% identity with the VIP sequence. They are expressed in nerves in various organs throughout the body (small and large intestines, pancreas, thyroid, lung, urogenital system, and central nervous system). Vasoactive intestinal polypeptide/peptide histidine-isoleucin-containing nerves are localized both in the submucosal and the myenteric layers of the entire gastrointestinal tract, with a particularly dense accumulation in the sphincteric regions. The VIP/PHI nerves seem to be intrinsic to the gut. The neuropeptides are released following cholinergic activation but are inhibited by adrenergic activation, opioids, and motilin. It has been hypothesized that VIP/PHI nerves are common pathways for various extrinsic regulators. Circulating levels of these neuropeptides are extremely low and unaffected by meal intake, consistent with their role as local neurotransmitters. The circulating half-life of exogenously administered vasoactive intestinal polypeptide is less than 1 minute. A high-affinity VIP receptor shown to be of the G protein-coupled seven transmembranous domain type with 459 amino acids and coupled to adenylate cyclase and phospholipase C has been identified. This receptor, which shows equal affinity for pituitary adenylate cyclase-activating polypeptide (PACAP), is expressed in smooth muscle cells in the gastrointestinal tract and in the vascular bed, as well as in exocrine and endocrine cells in the pancreas.

Vasoactive intestinal polypeptide and peptide histidine-isoleucin exert a variety of actions; however, the lack of specific VIP/PHI antagonists has complicated conclusions on the physiological significance of these actions. First, vasoactive intestinal polypeptide relaxes smooth muscle in the gastrointestinal tract, which relaxes the sphincters and prolongs intestinal transit time. Second, vasoactive intestinal polypeptide induces vasodilatation, which induces intestinal hyperemia in the gut. Third, vasoactive intestinal polypeptide stimulates intestinal and exocrine pancreatic secretion and insulin and glucagon secretion. The stimulation of intestinal secretion is a very prominent effect, which is obvious in subjects with VIP-producing tumors. It is an isotonic secretion caused by a direct cyclic AMP-dependent action on the enterocytes. It may be hypothesized that vasoactive intestinal polypeptide is of importance for digestion by activating intestinal and pancreatic responses following a meal intake. However, the exact functional role of the VIP/PHI nerves remains to be established.

VIP-producing tumors originate in 90% of cases from the pancreas. It is a rare tumor: the incidence is <1 per 10 million per year. In approximately half of the cases, peptide histidine methionine is also produced. Almost all of the subjects with VIPoma exhibit extremely severe secretory diarrhea (sometimes called pancreatogen or endocrine cholera) that is isotonic and caused by the stimulation of intestinal secretion by vasoactive intestinal polypeptide. They also experience hypokalemia due to the loss of bicarbonate and potassium in the stools. The secretory diarrhea in particular can be quite dramatic, with losses of >3 liters of isotonic watery stool daily possible. Approximately 50% of the subjects also exhibit hypotension, which is due to the vasodilatory action of the peptide, and hyperglycemia, due to stimulation of glucagon secretion. In addition, 75% of the subjects have hypochlorhydria, 20% observe flushing, and some subjects have hypercalcemia. These latter effects may be caused by vasoactive intestinal polypeptide and/or PHM, but they may also be due to a concurrent release of other bioactive peptides from the tumors. In more than 50% of the subjects, VIPomas have already metastasized at the time of diagnosis, mainly to the liver and lymph nodes. The treatment relies on a combination of surgery, embolization of the liver, and medical treatment with somatostatin analogues or a-interferon.

Galanin

Galanin is a 30-amino acid peptide exclusively localized to nerves. It is processed from a 124-amino acid precursor molecule, and it is expressed together with a 60-amino acid sequence called galanin message-associated peptide. It is ubiquitously distributed throughout the body and occurs in nerves, such as in the gastrointestinal and urogenital tracts, and the pancreas, lung, spinal cord, and central nervous system. In the gastrointestinal tract, galanin nerves occur in the submucosal and myenteric plexa along the entire tract, from the stomach to the colon, with a particularly dense accumulation in the small intestine. The galanin nerves are most likely intrinsic, although extrinsic galanin nerves may also occur since galanin is produced in the celiac ganglion. Some galanin nerves are exceptionally long, projecting a great distance along the intestinal tract. This has led to the hypothesis that galanin nerves coordinate different segments of the gut. Galanin is sometimes colocalized with vasoactive intestinal polypeptide, neuropeptide Y, substance P and/or calcitonin gene-related peptide in nerve terminals.

Galanin has profound influences on the contraction of smooth muscle cells of the gastrointestinal tract, making it likely that the neuropeptide is involved in the regulation of intestinal contractility. The influence of galanin is, however, different in different segments of the gastrointestinal tract. The net effect of galanin is the inhibition of gastric emptying and the slowing of colonic transit time.

Galanin also relaxes the lower esophageal sphincter and the internal anal sphincter tone and inhibits peristalsis. In addition, it inhibits pancreatic amylase secretion and insulin secretion. The physiological effect of galanin, however, remains to be established.

Substance P

Substance P is an 11-amino acid peptide that is a neurotransmitter expressed in nerves both in the central nervous system and in nerves in several peripheral organs. The gastrointestinal tract – all segments from the esophagus to the rectum – harbors substance P-containing nerves, which are mainly concentrated in the myenteric and submucosal plexa. It is thought that the substance P-containing nerves are intrinsic to the gastrointestinal tract, and that the activity of these nerves with release of substance P is regulated by the extrinsic nerves, mainly the parasympathetic nerves. The main action of substance P is to stimulate contraction in the smooth muscle cells of the gastrointestinal tract; both phasic and tonic contractions of the gut are initiated by substance P. At the same time, substance P initiates so-called intestino-intestinal reflexes, causing relaxation of distally located gut segments. Substance P is therefore thought to be of importance for the peristaltic movement of gut content. Substance P has also been shown to increase local blood flow in the gut.

Besides its localization to enteric nerves, substance P is also expressed in the intestinal EC cells, and it is often overexpressed in midgut carcinoids. In many subjects with this disease, circulating substance P is therefore increased, although it is still a matter of controversy whether substance P contributes to the clinical features of the carcinoid syndrome.

Gastrin releasing peptide

Gatrin releasing peptide is a 27-amino acid peptide that bears a resemblance to the amphibian peptide, bombesin. It is derived from a 145-amino acid precursor and is expressed in nerves in several locations, such as the central nervous system, the lung, the pancreas, and the gastrointestinal tract. In the gastrointestinal tract, the GRP nerves are localized from the fundus of the stomach to the distal colon. The nerves are distributed in the muscular submucosal as well as in the mucosal layers of the tract. There is a particularly rich innervation in close association with the gastrin cells in the stomach. Although its physiological function remains to be established, gastrin releasing peptide exerts a variety of actions in the gastrointestinal tract: it stimulates the secretion of gastrin, gastric inhibitory peptide, cholecystokinin, glucagon-like peptide 1, and vasoactive intestinal polypeptide, and it also stimulates the secretion of insulin and glucagon from the endocrine pancreas. Furthermore, gastrin-releasing peptide stimulates pepsin secretion and motor activity of several different segments of the stomach and gut and also promotes growth of the gut and pancreas. It is thereby thought that GRP nerves are of importance both for the short-term regulation of gastrointestinal functions after food intake as well as for the long-term regulation as a

trophic factor. At least two types of GRP receptors exist. One type is expressed mainly in the central nervous system and the pancreas, whereas another receptor type is expressed in the gastrointestinal tract. These receptors are both of the seven transmembraneous domain type linked with IP_3 formation with approximately 400 amino acids; they show 56% identity to each other.

Neuropeptide Y

Neuropeptide Y is a 36-amino acid peptide derived from a 97-amino acid precursor. It shows structural similarities to peptide YY and pancreatic polypeptide. Neuropeptide Y is expressed exclusively in nerves, most of which are adrenergic and therefore belong to the sympathetic nervous system. In fact, neuropeptide Y is one of the most ubiquitously distributed neuropeptides in the body. In the gastrointestinal tract, neuropeptide Y nerves occur in all its layers from the fundus to the rectum. In the submucosa, it has been shown that neuropeptide Y nerves are closely associated with the blood vessels, whereas in the mucosa, the fibers form a network. It has been shown that three different types of neuropeptide Y nerves exist in the gastrointestinal tract: one type is extrinsic and adrenergic, in which neuropeptide Y is co-localized with tyrosine hydroxylase and noradrenaline; another type is intrinsic, innervating smooth muscle cells; and a third type is intrinsic, innervating blood vessels.

At least six different NPY receptor subtypes have been described, all of which are of the G protein-coupled seven transmembranous domain type. They are expressed in various tissues; the receptor subtypes of interest in the actions of NPY on gastrointestinal function are the Y1 and Y2 receptors. Neuropeptide Y exerts a variety of effects on gastrointestinal functions. Neuropeptide Y induces vasoconstriction, both by itself and by potentiating the vasoconstriction induced by noradrenaline. Furthermore, neuropeptide Y has also been shown to inhibit gut motility, and, finally, it also affects mucosal function by stimulating ion absorption. Therefore, neuropeptide Y could be involved in the regulation of blood flow, motility, and absorption of the gastrointestinal tract.

Calcitonin gene-related peptide

Calcitonin gene-related peptide (CGRP) is a 37-amino acid peptide processed in nerves from the calcitonin gene. Calcitonin gene-related peptide nerves are distributed in all portions of the gastrointestinal tract. In the esophagus and the stomach, the calcitonin gene-related peptide nerves are extrinsic and sensory and occur mainly in the mucosa, submucosa, and the muscle layer. Calcitonin gene-related peptide inhibits gastric acid secretion and stimulates somatostatin secretion. In the intestine, the calcitonin gene-related peptide nerves seem to be intrinsic, occurring in the muscle layer from the duodenum to the colon. The intestinal calcitonin gene-related peptide nerves may therefore be of importance for gut contractility; and, interestingly, calcitonin gene-related peptide exerts a dual action on gut motility, as it induces both contraction and relaxation depending on the dose of peptide and potential interaction with other nerves. Hence, intestinal calcitonin gene-related peptide nerves may be involved in the regulation of gut peristalsis.

Pituitary adenylate cyclase-activating polypeptide

Pituitary adenylate cyclase-activating polypeptide (PACAP) was initially described as a hypothalamic peptide that stimulated adenylate cyclase in the pituitary, however the peptide was later demonstrated to be ubiquitously distributed in nerves throughout the body. PACAP consists of two forms, with 27 and 38 amino acids, respectively. It shows a structural similarity to vasoactive intestinal polypeptide, and, furthermore, cross-reacts with the VIP receptor (which is now termed the VIP-PACAP 2 receptor). A specific PACAP receptor has also been cloned (the PACI receptor). In the gastrointestinal tract, PACAP has been localized to nerves in all layers of the gut, from the stomach to the colon; a particularly dense PACAP expression occurs in submucous and myenteric ganglia. Although the physiological influence of PACAP has not been established, it exerts VIP-like actions, that is, it induces muscle relaxation and vasodilatation in addition to stimulating exocrine pancreatic, insulin, and glucagon secretion.

Table 65.2 Influence exerted by the gastrointestinal regulatory peptides

Process	Stimulatory action	Inhibitory action
Gastric acid secretion	Gastrin	GIP
		GLP-1
		CGRP
		Somatostatin
Gastric emptying		CCK
		GLP-1
		GIP
		VIP
Pancreatic enzyme secretion	CCK	PYY
	GRP	Somatostatin
Pancreatic bicarbonate/ water secretion	Secretion	Somatostatin
Gut peristalsis	Substance P	Somatostatin
	CGRP	
	VIP	
	NPY	
	Galanin	
	Motilin	
Glucose absorption		Somatostatin
Absorption of sodium, chloride	NPY	
Intestinal blood flow	CGRP	
	VIP	
Insulin secretion	GIP	Somatostatin
	GLP-1	Galanin

Processes regulated by regulatory peptides

Gastrointestinal regulatory peptides exert a variety of influences on gastric acid, pancreatic and intestinal secretion, gastrointestinal motility, blood flow, and insulin secretion (Tab. 65.2). Many processes are redundantly regulated by several peptides, which allows for finely tuned regulation. In most cases, however, the detailed physiology of the peptides remains to be established.

Role of gastrointestinal regulatory peptides in disease processes

The role of the various regulatory peptides in the gastrointestinal tract in disease states is far from established. Circulating levels of some of the peptides are altered in diseases, such as the reduction of secretin, cholecystokinin, and gastric inhibitory peptide in celiac disease, and the elevation of motilin in diarrhea and ulcerative colitis. Some of those changes in concentrations may be of pathophysiological importance, and some may be compensatory mechanisms to adjust to a disease state. Finally, tumors producing the gastrointestinal peptides are associated with grossly elevated levels, such as the gastrin produced in gastrinoma, vasoactive intestinal polypeptide in VIPoma, and somatostatin in somatostatinoma.

GUT HORMONE-PRODUCING TUMORS

Gut hormone-producing tumors occur in the gut and in the pancreas, hence they are grouped together as gastro-entero-pancreatic tumors. In general, gastro-entero-pancreatic hormone-producing tumors are rare, with an annual incidence of approximately 15 to 20 new cases per million people. The most common of these tumors are the carcinoids, which constitute 90 to 95% of all endocrine tumors of the gut and the pancreas. Less common are the tumors producing gastrin, vasoactive intestinal polypeptide, somatostatin, pancreatic polypeptide, glucagon, and insulin. In addition, there are nonfunctioning endocrine tumors that do not seem to produce any specific hormone, but their tumor cells show characteristic endocrine patterns. The classification of the gastro-entero-pancreatic tumors is sometimes difficult, since they may consist of more than one cell type producing more than one hormone. In most cases, however, a single hormone is responsible for the clinical picture, justifying a clinical diagnostic name based on this hormone.

Carcinoid tumors most commonly occur in the gut, primarily in the jejunum and ileum, whereas the other tumors commonly occur in the pancreas. Approximately 25% of the gastro-entero-pancreatic tumors, most often the gastrin-producing tumors and non-functioning tumors, occur in association with the MEN-1 syndrome. MEN-1 is an autosomal dominant syndrome that, in addition to the gastro-entero-pancreatic tumors, most commonly involve parathyroid adenoma and less commonly pituitary tumors. Its genetic basis is a deletion in the q13 region of chromosome 11.

Most cases of gastro-entero-pancreatic tumors are malignant. Malignancy is more common in the sporadic cases (approximately 75%) than among those associated with the MEN-1 syndrome (approximately 50%). The common sites for metastases are the regional lymph nodes and the liver. Less common metastatic sites are the lung, the brains, and the adrenals.

The gastro-entero-pancreatic tumors are usually small with a slow growth rate. Since endocrine symptoms before metastases occur are usually rare, it is common that patients have had their disease for many years before diagnosis. Furthermore, due to the slow growth rate of the tumors, the prognosis is usually better than in other types of malignancies. The improved prognosis is true even for cases where malignant tissue is retained after surgery, provided that treatment is directed both toward reduction of the tumor growth as well as to inhibition of the secretion of hormones from the tumors.

The gastro-entero-pancreatic tumors show characteristic symptoms due to the production of their hormones, and these differences form the basis for the clinical division of the tumors. The most common tumors are the *carcinoid* tumors (approximately 15 cases per million per year), which are distinguished in the foregut, midgut, and hindgut carcinoid tumors, depending on the anatomical origin. Most common are midgut carcinoids, occurring in the small intestine and ascending colon (approximately 90% of all carcinoid tumors). In this location, it originates in the EC cells, usually producing substance P and 5-hydroxytryptamine. The tumors are slowly growing. A common presenting symptom is obstruction of the small intestines. Carcinoid tumors are therefore commonly diagnosed during an emergency operation of a small intestine obstruction. After producing metastases in the liver, the carcinoid syndrome occurs, since then substance P and 5-hydroxytryptamine reach the general circulation, although the molecular basis of the carcinoid syndrome is still under debate. The carcinoid syndrome consists of intense flushing and diarrhea; and in long-standing cases, fibrosis of the heart valves occurs, with the development of tricuspid insufficiency as the dominating symptom. The carcinoids are diagnosed by measuring 5-hydroxyindole-acetic acid (the metabolite of 5-hydroxytryptamine) in the urine.

The incidence of *gastrinoma* (Zollinger-Ellison syndrome) is approximately 1 to 2 per million per year. Approximately 60% are malignant, and in 30% of the cases, metastases are already seen at the time of diagnosis. Thirty percent of gastrinoma are part of the MEN-1 syndrome. Approximately 80% of all gastrinomas occur within the pancreas, and most of the remaining gastrinomas are seen in the duodenum. Dominating symptoms of gastrinoma are ulceration (severe, multiple, unusual location), secretory diarrhea, and in advanced cases, weight loss. The diagnosis is based on symptoms in combination with elevated circulating levels of gastrin. In suspected cases with normal circulating gastrin, an exaggerated gastrin response to intravenous secretin is usually found.

The *somatostatinomas, VIPomas, PPomas,* and *glucagonomas* are very rare gastro-entero-pancreatic tumors (annual incidence of approximately 1 case per million). *Somatostatinomas* occur in 50% of cases in the pancreas and in 50% in the gut, and more than 90% of the reported cases have been malignant. Usually somatostatinomas present with local symptoms (intestinal obstruction, obstructive jaundice, or gastrointestinal hemorrhage). Common hormone-related symptoms include dyspepsia, steatorrhea, diarrhea, gallstones, goiter, and mild diabetes. *VIPomas* are most commonly seen in the pancreas, and only 10% of all VIPomas described have been localized to the gut. Approximately 50% of VIPomas are malignant and have already given rise to metastases at the time of diagnosis. VIPomas usually present with severe watery diarrhea, sometimes profuse, exceeding 3 liters of fluid per day. This results in dehydration, hypotonia, weakness, and hypokalemia. Hyperglycemia is also a common symptom. *PPomas* are a type of "nonfunctioning" gastro-entero-pancreatic tumor that produce pancreatic polypeptide. They are found in the pancreas. The yearly incidence is approximately 1 to 2 per million. Besides tumor-associated symptoms, no or only few endocrine symptoms exist. Most cases of PPomas are highly malignant. Finally, *glucagonomas* are uncommon, with a reported annual incidence of only 1 per 10 million. They occur primarily in the pancreas, although extrapancreatic glucagonomas have been described. Approximately 80% of the glucagonomas are malignant, and more than 50% of the cases already have metastases at the time of diagnosis. The most common initial symptom is a characteristic rash, the necrolytic migratory erythema. Other common symptoms are mild diabetes, weight loss, and mental symptoms. A high circulating level of glucagon is the main laboratory finding.

Insulinoma occurs in approximately 1 to 2 cases per million per year. Only 10% are malignant. It usually presents with hypoglycemic episodes, the characteristic symptoms being headache, drowsiness, confusion, and in severe cases, coma. Other symptoms include hunger, tachycardia, tremor, and profuse sweating. The insulinoma usually consists of a single, slowly growing tumor. The diagnosis is documented by measuring fasting hypoglycemia in combination with elevated levels of insulin and C-peptide. A prolonged (up to 72-hour) fast could be performed in hospitalized patients to aid the diagnostic work.

Clinical findings

The gastro-entero-pancreatic tumors are usually discovered either incidentally during operations for intestinal obstruction or by presenting with typical endocrine symptoms in combination with determined elevated levels of the hormone in question. Following this diagnosis, a preoperative localization procedure is required, which is usually performed by ultrasonography and CT scan. If in doubt, angiography or venous catheterization with a determination of local levels of the hormone in question may be performed, although in most cases an intraoperative ultrasonography is the best localization procedure. A newly developed procedure is scintigraphy with the use of ^{111}In-labeled octreotide, which binds to somatostatin receptors in the tumors. A final characterization of the tumors is the microscopical characterization of the tumor tissue with specific staining techniques.

Treatment

The basis for the treatment of gastro-entero-pancreatic tumors is the surgical removal of the primary tumor and removal of as much tumor mass as possible. The debulking procedure not only improves symptoms, but it also improves the prognosis. When tumors are left after surgery, radiological embolization of the metastases provides palliation. The rationale behind embolization is that the hepatic metastases are supplied only by the arteries, whereas the normal liver parenchyma is supplied by the portal vein as well. Therefore, embolization of the arterial tree results in tumor devascularization, whereas the circulation of the normal liver tissue remains. Finally, cases with remaining metastases can be treated with somatostatin analogues, mainly octreotide, which both inhibit hormone production, thereby improving the symptoms of the patients and inhibiting the tumor growth rate. Other medical treatments have also been tried, such as α-interferon with a combination of 5-fluoro-uracil and streptozotocin. During recent years, treatment with radiolabeled somatostatin analogues is being developed.

Prognosis

Gastro-entero-pancreatic tumors have a better prognosis than other types of malignancies, such as pancreatic adenocarcinoma, but the mortality rate is nevertheless high. For example, in the most common of the gastro-entero-pancreatic tumors, the carcinoids, a five-year survival rate of approximately 20% is a common figure. In other types of gastro-entero-pancreatic tumors, such as PPomas and glucagonomas, the prognosis is even worse.

Suggested readings

AHRÉN B, KARLSSON S. Pancreatic endocrine physiology. In: Clark OH, Duah QY (eds). Textbook of endocrine surgery. Philadelphia: WB Saunders, 1997;562-75.

AHRÉN B. Regulatory peptides of the gastrointestinal tract. In: Jensen SL, Gregersen H, Moody F, Shokouh-Amiri MH, eds. Essential of experimental surgery: gastroenterology and endocrinology. London, Paris, New York, Melbourne: Harwood Academic, 1996;1-24.

BLOOM S, HAMMOND P. Endocrinology of the gastrointestinal tract. In: Besser GM, Thorner MO (eds). Clinical endocrinology. London: Wolfe, 1994;19:1-6.

BLOOM SR, POLAK JM. The endocrine gastrointestinal tract: physiology. In: Becker KL (ed). Principles and practice of endocrinology and metabolism. Philadelphia: Lippincott, 1985;1499-512.

BRAND SJ, SCHMIDT WE. Gastrointestinal hormones. In: Yamada T (ed). Textbook of gastroenterology. 2nd ed. Philadelphia: Lippincott, 1995;25-71.

FURNESS JB, COSTA M. The enteric nervous system. London: Churchill-Livingstone, 1987.

HOLST JJ, FAHRENKRUG J, STADIL F, REHFELD JF. Gastrointestinal endocrinology. Scand J Gastroenterol 1996; (Suppl) 216:27-38.

HOLST JJ, SCHMIDT P. Gut hormones and intestinal function. Ballières Clin Endocrinol Metab 1994;8:137-64.

LLOYD KC. Gut hormones in gastric function. Ballières Clin Endocrinol Metab 1994;8:111-36.

WYNICK D, BLOOM SR. Diagnosis and medical management of gastroenteropancreatic tumors. In: Lynn J, Bloom SR (eds). Surgical endocrinology. Oxford: Butterworth Heinemann, 1993;487-93.

Prostaglandins and other eicosanoids

Bianca Rocca, Carlo Patrono

Arachidonic acid metabolic pathways and their regulation

Eicosanoids are biologically active metabolites that are derived from arachidonic acid. Arachidonic acid is released from membrane phospholipids in response to a variety of cellular activation processes through the action of phospholipases. Arachidonic acid can then be converted to prostaglandin (PG)H_2 by PGH-synthase-1 or -2 (also referred to as cyclo-oxygenase or COX-1 and -2), which catalyzes a two-step reaction: first it cyclizes arachidonic acid to form PGG_2, and second, it reduces the 15-hydroperoxy group to form PGH_2. Cell-specific isomerases or reductases catalyze the conversion of PGH_2 to biologically active end-products, which include PGE_2, $PGF_{2\alpha}$, PGD_2, PGI_2, and thromboxane (TX) A_2; these are known collectively as prostanoids (Fig. 66.1). In addition, arachidonic acid can be metabolized by different lipoxygenases and converted to leukotrienes, 12-hydroxyeicosatetraenoic acid, or 15-hydroxyeicosatetraenoic acid (Fig. 66.1). Eicosanoids are produced "on demand" in the cell of origin, act locally, and their biological half-lives are very short. In contrast to classical circulating hormones, prostanoids act primarily as autacoids on the parent and/or neighboring cells. A novel class of prostaglandin-like compounds (isoprostanes), which are produced in vivo in humans by a noncyclo-oxygenase mechanism, may be of considerable importance as in vivo markers of lipid peroxidation and as mediators of oxidant injury in various clinical disorders.

For many years the rate-limiting step in the production of prostaglandins was thought to be the activation of phospholipases to release membrane-bound arachidonic acid (Fig. 66.1). The discovery of COX-2 and the different regulatory mechanisms for the two COX isoforms indicates that an additional rate-limiting step in prostaglandin biosynthesis is the inducible conversion of arachidonic acid to PGH_2 by COX-2 (Fig. 66.1).

One of the most significant recent developments in this field is the identification of an inducible form of COX, designated as COX-2, the constitutive isozyme being COX-1. These isozymes catalyze the same reactions, but they are encoded by two different genes located in different chromosomes and serve different functions even within the same cell type. COX-1 is thought to serve a number of physiologic "housekeeping" functions, such as generation of TXA_2 by platelets, production of cytoprotective prostanoids in the gastric mucosa, and nephron-comparti-

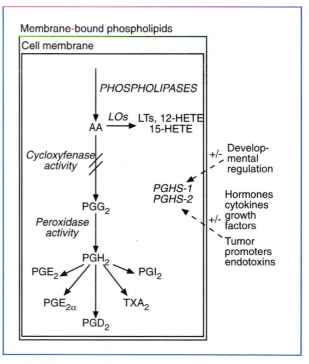

Figure 66.1 Metabolic transformations of arachidonic acid. (AA = arachidonic acid; PG = prostaglandin; TX = thromboxane; LO = lypoxygenase; HETE = hydroxyeicosatetraenoic acid; PGHS = PGH-synthase; LT = leukotriene; + = activation; − = inhibition.)

mentalized synthesis of prostanoids. It has been shown to be developmentally regulated in many tissues; its concentration remains relatively stable, but small changes in expression can occur after stimulation with hormones or growth factors. In contrast, COX-2 is virtually undetectable under physiological conditions, but its expression is induced in macrophages, fibroblasts, and vascular endothelial and smooth muscle cells by various cytokines, endotoxins, growth factors, or tumor promoters; this indicates that COX-2 plays a role in inflammation and cell proliferation. Constitutive expression of COX-2 has been found in certain regions of the brain, reproductive tissues and kidney. Glucocorticoids downregulate COX-2 gene expression in different cellular systems and in response to a variety of inducers. Experiments in adrenalectomized animals suggest that endogenous glucocorticoids modulate COX-2-dependent prostaglandin biosynthesis.

Prostanoids in physiology and pathology, and pharmacological regulation

Prostanoids exert a wide spectrum of actions on ubiquitous targets via specific cell surface, G protein-linked receptors. Prostaglandin receptors are classified into five basic types on the basis of their sensitivity to five primary prostanoids: that is, PGE_2, PGI_2, TXA_2, PGD_2 and $PGF_{2\alpha}$, and termed EP, IP, TP, DP and FP, respectively. Furthermore, EP is subdivided into four subtypes – EP1, EP2, EP3, EP4 – on the basis of their responses to various agonists and antagonists. PGD_2 and its derivative PGJ_2 have been shown to bind and activate a different class of nuclear receptors. These are peroxisome proliferator-activated receptors, which are members of the nuclear receptor superfamily of ligand-activated transcription factors that include the steroid, retinoid, and thyroid hormone receptors. In particular, PGJ_2 and its derivatives activate peroxisome proliferator-activated receptors α and γ. Peroxisome proliferator-activated receptor α, which is primarily expressed in the liver, is implicated in lipid homeostasis, while peroxisome proliferator-activated receptor α is a major initiator of adipocyte differentiation.

Prostanoids mediate a wide variety of cellular interactions in physiological and pathological processes, such as hemostasis/thrombosis, glomerular filtration and water balance, ovulation, embryo implantation and development, the initiation of labor/abortion, inflammation, and the activation and/or suppression of immunological responses. 12-Hydroxyeicosatetrenoic acid has been proposed to modulate angiotensin-induced aldosterone secretion in the adrenal gland and glucose-induced insulin secretion in the pancreas. Bartter's syndrome, characterized by hypokalemia and hypochloremic metabolic alkalosis, is associated with and dependent upon enhanced renal prostaglandin synthesis for full expression of its metabolic abnormalities, though this increased prostaglandin biosynthesis is not the primary genetic defect. COX inhibitors, such as ibuprofen or indomethacin, partially correct the metabolic abnormali-

ties promoting sodium and chloride retention. The same eicosanoid may therefore serve physiologic and pathologic functions, depending upon the rate of its biosynthesis in vivo, as affected by pathophysiologic stimuli acting on substrate availability and/or COX modulation. For example, TXA_2 promotes physiologic hemostasis and participates in atherothrombosis, and renal prostaglandins modulate medullary and cortical function under physiologic circumstances and contribute to electrolyte abnormalities in Bartter's syndrome.

Aspirin and nonsteroidal anti-inflammatory drugs (NSAIDs) inhibit COX activity and consequently prevent the formation of prostanoids. COX-inhibitors may have "desired" and "undesired" effects depending upon the role played by a given eicosanoid in the individual clinical setting. Examples of this are aspirin preventing thrombosis versus causing gastrointestinal or cerebral bleeding, and indomethacin correcting the abnormalities of Bartter's syndrome versus deteriorating renal function and/or raising blood pressure in elderly people. Individual NSAIDs show variable potencies against COX-1 compared to COX-2, although none of the commercially available inhibitors show greater than 20-fold preference for COX-2. This may explain, at least in part, the variable incidence of side effects of different NSAIDs, as well as the variation in therapeutic effects seen with different compounds or even using different doses of the same drug. One would predict that drugs with high selectivity (i.e., ≥ 100-fold) for COX-2 would have antiinflammatory activity with fewer gastrointestinal and bleeding complications than conventional NSAIDs. Highly selective COX-2 inhibitors (e.g., celecoxib, rofecoxib) have been developed and results of phase-3 studies are consistent with these theoretical expectations.

PROSTAGLANDINS IN OVARIAN AND UTERINE PROCESSES

Prostaglandins, primarily of the E and F series, appear to be important for ovulation, luteolysis, embryo implantation, labor, delivery, and postpartum in different animal species, including humans.

Ovulation

Prostaglandins appear to be involved in the process of follicular rupture, as suggested by the observation that NSAIDs inhibit ovulation if the drug is administered during the first 80% of the ovulatory process. Prostaglandins of the E and F types increase in ovarian follicles during the first several hours of the ovulatory process, they reach a peak at about the time the follicle begins to rupture, and shortly thereafter their ovarian levels decline toward preovulatory values. Interleukin 1β (IL-1β) and tumor necrosis factor α play a central role in the mature follicle. They may induce an acute rise in prostaglandins immediately prior to ovulation, which would contribute to the rupture of the follicle (Fig. 66.2). Based on this inflammatory-like model of ovulation, one would anticipate that COX-2 may play an important role in this phenomenon.

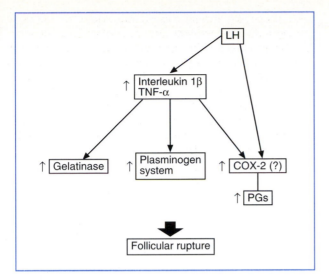

Figure 66.2 Potential pathways utilized by luteinizing hormone in ovarian follicular rupture. (LH = luteinizing hormone; TNF = tumor necrosis factor; COX = cyclooxygenase; PG = prostaglandin; ↑ = induction/increased production.)

In support of this hypothesis, COX-2-deficient mice were infertile and showed major ovarian abnormalities. In addition, in vitro studies showed that luteinizing hormone directly up-regulates COX-2 expression in mouse ovarian granulosa cells.

Embryo implantation, labor, and delivery

Prostaglandins act as important mediators of localized vascular permeability at the time of embryo implantation.

The use of NSAIDs and the measurement of uterine prostaglandins during early pregnancy in rodents provide futher evidence that PG are involved in implantation and decidualization. Moreover, the localization of PG synthesis in uterine cells changed markedly during the implantation process. Recently it has been shown that COX-1 and -2 in the mouse uters are differentially regulated in the peri-implantation period: COX-1 is expressed in the uterine epithelium and is influenced by ovarian steroids, while COX-2 is upregulated exclusively in the uterine tissues (epithelium and stroma) surrounding the implanting blastocyst. Furthermore, COX-2 deficient mice show major defects in implantation.

The different lines of evidence supporting an important role of prostaglandins in the initiation and maintenance of labor in humans include: (1) prostaglandins stimulate uterine contractility in vitro; (2) prostaglandin levels in maternal urine and amniotic fluid increase with labor progression; (3) blocking prostaglandin synthesis delays labor onset, reduces uterine contractions, and prolongs the duration of labor; and (4) the administration of PGE_2 and $PGF_{2\alpha}$ during the period of midpregnancy to term induces labor. The mechanism(s) responsible for changes in prostaglandin production and their regulation in late gestation remain to be clarified, though it is known that COX-2 is expressed at high levels in

human fetal tissues, while COX-1 is mainly expressed in the maternal decidua.

However the mechanism(s) responsible for changes in prostaglandin production and their regulation remains to be clarified. Induction of labor was lacking in Fp-deficient mice and they did not show the typical decline of progesterone concentration in maternal plasma, which usually precedes parturition in mammals. In addition, these animals failed to express oxytocin receptors in the uterus at term. These findings suggest a role for $PGF_{2\alpha}$ and its receptor upstream of oxytocin release. $PGF_{2\alpha}$ is involved in the process of luteolysis through apoptosis of luteal cells. This event appears to precede the expression of oxytocin receptors and the increase in myometrial contractility. Possible mechanisms of action of $PGF_{2\alpha}$ in inducing labor are depicted in Figure 66.3.

PROSTAGLANDINS IN CELL PROLIFERATION AND CANCER

Cell proliferation

Prostaglandins, PGE_2 and $PGF_{2\alpha}$ in particular, can act as in vivo growth-modulating factors in regenerating tissues such as the liver; they can also act as co-mitogenic growth factors, making hepatocytes more responsive to concomitant or subsequent exposure to complete growth factors. Under certain circumstances, prostaglandins can act alone as mitogens. Furthermore, $PGE_{2\alpha}$ evokes extracellular Ca^{++} influx and induces c-myc, c-fos, and Egr-1 mRNAs, which are growth-associated early genes, suggesting that PGE_2 plays an important role in growth regu-

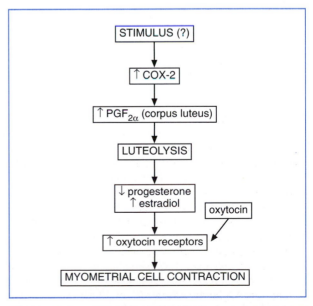

Figure 66.3 Potential mechanism(s) of prostaglandin (PG)$F_{2\alpha}$ in inducing labor. (COX = cyclooxygenase; ↑ = upregulation/increased production; ↓ = decreased production.)

lation. Moreover, growth-promoting and -inhibiting activities of TXA2 and PGE_2, respectively, have been described in vascular smooth muscle cells and glomerular mesangial cells.

Carcinogenesis

In vitro, ex vivo, and in vivo studies indicate a possible involvement of PGH-synthases and/or prostaglandins in carcinogenesis. Different lines of evidence suggest a protective effect of aspirin and other NSAIDs against colorectal cancer. Several studies have shown that different NSAIDs prevent or inhibit chemically-induced adenomas and carcinomas of the rodent colon by reducing the incidence, the number and size of tumors. At least in this animal model, NSAIDs seem to affect tumor promotion, and the mechanism of tumor inhibition involves suppression of prostaglandin biosynthesis. Several case reports and small randomized clinical trials of the NSAID sulindac in patients with familial adenomatous polyposis showed a regression of adenomas associated with this treatment. Retrospective – and all but one of the prospective observational – studies in the general population provide evidence that aspirin and possibly other NSAIDs have a protective effect against the development of colorectal cancer, lowering the relative risk by about 40 to 50%. Furthermore, some of these studies found a time-dependent relationship with a lower risk of disease in subjects with more prolonged or more frequent use of NSAIDs. Although the above mentioned studies differ in the design, study population, outcome (adenomatous polyps, cancer incidence, cancer mortality), evaluation of NSAIDs exposure (dose and length), evaluation of the outcome diagnosis, nevertheless the results appear consistent. Carefully designed, randomized clinical trials are needed to directly test the protective effect of NSAIDs against colorectal cancer and to answer the many unsolved questions such as the risk/benefit profile of a prolonged treatment, which patient population may derive the largest absolute benefit from this preventive treatment, the potential advantage of using selective COX-2 inhibitors, the dose- and time-requirement for this protective effect to become apparent, and the stage in carcinogenesis mainly affected by the NSAIDs. It is presently unclear whether the inhibition of COX-1 or -2 activities or other mechanism(s) independent of prostaglandin formation and/or COX are responsible for the protective effect of NSAIDs in carcinogenesis. The cyclo-oxygenase-independent mechanisms include: (1) the peroxidase activity of COX, which has a broad specificity and may activate substrates other than PGG_2 (such as chemical carcinogens); (2) malondialdehyde, which is known to be involved in tumor initiation, is generated by enzymatic as well as a nonenzymatic breakdown of PGH_2; and (3) certain NSAIDs induce apoptosis and arrest tumor growth independently of the inhibition of COX activity. Several experimental data suggests that COX-2 may play an important role in the early stages of colorectal tumorigenesis (Tab. 66.1). The possible sites of COX, prostaglandin, and NSAID action in the multistage colo-carcinogenic process are depicted in Figure 66.4.

Finally, the production of PGE_2 and other prostaglandins is often increased in colorectal and lung cancer tissues. PGE_2 has been demonstrated to inhibit the ability of human natural killer cells to bind to tumor cells, resulting in impaired tumor cell death (Fig. 66.4). A reduced host immunity may contribute to tumor growth and its metastatic potential.

PROSTANOIDS IN HEMOSTASIS AND THROMBOSIS

Prostanoids play a fundamental role in modulating the local interactions between platelets and endothelial cells in physiological and pathological kemostasis.

Platelet agonists – such as collagen, thrombin, epinephrine, and serotonin – induce phospholipase A2-mediated hydrolysis of arachidonic acid and synthesis of TXA_2 via COX-1 and TX synthase. TXA_2 binds to specific platelet receptors to further amplify the platelet aggrega-

Table 66.1 COX-2 and colorectal cancer

Experimental design / setting	Results
Expression of COX-2 in human colorectal adenocarcinomas and adjacent colonic mucosa but not in normal tissues	Upregulation of COX-2 in 85-90% of adenocarcinomas
Expression of COX-2 in rodent colonic tumors developed after carcinogen treatment	Upregulation of COX-2 mRNA
Analysis of adenoma tissues taken from Min mice (murine model of familial polyposis)	Upregulation of COX-2 mRNA
Carcinogen-treated rats given selective COX-2 inhibitors	40-49% reduction in aberrant crypt formation
COX-2 expression in carcinomas by in situ hybridization	COX-2 expression in carcinoma epithelial cells, but not in the normal colonic epithelium
Phenotypic analysis of non-transformed epithelial cells over-expressing COX-2	Cell phenotype: resistance to apoptosis, increased adherence to extracellular matrix components
APCΔ^{716} mice (rodent analog for human familial adenomatous polyposis) bred with COX-2 null mice	Gene dosage-dependent reduction in tumor multiplicity
Growth of human colon cancer cell lines constitutively expressing COX-2 transplanted in nude mice, plus or minus selective COX-2 inhibitor treatment	In the presence of COX-2 inhibitor, implanted tumor cells showed 85-90% reduction of tumor growth

tion process, and it promotes vasoconstriction by interacting with vascular smooth muscle cell receptors. These phenomena may lead to the formation of an occlusive thrombus at the site of vascular injury. In contrast, PGI_2 and nitric oxide produced by the endothelial cells exert opposing actions, promoting vasorelaxation and inhibition of platelet aggregation. Moreover, COX-2 expression in vascular endothelial cells is upregulated by laminar shear stress but not by turbulent shear stress, hence it has been suggested that COX-2 may function as an "athero-protective" gene.

Aspirin is still considered the "golden standard" of antithrombotic therapy for the secondary prevention of occlusive vascular diseases. Saturation of the antithrombotic effect at low doses (50-75 mg daily) suggests that the effect is largely due to platelet cyclo-oxygenase inactivation.

Prostanoids and diabetes

Both micro- and macroangiopathies characterize the natural history of diabetes mellitus. Increased biosynthesis of TXA_2 in vivo has been reported in patients with type II diabetes mellitus who had macrovascular complications, reflecting in vivo platelet activation. Metabolic control may influence the determinants of platelet activation. In addition, in peripheral arterial disease, diabetes mellitus is independently associated with persistent platelet activation in vivo, while no activation has been found in patients with similar vascular involvement without any major cardiovascular risk factors. These studies indicate that diabetes per se can influence in vivo platelet function.

The potential protective effect of prolonged antiplatelet therapy on cardiovascular endpoints in diabetics with clinically evident vascular disorders (secondary prevention) is available from the second meta-analysis of the Antiplatelet Trialists' Collaboration, which examined the protective effect of a prolonged antiplatelet regimen in diabetic and non-diabetic patiens enrolled in 29 randomized clinical trials. Treatment produced similar propor-

tional risk reductions in diabetics and nondiabetics. Because diabetics were at a higher than average risk of vascular events, the overview suggests that the absolute benefit of antiplatelet therapy may have been greater than average among them. Recently, enhanced formation of the F_2-isoprostane 8-epi-$PGF_{2\alpha}$ has been reported in patients affected by both type I and type II diabetes mellitus. Moreover, high glucose concentrations enhance 8-epi-$PGF_{2\alpha}$ release from vascular smooth muscle cells. One could speculate that the biological effects of isoprostanes and other iso-eicosanoids may provide a biochemical link between lipid peroxidation and specialized forms of cellular activation, such as platelet activation and smooth muscle cell proliferation (Fig. 66.5).

PROSTANOIDS AS IMMUNOMODULATORS

Eicosanoids can modulate various steps of the mature T-cell-mediated immune response, as well as T-cell development within the thymus. PGE_2 modulates the cytokine secretion of two human CD4+ T-lymphocyte subsets inflammatory CD4– T cells (Th1), which secrete interferon-γ and interleukin-2, and helper CD4+ T cells (Th2) which secrete interleukin-4, -5 and -6 PGE_2, which is synthesized by antigen presenting cells at the site of immune response, inhibits Th1-associated cytokines, whereas the production of Th2-associated cytokines is enhanced. Interleukin-4 in particular induces selective isotype switching to IgE and IgA of B-lymphocytes. In addition, PGE_2 directly increases IgE secretion by directly enhancing isotype switching to the heavy chain locus. These effects are mediated by the EP2 and EP4 receptor subtypes that are co-expressed in nature B-lymphocytes. These immunoregulatory effects of PGE_2 can be of particular interest because increased PGE_2 production has

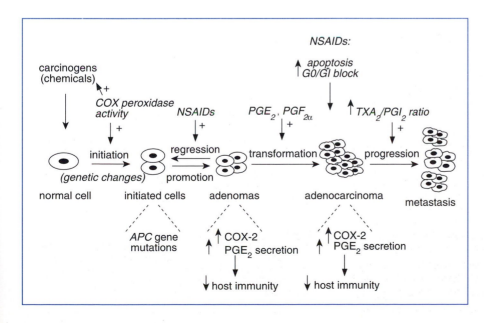

Figure 66.4 Possible interventions of prostaglandins, cyclooxygenases, and nonsteroidal anti-inflammatory drugs in the multistage carcinogenic process. (NSAIDs = nonsteroidal anti-inflammatory drugs; + = activation; ↑ = induction/increased production; ↓ = inhibition; PG = prostaglandin; TX = thromboxane; COX = cyclooxygenase.)

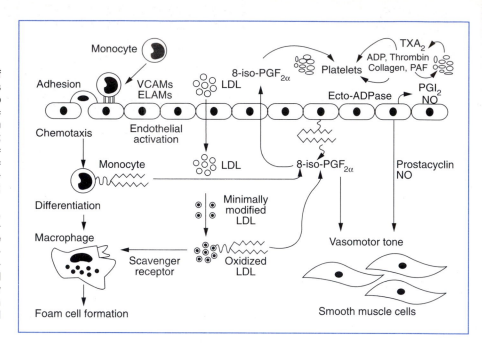

Figure 66.5 Potential sites of formation and cellular targets of 8-iso-PGF$_{2\alpha}$ of relevance to atherothrombosis. (ELAM = endothelial leukocyte adhesion molecule; NO = nitric oxide; PGI$_2$ = prostacyclin; PAF = platelet-activating factor; TX = thromboxane; VCAM = vascular cell adhesion molecule; LDL = low density lipoprotein.) (From Chakraborty I, Das SK, Wang J, Dey SK. Developmental expression of the cyclooxygenase 1 and cyclooxygenase 2 genes in the peri-implantation mouse uterus and their differential regulation by the blastocyst and ovarian steroids. J. Mol Endocrinol 1996;16:107.)

been reported in immunological disorders characterized by elevated Th2 and/or IGE responses such as AIDS, allergy hyper-IgE syndrome and autologous bone-marrow transplantation.

Several observations implicated PGs in the development of the T-cell lineage: thymic expression of various PG biosynthetic enzymes and receptors has been detected in human and rode in thymus. Thymus and non-lumphoid thymic stromal cell lines have been shown to secrete PGs *in vitro*. We have recently investigated the role of COX-1

and -2 as well as PGs in murine T-lymphocyte development. The two isozymes appear to be differentially expressed in embryonic and adult thymus. In addition, COX-1, PGE$_2$ and the EP2 receptor subtype appear to regulate the formation of the CD4+CD8+ thymocytes, while COX-2, PGE$_2$ and EP3 receptor seem to be involved in proliferation of early thymic lymphoid progenitors and the positive selection of CD4– T-cells. Whether similar mechanism(s) are relevant to human T-cell development remains to be established.

Suggested readings

CHAKRABORTY I, DAS SK, WANG J, DEY SK. Developmental expression of the cyclooxygenase 1 and cyclooxygenase 2 genes in the peri-implantation mouse uterus and their differential regulation by the blastocyst and ovarian steroids. J Mol Endocrinol 1996;16:107.

DAVI G, GRESELE P, VIOLI F, et al. Diabetes mellitus, hypercholesterolemia and hypertension but not vascular disease per se are associated with persistent platelet activation in vivo. Circulation 1997;96:69.

DINCHUK J, CAR BD, FOCHT RJ, et al. Renal abnormalities and an altered inflammatory response in mice lacking cyclooxygenase II. Nature 1995;378:406.

FEDYK ER, PHIPPS RP. Prostaglandin E$_2$ receptors of the EP2 and EP4 subtypes regulate activation and differentiation of mouse B lymphocytes to IgE-secreting cells. Proc Natl Acad Sci USA 1996;93:10978.

GIBB W, SUN M. Localization of prostaglandin H synthase type 2 protein and mRNA in term human fetal membranes and decidua. J Endocrinol 1996;150:497.

HILKENS CMU, VERMEULEN H, VAN NEERVEN RJJ, et al. Differential modulation of T helper type 1 (Th1) and T helper type 2 (Th2) cytokine secretion by prostaglandin E2 critically

depends on interleukin 2. Eur J Immunol 1995;25:59.

LIM H, PARIA BD, DAS SK, et al. Multiple female reproductive failures in cyclooxygenase-2- deficient mice. Cell 1997;91:197.

O'BRIEN WF. The role of prostaglandins in labor and delivery. Clin Perinatol 22:973, 1995.

PATRONO C. Aspirin as an antiplatelet drug. N Engl J Med. 1994;330:1287.

PATRONO C, FITZGERALD GA. Isoprostanes: potential markers of oxidant stress in atherothrombotic disease. Arterioscler Thromb Vasc Biol 1997;17:2309.

ROCCA B, SPAIN LM, PURE E, LANGENGACH R, PATRONO C, FITZGERALD GA. Distinct and coordinated roles of prostaglandin H synthases 1 and 2 in T-cell development. J Clin Invest 1999;103:1469-77.

SMALLEY WE, DUBOIS RN. Colorectal cancer and nonsteroidal anti-inflammatory drugs. Adv Pharmacol 1997;39:1.

SUGIMOTO Y, YAMASAKI A, SEGI E, et al. Failure of parturition in mice lacking the prostaglandin F receptor. Science 1997;277:681.

USHIKUBI F, HIRATA M, NARUMIYA S. Molecular biology of prostanoid receptors, an overview. J Lipid Med Cell Sign 1995;12:343.

WILLIAMS CS, DUBOIS RN. Prostaglandin endoperoxide synthase, why two isoforms? Am J Physiol 1996;1270:G393.

67

Endocrine kidney, endocrine lung, endocrine heart

Giuseppe Opocher, Franco Mantero

ENDOCRINE KIDNEY

THE RENIN-ANGIOTENSIN SYSTEM

The renin-angiotensin system is the most important and well-characterized endocrine system in the kidney. The site of production of renin is the juxtaglomerular apparatus, localized where the afferent arteriole enters the glomerulus. The juxtaglomerular cells are smooth muscle cells modified to perform a secretory function. Adjacent to these cells there is another group of cells, the macula densa, which is located within the terminal position of the thick ascending limb of the Henle loop; it exerts tubular control of renin secretion and of the tubuloglomerular feedback mechanism.

Renin acts on a substrate, an α-globulin (angiotensinogen) secreted by the liver, to cleave a decapeptide, angiotensin I, which is then converted to the octapeptide angiotensin II by angiotensin-converting enzyme. Biochemical characteristics, mechanisms of regulation, and biological activity of all of the components of the renin-angiotensin system – as well as the multiple systemic activities of the final product, the biologically active angiotensin II, and its receptors – have been illustrated exhaustively in Chapter 34.

The main actions of the renin-angiotensin system are the vasoconstriction of peripheral arterioles, inducing an increase of total peripheral resistances; stimulation of aldosterone secretion by the zona glomerulosa of the adrenal cortex; and direct intrarenal sodium retention. The latter is achieved both by preferentially constricting efferent arterioles, thus maintaining perfusion pressure, and by reducing peritubular hydrostatic pressure. This facilitates proximal tubule sodium reabsorption, which is also directly driven by angiotensin II.

VASODILATING NATRIURETIC SYSTEMS

The kidney also produces vasodilating and natriuretic substances (kallikrein-kinins, prostaglandins). Kallikrein is an enzyme that catalyzes the production of the potent vasodilating peptide, kinin. The angiotensin-converting enzyme also has inactivating properties on bradykinins (and is also called kininase II).

PROSTAGLANDINS

The kidney is among the most active tissues in synthesizing prostaglandins (PG), that is, all of the compounds derived from the metabolism of arachidonic acid. This metabolic pathway leads to the synthesis of PGE_2, $PGF_{2\alpha}$ thromboxane (Tx) A_2, and prostacyclin (PGI_2), via a cascade of multienzymatic sequences, in which cyclooxygenase is the initiating event. PGI_2 is probably the most important prostaglandin for the maintenance of glomerular filtration and flow, however the exact physiological role of these compounds remains elusive.

THE KIDNEY AS A SOURCE OF DOPAMINE

The effect of dopamine on renal function, which consists of a potent increase of cortical blood flow and of sodium and water content in urine, is well-described, though, renal dopamine neurons were only first documented in the late 1970s. Kidney dopamine neurons only have the aromatic L-amino acid decarboxylase (L-AAAD) and synthesize dopamine from L-dopa, but they are unable to proceed further to form catecholamines. While dopamine neurons have been localized over the renal tubules, the L-AAAD enzyme has also been found in renal cortical cells, particularly near the proximal convoluted tubules. It has been suggested that renal cells can take up L-dopa from blood circulation tubules and synthesize dopamine. Therefore, the kidney has a complex dopaminergic system: urinary free dopamine is derived from the deconjugation of circulating dopamine, a release from dopamine renal neurons, and local biosynthesis from L-dopa-containing cells.

Renal dopaminergic activity is depressed in essential hypertension: whether this is the result or the cause of hypertension is not clear. It is possible that the decrease in renal dopaminergic activity has a role in the pathogenesis of hypertension.

THE KIDNEY AS A REGULATOR OF MINERALOCORTICOID FUNCTION: TYPE 2 11β-HYDROXYSTEROID DEHYDROGENASE

Type 2 11β-hydroxysteroid dehydrogenase (11β-HSD2) has an important role in cortisol metabolism since it dehydrogenates cortisol to cortisone. It is of particular interest in the regulation of mineralocorticoid hormone effects in the kidney. In fact, 11β-HSD2 protects the receptor from the potential effect of cortisol as a mineralocorticoid hormone, by dehydrogenating cortisol to cortisone, since cortisone has no binding capacity to mineralocorticoid hormones receptors. A failure of this protective action of 11β-HSD2 is responsible for the apparent mineralocorticoid excess syndrome, a congenital disease that results in severe hypertension, hypokalemia, and hypoaldosteronemia.

Recently, the gene encoding 11β-HSD2 was cloned (HSD11B2) and the molecular basis of apparent mineralocorticoid excess elucidated. Although mutations of 11β-HSD2 are rare, this gene may have a pathogenetic role in essential hypertension. No data on the frequency of heterozygous mutations are currently available, and studies on the polymorphism of the gene and its promoter are in progress.

ENDOCRINE LUNG

ENDOCRINE PULMONARY SYSTEM

The endocrine system of the lung is fundamentally a component of the diffuse endocrine system that acts in concert with the nervous system and the general endocrine regulation. The endocrine activity of the lung in physiological conditions is uncertain, though it is clear it has a role in pathological conditions, such as chronic pulmonary diseases and neoplastic diseases.

ENDOCRINOLOGY OF NON-NEOPLASTIC LUNG

The secretory function of the lung seems to be located at the level of innervated cell clusters known as neuroepithelial bodies, which are concentrated where the airways branch. Chemoreception is the central role of neuroepithelial pulmonary cells, and prolonged exposure to hypoxia causes an increase in neuroepithelial bodies.

In a normal human lung, endocrine pulmonary cells principally secrete calcitonin, calcitonin gene-related peptide, serotonin, and gastrin-releasing peptide. The secretory activity is increased in chronic pulmonary diseases, where ectopic secretion is also present. Indeed, in many pulmonary disorders such as bronchial asthma and chronic bronchitis, a proliferation of endocrine pulmonary cells is observed; if the pathological stimulus persists, they eventually assume the aspect of nodular aggregates protruding into the airways. The amount of secreted hormones is often very low or undetectable in plasma and is thus unable to give rise to clear-cut clinical pictures. In some pneumopathies, adrenocorticotropic hormone (ACTH), arginine vasopressin, leuenkephalin, somatostatin, human growth hormone, and vasoactive intestinal peptide may be produced by the lung. Adrenomedullin, a potent hypotensive peptide recently discovered in extracts of human pheochromocytoma, has been recognized in normal and tumoral lung and is produced by both endothelial and smooth muscle cells of the airways.

The secretory activity of lung endothelium has an important role in the pathophysiology of pulmonary hypertension and in mediating the responses to acute or chronic hypoxia. Hypoxic pulmonary vasoconstriction activates the lung vasoregulatory system to match ventilation and perfusion in order to maintain arterial oxygenation. Endothelin-1, largely secreted from the pulmonary endothelium, mediates chronic hypoxic pulmonary hypertension, though its role in acute hypoxia is less clear. In chronic hypoxia, increased nitric oxide synthesis probably attenuates the vasoconstriction. An impaired balance between different substances with contrasting effects on vascular smooth muscle cells of the lung may constitute one mechanism underlying pulmonary hypertension.

The endothelial activity of the lung is important in the modulation of the physiological effects of circulating vasoactive substances. Pulmonary endothelial cells take up and degrade vasoactive amines as norepinephrine and serotonin. Pulmonary endothelial cells contain and secrete large amounts of angiotensin-converting enzyme, which catalyzes angiotensin II formation. Endothelial cells also contain neutral endopeptidase to degrade enkephalin and other short peptides, including tachykinin.

ENDOCRINOLOGY OF NEOPLASTIC LUNG

The classic clinical examples of hormonal overproduction in the lung are found in pulmonary tumors: carcinoid syndrome, Cushing's diseases, and the syndrome of inappropriate secretion of antidiuretic hormone (SIADH).

Most endocrine pulmonary neoplasms belong to the neuroendocrine neoplasm group, ranging from typical carcinoids tumors to largely undifferentiated neoplasms. Neuroendocrine neoplasms of the lung can be divided into four categories, in order of increasing aggressiveness: (1) carcinoid tumors; (2) atypical carcinoids or well-differentiated neuroendocrine tumors (WDNC); (3) intermediate-cell neuroendocrine or large-cell undifferentiated carcinomas; and (4) small-cell lung carcinomas. The differential diagnosis between neuroendocrine lung neoplasm and the other lung cancers is mostly based on immunostaining for neuronal specific enolase, on chromogranin, and on flow cytometry.

Typical paraneoplastic endocrine syndromes (for detailed descriptions of these syndromes, see the relative chapters) are not frequently observed. They may become apparent in patients with hepatic metastases of carcinoid tumors and constitute a clinical sign of secondary localization of the tumor, resulting in a worse prognosis.

Ectopic ACTH syndrome is related to small-cell lung carcinomas (60% of cases), as well as carcinoid tumors; only in rare cases has ectopic secretion of corticotropin-releasing hormone been reported. Marked increases of plasma immunoreactive ACTH levels are detected in only half of the cases, while increased levels of cortisol are always found. Clinical symptoms partially overlap with those of classic Cushing's syndrome with more severe metabolic abnormalities, such as hypokalemia.

The syndrome of inappropriate secretion of antidiuretic hormone is caused mainly by small-cell lung carcinomas. In 80% of cases there is evidence of increased arginine vasopressin secretion. The diagnosis is based on the findings of hyponatremia (<130 mEq/l), reduced plasma osmolality, and increased urinary osmolality (>300 mmol/kg). The symptoms are nonspecific and include fatigue, impaired attention, vomiting, and headache; in severe hyponatremia, major neurological disturbances including coma can be present. The correction of hyponatremia can require hydric restriction, hypertonic saline, demeclocycline (600-1200 mg qd), lithium, or Dilantin. A rapid correction of hyponatremia must be avoided because of the risk of pontine lysis.

Gynecomastia due to ectopic human chorionic gonadotropin secretion has also been described in lung carcinoma. Ectopic acromegaly can be associated with several neoplasms, including carcinoid tumors of the lung: it is caused mainly by growth hormone-releasing hormone production.

Non-neuroendocrine lung neoplasms rarely cause paraneoplastic syndromes such as SIADH or gynecomastia. Hypercalcemia of malignancy is usually related to squamous cell bronchial carcinoma and is not usually found in neuroendocrine neoplasms. Hypercalcemia of malignancy is caused by parathyroid hormone-related peptide. Less frequently, a local osteolytic hormone is involved in its pathogenesis, and in even fewer cases authentic parathyroid hormone or vitamin D analogs can also be secreted. Hypercalcemia of malignancy is usually a late manifestation of the neoplasm and is more frequently observed close to death. A sequence of hydration, furosemide, biphosphonates (pamidronate), and calcitonin administration constitutes the usual treatment.

ENDOCRINE HEART

The concept that the heart is a complex endocrine gland is now an acquired notion: after the discovery of atrial natriuretic peptides, significant evidence has also accumulated regarding the importance of a local cardiac renin-angiotensin system acting with paracrine mechanisms. The effects of atrial natriuretic peptides and a local cardiac renin-angiotensin system are mainly involved in the protection of cardiac integrity and function.

ATRIAL NATRIURETIC PEPTIDES

The identification of atrial natriuretic peptides is relatively recent. The isolation and identification of atrial natriuretic peptides was soon followed by the demonstration of other peptides with a high homology of structure, such as brain natriuretic peptide, which was first isolated in porcine brain but was subsequently found to be primarily produced by cardiac cardiocytes. More recently, C-type natriuretic peptide has been isolated as well, which is the most conserved member of the atrial natriuretic peptide family among different species and is produced almost exclusively by the brain.

Atrial natriuretic peptide is a 28-amino acid peptide with a disulfide bridge between cysteine residues at positions 7 and 23, which is responsible for its characteristic ring conformation.

Both brain natriuretic peptide and C-type natriuretic peptide are generated by a gene structure and processing similar to atrial natriuretic peptides. Brain natriuretic peptide is a 32-amino acid peptide with a disulfide bridge between residues 10 and 26. Atrial natriuretic peptides and brain natriuretic peptide share 14 amino acids. C-type natriuretic peptide is a 22-amino acid peptide with a disulfide bridge between residues 6 and 22. C-type natriuretic peptide shares 14 amino acids with brain natriuretic peptide and 11 with atrial natriuretic peptides.

Atrial natriuretic peptide mRNA is mainly produced in atrial cardiocytes, where it represents 1% of the mRNA contained in the atrium. Atrial tissue is the primary, though not the only, source of atrial natriuretic peptides. Indeed, mRNA encoding pre-pro atrial natriuretic peptides has been discovered in extra-atrial tissues including the heart ventricles, brain, pulmonary veins, lung, adrenal medulla, hypothalamus, and anterior pituitary gland.

Brain natriuretic peptide mRNA is expressed predominantly in the heart ventricles. Extra-cardiac expression has been localized in the adrenal medulla, brain, and, more recently, in the amnion tissue, where large amounts of brain natriuretic peptide have been documented.

The level of expression of C-type natriuretic peptide in the heart is very low. Higher levels have been documented in the brain, principally in the cerebellum and spinal cord, and in lower levels in the kidney and testis.

Three different subtypes of atrial natriuretic peptides receptors have been identified so far. The atrial natriuretic peptide-A receptor recognizes the intact 1-28 sequence: the hormone-receptor interaction activates the guanylate cyclase activity and expresses the biological action. Atrial natriuretic peptide-B receptor is similar to atrial natriuretic peptide-A (70% homology in the intracellular domain that activates the guanylate cyclase) but seems to be more selective for C-type natriuretic peptide. Atrial natriuretic peptide-C receptor binds the intact sequence, as well as several fragments of atrial natriuretic peptide, C-type natriuretic peptide, or brain natriuretic peptide, but it does not activate the guanylate cyclase. Atrial natriuretic peptide-C receptor is a clearance receptor, which removes atrial natriuretic peptides from the plasma by means of uptake, internalization, and degradation of the peptide.

Atrial natriuretic peptide receptors are found in the kidney, adrenal gland, heart, adipose tissues, eye, and vascular endothelium. Different types of receptors and the wide distribution confers considerable variability of response to atrial natriuretic peptides to the organs.

The main physiological stimulator of atrial natriuretic peptide secretion is the increase in atrial transmural pressure. Supine posture, head-out water immersion, acute or chronic sodium load, volume expansion, exercise, tachycardia, hypoxia, and myocardial ischemia can induce a rapid and marked release of atrial natriuretic peptides. The acute secretion of atrial natriuretic peptide is coupled to the effect of mechanical forces and is primarily due to atrial storage depletion. By contrast, the chronic atrial natriuretic peptide secretion that occurs in the presence of hypertension, cardiac hypertrophy, and chronic cardiac failure is secondary to an increase in atrial natriuretic peptide mRNA expression in atrial and ventricular cardiocytes.

Atrial natriuretic peptide mainly acts on the kidney, the cardiovascular system, and the hormones that regulate sodium and water homeostasis. Low-dose atrial natriuretic peptide injection is followed by natriuresis, systolic arterial pressure decrease, inhibition of plasma renin activity, and aldosterone. Atrial natriuretic peptide inhibits sodium transport in the inner medullary collecting ducts, but it may also inhibit angiotensin II-mediated sodium resorption in the proximal tubule and antidiuretic hormone-mediated water resorption. Atrial natriuretic peptides have a significant action on the cardiovascular system: they cause a rapid reduction of blood pressure without an increase in heart rate, they cause a decrease in cardiac filling pressure, a reduction of peripheral vascular resistance, and a reduction of intravascular volume. Most of these effects are due to the stimulation of the parasympathetic system, reduction of preload secondary to capacitance vein dilatation, and to an increase in transcapillary flow. Atrial natriuretic peptide can inhibit vasopressin production and renin secretion, it antagonizes the vasoconstrictor activity of angiotensin II, and blunts angiotensin II-stimulated aldosterone secretion. Finally, atrial natriuretic peptide itself or C-type natriuretic peptide can affect pituitary secretion both at corticotropin-releasing factor and ACTH levels.

The measurement of atrial peptides is of potential interest in many human diseases. An alteration of atrial natriuretic peptide or brain natriuretic peptide levels has already been demonstrated in chronic heart failure, pulmonary hypertension, primary aldosteronism, SIADH, and diabetes mellitus. In particular, increased atrial natriuretic peptide or brain natriuretic peptide levels may be an early marker of left ventricular insufficiency, a powerful prognostic factor in the early or subacute phase of myocardial infarction, and good predictors of mortality in the elderly.

A specific therapeutic approach was developed with the use of inhibitors of neutral endopeptidase 24.11, which are partly responsible for the degradation of atrial natriuretic peptides in vivo. Several neutral endopeptidase inhibitors reduce pulmonary hypertension, and in some cases they also affect cardio-pulmonary remodeling in animal models.

RENIN-ANGIOTENSIN SYSTEM: THE LOCAL CARDIAC SYSTEM

Substantial evidence has accumulated regarding the presence of a locally produced renin-angiotensin system acting by paracrine or autocrine mechanisms in the heart. Whether the different components of the renin-angiotensin system found at the cardiac level are the result of local gene expression or are taken up from plasma is still unsettled.

Local generation of renin mRNA, although at very low levels, has been observed in the normal heart. In experimental models of myocardial infarction, however, a great increase of renin mRNA was observed in the border zone of the infarction area, particularly in myofibroblasts. These cells, which have a key role in the cardiac tissue repair mechanism, also express angiotensin-converting enzyme mRNA. Moreover, cardiac cells synthesize and contain both types of angiotensin II receptors, that is, AT1 and AT2 receptors.

The role of the renin-angiotensin system in cardiac disease has recently received considerable attention because of the capability of angiotensin II to regulate cell growth, induce cardiac hypertrophy, and regulate cardiac cell apoptosis.

Suggested readings

DE BOLD AJ, BRUNEAU B, KUROSKI DE BOLD ML. Mechanical and neuroendocrine regulation of the endocrine heart. Cardiovascular Res 1996;31:7-18.

ESPINER EA. Physiology of natriuretic peptides. J Intern Med 1994;235:527-41.

GOSNEY JR. Pulmonary endocrine pathology: endocrine cells and endocrine tumors of the lung. Woburn: Butterworth-Heinemann, 1992.

RUZICKA M, LEENEN FHH. Update on local cardiac renin-angiotensin system. Curr Op Cardiol 1997;12:347-53.

SHEARD JDH, GOSNEY JR. Endocrine cells in tumor-bearing lungs. Thorax 1996;51:721-6.

WALLEN T, LANDHAL S, HEDNER T, NAKAO K, SAITO Y. Brain natriuretic peptide predicts mortality in the elderly. Heart 1997;77:264-7.

WHITE PC, MUNE T, AGARWAL AK. 11β-Hydroxysteroid dehydrogenase and the syndrome of apparent mineralocorticoid excess. Endocrine Rev 1997;18:135-56.

Hormones
and cancer

Hormones and cancer

KEY POINTS

- Breast cancer is considered to be one of the leading causes of death – in conjunction with cancer of the lung, intestine, and prostate – in the Western Hemisphere. In the United States and Europe it has become the most common cancer among women and the second leading cause of female death.
- During the past 2 to 3 decades, significant progress has been made with the development of early detection techniques, less "radical" and morbid primary surgery aimed at breast conservation, the incorporation of radiation in primary therapy to lessen local recurrence, and the addition of adjuvant systemic therapy to control micrometastatic disease.
- Even more importantly, many of the genes involved in the pathogenesis of the disease have recently been identified. A number of breast cancers depend on estrogens for their growth; maneuvers to suppress endogenous estrogens have long been a mainstay in breast cancer treatment.
- Prostate cancer is the most frequently diagnosed cancer in men in North America and Europe and is the second cause of male cancer death. One in eight men will be diagnosed with prostate cancer during his lifetime.
- The androgens acting in the prostate originate from two sources of approximately equal importance: the testicles and the adrenals. This indicates the need for a combined androgen blockade.
- The efficacy of androgen deprivation in prostate cancer is at least one order of magnitude greater for localized than for metastatic disease, thus indicating the critical importance of early treatment.
- Androgen blockade is the only treatment shown in randomized clinical trials to prolong life in prostate cancer, both in localized and advanced stages of the disease.

BREAST CANCER

Angelo Raffaele Bianco, Roberto Bianco

Epidemiology, etiology, and risk factors

Breast cancer is exceptional before the age of 20 and seldom occurs below 30. The incidence rate rises steadily up to the age of 60 and then slows down, though continuing to rise and finally declining past 80. Mortality rates in western Europe and North America are on the order of 15 to 25×10^5 women per year, which is slightly more than one-third of the incidence rate of 50 to 60 new cases per 10^5 women per year. In the United States in 1997, breast cancer prevalence has been estimated to be approximately 2×10^6, which is approximately five times that of lung cancer. The death rate has remained constant. In 1976 the risk of dying of breast cancer was approximately 1:30. This figure changed very slightly to a risk of 1:28 over the following 10 years, even though an increase in incidence of nearly 20% occurred during the same period. The highest rates are in the Western Hemisphere (over 100 new cases per 10^5 women per year), the lowest in Asian countries (10 to 15 new cases per 10^5 women per year). When a low-risk population migrates to an area of high risk, the low-risk population gradually assumes the incidence of the high-risk population, although the shift may take one to two generations. Within a country, rates increase in urban areas relative to rural ones, correlate with pro-capita income, and can be associated with religious and cultural differences. These facts point to the critical importance of environmental and lifestyle factors. Such factors include diet, body habitus, hormonal and reproductive history, and previous radiation exposure. Breast cancer is more prevalent in families who have had previous breast cancer experience, and approximately 5% of breast cancers cluster very tightly in what appears to be a hereditary fashion. Major risk factors for breast cancer are listed in Table 68.1.

Etiopathogenesis

The specific cause for the malignant transformation of a normal ductal epithelial cell is unknown. Breast tissue and breast malignancies are dependent upon estrogen for growth. Many breast cancers express the estrogen receptor protein and, in general, these tumors are responsive to manipulations of the endocrine system. It is clear, however, that breast cancer gradually becomes hormone-independent, that is, it can sustain growth without the need for estrogenic stimulation. Estrogen stimulates cell growth by binding to the estrogen receptor. The receptor-hormone complex then migrates to the nucleus, binds to specific DNA sites and activates genes responsible for synthesizing growth factors. In the acquisition of hormone independence, it appears that some cells mutate their estrogen receptor, while others acquire the ability to secrete these growth factors – namely transforming growth factor alpha (TGFα) and epidermal growth factor (EGF) – without the need for estrogen stimulation. This biologic information has prognostic significance in the short-term. Tumors that express the EGF receptor or overexpress the Her-2/neu (c-erbB2) gene, which codes for a membrane protein structurally similar to the EGF receptor, have both been associated with poor prognosis.

Breast cancer is a genetic disease involving a number of gene alterations, including mutations in the oncogene family. It is likely that once the initial mutations have occurred additional mutations are facilitated, thus accounting for the genetic instability of tumor cells, as opposed to normal cells. Genetic instability is responsible for tumor population heterogeneity. In fact, karyotypic analyses have indicated that a truly diploid breast cancer cell may not exist. Ploidy and cell growth fraction appear to be prognostic indicators of outcome in breast cancer patients. They may help in identifying subsets of patients at risk of relapse after primary surgery such that adjuvant therapy could be tailored to their individual risk.

Table 68.1 Risk factors in breast cancer

Factor	Variable	Relative risk
Family history	One first-degree relative	1.5 - 2.0
	Two first-degree relatives	5.0
Diet	High fat	1.2
	Obesity, premenopausal	0.8
	Obesity, postmenopausal	1.2
Alcohol	Consumption	1.3
Oral contraceptives	Regular use	1.0
Postmenopausal HTR	Use	1.1 - 1.4
Oophorectomy	Prior to age 40	0.5
Age at menarche	Younger	Risk increase of 4.5% per yr
Age at menopause	Older	Risk increase of 4.5% per yr
Age at first child birth	≤ 20	1.0
	Multiparous	1.6
	Nulliparous ≥ 35	1.9
Breast feeding	Yes	0.8
Benign breast disease	Hyperplasia	1.5 - 2.0
	Atypia	3.0 - 5.0
Previous breast cancer	Yes	Risk increase of 0.7% per yr
Breast irradiation	Age 10 - 20	20
	20 - 30	15
	≥ 50	1.0

(HTR = hormone replacement therapy.)

The retinoblastoma gene, RB-1, a tumor suppressor gene, is reported to be mutated in 15 to 20% of breast cancers. The gene for p-53, a cell-cycle regulatory protein, is altered in a substantial proportion of breast cancer cells. The oncogene c-myc is amplified in approximately one-third of tumor specimens, and point mutations in the H-ras proto-oncogene have been demonstrated. Recently two genes, BRCA-1 and BRCA-2, have been identified, whose mutations are associated with a hereditary form of breast cancer.

Breast cancer, in common with other solid tumors, exhibits two additional biological properties that contribute to its lethal potential: an ability to metastasize, and an acquisition of resistance to antineoplastic drugs.

Familial and hereditary breast cancer

The risk of breast cancer increases if a first-degree relative (mother, sister, daughter) has been diagnosed with the disease. A postmenopausal diagnosis in the affected relative poses less of a risk than a premenopausal one (Tab. 68.2). The association of breast cancer cases within families does not necessarily imply a purely genetic transmission of the disease but might mean there has been a common risk exposure, or possibly a combination of both.

By performing linkage analysis of high-risk families, a gene of the long arm of chromosome 17 (17q21) has been identified as abnormal in these families. Mutations of this tumor suppressor gene, the BRCA-1 gene, are believed to be responsible for a large percentage of hereditary breast and ovarian cancers. Carriers of BRCA-1 mutations appear to have a risk of developing breast cancer of approximately 85% by the age of 70, and a 45% risk of developing ovarian cancer by the same age. Despite the high rate of cancer in carriers of the BRCA-1 mutation, the gene accounts for only half of the cases of hereditary breast cancers. In fact, a second gene, the BRCA-2 gene, has been recently mapped on chromosome 13. While BRCA-1 and BRCA-2 mutations are responsible for approximately 5% of all breast cancers, it is estimated that one in 200 to 400 women carry a mutated gene.

Identification and management of the high-risk patient

In the National Surgical Adjuvant Breast Project (NSABP) tamoxifen breast cancer prevention trial, a sliding scale of relative risk was used to identify high-risk individuals who would be eligible. In the so-called high-risk patients, some four possible actions may be taken, even simultaneously: (1) enhanced surveillance, (2) behavior modifications, (3) preventive strategies, and (4) prophylactic mastectomy.

Enhanced surveillance

The American Cancer Society recommends that a baseline mammogram be obtained at the age of 35 years. Between ages of 40 and 50, a mammogram should be obtained every 2 years, while annual surveillance is recommended past 50. In women at high-risk, surveillance should be increased. Breast self examination should be taught to women at high risk. While controversy exists whether this self examination reduces breast cancer mortality, several studies have shown that examiners present with smaller tumors and less frequent axillary node involvement.

Table 68.2 Relative risks associated with a family history of breast cancer

Family history	Relative risk
One first-degree relative	1.5 - 2.0
Two first-degree relatives	5.0
First-degree relative with bilateral, postmenopausal cancer	10.0
First-degree relative with bilateral, premenopausal cancer	20.0

Behavior modifications

Lifestyle factors, including obesity, a high-fat diet, and alcohol consumption, are small but measurable risk factors.

Prevention

Breast cancer patients who have taken tamoxifen for a minimum of 2 years have a significantly lower incidence of contralateral breast cancer than a control. Tamoxifen is a "non-pure" antiestrogen, possessing antiestrogenic as well as estrogenic effects. At mean follow-up of 4 years, tamoxifen prevented about half of both invasive and non-invasive breast cancer. Serious side effects included thromboembolic vascular events and endometrial cancer, but they where limited to women over 50. It is believed that the increased rate of endometrial cancer and vascular effects observed in postmenopausal women are caused by the estrogenic component of tamoxifen. Even more interesting is the significantly lower incidence of breast cancer among women taking long-term raloxifene, a tamoxifen analog, which is almost completely devoid of estrogenic effects.

Additional drugs, such as fenretinide (4-HPR), a synthetic retinoid, have shown promising results in breast cancer prevention.

Prophylactic mastectomy

Prophylactic simple mastectomy is probably the most controversial area in the management of high-risk breast cancer. Screening mammography is now readily available and highly sensitive, the treatment of a diagnosed cancer with lumpectomy and radiation therapy is cosmetically less disfiguring than simple mastectomy for prophylaxis, and genetic counseling is helping women to determine if they are at high risk for hereditary breast cancer, thus making prophylactic mastectomy seemingly unnecessary. Furthermore, while prophylactic mastectomy reduces the risk for developing breast cancer, it does not eliminate that risk. Therefore, prophylactic mastectomy should be performed with caution in the current management of breast cancer, and only in the well-selected patient, such as in women with demonstrated ductal atypia.

Presentation, diagnosis and screening

More than 85% of newly diagnosed breast cancers are detected as a lump in the breast. In about 80% of the cases, the patient discovers the thickening of the breast. Hemorrhagic nipple discharge, nipple retraction or erosion, skin dimpling, enlarged axillary nodes, and pseudo-inflammatory skin changes with ill-defined breast infiltration are less frequent complaints leading to diagnosis. In about 10% of the cases, breast cancer is diagnosed as a result of metastatic disease.

Early detection, primarily by mammography, reduces mortality. Modalities for early detection include breast self examination, periodic clinical examination, and imaging techniques. Both breast self examination and clinical examination are aimed at diagnosing breast cancer by drawing attention to a suspicious lump in the breast or the axilla. In these cases mammography and biopsy, either fine needle aspiration or open biopsy with histologic examination, can establish the diagnosis. Screening mammography can detect subclinical breast cancer and has proven to reduce mortality by approximately 30% in women over 50. The usefulness of screening mammography below 50 is controversial because of the lower incidence of the disease and also because of the lower efficacy of mammography in the premenopausal breast. Histologic examination by open biopsy or cytologic examination of fine needle aspirate are indicated whenever a lesion detected by an imaging procedure is not clearly benign. Ultrasonography of the breast has not proven useful in breast cancer detection. Its greatest accuracy (>95%) is in the diagnosis of breast cysts.

Pathophysiology

Several entities are defined through pathological examination.

Noninvasive breast carcinoma

• Lobular carcinoma in situ (LCIS) is a proliferative lesion limited to one or more mammary lobules and composed of truly neoplastic cells but without invasion of basement membrane. It occurs mainly in premenopausal women and is multicentric in 50 to 70% of the cases. The risk of developing invasive carcinoma following the diagnosis of LCIS not treated with mastectomy is approximately 10 to 15% at 10 years.
• Ductal carcinoma in situ (DCIS) identifies a group of lesions characterized by the proliferation of ductal cancer cells within the ducts and without invasion of surrounding stroma. DCIS includes comedo and noncomedo types. The comedo type is characterized by necrosis at the center of the ducts, and it has at higher risk of recurrence after surgery, especially after breast conservation. DCIS is multifocal in some 30% of the cases. The incidence of axillary lymph node metastasis is very limited, not exceeding 2 to 6%, and is probably the result of an invasive component within the lesion.

Invasive breast carcinoma

• Invasive *ductal* carcinoma is the commonest type of breast cancer, contributing to over 70 to 80% of all cases.
• Invasive *lobular* carcinoma represents 10 to 20% of all breast cancers.
The remaining 10% of breast cancers include the following:
• Medullary carcinoma: sharp tumor borders and lymphoid infiltration

• Mucoid carcinoma: large amounts of intracellular mucus
• Papillary/tubular carcinoma: has well-differentiated papillary/tubular architecture
• Inflammatory carcinoma: usually an invasive ductal carcinoma, poorly differentiated with extensive invasion of lymphatic vessels of the dermis. It accounts for 1 to 2% of all cases and bears a poor prognosis
• Paget's disease of the nipple: a variant of ductal carcinoma in situ in which tumor cells invade the ducts without infiltrating basement membrane and extend into the major ducts of the nipple and the epidermis of the areola. Invasive carcinoma is associated with this condition in 90% of patients.

Other rare cases of invasive cancers include adenoid cystic carcinoma, apocrine carcinoma, neuroendocrine type carcinoma, and carcinoma with squamous metaplasia. Malignant diseases of the breast, which could simulate breast cancer, include cystosarcoma phylloides, sarcoma, and malignant lymphoma, usually Hodgkin's or non-Hodgkin's lymphoma of the B cell type.

Most common nonmalignant conditions are fibrocystic disease (with or without atypia), fibroadenoma, and intraductal papilloma.

Staging and prognostic evaluation

About 90% of patients with breast cancer are diagnosed with operable disease, which implies that all clinical cancer is confined to the breast and the ipsilateral axillary lymph nodes. The extension of the disease from mammary gland to the overlying or the underlying soft tissues of the chest wall (T4) defines a stage of locally advanced disease. Overt metastases to supraclavicular lymph nodes or other organs are referred to as metastatic (M1) disease. The most widely used staging system for breast cancer is based upon the definition of primary tumor (T), local-regional nodes (N), and distant metastasis (M) (Tabs. 68.3 and 68.4).

Staging has important prognostic implications: the stage is a strong determinant of survival. Pre-surgical staging is accomplished by complete physical examination, diagnostic mammography, biochemical blood testing, chest X-ray, liver ultrasound, and bone scan. Whenever indicated, CT scans or nuclear magnetic resonance (NMR) scans may be used as well as X-rays for detailed hot spots on bone scans. The T category is determined by breast clinical examination, mammography or breast ultrasound; the N category is defined by clinical examination, ultrasound of the axilla, or CT scan of the chest for the detection of internal mammary nodes; and the M is assessed by clinical examination, chest X-ray, liver ultrasound, and isotope bone scan. Serum tumor marker determinations, including the measurement of carcinoembryonic (CEA), sialomucin (CA 15.3, MCA), tissue polypeptide antigen (TPA), may be useful for detecting clinically occult disease. Post-surgical ("pathological") staging is identified by the p prefix (pTNM).

In addition to the stage, a number of biological and pathological variables have been identified in the primary tumors of patients with breast cancer that can have an impact on prognosis. A list of established or putative prognostic and predictive factors for patients with limited stage (I-II-IIIA) breast cancer is provided in Tables 68.5 and 68.6, respectively. Of all of the identified prognostics factors, nodal involvement of the axilla and the number of involved nodes are the most relevant ones. As opposed to prognostic factors, "predictive" factors are useful in cases in which there is a qualitative or quantitative difference in response to a given treatment, thus allowing for an optimal use of all available therapeutic options.

Clinical findings

Local regional disease (M0)

Local regional disease includes (1) "early" breast cancer (TNM stages I-II-IIIA) and, (2) locally advanced disease (stage IIIB). A specific clinical-pathologic entity within stage IIIB merits consideration – inflammatory breast

---

Table 68.3 TNM classification of breast cancer

TNM Clinical classification
T Primary tumor

TX	Primary tumor cannot be assessed
T0	No evidence of primary tumor
Tis[1]	Carcinoma in situ: intraductal carcinoma or lobular carcinoma in situ or Paget's disease of the nipple with no tumor
T1	Tumor 2 cm or less in greatest dimension
	T1mic Microinvasion of 0.1 cm or less in greatest dimension
	T1a 0.5 cm or less in greatest dimension
	T1b >0.5 cm but not >1 cm in greatest dimension
	T1c >1 cm but not >2 cm in greatest dimension
T2	Tumor >2 cm but not >5 cm in greatest dimension
T3	Tumor >5 cm in greatest dimension
T4	Tumor of any size with direct extension to chest wall[2] or skin
	T4a Extension to chest wall
	T4b Edema (including *peau d'orange*) or ulceration of the skin of the breast or satellite skin nodules confined to the same breast
	T4c Presence of both T4a and T4b features
	T4d Inflammatory carcinoma

N Regional lymph nodes

NX	Regional lymph nodes cannot be assessed (for example, previously removed)
N0	No regional lymph node metastasis
N1	Metastasis to movable ipsilateral axillary node(s)
N2	Metastasis to ipsilateral axillary node(s) fixed to one another or to other structures
N3	Metastasis to ipsilateral internal mammary lymph node(s)

M Distant metastasis

MX	Presence of distant metastasis cannot be assessed
M0	No distant metastasis
M1	Distant metastasis (includes metastasis to supraclavicular lymph nodes)

pTNM Pathological classification
pT Primary tumor

The pathological classification requires the examination of the primary carcinoma with no gross tumor at the margins of resection. A case can be classified pT if there is only microscopic tumor in a margin
The pT categories correspond to the T categories

pN Regional lymph nodes

The pathological classification requires the resection and examination of lower axilla lymph nodes (level I). Such a resection will ordinarily include six or more lymph nodes.

pNX	Regional lymph nodes cannot be assessed (not removed for study or previously removed)
pN0	No regional lymph node metastasis
pN1	Metastasis to movable ipsilateral axillary node(s)
pN1a	Only micrometastases (none >0.2 cm)
pN1b	Metastasis to lymph nodes(s), any >0.2 cm
pN1bi	Metastasis in 1-3 lymph nodes, any >0.2 cm and all <2.0 cm in greatest dimension
pN1bii	Metastasis in 1-4 lymph nodes, any >0.2 cm and all <2.0 cm in greatest dimension
pN1biii	Extension of tumor beyond the capsule of lymph node metastasis <2.0 cm in greatest dimension
pN1biv	Metastasis to a lymph node > 2.0 cm in greatest dimension
pN2	Metastasis to ipsilateral axillary lymph nodes that are fixed to one another or to other structures
pN3	Metastasis to ipsilateral internal mammary lymph node(s)

[1] Paget's disease associated with a tumor is classified according to the size of the tumor.
[2] Chest wall includes ribs, intercostal muscles and serratus anterior muscle, but not pectoral muscle.

Table 68.4 Stage grouping of breast cancer			
Stage 0	Tis	N0	M0
Stage I	T1	N0	M0
Stage IIA	T0	N1	M0
	T1	N1*	M0
	T2	N0	M0
Stage IIB	T2	N1	M0
	T3	N0	M0
Stage IIIA	T0	N2	M0
	T1	N2	M0
	T2	N2	M0
	T3	N1	M0
	T3	N2	M0
Stage IIIB	T4	any N	M0
	any T	N3	M0
Stage IV	any T	any N	M1

* Prognosis of N1a patients is similar to that of pN0 patients.

Table 68.6 Predictive factors		
Factor	**Treatment**	**Effect**
ER/PgR	ET	+
c-erbB2	ET	−
	CT	−/+
Proliferative activity	ET	−
	CT	+
P53	ET	−
	CT	−
Ploidy	ET	−
	CT	+

(ET = endocrine therapy; CT = chemotherapy; ER = estrogen receptor; PgR = progesterone receptor.)

Approximately 35% of the patients will have obvious metastases at diagnosis. Mammography most often shows a generalized distortion of the mammary gland architecture rather than a well-identifiable nodule.

Metastatic disease (M1)

The clinical picture of systemic disease (stage IV) is a consequence of individual organ involvement. Skeletal lesions may be associated with bone pain in different body districts or pathological fractures of distinct, single, or multiple, bone segments; liver metastases may include pain in the right hypochondrium or epigastrium or jaundice; lung metastases may be associated with coughing and shortness of breath; central nervous system involvement may be associated with neurological dysfunction.

cancer – which can be considered the most aggressive form of nonmetastatic breast cancer. This accounts for only 1 to 4% of all cases and is characterized by the rapid enlargement and generalized induration of the breast, usually without a distinct mass within the organ. Erythema of the skin affecting greater than one-third of the breast has been indicated as the most distinctive clinical feature. Flattening and retraction of the nipple with diffuse breast warmth and "peau d'orange" are common, and most patients present with palpable lymphadenopathy.

Treatment

The current multidisciplinary approach to operable disease involves the sequential use of surgery, irradiation of the residual breast in case of limited surgery, and adjuvant systemic therapy. Locally advanced disease requires systemic treatment, which represents the primary approach. The therapeutic attitude toward metastatic disease takes into account the fact that at this stage the disease is considered to be largely incurable; mainstays of treatment should follow the principle of the maximum prolongation of survival and of the maintenance of an optimal quality of life at the minimum cost in terms of side effects.

Table 68.5 Prognostic factors		
Clinical	**Pathological**	**Biological**
Age	T category	ER, PgR
Menopausal status	Lymph node metastases	Ploidy, S-phase
Performance status	Local extension	Labeling index
Stage (TNM)	Grade (nuclear, histologic)	Cathepsin D
	Vascularity	HER-2/neu (c-erbB2)
	Mitotic index	p53
	Vascular/lymphatic invasion	Heat shock proteins
		BCL2
		EGFR

(ER = estrogen receptors; PgR = progesterone receptor; EGFR = epidermal growth factor receptor.)

Local regional disease

With surgery alone, long-term disease-free survival and possibly cure can be expected in a substantial proportion of patients. The following modalities of the treatment program should be given consideration:

- Breast surgery should primarily be utilized when tumors present at stages T<4 and N<2. In selected T3 lesions, the use of primary ("neoadjuvant") systemic chemotherapy should be considered, although its role as initial treatment for patients with operable disease is still investigational.
- Postoperative radiation therapy to the residual breast is generally indicated for patients undergoing a breast-conserving procedure. Routine postoperative radiation to the chest wall or the axilla after "radical" mastectomy and axillary dissection, respectively, is to be avoided.
- Adjuvant ("postoperative") systemic therapy should be considered for all patients with invasive breast cancer whose risk of relapse exceeds 10 to 20% at 10 years.
- Locally advanced disease (T4 lesions, N2/N3) is not initially amenable to surgery and should be primarily treated with neoadjuvant ("preoperative") chemotherapy prior to definitive surgery.

Surgery should consist of standard modified radical mastectomy or even conservative surgery (quadrantectomy/lumpectomy) with axillary node dissection in cases of chemotherapy-induced significant tumor regression. Under these conditions, optimal primary chemotherapy, in general combination chemotherapy, can be expected to yield tumor regression (partial + complete responses) in up to 90% of the patients. In cases of a lack of significant tumor regression, radiation therapy is indicated. In patients with involvement of ipsilateral internal mammary nodes (N3) and with significant tumor response after neoadjuvant chemotherapy; surgery, either mastectomy or conservative surgery with axillary node dissection, should be followed by radiation therapy of the initially involved internal mammary nodes.

Surgery Surgery has a central role in the removal of local regional disease. Breast conservation and radical mastectomy have been demonstrated in a number of randomized clinical trials to produce equivalent survival. In general, proper breast conservation, defined as complete tumor excision followed by whole breast irradiation, should be offered to most women with operable disease and with tumors not exceeding 3 cm in diameter. Omitting radiation carries a risk of developing intra-breast relapse of approximately 30%, which, being generally approached by mastectomy, nullifies the advantage of initial conservative surgery. Routine irradiation of the dissected axilla or of additional uninvolved draining lymph node stations (ipsilateral internal mammary, supra-/subclavicular) does not improve local control while increasing morbidity.

Complete axillary node dissection is usually preferred to other partial techniques ("sampling", removal of level I-II nodes only). It provides the most significant staging and prognostic information and prevents disease progression in the axilla. Sentinel node biopsy has recently been shown to be an excellent predictor of the axillary status and may prevent the morbidity of an unnecessary axillary clearance in a significant proportion of patients.

Radiation therapy after limited surgery ("adjuvant") Radiation therapy of the conserved breast significantly reduces local relapses. The efficacy of radiotherapy is unchanged whether it is administered concurrently with or delayed 3 to 6 months after completion of the adjuvant chemotherapy.

Follow-up after local treatment Follow-up after primary therapy should include periodic physical examinations and mammography to detect early recurrence or the emergence of a second primary tumor in the operated or in the contralateral breast. The routine use of bone scans, chest X-ray, liver ultrasound, and blood tests does not improve survival in the asymptomatic patient. The role of circulating tumor markers (mainly CEA, TPA, CA15.3, MCA) is still controversial. The frequency of visits should be determined according to the risk of relapse and the preference of the individual patient.

Adjuvant systemic therapy Although early breast cancer is a potentially curable disease, approximately 55% of breast cancer patients who become disease-free after local-regional treatment subsequently relapse and die of metastatic disease. The current paradigm ascribes failure of cure to distant occult micrometastatic tumor foci already present at the time of the initial diagnosis and surgery. This hypothesis has received indirect support from the results of clinical trials that have shown no additional advantage in terms of survival from more aggressive local-regional therapy. To avoid unnecessary overtreatment in an attempt to eradicate micrometastatic disease, the application of adjuvant therapy, either chemotherapy or endocrine therapy, implies prior identification of patients at risk of relapse after removal of local-regional disease who might benefit from the therapy.

Traditionally the major indication for systemic adjuvant therapies in breast cancer has been the histologically confirmed metastatic involvement of axillary nodes (N+ state). However, it must be appreciated that an average risk of relapse on the order of 30% at 5 years also applies to patients with negative nodes. Guidelines have been established for the classification of the risk of relapse in node-negative patients (Tab. 68.7).

Table 68.7 Risk categories for node-negative patients

Prognostic factor	Minimal/low risk*	Intermediate risk	High risk**
Tumor size	≤ 1 cm	1.1-2 cm	>2 cm
ER/PgR	Positive	Positive	Negative
Tumor grade	1	1-2	
Age	> 35		

* Simultaneous presence of all factors.
** Presence of at least one factor.
(ER = estrogen receptor; PgR = progesterone receptor.)

Almost all information relative to the benefits of adjuvant systemic treatments derives from randomized trials. Treatment benefits have been defined as the capability to improve disease-free survival (DFS), that is, the time elapsed from initial surgery to the time of first recurrence, and overall survival (OS). In the majority of studies, patient allocation to different treatments was done on an intention-to-treat basis. Diagnosis of contralateral breast cancer was considered disease recurrence. Two major types of systemic treatment have been employed: (1) endocrine therapy, which includes administration of the antiestrogen tamoxifen and ovarian ablation, and (2) cytotoxic chemotherapy.

Although prospective randomized trials of systemic adjuvant therapy were first initiated some 35 years ago, considerable controversy has existed even throughout recent years as to the time benefits of such treatments. These uncertainties were largely a result of the apparently modest absolute benefits of the adjuvant systemic therapies as well as the significant heterogeneity in the clinical course of early breast cancer. To establish whether a specific therapeutic modality had a clinically worthwhile benefit, the Early Breast Cancer Trialists Collaborative Group (EBCTCG) undertook an overview ("meta-analysis") of all worldwide randomized clinical trials that began before 1985 and, sub-

---

Table 68.8 Results of the "meta-analysis" performed by the Early Breast Cancer Trialists Collaborative Group on worldwide randomized clinical trials concerning specific therapeutic modalities for breast cancer

Type of trial	Number of trials/patients	Results
Adjuvant tamoxifen	55 trials/37 000 women	• Tamoxifen significantly improves both DFS and OS at the dose of 20 mg per day. Optimal duration of tamoxifen administration is five years • The effect of tamoxifen is independent of age and menopausal status but is strictly related to the presence of estrogen receptors (ER) in the primary tumor, being negligible for patients with ER-negative tumors. It is equally effective in node-positive and in node-negative patients • Five years of tamoxifen, when administered to patients with ER-positive tumors, reduces the annual risk of relapse and of death by 50% and 28%, respectively • Tamoxifen effect is unchanged in the presence or in the absence of chemotherapy (lack of interaction between tamoxifen and cytotoxics). That is, when the same patient has received both tamoxifen and chemotherapy the effect of tamoxifen is additive to that of chemotherapy • Five years of tamoxifen reduces the risk of developing cancer in the contralateral breast by 47%. However, the risk of endometrial cancer is increased fourfold
Ovarian ablation	12 trials/3500 women	• In women below 50, ovarian ablation, either surgical or radiation-induced, significantly reduces the annual risk of relapsing or of dying by 25% and by 24%, respectively. The addition of chemotherapy does not result in additional significant benefit • Studies of ovarian suppression by the use of LHRH superagonists are still in progress but preliminary data have shown effects comparable to those produced by surgical oophorectomy
Chemotherapy	69 trials/30 000 women	• Overall, combination chemotherapy reduces relative risk of relapsing or dying by 23.5% and 15.3%, respectively. The effect of chemotherapy is age-related, being highest in patients below 50 and lower, but still significant, above 50. The annual risk reduction of relapse in patients receiving adjuvant chemotherapy as opposed to controls is 37%, 34%, 22%, 18% in the different age categories of years <40, 40-49, 50-59, 60-69, respectively. The annual risk reduction of death is 27%, 27%, 15%, 8%, respectively • The effect of chemotherapy is independent of axillary nodal status and of presence/absence of ER in primary tumor • Chemotherapy is equally effective in the presence as well as in the absence of tamoxifen, indicating that the two treatment modalities have as additive effect if administered together (chemotherapy + tamoxifen superior to either used alone) • Chemotherapy regimens including anthracyclines seem to produce additional though small benefit, on both DFS and OS, as compared to CMF (Cyclophosfamide-Methotrexate-Fluorouracil)-based combinations

(ER = estrogen receptor.)

sequently, before 1990. The results of the latest overview, held in Oxford in 1996, have recently been published. The group's conclusions are summarized in Table 68.8.

The results of the 1996 overview can be summarized as follows: 5 years of tamoxifen reduces the annual risk of dying by 28% in patients with estrogen receptor positive (ER+) tumors; ovarian ablation reduces that risk by 24% in women below 50; and polychemotherapy reduces the annual risk of death by 27.3% in women below 50 and by 11.3% in patients above 50.

The results of the 1996 overview were translated into treatment choice recommendations for different risk categories at a consensus conference held at S. Gallen, Switzerland, in 1998. These conclusions are summarized in Table 68.9.

Metastatic ("systemic") disease

Since the major goal of therapy for metastatic disease is not to provide a cure but rather a reduction of tumor mass and its related symptoms, treatments are defined by their efficacy to provide palliation. Survival may range from a few weeks to several years, with an average of about 2 years. Therefore, a correct choice of treatment should take into consideration the extent of disease, the type of metastatic sites and its related symptoms, and the estimated survival. Ideally, optimal therapy should aim at maximally increased survival with no or few disease-related symptoms, with minimal side effects related to treatment.

When selecting treatment, one should also take into consideration certain biological features that define the aggressiveness of the disease and its chances for response. Shorter disease-free survival, low or absent receptor content in the tumor cells, and multiple organ involvement are indicators for aggressive disease and short survival. Host-related prognostic factors, mainly performance status, also influence prognosis (Tab. 68.10). An algorithm

Table 68.10 Prognostic and predictive factors in metastatic breast cancer

Age, menopausal status

Disease-free survival

Estrogen and progesterone receptors

Prior therapy and response

Number and sites of metastasis

Performance status

Psychological factors

that involves several of these factors for the selection of the type of initial therapy is shown in Figure 68.1.

The subjective attitude of the patient and the physician towards systemic treatments such as chemotherapy and its related side effects, and consideration about quality of life, must also guide treatment selection.

Time to response should also influence the choice of therapy: endocrine manipulations require an average of 6 to 12 weeks, while chemotherapy has a much shorter lag interval. It is generally accepted that treatment should be initiated shortly after diagnosis of metastasis in an attempt to prevent the emergence of the disease-related symptoms or to afford their control within the shortest time.

Before starting systemic therapy – either first-, second-, or third-line – it is important to evaluate (generally with imaging techniques) the number and size of disease sites, which provides the basis for accurate evaluation of tumor

Table 68.9 Guidelines for the adjuvant therapy of breast cancer

Patients	N⁻			N⁺
	Low risk	Intermediate risk	High risk	
PREMENOPAUSAL				
ER⁺ or PgR⁺	Nil or TAM	TAM + CT	CT + TAM Oophorectomy LHRHa1	CT + TAM LHRHa[1] CT± LHRHa+TAM[1]
ER⁻ and PgR⁻			CT	CT
POSTMENOPAUSAL				
ER⁺ or PgR⁺	Nil or TAM	TAM ± CT	TAM ± CT	TAM + CT
ER⁻ and PgR⁻			CT	CT
ELDERLY				
ER⁺ or PgR⁺	Nil or TAM	TAM ± CT	TAM ± CT	TAM ± CT
ER⁻ and PgR⁻			CT	CT

[1] Treatment to be considered still investigational.
(CT = chemotherapy; TAM = tamoxifen; LHRHa = LHRH analogs; N⁻ = axillary nodes, pathologically uninvolved; N⁺ = pathologically metastatic axillary nodes; ER⁺ = estrogen receptor-positive; PgR⁺ = progesterone receptor-positive; ER⁻ = estrogen receptor-negative; PgR⁻ = progesterone receptor-negative.)

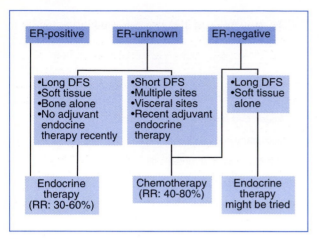

Figure 68.1 Algorithm for the selection of the type of initial therapy in metastatic disease based upon prognostic/predictive factors. (RR = response rate.)

response. Serial determination of serum tumor markers (primarily CEA, TPA, CA15.3 and MCA) might be of use in monitoring the response, but only in the context of the whole clinical picture.

Measurable objective tumor response (Tab. 68.11) is important for the assessment of the effectiveness of anticancer drug therapy. In clinical metastatic breast cancer, the existence of a correlation between response and survival is still controversial.

If associated with acceptable quality of life, stable disease could be considered a valuable response, particularly if obtained with endocrine therapy.

Endocrine therapy Endocrine therapy is generally well-tolerated and therefore, whenever indicated, it should be offered as a primary option to the patient. The major hor-

Table 68.11 Classification of objective response to therapy

Complete response
Disappearance of all measurable or evaluable disease, signs, symptoms and biochemical changes related to tumor for >4 weeks

Partial response
>50% reduction in the sum of the products of the 2 perpendicular diameters of all measurable lesions, lasting >4 weeks

Stable disease
<50% reduction and <25% increase in the sum of the products of the two perpendicular diameters of all measurable lesions

Progression
Increase in the product of two perpendicular diameters of any measurable lesion by >25% and/or the appearance of new metastases

Table 68.12 Hormonal agents

Premenopausal patients
LHRH agonists
Goserelin
Buserelin
Leuprolide

Postmenopausal patients
Aromatase inhibitors
First generation: aminoglutethimide, roglethimide
Second generation: steroidal (formestane)
Third generation: nonsteroidal (anastrozole, letrozole, vorozole); steroidal (exemestane)
Progestins
Medroxyprogesterone acetate
Megestrol acetate
Androgens
Fluoxymesterone

All ages
Antiestrogens
Nonsteroidal ("non-pure"): tamoxifen, toremifene, raloxifene, droloxifene
Steroidal ("pure"): faslodex
Corticosteroids

monal agents commonly used for the treatment of metastatic breast cancer are summarized in Table 68.12.

The following items should be emphasized:
- About one-third of unselected patients should be expected to respond, with a median duration of response of 8 to 14 months. Response rates are approximately 50 to 60% in patients whose primary tumor is ER-rich. Responses are more frequent in patients with prolonged disease-free survival (>2 years) and with metastatic presentation in soft tissues or bone.
- Response to one endocrine therapy predicts a higher chance of response to subsequent, second-line hormonal manipulation.
- Discontinuation of one endocrine therapy, such as progestins and antiestrogens at the time of disease progression, usually following an initial response, might induce a subsequent response ("withdrawal" response).
- Initiation of endocrine therapy may be accompanied in 3 to 9% of patients by an exacerbation of tumor-related symptoms ("flare"), which could develop within hours or days and last for several days or a few weeks. Flare, which is often followed by an objective response, has been observed with estrogens, tamoxifen, androgens, and progestins, but not with aromatase inhibitors.

Endocrine therapies have been developed to cover different endocrine-related mechanisms controlling tumor growth. Many of those mechanisms include the suppression of estrogens or of estrogen-mediated cell proliferation.

Other mechanisms include direct cytotoxicity on tumor cells, growth factor-mediated effects (such as increased production of the growth-inhibitor transforming growth factor beta [TGFβ] or reduced expression of insulin-like growth factor I [IGF-I]), and antiangiogenetic effects.

With the exception of ovarian ablation – which for premenopausal women remains a permanent treatment option

– the other forms of surgical endocrine ablation used in the past, such as adrenalectomy and hypophysectomy, have been made obsolete by the development of molecules that mimic the hormonal effect of such surgical treatments and have less side effects (luteinizing hormone-releasing hormone [LHRH] agonists, aromatase inhibitors).

Tamoxifen belongs to the family of synthetic nonsteroidal antiestrogens, which also includes toremifene, raloxifene, and droloxifene. The drug binds by competition to the estrogen receptor, altering the effects of the receptor-hormone complex and inducing arrest of growth. Additional mechanisms of growth inhibition have been ascribed to tamoxifen-induced TGFβ production and to the inhibition of tumor angiogenesis. Similarly to other antiestrogens of the same class, tamoxifen behaves as an antagonist (antiestrogen) or agonist (estrogen-like), depending on the target organ or tissue: the antiestrogenic effect is preminent on mammary glands, either normal or neoplastic, and the estrogenic effect prevails on the endometrium and on bone and lipid metabolism. Physiologic effects of tamoxifen on the hypothalamic-pituitary axis are estrogenic in postmenopause (lowering of circulating luteinizing hormone [LH] and follicle-stimulating hormone [FSH]) and antiestrogenic in premenopause (normal LH and FSH in the presence of elevated serum estrogen). Side effects of tamoxifen include amenorrhea, hot flashes, and vaginal discharge in a small proportion of patients, and, rarely, nausea and vomiting. It has been reported to modestly increase the risk of thromboembolic phenomena; its chronic use is associated with a two- to threefold increased risk of endometrial cancer in postmenopausal women.

The use of tamoxifen in premenopausal women may precede ovarian ablation or be associated with it. There is evidence that the combination of tamoxifen and goserelin, an LHRH analog, is superior to goserelin alone. For the postmenopausal woman, tamoxifen is considered first-line therapy. In case of response and subsequent relapse, progestins or an aromatase inhibitor of third generation is recommended.

Tamoxifen is usually administered at a daily dose of 20 mg. Its half-life after continuous administration is in excess of 200 hours; it requires 4 weeks or longer to achieve steady state blood levels, and these remain detectable for 6 to 12 weeks after discontinuation of treatment. Plasma levels at steady state are cytotoxic for breast cancer cell lines in vitro, while lower levels may only be cytostatic. Higher daily doses are not beneficial and may be associated with serious adverse effects (impaired visual acuity and retinopathy).

Progestins are an effective therapy in metastatic breast cancer. They work via a receptor-mediated mechanism as well as via interference with the pituitary-ovarian and pituitary-adrenal axes. Medroxyprogesterone acetate is administered at a dose of 500 mg per day; the dose for megestrol acetate is 160 mg once daily. Side effects are primarily weight gain, water retention, and other glucocorticoid-like effects.

Corticosteroids induce responses in 10 to 20% of the patients. They provide palliation, especially for bone pain and dyspnea, and are therefore particularly useful in terminal care.

The progenitor of the aromatase inhibitor family is aminoglutethimide. Its administration functions as a medical adrenalectomy, and patients receiving relatively high doses (1 gm daily) may need maintenance hydrocortisone and/or mineralocorticoid. Toxicity includes mild neurologic (mainly lethargy) and dermatologic (rash) symptoms. On rare occasions, reversible leukopenia and thrombocytopenia have been observed.

More recent steroidal and nonsteroidal new-generation aromatase inhibitors, with higher selectivity (no effect on adrenal steroidogenesis), are significantly less toxic and have improved aromatase inhibitory capacity. They include the steroidal aromatase inhibitors formestane and exemestane and the nonsteroidal ones anastrazole, vorozole, and letrozole. Aromatase inhibitors are reserved to postmenopausal women or women with prior ovarian ablation. The dose for anastrozole is 1 mg once a day and 2.5 mg daily for letrozole.

Agonists of luteinizing hormone-releasing hormone (LHRH analogs) primarily include goserelin, buserelin, and leuprolide. Their chronic administration (generally in depot formulation) depresses circulating estrogens to castrate levels, thus mimicking the effects of oophorectomy. However, while castrated women have high levels of circulating FSH and LH, women treated with LHRH superagonists have markedly low levels of gonadotropins.

Chemotherapy Cytotoxic antineoplastic drugs are indicated in patients whose aggressive disease requires a quick objective tumor response. Overall response rates for combination chemotherapy range from 40 to 90%, with complete responses in 5 to 35% (Tab. 68.13). The most commonly used drugs include cyclophosphamide, doxorubicin, epirubicin, methotrexate, fluorouracil, mitomycin C, mitoxantrone, taxanes (docetaxel, paclitaxel), and vinorelbine (Tab. 68.14).

The median time to maximal response to chemotherapy varies between 7 and 14 weeks, and the median duration of response ranges between 6 and 12 months. A small proportion of treated patients achieving a complete response (about 5%) are long-term survivors and might be cured.

Whether chemotherapy actually prolongs survival is controversial. Undoubtedly, the most significant factor for improved survival, as for improved quality of life, is

Table 68.13 Responses to first-line polychemotherapy

Overall response rate (%)	45 - 90
Complete response (%)	5 - 35
Median time to response (weeks)	4 - 8
Median duration of response (months)	5 - 13
Median survival of responders (months)	15 - 33

Table 68.14 Commonly used cytotoxic agents grouped by activity

Very active (>50% response rate)
Docetaxel
Doxorubicin
Epirubicin
Paclitaxel
Vinorelbine

Moderately active (20-50% response rate)
Cyclophosphamide
5-Fluorouracil
Methotrexate
Mitomycin C
Mitoxantrone
Vinblastine
Vincristine
Cisplatin

Weakly active (<20% response rate)
Actinomycin D
Carboplatin
Carmustine (BCNU)
Irinotecan
Etoposide
Gemcitabine
Idarubicin
Lomustine (CCNU)
Melphalan
Vindesine

response to treatment, complete response in particular. As with hormonal therapy, patients who benefit from chemotherapy may be treated successfully with other regimens at the time of progression. However, chances of response decrease about half with each subsequent treatment. After the best drugs are used to maximum effect, the remaining agents offer little benefit. Sometimes, however, the same drug that worked previously may have an effect later on. This is especially true if a significant period of time has elapsed and if a different schedule of administration is used. Combination chemotherapy has demonstrated a significantly higher response rate as compared to single agent chemotherapy in the majority of clinical trials.

The most frequently used drugs include cyclophosphamide, antracyclines, methotrexate, and 5-fluorouracil, which are all used in first-line combination regimens; and mitomycin C, mitoxantrone, taxanes, and vinorelbine. Taxanes and vinorelbine were shown to be very effective for patients with advanced cancer, and they have recently been incorporated in adjuvant trials.

Although it is reasonable to continue endocrine therapy until disease progression, the optimal duration of chemotherapy is unknown. A maximal useful duration of 6 months is indicated by clinical trials.

High-dose chemotherapy with hematopoietic growth factor support or megadose chemotherapy, followed by autologous bone marrow or peripheral blood progenitor cell reinfusion, have shown a significant rate of complete responses. However, many patients so-treated relapse and

Table 68.15 Therapy of specific metastatic sites

Site	Standard therapy	Open questions
Local-regional recurrence	Surgery if limited. Radiation controls about half of cases. Significant response rates (60-80%) with systemic therapy (chemotherapy or endocrine therapy if ER⁺)	Role of radical surgery. Role of adjuvant chemotherapy uncertain. Positive role of adjuvant tamoxifen in ER⁺ disease
Breast recurrence after breast-conserving surgery	Mastectomy. Lumpectomy in selected cases	Adjuvant systemic therapy
Contralateral breast	Usually as a new primary tumor	Adjuvant systemic therapy
Bone metastases	Systemic therapy. Radiation for localized pain and risk of fractures. Surgery might be considered for weight-bearing structures (femur, humerus)	Routine use of biphosphonates for reducing osteolysis and preventing fractures
Brain metastases	High-dose corticosteroids and radiation. Surgery for single accessible metastasis	Concurrent systemic and radiation therapy. High-dose chemotherapy
Spinal cord compression	High-dose corticosteroids. Radiotherapy. Laminectomy to relieve acute compression	Combination of systemic therapy and radiotherapy
Symptomatic malignant effusion	Drainage and systemic therapy. If pleural effusion, surgical pleurodesis in cases of relapse	Local administration of biological agents (interferons, interleukins)

(ER⁺ = estrogen receptor positive.)

die of the disease, and therefore this treatment modality should still be considered investigational.

Patients who fail to respond to conventional chemotherapy may be eligible for research protocols. These include new chemotherapeutic agents, new hormonal agents (e.g., "pure" antiestrogens such as faslodex), biologic therapies (antiangiogenetic factors, monoclonal antibodies to growth factor receptors, vaccines), and other treatments that have shown to be promising in preclinical models. Monoclonal antibodies to the putative growth factor receptor HER2/new can cause prolonged regression of HER2-positive advanced breast cancer, and combination with chemotherapy (taxol, adriamycin) is markedly superior to chemotherapy alone. Monoclonal antibodies against the epidermal growth factor receptor, tyrosine kinase, and protein kinase A inhibitors seem to be other promising agents.

Therapeutic issues related to special metastatic sites The treatment of metastatic disease is influenced by the involvement of distinct anatomical sites. Table 68.15 describes the issues related to the treatment of special sites.

PROSTATE CANCER

Fernand Labrie

Endocrinology of prostate cancer – intracrinology

Prostate cancer is very sensitive to androgen deprivation. However, although the first evidence of a positive response to androgen blockade was obtained in advanced disease, it is now clear that localized disease is much more sensitive to androgen deprivation. Despite the fact that the androgen blockade used by Huggins as primary treatment was only partial and limited to the blockade of androgens of testicular origin (approximately 50% of total androgens), the positive results obtained led to the use of orchiectomy or medical castration with high doses of estrogens as the standard treatment of metastatic prostate cancer for the next 50 years.

The next most important advance in our understanding of the endocrinology of prostate cancer was the observation that humans and some other primates are unique among animal species in having adrenals that secrete large amounts of the inactive precursor steroids dehydroepiandrosterone (DHEA), its sulfate DHEA-S, and some androstenedione (4-dione), which are converted into potent androgens in a large number of peripheral tissues, including the prostate (Fig. 68.2). In fact, plasma DHEA-S levels in adult men are 100 to 500 times higher than those of testosterone, thus providing high levels of the substrate required for conversion into androgens in the prostate as well as in other peripheral intracrine tissues.

Although orchiectomy, estrogens, or LHRH agonists or antagonists (through blockade of bioactive LH secretion) cause a 90 to 95% reduction in testosterone concentration in the circulation, a much smaller effect is seen on the only parameter directly reflecting androgenic action, namely the intraprostatic concentration of the potent

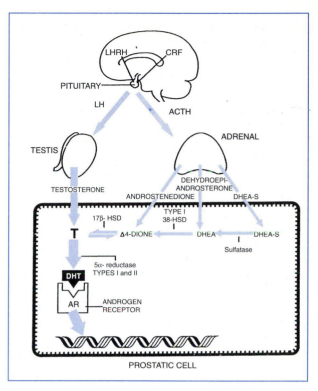

Figure 68.2 Intracrine activity in the human prostate or biosynthetic steps involved in the formation of the active androgen dihydrotestosterone (DHT) from testicular testosterone as well as from the adrenal precursors dehydroepiandrosterone (DHEA), DHEA-sulfate (DHEA-S), and androstenedione (4-dione) in human prostatic tissue. The widths of the arrows indicate the relative importance of the sources of DHT in the human prostate: approximately 60% of total intraprostatic DHT originates from the testes, while 40% is from adrenal origin in a 65-year-old man. The testis secretes testosterone (T), which is transformed into the more potent androgen DHT by 5α-reductase in the prostate. Instead of secreting T or DHT directly, the adrenal secretes very large amounts of precursors of DHT, namely DHEA and DHEA-S, as well as some androstenedione (4-dione), which are transported in the blood to the prostate and other peripheral tissues. These inactive precursors are then transformed locally into the active androgens T and DHT by intracrine activity. In fact, the enzymatic complexes DHEA sulfatase, 3β-HSD, 17β-HSD and 5α-reductase are all present in the prostatic cells, thus providing 40% of total DHT in this tissue. (17β-HSD = 17β-hydroxysteroid dehydrogenase; 3β-HSD = 3β-hydroxysteroid dehydrogenase/Δ5-Δ4-isomerase.)

androgen DHT. In fact, intraprostatic DHT levels are reduced by only 50 to 70% following medical or surgical castration.

The amounts of androgens synthesized from DHEA-S, DHEA, and 4-dione in each cell and tissue depend upon the relative levels of expression of the different steroidogenic enzymes, specifically, steroid sulfatase, 3β-hydroxysteroid dehydrogenase/Δ5-Δ4-isomerase, 17β-hydroxysteroid dehydrogenase, and 5α-reductase.

Combined androgen blockade

Metastatic disease

As indicated above, the discovery that the adrenals contribute 30 to 50% of total androgens in the human prostate through the local transformation of DHEA of adrenal origin into the potent androgen DHT clearly indicates that the most efficient androgen blockade should be a two-way approach. This approach should include: (1) the elimination of testicular androgens by orchiectomy or an LHRH agonist, combined at the start of treatment with (2) blockade of the action of DHT made locally in the prostate cancer using a pure antiandrogen, such as flutamide or one of its derivatives, namely nilutamide or bicalutamide at the appropriate dose.

Following our initial data, a series of prospective, randomized, and controlled clinical trials have demonstrated, for the first time in the field of prostate cancer, a prolongation of life by combined androgen blocking (CAB). Although the clinical data are not yet available for bicalutamide, the two antiandrogens flutamide and nilutamide have been shown, in prospective and randomized studies, to prolong life, to increase the number of complete and partial responses, to delay progression, and to provide better pain control (thus improving quality of life) in metastatic prostate cancer when added to surgical or medical castration compared to castration alone.

Discussion and controversy about the benefits of CAB should now be something of the past, since it has been determined that CAB adds an average of 6 to 12 months of cancer-specific survival in patients with metastatic disease. To the living population of males in the United States, where 3.0 million are expected to die from prostate cancer, 6 additional months of life correspond to the addition of 1.5 million years of life.

Intermittent androgen blockade is largely based upon the control of prostate-specific antigen (PSA). One should realize, however, that PSA, especially in localized disease, is exquisitely sensitive to androgen blockade. Its use can be extremely misleading and lead to a premature arrest of androgen blockade well before the cancer itself is under control.

CAB in localized disease

It is well-recognized that the only possibility of a significant reduction in prostate cancer death is treatment of localized disease.

Table 68.16 Clinical staging of prostate cancer

Description	TNM	Whitmore-Jewett
Incidental finding, no palpable tumor		
Local tumor cannot be evaluated	TX	
No local tumor detectable	T0	
Tumor found by chance in <5% of excised tissue	T1a	A1
Tumor found by chance in >5% of excised tissue	T1b	A2
Tumor diagnosed following elevated PSA	T1c	
Intracapsular tumor		
Tumor limited to half of one lobe or less	T2a	B1
Tumor has spread to more than half or one lobe but not to both	T2b	B2
Tumor has spread to both lobes	T2c	B3
Extracapsular tumor		
Unilateral extracapsular spread	T3a	C1
Bilateral extracapsular spread	T3b	
Tumor has spread to one or both seminal vesicles	T3c	C2
Tumor is attached to or has invaded adjacent structures other than the seminal vesicles	T4	
Disseminated tumor		
Local regional lymph nodes cannot be evaluated	NX	
No lymph node involvement	N0	
Lymph nodes <2 cm in diameter	N1	D1
One node only >2 cm or <5 cm; multiple nodes <5 cm	N2	
Distant metastases cannot be evaluated	MX	
No distant metastases	M0	
Distant metastases present	M1	D2
Lymph nodes other than regional nodes		
Skeletal		
Other sites		
Resistant to hormonal therapy		D3

(Adapted from Vogelsang NJ, Scardino PT, Shipley WU, Cossey DS, eds. Comprehensive textbook of genitourinary oncology. Baltimore: Williams & Wilkins, 1999;714-15.)

Screening strategy and staging of disease With the available technology, close to 100% of prostate cancers can now be diagnosed at the clinically localized stage, when cure is a possibility. This practically eliminates the diagnosis of metastatic and noncurable disease (Fig. 68.3 and Tab. 68.16). Instead of being medically nonsignificant, the fact is that at least 50% of the cancers diagnosed by screening have already migrated outside the prostate at the time of diagnosis and have already reached the stage of being noncurable by the standard approaches of surgery and radiotherapy. The appropriate treatment of these patients thus includes systemic endocrine therapy.

The most powerful tool by far for the early diagnosis of prostate cancer is PSA. Following rigorous scientific evaluation, the correlation established between serum PSA and the presence of prostate cancer shows *that 3 ng/ml and not 4 ng/ml should be used as the upper limit of normal serum PSA*. Accordingly, a serum PSA value above 3.0 ng/ml indicates a relatively high risk of prostate cancer. In fact, at first screening of men aged between 45 and 80 years, a serum PSA value above 3.0 ng/ml corresponds to a risk of approximately 20% of having detectable prostate cancer, while the risk decreases to only 1% for men having serum PSA at or below 3.0 ng/ml.

When screening is performed in the general population, digital rectal examination should be done at the first visit, in addition to serum PSA. If serum PSA is above 3.0 ng/ml (Hybritech test or its equivalent), trans-rectal ultra-sound (TRUS) is the next most important diagnostic approach. Trans-rectal ultrasound, however, is indicated only if serum PSA is above 3.0 ng/ml or if the digital rectal examination is abnormal (Fig. 68.3).

The Whitmore-Jewett and TNM classification systems are illustrated in Table 68.16. In fact, the TNM system is rapidly becoming the more widely used.

Choice of treatment of localized disease Despite the fact that clinically localized prostate cancer has become by far the predominant stage at diagnosis, there is no randomized and prospective comparison of the efficacy of the available treatments. The only exception is the recent and most important demonstration that the addition of androgen blockade to radiotherapy prolongs disease-free survival and overall survival compared to radiotherapy alone in stage T3 patients.

The lack of sufficient scientific information makes the choice of treatment difficult for localized disease. However, based upon the most rigorous evaluation of the data available in the literature and on our own experience, we will make the suggestions that in our opinion provide the best prospect for controlling the cancer while minimizing the risk of progression to metastatic disease, thus avoiding death from prostate cancer.

The treatment options for localized disease are radical

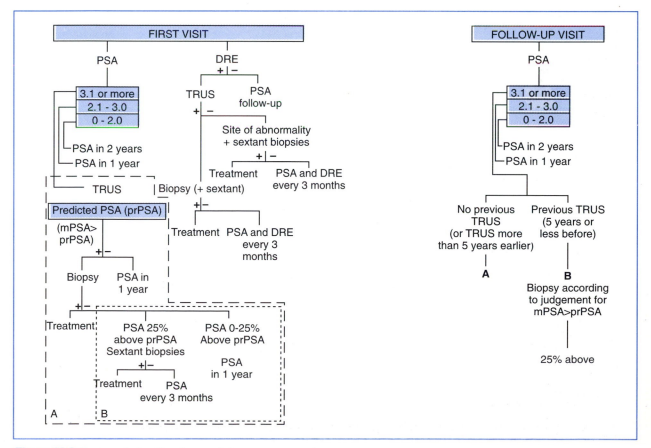

Figure 68.3 Proposed algorithm for prostate cancer screening.

prostatectomy, external beam radiotherapy, brachytherapy and hormone therapy alone, a combination of hormone therapy with surgery, radiotherapy, brachytherapy, or even – in rare cases – deferred treatment (watchful waiting). Life expectancy rather than the age of the patient should be the factor considered in treatment selection.

CAB in localized disease: high efficacy and duration of treatment It is pertinent to indicate that CAB alone is highly efficient in keeping localized prostate cancer under control. In fact, in 26 stage T2-T3 patients who received flutamide and an LHRH agonist for up to 12 years (median = 7.1 years), the first PSA rise occurred in only one patient after 7 years and 4 months of treatment. Such data obtained with continuous treatment with CAB alone in localized disease are superior to those obtained in comparable groups of patients treated by surgery or radiotherapy alone.

Such data combined with those of the 3-year treatment period of Bolla et al. (1997) – and the results obtained following 10.5 months versus 3 months of CAB associated with radiotherapy – indicate the importance of administering CAB as neoadjuvant (before surgery or radiation therapy) and/or adjuvant for a continuous period of a few years, probably five years.

CAB alone is a valid alternative, especially for patients aged 70 years or more and for those having a life expectancy of less than 10 years. In fact, in men unable to receive curative therapy and those having a less than 10-year life expectancy, CAB alone appears as a highly efficient means of controlling localized prostate cancer. For younger men having a more than 10-year life expectancy, the best approach, however, is likely to be the association of long-term CAB (probably 5 years) with surgery, radiotherapy, or brachytherapy. Because the aim of androgen blockade is to cause a maximal reduction in prostatic androgen levels in order to induce maximal atrophy, apoptosis, and death of prostate cancer cells; CAB using a pure antiandrogen in association with an LHRH agonist or surgical castration is the most logical approach instead of monotherapy, which only blocks 50 to 60% of androgens.

Suggested readings

AMERICAN JOINT COMMITTEE ON CANCER. Manual for staging of cancer. Fleming ID, Cooper JS, Henderson DE, et al (eds). Philadelphia: JB Lippincott, 1997.

BOLLA M, GONZALEZ D, WARDE P, et al. Improved survival in patients with locally advanced prostate cancer treated with radiotherapy and goserelin. N Engl J Med 1997;337:295-300.

DE PLACIDO S, DE LAURENTIIS F, PERRONE F, BIANCO AR. Carcinoma della mammella. In: Bianco AR (ed). Manuale di oncologia clinica. Milano: McGraw-Hill Libri Italia, 1996;103-29.

CAUBET JF, TOSTESON TD, DONG EW, et al. Maximum androgen blockade in advanced prostate cancer: a meta-analysis of published randomized controlled trials using nonsteroidal antiandrogens. Urology 1997;49:71-8.

EARLY BREAST CANCER TRIALIST'S COLLABORATIVE GROUP. Ovarian ablation in early breast cancer: overview of the randomized trials. Lancet 1996;348:1189-96.

EARLY BREAST CANCER TRIALIST'S COLLABORATIVE GROUP. Tamoxifen for early breast cancer: an overview of the randomized trials. Lancet 1998;351:1451-67.

EARLY BREAST CANCER TRIALIST'S COLLABORATIVE GROUP. Polychemotherapy for early breast cancer: an overview of the randomized trials. Lancet 1998;352:930-42.

FISHER B, COSTANTINO JP, WICKERHAM DL, et al. Tamoxifen for prevention of breast cancer: Report of the national surgical adjuvant breast and bowel project P-1 study. J Nat Cancer Inst 1998;90:1371-88.

HARRIS J, MORROW M, NORTON L. Malignant tumors of the breast. In: Devita VT, Hellman S, Rosenberg SE (eds). Cancer: principles and practice of oncology. Philadelphia, New York: JB Lippincott & Raven, 1997;1577-616.

LABRIE F, BÉLANGER A, CUSAN L, et al. Antifertility effects of LHRH agonists in the male. J Androl 1980;1:209-28.

LABRIE F, CANDAS B, CUSAN L, et al. Diagnosis of advanced or noncurable prostate cancer can be practically eliminated by prostate-specific antigen. Urology 1996;47:212-7.

LABRIE F, CUSAN L, GOMEZ JL, DIAMOND P, BÉLANGER A. Long-term neoadjuvant and adjuvant combined androgen blockade is needed for efficacy of treatment in localized prostate cancer. Mol Urol 1997;1:253-63.

LABRIE F, DUPONT A, SUBURU R, et al. Serum prostatic specific antigen (PSA) as prescreening test for prostate cancer. J Urol 1992;147:846-51.

LABRIE F, LUU-THE V, LIN SX, et al. The key role of 17β-HSDs in sex steroid biology. Steroids 1997;62:148-58.

LAVERDIERE J, GOMEZ JL, CUSAN L, et al. Beneficial effect of combination therapy administered prior and following external beam radiation therapy in localized prostate cancer. Int J Radiat Oncol Biol Phys 1997;37:247-52.

CHAPTER
69

Carcinoid tumors

Aaron I. Vinik

Carcinoid tumors, the most frequently encountered tumors of the gastroenteropancreatic axis, are also found in extra-gastroenteropancreatic sites.

Epidemiology

More than 50% of neuroendocrine tumors in clinical practice are of the so-called carcinoid variety. The remaining distribution is approximately 50% gastrinomas, 30% insulinomas, 13% vipomas, 5 to 10% glucagonomas, and <5% neurotensinomas, somatostatinomas, and ectopic hormone-secreting tumors. Nonsecretory tumors were at one time thought to make up the bulk of pancreatic tumors. However, with better immunohistochemical stains for endocrine cells – especially for neuron-specific enolase, chromogranin, synaptophysin, and receptors for somatostatin – there is increasing recognition that tumors masquerading as carcinomas of liver, small cell carcinoma of the lung and the like, are, in effect, endocrine tumors. The majority of these "nonsecretory" tumors actually store and secrete pancreatic polypeptide, but because pancreatic peptide has so little biologic activity, the tumors remain silent.

The incidence of carcinoid tumors is estimated to be approximately 1.5 cases per 100 000 of the general population, that is, about 2500 cases per year in the United States. Nonetheless, they account for 13 to 34% of all tumors of the small bowel and 17 to 46% of all malignant tumors of the small bowel. The most frequent sites for carcinoid tumors are the gastrointestinal tract (73%) and the bronchopulmonary system (27%). Within the gastrointestinal tract, most tumors are found in the small bowel (28.7%), appendix (18.9%), and rectum (12.6%). Of great interest and importance to patient surveillance was a finding that associated noncarcinoid tumors were frequent in conjunction with small intestine (16.6%), appendiceal (14.6%), and colonic carcinoids (13.1%). Whether or not these tumors are dependent upon the tumor products of carcinoids or cosegregate in the same individuals needs to be explored.

Carcinoids are derived from a primitive stem cell and are generally found in the gut wall. Carcinoids may, however, occur in the pancreas, rectum, ovary, lung, and else-where. The tumors grow slowly and are often clinically silent for many years before becoming manifest, usually when metastases have occurred. They frequently metastasize to the regional lymph nodes, the liver, and less commonly to bone. The likelihood of metastases is related to tumor size: the incidence of metastases is less than 2% with a carcinoid tumor less than 1 cm in size, but it rises to 100% with tumors greater than 2 cm in diameter. These tumors may be only episodically symptomatic and their existence may go unrecognized for many years. The average time from the onset of symptoms attributable to the tumor and diagnosis is a little over 9 years and is usually made only when the carcinoid syndrome occurs, however the syndrome only occurs in less than 10% of patients with carcinoid tumors. The syndrome is especially common in tumors of the ileum and jejunum, but it also occurs with bronchial, ovarian, and other carcinoids. One of the more clinically useful characterizations of carcinoid tumors is to classify them according to the division of the primitive gut from which the tumor cells arise. There are two types of foregut carcinoid tumors: sporadic primary tumors and tumors secondary to achlorhydria. Sporadic primary foregut tumors include carcinoids of the bronchus, the stomach, the first portion of the duodenum, and the pancreas. Midgut carcinoid tumors derive from the second portion of the duodenum, the jejunum, ileum, and right colon. Hindgut carcinoid tumors include those of the transverse colon, left colon, and rectum. This distinction assists in distinguishing a number of important biochemical and clinical differences between carcinoid tumors, since the presentation, histochemistry, and secretory products are quite different (Tab. 69.1).

Foregut carcinoids are argentaffin-negative. They have a low content of serotonin (5-hydroxytryptamine, 5-HT). They often secrete the serotonin precursor 5-hydroxytryptophan (5-HTP) and histamine and a multitude of polypeptide hormones. Their functional manifestations include atypical carcinoid syndrome, gastrinoma syndrome, acromegaly, Cushing's disease, and a number of other endocrine disorders. Furthermore, they are unusual in that the flush that occurs tends to be of protracted duration, is often of a purplish or violaceous hue rather than the usual pink-red color, and frequently leaves permanent telangiectasia and skin hypertrophy of the face and upper neck. The face assumes a leonine characteristic after repeated episodes. It is not unusual for these tumors to metastasize to bone. Gastric carcinoids may have a distinctive pathogenesis and clinical relevance compared with other foregut carcinoids. It seems that long-standing hypergastrinemia per se does not lead to gastric carcinoid formation (for example, in the gastrinoma syndrome in the absence of an associated abnormality such as multiple endocrine neoplasia [MEN] syndrome). Rather, multiple small tumors of low malignant potential are found in the gastric fundus/body of patients with atrophic gastritis type A in which hypergastrinemia coexists with atrophic gastritis and pernicious anemia.

Midgut carcinoids, in contrast, are argentaffin-positive, have a high 5-HT content, rarely secrete 5-HTP, and often produce a number of other vasoactive compounds such as kinins, prostaglandins, and substance P. The clinical syndrome that results is the classic carcinoid syndrome. These tumors may produce adrenocorticotropic hormone (ACTH), albeit rarely, and very infrequently metastasize to bone.

Hindgut carcinoids are argentaffin-negative. They rarely contain 5-HT, rarely secrete 5-HTP or other peptides, and are usually silent in their presentation, but they may metastasize to bone.

A further point of interest is the finding that if a carcinoid tumor coexists with multiple endocrine neoplasia type I (MEN-I), more than two-thirds of the time in males the tumor is in the thymus, whereas greater than 75% of the time in females it is in the lung.

Prior to 1980 most of these tumors were found inci-dentally at post mortem. Indeed, two-thirds were found in the appendix or adjacent ileocecal region because of the tendency for surgeons to excise the appendix during laparotomy in which incidental carcinoid tumors were found. With increasing sophistication, this number has fallen to about one-third. A near 25% frequency of lung tumors has replaced the frequency of the small intestine tumors. This may not be due to a real growth in the number of these tumors, but rather the evolution of recognition because of improved immunohistochemistry. Many tumors previously identified as small or squamous carcinomas of the lung have turned out to be carcinoid tumors. It is important to make this distinction because of the very different prognosis. A similar trebling in the frequency of ovarian carcinoid has occurred over the same time period, which is probably also due to improved immunohisto-chemistry (Tab. 69.2).

Age distribution

The distribution of carcinoids is gaussian in nature. The peak incidence occurs in the sixth and seventh decades but includes patients as young as 10 years of age as well as people in their ninth decade. Males and females are affected almost equally.

The natural history

Carcinoid tumors are slow growing and may be present for years without overt symptoms. In the early stages, vague abdominal pain goes undiagnosed and is invariably ascribed to irritable bowel or spastic colon. Fully one-third of patients with carcinoid tumors present with years of intermittent abdominal pain (Fig. 69.1).

Table 69.1 Clinical and biochemical characteristics of carcinoid tumors

Location	Clinical	Biochemical
Gastric Primary sporadic Secondary to achlorhydria	Same as foregut Pernicious anemia, atrophic gastritis, gastric polyps, gastrin >1000 pg/ml	Same as foregut Totipotential
Foregut Bronchus Stomach Proximal duodenum	Atypical carcinoid, protracted flushing, wheezing, ZE, Cushing's, acromegaly, hyponatremia, heart disease, moderate to high metastatic potential (25% liver/bone)	Elevated 5-HTP (high MAO, low aromatic acid decarboxylase activity), histamine, multiple peptides: hCG, ACTH, GH, GHRH, gastrin, tachykinins
Midgut Distal duodenum, jejunum, ileum, appendix, right colon. Argentaffin and argrophil +tive	Classical carcinoid syndrome (80%), typical flush, hypotension, diarrhea, wheezing, heart disease. Metastatic potential, liver (60-80%)	5-HT, bradykinin, substance P, CGRP, neurokinin, others
Hindgut Transverse colon to rectum Argyrophil +tive	Silent, may contain 5-HT, SRIF, GLI, PYY neurotensin and tachykinins. Metastases 5-40%	Usually nonsecretory

(Modified from Perry and Vinik Annual Rev Med 1996:57-68). (Argentaffin+tive = precipitation of silver in absence of reducing agent; argyrophil+tive = precipitation of silver only in presence of reducing agent; SRIF = somatotropin release-inhibiting factor (somatostatin); PYY = peptide tyrosine; tyrosine; 5-HT = 5-hydroxytryptamine; 5-HTP = 5-hydroxytryptophan; GH = growth hormone; GHRH = growth hormone-releasing hormone; ADH = vasopressin; ACTH = adrenocorticotropin; MAO = monamineoxidase; CGRP = calcitonin gene-related peptide; GLI = glucagon like immunoreactivity.)

Table 69.2 Sites of primary carcinoid tumors

Primary site	Percent
Intestinal	
Small intestine	28
Ileocecal/appendix	22
Pancreas	17
Colon	9
Stomach	4
Hepatobiliary	4
Duodenum	3
Esophagus, rectum, other	10
Extraintestinal	
Lung	9
Thymus	<1
Ovary	20

Clinical findings

In more than one-third of patients, the major clinical manifestations of carcinoid syndrome, after years of vague abdominal pain, include cutaneous flushing (84%), gastrointestinal hypermotility with diarrhea (70%), and heart disease (37%). In addition, bronchial constriction (including asthma and dyspnea) occurs in 17%, a proximal myopathy in 7%, and an abnormal increase in skin pigmentation in 5% of the cases. With extensive metastases, about one-third of the patients will present with hepatomegaly, 25% with weight loss, and 20% with marked edema. With the introduction of a better means of treatment of the condition, patients are living longer, and thus a greater prevalence of carcinoid cardiopathy (17-37%) is emerging, as well as hypertrophic osteoarthropathy (1-2%) and teleangiectasia with overgrowth of certain facial features (10%).

Intestinal tumors predominantly metastasize to the liver (80%), lymph nodes (44%), the peritoneum, and mesentery (20%); they also metastasize to lung, bone, adrenal, skin, and many other unusual places, such as the pituitary, thyroid, and breast. Extraintestinal tumors, on the other hand, can produce the clinical syndrome without metastasizing since the hormones are delivered directly to the systemic circulation. When they do spread, the liver is the target 60% and the lymph nodes 25% of the time. These tumors have twice the likelihood of metastasizing to lung, bone, skin, and adrenal.

Diagnosis

The diagnosis of carcinoid tumors is based upon a strong clinical suspicion in patients who present with flushing, diarrhea, wheezing, myopathy, and right heart disease, and includes appropriate biochemical and localization studies.

Biochemical studies The rate-limiting step in carcinoid tumors for the synthesis of serotonin is the conversion of tryptophan into 5-hydroxytryptophan (5-HTP). In midgut tumors, 5-HTP is rapidly converted to 5-hydroxytryptamine (5-HT). Circulating 5-HT is then largely converted into the urinary metabolite 5-hydroxyindoleacetic acid (5-HIAA). In patients with foregut tumors, the urine contains relatively little 5-HIAA but large amounts of 5-HTP. For midgut carcinoids, the gold standard remains urinary 5-HIAA. The normal range for 5-HIAA secretion is 2 to 8 mg per 24 hours. False-negatives may be obtained in patients taking salicylates or L-Dopa; 24-hour urinary 5-HIAA has a sensitivity of 75% and >90% specificity. In

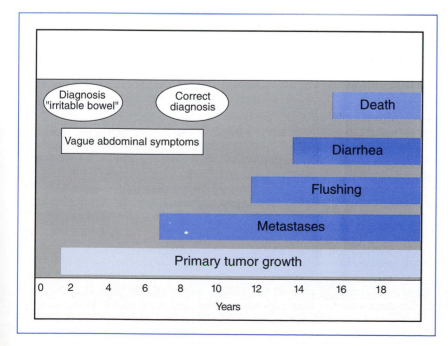

Figure 69.1 The natural history of carcinoid tumors. (From Vinik AI, Moattari AR. Use of somatostatin analogue in the management of carcinoid syndrome. Dig Dis Sci 1989; 34:14s.)

carcinoid tumors, neurotensin is elevated in 43%, substance P in 32%, motilin in 14%, somatostatin in 5% of cases, and vasoactive intestinal polypeptide (VIP) rarely.

Localization studies   A chest X-ray or CT suffices to detect bronchial carcinoids. In contrast, carcinoids of the cecum, right colon, and hindgut are usually demonstrable by endoscopy or barium enema examination. The greatest problems encountered are in localizing small bowel carcinoids (which may be small), and carcinoids in extra-intestinal sites. Abdominal CT scans and ultrasounds are usually not helpful because the primary tumors are below the resolution capacity of even the most sophisticated scanning apparatus, though superior mesenteric angiography may be of help.

Barium examinations are rarely diagnostic, but they may demonstrate fixation, separation, thickening, and angulation of the bowel loops. Computer tomography is the primary diagnostic procedure for tumor staging; it allows for the assessment of the extent of tumor spread to the mesentery and bowel wall, as well as metastases to the lymph nodes and liver.

Magnetic resonance imaging (MRI) is a very sensitive technique for the detection of liver metastases, but it appears to be less sensitive for the diagnosis of extrahepatic disease. MRI can, however, visualize bronchial carcinoids that have been missed by CT.

The role of angiography in the diagnosis of carcinoid tumors has been decreased by the availability of the new imaging methods. Diagnostic angiography is generally employed when noninvasive imaging studies are equivocal and surgery is contemplated. Positron-emission tomography (PET) has been used, but the experience thus far is very limited.

The sensitivity of ^{111}In-DTPA Octreotide scintigraphy for the detection of primary and metastatic carcinoid tumors approaches 80 to 90%. It may reveal unsuspected metastases or those not detected by other imaging methods in up to two-thirds of patients. A positive scan predicts a positive symptomatic response to Octreotide treatment and thus a better prognosis, whereas a negative scan suggests a more malignant tumor that may be better treated with chemotherapeutic agents such as cisplatinum and/or etoposide. However, the technique appears to be insensitive in detecting tumors less than 1cm in diameter or in detecting liver metastases, particularly when they are small. There are a host of conditions and sites in which the accumulation of ^{111}In-DTPA-d-Phe1 Octreotide may occur: non-small cell and small cell lung cancer (100%), other non-carcinoid endocrine tumors (55-90%), meningiomas (100%), breast cancer stages I and II (>60%), granulomatous diseases (sarcoidosis, TB, systemic mycoses), renal carcinomas, external lung radiation, bleomycin-induced pulmonary fibrosis, recent operation sites, and in the nasal region. This must serve as a caveat for adopting the attitude that a positive scan is diagnostic of a carcinoid tumor.

Thus, Octreotide scintigraphy, although useful, is likely to be of limited benefit in identifying small primary tumors and liver metastases. This imaging technique may prove to be most valuable in identifying metastatic disease to extra-abdominal sites. In addition to tumor imaging, Octreotide scanning may be useful in predicting responses to Octreotide. Further enhancements of the technique has been the development of the intraoperative use of a hand-held gamma camera that allows one to locate tumors <10 mm in size.

In the remaining cases in whom the tumor has not been identified by the above techniques, total body venous sampling with measurement of a peptide hormone that is produced may be considered. Measurements of serotonin may be misleading, but measurements of substance P may well direct attention to the source of overproduction of the peptide. This has proved useful in substance P-producing tumors.

Carcinoid syndrome   Carcinoid syndrome occurs in less than 10% of patients with carcinoid tumors. The principal features of carcinoid syndrome include flushing, sweating, wheezing, diarrhea, abdominal pain, cardiac fibrosis, and pellagra dermatosis. Diarrhea is found in 83% of cases, flushing in 49%, dyspnea in 20%, and bronchospasm in 6%. The specific etiologic agent(s) for each of the protean manifestations of the carcinoid tumors are not known. Serotonin, prostaglandins, 5-hydroxytryptophan, substance P, kallikrein, histamine, dopamine, and neuropeptide K are thought to be involved in the clinical manifestations of carcinoid tumors. In addition, symptoms may be related to overproduction of peptides of the proopiomelanocortin family, such as endorphin and enkephalin. Pancreatic polypeptide and motilin levels are often raised; they may be important markers of tumor activity and may provide a means of monitoring tumor growth and response to therapy rather than contributing to specific symptomatology.

Serotonin – which is measured either as its urinary metabolite, 5-HIAA, or as whole blood serotonin – is raised in 84% of patients with carcinoid tumors. Urinary 5-HIAA alone had a 73% sensitivity and 100% specificity. Neurotensin and substance P are raised in 43 and 32% of patients with specificity values of 60 and 85%, respectively. Motilin and somatostatin are raised in 14 and 50%, respectively. It appears that a high serotonin level is a predictor of the development of carcinoid heart disease and of poor prognosis.

Diarrhea   The diarrhea syndrome that occurs with carcinoid tumors is usually of a secretory nature. Diarrhea persists with fasting or fails to disappear when feeding has been curtailed and sustenance is given by the intravenous route. There are, however, a number of other causes of secretory diarrhea, but virtually all endocrine diarrheas are secretory in nature (Tab. 69.3).

Flushing   Flushing in carcinoid syndrome is of two varieties. With a midgut carcinoid, the flush is usually of a faint pink to red color and involves the face and upper trunk as far as the nipple line. The flush is initially provoked by alcohol and food-containing tyramines such as

Table 69.3 Causes of secretory diarrhea

Carcinoid syndrome
Medullary cancer of the thyroid (MCT)
Watery diarrhea, hypokalemia, hypochlorhydria,
  acidosis syndrome (WDHHA), e.g., vipomas
Gastrinoma syndrome (Zollinger Ellison)
Secreting villous adenoma of the rectum
Surreptitious laxative ingestion
Idiopathic

blue cheese, chocolate, red sausage, and red wine. With time the flush may occur spontaneously without provocation. It is usually ephemeral, lasting only a few minutes, and it may occur many times per day but does not usually leave permanent discoloration. In contrast, the flush of foregut tumors is often more intense, of protracted duration, lasting hours, purplish in hue, is frequently followed by telangiectasia, and involves not only the upper trunk but also the limbs. The limbs may become acrocyanotic, and the nose resembles that of rhinophyma. The skin of the face often thickens with the appearance of a leonine facies that resembles the features seen in leprosy and acromegaly.

Flushing cannot always be attributed to a carcinoid syndrome. The differential diagnosis of flushing includes: the postmenopausal state, simultaneous ingestion of chlorpropamide and alcohol, panic attacks, medullary carcinoma of the thyroid, autonomic epilepsy, autonomic neuropathy, and mastocytosis (Tab. 69.4).

Flushing in carcinoid syndrome has been ascribed to prostaglandins, kinins, and serotonin (5-HT), and other neurohumors, including: serotonin, dopamine, histamine and 5-HIAA, kallikrein, substance P, neurotensin, motilin, somatostatin, vasoactive intestinal polypeptide, prostaglandins, neuropeptide K, and gastrin-releasing peptide.

Carcinoid heart syndrome

Carcinoid heart disease is a heart disease uniquely associated with this cancer; it may be seen in up to 60% of patients with metastatic carcinoid. Valvular disease is the most common pathologic feature; tricuspid damage is found in 97%; and pulmonary valve disease in 88%, with 88% displaying insufficiency and 49% stenosis. Ovarian carcinoids are a rare variety in which cardiac involvement occurs without metastases to the liver because of the direct drainage of the ovarian veins into the systemic circulation. Carcinoid heart disease is the only condition in

Table 69.4 Distinction between flushing syndromes

Flushing syndrome	Associated features	Diagnostic tests	Treatments
Carcinoid	Diarrhea, wheezing, myopathy	Urine 5-HIAA, 5-HTP, substance P, chromogranin, NKA	Octreotide, peptide antagonists, decrease tumor bulk
Medullary cancer of thyroid	Mass in the neck, FH	Calcitonin, pentagastrin stimulation test TCT	Thyroid ablation
Pheochromocytoma	Paroxysmal hypertension, tachycardia	VMA, catecholamines	Tumor extirpation alpha and beta-blockers
Diabetes	Chlorpropamide, alcohol ingestion, autonomic neuropathy	FPG > 126 mg/dl	Avoid alcohol and chlorpropamide, scopolamine patches
Menopause	Cessation of menses	FSH	Estrogen, clonidine
Mastocytosis	Dyspepsia, ulcer disease, dermatographia	Plasma histamine, tryptase	$H_1 + H_2$ blockers or cromolyn
Diencephalic seizures	Autonomic epilepsy	EEG	Antiepileptic drugs
Panic syndrome	Phobias, anxiety, underlying condition	Pentagastrin stimulation test for ACTH	Sertroline or alprazolam
Drugs Niacin, Ca^{++} antagonists, iv contrast, disulfuram, alcohol+chlorpropamide or disulfuram		None	Use slow release agents, titrate slowly, add aspirin
Idiopathic	None	None	H_1 or H_2 blockers, Octreotide

(FSH = follicle-stimulating hormone; Ca^{++} = calcium; iv = intravenous.)

which both right-sided valves are involved and the combination of pulmonary stenosis and tricuspid regurgitation occur. The development of pulmonary stenosis favors the development of tricuspid regurgitation. In approximately 20% of patients with carcinoid disease, the presenting symptom may be attributable to heart failure (Tab. 69.5).

The dismal prognosis of patients with carcinoid heart disease of < 20% 5-year survival compared with > 66% in patients with tumors treated with Octreotide dictates a need for a much more aggressive approach to management. Up until 1995, 38 patients had been reported in either single case studies or within a small series of patients who had undergone valve replacement. There were no significant differences in the survival of patients with bioprosthesis versus a mechanical prosthesis in the tricuspid valve position. Long-term survival was predicated by low serotonin values, and none of the patients <60 years died early. All who survived had symptomatic improvement. Balloon valvulotomy has had mixed results.

Thus, if the distinction between symptoms due to cardiac disease are recognized early, before there is marked elevation of the serotonin levels (especially in patients under the age of 60 years and without EKG evidence of low voltage), it is probably prudent to aggressively replace the tricuspid and pulmonary valves. Prolongation of life can be achieved and, more importantly, the quality of life is greatly enhanced for the remaining years.

Treatment

Medical treatment

Different therapeutic agents have been used with variable success, but eventual relapse with increasing resistance to drugs is usually encountered. Since a carcinoid is a slow growing tumor, even patients with extensive metastatic disease can enjoy a normal quality of life so long as the endocrine syndrome is quiescent. Different chemical agents such as antagonists of 5-HT$_1$, (methysergide), 5-HT$_2$ (ketanserin), cyproheptadine, heparin, phenothiazines, alpha-adrenergic antagonists, corticosteroids, H$_1$ and H$_2$ anti-histamine blockers, symptomatic treatment of diarrhea with opioids, and codeine have been tried with

variable results. Bronchodilators may be helpful if there is bronchoconstriction. However, progressive pulmonary fibrosis can cause dyspnea that is refractory to almost all forms of intervention. Niacin may be needed for the pellagra syndrome due to a deficiency created by enhanced synthesis of serotonin from tryptophan using niacin as a cofactor. Since somatostatin has very broad inhibitory effects, somatostatin-14 has been used successfully to suppress diarrhea and flushing in patients with carcinoid tumors, but its clinical use is limited by its short half-life, with the resulting need for continuous intravenous infusion. With the advent of the long-acting somatostatin analogue, Octreotide, it has been used in the treatment of different neuroendocrine tumors, including carcinoids.

Serotonin is the major product of carcinoid tumors, but its action explains only part of the symptom complex. Undoubtedly many of the features are ascribable to a variety of other amines and peptides produced by these tumors (Tab. 69.1).

Various chemotherapeutic agents, including parachlorophenylalanine, cyproheptadine, methotrimeprazine, corticosteroids, aprotinin, phenoxybenzamine, ketanserin, H$_1$ and H$_2$ histamine antagonists such as diphenhydramine, cyproheptadine, cimetidine, sodium cromoglycate, aprotinin, and numerous antineoplastic agents have been used in carcinoid syndrome with variable success. These medications either inhibit serotonin synthesis, act as systemic antagonists of serotonin, or block kallikrein release. Others neutralize histamine that is either co-secreted by the tumor or potentiated by serotonin. Cromoglycate inhibits histamine release, and steroids and aprotinin inhibit bradykinin synthesis. A number of peptide antagonists have been developed but are in the early stages – phase 1 or 2 – of research. Most recently, somatostatin 14 and its long-acting analog, Octreotide, have been used successfully to control symptoms of diarrhea and flushing in the carcinoid syndrome, but they may be less effective for bronchospasm and appear not to influence the course of cardiac disease. Objective improvement in the symptom complex, a 50% reduction in tumor markers, a decrease in tumor bulk and in symptoms occurs in >70% of patients for a median duration of 12 months and was reported to prolong survival threefold when compared with historical data. Although Octreotide can shrink both the primary and secondary tumors, the effect is not pronounced. It acts by direct antimitotic action; and it may be additive with cytotoxic actions in vitro, alter angiogenesis, or modulate immunological activity. Occasionally massive tumor necrosis occurs. The prediction of a successful response may be predicated by a positive Octreotide scan. Loss of responsiveness is now well-recognized. When it occurs early it is thought to be due to the down-regulation of receptors, which is restorable with a short period of abstinence from the drug. However, loss of responsiveness that progresses with time may be due to the development of alternate receptors that do not bind to Octreotide or receptor-negative clones.

Octreotide is usually administered three times daily by subcutaneous injection. Starting doses are usually on the order of 150 µg tid, but dose escalation may be necessary;

Table 69.5 Distinguishing features of carcinoid heart syndrome and carcinoid symptoms

Carcinoid heart symptoms	Carcinoid symptoms
Dyspnea	Flushing
Fatigue	Diarrhea
Ascites	Bronchospasm
Anorexia	Hypotension
Edema	Tachycardia

the maximum daily dose is 1500 µg. Side effects of the drug are minimal and usually only occur with doses >500 µg per day. Anorexia, nausea, and vomiting may occur but can usually be avoided if the dose is titrated carefully. Diarrhea or steatorrhea can be confusing, since this is often the symptom that is being treated. The diarrhea induced by somatostatin is due to fat malabsorption; thus; a fecal fat content of >25 g can thus be helpful since the diarrhea of carcinoids is not due to fat malabsorption. Of greater difficulty in decision-making is the propensity to develop gallstones because of the inhibition of gallbladder contraction. Gallstones occur in about 20% of patients treated for >1 month. It is advisable to obtain a gallbladder ultrasound before starting therapy and if stones are present to do a prophylactic cholecystectomy.

Surgical treatment

Carcinoid tumors

Surgical removal of the primary tumor is the treatment of choice for small and localized tumors and for the alleviation of any obstructive symptoms, but surgical cure of carcinoids is almost impossible in the presence of intra-abdominal and hepatic metastases. Appendiceal tumors <1 cm can be treated by simple appendectomy, whereas those >2 cm require right hemicolectomy and regional lymph node removal. In other situations, the extent of surgery is dictated by tumor size. Nonetheless, it is often salutary to debulk tumors to relieve obstructive symptoms and induce responsiveness to chemotherapeutic intervention. Careful evaluation of symptoms and signs of cardiac involvement dictates an aggressive approach to tricuspid and pulmonary valve replacement or pulmonary valvulotomy. After the age of 60 the perioperative mortality for valvular surgery is as high as 50%, which must be considered in decision-making.

Gastric carcinoids

No simple straightforward approach to surgical treatment of gastric carcinoids has evolved. For the patient with Type A chronic atrophic gastritis, endoscopic resection and surveillance for patients with less than five tumors that are <1 cm size are recommended. If the gastrin level is >1000 pg/ml, however, there are more than five tumors, or there is recurrence, we advocate antrectomy to remove the source of gastrin. Excision and antrectomy are also recommended for tumors >1 cm, and gastrectomy is advised if there is local invasion or lymph node metastases. For the patient with sporadic nonatrophic gastritis-related gastric carcinoid, aggressive surgery is recommended because of the highly malignant potential. Multicentric carcinoids found as part of the MEN syndrome can be watched and treated surgically only if they develop into macrocarcinoids.

Bronchial carcinoids

For the most part a conservative tumor excision is all that is necessary.

Rectal carcinoids

Although surgical excision is mandated for rectal carcinoids, there remains a relatively high rate of mortality even after removal of the lesion. It would seem that a more aggressive form of treatment should be considered.

Surgery may also be considered in patients with localized metastasis or when the metastasis has been shown angiographically to have a single large vascular feeder. Reports of cure in 10 to 25% of these cases may be achieved with hepatic artery embolization using Gelfoam or Ivalon particles (<250 µ) or by surgical resection. Great care should be exercised when preparing a patient for embolization, since the tissue necrosis that occurs is often accompanied by a release of a variety of vasoactive peptides and amines that can result in a carcinoid crisis with profound hypotension. It is thus advisable to prepare the patient beforehand as if they had a crisis (see below). Palliative debulking of tumors may substantially reduce symptoms and render tumors responsive to chemotherapy. There is limited experience with hepatic and/or multiple organ transplantation, but a survival time of 13 months has been reported.

Prognosis

The general prognosis for carcinoid tumors is excellent in comparison to other visceral cancers. Based upon a world literature of some 8305 cases, the median 5-year survival for all cases is 82%. If the tumor is localized the 5-year survival is 94%, decreasing to 64% with regional lymph node involvement and to 18% with distant metastases. The major causes of death are carcinoid heart disease (43%) and cachexia due to mesenteric vascular entrapment (35%). Median survival is 11 years in patients with irresectable metastases, 7 years with liver metastases, and 1 year with extra-abdominal spread. Metastatic potential is linked to tumor size; in hindgut tumors the risk is less than 2% for tumors <1 cm in maximum diameter and over 80% in tumors >2 cm.

Evaluation of responses to Octreotide (Fig. 69.2)

Flushing There is often a dramatic response of flushing during treatment with somatostatin, with a clear decrease in this symptom with doses of Octreotide 6 to 20 µg/kg per day. In no instance has there been a resistance to the drug. Tachyphylaxis does not occur, and withdrawal of the drug or substitution with distilled water is always followed by recurrence of the symptom complex. However, in certain patients the severity decreases only slightly and the duration of each episode is essentially unchanged.

Carcinoid crisis The extreme example of flushing is the carcinoid crisis, in which there is a profound fall in blood pressure, or a hypertensive crisis, with or without severe bronchospasm. Precipitating factors include anesthesia, fine needle aspiration, and tumor embolization. It is deemed unwise to submit a patient to anesthesia or to an operation without premedication with a combination of adrenergic blockade, steroids, Thorazine, and aspirin. Preoperative use of Octreotide may also help prevent a carcinoid crisis. Octreotide at a dose of 150 to 500 μg can be given subcutaneously as prophylaxis or even during or after the procedure. In the event of a crisis, 50 to 100 μg can be given intravenously. Anesthetists should be warned that the use of sympathetic vasoconstrictors is contraindicated since they are likely to aggravate the crisis.

Responses of diarrhea In our experience, diarrhea occurs in 86% of patients and responds variably to Octreotide. Only 58% of patients with diarrhea have complete remission, while improvement is found in 76% of patients. This could be due to the fact that diarrhea in patients with carcinoid tumors has multiple etiologies. The diarrhea may even appear to worsen with the appearance of steatorrhea, and the physician is frequently faced with the confounding situation of not knowing to what to attribute the symptom.

Perioperative management

Carcinoid and other gastroenteropancreatic tumors can be a major therapeutic problem perioperatively when vast quantities of active peptides are released into the circulation because of the manipulation of tumors. Octreotide has been shown to be an effective suppressor of the release and action of peptide hormones during surgery. It has been shown that profound refractory hypotension in carcinoid syndrome can be rapidly reversed by Octreotide, as well as gastric acid secretion and fistula drainage.

Biochemical responses There are conflicting reports regarding the biochemical responses of carcinoid patients

to Octreotide. In our patients, urinary 5-HIAA dropped in almost all patients and normalized in one-third of the patients. Four out of eight patients normalized their 24-hour 5-HIAA levels. Although few of our patients had a fall in their blood serotonin level, the overall post-Octreotide values were not significantly lower than pre-treatment values.

Responses of tumor growth and metastases to Octreotide Due to the slow growth of carcinoid tumors, it is difficult to assess the effect of Octreotide on the rate of tumor growth or regression. It appears that cessation or reversal of growth occurs in about two-thirds of patients with carcinoid tumors treated with Octreotide.

Short of an effective curative or palliative agent, Octreotide can control flushing and wheezing in most and diarrhea in some patients with carcinoid tumors, with improvement in their general condition. The effects of Octreotide on tumor growth need to be further evaluated in relation to the slow progression and indolent nature of these tumors. Octreotide increases the median survival of patients with metastatic carcinoid from 11 to 33 months.

When there is clear evidence that tumor growth is not contained by Octreotide, alternative forms of treatment should be considered. Clinical trials are now underway with a microsphere-encapsulated slow-release formulation of a newer analog called lanreotide. These analogs also target the type 2 receptor subtype but bind to subtype 5 equally well and to a lesser extent subtype 4. This confers an advantage over Octreotide, as does the half-life time of 3 to 4 days, allowing treatment by intramuscular injection every 10 to 14 days.

Dearterialization Hepatic artery embolization has proved to be a relatively safe procedure for palliation of the carcinoid syndrome related to an excessive hormone production from hepatic carcinoid metastases. Gelfoam powder (particle sizes 80-200 μ) and Ivalon particles (sizes 149-250 μ) are the frequently used agents for devascularization of the hepatic metastases. Although hepatic artery

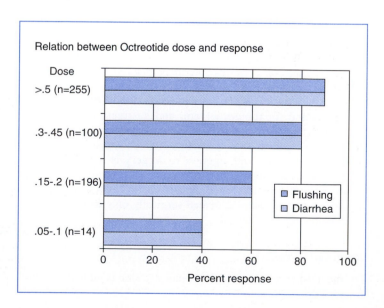

Figure 69.2 Relation between Octreotide dose and resolution of diarrhea and flushing.

occlusion may produce subjective and objective responses in the majority of highly selected patients, the toxicity and duration of responses resulting from this therapy generally do not support its routine use.

Radiation therapy   There are no data available to support the use of radiation therapy in patients with metastatic carcinoids unless they have symptomatic bone metastases or spinal cord compression, which are amenable to this modality.

Chemotherapy   In malignant carcinoid tumors, chemotherapy has not been shown to be effective for the majority of patients, and this approach should still be considered investigational. Responses are generally short-lived, and median survival times compare poorly with Octreotide and the inteferons. The agent most studied in carcinoids is 5-fluorouracil, which has accounted for observed response rates of 26 and 18% in single institution and multi-institutional trials, respectively. Few responses were observed following intravenous doxorubicin (60 mg/m^2) every 3 to 4 weeks. Dacarbazine and dactinomycin have little activity against metastatic carcinoids. Phase 2 studies in evaluable patients with carcinoids have shown rare objective responses to either cisplatin or etoposide. No responses to carboplatinum were seen in a series of twenty patients.

Interferons   Interferons are reported to improve diarrhea, flushing, and bronchospasm in about 60% of patients, reduce tumor size in 15%, and curtail growth in 39%, with a median duration of response of 34 months. The encouraging results of some trials with interferon must be interpreted with caution, however, considering that others have had less favorable results. The major drawbacks to using inteferons are the severe constitutional upset, the flu-like syndrome, and the hematologic abnormalities, which most patients will not tolerate albeit their transitory nature.

Adjuvant therapy   Combined modality therapy, such as the use of adjuvant chemotherapy prior to or following surgery, remains undefined for metastatic carcinoids. In the absence of well-established activity for chemotherapy in this disease, there is no rationale to support the use of adjuvant chemotherapy. In contrast, the preliminary results of the prospective experience of sequential hepatic artery occlusion and alternating combination chemotherapy at the Mayo Clinic is of some interest. Following hepatic artery occlusion by surgical ligation or percutaneous embolization, twenty-one patients were treated with dacarbazine (250 mg/m^2) daily for 5 days, plus doxorubicin (60 mg/m^2) alternating every 4 to 5 weeks with 5-fluorouracil (400 mg/m^2) daily for 5 days, plus streptozotocin (500 mg/m^2) daily for 5 days, until the maximum response was observed. Using this combined modality approach, Moertel reported a hormonal response rate of 86% with a median duration of response of 2 years.

Tumor growth   The role of Octreotide in the treatment of carcinoid tumors is still not well-established. Due to the clear evidence of symptomatic relief (e.g., flushing, wheezing, diarrhea), it has established a place in the treatment of gastroenteropancreatic tumors, both pre- and postoperatively. Perioperative use can prevent fatal episodes of rapid extreme increases of hormones in the circulation. There is enough evidence of the control of

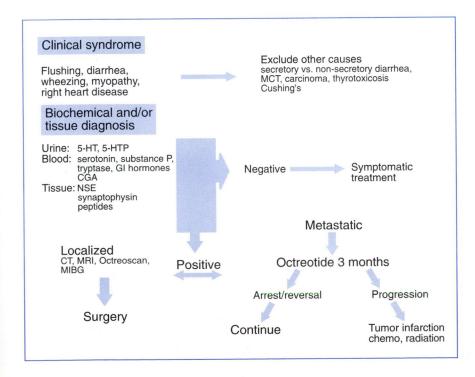

Figure 69.3 Proposed algorithm for the management of carcinoids. For abbreviations see Table 69.1. (Studies of Vinik AI, reported here, were supported by a grant from the Diabetes Institutes Foundation.)

tumor growth that primary treatment of select metastatic tumors, with proper monitoring of tumor growth, is recommended.

Chemotherapy of metastatic carcinoid tumors

Hepatic artery embolization with polyvinyl alcohol parti-cles has been used in patients with metastatic pancreatic endocrine tumors, and partial remission of measurable hepatic tumors was achieved in some evaluable patients. This suggests that this modality can be used for prolonged palliation in selected patients.

In conclusion, much remains unsolved, requiring diligent research and evaluation, if we are ultimately to include carcinoid tumors among the curable cancers. An outline of the current approach to management of the patient suspected of harboring a carcinoid tumor is depicted in Figure 69.3.

Suggested readings

JANSON ET, OBERG K. Long-term management of the carcinoid syndrome. Treatment with Octreotide alone and in combination with α-interferon. Acta Oncol 1993;32:225-9.

JANSON ET, WESTLIN JE, ERIKSSON B, AHLSTROM H, NILSSON S, OBERG K. [^{111}In-DTPA-D-Phe1] Octreotide scintigraphy in patients with carcinoid tumors: the predictive value for somatostatin analogue treatment. Eur J Endocrinol 1994;131:577-81.

OBERG K. The use of chemotherapy in the management of neuroendocrine tumors. Endocrinol Metab Clin North Am 1993;22:841-952.

PERRY RR, VINIK AI. Endocrine tumors of the gastrointestinal tract. Ann Rev Med 1996;47:57-68.

STRODEL WE, VINIK AI, THOMPSON NW, ECKHAUSER FE, TALPOS GB. Small bowel carcinoid tumors and the carcinoid syndrome. In: Thompson NW, Vinik AI (eds). Endocrine surgery update. New York: Grune & Stratton, 1983.

TSAI ST, ECKHAUSER FE, THOMPSON NW, STROEDEL WE, VINIK AI. Perioperative use of long-acting somatostatin analogue (SMS 201-995) in patients with endocrine tumors of the gastroenteropancreatic axis. Surgery 1986;100:788-95.

VINIK AI, ACHEM-KARAM S, OWYANG C. Gastrointestinal hormones in clinical medicine. In: Cohen MP, Foa PP (ed). Special topics in endocrinology and metabolism. Vol. 4. New York: Alan R. Liss, 1983.

VINIK AI, MOATTARI AR. Use of somatostatin analogue in the management of carcinoid syndrome. Dig Dis Sci 1989;34:14s-27s.

VINIK AI, MOATTARI AR, FAJANS SS, VINIK A. Treatment of endocrine tumors of the pancreas. Endocrinol Metab Clin North Am 1989;18:45-74.

VINIK AI, PAVLIC-RENAR I. Carcinoid tumors. Diabetologia Croatica 1995;23-4:123-30.

VINIK AI, PERRY RR. Neoplasms of the gastroenteropancreatic endocrine system. In: Holland JF, Bast RC, Morton DL, Frei E, Kufe DW, Wichselbaum RR (eds). Cancer medicine. Baltimore: Williams & Wilkins, 1997.

VINIK AI, STRODEL WE, O'DORISIO TM. Endocrine tumors of the gastroenteropancreatic axis. In: Santen RJ, Manni A (ed). Diagnosis and management of endocrine-related tumors. Boston: Martinus Nijhoff Publishers, 1984.

VINIK AI, TSAI S, MOATTARI AR, CHEUNG P, ECKHAUSER F, CHO K. Somatostatin analogue (SMS 20-995) in the management of gastroenteropancreatic tumors and diarrhea syndromes. Am J Med 1986;81:23-23.

WYNICK D, WILLIAMS SJ, BLOOM RS. Symptomatic secondary hormone syndromes in patients with established malignant pancreatic endocrine tumors. N Engl J Med 1988;319:605-7.

70

Paraneoplastic endocrine syndromes

Stefano Mariotti, Leonardo Sammartano

◼ KEY POINTS ◼

- Endocrine paraneoplastic syndromes are conditions resulting from the abnormal production of hormones or hormone-like substances from tumors.
- The paraneoplastic syndromes most frequently observed include: Cushing's syndrome, hypercalcemia, the syndrome of inappropriate production of antidiuretic hormone, hypoglycemia, and acromegaly. Hyperthyroidism, Zollinger-Ellison syndrome, and other conditions related to ectopic secretion of gastrointestinal polypeptides are rarely observed.
- The mechanisms involved in paraneoplastic hormones still remain to be fully elucidated. It is well established that tumors produce only polypeptide and protein hormones in a non-random association. The hypotheses presently considered to explain this phenomenon are: (1) there is a common origin of tumors from neuroendocrine cells with "amine precursor uptake and decarboxylation" characteristics; (2) alterations of cellular differentiation occur (de-differentiation and dys-differentiation); (3) hyperexpression of normal genes occurs; (4) oncogenes and growth factors are involved.
- Criteria for the diagnosis of endocrine paraneoplastic syndromes are both clinical and investigational. One must first exclude coexistent primary endocrine diseases and closely examine the temporal relationship between clinical and biochemical endocrine disturbances and the eradication or relapse of the tumor. Biochemical examination should include analysis of the arteriovenous hormone gradient across the tumor, the demonstration of protein/peptide, mRNA, and in vitro synthesis of the specific hormone in tumoral tissue.
- Paraneoplastic endocrine syndromes (especially hypercalcemia, the syndrome of inappropriate production of antidiuretic hormone, and Cushing's syndrome) are rather frequent in oncologic patients, and their early recognition has important clinical implications, particularly due to the increasing number of cancer patients in the general hospital population.

In addition to signs and symptoms related to primary tumors and their metastases, cancer patients may show clinical manifestations that result from abnormalities unrelated to the mass effect of neoplasias, termed paraneoplastic syndromes.

Paraneoplastic syndromes can involve almost any organ or system, of which a comprehensive discussion is beyond the scope of this chapter. The most common syndromes involve neurologic dysfunctions, hematological abnormalities, and abnormal hormone production. Paraneoplastic syndromes in general occur often in cancer patients: their prevalence has been estimated at 20% at any time period and up to 75% at some time during the course of disease. Early recognition of these syndromes has important clinical implications due to the increasing incidence of cancer patients in the hospital population. The pathogenesis of several paraneoplastic syndromes remains to be clarified, but in many instances they are the consequence of abnormal qualitative or quantitative production of bioactive soluble factors by tumors.

Endocrine paraneoplastic syndromes are conditions related to the abnormal hormone production of tumors. This concept stems from a series of clinical observations, followed by the direct demonstration of the synthesis and secretion of biologically active hormones by tumors. Historically, the hypothesis that tumoral hormone secretion could produce endocrine dysfunction was first proposed by Albright in 1941 to explain the presence of hypercalcemia and hypophosphatemia in a patient with renal carcinoma. Subsequent studies confirmed this concept, and the term "ectopic hormone production" was later proposed by Liddle. The term ectopic was proposed in contrast to the conventional endocrine disturbances resulting from "eutopic" hormone secretion by the endocrine glands. As discussed in the next paragraph, however, it has been subsequently recognized that hormone production by tumors cannot always strictly be considered "ectopic," since small amounts of polypeptide hormones are found in many normal tissues. However, the term "ectopic hormone production" is still currently used to define the main mechanism underlying endocrine paraneoplastic syndromes and will be used in this chapter. Other synonymous terms referring to this group of disorders include "paraendocrine tumors," "endocrine phenocopies," and "production of hormones by non-endocrine tumors."

The endocrine clinical syndromes most frequently observed in association with non-endocrine tumors and the respective hormones secreted by them are summarized in Table 70.1.

Although the number of hormone types produced by tumors is very large, it should be noted that in virtually all cases they are polypeptide hormones. Tumors may also produce peptides closely related to the native hormone but devoid of biological activity. In these cases, no clinical symptoms are observed, but the hormone-like substance synthesized by tumors and detected in plasma may be employed as a tumor marker. Interestingly, amino acid hormones, such as thyronines or steroid hormones, are not produced by tumors, probably because the strictly specific

Table 70.1 Principal clinical syndromes sustained by ectopic tumoral production

Clinical syndrome	Hormones involved	Frequent tumor type
Cushing's syndrome	ACTH CRF POMC-derived peptides	Small cell lung carcinoma, pheochromocytoma, medullary thyroid carcinoma, pancreatic adenocarcinoma, carcinoids (thymic, bronchial)
Hypercalcemia	PTH-related protein (PTHrP) PTH TGFα, IL-1β, TNF-β, 1,25-dihydroxyvitamin D, prostaglandins	Breast, lung (squamous), endocrine pancreas carcinoma; lymphomas; ovary and uterus carcinoma; carcinoma of the gastrointestinal tract (liver, bladder)
Syndrome of inappropriate antidiuretic hormone (SIADH) secretion	ADH Atrial natriuretic peptide (ANP)	Small cell and non-small cell carcinomas of the lung, carcinomas of the pancreas, adrenal and gastrointestinal tract, thymoma, lymphomas, lymphosarcomas, sarcomas, laryngeal carcinoma, malignant histiocytosis, neuroblastoma
Acromegaly	GH, GHRH	Pancreatic endocrine tumors, lung carcinomas, carcinoids
Hypoglycemia	Insulin Insulin-like growth factors I and II (IGF-I, IGF-II)	Mesodermal and mesenchymal tumors; bronchogenic, gastric, hepatocellular carcinomas
Gynecomastia, precocious puberty	hCG	Pancreatic adenocarcinoma, islet cell carcinoma, carcinoids, trophoblastic diseases
Hyperthyroidism	hCG	Trophoblastic diseases
Zollinger-Ellison syndrome	Gastrin, gastrin-releasing peptide (GRP)	Undifferentiated lung carcinoma, carcinoids, pancreatic and ovarian carcinomas, duodenal adenocarcinoma
Verner-Morrison syndrome	Vasoactive intestinal peptide (VIP) Somatostatin	Lung carcinomas, carcinoids, pheochromocytoma, pancreatic carcinoma

and coordinate enzymatic pathways required for thyroid and steroid hormone synthesis cannot be replicated in neoplastic tissues. Although neoplasms do not directly secrete steroid hormones, they may express abnormal amounts of enzymes normally involved in steroid hormone metabolism and activation. A typical example is represented by the increased conversion of vitamin 25-OH-D$_3$ to 1,25-(OH)$_2$-D$_3$ by lymphomas.

For the unequivocal identification of ectopic hormone production by a non-endocrine tumor, several criteria must be fulfilled (Tab. 70.2). Clinical criteria are sufficient for a presumptive diagnosis, but investigational criteria are often needed for the definitive establishment of ectopic hormonal production. The coexistence of an endocrine syndrome with a non-endocrine cancer should always be considered in the differential diagnosis. This is best exemplified by primary hyperparathyroidism, which occurs in cancer patients with a frequency greater than that expected by chance. Endocrine syndromes due to ectopic tumoral production of releasing hormones such as corticotropin-releasing hormone (CRH) and growth hormone-releasing hormone (GHRH) may be erroneously attributed to tumoral production of the corresponding pituitary hormone. In some cases tumors may produce endocrine disturbances by mass effects, such as when lung cancer causes altered intrathoracic pressure and leads to inappropriate antidiuretic hormone (ADH) secretion via stretch receptor stimulation. Even the finding of increased hormone concentration in non-endocrine tumoral tissues cannot be considered a definitive criterion, since some tumors may concentrate hormones from the circulation.

MECHANISMS INVOLVED IN ECTOPIC HORMONE PRODUCTION

Several theories have been put forward to explain hormone production by tumors, but the precise mechanisms involved remain to be fully elucidated. Before discussing in more detail the current hypotheses, it is important to review some established points that should be considered in any etiologic theory. First, tumors produce only polypeptide and protein hormones, which are structurally closely related to their eutopically secreted counterparts. Interestingly, tumors may produce pro-hormones, hormone subunits, or hormone fragments, but they do not synthesize new proteins that have not been identified in physiological conditions. The second important point is that, although multiple hormones may be produced by single tumors and the same hormone may be secreted by different neoplasms, ectopic hormone production is not a random phenomenon. A thorough classification based on the association between different tumors and specific clinical syndromes has been proposed by Levine and Metz and is reported in Table 70.3. According to this classification, most tumors can be subdivided into two main groups according to their embryological, morphological, and hormone-producing characteristics: tumors of group I are derived from neuroectoderm cells, while group II includes neoplasias derived from endoderm and mesoderm. A smaller group of tumors (transitional group) derived form the neural crest that share several embryological and histological features with group I neoplasias may produce hormones of both groups I and II.

Gene mutation and sponge theory

According to the gene mutation theory, ectopic hormone production should result from genomic DNA alterations as a consequence of the neoplastic process, leading to the synthesis of new protein hormones. As stated before, this event has never been demonstrated; furthermore, this hypothesis would not explain the nonrandom nature of ectopic hormone production and is therefore presently considered only of historical interest.

The "sponge hypothesis" was proposed in 1964 by Unger, who suggested that tumors may concentrate hormones from the bloodstream and then release them back into it. Although circumstantial evidence for this mechanism has been obtained in some cases, direct proof of hor-

Table 70.2 Criteria for the identification of paraneoplastic endocrine syndrome

Clinical

Recognition of an endocrine syndrome associated with a non-endocrine tumor

Increased serum/urinary concentrations of the hormone responsible for the syndrome in the absence of primary disease of the relevant endocrine gland

Disappearance and/or remission of the endocrine syndrome after effective treatment of the primary tumor; recurrence of the syndrome with tumor relapse

Normalization of serum/urinary hormone concentrations after successful therapy of the tumor, and recurrence of high hormone levels with tumor relapse

Investigational

Demonstration of an arteriovenous gradient in hormone concentrations across the tumor, with higher levels on the venous side

Extraction of the hormone involved from neoplastic tissue, followed by:
- determination of hormonal activity by biological, immunological, radioimmunological or radioreceptor assay
- biochemical characterization of the peptides produced by the tumor

Demonstration of in vitro hormone synthesis by the tumor cells

Identification of hormonal mRNA in tumoral tissue or cultured cells

Reproduction of the clinical and biochemical syndrome in animals after transplantation of the tumor cells

Table 70.3 Classification of tumors causing paraneoplastic endocrine syndromes (according to Levine and Metz)

	Tumors	Hormones
Group I (APUD)	Carcinoids, oat-cell lung carcinoma, islet cell tumors, thymomas, medullary thyroid carcinoma	ACTH/POMC, ADH, gastrin, calcitonin
Group II	Hepatomas, cholangiomas, Wilms' tumors, hypernephromas, connective and mesodermal tumors, reticuloendothelial tumors, pancreatic adenocarcinomas, and other gastrointestinal tumors	PTHrP, PRL, GH, IGFs, hPL, hCG, renin, erythropoietin
Transitional	Pheochromocytomas, melanomas	PTHrP, erythropoietin, ACTH, biogenic amines, calcitonin, hPL, glucagon

mone synthesis and secretion by tumors is now available for most of the hormones listed in Tables 70.1 and 70.3.

Amine precursor uptake and decarboxylation (APUD) cell hypothesis

The amine precursor uptake and decarboxylation cell hypothesis represents the first and still the most cogent attempt to explain the nonrandom nature of ectopic hormone production. In this view, originally proposed by Pearse and colleagues, hormone-secreting tumors may originate from cells of neuroectodermal origin widely distributed throughout the body. These cells share the common functional characteristic of concentrating amine precursors, decarboxylating them, and finally converting them into biogenic amines (hence the name "amine precursor uptake and decarboxylation," or APUD). Histologically, APUD cells display the presence of typical neurosecretory granules associated with the storage and secretion of peptide hormones and amines. Cells with APUD characteristics include thyroid parafollicular (C) cells, adrenal medullar cells, anterior pituitary cells, pancreatic islets and other neuroendocrine cells of the gastrointestinal tract, neuroendocrine cells of the thymus, and cells scattered in the bronchial mucosa (Kultschitsky cells). According to Pearse's view, APUD cells represent a "diffuse neuroendocrine system," a branch of the central nervous system. This hypothesis has recently been challenged by the demonstration that not all APUD cells are of neuroectodermal origin: gastrointestinal, pancreatic and possibly bronchial APUD cells may derive from the endoderm; parathyroid cells, which share several neuroendocrine characteristics and have been advocated to be included in the APUD system, have different cytochemical properties and are not of neuroectodermal origin. However, the concept that ectopic hormone production is sustained by APUD cells present within the tumors provides the best explanation for the endocrine syndromes observed in group I neoplasias of the Levine-Metz classification. On the other hand, the APUD hypothesis does not explain the hormone production by Levine-Metz group II

tumors, nor the frequent production of "APUD" hormones by group II tumors. It should be underlined, however, that while the bioinactive adrenocorticotropic hormone (ACTH) precursor proopiomelanocortin is produced by many tumors, only APUD cell carcinomas of group I are actually associated with clinically overt hypercortisolism. This phenomenon is probably due to the presence in APUD cells of convertases and other processing enzymes that allow for the secretion of bioactive hormones. In this view, the APUD characteristics would identify cytochemical and structural features associated with the capacity of processing and secreting active hormones rather than with the mere capacity of synthesizing hormonal peptides.

Gene derepression and cellular de-differentiation

Under normal conditions more than 90% of the genome is repressed. According to the de-repression hypothesis, different portions of cellular DNA may become "de-repressed" during the process of neoplastic transformation, consequently activating genes coding for specific hormones. The main objection to this hypothesis is that ectopic hormone production is a nonrandom phenomenon, while de-repression should be an entirely casual process. An extension of this hypothesis is the cellular de-differentiation hypothesis: according to this theory, tumor cells may regress from a differentiated to a less differentiated or totally undifferentiated state. During this process tumor cells could produce fetal proteins or hormones normally present in immature cells (e.g., human chorionic gonadotropin [hCG]). This hypothesis would account for the production of some, but not all, hormones involved in paraneoplastic syndromes. Furthermore, direct evidence for a de-differentiation process in tumor cells is still lacking.

Dys-differentiation theory

This hypothesis, proposed by Baylin and Mendelsohn, is an extension of the de-differentiation theory. According to this view, every tissue in the body contains continuously renewing stem cells with totipotential or undifferentiated features, a model similar to that currently accepted for the hematological system. Epithelial tumors could result from clonal expansion of a particular cell stage along the pathway of normal differentiation. At each stage the differentiating cell may express a variety of phenotypes and protein syntheses, including APUD characteristics and hormone (or fetal protein) production. This hypothesis accounts for several characteristics of tumoral tissues, such as phenotypic and functional heterogeneity, and also provides a basis from which to understand the nonrandom association of certain hormone production with specific tumors.

Normal gene hyperexpression

Low levels of hormone production may be demonstrated in the majority of non endocrine tissues, possibly due to incomplete genomic repression. It has therefore been hypothesized that the ectopic hormone production of tumors may represent hyperexpression of normal genes in proliferating cells. As suggested by Odell, peptide synthesis could be a "universal concomitant of neoplasia" with clinical syndromes occurring when bioactive hormones are produced.

Oncogenes and growth factors

A key step in the initiation and the maintenance of the neoplastic state is represented by one or more genomic mutations involving the activation of oncogenes or the inactivation of onco-suppressor genes. Oncogenes are aberrant forms of normal genes (called proto-oncogenes) involved in the growth and differentiation process and generally encode growth factors (e.g., sis, encoding platelet-derived growth factor [PGDF]), growth-factor receptors (e.g., erb-B, encoding a structure related to epidermal growth factor [EGF] receptor; or ret, encoding a protein kinase-linked receptor), or cellular effector systems coupled to growth factor receptors (e.g., sarc, encoding a tyrosine kinase). Tumor-suppressor genes (e.g., p-53) are normally involved in inhibiting cell growth and may be inactivated by mutation or deletion.

The hypothesis linking oncogenes and ectopic hormone production stems from the concept that hormones could act as autocrine growth factors needed for the survival and growth of the tumor. A possible example of this relationship is demonstrated by the gastrin-releasing peptide, the mammalian counterpart of the amphibian bombesin. Gastrin-releasing peptide/bombesin, which may be secreted by oat-cell carcinoma of the lung, has been shown to stimulate cell replication via specific receptors. Further studies are needed to clarify whether and to what extent other hormones produced by tumors may act as autocrine growth factors.

SYNDROMES DUE TO ECTOPIC HORMONE PRODUCTION BY TUMORS

Ectopic ACTH syndrome

Hypercortisolism due to the ectopic production of ACTH and its related peptides accounts for 13 to 20% of all cases of Cushing's syndrome. As listed in Table 70.4,

about 75% of tumors associated with ectopic Cushing's syndrome are located in the overdiaphragmatic region, while the remaining arise in the abdominal cavity. In over 80% of cases, ACTH-producing tumors show cyto-morphological APUD characteristics.

Overt hypercortisolism is present only in a small minority of the above-mentioned tumors, the highest proportion (up to 2 to 5%) being observed in oat-cell carcinoma of the lung. High immunoreactive serum concentrations of peptides related to proopiomelanocortin/ACTH molecules in the absence of a definite clinical syndrome are found in a larger proportion (25 to 75%) of cases; not infrequently biochemical evidence of subclinical hypercortisolism (a slight elevation of serum cortisol with incomplete suppression after high doses of dexamethasone) is observed in these patients.

This state is due to tumoral release of abnormal proopiomelanocortin/ACTH molecules with lower or absent biological activity. Differences both in length and kilobase content have been observed between proopiomelanocortin mRNA derived from normal pituitary, and from non-pituitary normal tissues and tumoral cells. A different post-translational process of proopiomelanocortin/ACTH molecules is also involved in the generation of peptides with variable biological activity. Large immunoreactive ACTH-like molecules are typically found in tumors from patients without overt hypercortisolism. Tumors involved in ectopic Cushing's syndrome may produce CRH, which is generally cosecreted with ACTH but is occasionally the only ectopic hormone produced.

Clinical findings

Due to the rapid course of the tumors, ectopic ACTH secretion syndrome is rarely associated with florid Cushing's features, even in the presence of high plasma ACTH and cortisol concentrations. The syndrome often has acute onset with profound weakness, psychosis, pitting edema of the lower extremities, hyperpigmentation,

Table 70.4 Tumors associated with ectopic ACTH syndrome

Tumor type	Frequency
Oat-cell carcinoma of lung	45-60%
Thymic tumors (including carcinoids)	10-20%
Islet-cell carcinoma	5-10%
Bronchial adenoma (carcinoid type)	5-10%
Miscellaneous: pheochromocytoma, medullary thyroid carcinoma, ovarian carcinoma, abdominal carcinoids, others	10-15%

hypertension, diabetes, and marked hypokalemia.

Less frequently, ectop,ic ACTH production may be observed in patients with typical Cushing's clinical manifestations, becoming evident only after months or years of sustained hypercortisolism; these features may be observed in patients with ectopic ACTH production due to slow-growing tumors such as carcinoids, pheochromocytomas, thymomas, or medullary thyroid carcinoma. In these cases a history of Cushing's syndrome may be present for a long time before the identification of the tumor responsible for the ACTH hyperproduction.

Signs dependent on hypercortisolism may be variously associated with those of a tumor, which may confound the clinical picture. An example is weight loss, which is frequently observed in cancer patients, rather than the weight gain of typical Cushing's disease.

Diagnostic procedures

High-dose dexamethasone suppression test This test can be performed either in a single overnight dexamethasone administration (8 mg orally at 23:00), or, alternatively, in the classic fashion (2 mg of dexamethasone orally qid for 2 days). ACTH and cortisol suppression after a high-dose dexamethasone suppression test is observed in patients with pituitary Cushing's disease, while no suppression should occur in patients with ectopic ACTH secretion. However, some degree of suppression after a high-dose test may be observed in a substantial minority of patients with ectopic ACTH production, especially when benign (e.g., bronchial carcinoid) or CRH-producing tumors are involved. The high-dose dexamethasone suppression test therefore has limited value as a single test in the differential diagnosis of ACTH-dependent Cushing's syndrome, and other techniques must be added to achieve satisfactory diagnostic accuracy.

Corticotropin-releasing hormone test ACTH stimulation with CRH (1 mg/kg iv as bolus) has been proposed as a pivotal test in differentiating ectopic from pituitary causes of Cushing's syndrome. In patients with pituitary Cushing's disease, iv administration of CRH induces a further increase in plasma ACTH and cortisol levels; in contrast, no response is expected in patients with ectopic ACTH production. Similarly to the high-dose dexamethasone test, the specificity of the CRH test is not absolute, as a positive ACTH response after CRH administration may also be observed in ectopic ACTH syndrome.

Metyrapone test Metyrapone, an inhibitor of cortisol synthesis, has been widely used in the past and is still employed in the differential diagnosis of Cushing's syndromes. The rationale of this test is the rise in plasma ACTH and 17-deoxycortisol (or urinary 17-corticoids) induced from removal of the negative feedback exerted by cortisol. In ACTH-independent Cushing's syndrome and in ectopic ACTH-secreting tumors, no response to metyrapone should be observed. When tumoral CRH production occurs, ACTH may rise after metyrapone administration, even in cases unresponsive to exogenous CRH.

Bilateral inferior petrosal sinuses sampling A high diagnostic accuracy is reached by bilateral inferior petrosal sinuses sampling, which was originally proposed for lateralizing small pituitary secreting adenomas. In short, a sample is taken from catheters introduced by femoral vein route into both petrosal sinuses. Blood samples for ACTH are collected at basal time and after 2, 5, and 10 minutes after CRH stimulation, either in petrosal sinuses or peripherally at various anatomical sites. A basal petrosal/peripheral ratio of plasma ACTH concentration >2, increasing further after CRH administration, excludes ectopic ACTH production with a sensitivity and specificity of 100%. Ectopic CRH production cannot be definitively ruled out by this procedure, since corticotropic hyperplasia may mimic pituitary Cushing's disease. In the absence of increased basal and CRH-stimulated petrosal/peripheral plasma ACTH ratio, ectopic ACTH production is almost conclusively established. Assays of ACTH in blood samples collected at specific anatomical sites during the catheterization may aid in localizing the source of ectopic ACTH release.

Imaging studies

Because a common cause of ectopic ACTH syndrome is small cell carcinoma of the lung, careful evaluation of the chest by X-ray or CT-scan may reveal direct or indirect signs of neoplasia. In all other cases, localization of primary ACTH-secreting tumors relies on echographic or radiographic diagnostic procedures, often associated with angiography, as in the case of pancreatic tumors. (^{111}In-DTPA-D-Phe)-Octreotide scintigraphy (Octreoscan®), which detects neuroendocrine tumors expressing somatostatin receptors, is an additional sensitive and reliable tool to localize ACTH-producing neoplasias (Fig. 70.2, see Color Atlas).

Differential diagnosis

The differential diagnosis of hypercortisolemic conditions is detailed elsewhere in this book. Briefly, the presence of hypercortisolism in patients with suspected ACTH syndrome may be established on the basis of high 24-hour free cortisol excretion and a negative low-dose dexamethasone suppression test. In exceptional cases, normal urinary free cortisol excretion and/or cortisol suppression by low-dose dexamethasone administration may be observed in patients with ectopic ACTH syndrome. This is due to periodic remissions of hypercortisolism, which may occur either in ectopic or pituitary Cushing's disease.

The most important indication for the diagnosis of ectopic ACTH syndrome is the presence of markedly increased plasma ACTH concentrations that are unsuppressible with high doses of dexamethasone. This greatly facilitates the differential diagnosis of ACTH-independent syndromes, as the latter are associated with low or undetectable plasma ACTH concentrations either before and after dexamethasone administration. Plasma ACTH levels in patients with ectopic ACTH syndrome are often much higher than those observed in patients bearing a pituitary ACTH-secreting adenoma. In the latter condition, normal to moderately elevated (20 to 500 pg/ml, or 4.4 to 110 pmol/l) plasma ACTH levels are commonly observed. Values >500 pg/ml (110 pmol/l) are very suggestive of ectopic ACTH production, although in about at least 50% of patients with this condition, plasma ACTH concentrations overlap those found in pituitary Cushing's disease.

A further diagnostic indication of ectopic ACTH syndrome may be the demonstration of increased plasma or urine concentrations of the substances specifically secreted by the tumors involved, such as serum serotonin or urinary 5-hydroxyindolacetic acid in carcinoids, plasma and/or urinary catecholamines in pheochromocytomas, and serum calcitonin in medullary thyroid carcinomas.

The differential diagnosis between ectopic and pituitary ACTH-dependent Cushing's syndrome primarily relies on the use of dynamic tests (Fig. 70.1). The rationale of these tests is based on the assumption that pituitary ACTH-producing adenomas retain some degree of responsiveness to both negative and positive stimuli, while the ectopic ACTH production in tumors is not responsive. Exceptions to these assumptions, however, may be observed, which make the unequivocal identification of ectopic ACTH production a difficult task. The dynamic tests employed for the diagnosis of ectopic ACTH syndrome include the high-dose dexamethasone

suppression test, and other procedures evaluating the normal ACTH secretion pathway, such as testing by CRH or metyrapone administration.

Treatment

Therapy of patients with ectopic ACTH-producing tumors depends primarily on the biological behavior of the neoplasia. Pheochromocytomas, bronchial carcinoids, thymomas, and paragangliomas often having a benign clinical course may be surgically removed. Successful surgical treatment of these tumors is associated with acute postoperative adrenal gland failure, demonstrating the complete removal of the ectopic ACTH source. In contrast, the postoperative persistence of high or even normal plasma cortisol suggests residual tumor. An intraoperative ACTH measurement may help to evaluate the effectiveness of surgical therapy.

Unfortunately, most of the other malignancies sustaining ACTH production are unresectable due to tumor diffusion and/or metastases at the time of diagnosis. When the tumor cannot be surgically removed, controlling the patient's hypercortisolism may be the only way to improve, at least transiently, the clinical course. To this end, bilateral adrenalectomy or pharmacological agents may be employed. Bilateral adrenalectomy is effective but

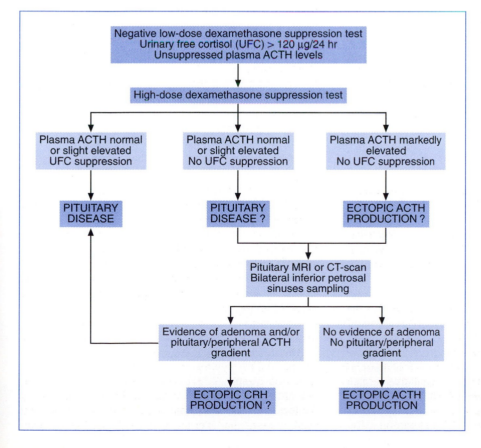

Figure 70.1 Diagnostic flowchart in suspected ectopic ACTH syndrome (see text for details.)

is associated with a high rate of morbidity and mortality. Pharmacological agents for the treatment of ectopic ACTH syndrome include adrenolytic agents such as mitotane, and inhibitors of cortisol synthesis such as aminogluthetimide and metyrapone.

Mitotane (*o,p'*-DDD) has a specific cytotoxic effect on adrenocortical cells, but it has rarely been employed in the treatment of ectopic ACTH syndromes due to the side effects and its slow onset of action. Aminogluthetimide impairs the cortisol synthesis by blocking the conversion of cholesterol to pregnenolone and has been used at doses of 1-3 per day in several ACTH-producing tumors. Frequent side effects include skin rash, dizziness, ataxia, sedation, and gastrointestinal irritation. This drug is used best in controlling hypercortisolism in patients bearing benign tumors (e.g., carcinoids) before surgical therapy, while less satisfactory results have been obtained in malignant neoplasias. Metyrapone is an inhibitor of the conversion of 11-deoxycortisol to cortisol via the enzymatic blockade of 11β-hydroxylase. When administered alone, the dose effective in inducing biochemical and clinical improvement is between 2.25-4.0 per day. Ketoconazole, usually employed as an antimycotic drug, inhibits P450 cytochrome oxydase, which blocks all the enzymes involved in the biosynthetic processes of the adrenal cortex. This drug has been widely employed in controlling hypercortisolism due to pituitary Cushing's syndrome and adrenal adenomas. The effectiveness of ketoconazole in ectopic ACTH syndrome is still controversial, although good results have been reported at doses ranging from 400-1200 mg per day.

Medical therapy aimed to inhibit ACTH production has been recently proposed after the introduction of Octreotide, a long-acting somatostatin analogue, to clinical practice. The best results with this drug have been observed in ACTH-producing carcinoids and gastrinomas at doses between 100 and 600 mg per day.

Syndrome of inappropriate antidiuretic hormone secretion (SIADH)

As shown in Table 70.5, lung carcinoma is the tumor most commonly associated with the syndrome of inappropriate antidiuretic hormone secretion (SIADH), accounting for >80% of cases; less frequently, this syndrome is associated with other malignancies, including gastrointestinal, laryngeal, and central nervous system neoplasias or lymphomas.

Immunoreactive ADH is frequently detected in tumoral tissues (surgical specimens and cell cultures) even in the absence of clinically overt SIADH. The biosynthetic pathway leading to neoplastic ADH production is similar to that followed in the hypothalamus. Briefly, a 21 kDa precursor (provasopressin) is synthesized, which consists of ADH, its carrier protein (neurophysin), and a glycoprotein fragment. Provasopressin is incompletely cleaved before secretion by tumor cells, resulting in detectable circulating precursor molecules, neurophysin and glycoprotein.

Table 70.5 Tumors associated with the syndrome of inappropriate antidiuretic hormone secretion

Tumor type	Approximate frequency
Carcinoma of the lung	80%
Lymphoma	< 5%
Pancreatic carcinoma	< 5%
Laryngeal carcinoma	~1%
Duodenal carcinoma	~1%

Miscellaneous:
  sarcomas, lymphosarcomas,
  reticulosarcomas, mesotheliomas,
  thymomas; bladder, prostate,
  colon, uterus (cervix) carcinomas
	10%

In contrast, ADH hypersecretion derived from the posterior pituitary is not associated with measurable circulating provasopressin, due to complete cleavage of the precursor. Thus, the detection of provasopressin in the serum is considered strong evidence for ectopic tumoral ADH production. The activation of ADH biosynthesis is an extremely frequent phenomenon in small cell lung carcinomas: plasma ADH is elevated in up to 60% of patients with this tumor, and 20 to 40% of them exhibit the clinical syndrome.

Inappropriate secretion of ADH in cancer patients is not necessarily due to ectopic ADH production, as it may be the consequence of abnormally regulated eutopic secretion. Interference with the normal release of ADH in cancer patients may in fact result from mechanisms acting at the baroceptorial level (vena cava obstruction), from nonspecific vagus nerve fiber stimulation (mass effect), carcinomatous neuropathy, or hypothalamic metastases. It should be noted that similar mechanisms may be involved in the inappropriate ADH secretion observed in several non-neoplastic conditions such as acute porphyria, systemic erythematous lupus, cerebrovascular disease, and central nervous system and pulmonary infections. Some drugs administered for primary neoplasias such as cisplatin, doxorubicin, vinblastine, cyclophosphamide, bleomycin, and morphine may also cause inappropriate ADH secretion in cancer patients.

Recent data provide evidence that suggests there can be ectopic production of atrial natriuretic peptide by small cell carcinomas of the lung. Abnormal atrial natriuretic peptide production could contribute to hyponatremia observed in SIADH, but further studies are needed to clarify the clinical relevance of ectopic atrial natriuretic peptide production.

Clinical findings

When the syndrome develops slowly or when hyponatremia is not severe (130-135 mmol/l), anorexia, nausea, vomiting, abdominal cramps, and bloating are the most frequent symptoms. Marked hyponatremia (<120 mmol/l)

is characterized by the sudden appearance of neurological signs and symptoms of water intoxication (irritability, restlessness, extrapyramidal signs, confusion, pseudobulbar palsy, lethargy, and coma). The considerable amount of water retained (4-5 liters) leads to body weight increase, but edema is typically absent because excess water is equally distributed among extracellular and intracellular spaces. In the presence of an intact thirst mechanism, the patient may tolerate well moderate ADH excess by spontaneous reduction of water intake. However, if fluid balance is suddenly increased (e.g., by saline intravenous administration), severe symptoms of water intoxication may rapidly develop.

Differential diagnosis

Diagnosis may be suspected in cancer patients showing the above clinical manifestations and hyponatremia, and other significant signs of hemodilution (reduced BUN, creatinine, uric acid, and albumin) associated with reduced plasma (<180 mOsm/kg) and inappropriately increased urinary osmolality. The differential diagnosis of SIADH is based on the exclusion of other hyponatremic conditions such as hypovolemia, edematous states, hypothyroidism, and adrenal insufficiency. Inappropriate ADH secretion may be directly confirmed by the measurement of plasma ADH by radioimmunoassay, although this determination is often unnecessary for establishing the diagnosis. When available, measurement of serum provasopressin or neurophysin may be useful, since these molecules are detected in the circulation only in patients with tumoral production of ADH.

Restriction of water intake to <1 l/day is a useful diagnostic and therapeutic procedure in patients with SIADH. A prompt weight loss of 3 to 4 kg is observed over a 3-day period, associated with the gradual correction of hyponatremia and urinary sodium loss.

Treatment

Severe hyponatremia may require hypertonic saline infusion; in this case, it is necessary to promote free water clearance to avoid the further increase of body water content and subsequent congestive heart failure and hypertension. To this end, furosemide administration is useful to correct hyponatremia without the expansion of extracellular fluid volume. During therapy with hypertonic infusion, attention should be paid in monitoring the plasma sodium concentration, and the infusion rate should be reduced when plasma sodium levels reach 130 mEq/l.

Several drugs may be used in the medical treatment of SIADH, including demeclocycline, lithium carbonate, and urea. The first, a tetracycline antibiotic, inhibits cAMP formation and action at the level of the renal tubule collecting ducts, producing nephrogenic diabetes insipidus. The starting dose is 1200 mg per day, followed by gradual reduction when urine osmolality decreases. When serum sodium reaches the normal range, patients must intake a sufficient amount of water to avoid dehydration. Unfortunately, the use of this drug is often limited by its nephrotoxicity. Lithium carbonate also acts via induction of nephrogenic diabetes insipidus at doses of 900-2100 mg per day. Its effectiveness is inferior to that of demeclocycline, and its use is associated with more side effects. Exogenous urea, given in a single daily dose of 30 g, acts as an osmotic diuretic, increases free water clearance, and allows free access to water intake by the patient. Urea also lowers urinary sodium excretion, which resolves hyponatremia. The main risk related to urea use is dehydration, which can be prevented by adequate fluid intake.

Hypercalcemia in malignancies

Hypercalcemia has long been recognized as a frequent complication of neoplastic disease. The concept of tumoral hypercalcemia independent from bone metastases was first put forward by Albright in 1941, who suggested that cancer may produce a substance(s) with biological activity similar to that of parathyroid hormone. This concept remained controversial for several decades until the recent identification of parathyroid hormone-related protein as the major humoral factor responsible for paraneoplastic hypercalcemia.

Pathology

Hypercalcemia is the most common paraneoplastic syndrome, being observed in up to 10 to 20% of patients with advanced cancer. As listed in Table 70.6, of several tumors associated with paraneoplastic hypercalcemia, squamous carcinomas of the upper body region (lung, breast, neck and head) are most frequently involved (50%). Other malignancies found are multiple myelomas, lymphomas, renal and ovarian carcinomas, and mesenchymal cell-derived tumors.

Several mechanisms are potentially responsible for neoplastic hypercalcemia: the first and more frequently seen is the direct invasion of bone by tumor, which cannot

Table 70.6 Tumors associated with paraneoplastic hypercalcemia

Tumor type	Frequency
Breast carcinoma	10-35%
Lung carcinoma	15-35%
Renal carcinoma	5-25%
Hematological neoplasias	5-15%
Miscellaneous: genital, neuroendocrine, bone, mesenchymal-derived neoplasias, melanoma	5-10%

be considered sensu strictu a paraneoplastic manifestation. However, recent evidence has shown that even when tumor cells are physically present in bone tissue, bone lysis is mediated by one or more soluble factors such as prostaglandins, osteoclast-activating factor (OAF) or other cytokines, which have been implicated in other forms of neoplastic hypercalcemia (see below).

A second mechanism involved is the production of parathyroid hormone (PTH) or parathyroid hormone-related protein (PTH-rp) by the tumor. While the production of PTH has been reported in rare cases only, the secretion of PTH-rp is now well-documented in most solid tumors. PTH-rp is structurally different from PTH and exists in three isoforms of 139, 141 and 173 amino acids, differing only at their carboxyl terminus. PTH-rp shares almost all of the biological activities of parathyroid hormone in respect to calcium metabolism due to sequence homology in the 13 amino-terminal amino acids. PTH-rp is not an abnormal substance produced by tumors, but a physiological hormone synthesized by parathyroid cells, whose functions still remain to be fully elucidated. Despite intensive investigation to detect a specific PTH-rp receptor, a single adenylate cyclase-coupled receptor appears to mediate the action of both PTH and PTH-rp. Prenatally, PTH-rp is essential for skeletal development of the fetus; deletion of the PTH-rp protein gene is lethal. Postnatal functions of this hormone may include paracrine functions on keratinocytes and other epithelial cells. Interestingly, PTH-rp and its mRNA are detectable in the majority of normal cells from which tumors commonly associated with paraneoplastic hypercalcemia are derived.

A third mechanism leading to neoplastic hypercalcemia is related to the tumoral production of calcium-mobilizing substances such as prostaglandins and cytokines. Prostaglandins of the E series (prostaglandin Es) are able to stimulate in vitro osteoclastic bone resorption and able to increase cAMP production; furthermore, there is evidence that high plasma and tumor concentrations of prostaglandin Es are present in neoplastic hypercalcemia. However, since prostaglandin E is extensively metabolized during its first pass through the lung and liver, it has been calculated that the venous prostaglandin E concentration to give the minimal arterial level necessary to increase bone resorption should have been at least tenfold greater than that observed in hypercalcemic patients with tumors. Increased circulating prostaglandins are therefore not associated with paraneoplastic hypercalcemia; in contrast, local prostaglandin production is an important factor leading to osteolysis. This mechanism seems to be particularly involved in hypercalcemia associated with multiple myeloma and with metastatic lung and breast cancers. Osteolytic hypercalcemia is also mediated by other local factors produced by tumors, including OAF, tumor growth factor (TGF), and cytokines such as interleukin 1 (IL-1), interleukin 6 (IL-6), and tumor necrosis factors alpha (TNF-α or cachectin) and beta (TNF-β or lymphotoxin).

A distinct mechanism responsible for hypercalcemia has been identified in Hodgkin's disease and in other non-Hodgkin's lymphomas. In these conditions excessive tumoral 1α-hydroxylase activity leads to unregulated conversion of 25-OH-D_3 to the active 1,25$(OH)_2$-D_3 form (calcitriol).

It should be kept in mind that many tumors (in particular breast cancer) may produce hypercalcemia through a combination of systemic, humoral, and local osteolytic mechanisms, and that multiple biologically active substances may be involved in hypercalcemia observed in individual cancer patients.

Clinical findings

Hypercalcemia is a frequent complication of tumors, often observed as a late and sometimes pre-terminal manifestation. In most cases, death occurs within 3 months after diagnosis. The signs and symptoms of paraneoplastic hypercalcemia are similar to those observed in other hypercalcemic conditions. In patients with milder forms of hypercalcemia (<7.0 mEq/l), they include nonspecific general disturbances such as weakness, fatigue, headache, and behavioral abnormalities. Patients with more severe hypercalcemia (>7.0 mEq/l) often present with anorexia, nausea, vomiting, constipation, and abdominal pain associated with neurological manifestations (drowsiness, visual abnormalities, confusion, lethargy, stupor, and coma). Hypercalcemia may alter the kidney tubular function, producing a nephrogenic diabetes insipidus that results in polyuria, polydipsia, and possible marked dehydration if fluid intake is insufficient. In severe hypercalcemia, cardiac abnormalities may be found such as short Q-T intervals and arrhythmias.

Differential diagnosis

Diagnosis is based on the recognition of the clinical syndrome and on appropriate biochemical tests. Patients with paraneoplastic hypercalcemia must be differentiated from those with primary hyperparathyroidism or from those with other hypercalcemic conditions. The first diagnostic procedure should be aimed at excluding osteolytic metastases. A bone scan is the most sensitive test for this purpose, followed by radiological study of suspected areas. If no evidence of bone metastases is found, the determination of serum PTH concentrations help to exclude a diagnosis of primary hyperparathyroidism. Clinical and laboratory features of primary hyperparathyroidism and paraneoplastic hypercalcemia are compared in Table 70.7. Paraneoplastic hypercalcemia and primary hyperparathyroidism display several common biochemical abnormalities such as increased serum calcium concentrations, reduced serum phosphate levels, and increased urinary nephrogenic cAMP concentrations. However, other biochemical parameters are differentially altered in these two conditions. When compared to primary hyperparathyroidism, paraneoplastic hypercalcemia causes a higher urine/serum calcium ratio, lower serum chloride and lower serum 1,25$(OH)_2$-D_3 concentrations. These discrepancies are probably due to other humoral factors or to nutritional/metabolic abnormalities of cancer patients.

Table 70.7 Principal differences between primary hyperparathyroidism and paraneoplastic hypercalcemia

	Primary hyperparathyroidism	Paraneoplastic hypercalcemia
Sex	>50% female	>70% male
History	Long asymptomatic phase	Short, rapid, progressive
Symptoms	Bilateral nephrolithiasis, pancreatitis, peptic ulcer, bone pain	Weight loss, nausea, vomiting, neurologic disturbances, polyuria
Serum PTH	Normal or increased	Low
Serum PTHrP	Low	Elevated
Serum calcium	Often <7 mEq/l	Often >7 mEq/l
Serum chloride	Often >102 mEq/l	Often <102 mEq/l
Urine/serum calcium	Lower	Higher
Alkaline phosphatase	Often normal	Often elevated
Bone biopsy	Coupled resorption/formation (high osteoclastic resorption with high osteoblastic bone formation)	Uncoupled resorption/formation (high osteoclastic bone resorption with reduced osteoblastic bone formation)

Serum intact PTH is increased in primary hyperparathyroidism, while it is completely suppressed in paraneoplastic hypercalcemia due to PTH-rp. Older parathyroid hormone radioimmunoassays specific for amino- and carboxyl-terminal regions provide a lower specificity since PTH immunoreactive forms are not always fully suppressed. Recently, PTH-rp assays have been developed and introduced for clinical use. Detectable serum PTH-rp is found in most patients with paraneoplastic hypercalcemias, though the actual relevance of PTH-rp determination remains to be defined. If serum PTH is elevated, the coexistence of primary hyperparathyroidism should be considered, since this condition is more frequent in patients with tumors, and PTH production by tumors has been reported only in rare cases. If both PTH and PTH-rp are normal or reduced, calcitriol- or prostaglandin-dependent hypercalcemia is the most probable diagnosis. The first possibility can be confirmed by the direct measurement of increased serum $1,25(OH)_2\text{-}D_3$ concentrations. Administration of indomethacin (a powerful prostaglandin synthesis inhibitor) can be used as a diagnostic and therapeutic tool, since a decrease in serum calcium concentration after indomethacin administration provides the best evidence of prostaglandin-mediated hypercalcemia.

Treatment

The management of paraneoplastic hypercalcemia is based on the treatment of the underlying tumor and on measures aimed to reduce serum calcium concentrations. In many cases, the correction of hypercalcemia is immediately required and must precede the completion of the diagnostic work-up, although a precise diagnosis is useful to direct a more effective therapy. Nonspecific procedures currently employed in all cases of tumoral hypercalcemia include hydration, which expands intravascular volume, decreases serum calcium, and promotes urinary calcium excretion. This may be performed by infusion of isotonic NaCl solution at a rate of 200-300 ml/h, although higher infusion rates of up to 10-20 l/day have also been advocated. In the latter case, careful central venous pressure monitoring is needed to avoid volume overload. If saline infusion is not sufficient to lower serum calcium levels, diuretics such as furosemide (40-60 mg 2-4 times/day) or ethacrynic acid may be added, noting urinary potassium loss and providing appropriate replacement. This therapy is ineffective in the presence of severely impaired renal function independent of volume contraction: in this case, first-line therapy is represented by dialysis, possibly against a zero or low calcium dialysate.

The effectiveness of hydration and diuretic administration may be increased by association with drugs inhibiting bone resorption, such as biphosphonates, calcitonin, mithramycin, glucocorticoids, and gallium nitrate.

Biphosphonates directly inhibit osteoclast function and hydroxyapatite crystal dissolution. Currently available agents for first-line anti-absorptive therapy in paraneoplastic hypercalcemia are pamidronate and etidronate. Pamidronate is administered at a daily dose of 30-90 mg via 24-hour infusion. Etidronate is administered at a daily dose of 7.5 mg/kg, employing a 4-hour iv infusion. Although both agents are effective, pamidronate appears to be more potent and possibly less toxic than etidronate.

Both human and salmon calcitonin inhibit osteoclastic bone resorption and increase urinary calcium excretion. At a dosage of 4-8 UI/kg every 6-12 h sc or iv, calcitonin produces a fairly rapid decrease of serum calcium, though its effect is short-lived. Calcitonin should therefore be employed as a primary therapeutic modality only in mild to moderate hypercalcemia.

Mithramycin is a very effective and quick calcium-lowering agent, but its use is limited by severe adverse effects that include hepatotoxicity, nephrotoxicity, and thrombocytopenia. Gallium nitrate can be considered in the management of severe hypercalcemia unresponsive to conventional treatment. This drug is administered as a continuous iv infusion at a dosage of 200 mg/m^2 for 5 consecutive days, however its use is limited by severe nephrotoxicity.

Glucocorticoids (at daily doses equivalent to 200-300 mg of hydrocortisone for 5 consecutive days) represent the therapy of choice for calcitriol-induced hypercalcemia, while in other hypercalcemic conditions they are of limited utility. In rare cases of patients bearing prostaglandin-mediated hypercalcemia, indomethacin or other prostaglandin synthesis inhibitors may be effective.

Hypoglycemia in malignancies

After the first description by Nadler in 1929, several patients bearing noninsular neoplasias have been reported in whom fasting hypoglycemia remitted after surgical treatment of the tumor. More recently, it has been recognized that tumors may produce hypoglycemic factors and that paraneoplastic hypoglycemia, although a rare event, is a distinct clinical entity.

Pathology

Tumors associated with paraneoplastic hypoglycemia are listed in Table 70.8. In the majority of cases (60%), they are located in the abdominal cavity (often in the retroperitoneum) and are frequently large in size. One-half of these tumors are of mesenchymal origin with a poorly differentiated histotype, although a benign behavior may be rare.

The principle phenomenon involved in paraneoplastic hypoglycemia is a combination of increased peripheral glucose uptake/metabolism and decreased glucose hepatic production. Increased tumoral glucose utilization was originally proposed to explain hypoglycemia occurring in patients with large retroperitoneal neoplasias, but it has been subsequently documented that in cancer patients with hypoglycemia the glucose uptake is increased in all tissues. In any case, increased peripheral utilization of glucose should be easily compensated by hepatic glucose production, unless the latter is markedly impaired. Decreased glucose production may derive from massive liver destruction due to tumoral invasion or metastases, though rarely in the absence of direct liver involvement, reduced glucose hepatic production could result from circulating substances affecting hepatic glycogenolytic or neoglucogenetic processes, or from interfering with the counterregulatory hormonal response to hypoglycemia. In keeping with this concept, residual non-suppressible insulin-like activity has been detected in sera of hypoglycemic cancer patients after neutralization of endogenous insulin with anti-insulin antibodies. Further studies have provided evidence that non-suppressible insulin-like activity is mainly constituted by insulin-growth factors (IGF-I and IGF-II), IGF-II being the most important hypoglycemic factor. IGF-II is secreted by tumors in a precursor form due to abnormal post-translational processing, but it maintains its biological activity. Alternatively, IGF-II precursor is unable to bind plasma carrier proteins: this leads to high free circulating IGF-II concentrations and widespread reactions throughout the body.

Clinical findings and differential diagnosis

The clinical manifestations and the differential diagnosis of fasting hypoglycemia are discussed elsewhere in this book. In patients with non-islet cell tumors hypoglycemia, neuroglycopenic rather than sympathomimetic symptoms predominate, since the rate of blood glucose decline is generally slow. In addition to hypoglycemia, clinical signs and symptoms result, which are dependent on the size and the anatomical site of tumor. Large mesenchymal neoplasias are mostly located in the retroperitoneal, abdominal, or thoracic regions. Thus, abdominal pain or fullness associated with a palpable abdominal mass, dyspnea, cough, and peripheral neurologic symptoms are often present. Since hepatomas account for the second-most common cause of paraneoplastic hypoglycemia, weakness, anorexia, fever, jaundice, and hepatomegaly are commonly observed. A distinctive diagnostic feature of paraneoplastic hypoglycemia is that plasma insulin concentrations are suppressed in spite of low serum glucose levels. High serum IGF-II concentrations could represent a helpful diagnostic aid, though assays for IGF-II are generally not available.

Table 70.8 Tumors types associated with hypoglycemia

Tumor type	Approximate frequency
Mesenchymal (often fibrosarcoma)	50%
Hepatoma	20%
Adrenal carcinoma	10%
Lymphoma	6%
Intestinal carcinoma	< 5%
Miscellaneous: neuroectodermal tumors, teratomas, hypernephroma, melanoma, cholangiocarcinoma	~15%

When possible, a surgical approach directed against tumors is the most effective therapy. In addition to surgical management, radiotherapy or polychemotherapy may be helpful. The prognosis for the patient with tumors causing paraneoplastic hypoglycemia is generally poor due to the frequent local recurrence and mass effect of the tumors. Medical therapy is often utilized to counterbalance hypoglycemia; frequent feedings, glucose infusion, growth hormone, glucagon, and glucocorticoids may help in reducing symptoms.

Ectopic growth hormone-releasing hormone (GHRH) and growth hormone (GH) secretion

GH-like immunoreactive substances are frequently detected in both normal and tumoral extra-pituitary tissues, while clinical or biochemical evidence of GH excess in cancer patients is a rare event.

To date, full-blown acromegaly due to unequivocally proven ectopic GH secretion has been reported in only one islet-cell tumor case. In contrast, increased serum GH levels and acromegaly due to ectopic GHRH secretion have been documented in many patients with neuroendocrine tumors (carcinoids, islet-cell carcinomas, small cell lung carcinomas, sympathetic neural tumors, and adrenal adenomas). Overall, ectopic acromegaly is a rare condition, accounting for <1% of all acromegalic patients.

Clinical findings

Clinically, ectopic acromegaly is characterized by classical acromegalic features associated with other abnormalities typical of the primary tumor. These include hypoglycemia due to islet-cell tumor and hypertension due to pheochromocytoma; hyperparathyroidism and Zollinger-Ellison syndrome may be observed, since multiple endocrine neoplasia type I syndrome can result from tumors involved in GHRH production. The delay between the onset of disease and the appearance of acromegalic features is variable, with a prolonged lag phase when the underlying tumor is slowly growing (e.g., carcinoids), or short in the case of pancreatic islet-cell carcinomas or other aggressive malignancies.

Differential diagnosis

Clinical presentation of acromegaly due to GHRH-producing tumors does not differ from that seen in pituitary GH-secreting adenoma. Thus, the correct diagnosis in these patients is often made after an unsuccessful neurosurgical therapy for GH adenoma, showing at histology only somatotroph hyperplasia.

Common diagnostic tests used to assess acromegaly are of no value in differentiating the ectopic source of GHRH from GH-secreting adenoma. In both cases, lack of GH suppression after an oral glucose tolerance test,

and a paradoxical increase of GH after the glucose test or TRH administration may be frequently found. A stimulation test with GHRH may be of some help, since some patients with ectopic GHRH production do not show any further increase of serum GH after exogenous GHRH administration. The best tool to distinguish the two conditions is the direct measurement of serum GHRH concentration, which is markedly increased in patients with GHRH-producing tumor, but this assay is seldom available in routine clinical settings. In addition to biochemical evaluation, imaging techniques such as CT-scan or MRI are useful in localizing the primary tumor and possible metastases. Whole body Octreoscan® may further aid in the recognition of these tumors, which often express somatostatin receptors.

Treatment

Surgical removal of primary neoplasm is the most effective therapy and improves the clinical course even in the presence of metastases. Restoration of the GH secretory dynamic is observed when surgery has accomplished complete removal of the tumor. In some cases, medical therapy with long-acting somatostatin analogs is able to inhibit both GHRH secretion by the tumor and GH release by hyperplastic pituitary somatotrophs.

Ectopic production of human chorionic gonadotropin (hCG)

The dimeric protein hCG is normally secreted by trophoblastic tissue, which is constituted by α- and β-subunits noncovalently bound. The α-subunit is similar in amino acid sequence to that of other pituitary glycoproteins TSH, LH, and FSH. Serum hCG increases during the first trimester of pregnancy, and extremely elevated concentrations are found in patients with trophoblastic tumors (vesicular mola and choriocarcinoma).

Detectable hCG was frequently reported in sera from cancer patients using early radioimmunoassays. This finding was not confirmed after the introduction of sensitive and specific assays for the hCG β-subunit, showing that serum hCG is generally not increased in nontrophoblastic tumors, with rare exceptions characterized by the production of high amounts of biologically active hormone (Tab. 70.9). In these cases, the clinical manifestations include isosexual precocious puberty in young boys and gynecomastia in adult males.

Hyperthyroidism is a distinct endocrine manifestation of tumoral hCG production. This frequently occurs in association with "eutopic" hCG hypersecretion by choriocarcinoma and vesicular mola, but in rare cases it has also been reported in nontrophoblastic tumors such as mesothelioma or bronchogenic carcinoma. Human chorionic gonadotropin exerts its thyrotrophic action via TSH receptor-mediated adenylate cyclase activation, with a subsequent increase in thyroid hormone production. The degree

Table 70.9 Neoplasias associated with ectopic production of HCG

Tumor type	Approximate frequency
Bronchogenic carcinoma	40%
Hepatoma or hepatoblastoma	
Pancreatic carcinoma	30%
Intestinal carcinoma	
Breast carcinoma	20%
Miscellaneous: melanoma, carcinoid tumors, others	10%

of thyrotoxicosis is generally mild, due to the low intrinsic thyroid stimulation activity of hCG. Goiter may be present, but other signs of Graves' disease, such as ophthalmopathy or dermopathy, are consistently absent. Hyperthyroidism disappears after removal of the primary tumor, though in some cases treatment with antithyroid drugs may be needed before performing surgical intervention.

Ectopic production of human placental lactogen (hPL)

Human placental lactogen (hPL), normally produced by syncytiotrophoblasts of the placenta during pregnancy, shows structural, immunological, and biological similarities with pituitary GH. "Eutopic" hypersecretion of hPL occurs in trophoblastic-derived tumors, while ectopic hPL production, behaving identically to native placental hPL in radioimmunologic assay, may occasionally be observed in some nontrophoblastic neoplasias (mostly ovarian, uterine, gastrointestinal, lung and prostate carcinomas). In these tumors, serum hPL immunoreactivity can be detected in 9 to 14% of cases, and in about 50% of tumoral specimens hPL is detected by immunohistochemistry. Immunoreactive hPL may also be found in a minority of patients affected by benign breast diseases, but not in normal breast tissue. However, the sensitivity and specificity of serum hPL assay is too low to be clinically relevant in nontrophoblastic malignancies.

Tumoral production of hPL is not associated to any clinical manifestation, with the possible exception of rare cases of gynecomastia.

Ectopic production of prolactin

Immunoreactive prolactin has been detected in some tumoral tissues and cell lines, but significant in vivo ectopic prolactin synthesis and secretion is a rare event, and its clinical impact in cancer patients is very limited. In several oncologic series, true ectopic prolactin secretion accounts for only 1% of all cases of hyperprolactinemia, and it is not associated to clinical findings.

Ectopic production of calcitonin

Calcitonin, the product of the secretion of thyroid C cells in mammals, is a hormone mainly acting to reduce serum calcium concentrations. Markedly increased eutopic calcitonin production is observed in both sporadic and inherited forms of medullary thyroid carcinomas, thus making calcitonin determination a very useful marker for diagnosis and follow-up in these patients.

A mild to moderate increase of serum calcitonin may also be observed in about one-third of other tumors, such as carcinomas arising from the lung, colon, breast, pancreas, or stomach. The highest prevalence of increased serum calcitonin is observed in patients with small-cell carcinoma of the lung. Ectopic calcitonin production is strictly associated to tumors showing APUD characteristics. Chromatographic analysis of tumoral extracts and in vitro studies on cultured tumor cells provide evidence that calcitonin produced by nonmedullary thyroid tumors has a molecular weight higher (7-14 kD) than that of the native hormone (3.5 kD).

Serum calcitonin markedly increases after pentagastrin administration in patients with medullary thyroid carcinoma, while the response to pentagastrin is blunted in patients with other tumors.

Since serum calcitonin excess does not cause clinical symptoms, hypercalcitoninemia per se is not associated to a well-defined clinical schema.

Ectopic production of erythropoietin

Erythropoietin is produced physiologically by the liver and the kidney. Erythropoietin hypersecretion with polycythemia are observed in both benign and malignant diseases arising from these organs. In renal neoplastic conditions, erythropoietin hypersecretion occurs in more than 50% of patients, but in only a minority of them (<5%) is polycythemia recognizable.

In addition to eutopic production of this hormone, ectopic erythropoietin production has been observed in other neoplasias, such as cerebellar hemangioblastoma, ovarian, uterine and adrenal tumors, hepatomas, and, more rarely, pheochromocytomas. In these tumors, polycythemia is reported with a greater prevalence (10 to 20%) than is observed in renal cancer patients. It has been suggested that in some patients with paraneoplastic erythropoietin production, polycythemia may also result from different mechanisms, such as glucocorticoid and androgen secretion occurring in adrenal or ovarian tumors.

Diagnosis relies on an elevated hematocrit value associated with increased total red cell mass, after the exclusion of dehydration conditions. Polycythemia vera is easily excluded on the basis of increased white cell and platelet counts, while polycythemia secondary to hypoxia is characterized by low partial oxygen pressure in the blood. Serum erythropoietin concentration is normal or suppressed in polycythemia vera, and it is increased both in hypoxic and paraneoplastic conditions.

Surgical treatment of primary tumors is able to reverse the clinical condition of the patient and to decrease serum erythropoietin levels. When the tumor is unresectable, phlebotomy may ameliorate symptoms related to polycythemia.

Oncogenic osteomalacia

Hypophosphatemic osteomalacia is a very rare paraneoplastic syndrome (generally observed in tumors of mesenchymal origin: hemangiopericytomas, fibromas, hemangiomas, fibroangiomas, osteoblastomas, chondromas, chondroblastomas, and fibrous xanthonomas) and is often localized at the extremities. Carcinoma of the prostate, small cell carcinoma of the lung, and hematological neoplasias may also be observed.

The biochemical abnormality underlying this condition is the impaired conversion of 25-OH-vitamin D to its active form, leading to renal hyperphosphaturia with osteomalacia. The pathophysiologic mechanism responsible is still undefined. The presence of tumor-derived humoral factor(s) have been hypothesized on the basis of the disappearance of this syndrome after complete removal of the primary tumor.

Clinical features include bone pain and, less frequently, muscular weakness, myalgias, and fractures of the long bones. The diagnosis must rule out all other causes of osteomalacia with hypophosphatemia and hyperphosphaturia, such as nutritional deficits, malabsorption diseases, chronic renal failure or familial renal phosphate transfer defects, antacid drug abuse, Fanconi's disease, and cystinosis.

In addition to surgical removal of the tumor, the medical therapy is the administration of $1,25(OH)_2\text{-}D_3$. Because of the frequent benign behavior of the underlying neoplasia, the prognosis for this condition is good.

Miscellaneous endocrine paraneoplastic syndromes

Excessive production of vasoactive intestinal peptide may be associated with non-β-cell pancreatic tumors (also called vipomas), lung carcinoma, and, more rarely, adrenal ganglioneuroblastoma or pheochromocytoma. Clinical manifestations are typically watery diarrhea, hypokalemia, and achlorhydria. When possible, surgical resection of the tumor reverses this clinical condition, and a fall in plasma vasoactive intestinal peptide levels can be observed. When the primary tumor is not operable, long-acting somatostatin analogue therapy may be effective in controlling vasoactive intestinal peptide secretion by the tumor.

Ectopic glucagon production with overt clinical symptoms has been occasionally reported in non-small-cell lung carcinomas and in renal carcinomas; immunoreactive glucagon has also been demonstrated in ovarian carcinomas in the absence of clinical manifestations.

Zollinger-Ellison syndrome due to ectopic gastrin production has been documented in patients with pancreatic and ovarian cystoadenocarcinomas.

Somatostatin production by non-islet-cell cancers has been reported in neuroectodermal tumors such as small-cell lung carcinoma or carcinoids, and in some instances it has been associated with ectopic ACTH secretion.

Ectopic production of renin has been reported in lung carcinomas (small-cell and adenomatous type), hepatomas, and pancreatic and ovarian carcinomas. Renin production occurs eutopically in the juxtaglomerular region, and some renal neoplasms such as hemangiopericytoma, Wilms' tumor, or renal cell carcinoma may secrete renin or its precursor form. Clinically, mild to moderate hypertension with secondary hyperaldosteronism may be present in association with hypokalemic alkalosis and elevated plasma renin activity; in some cancer patients hypertension may be absent because of the tumoral secretion of inactive renin. Differential diagnosis of hyperreninemic conditions includes nephrovascular hypertension and malignant hypertension. Surgical treatment of the primary tumor resolves the hypertension, while administration of angiotensin-converting enzyme inhibitors may be useful in the treatment of unresectable neoplasms.

In patients with lung carcinoma, bronchial and other carcinoids, medullary thyroid carcinoma, and pheochromocytoma, the ectopic production of gastrin-releasing peptides has been documented by plasma gastrin-releasing peptide measurements, although no clinical manifestations have been reported.

Suggested readings

AGARWALA SS. Paraneoplastic syndromes. Med Clin North Amer 1996;80:173-84.

ARON DC, RAFF H, FINDLING JW. Effectiveness versus efficacy: the limited value in clinical practice of high dose dexamethasone suppression testing in the differential diagnosis of adrenocorticotropin-dependent Cushing's syndrome. J Clin Endocr Metab 1997;82:1780-5.

BALL DW, BAYLIN SB, DE BUSTROS AC. Ectopic production of hormones. In: Moore WT, Eastman RC (eds). Diagnostic endocrinology. 2nd ed. St. Louis: Mosby-Year Book 1996; 493-507.

BECKER M, ARON DC. Ectopic ACTH syndrome and CRH-mediated Cushing's syndrome. Endocrinol Metab Clin North Am 1994;23:585-606.

BLIND E. Humoral hypercalcemia of malignancy: role of parathyroid hormone-related protein. Recent Results Cancer Res 1994;137:20-43.

BRAUNSTEIN GD. Ectopic hormone production. In: Felig P, Baxter JD, Frohman LA (eds). Endocrinology and metabolism. 3rd ed. New York: McGraw-Hill 1995;1733-83.

EDELSON GW, KLEEREKOPER M. Hypercalcemic crisis. Med Clin North Am 1995;79: 79-92.

FAGLIA G, AROSIO M, BAZZONI N. Ectopic acromegaly. Endocrinol Metab Clin North Am 1992;21:575-95.

MIDGETTE AS, ARON DC. High-dose dexamethasone suppression testing versus inferior petrosal sinus sampling in the differential diagnosis of adrenocorticotropin-dependent Cushing's syndrome: a decision analysis. Am J Med Sci 1995;309:162-70.

MUNDY GR. Ectopic production of calciotropic peptides. Endocrinol Metab Clin North Am 1991;20:473-87.

ODELL WD, APPLETON WS. Humoral manifestations of cancer. In: Wilson JD, Foster DW (eds). Williams' textbook of endocrinology. 8th ed. Philadelphia: WB Saunders 1992;1599-616.

SHERWOOD LM. Paraneoplastic endocrine disorders (ectopic hormone syndromes). In: DeGroot LJ, et al (eds). Endocrinology. 3rd ed. Philadelphia : WB Saunders 1994;2754-802.

STREWLER GJ. Humoral manifestations of malignancy. In: Greenspan FS, Baxter JD (eds). Basic and clinical endocrinology, 4th ed. East Norwalk: Lange Medical Publishers 1994;703-12.

TSIGOS C, PAPANICOLAOU DA, CHROUSOS GP. Advances in the diagnosis and treatment of Cushing's syndrome. Baillière Clin Endocrinol Met 1995;9:315-36.

WYSOLMERSKI JJ, BROADUS AE. Hypercalcemia of malignancy: the central role of parathyroid hormone-related protein. Annu Rev Med 1994;45:189-200.

Special topics
in endocrinology

Multiple endocrine neoplasia

Robert F. Gagel, Douglas B. Evans, Jeffrey E. Lee

█ KEY POINTS █

- Multiple endocrine neoplasia type 1 (MEN 1) is caused by inactive mutations of menin; there is no correlation between genotype and phenotype.
- Hereditary medullary thyroid carcinoma and multiple endocrine neoplasia type 2 are caused by mutations of the Ret proto-oncogene.
- There is a specific correlation between genotype and phenotype: mutations of specific codons of the Ret proto-oncogene cause specific phenotypes.
- Mutations of the Ret proto-oncogene can be identified easily by molecular genetic techniques, which can be then be used as guides in the clinical management of families at risk for the conditions they cause.
- Children who have Ret proto-oncogene mutations causative for hereditary medullary thyroid carcinoma should have a thyroidectomy performed at an early age.

The multiple endocrine neoplasia syndromes form a distinct group of genetic tumor syndromes. Multiple endocrine neoplasia types 1 and 2, von Hippel-Lindau syndrome, neurofibromatosis, and several other less common disorders provide challenging diagnostic and clinical management problems for endocrinologists. Recent advances in our understanding of the molecular basis for these syndromes have propelled these syndromes into the spotlight as models of neoplasia.

MULTIPLE ENDOCRINE NEOPLASIA TYPE 1

The association of the parathyroid glands, pancreatic islets, and pituitary hyperplasia or neoplasia is called multiple endocrine neoplasia type 1 (MEN 1). Recent reassessment of the associated clinical features, however, suggests that adrenal cortical abnormalities may be more common than pituitary tumors. The clinical syndrome is transmitted as autosomal dominant and most commonly develops in the context of a known kindred with MEN 1, although de novo mutations do occur.

Management of patients with MEN 1 is always challenging and requires an appreciation of several important points: First, tumors associated with MEN 1 are almost always multicentric. Therefore, removal of a single tumor rarely results in clinical cure. Second, each gene carrier can be expected to undergo at least three to six surgical procedures related to MEN 1 during his or her life; it is therefore important to time these procedures to derive the maximum benefit with the fewest surgical interventions. Third, and most importantly, is the necessity to balance the clinical sequelae of hormone excess (caused by the tumor syndrome) with the risk of hormone deficiency (caused by removal of a gland) when considering the overall management of the patient.

Etiology

The localization of the causative gene for MEN 1 to chromosome 11q in 1988 initiated an almost decade-long search that culminated in the identification of a new gene, that encodes menin, in 1997 (Fig. 71.1). In kindreds with

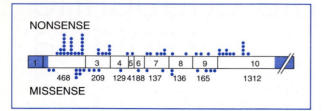

Figure 71.1 Mutations of the MEN 1 gene (menin). Over 75 different mutations of menin, most inactivating, have been identified in MEN 1. The greatest mutation frequency (shown as closed circles above or below the protein structure) is found in exons 2 and 10. Germline mutations of menin are inherited; the acquisition of a second somatic mutation in the other allele of menin initiates neoplastic change. Exons are numbered 1 to 10. The number of nucleotides per exon is shown below each numbered exon. (From Agarwal et al. Hum Mol Genet.1997;6:1169-75; Lemmens et al. Hum Mol Genet.1997;6:1177-83.)

MEN 1, a germline inactivating mutation is inherited (or a *de novo* mutation occurs, though this is rare); the other copy is lost in a single cell through somatic mutation. More than 75 different inactivating mutations distributed throughout the gene have been described (Fig. 71.1). Genetic testing is currently being performed in research laboratories and will likely be available in commercial laboratories within 2 years. Somatic mutations affecting the MEN 1 gene have also been identified in patients with parathyroid and other tumors.

HYPERPARATHYROIDISM

Clinical findings

The clinical features of hyperparathyroidism in MEN 1 are identical to the more common form of sporadic hyperparathyroidism. Hypercalcemia has been reported in gene carriers of MEN 1 as young as 17 years of age, and it develops in more than 90% before the age of 40 years. Other familial disorders such as familial hypercalcemic hypocalciuria, MEN 2A, parathyroid hormone-related protein production by an islet cell or carcinoid tumor, and the familial parathyroid tumor/jaw tumor syndrome should be considered in the differential diagnosis of familial hypercalcemia, especially when there is no clear family history of MEN 1.

Treatment

Surgical removal of adenoma(s) or multiple hyperplastic glands is the treatment of choice: the major question is when to operate. There is general agreement that operative intervention is indicated in patients with a serum calcium higher than 3.0 mm/l (12 mg/dl), renal nephrolithia-

sis or calcification, a decreased bone density, or an elevated serum gastrin (normalization of the serum gastrin will occur in more than one-half of patients in whom the serum calcium is normalized). Two different operative approaches have been recommended: (1) the complete removal of all parathyroid tissue from the neck with transplantation of tissue to the nondominant arm, and (2) subtotal parathyroidectomy. Approximately two-thirds of patients will have recurrent hyperparathyroidism within 6 to 10 years. The major advantage of total parathyroidectomy and autotransplantation to the arm is the elimination of the inevitable subsequent operative procedures.

ISLET CELL TUMORS

Clinical findings

Pancreatic islet cell abnormalities occur in approximately 80% of MEN 1 gene carriers. The abnormalities include hyperplasia of individual islets, small adenomas, large adenomas, and carcinomas with or without metastasis. Most commonly *multiple* islet cell tumors are identified within the pancreas of a gene carrier. It is also common for the islet cell tumors to produce multiple hormones. Elevated serum pancreatic polypeptide is the most common hormonal abnormality, although overproduction of glucagon, somatostatin, gastrin, insulin, vasoactive intestinal peptide, gastric inhibitory peptide, and neurotensin may be found. Tumors that produce several hormones are common.

Diagnostic procedures

The most sensitive test for detecting early islet cell hyperplasia is the measurement of serum pancreatic polypeptide following a standardized meal (Tab. 71.1). Routine screening for islet cell tumors by this approach has resulted in earlier detection of tumors. Clinically recognizable hormonal syndromes develop when the secretion of a single peptide hormone – such as gastrin, insulin, vasoactive intestinal polypeptide, or corticotropin-releasing hormone – predominates.

Imaging studies

Several diagnostic imaging approaches have been applied to the diagnosis of islet cell tumors. Traditional computed tomography (CT) and magnetic resonance imaging (MRI) are of limited usefulness for the detection of small islet cell tumors and will almost never identify duodenal wall tumors. Preliminary studies combining high resolution helical or spiral CT performed at the time of maximal contrast enhancement has greatly improved image quality and resolution. A second approach that is useful for the detection of small tumors in the duodenal wall or head of the pancreas is endoscopic ultrasound. Octreotide scanning is useful for the detection of pancreatic islet tumors greater than 1 cm in size and for extrapancreatic metastasis, but it is rarely useful for detecting small pancreatic islet cell tumors.

Screening for pancreatic islet cell tumors should focus on historical features (symptoms of ulcer disease [gastrinoma], hypoglycemia [insulinoma], skin rash [glucagonoma], and watery diarrhea [vasoactive intestinal peptide-producing tumor]), combined with measurements of pancreatic polypeptide basally or after a meal stimulation test (Tab. 71.1). It is appropriate to perform a CT or MRI every 5 years after the age of 20 to detect an islet cell tumor.

ZOLLINGER-ELLISON SYNDROME

Zollinger-Ellison syndrome or gastrinoma is characterized by gastrin-induced gastric acid secretion.

Clinical findings

The clinical features of Zollinger-Ellison syndrome include excessive acid secretion, peptic ulceration, reflux esophagitis, and diarrhea. Over 60% of MEN 1 patients with functional islet cell tumors have increased gastrin production (a value greater than 171 pmol/l or 300 pg/ml). In patients with symptoms and clinical findings of Zollinger-Ellison syndrome (increased gastric acid secretion and peptic ulceration of the stomach, duodenum, or small bowel) and borderline abnormalities of serum gastrin concentration, the diagnosis can be confirmed by the finding of an abnormal gastrin response (greater than 114 pmol/l) after either calcium or secretin infusion (Tab. 71.1). The differential diagnosis of hypergastrinemia includes atrophic gastritis, retained gastric antrum, gastric outlet obstruction, near complete small bowel resection, hypercalcemia, and omeprazole administration. Increased gastrin production in patients with MEN 1 is caused by multiple neuroendocrine tumors located in the duodenal wall and throughout the pancreas.

Treatment

Treatment of gastrinoma in the context of MEN 1 has changed several times over the past 3 decades. Initially Zollinger and Ellison recommended total gastrectomy

---

Table 71.1 Procedures used to evaluate endocrine tumor syndromes

Test	Purpose	Brief description	Interpretation
Secreting test	Diagnose gastrinoma	Infuse secretin (2 U/kg) as iv bolus with measurement of serum gastrin at 0, 2, 5, 10, and 15 min	Normal response is <50% increase of serum gastrin over basal value
Calcium stimulation	Diagnose gastrinoma	15 mg/kg of calcium in 500 ml normal saline infused over 3 h. Measure serum gastrin at 0, 1, 2, and 3 h	Normal response is <50% increase of serum gastrin over basal value
Meal stimulation test for pancreatic polypeptide and gastrin	Diagnostic test for islet cell tumor in MEN 1	Consume 560 kcal meal rich in carbohydrates (66 g) and low in protein (18 g) and fat (22 g) over 20 min. with measurements of serum gastrin and pancreatic polypeptide at 0, 10, 20, and 60 min	Normal response is a serum pancreatic polypeptide or gastrin level less than 2 times the basal level. False positive rate approximately 12%
Selective arterial calcium injection with hepatic venous sampling	Localize hormone-secreting tumor, most commonly insulinoma, to specific pancreatic arterial distribution	Selective injection of calcium into specific pancreatic arteries with sampling of hepatic venous effluent for insulin or other peptides after each injection	An increase in the hepatic venous (0, 30, 60, and 120 s) serum peptide (insulin) concentration after selective arterial injection likely indicates a tumor in the distribution of the artery
Pentagastrin test	Diagnose MTC	Infuse pentagastrin (0.5 µg/kg body weight) over 10 s with measurement of serum calcitonin basally and at 2, 5, 10, and 15 min	Normal response is calcitonin radioimmunoassays the peak assay-dependent, but in most calcitonin is <30 pg/ml in females and <100 pg/ml in males
Combined calcium-pentagastrin test	Diagnose MTC	Infuse calcium gluconate (2 mg/kg) over 1 min followed immediately by pentagastrin (0.5 µg/kg body weight) over 5 s. Measure serum calcitonin basally and at 1, 2, 3, and 5 min	Normal response is calcitonin radioimmunoassays the peak assay-dependent, but in most calcitonin is <50 pg/ml in females and <150 pg/ml in males

(MEN = multiple endocrine neoplasia; MTC = medullary thyroid carcinoma.)

because of the difficulty of identifying all gastrin-producing tissue. Subsequently there was enthusiasm for surgical resection of gastrin-producing islet cell tumors in MEN 1 as localization procedures improved. The low rate of surgical cure and the high rate of clinical recurrence – combined with the introduction of H2 receptor antagonists in the 1970s and proton pump inhibitors in the 1980s – led to the suggestion that medical therapy be substituted for surgical intervention. The recognition over the past decade that duodenal wall carcinoid-like tumors are present in the majority of patients with Zollinger-Ellison syndrome in MEN 1, and the development of techniques for intraoperative identification of these tumors, has markedly improved the success of surgery and forced caregivers to rethink management of these patients. In MEN 1 patients with Zollinger-Ellison syndrome and no evidence of hepatic metastasis, our preferred operative procedure is distal pancreatectomy, enucleation of tumors in the pancreatic head, duodenotomy with resection of all duodenal tumors, and regional lymphadenectomy.

In patients in whom a gastrinoma is not identified or for those with evidence of metastatic disease, medical therapy with either H2 receptor antagonists or proton pump inhibitors is effective for the control of peptic acid symptoms.

INSULINOMA

Approximately one-third of patients with functional islet cell neoplasms in the context of MEN 1 have evidence of excessive and unregulated insulin secretion associated with hypoglycemia. The identification of hypoglycemia and an inappropriate elevation of serum insulin or C-peptide concentration confirms the diagnosis of an insulin-secreting neoplasm. Insulinomas are frequently small, difficult to identify, and can occur throughout the pancreas. Treatment is further complicated in MEN 1 by the presence of multiple islet cell tumors of other types. Identification and removal of the specific tumor causing excessive insulin secretion can be a challenge. Two approaches have been utilized. The first is to thoroughly evaluate the pancreas preoperatively by use of high resolution helical CT scanning, endoscopic ultrasound, and selective arterial infusion of calcium with hepatic venous sampling in order to localize the insulin-producing tumor to a specific pancreatic arterial distribution (Tab. 70.1). An alternative approach, and the one preferred by the authors, is to image the pancreas with high resolution helical CT scanning and then proceed directly to surgical evaluation of the pancreas, utilizing intraoperative ultrasound examination to identify the tumor. Those who utilize the latter approach identify approximately 90% of islet cell tumors, and thus one can argue that the more detailed and costly evaluation should be reserved for those patients in whom a tumor is not identified during the primary surgical procedure. Subtotal (60%) pancreatectomy is appropriate in patients with multiple small tumors. In patients with hepatic metastasis from insulino-

ma, continuous infusion of glucagon or 10 to 20% glucose has been used successfully to control hypoglycemia; octreotide therapy has been successfully used in only a small percentage of these patients.

GLUCAGONOMA

Increased production of glucagon by a pancreatic islet cell tumor produces a rare but distinctive syndrome characterized by hyperglycemia, an erythematous and necrolytic skin rash localized to the inguinal and axillary regions and the extremities, glossitis, anorexia, occasional diarrhea, and venous thrombosis. There is compelling evidence that glucagon is involved in the genesis of the syndrome. Intravenous infusion of glucagon has been shown to cause the skin lesions, and normalization of the plasma glucagon by octreotide therapy or surgical removal has been shown in most cases to improve them. Hepatic metastasis occurs frequently; palliative management approaches include hepatic artery embolization, chemotherapy, and somatostatin analogues (octreotide or lanreotide).

VERNER-MORRISON SYNDROME

Verner-Morrison syndrome is the association of watery diarrhea, hypokalemia, hypochlorhydria, and acidosis. In the context of MEN 1, this syndrome may occur with either carcinoid or pancreatic islet cell tumors. Increased production of vasoactive intestinal peptide is the most common hormonal abnormality found in this group of patients, although the increased production of gastric inhibitory peptide and calcitonin has occasionally been described in patients.

Surgical excision of either a pancreatic islet or carcinoid tumor may be curative. Treatment for patients with hepatic metastasis may include systemic chemotherapy, hepatic artery embolization, or chronic octreotide therapy. Although mortality related to the cholera-like diarrhea was high in the past; the introduction of somatostatin analogue therapy, and the more frequent use of outpatient intravenous fluid replacement, combined with intermittent hepatic artery embolization/chemotherapy, has improved the clinical outcome in these patients.

PITUITARY NEOPLASIA

Pituitary tumors occur in one-half of MEN 1 gene carriers. These tumors are frequently multicentric and may produce excessive prolactin, growth hormone, adrenocorticotropic hormone (ACTH), or the alpha subunit of the pituitary glycoprotein hormone. The most common mechanism of clonal tumor formation is the functional loss of both copies of the menin gene. Production of a trophic hormone by another endocrine tumor that stimulates further tumor growth is a second, and probably less common, mechanism. For example, production of corticotropin-releasing hormone or growth hormone-releasing hormone (GHRH) by islet cell or carcinoid tumors may accelerate the development of

ACTH- or growth hormone (GH)-producing tumors. There is also some evidence that pituitary tumors may produce a member of the fibroblast growth factor-like family of peptides that contributes to parathyroid growth.

PROLACTINOMA

Prolactinoma is the most common pituitary neoplasm, accounting for more than one-half of all pituitary tumors in MEN 1. The tumors are almost always multicentric and frequently large, and they produce galactorrhea and amenorrhea in women and hypogonadism in males (see Chap. 40). There are rare MEN 1 kindreds in which prolactinoma is the predominant manifestation.

Treatment with dopamine agonist therapy (bromocriptine, pergolide, quinagolide, or cabergoline especially when applied early in the clinical course of these tumors, is generally effective therapy. Transphenoidal or transfrontal surgical excision is used in those patients with large tumors, dopamine agonist-unresponsive tumors, or those producing compressive symptoms. Radiotherapy (external irradiation, proton beam, or gamma knife) following surgical decompression is reserved for those patients with large tumors and/or for those who are unresponsive to dopamine agonist therapy.

ACROMEGALY

Growth hormone-producing tumors are the second most common pituitary neoplasm and represent approximately one-fourth of all pituitary neoplasms in MEN 1. Although growth hormone-releasing hormone stimulation of pituitary tumor formation is not common, this possibility should be considered in MEN 1-related acromegaly. The diagnosis is confirmed by the finding of a nonsuppressible GH and an elevated somatomedin C concentration. The greater awareness of this clinical syndrome in MEN 1 has led to the recognition of patients with earlier manifestations of acromegaly and some patients with only GH and/or somatomedin C abnormalities. Early intervention in these patients is appropriate to prevent the long-term complications of GH excess.

Surgical excision of a GH-producing neoplasm, most commonly by a transphenoidal procedure, is the preferred form of primary therapy. In patients who are not cured by surgical therapy, two approaches are currently used: (1) In patients with a small residual tumor with minimal GH and somatomedin C elevations postoperatively (generally a GH <15 ng/ml), long-term therapy with somatostatin analogue therapy (octreotide or lanreotide) may be effective. (2) In patients with higher values, radiation therapy (external beam, proton beam, or gamma knife) will result in normalization of the GH and somatomedin C values, although 3 to 10 years may be required, and concurrent therapy with somatostatin analogues may be necessary.

In patients with a carcinoid or islet cell tumor and elevated GH or somatomedin C, production of GHRH by a carcinoid or islet cell tumor should be considered. Excision of the GHRH-producing tumor may normalize the growth hormone.

CUSHING'S SYNDROME

Cushing's syndrome in the context of MEN 1 can be caused by an ACTH-producing pituitary tumor, ectopic production of ACTH, or corticotropin-releasing hormone production by a carcinoid or islet cell tumor. The etiology of Cushing's syndrome may be further confounded by the presence of adrenal cortical adenoma, a frequent finding in MEN 1. However, these adenomas are rarely functional in the absence of excessive ACTH production. It is important to consider the entire spectrum of causes for Cushing's syndrome in MEN 1 patients (as outlined in Chap. 29).

CARCINOID TUMORS

Carcinoid tumors do not occur frequently in MEN 1. They appear to cluster in certain families. Foregut carcinoids (thymus in men and lung in women) account for two-thirds of these tumors. Approximately one-half of these tumors are malignant with local or distant metastasis. Hepatic metastasis and symptoms of flushing, diarrhea, and bronchospasm are less common in MEN 1-associated carcinoid tumors; somatostatin analogues are generally effective in the rare patient with these symptoms.

CUTANEOUS MANIFESTATIONS

Lipomas occur in a high percentage of MEN 1 patients. The most common location is in subcutaneous or omental fat. Cutaneous angiofibromas occur with a high frequency in MEN 1 patients.

OTHER MANIFESTATIONS OF MEN 1

Nodular adrenal cortical hyperplasia or adenomas occur in approximately 50% of MEN 1 patients. Malignant transformation rarely occurs, although surgical excision may be appropriate in those with cortical tumors greater than 4 to 5 cm. These tumors may be functional in a patient with excessive ACTH production.

A handful of adrenal medullary tumors have been described in the context of MEN 1, suggesting a frequency greater than would occur by chance. This possibility should be considered in the differential diagnosis of a patient with an adrenal mass or with symptoms and signs of catecholamine excess.

MULTIPLE ENDOCRINE NEOPLASIA TYPE 2

Multiple endocrine neoplasia type 2 (MEN 2) is a syndrome characterized by medullary thyroid carcinoma (MTC), pheochromocytoma, and parathyroid hyperplasia (Tab. 71.2). It is inherited as an autosomal dominant trait;

Table 71.2 Genetic syndromes with endocrine neoplastic components

Syndrome	Neoplastic features
MEN 1	Pituitary Parathyroid glands Pancreatic islets Adrenal cortex Cutaneous angiofibromas Lipomas
MEN 2A	C-cell of the thyroid (MTC) Adrenal medulla (pheochromocytoma) Parathyroid glands
MEN 2B	C-cell of the thyroid (MTC) Adrenal medulla (pheochromocytoma) Intestinal ganglioneuromatosis Marfanoid features
Von Hippel Lindau syndrome	Adrenal medulla (pheochromocytoma) Pancreatic islets Hemangioblastoma of the central nervous system Retinal angiomas Renal cell carcinomas Visceral cysts
Neurofibromatosis type 1	Neurofibromas Inconstant development of endocrine tumors Adrenal medulla (pheochromocytoma) C-cell (MTC) Parathyroid neoplasia Somatostatin-producing carcinoid tumors
Cowden disease	Thyroid hamartomas or carcinoma Breast Intestinal Skin
Carney complex	Pituitary Thyroid Testicular Adrenal cortex Myxomas of heart, breast, and skin Cutaneous spotty pigmentation

(MEN = multiple endocrine neoplasia; MTC = medullary thyroid carcinoma.)

Etiology

The identification of mutations in the c-ret proto-oncogene, a tyrosine kinase receptor, culminated a decade-long search for the causative gene of MEN 2. The Ret tyrosine kinase receptor and a membrane-linked protein (termed the GDNF-alpha receptor) form a receptor complex for glial cell-derived neurotrophic factor (GDNF; Fig. 71.2). This ligand-receptor complex is important for normal differentiation of the gastrointestinal neuronal system, parts of the sympathetic nervous and neuroendocrine systems, and for renal development.

The activating mutations of c-ret that cause MEN 2 affect 2 major regions of the Ret receptor (Fig. 71.2). The first is a cysteine-rich extracellular domain where mutations of cysteines at codons 609, 611, 618, 620, 630, and 634 cause receptor dimerization in the absence of ligand and cause transformation. Codon 634 mutations are found most commonly, accounting for approximately 80% of mutations and are associated most frequently with classic MEN 2A (Sipple's syndrome), although a small percentage of families have only familial medullary thyroid carcinoma. Ten to 15% of hereditary medullary thyroid carcinoma kindreds have codon 609, 611, 618, 620, or 630 extracellular domain mutations (Fig. 71.2). The clinical phenotype most commonly associated with these muta-

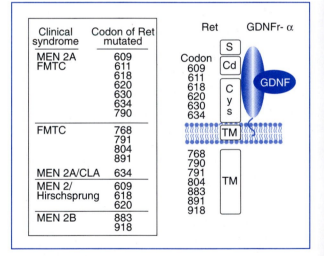

Figure 71.2 Mutations of the c-ret proto-oncogene causative for hereditary medullary thyroid carcinoma. Glial cell-derived neurotrophic factor (GDNF) binds to a receptor complex composed of the GDNF-α receptor and the Ret tyrosine kinase receptor. Mutations of the cysteine-rich extracellular domain are associated with multiple endocrine neoplasia type 2A (MEN 2A) and familial medullary thyroid carcinoma. Mutations of the intracellular domain associated with familial medullary thyroid carcinoma include codons 768, 804, 790, 791, and 891. Mutations of codons 790 and 791 have been identified in MEN 2A. Multiple endocrine neoplasia type 2B is associated most commonly with a codon 918 mutation and rarely with a codon 883 mutation. (S = signal peptide; Cd = cadherin-like region; Cys = cysteine-rich extracellular domain; GDNF = glial cell-derived neurotrophic factor; TK = tyrosine kinase domain; MEN 2A/CLA = MEN 2A and cutaneous lichen amyloidosis.)

children of an affected individual have a 50% probability of inheriting the causative gene. Two major subcategories have been identified. Multiple endocrine neoplasia type 2A or classic Sipple's syndrome is a combination of medullary thyroid carcinoma, pheochromocytoma, and parathyroid hyperplasia. Multiple endocrine neoplasia type 2B includes medullary thyroid carcinoma, pheochromocytoma, gastrointestinal mucosal neuromas, and a characteristic marfanoid habitus with long arms and legs and thin fingers. Other marfanoid features, such as lens abnormalities or aortic aneurysm, do not occur in MEN 2B.

tions is familial MTC, although some have classic MEN 2A. Kindreds with MEN 2A and cutaneous lichen amyloidosis, a characteristic pruritic skin lesion that in all cases is located over the upper back, have codon 634 mutations. A second group of intracellular Ret receptor mutations affect codons 768, 790, 791, 804, 891, and 918 (Fig. 71.2). Mutations of codons 768, 804, and 891 have been associated exclusively with familial MTC. Mutations of codons 790 and 791 have been identified in German kindreds with MEN 2A (790) or familial MTC (790 and 791). MEN 2B is most commonly associated with a germline codon 918 mutation, although a handful of patients with MEN 2B have a codon 883 mutation.

MEDULLARY THYROID CARCINOMA

The greatest concentration of C cells is normally located in the central upper portion of each thyroid lobe. Neoplastic transformation of the C cells in hereditary medullary thyroid carcinoma (MEN 2A, MEN 2B, or familial MTC) is bilateral and proceeds through a predictable series of histologic stages: from normal → hyperplasia → microscopic → macroscopic carcinoma. Although activating mutations of the Ret tyrosine kinase initiate the transformation process, additional mutational events are likely required for the development of a malignant tumor. It is unclear at what stage of development metastasis occurs, although tumors spreading to central, cervical, or upper mediastinal lymph nodes occurs in more than 50% of tumors greater than 2 cm in diameter.

Medullary thyroid carcinoma produces several unique tumor markers. The most distinctive are the calcitonin gene products, including calcitonin and calcitonin gene-related peptide (discussed below). Carcinoembryonic antigen is a third tumor marker.

In an abrupt paradigm shift, genetic testing for c-Ret proto-oncogene mutations has largely replaced calcitonin measurements for the diagnosis of gene carrier status in MEN 2 kindreds. Genetic testing is simple and reliable (in those kindreds where a c-Ret mutation has been identified). Genetic testing should be performed at the earliest age at which treatment for medullary thyroid carcinoma would be considered (discussed below), most commonly by the age of 5 years. These tests are commercially available through a variety of sources in Europe and North America. It is important that the clinician ordering these tests be aware of the possibility of sample mix-up or technical error (contamination by DNA carrying a mutation or polymerase chain reaction error). It is prudent to repeat the analysis on a separate sample from an independent blood draw before considering a test result to be positive or negative.

Approximately 5% of kindreds with proven hereditary transmission of medullary thyroid carcinoma have no identifiable c-ret mutation. In these families, continued screening by pentagastrin or combined calcium-pentagastrin testing will be necessary.

Sporadic or unifocal medullary thyroid carcinoma accounts for more than 75% of all medullary thyroid carcinoma. However, recent reports have shown that approximately 6% of patients with apparent sporadic medullary thyroid carcinoma have germline mutations of the c-Ret proto-oncogene indicative of hereditary medullary thyroid carcinoma, and are the possible propositi for new kindreds. All first degree relatives of the mutant gene carrier should be genetically tested in an attempt to identify other carriers and detect medullary thyroid carcinoma prior to the development of metastatic disease. One of the biggest surprises resulting from the elucidation of the molecular defects in MEN 2 and familial MTC has been the large number of previously undetected kindreds that have surfaced.

Treatment

The management of medullary thyroid carcinoma in the context of MEN 2 can be divided into two treatment areas: the first is prophylactic thyroidectomy for early medullary thyroid carcinoma, the second is management of macroscopic disease.

Management of early medullary thyroid carcinoma

For the past 25 years, management of MEN 2A-associated medullary thyroid carcinoma has been based on measurement of serum calcitonin following annual provocative stimulation by pentagastrin or combined calcium and pentagastrin (Tab. 71.1). This approach resulted in the identification of mutant gene carriers at an earlier age (mean of 10 to 13 years, versus 35 years before pentagastrin testing) and the identification of C cell abnormalities in a preneoplastic (50%) or early carcinomatous stage before identifiable metastasis (50%). This led to the belief that thyroid surgery at these ages would be curative. Long-term follow-up of MEN 2A kindreds, who were screened annually and treated with thyroidectomy at the time of the first abnormal test result, has confirmed that surgery was curative in the majority of patients. It is also clear, however, that 5 to 15% of children followed for 20 years have evidence of disease recurrence.

The finding of tumor recurrence in a small number of patients thought to be adequately treated has forced a reexamination of early detection and screening. If our goal is to cure 100% of children at risk, it will be necessary to consider earlier and/or more complete surgery, a concept for which consensus is building. The age at which thyroidectomy should be performed is unclear; the finding of metastasis in a 6 year-old child with a codon 634 c-ret mutation is the youngest age of known metastatic disease and is instructive. Most clinicians and surgeons who manage this disease now consider thyroidectomy at age 5 to 6 years reasonable since children tolerate surgery at this age well, the anatomical structures in the neck are clearly defined, and the children are old enough to take thyroid hormone pills with parental encouragement. Available information suggests that the risk of hypoparathyroidism and recurrent laryngeal nerve damage at this age is no greater than in adults. A total thyroidectomy with complete removal of the posterior capsule should be performed. Consideration should be given to central lymph node dissection, and any devascularized parathyroids should be autografted to the nondominant forearm. Permanent hypoparathyroidism should not be a complication of prophylactic thyroidectomy.

Whether this treatment approach will result in a cure of medullary thyroid carcinoma in more children is unclear and will require another 15 to 25 years of follow-up. At this point it seems reasonable to consider earlier thyroidectomy, although it is important to include parents in a discussion of the risks and benefits of therapy. Most, but not all, parents will embrace earlier surgery.

Children with MEN 2B should have a thyroidectomy performed at the earliest possible point following birth. Metastasis has been described during the first month of life in MEN 2B and surgical cure is rare. Total thyroidectomy and compartment-oriented lymph node dissection should be performed in all patients, even those with early disease.

Management of established medullary thyroid carcinoma, hereditary or sporadic

Total thyroidectomy and lymph node dissection remain the treatment of choice for all patients with palpable medullary thyroid carcinomas. There are several reasons for this recommendation. First, it is difficult to differentiate between hereditary (hence bilateral) and sporadic disease. The second compelling reason for total thyroidectomy relates to the long-term management of the patient. Persistent calcitonin elevations following primary surgery, usually indicative of metastatic disease, are quite common in patients with palpable medullary thyroid carcinoma. If a unilateral thyroidectomy is performed and there is a persistent elevation of the serum calcitonin following surgery, it will be unclear whether the residual tumor is located within the other thyroid lobe, in local lymph nodes (a 50% probability of local nodal metastasis with a tumor >2 cm), or in occult distant metastases. Total thyroidectomy and compartment-oriented lymph node dissection at the primary surgical operation offers the patient the greatest chance of cure, maximizes local-regional tumor control, simplifies follow-up, and may avoid the complications of recurrent laryngeal nerve injury and permanent hypoparathyroidism that frequently accompany reoperative cervical procedures. Other possible procedures are following.

Management of persistent postoperative calcitonin measurements
A vexing problem for clinicians is the persistence of calcitonin elevation following primary surgical management. The major question is whether reoperation to remove all identifiable lymph nodes in the neck (compartment-oriented dissection) has value. A recent body of experience has accumulated regarding reoperative strategies in patients with persistent disease. In the selection of

these patients, it is important to perform a careful search for distant metastatic disease and to exclude hepatic, bone, and pulmonary metastasis by appropriate imaging studies. Some perform laparoscopy with direct hepatic visualization, or selective catheterization of the arterial and venous supply of the liver with measurement of pentagastrin-stimulated calcitonin in hepatic venous effluent, in order to exclude hepatic metastasis. In patients with no evidence of distant metastatic disease, reoperative compartment-oriented lymphadenectomy may be appropriate. Approximately 1 of 5 carefully selected patients will have their serum calcitonin normalized following microsurgical dissection (nondetectable calcitonin values following pentagastrin). There are no long-term follow-up studies in this group of patients to determine whether this type of surgical intervention affects morbidity or mortality related to medullary thyroid carcinoma, yet the lack of other effective therapy for this disease makes it a reasonable consideration.

Management of patients with distant metastasis
In patients with evidence of distant metastatic disease, reoperation in the neck is generally indicated only when a tumor mass or lymph node threatens to compromise laryngeal, tracheal, or esophageal function; or if there is a belief that removal of tumor bulk will improve diarrheal symptoms.

In most patients with distant metastasis, the disease will progress slowly over decades and little benefit will accrue from early active intervention with chemotherapy or radiation. In patients with rapidly progressive disease, recent experience from several centers indicates 25 to 30% of patients treated with chemotherapeutic regimens that include dacarbazine (5-fluorouracil and dacarbazine or adriamycin, vincristine, cyclophosphamide, and dacarbazine) have tumor regression, and in 1 to 5% there is evidence of long-term durable remission. Dacarbazine appears to be the most active chemotherapeutic agent. If there is no evidence of objective tumor regression after 3 to 6 cycles of chemotherapy, consideration should be given to alternative therapeutic approaches. The use of neck and mediastinal radiation therapy is controversial. Some reports indicate that local recurrence of disease is less in patients treated with external-beam radiation therapy, although there is little effect on overall survival duration.

PHEOCHROMOCYTOMA

Pheochromocytomas occur in approximately 50% of patients with MEN 2A. Pheochromocytomas develop most frequently in patients with codon 634 *c-ret* proto-oncogene mutations; they are also sometimes observed in patients with codon 611, 618, 620, 790, or 791 mutations; and they have not been reported in patients with 609, 768, 804, or 891 mutations. Pheochromocytomas are found in approximately 50% of patients with MEN 2B (codon 883 or 918 mutations). There is a histological progression from adrenal medullary hyperplasia → nodular hyperplasia → pheochromocytoma. Careful histologic examination of the adrenal medulla in most patients with codon 634 mutations would reveal some histologic abnormalities. Although adrenal capsular invasion occurs frequently, metastatic pheochromocytoma is rare.

Clinical findings

The clinical syndrome associated with pheochromocytoma in MEN 2 differs from that observed in sporadic pheochromocytoma. Most commonly, the intra-adrenal pheochromocytomas associated with MEN 2 produce a relative excess of epinephrine and a pattern that contrasts with predominant norepinephrine production in sporadic pheochromocytomas. Thus, the clinical syndrome associated with MEN 2-related pheochromocytomas is characterized initially by palpitations, nervousness, and intermittent headaches. In patients with larger tumors; hypertension, weight loss, cardiac arrhythmias, and sudden death may occur.

Diagnostic procedures

The diagnosis of pheochromocytoma is established by the measurement of either plasma or urine catecholamines or metanephrine. The most commonly employed screening strategy is annual urine catecholamine and metanephrine testing. The most sensitive indicator of adrenal medullary abnormality in MEN 2 is either an increased 12- or 24-hour urine epinephrine or an abnormal urine metanephrine. The goal is to detect excessive catecholamine secretion at a point before it is life-threatening.

Imaging studies

Magnetic resonance imaging of the adrenal medulla with T2-weighted images is the most specific method for the detection of adrenal medullary abnormalities and should be performed in patients with catecholamine or metanephrine abnormalities. CT is equally sensitive, but it is less specific because it is difficult to differentiate adrenal cortical nodules from adrenal medullary nodules. Radiolabeled meta-iodobenzylguanidine or octreotide scanning may be helpful in determining a surgical strategy in patients with elevated urinary catecholamines and bilateral adrenal abnormalities on MRI. Special attention should be placed on surveillance in pregnant women because of reported deaths at the time of delivery.

Treatment

The challenge confronting the physician caring for these patients with MEN 2 is to recommend surgical removal of one or both adrenal glands at an appropriate time in the clinical course of their disease. There is a necessity to balance the risks of catecholamine excess with those associated with adrenal insufficiency. Cardiac arrhythmias, stroke, and sudden death are well-known sequelae of pheochromocytoma; however, at least 2 deaths directly attributable to adrenal insufficiency related to bilateral adrenalectomy in the context of MEN 2 have been described.

All physicians generally agree that the patient with abnormal urine catecholamines, symptoms or signs of pheochromocytoma, and unilateral or bilateral adrenal masses should have surgical excision. It is probably also prudent to consider surgical excision of a nodular adrenal gland in young women of childbearing age with borderline urine catecholamine values because of the risks associated with pregnancy and childbirth. Finally, surgical excision of the adrenal gland(s) may be appropriate in the rare family with a history of adrenal medullary malignancy.

It is less clear what to do with a patient who has a small adrenal abnormality with no symptoms or catecholamine abnormalities. Experience in this group of patients over the past 25 years has shown that the risk of stroke or cardiac arrhythmia is low, provided that annual screening to detect catecholamine/metanephrine abnormalities is continued.

Patients should be blocked prior to surgery with combined alpha- and beta-adrenergic receptor antagonists and/or inhibition of catecholamine synthesis with alpha-methyltyrosine for at least 7 to 10 days prior to surgery.

Several different types of surgical procedures have been used in patients with pheochromocytoma in the context of MEN 2. Most surgeons remove only the affected adrenal gland via an anterior or posterior approach, leaving the unaffected adrenal gland untouched. Long-term studies have shown that 50% of patients so treated will develop a contralateral pheochromocytoma, on average 8 to 10 years later. The availability of high quality MRI examination makes it generally unnecessary to examine the contralateral adrenal gland intraoperatively and hence makes a posterior unilateral approach suitable for most patients. Laparoscopic adrenalectomy is being used with increasing frequency, and early experience suggests its use is appropriate for small tumors.

In patients with bilateral adrenal masses thought to represent pheochromocytomas, several different surgical approaches have been utilized. Bilateral adrenalectomy is the most commonly used procedure. In situations where maintenance of adrenal cortical function is desirable or essential; unilateral adrenalectomy, combined with a contralateral cortical sparing adrenalectomy, provides an attractive alternative with a reasonable probability of adequate postoperative adrenal cortical function.

HYPERPARATHYROIDISM

Hyperparathyroidism occurs in 15 to 20% of patients with MEN 2, most commonly in association with a codon 634 c-ret proto-oncogene mutation. The clinical features of hyperparathyroidism in MEN 2 do not differ from those found in the more common sporadic hyperparathyroidism (see Chap. 19). Hyperparathyroidism associated with MEN 2 most commonly involves multiple glands, is usually diagnosed during the third and fourth decades, and the tumors are almost never malignant. Unlike hyperparathyroidism associated with MEN 1, recurrent hyperparathyroidism is rare.

Indications for surgery do not differ from those for sporadic hyperparathyroidism. Two different surgical approaches have been employed. The first is subtotal parathyroidectomy; leaving approximately 50 mg of clearly marked parathyroid tissue in place is done most commonly. In the rare kindred with a history of recurrent hyperparathyroidism, total parathyroidectomy and transplantation to the nondominant arm will facilitate reoperation.

OTHER WELL-DEFINE MULTIPLE ENDOCRINE NEOPLASIA SYNDROMES

VON HIPPEL-LINDAU SYNDROME

Von Hippel-Lindau syndrome (VHL) is an autosomal dominant neoplastic syndrome characterized by hemangioblastomas of the central nervous system, retinal angiomas, renal cell carcinomas, visceral cysts, pheochromocytomas, and islet cell tumors. The causative gene, a tumor suppressor, is located on chromosome 3p25.3 and was identified in 1993 by positional cloning. In Von Hippel-Lindau syndrome, one inactivated copy of the gene is inherited, and a loss of function mutation in the other copy initiates transformation. Somatic inactivating mutations of the VHL gene have been implicated in the causation of sporadic pheochromocytomas and islet cell tumors.

Twenty-five to 35% of Von Hippel-Lindau syndrome kindreds will develop pheochromocytomas, and 15 to 20% will develop islet cell tumors. A careful examination of family history for central nervous system tumors and renal cell carcinoma should be pursued in all patients with pheochromocytoma or islet cell neoplasms. Mutations of codon 238 of the VHL gene have been identified in approximately 40% of families with pheochromocytoma, suggesting that families with a mutation in this codon should be routinely screened for pheochromocytoma. A large number of inactivating mutations have been described in the VHL gene.

Those planning the clinical management of pheochromocytoma and islet cell tumors in patients with Von Hippel-Lindau syndrome should consider the impact of treatment on the neurologic and renal neoplastic manifestations of this syndrome. It may be appropriate, for example, to pursue a cortical-sparing adrenalectomy in a patient with pheochromocytoma if the patient also has a renal cell carcinoma requiring chemotherapy. Otherwise, clinical management of pheochromocytomas or islet cell tumors does not differ from that described in earlier sections of this chapter.

NEUROFIBROMATOSIS TYPE 1

A variety of neoplastic endocrine manifestations have been described in neurofibromatosis type 1, including hyperparathyroidism, pheochromocytoma, medullary thyroid carcinoma, and somatostatin-producing carcinoid tumors of the duodenal wall. Indirect endocrine manifestations such as precocious puberty may occur as a result of hypothalamic or optic nerve tumors. The causative gene, neurofibromin, is a member of the *ras* GTPase-activating protein family, which enhances GTP hydrolysis. Loss of function results in uncontrolled activation of p21 Ras. Endocrine tumors occur with some regularity in neurofibromatosis type 1. A heightened awareness of this possibility is appropriate, though routine screening for these tumors other than by history and physical examination is generally not performed.

COWDEN DISEASE

Cowden disease is a rare autosomal dominant cancer syndrome characterized by breast, thyroid, intestinal, and skin tumors (Tab. 71.1). Most commonly patients with this syndrome develop hamartomas, which are differentiated but disorganized cells derived from the specific tissue. Carcinoma may develop in the breast and thyroid (approximately 10% of affected individuals). Missense or nonsense (presumed inactivating) mutations of PTEN or MMAC1, a protein tyrosine phosphatase, have been identified in 80% of families. The important clinical point for endocrinologists is to note the potential for the development of differentiated thyroid carcinoma. Cowden family members with a thyroid nodule should have fine needle aspiration of the nodule to exclude carcinoma.

CARNEY COMPLEX

Carney complex is a rare autosomal dominant genetic syndrome characterized by myxomas of several tissues (heart, breast, and skin), dermatologic spotty pigmentation, and tumors of multiple endocrine organs (pituitary, thyroid, testicular, adrenal). The gene for this disorder has been mapped to chromosome 2p11. These tumors can sometimes produce hormonal syndromes, necessitating evaluation and treatment.

Suggested readings

BURGESS JR, SHEPHERD JJ, PARAMESWARAN V, HOFFMAN L, GREENAWAY TM. Spectrum of pituitary disease in multiple endocrine neoplasia type 1 (MEN 1): clinical, biochemical, and radiological features of pituitary disease in a large MEN 1 kindred. J Clin Endocrinol Metab 1996;81:2642-6.

CHANDRASEKHARAPPA SC, GURU SC, MANICKAM P, et al.

Positional cloning of the gene for multiple endocrine neoplasia-type 1. Science 1997;276:404-7.

CHEN F, KISHIDA T, YAO M, HUSTAD T, et al. Germline mutations in the von Hippel-Lindau disease tumor suppressor gene: correlations with phenotype. Hum Mutat 1995;5:66-75.

ENG C, CLAYTON D, SCHUFFENECKER I, et al. The relationship between specific Ret proto-oncogene mutations and disease phenotype in multiple endocrine neoplasia type 2.

International Ret mutation consortium analysis. JAMA 1996;276:1575-9.

GAGEL RF, TASHJIAN AH JR., CUMMINGS T, et al. The clinical outcome of prospective screening for multiple endocrine neoplasia type 2a: An 18-year experience. N Engl J Med 1988;318:478-84.

LEMMENS I, VAN DE VEN WJ, KAS K, et al. Identification of the multiple endocrine neoplasia type 1 (MEN 1) gene. The European Consortium on MEN 1. Human Molecular Genetics 1997;6:1177-83.

LIAW D, MARSH DJ, LI J, et al. Germline mutations of the PTEN gene in Cowden disease, an inherited breast and thyroid cancer syndrome. Nature Genetics 1997;16:64-7.

LIPS CJ, LANDSVATER RM, HOPPENER JW, et al. Clinical screening as compared with DNA analysis in families with multiple endocrine neoplasia type 2A. N Engl J Med 1994;331:828-35.

MARX SJ, VINIK AI, SANTEN RJ, FLOYD JC, JR, MILLS JL, GREEN J III. Multiple endocrine neoplasia type I: assessment of laboratory tests to screen for the gene in a large kindred. Medicine (Baltimore). 1986;65:226-41.

MULLIGAN LM, KWOK JB, HEALEY CS, et al. Germ-line mutations of the Ret proto-oncogene in multiple endocrine neoplasia type 2A. Nature 1993;363:458-60.

SKOGSEID B, RASTAD J, OBERG K. Multiple endocrine neoplasia type 1. Clinical features and screening. Endocrinol Metab Clin North Am 1994;23:1-18.

STRATAKIS CA, CARNEY JA, LIN JP, et al. Carney complex, a familial multiple neoplasia and lentiginosis syndrome. Analysis of 11 kindreds and linkage to the short arm of chromosome 2. Journal of Clinical Investigation 1996;97:699-705.

WELLS SA, CHI DD, TOSHIMA K, et al. Predictive DNA testing and prophylactic thyroidectomy in patients at risk for multiple endocrine neoplasia type 2A. Ann Surg 1994;220:237-50.

WOHLLK N, COTE GJ, BUGALHO MMJ, et al. Relevance of Ret proto-oncogene mutations in sporadic medullary thyroid carcinoma. J Clin Endocrinol Metab 1996;81:3740-5.

Endocrine immunology

Anthony P. Weetman

KEY POINTS

- Humoral and cell-mediated autoimmune responses cause a variety of endocrinopathies due to the failure of central and peripheral tolerance mechanisms, which are determined by genetic and environmental factors.
- Autoimmune endocrinopathies occur together more often than expected, and they are frequently associated with other autoimmune disorders such as vitiligo, alopecia, and pernicious anemia.
- Autoimmune polyglandular syndrome type 1 is a rare autosomal recessive disorder and is comprised of hypoparathyroidism, Addison's disease, and chronic mucocutaneous candidiasis, usually with onset in childhood or adolescence. Other endocrine disorders, especially gonadal failure and ectodermal dysplasia, also occur.
- Autoimmune polyglandular syndrome type 2 is a common, autosomal dominant disorder in which there is a co-existence of two or more autoimmune endocrinopathies in the same patient. There is a strong association with HLA-DR3.
- Other autoimmune syndromes include endocrinopathies less frequently, particularly the "polyneuropathy, organomegaly, endocrinopathy, monoclonal gammopathy and skin changes syndrome" and type B insulin resistance.

Autoimmunity is a common, well-established cause of endocrine disease (Tab. 72.1). In addition to the more well-known disorders, autoimmunity also causes, or is postulated to cause, a wide variety of other endocrinopathies (Tab. 72.2). The etiology and pathogenesis of these conditions is becoming clearer. It is also well-established that autoimmune endocrinopathies occur together more frequently than expected by chance. The first part of this chapter provides an overview of the basis for endocrine autoimmunity, and the second part of the chapter details the important clinical features of the so-called autoimmune polyglandular syndromes into which the endocrinopathies group.

TOLERANCE AND AUTOIMMUNITY

Autoimmune endocrine disease arises from a specific response against a target organ containing one or more autoantigens. There are two broad classes of response: humoral, mediated by antibodies; and cellular, mediated primarily by T cells (Tab. 72.3). Both responses are also utilized for the primary effector role of the immune system: defense against infection. In essence, autoimmunity is a consequence of the need to have an enormous diversity of T and B lymphocytes capable of responding to all the micro-organisms an individual will encounter. This prodigious diversity inevitably results in the chance

Table 72.1 Major autoimmune endocrinopathies and approximate frequency in caucasian women; frequencies are 4- to 10-fold lower in men

Autoimmune endocrinopathy	Approximate frequency
Graves' disease	1:100
Autoimmune hypothyroidism (primary myxedema or Hashimoto's thyroiditis)	1:100
Post partum thyroiditis	1:20
Type 1 diabetes mellitus	1:500
Addison's disease	1:10 000
Premature ovarian failure (associated with Addison's disease)	1:100 000

Table 72.2 Endocrinopathy cases believed to be due to autoimmunity, or in which the autoantigens have not been established

Thyroid
Silent thyroiditis

Pituitary
Lymphocytic hypophysitis
Isolated ACTH deficiency
Other anterior pituitary hormone deficiencies
Lymphocytic infundibuloneurohypophysitis
Idiopathic diabetes insipidus

Pancreas
Insulin autoimmune syndrome

Parathyroid
Idiopathic hypoparathyroidism
Parathyroiditis with hyperparathyroidism

Testis
Idiopathic orchitis

Ovary
Premature ovarian failure not associated with Addison's disease

Heart
Antibodies altering ANP secretion

occurrence during development of some lymphocytes being capable of recognizing autoantigens. In healthy individuals, such autoreactive lymphocytes are either successfully eliminated or at least held in check. Autoimmune disease results from a failure of these protective mechanisms.

Central tolerance and ignorance

The protective mechanisms against autoimmunity can be viewed in a descending order of effectiveness (Fig. 72.1). Most autoreactive T cells are eliminated in the thymus during development; this is accomplished by apoptosis via contact with cortical epithelial cells or medullary antigen presenting cells expressing self-antigens. However,

not all autoantigens can be expressed by these thymic cells, and therefore some target autoantigens in endocrine autoimmunity may not have the chance to eliminate T cells capable of recognizing them. Additionally, in some cases, intrathymic contact with self-antigens results not in clonal elimination, but in *anergy*, whereby the T cell is paralyzed and unable to respond when it comes into contact with the antigen. Anergy can be overcome in certain circumstances, such as by the provision of high concen-

Table 72.3 Characteristics of humoral and cell-mediated autoimmunity

Humoral immunity	Cell-mediated immunity
Antibodies, usually against conformational epitopes on autoantigen, found in all patients	T cells, reactive against short linear epitopes of autoantigen, found in all patients
Antibody localized to target organ	T cell infiltrate in target organ
Neonatal disease due to transplacental transfer of antibodies	No neonatal disease
Transferred in animal models by antibody	Transferred in animal models by T cells
Treatment lowering antibody levels lessens disease	Treatment against autoreactive T cells lessens disease
Disease produced by antibody capable of complement-fixation, antibody-dependant cell-mediated cytotoxicity (ADCC), receptor stimulation, or blocking or altering enzyme activity	Disease produced by cytotoxic T cells releasing TNF-β or perforin or by Fas-Fas ligand interaction

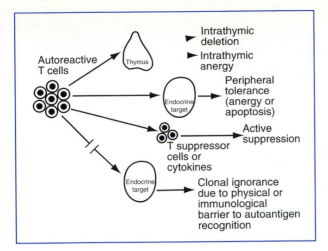

Figure 72.1 Hierarchy of tolerance mechanisms preventing autoreactive T cells from producing autoimmune disease. The most secure mechanisms are at the top of the figure, the least secure at the bottom.

trations of the cytokine interleukin 2 (IL-2), which is crucial to T cell division and differentiation. As IL-2 is released at sites of inflammation, anergy is clearly less efficient in controlling autoreactivity than deletion. An alternative protective mechanism is *clonal ignorance*: the pathologically harmless presence of autoreactive lymphocytes as there is no anatomical access to the autoantigen (e.g., blood-brain barrier, Sertoli cells). This occurs because antigen presenting cells are absent or defective at this site, or because the T cells have a defect in homing ability.

Peripheral tolerance

Clearly, for autoimmune endocrinopathies to occur, central (thymic) tolerance (imposed by apoptosis or anergy) and clonal ignorance must fail. (The reasons for this failure are discussed in the next section.) However, failure is still insufficient to necessarily cause tissue damage, because peripheral mechanisms exist to control autoreactivity. Most endocrine tissues have resident antigen presenting cells such as dendritic cells that could activate any autoreactive T cells that gain access. One way to control these is with peripheral tolerance mediated through the expression of major histocompatibility complex (MHC) class II molecules, such as HLA-DR, by endocrine tissues. MHC class II molecules are constitutively expressed by antigen presenting cells and play a fundamental role in presenting autoantigen fragments to CD4+ (helper) T cells, which recognize this bi-molecular complex by means of an antigen-specific T cell receptor. However, a second, co-stimulatory signal is also required in most circumstances for the initial activation of CD4+ T cells. The most important of these signals is provided by B7-1 (CD80) and B7-2 (CD86) on the antigen presenting cells, which interact with CD28 or CTLA-4 on the T cell.

Endocrine cells express class II but not B7 molecules when stimulated by cytokines, particularly interferon gamma (IFN-γ). When MHC class II molecules present

autoantigenic peptide to a naive T cell in the absence of B7-mediated co-stimulation, anergy or even apoptosis results. As cytokines capable of inducing such class II expression are released during inflammation, such as during viral infection of an endocrine organ, this method of peripheral tolerance can operate at precisely the right time to prevent autoimmunity; that is, when previously ignorant and untolerised T cells might gain access to the tissue. However, peripheral tolerance is double-edged, as B7-mediated co-stimulation is not important for the activation of certain CD4+ T cells, particularly those previously exposed to B7 provided by constitutive antigen presenting cells. Any such T cells, if they are specific for the appropriate autoantigen, can therefore be stimulated by class II-positive endocrine cells. In an ongoing response, when locally-released cytokines cause expression of class II, this could be an important mechanism by which the autoimmune process is upregulated.

Other peripheral mechanisms can control potentially harmful autoreactivity as well. For many years, the existence of a poorly defined subpopulation of T cells capable of mediating suppression of antigen-specific responses has been suggested by a variety of techniques. The CD8+ T cell population, in addition to containing cytotoxic effector cells, has been widely regarded as an important source of suppressor T cells. However, as CD8 knockout mice without CD8+ T cells do not develop autoimmune disease, this population now appears unlikely to be essential to maintaining self-tolerance. Instead, suppression seems to be a much more complex phenomenon, particularly with the recognition of two broad types of CD4+ T cells (Tab. 72.4) that display reciprocal regulation via their distinctive patterns of cytokine release. For example, the T helper-type 1 cytokine IFN-γ helps mediate delayed-type hypersensitivity reactions and inhibits T helper-type 2

Table 72.4 Characteristics of CD4$^+$ helper T cell subsets

	T helper-1	T helper-2
Major cytokines released	IL-2, IFN-γ, TNF	IL-4, IL-5, IL-6 IL-10, IL-13
Major roles	Delayed type hypersensitivity; killing of intracellular pathogens	B cell help; antibody production
Cytokines directing T helper cell differentiation	IL-12	IL-4
Cytokines inhibiting T helper cell response	IL-4, IL-10, IL-10	IFN-γ

(IL = interleukin, IFN-γ = interferon-gamma, TNF = tumor necrosis factor.)

responses, whereas IL-4 stimulates the T helper-2 response and promotes B cell activation, but it inhibits T helper-1 proliferation and counters some of the effects of IFN-γ.

Thus, the balance between T helper-1 and T helper-2 cells is critical in determining whether (and what type of) an immune response occurs. This balance in turn is determined by genetic factors, the concentration of antigen, the type of antigen presenting cell, and the co-stimulatory signals being delivered. For cell-mediated destructive responses dependent on T helper-1 cells, such as occur in many autoimmune endocrinopathies, T helper-2 cells therefore have a protective effect and may have been responsible for some previously observed suppressor effects. However, it is highly likely that other T cell regulatory pathways operate to prevent autoimmunity, including veto cells and idiotype-anti-idiotype interactions that are mediated via specific T cell receptors, but their relative importance and full characterization are presently unknown.

The processes involved in B cell tolerance are similar to those described above in T cells. Autoreactive B cells are eliminated or rendered anergic in the bone marrow. There is the potential for further tolerance before or after activation in peripheral lymphoid tissues. Furthermore, autoreactive B cells can to some extent be considered harmless, provided autoreactive CD4+ T cells are not allowed to escape tolerance and provide the necessary help for B cell proliferation and differentiation. Again, however, this state of affairs may prove ultimately disastrous, as B cells are highly efficient antigen presenting cells. B cells are capable of capturing specific antigen via surface immunoglobulin and presenting multiple fragments (or epitopes) of this to CD4+ T cells recognizing the same antigen, thus diversifying the response. Failure to remove autoreactive B cells (or anything reversing anergy in such cells) is therefore another point at which autoimmune disease can emerge.

Breaking tolerance and emergence of autoimmunity

Given the complexity of these mechanisms, it hardly seems surprising that occasional failures occur and autoimmune diseases result. Thymic tolerance is now recognized to be incomplete for many autoantigens, and an individual's tolerance may be genetically determined. The more autoreactive T cells that there are escaping to the periphery, the more likely subsequent autoimmune disease will be. Such genetic differences result from the differing abilities of allelic MHC class II molecules to present antigen to T cells, resulting in deletion or anergy, and possibly arise from differences in expression of autoantigens within the thymus.

Other factors in autoimmunity

Genetic differences also appear to regulate the efficiency of peripheral tolerance mechanisms. Environmental factors are likely to have a major role in the evolution of the autoimmune process. For instance, infections could result in autoimmunity through a number of mechanisms: (1) modification of self-antigen results in a novel autoantigen for which tolerance does not exist; (2) exposure of cryptic antigens overcomes clonal ignorance; (3) molecular mimicry, whereby an antigenic epitope in the infecting organism closely resembles a self-epitope, leads to an immune response against the former being directed against the latter; (4) non-specific immunological stimulation, such as by inducing local cytokine release during the immune response to the infection, could overcome anergy in autoreactive T cells; some micro-organisms express "superantigens" capable of non-specifically stimulating T cells, including those with autoreactivity; (5) direct effects on the target cell induce expression of immunologically relevant molecules, such as MHC class II, which could enhance a previously minor autoimmune response.

As well as environmental factors, endogenous factors such as aging, sex hormones, and the neuroendocrine response to stress have a variety of effects on the balance between regulatory T cells, and thus contribute to the emergence of autoimmunity. This would account for the increased frequency of many autoimmune endocrinopathies in women and in the elderly, but all such factors operate against a genetic background that determines susceptibility or resistance to autoimmunity (Fig. 72.2), so that only the appropriate combination of circumstances results in an autoimmune disease.

PATHOGENESIS OF AUTOIMMUNITY

Most autoimmune endocrinopathies arise from tissue destruction, best seen in the attack exclusively on the beta

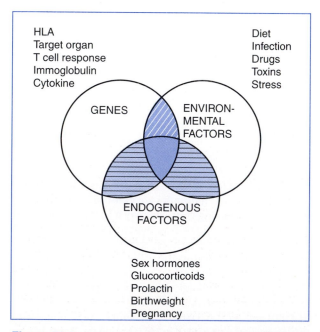

Figure 72.2 Interaction of genetic, environmental, and endogenous factors in autoimmune disease. Individuals with two or three risk factors (shaded area) are more likely to develop disease than those with one or no risk factor.

cells within the islets of Langerhans in type 1 diabetes mellitus. The specificity of this response implies the involvement of cytotoxic T cells or autoantibodies that recognize only target cell autoantigens. However, this does not mean that the non-specific effectors of the immune system, such as macrophages and natural killer cells, have no role in autoimmunity, as they may well be important in amplifying the local immune response.

T cell-mediated cytotoxicity

There is considerable evidence from animal models of autoimmune endocrinopathies that CD8+ cytotoxic T cells are involved in the final destructive phase of disease, following accumulation of a mixed (CD4+ and CD8+) lymphocytic infiltrate into the target site. Similarly, human insulitis or thyroiditis may be detected for months or years prior to the clinical presence of diabetes or hypothyroidism. This reflects both the presence of defense mechanisms within the tissue preventing destruction, and the lack of sufficient cytotoxic effectors. Cytotoxic CD8+ T cells recognize tissue-specific antigens presented by MHC class I molecules on the surface of the endocrine cell; this interaction also requires adhesion molecules that bring the T cell and its target into close proximity and which may also co-stimulate the T cell. It is therefore noteworthy that endocrine target cells upregulate MHC class I and adhesion molecule expression as a consequence of cytokine production by the infiltrating lymphocytes, thereby enhancing the potential for their attack by cytotoxic T cells.

Target cells are killed by degranulation of the cytotoxic T cell, releasing the pore-forming protein perforin, which shares many features with complement components C8 and C9. Like them, perforin inserts into the target cell membrane, and if sufficient pores are formed, lysis follows. Perforin-independent cytotoxicity also occurs, at least in part mediated by the cytokine lymphotoxin (tumor necrosis factor[TNF]-β). Cytotoxic CD4+ T cells in vitro kill target cells in a MHC class II-restricted fashion; their importance in endocrine autoimmunity is unknown. However, CD4+ T helper-1 cells are likely to be involved in destructive endocrinopathies, at least indirectly, by producing the appropriate cytokines to allow for the development of specific CD8+ cytotoxic T cells and to activate macrophages that contribute to tissue damage.

Humoral mechanisms

Antibodies can produce autoimmune disease by a number of mechanisms (Tab. 72.3). Complement-fixing antibodies, such as those against the key thyroid enzyme thyroid peroxidase, can destroy thyroid cells in vitro in the presence of complement. The thyroid cells, however, are able to protect themselves to some extent by expressing regulatory proteins (e.g., CD59) that prevent the insertion of complement membrane attack complexes into the cell membrane. Sub-lethal complement attack may nonetheless impair the metabolic function of the attacked cell and

lead to the release of inflammatory mediators, such as cytokines, by the target cell. In turn these mediators could exacerbate the ongoing autoimmune response and therefore serve as an amplification mechanism. It is also important to appreciate that complement activation takes place in the absence of autoantibodies through the alternative pathway, thus making it possible for these effects to occur at any site of autoimmune damage.

Autoantibodies may also lead to tissue damage via antibody-dependent cell-mediated cytotoxicity. In this, the Fc portion of the antibody bound to a target cell is recognized by Fc receptors on natural killer cells, which then destroy the target via perforin and lymphotoxin. Antibody-dependent cell-mediated cytotoxicity is thus able to confer tissue-specificity on the activity of natural killer cells and may be an important mechanism whereby non-complement fixing autoantibodies, such as those against thyroglobulin, can effect tissue injury.

Autoantibodies can also have a number of direct effects on target cells. The best examples are those involving antibodies against receptors, of which the thyroid-stimulating antibodies causing Graves' disease are the archetype. Most receptor antibodies, however, appear to block receptor function. Several postulated receptor antibodies remain poorly characterized. Other autoantibodies, directed against enzymes as autoantigens, can inhibit enzyme function, at least in vitro. How important this is in vivo is currently unknown. The fact that such enzymes are usually intracellular is not the problem it appears to be in postulating the involvement of enzyme antibodies in pathogenesis, as there are now several clear examples of the penetration of autoantibodies into living cells. This opens up a new series of possibilities in the involvement of autoantibodies in endocrine disease.

Cytokine-mediated diseases

In addition to the two classical pathways for disease pathogenesis described here, cytokines may play a critical role that is not dependent on their ability to cause cytotoxicity. For example, it now seems very likely that the thyroid-associated ophthalmopathy that frequently accompanies Graves' disease is caused by the production of cytokines (IL-1, TNF, and IFN-γ) within the extra-ocular muscles. These cytokines lead to the stimulation of fibroblasts, increased production of glycosaminoglycans and water trapping, and result in muscle swelling and well-known clinical features. Eventually fibrosis occurs due to cytokine-stimulated collagen production. In this case there is little if any tissue destruction, at least during the initial phase of disease. This type of pathogenesis is therefore separate from the two types considered above.

Cytokines have a number of other important effects on endocrine tissues, some of which have already been mentioned, such as the stimulation of MHC class I and II expression and the upregulation of adhesion molecules. In addition, cytokines can stimulate or inhibit endocrine cell proliferation or function. The diverse array of cytokines produced by the gland infiltrate in endocrine autoimmunity is certain to contribute in these ways to pathogenesis, although the relative importance of this pathway, compared to the cell-mediated and humoral pathways, has not been established.

AUTOIMMUNE POLYGLANDULAR SYNDROMES

The previous section has outlined the mechanisms by which autoimmune endocrinopathies arise. Currently these appear to be similar in each disorder, with the exception of the stimulatory role thyroid-stimulating hormone (TSH) receptor antibodies play in Graves' disease. Even so, a significant proportion of Graves' patients develop spontaneous hypothyroidism after entering remission induced by antithyroid drugs. The majority of these patients have features shared with autoimmune hypothyroidism, particularly the presence of autoantibodies against thyroglobulin and thyroid peroxidase. Because of this similar pathogenesis, it is not surprising that autoimmune endocrinopathies cluster within individuals and within families, giving rise to the so-called autoimmune polyglandular syndromes (APS). Furthermore, these endocrinopathies are frequently associated with other disorders presumed or accepted to have an autoimmune basis, such as vitiligo, alopecia, and pernicious anemia. Part of the similarity in pathogenesis may depend on the sharing of immunogenetic or even environmental risk factors; there is also evidence that some autoantigens may share cross-reactive epitopes, such that a response against one antigen will provoke a response against the second.

There are two clearly identified types of APS, one rare and one common, both of which have Addison's disease as an important component. Other forms of polyendocrine autoimmune endocrinopathy are considered after these.

APS Type 1

Autoimmune polyglandular syndrome type 1 is an autosomal recessive disorder that has also been termed Blizzard's syndrome and autoimmune polyendocrinopathy-candidiasis-ectodermal dystrophy. In this syndrome, patients have at least two of three distinct conditions: chronic mucocutaneous candidiasis, Addison's disease (primary autoimmune adrenal failure), and/or hypoparathyroidism (Tab. 72.5). Children with apparently only one of these components should be screened carefully for one of the other components, and also for ectodermal dysplasia.

Epidemiology

The exact prevalence of this type 1 syndrome is unknown. The highest frequency is probably in Finland, where the prevalence is approximately 1:25000. Other clusters have been reported, such as in Iranian Jews and in Sardinians.

Table 72.5 Clinical features of autoimmune polyglandular syndrome type 1

	Approximate frequency
Major components	
Chronic mucocutaneous candidiasis	80-100%
Hypoparathyroidism	80%
Addison's disease	70%
Other endocrinopathies	
Gonadal failure	10% men
	60% women
Insulin-dependent diabetes mellitus	10%
Hypothyroidism	10%
Other features	
Enamel hypoplasia	80%
Nail dystrophy	50%
Keratopathy	40%
Tympanic membrane calcification	30%
Vitiligo	30%
Alopecia	30%
Malabsorption	20%
Pernicious anemia	10%
Chronic active hepatitis	10%

Aside from these clusters, however, APS type 1 is rare. As sporadic cases apparently occur, it is probable that new mutations are responsible in some instances. A founder gene effect may explain the observed clusters.

Pathophysiology

The genetic locus controlling APS type 1 lies on chromosome 21q22.3 as determined by linkage analysis, and the gene has recently been cloned. HLA genes may have a minor modifying role in the expression of different components of the syndrome. The exact function of the gene responsible for APS type 1 is unknown, though it is reasonable to speculate that it must influence T cell behavior during early life. Since there are similarities between APS types 1 and 2, it is possible that the gene responsible for APS type 1, or factors affecting its product, could be involved in the etiology of other endocrinopathies.

The three manifestations of APS type 1 suggest that there is a T cell defect that both impairs the response of T cells to candidal antigens and increases the likelihood of autoreactive T cells developing. Polyendocrinopathies can be produced in animal models by T cell manipulations such as thymectomy and irradiation, perhaps mirroring this T cell dysfunction. A defect at the T cell level in the response to candidal antigens has been described. This presumably accounts for the chronic mucocutaneous candidiasis, but the immune response toward *Candida* is complex and involves neutrophils, macrophages, and humoral immunity. The antibody response to candidal antigens is known to be intact in APS type 1; this probably explains the superficial nature of the candidiasis; systemic infection is very rare.

Considerable progress has been made recently in understanding the basis for autoimmune Addison's disease in both types of APS, as well as in the isolated form. The adrenal autoantibody response is typically more diverse in APS type 1 than in the other forms of adrenal failure; in the latter, the predominant reactivity is against the cytochrome enzyme 21-hydroxylase (P450c21). Although antibodies against P450c21 also occur in 60 to 70% of APS type 1 patients with Addison's disease, there are additional antibodies against 17α-hydroxylase (P450c17) and side-chain cleaving enzyme (P450scc), each in approximately 40 to 50% patients. Usually these antibodies occur with those against P450c21, though some patients have isolated antibodies against only one of the cytochromes.

P450c17 and P450scc are found in adrenal, gonadal, and placental cells synthesizing sex hormones. Antibodies against these, which cross-react with the adrenal cortex, were previously called steroid cell antibodies before their identity was known. Autoimmunity against these diverse steroid cells, based on their content of P450c17 and/or P450scc, most likely accounts for the frequency of gonadal (especially ovarian) failure in APS type 1. Premature ovarian failure also occurs in isolated or APS type 2 Addison's patients on a similar basis, but it occurs less frequently due to the much lower prevalence of P450c17 and P450scc antibodies. It still remains unclear if and how these cytochrome antibodies are involved in the pathogenesis of adrenal and ovarian failure. As mentioned previously, autoantibodies can gain access to intracellular antigens and therefore have a primary role in causing disease. Alternatively, the production of cytochrome autoantibodies could be a secondary phenomenon due to adrenal or ovarian damage arising through T cell-mediated cytotoxicity directed against the same antigens. Certainly the pathology of Addison's disease resembles Hashimoto's thyroiditis, suggesting that a similar pathogenesis is likely.

The other defining condition, hypoparathyroidism, almost certainly has an autoimmune basis, but less is known about this. In a recent study, just over half of the surveyed patients with idiopathic hypoparathyroidism had antibodies against the calcium-sensing receptor. Of these, a subgroup had APS type 1, and 35% of these had calcium-sensing receptor antibodies. This suggests either that there are other autoantigens besides calcium-sensing receptors involved in hypoparathyroidism, or that calcium-sensing receptor autoantibodies have a minor or secondary role in pathogenesis. A variety of other autoantibodies have been described in APS type 1, including those directed against beta cell antigens – glutamic acid decarboxylase and aromatic-L-amino acid decarboxylase – which account for the association of APS type 1 with diabetes mellitus. Chronic active hepatitis is another associated complication, and antibodies against the hepatic cytochrome P450 1A2 have been identified in some patients.

Clinical findings

The first manifestation of APS type 1 is usually chronic mucocutaneous candidiasis (Fig. 72.3), which usually

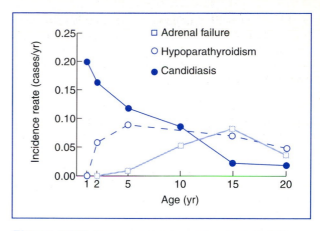

Figure 72.3 Incidence rates of adrenal failure, hypoparathyroidism, and chronic mucocutaneous candidiasis in APS type 1. (From Ahonen P, et al., Clinical variation of autoimmune polyendocrinopathy-candidiasis-ectodermal dystrophy [APECED] in a series of 68 patients. N Engl J Med 1990;322:1829-36.)

appears in childhood though can first appear as late as the third decade of life, and can run an intermittent course. The most common site is periungual, occurring in approximately 70% of patients, with dermal candidiasis occurring in around 10% (generally affecting less than 5% of the skin). In the remainder, candidiasis is oro-pharyngeal or esophageal, and may present with retrosternal pain resolving after antifungal treatment.

Hypoparathyroidism is the most common endocrinopathy and, as with mucocutaneous candidiasis, usually appears early in childhood though can become apparent as late as age 40. The clinical features are those of hypocalcemia and hyperphosphatemia. In particular, there is an increase in neuromuscular excitability, with symptoms ranging from paraesthesiae (especially circumoral) to tetany with carpopedal spasm, and even seizures. Mental changes including depression may be prominent, and in young children there may be congestive heart failure. Cataracts, basal ganglia calcification, and prolonged Q-T interval on ECG are important signs of all types of hypoparathyroidism.

Addison's disease usually appears 5-10 years after hypoparathyroidism, and again can first appear in the fourth or even fifth decade. Usually both cortisol and aldosterone deficiencies occur together, though either may precede the other (in equal proportion) in 20% of patients. The signs and symptoms of hypoadrenalism are 27; there are no special features of the form associated with APS type 1. Onset may be acute (Addisonian crisis) or chronic, with weakness, easy fatigability, anorexia, vomiting, non-specific abdominal pain, altered bowel habit, and/or postural symptoms. Loss of weight and an increase in pigmentation are nearly universal signs. Low serum sodium and raised potassium are useful clues to the diagnosis. There should be a low threshold for testing an APS type 1 patient with non-specific symptoms.

The other endocrinopathies and immune disorders associated with APS type 1 are less frequent (Tab. 72.5) and have no distinguishing clinical features compared to sporadic forms of these conditions. Gonadal failure is noteworthy, occurring in 60% of women and 10% of men. It occurs before the age of 30 and is generally primary. There is a close association with Addison's disease, as expected from the pathophysiology discussed above. Hypoparathyroidism is present in almost all patients with malabsorption, and the latter worsens with hypocalcemia.

The cause of the ectodermal signs is unknown. Nail dystrophy, in which scattered pits of 0.5 to 1mm appear in some (but never all) of the nails, is independent of candidal infection and may resolve spontaneously. Keratopathy and enamel hypoplasia are independent of hypoparathyroidism. The enamel defect does not affect the deciduous teeth. Tympanic membrane calcification occurs in plaques, usually in the posterior part of the membrane.

The most common causes of mortality have been unrecognized hypocalcemia and hypoadrenalism, though wider awareness and current replacement regimens should now make these far less of a problem. Fulminant hepatic failure is a significant cause of death, presumably related to chronic active hepatitis. Cases of carcinoma of the oral mucosa have been described; it is possible that chronic candidiasis is carcinogenic. Pure red cell aplasia has also been reported as a rare but serious complication. Infertility is also a significant problem affecting these patients. Other associated conditions, particularly recurrent or extensive gastrointestinal candidiasis and severe keratopathy, can lead to considerable morbidity.

The diagnosis of APS type 1 is based on the presence of particular clinical features, and as this syndrome can occur in childhood, it would be prudent to screen any infant or child with one of the three identifying conditions (Tab. 72.5). However, apparently isolated Addison's disease in adolescence or beyond is very unlikely to be associated with APS type 1, but may be associated with APS type 2, which is described in the following section. All Addisonian patients should be screened for autoantibodies to identify those at risk for the other components of the type 1 syndrome. Adrenal, islet, and parietal cell antibody assays are generally available and are based on the indirect immunofluorescence technique. Thyroid peroxidase plus thyroglobulin antibodies can be measured by hemagglutination or enzyme-linked immunosorbent assay. Recently developed immunoprecipitation assays, using in vitro translated recombinant autoantigens, can now detect the specific adrenal and islet cell autoantigens discussed under the section on pathogenesis, and may improve the predictive value of conventional antibody assays. Biochemical diagnosis of each of the endocrinopathies in Table 72.5 follows the same protocol described for the isolated form described elsewhere in this book. All APS type 1 patients should have annual tests of liver function to identify chronic active hepatitis. Once the type 1 syndrome is diagnosed in a family, all siblings should be screened for the disorder.

Treatment

Treatment of Addison's disease and hypoparathyroidism follows standard regimens. Intermittent malabsorption, in some cases with intestinal lymphangiectasia, can cause difficulty in tailoring replacement therapy. Ketoconazole has transformed the treatment of candidiasis in these patients, but often repeated and extended courses need to be given. It is important to bear in mind that this drug can inhibit glucocorticoid synthesis in those patients who still have intact adrenal function, and this could lead to errors in the diagnosis of Addison's disease. Hepatotoxicity is another significant problem with this drug. All patients require careful counseling in view of the need for lifelong endocrine replacement therapy and repeated screening to detect new components of the syndrome.

APS type 2

There is no universally accepted definition of autoimmune polyglandular syndrome type 2. Some authorities consider it to be equivalent to Schmidt's syndrome, given the presence of Addison's disease in a patient together with autoimmune thyroid disease (either hypothyroidism or Graves' disease) and/or type 1 diabetes mellitus; though they acknowledge that other autoimmune disorders are frequently associated. This seems too narrow a definition, however, as many patients have multiple endocrine disorders without necessarily having Addison's disease. Patients with any one of the endocrinopathies listed in Table 72.6, together with one of the other disorders in the same table, are viewed by some as having APS type 2. This seems too broad a definition, as some of the disorders are not endocrine, and therefore the patient does not have a truly polyglandular syndrome. Calling this type of cluster APS type 3 has not been generally accepted. Further

---

Table 72.6 Clinical features of autoimmune polyglandular syndrome type 2

Major endocrinopathies
Autoimmune thyroid disease (Graves' disease, primary myxedema, Hashimoto's thyroiditis, post partum thyroiditis)
Type 1 diabetes mellitus
Addison's disease
Premature ovarian failure

Other endocrinopathies
Lymphocytic hypophysitis
Isolated ACTH or gonadotropin deficiency
Lymphocytic infundibuloneurohypophysitis

Other features
Vitiligo
Alopecia or leucotrichia
Pernicious anemia
Coeliac disease/dermatitis herpetiformis
Myasthenia gravis
Serositis
Cardiac antibodies with hypertension

complications arise in those patients who have an endocrinopathy plus another autoimmune disorder (e.g., type 1 diabetes mellitus and celiac disease) or who have serological but not biochemical evidence of another endocrinopathy (e.g., thyroid autoantibodies). A reasonable compromise is to regard APS type 2 as the presence of two or more of any of the endocrinopathies listed in Table 72.6 in a patient, while the occurrence of one endocrinopathy in addition to one or more of the other features suggests that there is a risk of APS type 2 developing. Follow-up for the development of other endocrinopathies would be as for APS type 2.

Epidemiology

The overall prevalence in the community is not known, because the definition is variable between studies and the frequency depends on which component of the syndrome is analyzed. Thus, if one takes patients with type 1 diabetes mellitus, around 5% will have autoimmune thyroid disease and 0.1% will have Addison's disease, whereas 10 to 20% of patients with Addison's disease have type 1 diabetes and at least 25% have clinical or subclinical autoimmune thyroid disease. Indeed, APS type 2 occurs in around 50% of patients with Addison's disease. It is clear that APS type 2 is far more common than APS type 1.

Pathophysiology

There is nothing unique to the pathogenesis of the individual features of the syndrome when compared to the isolated disorders. However, there seems to be a much stronger genetic component to susceptibility, as there is a high frequency of other endocrinopathies in other family members. In many families (particularly when Addison's disease is a component), APS type 2 appears to be inherited as an autosomal dominant disorder with incomplete penetrance. Unlike APS type 1, there is a strong association with HLA genes. Only 5% of affected siblings share neither HLA haplotype of the proband (compared to an expected 25%). The HLA association is strong, particularly with the HLA-A1, -B8, -DR3 haplotype, although the strength of this association varies with disease components. For instance, HLA-DR4 is increased in APS type 2 patients with diabetes.

Clinical findings and treatment

Clinical manifestations and therapy are identical to those in patients with the individual, isolated endocrinopathies. It is important to remember that unexpected improvement in glycemic control (a drop in insulin requirement) in a diabetic patient provides an important clue that Addison's disease is developing.

Therapy for the endocrinopathies is also standard. One rare situation where special care is needed is in the treatment of hypothyroidism in an individual with unsuspected Addison's disease: unduly vigorous thyroxine replacement could theoretically precipitate an Addisonian crisis. In anyone suspected of Addison's disease, the diagnosis should be established and glucocorticoid therapy initiated prior to commencing thyroxine. Several patients with premature ovarian failure have been described in whom recognition and treatment of Addison's disease led to the resumption of menses, which could be due to the beneficial effects of glucocorticoids on the immune system. Reduced thyroid function may also improve with treatment of hypoadrenalism.

Screening

Because of the frequency of APS type 2 in patients with Addison's disease, it is worth assessing such patients regularly for other autoimmune disorders. A minimum screen would include annual assessment of thyroid antibodies and TSH, glucose, full blood count, and an inquiry about menstrual status in women. If readily available, islet cell and other antibodies may also be included, but the cost-effectiveness of this has not been established. Perhaps of even greater importance is the need to counsel these patients, and any patients with established APS type 2, about the possibility of developing other disorders so that they will seek medical advice when appropriate between annual visits.

The frequency of APS type 2 in patients with autoimmune thyroid disease or type 1 diabetes mellitus is probably insufficient, in the absence of clinical evidence, to warrant screening all such patients for other endocrinopathies. One exception is the high frequency of postpartum thyroiditis (10-15%) that occurs in women with type 1 diabetes mellitus. All such women should have thyroid peroxidase antibody estimation in the first trimester of pregnancy to detect those at risk of developing postpartum thyroiditis. Gonadal failure and lymphocytic hypophysitis are often associated with other endocrinopathies, such that these patients should probably be investigated with at least an autoantibody screen and measurement of glucose, TSH, and electrolytes.

Once APS type 2 is diagnosed in a proband, all first degree relatives should be offered a clinical examination, an autoantibody screen, and baseline biochemistry to determine those at risk. Because of incomplete penetrance, a single assessment is insufficient to exclude the syndrome in an individual family member, and regular follow-up is needed. For unaffected adolescents this could be at annual intervals, with less frequent testing in adult life if there is no evidence of the syndrome.

OTHER AUTOIMMUNE ENDOCRINOPATHY SYNDROMES

Some patients may not fall readily into the APS type 1 or 2 classification, particularly when idiopathic hypoparathyroidism occurs with another, non-adrenal endocrinopathy such as autoimmune thyroid disease. Given that

Addison's disease and other endocrinopathies are shared between the two syndromes, it is not surprising that hypoparathyroidism should occur more widely than in APS type 1. In the absence of chronic mucocutaneous candidiasis or ectodermal dystrophy, it would seem appropriate to include idiopathic hypoparathyroidism as a rare component of APS type 2. There is also an increase in autoimmune thyroid disease, and possibly in Addison's disease, in patients with thymoma, in whom myasthenia gravis is frequent. The reasons for these associations are unknown. Two other more or less distinct autoimmune syndromes occur, detailed below.

Type B insulin resistance

Type B insulin resistance is a syndrome that is the result of autoantibodies directed against the insulin receptor, causing severe insulin resistance, diabetes mellitus, and acanthosis nigricans. It is very rare. Most patients have been black women. In addition to often massive insulin requirements, distinctive features include leukopenia, hypergammaglobulinemia, hypocomplementemia, and positive antinuclear antibodies. Around one-third of these patients have systemic lupus erythematosus and alopecia. Vitiligo and hemolytic anemia each occur in 10 to 30% of

cases. Spontaneous remission has been reported, but in other patients diabetes persists despite enormous insulin doses.

POEMS syndrome

Polyneuropathy, organomegaly, endocrinopathy, monoclonal gammopathy, and skin changes (POEMS) syndrome (or Crow-Fukase syndrome) is a rare multi-system disease often associated with osteosclerotic bone lesions. The primary disorder is a plasma cell dyscrasia (IgA or IgG) with λ light chain restriction. The organomegaly in the acronym refers to splenomegaly, hepatomegaly, or lymphadenopathy, and the skin changes consist of thickening and increased pigmentation, as well as hypertrichosis, clubbing, and Raynaud's phenomenon. The endocrinopathies described in POEMS syndrome range from hypothyroidism and insulin-dependent diabetes mellitus (50% of patients) to the less frequent occurrence of hypogonadism, hypoadrenalism, hyperprolactinemia, and hypoparathyroidism. Autoantibodies against endocrine tissues are not usually found, and the etiological basis for the endocrine dysfunction remains unclear. It is possible that cytokines produced by the plasma cells, such as IL-2, IL-6, and TNF, are involved. There seems to be no clinical relevance in terms of survival from the plasma cell dyscrasia when comparing those individuals who have the POEMS syndrome from those who do not.

Suggested readings

AALTONEN J, BJÖRSES P, SANDKUIJL L, PERHEENTUPA J, PELTONEN L. An autosomal locus causing autoimmune disease: autoimmune polyglandular disease type I assigned to chromosome 21. Nat Genet 1994;8:83-7.

AHONEN P, MYLLÄRNIEMI S, SIPILÄ I, PERHEENTUPA J. Clinical variation of autoimmune polyendocrinopathy-candidiasis-ectodermal dystrophy (APECED) in a series of 68 patients. N Engl J Med 1990;322:1829-36.

ANDRÉ I, GONZALEZ A, WANG B, KATZ J, BENOIST C, MATHIS D. Checkpoints in the progression of autoimmune disease: lessons from diabetes models. Proc Natl Acad Sci USA 1996;93:2260-3.

BETTERLE C, PRESOTTO F, MAGRIN L, et al. The natural history of pre-type 1 (insulin-dependent) diabetes mellitus in patients with autoimmune endocrine diseases. Diabetologia 1994;37:95-103.

GOODNOW CC. Balancing immunity and tolerance: deleting and tuning lymphocyte repertoires. Proc Natl Acad Sci USA 1996;9:2264-71.

JANEWAY CA JR, BOTTOMLY K. Signals and signs for lymphocyte responses. Cell 1994;76:275-85.

LI Y, SONG Y-H, RAIS N, et al. Autoantibodies to the extracellular domain of the calcium sensing receptor in patients with acquired hypoparathyroidism. J Clin Invest 1996;97:910-4.

LIBLAU RS, SINGER SM, MCDEVITT HO. Th1 and Th2 CD4[+]T cells in the pathogenesis of organ-specific autoimmune diseases. Immunol Today 1995;16:34-8.

MONDINO A, KHORUTS A, JENKINS MK. The anatomy of T-cell activation and tolerance. Proc Natl Acad Sci USA 1996;93:2245-52.

MUIR A, MACLAREN NK. Autoimmune diseases of the adrenal glands, parathyroid glands, gonads, and hypothalamic-pituitary axis. Endocrinol Metab Clin North Am 1991;20: 619-44.

NEUFELD M, MACLAREN NK, BLIZZARD RM. Two types of autoimmune Addison's disease associated with different polyglandular autoimmune (PGA) syndromes. Medicine 1981;60:355-62.

REISER H, STADECKER MJ. Costimulatory B7 molecules in the pathogenesis of infectious and autoimmune diseases. N Engl J Med 1996;335:1369-77.

THODOU E, ASA SL, KONTOGEORGOS G, KOVACS K, HORVATH E, EZZAT S. Clinical case seminar. Lymphocytic hypophysitis: clinicopathological findings. J Clin Endocrinol Metab 1995; 80:2302-11.

VYSE TJ, TODD JA. Genetic analysis of autoimmune disease. Cell 1996;85:311-8.

WEETMAN AP. Autoimmunity to steroid producing cells and familial polyendocrine autoimmunity. Baillières Clin Endocrinol Metab 1995;9:157-74.

Hormones and athletic performance

Egil Haug, Kaare I. Birkeland

Scientific and medical interest in the physiological responses to exercise has grown as people have become increasingly active in recreational and competitive sports over the years. With the constant desire to perform better and to raise the limits of human achievement, some athletes have been prompted to use their sometimes limited knowledge of exercise physiology for the purpose of artificially enhancing genetic performance, that is, using drugs, or, "doping". Most of the drugs misused for doping purposes are hormones or hormone-like substances. It is therefore important for the physician to be aware of the influences of exercise on the endocrine system and on the outcome of endocrine tests. The physician should also realize that prescribing substances banned by sports organizations to athletes engaged in organized sports could have severe consequences for the athlete in a doping test in terms of their eligibility to compete or remain on their team. Moreover, the physician should be aware of the medical consequences and the adverse effects caused by the misuse of doping agents, since athletes may seek medical advice for these effects.

In this chapter we will briefly describe the endocrine adaptations to exercise, and then discuss in some depth the hormones most often used for doping purposes.

EFFECTS OF EXERCISE ON THE ENDOCRINE SYSTEM

During physical exercise, working skeletal muscles may increase the rate of energy expenditure as much as 300-fold. This amount of energy can only be supplied by local stores for a short time. Thereafter, energy delivery is adjusted by the nervous and endocrine systems. The four principle fuel-mobilizing hormones during exercise are catecholamines, glucagon, cortisol, and growth hormone. During long-term or repeated bouts of strenuous exercise, a balance must be achieved between the effects of these catabolic hormones and anabolic hormones (primarily insulin and the sex steroids) in order to not enter into a permanent catabolic state.

Fuel-mobilizing hormones

Plasma levels of catecholamines increase markedly shortly after the initiation of exercise. These hormones mobilize lipids and carbohydrates, making fuel available for the working muscle by inhibiting insulin secretion, thus promoting lipolysis from fat and glycogenolysis (and gluconeogenesis) from the liver. Strenuous exercise stimulates glucagon secretion, which increases hepatic glucose production through gluconeogenesis and glycogenolysis. After approximately 15 to 20 minutes, exercise also leads to a rise in serum cortisol levels. Cortisol acts synergistically with glucagon and catecholamines on hepatic glucose production and also increases lipolysis. Growth hormone (GH) rises profoundly during exercise, which is why exercise tests are utilized to assess GH secretion in children. Although this hormone is shown to have both glucogenic and lipolytic actions, its exact role in exercise metabolism remains unclear.

Pituitary hormones

In parallel with GH, serum prolactin rises with strenuous exercise in men and women. The GH and prolactin responses to exercise may be modulated by ambient temperature: a cold environment attenuates, while a warm environment has been shown to increase the responses. Serum corticotropin levels rise rapidly after starting exercise, preceding the rise in cortisol levels. Exercise usually has minor effects on the pituitary-thyroidal axis. Acute exercise seems to increase thyrotropin levels and also increase turnover rates of thyroxine (T_4) and tri-iodothyronine (T_3). Long-lasting strenuous exercise (such as a marathon run) may induce changes similar to those seen in non-thyroidal illness: reduced levels of free T_4 and T_3, increased reverse T_3, and at large unchanged levels of thyrotropin. Plasma vasopressin levels increase with exercise in men and women, dependent on intensity, duration, mode of exercise, and hydration status.

Gonadal hormones

Acute exercise increases the serum levels of both estradiol and progesterone. However, since secretion rates seem to be unaltered, these changes probably reflect reduced metabolic clearance. There has been considerable interest in examining the relationship between strenuous exercise and hormonal changes taking place during the normal menstrual cycle. The results from studies of the effects of the menstrual cycle phase on exercise performance are so far inconclusive. It has, on the other hand, become increasingly evident that engagement in competitive sports may lead to menstrual abnormalities, such as delayed menarche, oligomenorrhea, amenorrhea, or short luteal phases. The reason for these disturbances remains unclear, but the intensity and duration of exercise as well as the nutritional status, body weight, and body fat content of the individual are important factors. The menstrual irregularities are accompanied by an abnormal pattern of gonadotropin pulsatility and subnormal serum levels of estradiol and progesterone. These hormonal changes are readily reversible upon the reduction of training intensity. However, for women engaged in high intensity training for many years, the low estradiol levels may have negative effects on bone mineral content. Several reports show low bone mass and the increased prevalence of stress fractures in women with training-induced amenorrhea. Hence, despite the reversibility of the training-induced drop in sex hormone levels, there is a risk that these women may end up with reduced bone mass.

In men, serum testosterone usually increases during the initial phase of both heavy power and endurance exercise. During prolonged strenuous exercise and intense physical stress (e.g., a marathon run), however, testosterone levels in serum are usually depressed. The circadian variations in testosterone levels may modify these responses.

Other hormones

Strenuous exercise stimulates the renin-angiotensin-aldosterone system (RAAS). This is caused by a more than 10% decrease in effective blood volume during exercise, which stimulates stretch receptors in the renal afferent arterioles. Additionally, exercise-induced sweating and catecholamine release contribute to RAAS stimulation.

Serum insulin levels gradually decrease during exercise, mainly as a result of the α-adrenergic inhibition of β-cell function. Furthermore, muscle glucose uptake is increased during exercise, an effect that lasts for many hours after exercise. This has been described as an increase in insulin sensitivity, suggesting that regular training may have a long-lasting effect on glucose metabolism. The reduction in insulin levels and increase in insulin sensitivity during exercise seem to also be present in subjects with non-insulin-dependent diabetes. Some of the changes in serum hormone levels during acute exercise are summarized in Table 73.1.

HORMONES AND RELATED SUBSTANCES USED TO ENHANCE ATHLETIC PERFORMANCE

Anabolic-androgenic steroids

Anabolic-androgenic steroids (AAS) are naturally occurring androgens and synthetic derivatives of testosterone. In medicine, synthetic AAS are primarily used to treat hypogonadism in men. For many years, however, these steroids have been abused by bodybuilders, weightlifters, and other athletes. These substances are used with the expectation that they will enhance muscle mass and strength and are also used for the purpose of improving physical appearance.

The prevalence of AAS abuse is poorly documented in the literature. There are reports from North America and the United Kingdom suggesting that among college and high school male students, from 1 to 10% use or have used AAS. In the Scandinavian countries, recent data show that of the population between 14 and 25 years of age, including women, 1 to 2% admitted that they used or had used these substances. Among the users, only a small minority seem to be competing athletes. A recent study in the United Kingdom revealed that the prevalence of AAS misuse among people using private gymnasia on a regular basis was almost 40%, and that bodybuilders and weightlifters comprised more that 80% of the users. This

---

Table 73.1 Effects of acute exercise on hormonal levels

Hormone	Change from basal
Adrenaline	↑↑
Noradrenaline	↑↑
Glucagon	↑
Growth hormone	↑↑
Cortisol	↑
ACTH	↑
LH	↑↓
FSH	↑↓
Testosterone[1]	↑
Estradiol	↑
Insulin	↓
Prolactin	↑
Thyrotropin	↑
RAAS	↑
Vasopressin	↑

[1] In men testosterone usually increases during 1-3 hours of strenuous exercise, thereafter testosterone decreases. Testosterone also shows diurnal variation.
(RAAS = renin-angiotensin-aldosterone system; ↑↑ = profound increase; ↑ = increase; ↓ = decrease; ↑↓ = no change or variable.)

suggests that the large majority of abusers of AAS may be outside competitive sports.

Physiology

Anabolic-androgenic steroids have widespread effects on reproductive and non-reproductive tissues. The onset of puberty is marked by increased testosterone production responsible for the well-known pubertal alterations in primary sex structures, and also for the development of secondary sex characteristics. Testosterone is essential for sperm production and maturation. In hypogonadal men, testosterone replacement increases nitrogen retention and restores muscle mass and strength.

Do anabolic-androgenic steroids enhance athletic performance?

Although athletes have been using AAS in supraphysiologic doses for years, studies of the performance-enhancing effects of these substances have for different reasons been mostly inconclusive. Recently, however, a carefully conducted placebo-controlled study showed that injections of 600 mg testosterone weekly for 10 weeks significantly increased muscle size and strength in normal men 19 to 40 years of age. These effects were enhanced when combined with strength training. During the treatment period serum testosterone increased five- to sevenfold, and LH and FSH were suppressed, showing that the doses of testosterone used were in the supraphysiological range. Undoubtedly some athletes and bodybuilders use much higher doses; there are reports indicating the use of weekly doses of up to 3000 to 4000 mg. At this point in time, however, the optimal dose of AAS for use in the increase of muscle mass and strength is unknown.

The anabolic action of AAS is probably partly achieved by minimizing the catabolic effects of corticosteroids released during physical activity, and partly by maintaining a positive nitrogen balance by improving utilization of ingested protein. In addition, AAS also enhance training capabilities by counteracting the feeling of fatigue.

Anabolic-androgenic steroids drug regimens

The drug regimens used by a variety of athletes are based on anecdotal evidence, personal experience, financial factors, black market drug availability, and/or the "underground literature." Most athletes practice cyclic drug administration in which one steroid cycle typically takes between 4 to 12 weeks. At the end of the treatment period, athletes have usually reached a plateau in subjective benefits. During the cycle they also experience increasing side effects. The interval between steroid cycles vary from one user to the other: the most experienced users have shorter steroid-free gaps (4 to 6 weeks), while the less frequent users may remain steroid-free for several months.

Most athletes combine two or more different types of AAS (called "stacking"), because it is believed that this allows for the use of larger doses with less side effects, and that it also offers the possibility of obtaining synergis-

tic actions. Commonly used protocols include the use of oral and injectable preparations of short and long duration. Table 73.2 gives an example of an administration protocol.

Illicit drug use is usually not confined to AAS. Many athletes combine the use of AAS and non-steroid agents with anabolic properties such as growth hormone, clenbuterol (β_2-receptor agonist), and insulin. In addition, several other potent drugs are used by the athletes for various reasons.

Adverse effects

Numerous side effects have been associated with the abuse of AAS. Most athletes admit having adverse effects, but they are usually considered minor and acceptable to the user. The adverse effects may be divided into three categories: physical side effects, psychiatric side effects, and social side effects.

Physical side effects Liver enzyme derangement, altered serum lipids, hypertension, and clotting abnormalities (see below) are relatively common and are usually reversible upon cessation of AAS abuse. Acne, gynecomastia, striae, and testicular shrinkage frequently occur. Gynecomastia probably results from increased aromatization of androgens to estrogens, stimulating the growth of mammary glandular tissue. The high doses of AAS also cause suppression of the pituitary secretion of LH and

Table 73.2 Example of AAS treatment protocol

Treatment	Weeks of treatment			
	1 - 4	5 - 8	9 -12 (rest period)	13
Nandrolone im (mg/week)	200			
Testosterone propionate im (mg/week)		300		
Stanozolol im (mg/week)		150		
Tamoxifen po (mg/day)	20	20		
hCG im (U/at end of course)		6000		
Sustanon im[1] (mg/week)				500

(po = orally; im = intramuscularly.)
[1] Maintenance therapy until next cycle.

FSH, which leads to hypogonadotropic hypogonadism and oligospermia. Infertility clinics have in recent years experienced an increased number of men seen for infertility difficulties who have a history of AAS abuse. After stopping the misuse of AAS, it normally takes months and in some cases even years before normal testicular function is restored. Table 73.3 summarizes the most important laboratory changes caused by AAS abuse.

Recently, several case reports have appeared describing the occurrence of vascular catastrophic events such as myocardial infarction, cerebrovascular accidents, and pulmonary embolism in young AAS users. The reasons for this are not well understood, though it is known that AAS significantly decrease HDL-cholesterol and also activate the hemostatic system by increasing the generation of both thrombin and plasmin. The risk for having vascular catastrophes increases with the length of time of misuse; it is our experience that these accidents occur after many years of abuse. Case reports have also linked AAS misuse with liver tumors, tendon ruptures, and injection site problems.

Psychiatric side effects The bulk of available evidence suggests that the use and withdrawal of AAS may produce severe psychiatric effects. As many as one-third of AAS misusers are reported to experience mood syndromes such as mania, hypomania, or major depression. Psychotic features can occur. Aggressive and violent behavior also often accompany AAS-associated manic or hypomanic episodes, creating a serious problem for the misusers' families and other people in their surroundings. There are also data supporting the notion that the misuse of AAS may lead to psychological dependence.

Social side effects The Scandinavian studies and others have demonstrated that AAS misusers have a higher consumption of narcotics, alcohol, and nicotine than non-

users, and that they more often are involved in violent criminal behavior. Likewise, there are reports suggesting that AAS misusers are at a greater risk of engaging in sexual assault.

Methods for detection

The synthetic derivatives of testosterone (anabolic steroids) are easily detected in urine using a combination of gas chromatography and mass spectrometry. Testosterone and its biologically inactive epimer epitestosterone are both excreted in the urine. The urinary ratio testosterone/epitestosterone (T/E) is normally between 1 and 3. Testosterone in supraphysiological doses suppresses pituitary LH and FSH secretion to undetectable concentrations, and thereby also reduces the endogenous production of both testosterone and epitestosterone. The T/E-ratio is therefore increased after the administration of testosterone. The T/E ratio is used by "doping control laboratories" to detect testosterone doping, where T/E ratios of >6 are considered indicative of testosterone misuse. Urinary T/LH-ratios are also increased, allowing this ratio to be used to indicate testosterone doping as well. Testosterone administration decreases the hepatic production of sex hormone-binding globulin (SHBG) and thyroxin-binding globulin (TBG), such that low serum levels of SHBG and TBG may additionally indicate testosterone misuse (Tab. 73.3).

Growth hormone

Several peptide hormones, including growth hormone (GH), erythropoietin (EPO), corticotropin, and human chorionic gonadotropin (hCG) were banned by the International Olympic Committee in 1989. One of the reasons leading up to this was that out-of-competition testing for AAS had become routine, and athletes searched for new doping agents that were not so easily detected in standard doping control practices. At the same time, recombinant human growth hormone (rhGH) and erythropoietin (rhEPO) had become commercially available and were in use for medical purposes.

Physiology

There are two reasons why rhGH has been expected to improve performance in sports. First, exercise is a potent stimulus for GH secretion, as previously described. The magnitude of the GH response is mainly determined by the intensity and the duration of the exercise. Heavy exercise increases GH secretion after about 10 minutes, while an exercise level as low as 15% of the individual's VO_{2max} may give a GH response after 60 minutes. It also appears that long-term endurance training increases both basal and exercise-related GH production, though data on this are conflicting. While acute exercise has no convincing effect on insulin-like growth factor 1 (IGF-1), chronic exercise appears to increase IGF-1 levels.

Second, rhGH administration has been used to increase performance in sports because GH therapy in GH-deficient children and adults has been shown to reduce fat and increase muscle mass.

Table 73.3 Laboratory changes caused by AAS use

Serum concentration	Expected changes
LH	↓
FSH	↓
Testosterone[1]	↑↓
17-OH-Progesterone	↓
Estradiol[2]	↑
SHBG	↓
TBG	↓

[1] Increased in testosterone misusers, decreased in anabolic steroid misusers.
[2] Increased in male testosterone misusers.

Does rhGH enhance athletic performance?

Substitution therapy with GH to GH deficient adults increases lean body mass and probably muscle mass, muscle strength, and also (though not unequivocally proven) performance in endurance exercise. However, supraphysiological doses of GH given to athletes with intact endogenous GH production do not seem to increase muscle mass or muscle strength. Such treatment causes a modest increase in lean tissue, particularly connective tissue, and some reduction in fat mass. Skeletal muscle hypertrophy has not been demonstrated, and muscle strength is not increased. It is possible this is due to limitations caused by the side effects that follow the administration of high doses of GH.

Adverse effects

The adverse effects of GH treatment include muscle and joint pain, fluid retention, hypertension, and carbohydrate intolerance. The long-term use of high doses may result in acromegaly and may also increase the risk of malignancy.

Methods for detection

At the present time, there is no reliable method that can be applied as proof of rhGH misuse in doping control. Several parameters measured in blood and urine have been suggested to be used as markers of doping with rhGH, including IGF-1, ratio of IGF-1 to IGF-2, IGF-binding protein 3 (IGFBP-3), bone turnover markers (e.g., pyridinolines, osteocalcin), and others. Because the relative distribution between the 20 and 22 kD isoforms of GH may differ between endogenously produced GH and rhGH, the measurement of the isoforms has also been suggested as a tool to detect GH doping.

Erythropoietin

As soon as recombinant human erythropoietin (rhEPO) became available for treatment of EPO-deficient anemias, speculations started as to whether it could be used as a substitute for blood-doping in endurance sports. Not long after, rumors circulated in the lay press that some cases of unexpected death among professional cyclists might be attributed to the misuse of rhEPO. However, 5 to 10 years later, there is still little known about the prevalence of rhEPO misuse among athletes, except that it enhances most certainly performance in endurance sports and is being used for this purpose.

Physiology

Erythropoietin is produced in peritubular renal cells, circulates in the body, and stimulates precursor cells in the erythroid cell line to mature into erythrocytes. The main stimulus for erythropoietin production is reduced oxygen supply to the peritubular cells caused by anemia, reduced cardiopulmonary function, or low atmospheric pressure.

Does rhEPO enhance athletic performance?

There is good evidence that oxygen supply to the working muscle is one of the main limiting factors for performance in endurance sports. Several experiments with blood doping (transfusion of erythrocytes from 2 to 3 units of blood prior to exercise) have shown improvements in VO_2 max as well as in athletic achievements. In one unblinded clinical trial, the administration of 20-40 U rhEPO/kg body weight every second day for 4 to 6 weeks to 14 healthy volunteers increased VO_{2max} approximately 8%. Whether the same would hold true for top level athletes is not yet known.

Adverse effects

In patients with renal failure, severe hypertension sometimes follows the administration of rhEPO. It has been feared that this side effect would occur when rhEPO was used by healthy athletes, but it seems to be uncommon.

If hematocrit levels increase too rapidly to too high a concentration, thereby increasing whole blood viscosity, there may be an increase in the risk of thromboembolic disease. Anecdotal reports of severe thrombosis after doping with rhEPO exist, but the documentation of these events is poor.

Methods for detection

At the present time, several methods for the detection of doping with rhEPO are under investigation. The administration of rhEPO leads to an increase in reticulocyte count, and in the number of large erythrocytes with a low hemoglobin content (hypochrome macrocytes). Furthermore, the serum level of soluble transferrin receptor increases markedly, as do the levels of total fibrinogen degradation products, at least in patients with renal failure. All of these parameters may be used to indicate rhEPO administration, although none of them appear to be specific enough to serve as proof in a doping case.

A direct method to disclose rhEPO doping in blood and urine samples is under investigation. This method separates endogenously produced EPO from rhEPO due to the charge-differences between the two forms, which depend on variations in the carbohydrate moieties connected to the protein core.

Other hormones and hormone-like substances

Several other hormones are also misused as doping agents. Human chorionic gonadotropin is frequently used either together with AAS or between the AAS cycles. It is used to stimulate endogenous testosterone production, which is suppressed during the AAS administration. Clomiphene has been used for its LH-stimulating properties with the goal of re-establishing endogenous testosterone production after AAS use. Tamoxifen is being used by AAS misusers, not to enhance performance, but to avoid the gynecomastia that frequently follows. AAS misuse (Tab. 73.2). Clenbuterol and other oral β_2-agonists are being used for their anabolic properties. At least in some animal species, these agents increase muscle mass and reduce fat mass, but the data available do not support any major anabolic activity in humans. Amphetamine and ephedrine have adrenergic properties and are used mainly for their stimulating effects on the central nervous system. The dangerous side effect of cardiovascular collapse in athletes using amphetamines has been described. Insulin has been used for its anabolic actions, though hypoglycemic reactions probably limit its usefulness.

DOPING IN SPORTS

The word "dope" comes from South Africa. It was the name of a plant extract used as a stimulant. The Scandinavian Vikings used extracts prepared from mushrooms for the same reason, and the Indians in South America regularly used extracts containing cocaine.

It is probably correct to date the modern history of doping in sports back to the 1950s. Amphetamine misuse by athletes was first suspected at both the Summer and Winter Olympic Games in 1952. Amphetamine abuse was later linked to the death of one cyclist during the 1960 Summer Olympics in Rome and of another cyclist during the Tour de France in 1967.

In the early 1950s athletes from the United States and the Soviet Union started to use AAS. In the following years, the misuse of AAS in sports increased rapidly. Reports from the Olympic Games in Tokyo in 1964 indicated that the abuse was widespread among Olympic athletes.

International Olympic Committee's antidoping work

The impact of the information regarding the abuse of amphetamines and AAS stimulated the International Olympic Committee to start an antidoping program. The International Olympic Committee Medical Commission developed a list of banned substances and also formulated regulations for accrediting laboratories to conduct testing. Comprehensive testing was first performed at the Munich Summer Olympics in 1972, where the athletes were screened for the misuse of stimulants and opioids. Testing for AAS was introduced at the Olympic Games in Montreal in 1976. Since then, antidoping testing has been performed at all Olympic Games. The International Olympic Committee annually updates a list of doping agents and methods that are prohibited. This list is now, in some instances with minor revisions, approved by most sports organizations (Tab. 73.4).

The International Olympic Committee accredits the doping control laboratories, of which there are currently

Table 73.4 International Olympic Committee list of prohibited classes of substances and prohibited methods, 1997

Doping contravenes the ethics of both sport and medical science. Doping consists of (1) the administration of substances belonging to prohibited classes of pharmacological agents, and/or (2) the use of various prohibited methods.

I. **Prohibited classes of substances**
   A. Stimulants
   B. Narcotics
   C. Anabolic agents
      1. Anabolic-androgenic steroids
      2. β_2-agonists
   D. Diuretics
   E. Peptide and glycoprotein hormones and analogues

II. **Prohibited methods**
   A. Blood doping
   B. Pharmacological, chemical and physical manipulation

III. **Classes of drogs subject to certain restrictions**
   A. Alcohol
   B. Marijuana
   C. Local anesthetics
   D. Corticosteroids
   E. Beta-blockers

more than 20 throughout the world. They must follow the Committee's guidelines for good laboratory practice and are required to pass a re-accreditation test every year. The Committee's laboratories collaborate in the development of both new analytical tests and quality control systems.

Testing of athletes during and out of competition has become routine, and now more than 90 000 urine samples are collected every year. During the last few years, 1 to 2% of the samples were found to contain banned substances. Athletes testing positive are usually ruled by the sports authorities to abstain from participation in competition and organized training for a period of time dependent on the circumstances.

Council of Europe's antidoping work

In several countries governmental actions have also been taken to engage in controlling the misuse of ergogenic substances inside and outside sports. In 1989 the Council of Europe opened its Antidoping Convention for signature, which today has more than 30 contracting states. The Convention places a responsibility on the governments to act against doping, admitting that the problem cannot be solved entirely within sports itself. The contracting states are obliged to take the steps necessary to restrict the availability and use of banned doping agents and methods in sports. This means also that the contracting states in co-operation with the sports organizations shall facilitate the establishment of doping control laboratories.

APPENZELLER O. Sports Medicine. Fitness, training, injuries. 3rd ed. Baltimore-Munich: Urban & Schwarzenberg, 1988.

BHASIN S, STORER TW, BERMAN N, et al. The effects of supraphysiologic doses of testosterone on muscle size and strength in normal men. N Engl J Med 1996;335:1-7.

CUNEO RC, WALLACE JD. Growth hormone, insulin-like growth factors and sport. Endocrinology and Metabolism 1994;1:3-13.

DUCHAINE D. Underground steroid handbook II. Venice, Cal: HLR Technical Books, 1989.

EKBLOM B, BERGLUND B. Effect of erythropoietin administration on maximal aerobic power. Scand J Med Sci Sports 1991;1:88-93.

EVANS NA. Gym and tonic: a profile of 100 male steroid users. Br J Sports Med 1997;31:54-8.

HEMMERSBACH P, BIRKELAND KI. Blood samples in doping control. Oslo: On Demand Publishing, 1994.

INTERNATIONAL OLYMPIC COMMITTEE. IOC list of doping agents and methods 1997. Lausanne: IOC, 1997.

KICMAN AT, COWAN DA. Peptide hormones and sport: misuse and detection. Br Med Bull 1992;48:496-517.

POPE HG JR, KATZ DL. Psychiatric and medical effects of anabolic-androgenic steroid use. A controlled study of 160 athletes. Arch Gen Psychiatry 1994;51:375-82.

THOMAS JA. Drugs, athletes, and physical performance. New York: Plenum Medical Book Company, 1988.

WAGNER JC. Enhancement of athletic performance with drugs. An overview. Sports Med 1991;12:250-65.

WILSON JD. Androgen abuse by athletes. Endocr Rev 1988;9:181-99.

Endocrinology in AIDS

Guido Norbiato

▮ KEY POINTS ▮

- Abnormalities of the gonads, the thyroid, mineralocorticoid hormones, vaso-pressin, and α-melanocyte-stimulating hormone; and disturbances in carbohydrate, lipid and protein metabolism; are frequently associated with the human immunodeficiency virus (HIV) infection. Therapy for these disorders is being pursued, though the effects of these treatments on long-term disease progression are not yet known due to the lack of well-controlled studies.

- The pro-inflammatory cytokines interleukins (IL) 1 and 6 and interferon-γ, produced during acute immuno-reaction, may stimulate the hypothalamo-pituitary-adrenal axis function, causing the elevation of systemic glucocorticoid levels. Hypercortisolemia suppresses type 1 cytokines IL-2 and interferon-γ and stimulates type 2 cytokines IL-4 and IL-10. This common hypercortisolemic state increases susceptibility to infection and neoplasia in HIV patients.

- Hypercortisolemic HIV-infected patients may develop peripheral resistance to cortisol, leading to a shift from the type 2 cytokine profile to the type 1 and an increased susceptibility to autoimmune-inflammatory disease.

- Research indicates that the suppressive effect of hypercortisolism may be counteracted by manipulating cortisol with cortisol antagonists such as dehydroepiandrosterone and its metabolites.

- Testicular function may be impaired, which is often accompanied by decreased libido and diminished spermatogenesis. Sex hormone-binding globulin levels are often increased, thus resulting in normal levels of total testosterone but low free testosterone. In a hypogonadic man, free testosterone levels correlate with the loss of lean body mass, suggesting that loss of this anabolic steroid may be responsible, at least in part, for the wasting syndrome.

- Ovarian function is usually quite normal, although approximately 25% of women have amenorrhea.

- The most frequent alterations in thyroid function are as follows: exaggerated thyroid-stimulating hormone response to thyrotropin-releasing hormone, increased antibodies against peroxidase, elevation of thyroxine-binding globulin, depressed 3,5,3'-triiodothyronine (T_3), and increased reverse T_3 concentrations.

- Also frequent in HIV disease is the presence of an excess of water versus sodium ions, with consequent hyponatremia. While the inappropriate secretion of vasopressin is rarely responsible for hyponatremia, the increased release of vasopressin – stimulated by low pressure and/or volume, endotoxin, nausea, vomiting, or opiates – is a frequent cause.

The human immunodeficiency virus (HIV), responsible for the acquired immunodeficiency syndrome (AIDS), affects many organs and systems. As the viral load of HIV increases, an aggressive host response may have an adverse effect on organ function. The early phase of the illness is generally asymptomatic since the immune system actively contains the infection. When immune suppression does occur, usually due to the loss of CD_4 T helper cells, the disease becomes symptomatic with the onset of complications such as severe immunodeficiency, multiple opportunistic infections, and neoplasms. HIV infection is also accompanied by a number of endocrine and metabolic disturbances both 'in the early and later stages of the disease. Such alterations in the endocrine system may influence disease progression since the hormonal system, particularly the hypothalamo-pituitary-adrenal (HPA) axis, has important immunoregulatory functions. In addition, antibodies and cytokines or other molecules produced by HIV infection may interfere with hormonal function.

This chapter reviews hormonal and metabolic abnormalities reported in HIV disease, with specific attention paid to the relationship between these abnormalities and the immune function.

HYPOTHALAMO-PITUITARY-ADRENAL AXIS

Although the adrenal gland is frequently involved in cases of AIDS, and clinical manifestations of AIDS can be similar to those of adrenal insufficiency, a tissue dysfunction severe enough to cause adrenal insufficiency is rare.

The coexistence of conditions such as cachexia, weight loss, secondary infections, and secondary malignancies in the central nervous system (CNS) can potentially compromise hypothalamic and pituitary function. Despite this, frank hypopituitarism is rare in patients with AIDS. The most frequent infection found in the pituitary gland is cytomegalovirus, while tests for cryptococcosis, *Aspergillus*, toxoplasmosis, and *Pneumocystis carinii* are negative. Microadenomas are observed, but with the same frequency as in control group subjects. Provocative testing with adrenocorticotropic hormone (ACTH) or corticotropin-releasing hormone (CRH) suggests that about 50% of HIV-infected patients have some loss of either the pituitary or the adrenal reserve function.

CYTOKINES AND THE HYPOTHALAMO-PITUITARY-ADRENAL AXIS

Cytokine modulation of the hypothalamo-pituitary-adrenal (HPA) axis is a potential explanation for the hypercortisolemia seen in asymptomatic and symptomatic HIV patients. In vitro and animal experiments demonstrate that interleukin (IL) 1 and 6, tumor-necrosis factor, and interferon alpha (IFN-α) are all capable of influencing HPA function. The stimulatory effect of proinflammatory cytokines on the HPA axis produced during acute immune reaction mobilizes the CRH-ACTH-glucocorticoid cascade, thus causing an elevation of systemic glucocorticoid levels.

More specifically, IL-1 has been shown to increase hypothalamic CRH and pituitary ACTH production. The main effects of IL-1 include fever, anorexia, and catabolic metabolism, disturbances which often occur in HIV patients.

Interleukin 6, the principal endocrine cytokine, has been shown to stimulate both ACTH and cortisol in humans. IL-6 induces elevation of ACTH and cortisol levels well above those observed with maximal doses of CRH, suggesting that other secretagogues are also stimulated by this cytokine. However, glucocorticoids are known to suppress IL-6 production by decreasing the transcription rate of the gene for this interleukin.

IFN-α is a cytokine potentially capable of stimulating adrenal function. It may act directly on the adrenal gland or may be mediated by the pituitary ACTH release.

CORTISOL

Systemic hormone measurements have shown that serum and urinary levels of cortisol increase in HIV-infected patients at all stages of the disease. Corticotropin frequently increases together with cortisol in the early phase of the disease, suggesting increased HPA axis function. Patients with more advanced disease may have elevated serum cortisol concentrations but normal corticotropin concentrations, suggesting that other factors are responsible for increased cortisol production at later stages.

Increased ACTH and cortisol levels could result from the classic shift response in severe illness. In these cases, serotoninergic and other stimulatory neuropeptides cooperate in stimulating the production of corticotropin-releasing hormone (CRH). When the body is under stress, such as in severe illness, vasopressin synergizes with CRH to increase ACTH production.

ADRENAL ANDROGENS

Adrenal androgen production in HIV patients is lower than in seronegative subjects. The excretion of adrenal androgen metabolites also decreases even upon ACTH stimulation. In addition, the levels of dehydroepiandrosterone (DHEA) and its sulfate (DHEAS) in HIV-infected patients are below normal and decline in relation to decreasing CD4 cell counts. Consequently, a fall in DHEA levels predicts progression to AIDS.

MINERALOCORTICOIDS

Hyponatremia and hyperkalemia are common findings in AIDS patients, while the condition of aldosterone deficiency associated with elevated plasma renin is rare. The majority of patients studied have normal plasma aldosterone and a normal increase of this steroid in response to angiotensin infusion and postural stimulation. Other studies on AIDS patients have shown cases of impaired aldosterone response to ACTH stimulation. Hyporeninemic hypoaldosteronism can be caused by sulfamides used in the treatment of AIDS complications. A certain number of patients treated with trimethroprin-sulfamethoxazole, which impairs potassium secretion by inhibiting sodium channels in the distal nephron, may develop hyperkalemia. Finally, hyponatremia appears to be caused by drug toxicity or inappropriate vasopressin secretion rather than hypoaldosteronism.

DISTURBANCES IN HORMONE SYNTHESIS

In HIV-infected patients, a significant reduction in the 17-deoxy pathway steroids and a normal or increased production in the 17-hydroxy pathway steroids has been described. The shift from androgens to glucocorticoids is supported by the decrease in DHEA level and the increase in cortisol level frequently found in this disease.

GLUCOCORTICOID RECEPTOR AND CORTISOL RESISTANCE

At the cellular level, most known effects of glucocorticoids are mediated by an ~94 kD intracellular protein, the glucocorticoid receptor. Glucocorticoid receptors exhibit a complex structure. The N-terminal domain contains sequences responsible for activating target genes. The C-terminal (or ligand-binding domain) specifically binds the hormone. It contains heat-shock protein binding, and sequences for nuclear translocation, dimerization and transactivation, as well as sequences for silencing the receptor in the absence of the hormone.

In recent years, an acquired form of glucocorticoid resistance has been described in patients infected with HIV. The first case of resistance was observed as early as 1990, and later a number of HIV-infected patients were diagnosed to be resistant. Characteristics of cortisol-resistant patients are reported in Table 74.1.

A $[^3H]$-dexamethasone binding analysis of lymphomonocyte receptors was performed in cortisol-resistant AIDS patients. The results reveal the presence of a single class of binding sites with very low receptor affinity for glucocorticoids (K_d) and an increased number of receptors (Bmax) (Tab. 74.2). Recent data show that a low receptor affinity for glucocorticoids is also present in the early stages of infection. Thus, receptor alteration in HIV disease appears to be much more frequent than initially believed.

The HIV virus, the HIV-1 vpr gene, and the simultaneous effects of IL-2 and IL-4 cytokines combined seem to be the cause of the receptor defect.

GLUCOCORTICOIDS AND IMMUNE FUNCTION

The HPA axis and the immune system maintain a critical balance in the physiological state. An excessive HPA axis response produces a hypercortisolemic state and can lead to increased susceptibility to infections and neoplasia. A defective HPA axis response can lead to a glucocorticoid-deficient state and to increased susceptibility to autoimmune-inflammatory diseases.

Glucocorticoids and T helper cell function

Glucocorticoids are known to modulate T helper cell function. T helper cells are divided into T helper cells types 1 and 2 (Th1 and Th2) subclasses based on their function and cytokine production pattern (Fig. 74.1). In general, Th1-related cytokines promote Th1 activity (i.e., cell-mediated immunity) and inhibit Th2 activity (i.e., humoral immunity), and Th2-related cytokines do the opposite. Cell-mediated immunity is primarily stimulated by the type-1 cytokines IL-2 and interferon gamma, which promote the proliferation of Th1 cells. Humoral immunity is mainly promoted by the type-2 cytokine IL-4, the major growth factor of Th2 cells. Glucocorticoids inhibit the production of pro-inflammatory type-1 cytokines IL-2 and IFN-γ, and they favor the type-2 cytokine IL-4, thus they activate Th2 cells and suppress Th1 cells.

Recent studies demonstrate that HIV infection is associated with a progressive reduction in the type-1 cytokines IL-2 and IL-12, and associated with an increased production of type-2 cytokines IL-4, IL-6, and IL-10. Experiments performed on hypercortisolemic

---

Table 74.1 The syndrome of cortisol resistance in AIDS

Clinical presentation	Laboratory findings
Weakness	Increased plasma cortisol
Weight loss	Normal cortisol-binding globulin concentration
Hypotension	Increased urinary free cortisol
Chronic fatigue	Resistance to dexamethasone
Skin pigmentation	Maintenance of normal circadian pattern, but at higher levels, of ACTH and cortisol
	Increased interferon-α production

Table 74.2 Glucocorticoid receptor characteristics in AIDS

Increased concentration of glucocorticoid receptors on mononuclear leukocytes

Low receptor affinity for glucocorticoids

Defective glucocorticoid induced inhibition of $[^3H]$ thymidine incorporation into mononuclear leukocytes

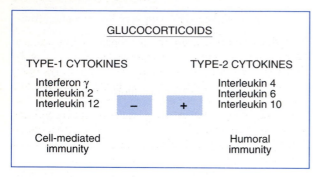

Figure 74.1 Proposed model of the possible interactions between glucocorticoids and type-2 cytokines.

AIDS patients with normal or low receptor affinity to glucocorticoids confirm these findings. They suggest that hypercortisolemia suppresses type-1 cytokine production and stimulates type-2 cytokine production, and that cortisol resistance reverses the immune response with a shift toward type-1 cytokine pattern.

These data suggest that cortisol has an important role in regulating T helper function in HIV-infected patients.

Glucocorticoids and IFN-α

Altered interferon alpha production is a characteristic feature of patients with HIV infection. Two principal types of cells produce IFN-α: dendritic cells and monocytes. In HIV-infected patients, there is a selective defect of IFN-α production by dendritic cells. Monocytes, however, are important hosts for HIV type-1, and retain their IFN-α-production capacity, which is about one-tenth of the total IFN-α production. A study in cortisol-resistant HIV patients shows that there is a marked increase in plasma IFN-α. In these subjects, one possible explanation of such an increase is that glucocorticoids fail to inhibit the virus-induced IFN-α release. The correlation found between the Kd of monocyte-glucocorticoid receptors and the level of circulating IFN-α suggests that the phenomenon is a direct consequence of the monocyte resistance to glucocorticoids. In the same study, glucocorticoids failed to inhibit IFN-α production in isolated monocytes from cortisol-resistant AIDS patients. These findings indicate that glucocorticoids and their receptors specifically regulate IFN-α production in AIDS patients. This may be important in HIV-infected patients, as IFN-α favors the induction and maintenance of Th1-like cells, thereby counteracting the suppressive effect of cortisol on the immune system.

GLUCOCORTICOIDS AND ANTIGLUCOCORTICOIDS

Clinical or subclinical alterations in the levels of cortisol and DHEA may produce an imbalance in type-1 and type-2 cytokine production that would then be self-perpetuating.

The androgen precursor DHEA is a hormone with a direct antiglucocorticoid effect, capable of balancing the glucocorticoid-induced immune suppression. The reduced levels of DHEA in HIV infection may favor the suppressive effect of cortisol on type-1 cytokine production. DHEA has already been shown to inhibit HIV replication and HIV-1 latency reactivation in vitro and also to reduce the viral load in patients not treated with anti-retroviral drugs. This underlines the importance of physiological cortisol antagonists such as DHEA and its derivatives, androstenediol, and androstenetriol, in the treatment of HIV disease.

In summary, the immune system of HIV patients can be induced to manifest a Th1 or Th2 response by manipulating cortisol. Thus, counteracting the immune-suppressive effect of cortisol with specific drugs could be beneficial in treating HIV infection.

TESTICULAR FUNCTION

Gonadal function might be impaired by a direct effect of HIV or HIV-related neoplasms, opportunistic infections, side effects of therapeutic agents, or effects of HIV-induced cytokines and antibodies on the pituitary-gonadal axis.

Sixty-seven percent of men with AIDS experience decreased libido. Absent or diminished spermatogenesis is common among AIDS patients, while hyalinization of the seminiferous tubules, diminished Leydig cell number, and interstitial mononuclear inflammation are infrequent findings.

Involvement of the testes with *Mycobacterium avium*, *Toxoplasma*, cytomegalovirus and disseminated tuberculosis has been found in up to 30% of patients. About 30 to 50% of men have subnormal serum free testosterone concentrations; half of these patients have inappropriately normal levels of gonadotropins, the other half have elevated follicle-stimulating hormone and luteinizing hormone values, suggesting primary hypogonadism. Sex hormone-binding globulin (SHBG) levels are elevated in about 40% of the men who have a normal total-testosterone level but low free testosterone. Recent data indicate that lean body mass and muscle mass correlate with androgen levels in hypogonadal patients. Patients with severe systemic illnesses have been shown to develop hypogonadotropic hypogonadism. This effect may be cytokine-mediated. IL-1 and tumor-necrosis factor may result in the reduced production of testosterone. Thus, cytokines and infections could lead to hypogonadism.

OVARIAN FUNCTION

There are few studies on the gonadal function of women with HIV infection. In the majority of cases, HIV infection does not induce menstrual irregularities or changes in hormone levels in either asymptomatic or symptomatic women. In one study, 26% of women had amenorrhea. Abnormalities in the female sex hormone axis seem to be related to immunodeficiency complications. The effects of drugs used to treat AIDS and related opportunistic infections on ovarian function have not been adequately studied.

THYROID FUNCTION

Thyroid dysfunction is uncommon in HIV patients. When it does occur, the thyroid gland or, less frequently, the hypothalamic-pituitary axis, is directly involved in opportunistic infections and neoplastic processes. Thyroid dysfunction may result from cytomegalovirus, *Cryptococcus neoformans*, *Mycobacterium avium*, or *P. carinii*. Thyroid involvement in fungal infection with *C. neoformans* and *Aspergillus fumigatus* has been described without significant alterations in the thyroid function. Kaposi's sarcoma, involving destruction of the thyroid and hypothyroidism, is rare. Recently, several cases of thyroiditis due to *P. carinii*, identified by needle biopsy, have been reported in association with thyrotoxicosis or hypothyroidism. Laboratory findings have confirmed the presence of subacute granulomatous thyroiditis. Subclinical primary hypothyroidism has also been reported, with minimally-elevated basal thyroid-stimulating hormone (TSH) levels and an exaggerated response to thyrotropin-releasing hormone (TRH). Also frequently found in HIV infection are elevated levels of antithyroid antibodies, particularly antibodies against peroxidase. Some medications, such as ketoconazole, rifampicin, and interferon, may be associated with an increased prevalence of autoimmune hypothyroidism. One of the most characteristic findings in HIV patients is an elevation of thyroxine-binding globulin, which is associated with the progression of the HIV infection and has been shown to correlate with the CD4 lymphocyte count. Thyroxine-binding globulin elevation is present in asymptomatic HIV-positive patients, both in adults and children, and increases with the progression of the disease. The cause of such alteration is still unknown. Owing to thyroxine-binding globulin elevation, total thyroxine may increase while free thyroxine remains normal or low.

As in other severe illnesses, AIDS patients, particularly those hospitalized, have depressed serum T_3 concentrations. A significant increase of reverse T_3 (rT_3) has also been identified in HIV-positive patients at all stages of the disease. Thyroid homeostasis can be influenced by cytokines produced in response to HIV infection. There are several reports of increased IL-6 in HIV infection, which might be responsible for decreased TSH and T_3 and increased rT_3 serum concentrations. These hormonal changes could also be caused by tumor-necrosis factor.

VASOPRESSIN

Hyponatremia is common in patients with the acquired immunodeficiency syndrome. About 40 to 60% of these patients have a serum sodium level below 130 nmol/l, which is the most important electrolyte imbalance found in hospitalized patients. Hyponatremia is due to an excess of water versus sodium ions in serum. Since spontaneous sodium loss without water loss is unlikely, hyponatremia may be linked to an inappropriate secretion of vasopressin and/or a reduction of glucocorticoid-induced renal water release. Thus, hyponatremia is a clear indication of excessive water retention in plasma. Hyponatremic patients can

be divided into two main groups: those with measurable vasopressin, and those with suppressed vasopressin. In the first case vasopressin is stimulated by pathways other than plasma osmolality, such as by low pressure and low volume, or by other stimuli such as endotoxin, nausea, vomiting, or opiates. In AIDS patients, severe volume depletion is common due to diarrhea and gastrointestinal fluid loss. Epidemiological studies show that most hyponatremic HIV patients are volume-depleted.

A certain number of AIDS patients develops the syndrome of inappropriate antidiuretic hormone (SIADH) due to the *P. carinii* infection. Pyrogenes and endotoxins may also stimulate vasopressin secretion in infected individuals, causing SIADH.

Hyponatremia with suppressed vasopressin is usually due to adrenal failure, reduced water excretion mediated by glucocorticoids, and consequent volume expansion. These forms of hyponatremia are rare in patients with AIDS as they rarely become Addisonian and are usually hypovolemic and/or hypotensive, which are situations that stimulate vasopressin release. HIV patients treated with high doses of Trimethoprim, an amiloride-like diuretic, develop low vasopressin hyponatremia (16% of hospitalized subjects) (Fig. 74.2).

α-MELANOCYTE-STIMULATING HORMONE

Experimental and clinical data indicate that α-melanocyte-stimulating hormone is a significant modulator of host reactions, including fever and inflammation. Patients infected with the HIV virus have greater plasma concentrations of α-melanocyte-stimulating hormone than seronegative patients. The α-melanocyte-stimulating hormone has been shown to prevent immune suppression induced by the gp 120 protein of the HIV-virus envelope

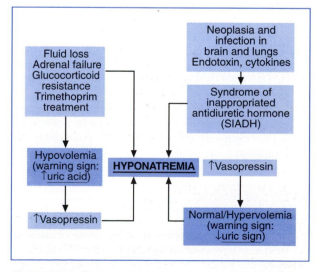

Figure 74.2 Pathogenesis of hyponatremia in HIV infection.

and to block production of the proinflammatory cytokine IL-1 in the brain.

α-Melanocyte-stimulating hormone, working together with ACTH and interferon alpha, is an important melanogenetic factor likely to be responsible for the intense skin pigmentation found in cortisol-resistant AIDS patients.

GLUCOSE METABOLISM

Symptomatic HIV-infected patients have higher rates of insulin clearance, increased peripheral sensitivity to insulin, and increased non-insulin-mediated glucose uptake when compared to normal subjects. Hepatic glucose production rates tend to increase, perhaps to maintain plasma glucose within the normal range, in spite of the increased disposal. Pentamidine, used in the prevention and treatment of *P. carinii*, can cause beta cell toxicity and reduce insulin and C-peptide production, which can lead to hyperglycemia and diabetes mellitus. In a subset of patients treated with pentamidine, insulin remains elevated, and they become hypoglycemic. Megestrol acetate, used to treat anorexia and cachexia in AIDS, may cause diabetes mellitus.

LIPID METABOLISM

Triglyceride levels may be elevated in asymptomatic HIV-infected patients, probably due to increased levels of very low density lipoproteins (VLDL). Lipoprotein lipase, the enzyme responsible for triglyceride clearance, is 27% lower in HIV patients. By contrast, de novo hepatic synthesis of fatty acids and plasma free fatty acid is higher.

In HIV patients elevated plasma triglyceride levels, increased fasting hepatic synthesis of fatty acids, and decreased triglyceride clearance correlate with circulating levels of interferon alpha. Although the exact role of interferon alpha in triglyceride metabolism is not known, antiretroviral therapy reduces both interferon alpha and triglyceride levels in patients with AIDS.

PROTEIN METABOLISM

Patients with weight loss and AIDS are usually reported to have an increased metabolic rate and a loss of lean tissue. This cachectic response carries a poor prognosis. The pathogenesis of the wasting syndrome in AIDS

remains unknown. Recent findings suggest that the production of anabolic factors such as androgens may be abnormally low in men with AIDS.

Opportunistic infections are the most important causes of weight loss in AIDS. Subjects with protozoal diarrhea have a decreased resting energy expenditure and decreased body fat. Patients with *P. carinii* pneumonia and those with *M. avium* have an elevated resting energy expenditure and decreased skeletal muscle mass. Patients with cytomegalovirus enteritis have a non-significantly elevated resting energy expenditure with non-significant loss of both fat and lean body tissue. These studies emphasize that hypermetabolism *per se* does not have a key role in weight loss. The failure to compensate for decreased caloric intake by adequately lowering resting energy expenditure leads to a negative energy balance. Therapies aimed to contrast anorexia and protein wasting are under investigation. Megestrol acetate induces increased appetite and weight gain, however it fails to increase lean body mass, probably because it decreases plasma testosterone levels. Insulin-like growth factor 1 (IGF-1) induces only transient increases in nitrogen balance. Growth hormone (GH) injected in a large series of patients with wasting syndrome induced a sustained increase in lean body mass, an increase in muscle power, a decrease in fat, and gave them an improved quality of life.

Hypercortisolemia, which is a frequent finding in AIDS patients, may assist in increasing protein wasting. Attempts are being made to counteract glucocorticoid-induced catabolism with glucocorticoid antagonists, such as DHEA and its metabolites.

Additional studies are needed to determine the efficacy of gonadal steroid replacement to increase lean body mass in this population.

CALCIUM METABOLISM

Hypocalcemia and hypercalcemia have both been reported in association with HIV infection. Parathormone levels usually decrease both at baseline and during EDTA-induced hypocalcemia. Magnesium is usually normal in these patients.

Hypercalcemia associated with AIDS-related lymphoma has been reported. These patients had elevated 1,25-dihydroxyvitamin D levels. The same findings were present in patients infected with *M. avium* and *P. carinii*. Hypocalcemia has also occurred during therapy with foscarnet, a pyrophosphate analogue used in the treatment of cytomegalovirus retinitis and following the administration of pentamidine. Ketoconazole reduces serum levels of 1,25-dihydroxyvitamin D and lowers total calcium levels.

Suggested readings

BAMBERGER CM, SCHULTE HM, CHROUSOS GP. Molecular determinants of glucocorticoid receptor function and tissue sensitivity to glucocorticoids. Endocrine Reviews 1996;17:245-61.

BEVILACQUA M. Hyponatraemia in AIDS. In: Norbiato G (ed). The endocrinology and metabolism of HIV infection. London: Baillière,1994;837-48.

CATANIA A, LIPTON JM. α-Melanocyte-stimulating hormone in the modulation of host reactions. Endocrine Rev 1993; 14:564-74.

CLERICI M, SHEARER GM. A Th1→Th2 switch is a critical step in the etiology of HIV infection. Immunol Today 1993; 14:107-11.

GRINSPOON SK, DONOVAN JR DS, BILEZIKIAN JP. Aetiology and pathogenesis of hormonal and metabolic disorders in HIV

infection. In: Norbiato G (ed). The endocrinology and metabolism of HIV infection. London: Baillière,1994; 735-55.

GRINSPOON S, CORCORAN C, LEE K, et al. Loss of lean body and
muscle mass correlates with androgen levels in hypogonadal
men. with acquired immunodeficiency syndrome and wasting.
J Clin Endocrinol Metab 1996;81:4051-58.

KAWA SK, THOMPSON EB. Lymphoid cell resistance to glucocorticoids in HIV infection. J Steroid Biochem Molec Biol.
1996;57:259-63.

LAMBERT M. Thyroid dysfunction in HIV infection. In: Norbiato
G (ed). The endocrinology and metabolism of HIV infection.
London: Baillière, 1994;825-35.

LORTHOLARY O, CHRISTEFF N, CASASSUS P, et al. Hypothalamo-
pituitary-adrenal function in human immunodeficiency
virus-infected men. J Clin Endocrinol Metab 1996;81:791-
96.

MAGGI M, FORTI G. Gonadal function in AIDS. In: Norbiato G,
ed. The endocrinology and metabolism of HIV infection.
London: Baillière, 1994;849-57.

NORBIATO G, BEVILACQUA M, VAGO T, et al. Cortisol resistance

in acquired immunodeficiency syndrome. J Clin Endocrinol
Metab 1992;74:608-13.

NORBIATO G, BEVILACQUA M, VAGO T, et al. Glucocorticoids and
immune function in the human immunodeficiency virus
infection: a study in hypercortisolemic and cortisol-resistant
patients. J Clin Endocrinol Metab 1997;82:3260-3.

PADGETT DA, LORIA RM. In vitro potentiation of lymphocyte
activation by dehydroepiandrosterone, androstenediol, and
androstenetriol. J Immunol 1994;153:544-52.

SELLMEYER DE, GRUNFELD C. Endocrine and metabolic disturbances in human immunodeficiency virus infection and the
acquired immune deficiency syndrome. J Clin Endocrinol
Metab 1996;17:518-32.

YANG JY, SCHWARTZ A, HENDERSON EE. Inhibition of 3'azido-
3'deoxythymidine-resistant HIV-1 infection by dehydroepiandrosterone in vitro. Biochem-Biophis-Res Commun
1994;201:1424-32.

Appendixes

Clinical trials

Silvano G. Cella, Eugenio E. Müller

In endocrinology, as in any other medical branch at the present time, the acceptance of new therapeutic modalities is conditioned upon a systematic approach to obtain convincing evidence. Such evidence should arise from adequately controlled clinical trials in which the efficacy and safety of a new treatment is tested against proven treatments or no treatment (placebo). All endocrinologists should therefore be able either to participate in therapeutic trials or to interpret their results.

To enter into the clinical phase of a drug trial, a new drug must have a long history behind it. Drug development is a complex, risky, expensive, and time-consuming process. From the discovery of a new drug to its marketing, it often takes more than ten years. The efficiency of the process is low. In fact, research on new chemical entities is abandoned without marketing approval in a substantial majority of cases. The costs of developing new drugs are critically dependent on the proportion of compounds that fail in pre-clinical or clinical testing, which, over time, seems to be rapidly rising. These overall costs are now calculated to be approximately 300 million US dollars.

The story of a putative new drug begins with its discovery. The goal is to identify new chemical entities endowed with high chances of providing therapeutic benefits. Once such a compound is identified, a series of investigations in animals and humans take place to demonstrate that it is effective and safe enough for use in people. The crucial problem is deciding whether or not to spend millions of dollars in the development of a new chemical entity in the hope that it will become a new drug. There are no easy or absolute answers to this question. The solution to this problem may arise only from the coordinate efforts of basic scientists, toxicologists, pharmaceutical chemists, clinical pharmacologists, clinicians, and government regulators.

This chapter will briefly provide the general rules that apply to the study of any new treatments or to the re-evaluation of "proven" treatments that, although their efficacy may have been demonstrated, may nevertheless require further studies concerning their long-term benefits versus their hazards. Peculiar features of some clinical trials in endocrinology will also be discussed.

PRE-CLINICAL DEVELOPMENT OF A NEW DRUG

The clinical study of a new drug begins only after adequate animal studies have been completed during the so-called pre-clinical phase. It involves multiple steps, of which detailed description is beyond the scope of this chapter.

During this phase, the new compound is tested in vivo and in vitro in different animal species in order to determine its pharmacokinetic and pharmacodynamic properties. The first goal is to screen a large number of compounds to identify those endowed with the highest activity and potency towards a particular target. The target could be a specific biochemical reaction, a receptor, or a more macroscopic effect, such as inhibition of a hormonal secretion. This field has become greatly aided by the application of molecular biologic techniques combined with a molecular computer graphic examination of cell surface pharmacological receptors and enzymes (target drug design).

Toxicology

Many factors may contribute to terminating further development of a new compound. Among them is a lack of efficacy or problems with developing an acceptable way to administer the drug to patients. The discovery of severe, undesired effects from the compound plays a prominent role in this context, since the drug would not be acceptable to patients. For this reason, during the pre-clinical phase, the toxicologic studies are of fundamental importance.

The duration of toxicologic studies varies. Usually single, very high-dose studies are done first. Later, studies of progressively longer duration are performed. Acute toxicologic studies are performed in which exponentially increasing single doses of the drug are administered to at least two animal species, one of which would be a non-rodent. In almost all cases the IV route of administration is used in order to ensure that the drug enters into the systemic circulation.

A minor aim of acute toxicologic studies is seeking possible antidotes to drug-induced mortality. The longest studies usually involve 2 years of daily dosing in order to detect carcinogenic effects in rodents. Exceptions to this are human recombinant peptide hormones, because non-human species may develop antibodies against them, making long-term delivery unfeasible. Generally, the periods of drug delivery to animals for prolonged toxicologic studies are shorter than those that will be used in humans for chronic therapies. However, considering that the duration of life in rodents is considerably shorter than in man, it can be assumed that the presentation of drug-induced reactions is also faster. Depending on what the eventual route of administration in humans is likely to be, other routes can also be tested in addition to the parenteral one.

Another aim of toxicologic studies is to determine the mutagenic and teratogenic potential of the drug. Teratogenic effects are usually studied in the rabbit (thought to be the most sensitive animal species to exhibit these effects); whereas mutagenesis is evaluated in vitro in microorganisms, mammalian cells, or in host-mediated systems. Toxicologic studies will not detect allergic or idiosyncratic reactions that might occur in humans, nor will they predict symptomatic or subjective experiences that might be produced in people.

Pharmacodynamics

The screening of biological effects is performed in progressively complex systems. The choice of an initial target system depends on the understanding of the pathogenesis of a particular disease for which treatment is sought. Approximations of human diseases (the so-called models of the diseases) can be induced in animals to test the ability of the investigational drug to cure a given pathological phenomenon. However, such models are imprecise reflections of human diseases and, therefore, are variably reliable in predicting the efficacy of drugs in humans even when the efficacy is seen in the model. On the contrary, the failure of a drug to affect the model does not necessarily preclude its value in humans.

The discovery of disease-specific drugs is heavily dependent on the understanding of basic molecular mechanisms of that disease. In some cases, instead of screening many compounds in one disease model, a specific molecule known to participate in certain biological processes is screened for use in a variety of diseases. In these instances, testing a new compound might lead to new discoveries in the pathogenesis and therapy of those diseases. The recent application of molecular biologic techniques to isolate and synthesize a wide variety of endogenous, biologically-active molecules has increased the interaction between the discovery of drugs and the discovery of molecular pathogenic mechanisms.

In addition to establishing that a new chemical entity has a desired pharmacologic effect in animals, its other pharmacologic effects must be determined. Knowing the full pharmacologic profile of a new drug allows us to anticipate its activity in man.

Another major purpose of pharmacologic testing is to define the dose-response relationship of the drug. The lowest dose that causes a definite pharmacologic effect must be determined. This is established in several animal species to identify the safe dose that can be used to initiate testing in humans. The shape (steepness) of the dose-response curve is also useful in the design of the first studies in humans. If the dose-response curve is steep, the drug may be difficult to give to humans without producing extreme effects. If the curve is shallow, the dose can be progressively increased to carefully establish the tolerated dose range.

Metabolism and pharmacokinetics

Knowing the metabolic profile of a drug in several species is a key element for understanding many quantitative aspects of that drug, such as the quantity of doses, the length of its action, and the interval required between administrations. It is also important to discover the drug's metabolites in humans. Once identified, major metabolites should be tested for their pharmacologic and/or toxicologic activity and then should be followed during testing in humans. Moreover, metabolic studies allow for the detection of potential pharmacometabolic interactions, since the metabolism of an index drug could be inhibited or induced by another drug, or even by itself.

The distribution of the drug throughout the body is determined in animals using a ^{3}H- or ^{14}C-radiolabeled drug. This information can alert investigators to look for effects that relate to organs where large concentrations of the drug may also reside in humans. Administration of the radiolabeled compound is also useful to identify its major elimination pathway(s).

Another aim of the pharmacokinetic studies is to calculate several relevant parameters useful to the clinical pharmacologist. Among them is its bioavailability, defined as the ratio between oral (or parenteral) and intravenous "areas under the time-concentration curves" (AUCs). A ratio equal to 1 indicates total bioavailability; ratios less than 1 indicate an incomplete absorption, attributable to the molecule or its formulation.

The data obtained from animal studies offer a reliable picture of the possible consequences derived from the clinical use of the compound. However, until the drug is administered to humans, it is very difficult to know which animal species will most mimic the full pharmacodynamic, pharmacokinetic, and toxicologic profile that will be seen in man.

An example is represented by studies with dehydroepiandrosterone (DHEA) and its sulfate derivative, DHEAS. These are two steroids produced in large amounts by the adrenals and are endowed with a scarce androgenic activity, but they are capable of being converted to testosterone and estradiol. The finding that a dramatic decline in the biosynthesis of DHEA and DHEAS occurs in humans during aging, though in only about 70% of subjects, has led to the idea that their decline may be (in concert with other hormones) among the pacemakers of aging. Studies in rodents in which the production of DHEA and DHEAS is very scarce or absent have shown beneficial effects on experimental models of obesity, diabetes, and neoplastic and cardiovascular diseases.

However, experiments in humans with pharmacological doses of these compounds have failed to show a real beneficial effect on some of the above parameters.

CLINICAL DEVELOPMENT OF A NEW DRUG

In the United States and Europe, no drug can be sold to the general population before approval by its government. A drug is approved for general use if adequately-controlled clinical trials show that it is safe and effective. After information has been collected in animals, a sponsor (usually a pharmaceutical company) willing to investigate a drug in humans must submit an application to the regulatory authorities seeking approval to start clinical trials in humans. The regulations in force dictate that – in addition to convincing evidence that the drug has a reasonable chance to be effective and safe – applications must contain a number of data. Among these are: the name of the drug; a description of the physical-chemical characteristics of its active principle; a full description of the intended studies, posologies, and typology; total number of the patients; ethical aspects (e.g., informed consent); inclusion/exclusion criteria; general criteria for the evaluation of the efficacy and tolerability; a list of the clinical centers involved in the studies; and the name of the firm responsible for the clinical study.

The drug must be formulated as a final product. Formulation is the process of mixing the active drug with a vehicle, allowing practical storage and administration. Thus, the drug must be mixed either in solution or in a matrix of solid, pharmacologically inert materials (excipient) that can be formed into a capsule or tablet. Solid forms must dissolve adequately in the gastrointestinal tract. In addition, the drug must be chemically stable to ensure that it will not rapidly degrade during storage. The length of time in which a substantial percentage of the drug will deteriorate (expiration time) must be well-described.

Once the request is approved to begin clinical trials in humans, the clinical pharmacologists set up the subsequent studies in man. If during clinical studies a potential beneficial but unexpected effect is observed, further animal testing may be required before additional studies proceed in humans. Throughout the world, clinical testing classically proceeds in at least three phases.

Phase 1

The methodology of phase 1 studies constitutes a highly-specialized branch of clinical pharmacology. During this phase, the clinical pharmacologist administers the drug to humans for the very first time. The major aims are: (1) to identify, at least approximately, the dose to be used, and (2) to detect potentially harmful adverse effects and the doses at which they occur. Since the effects of a given drug are never exactly alike in all individuals and all circumstances, it is necessary to think in terms of groups of subjects rather than in terms of individuals.

The initial dose is chosen based on the studies in animals, and it must be very small (e.g., one-hundredth of the dose per kilogram body weight that produced the first detectable effect in the most sensitive animal species tested). Subsequently, doses should be increased very slowly, using a geometric progression with a multiplication factor of 2-4. Single doses should always be tested before repeated doses. It is important to determine the dose that produces the first detectable effect, irrespective of the fact that such an effect is therapeutic or adverse.

Generally, young, healthy volunteers are recruited for this initial phase, since any potentially dangerous reaction to the drug is obviously more readily manageable in subjects in good health. Males are usually preferred, since in females the cyclic hormonal fluctuations may interfere with drug actions, and for safety reasons pregnancies need to be prevented.

Phase 1 also includes metabolic and pharmacokinetic studies, although these studies may be pursued during subsequent phases. Knowledge of the major pathways for eliminations of the drug, whether hepatic or renal, will be useful to predict necessary adjustments of dose that may be required in a particular subset of patients at risk (i.e., with hepatic or renal diseases).

Phase 2

During phase 2 of clinical investigations, the potential therapeutic usefulness of the drug is evaluated in rigorously conducted trials. Studies are performed for limited periods in a small number of selected patients. Several important conditions must be taken into account in the design of such trials. First of all, a reproducible definition of the disease is mandatory for the selection of the patients, which must be as homogeneous as possible. Moreover, the end-points to be measured to determine efficacy must be clearly defined.

Phase 3

Most of the drugs that enter phases 1 and 2 do not reach phase 3 clinical trials, either because a toxic effect appears that was not anticipated before, or because the expected beneficial effect did not emerge during the previous phases. In phase 3, administration of the drug is extended to a larger and more varied population of patients. The duration of the treatment is increased and may last up to 6 or 12 months. The efficacy of the study drug is assessed by comparing its effect with those of standard proven treatments.

Phase 4

Phase 4 begins after the new drug has been commercially available. One of the major goals is to detect, and possibly prevent, rare and serious adverse effects that have not been recognized in the previous clinical trials because of the smaller number of patients studied and the shorter duration of treatment. During phase 4 additional studies may be performed to investigate some other pharmacological effects of the drug in order to increase knowledge.

Post-marketing surveillance

The clinical evaluation of a drug prior to its release is limited for several reasons. First, the patients treated are highly-screened. They must meet certain criteria to enter clinical trials. Concomitant therapies are often eliminated in order to decrease the chance for drug interactions. The presence of concomitant diseases is also established as a criterion for being excluded from the study. Moreover, the limited size of the patient sample tested to support the approval of a drug limits the possibility of discovering uncommon adverse events.

After approval, most drugs will be used in millions of people and in a variety of ways. Patients given the drug after its approval will not be monitored as closely as patients in a pre-marketing clinical trial. They will have more concurrent diseases, they may be taking more concomitant medications, they may be younger or older or of a different sex, and so on. For such reasons, it is possible that new serious adverse events or new beneficial effects will occur that could not be detected sooner because they occur too infrequently or because they depend on a particular set of circumstances.

Mechanisms are in place around the world to collect data on drugs once they reach the marketplace. Methods are available to capture such information by post-marketing surveillance so that therapy can be improved. Post-marketing surveillance can be performed by patients, practicing or academic physicians, pharmacists, pharmaceutical companies, health authorities, or governmental agencies. Post-marketing surveillance can report events from the field (spontaneous recording), monitor large patient databases (record linkage), or work by a combination of these approaches.

PRINCIPLES OF CLINICAL TRIALS

The planning of a clinical trial should be a team effort with the participation of a clinician, a pharmacologist, a pharmacokineticist, a statistician, a quality assurance officer, and an ethics committee.

Since endocrinology is a highly-specialized field, a sound knowledge of the nosology of the illness treated, its clinical forms, prognostic factors, evaluation techniques, and the currently available therapies is mandatory for the accurate definition of patients and the collection of reliable, assessable and relevant data. However, it is also important to know some general principles of clinical trials that are applicable regardless of the type of disorder studied and may theoretically be used by any physician.

Since there are many specialized treatises in which these arguments are exhaustively considered, it is preferable to refer interested readers to them and only state briefly some basic rules.

Aim of the study

The first principle for drawing up the protocol could be defined as "One Question per Trial." Before undertaking a trial, a single, clear and explicit question must be formulated around which the trial will be built. The aim of the trial must be defined a priori in the protocol. It must be realistic and compatible with patient recruitment and the methodology available.

At the end of the study, the following questions will need to be answered in statistical terms: (1) Is the difference observed due to external factors unrelated to the treatment? and (2) Has chance favored one of the treatments evaluated? This can only be done properly if there are not too many questions to be answered in the course of the study. A trial can only answer the question it was designed for, and the greater the number of questions asked, the greater the chance of errors (false differences). For example, it is not possible, in the same trial, to evaluate the efficacy of the treatment, to study dosage and administration schedule, and to define precautions for use in all categories of subjects (children, older individuals, nephropathics, etc.). Designing a trial for each question should be considered. However, this does not exclude the possibility of asking subsidiary questions, such as regarding drug tolerability or acceptability.

Patients

Generally clinicians that undertake a trial feel that each patient is unique and are inclined to judge any treatment based on the results obtained in each individual patient. This reasoning must be changed. On the contrary, since the effects of a given therapeutic treatment are never exactly alike in all individuals and all circumstances, during a trial the efficacy of a treatment must be judged statistically, analyzing outcomes in terms of groups of patients rather than individuals. This will not eliminate the clinician's need, in many cases, for trying several treatments before finding the one that is most suitable for an individual patient, but at least he or she has a foundation on which to begin. If controlled clinical trials have been performed, they provide the physician with systematically collected data which, although specific for the population studied, nonetheless are generalizable to some degree. It is precisely because patients are individuals that a treatment must be assessed in terms of probable results, that is, by statistical reasoning derived from the study of a group. Patients differ from each other not only in their initial pre-treatment status, but also in their response to treatment. The greater the difference between individuals in a group, the more variable the anticipated difference between responses to therapy. Consequently, the more difficult it will be to draw general conclusions from the results observed in the group. It is therefore desirable to choose relatively homogeneous groups of patients in which there is as little variability as possible.

Eligibility and exclusion criteria

Since many factors can be considered as a source of variability affecting the outcome of a trial, it is important to list them so that they can be considered either for selecting the patients or for interpreting the results of the study. In other words, it is necessary to define precise and unambiguous eligibility and exclusion criteria. Eligibility criteria must include a clear definition of the disorder to be studied and its clinical forms. It must also include the patient's characteristics such as sex, age, body weight limits, occupation, extra-curricular activities, lifestyle habits (e.g., smoking, drinking, physical activity), compliance with treatments, and informed consent. The exclusion criteria include characteristics liable to jeopardize the evaluation of the results or the safety of the treatments compared; unassessable cases (e.g., scarcely reliable subjects in whom it is anticipated will be difficult to obtain compliance with treatment); contraindications to using one of the study treatments; associated disorders (such as renal insufficiency or hypertension, defined according to precise criteria); concomitant medications that are not compatible with the drug compared; pregnancy or possible pregnancy; and non-consenting subjects.

Sex

Among the sources of variability, sex represents an important factor. It is important not only for drug action, but also for adverse drug reactions independent of age and length of treatment. For example, women tend to have adverse events involving the gastrointestinal tract. On the other hand, men experience more blood dyscrasias. Women also develop more cutaneous allergic reactions, while their male counterparts are more likely to suffer complications of electrolyte disturbances. In certain instances, age and multiple drug use may interact with the factor of sex. There are several factors that might explain why sex would interfere with drug action, including: sex differences in pharmacokinetics and pharmacodynamics, differences in circulating hormone levels and use of medications that could inhibit drug metabolism in the liver (i.e., exogenous hormones), disproportionate rates of medication use in women, and, finally, a difference in reporting rates. Overall, women will achieve higher drug concentrations than men. Often body weight is not taken into account when determining the dose of a drug. Thus, at the most simplistic level, women generally receive a larger dose of a drug on a milligram per kilogram basis because they have a smaller body mass.

The amount of drug absorption will affect plasma concentrations. Absorption of a drug from the gastrointestinal tract depends on its acid/base and lipophilic properties as well as the physiology of the gastrointestinal tract. Differences between men and women in gastric acid secretion and gastric emptying exist, and they probably affect absorption. Although study results are conflicting, it appears that women secrete less gastric acid and have slower gastric emptying than men. The latter appears to be influenced by the levels of sex hormones. Thus, exogenous hormone use has been shown to influence the speed of gastric emptying.

The distribution of a drug is affected by its physicochemical properties, vascular and tissue volume of the distribution area, and the ratio of lean body mass to adipose tissue mass. Women tend to have lower ratios of lean body mass to adipose tissue mass.

The target organ for drug action is also important. It has been suggested that cerebral blood flow is higher in women, which would favor distribution of a compound to that organ. Such a mechanism might not only influence the efficacy of a compound but also affect the propensity for a medication to cause an adverse drug reaction.

Drugs are metabolized primarily in the liver, undergoing oxidation, reduction, hydrolysis, glucuronidation, or sulphonation. While genetic differences in enzyme activities probably have the greatest influence on drug metabolism, sex-related factors have been found to influence metabolism of several compounds, such as alcohol and propranolol.

Levels of hormones such as estrogen, progesterone, and testosterone may have varying effects on the efficacy of the drugs and on their potential for adverse drug reactions. These hormones may lead to differences in enzyme activity throughout the menstrual cycle. For instance, the activity of alcohol dehydrogenase changes across the menstrual cycle, with putatively less activity and higher resulting alcohol concentrations during the luteal phase of the cycle. This, coupled to the purported neuroactivity of progesterone metabolites via gamma-aminobutyric acid (GABA) type A receptors, may lead to inappropriate sedative effects. The activity of monoamine oxidase and hepatic microsomal oxidase may fluctuate with changing levels of progesterone and estrogen. In addition, exogenous hormone use (e.g., oral contraceptives) may influence drug metabolism, which is important to consider in designing a clinical trial.

Age

Among other characteristics of the patients in clinical trials, age represents an important factor. Thus, the appropriate age limits (upper and lower) must be clearly specified for each study. If the study is performed in aged subjects, it is important to remember that the pharmacokinetics, and in particular drug distribution, may be altered in older people. Because the lean body mass decreases and body fat increases in the elderly, in general the volume of distribution for water-soluble drugs decreases, and those for lipid-soluble drugs increases. These changes in volume of distribution can lead to higher or lower plasma concentrations when the dose is based on total body weight or surface area.

Another problem in the elderly is their compliance with treatment: between 25% and 50% of aged outpatients fail to take drugs as prescribed. It has been shown that in these instances of non-adherence, 90% of the cases were due to underuse, of which nearly 75% was intentional.

In the present day, life expectancy has increased from times past, which has lead to a larger interest in the elderly. Aging is characterized by a defective secretion of several hormones, and it has been found that elderly subjects may represent a useful model for studying the mechanisms underlying these endocrine defects. A number of studies are now underway that are aimed at clarifying the efficacy and appropriateness of hormone replacement therapies, and also to find new and more rationale therapeutic approaches to correct these age-related secretory defects.

An example is represented by the decline in growth hormone (GH) secretion, which afflicts most (approximately 70%) of older people. Twenty-four-hour GH secretion declines as a person ages, with resulting diminution in the circulating levels of insulin-like growth factor-I (IGF-I), the peptide that promotes most GH biological effects. Based on some similarities existing between the alterations in structure and function occurring with advancing age and those occurring in GH-deficient patients (such as osteopenia, muscle atrophy, and decreased exercise tolerance), it has been argued that defective GH secretion may be one of the pacemakers of aging. In addition, the term "somatopause" has been coined to indicate the age-related decline in the activity of the somatotropic axis. The possibility that GH hyposecretion may be responsible for many involutive aspects that connote aging has led to preliminary attempts to substitute the declining somatotropic function in the elderly by administering exogenous GH.

The precise mechanisms underlying the age-related reduction in circulating GH and IGF-I concentrations remains elusive: an age-dependent pituitary impairment in GH secretion does not account for the alterations as indicated by the demonstration of preserved pituitary GH content in old people. Animal studies have shown that the main cause of age-related decline in GH secretion appears to be an increasingly defective hypothalamic GH-releasing hormone (GHRH) function coupled to a relatively predominant effect of somatostatin. Noteworthy are some clinical trials in which the effects of intravenous or oral administration of relatively low doses of arginine combined with GHRH were assessed in elderly subjects either before or after 15 days of treatment with the respective combination. The results showed that the acute GH response to GHRH in the elderly was enhanced by even low intravenous doses of arginine and by the orally administered amino acid; the potentiating effect of arginine was not lowered by even 15 days of treatment. The potential usefulness of the combined treatment, also in view of curtailing the amount of neuropeptide needed, is envisaged.

Recently, the exciting possibility of stimulating GH secretion via pathways divorced from the classical, specific neuropeptides has been enlightened. Growth hormone-releasing peptides (GHRPs) are synthetic enkephalin-like peptides that specifically release GH in vitro and in vivo without concomitant, consistent release of other anterior pituitary hormones. The endogenous nature of these peptides has been suggested by the demonstration of specific binding sites in the pituitary and the hypothalamus. Growth hormone-releasing peptides release GH in a dose-dependent manner and are also effective in humans after acute oral or intranasal administration. Data in the elderly have shown that orally-administered GHRPs have a GH-releasing effect greater than that of intravenously administered GHRH.

It is too early to know whether the restoration of GH secretion in older people would be beneficial on a long-term basis or whether a reduced GH secretion connotes a physiologic adaptive event. However, where GH replacement therapy is indicated – based on the ability of the aged pituitary to respond normally to pharmacological maneuvers acting on the hypothalamus or the pituitary – stimulation of endogenous GH secretion in a physiologic, pulsatile manner would represent the most appropriate replacement.

Characteristics of the disease

Another source of variability is represented by several factors related to the characteristics of the disease under investigation. Thus, an operational definition of the disorder and its clinical forms must be given. A definition is operational when it enables unambiguous and reproducible selection based on readily identifiable symptoms in the patients. In particular, it is necessary to be precise with regard to the fate of marginal or borderline cases. In addition, this definition must exclude forms of the disorder that are too benign (the potential difference in therapeutic efficacy is small) or too serious (often resistant to all treatments). An example of the second instance is represented by the replacement of estrogen in menopausal women. Estrogen protects bone mass and offers significant protection against risk for osteoporotic fractures. The largest published experience has been with conjugated estrogens, for which it appears that 0.625 mg per day is a minimally effective dose, whereas there has been less experience with the 17β-estradiol transdermal patch. The use of estrogen for skeletal protection requires long-term therapy. Some evidence suggests that fracture risk is reduced only after 5 years of treatment. Since the rate of bone loss increases during the first few years after menopause, the optimal time period to evaluate the efficacy of the replacement therapy is as close to the cessation of ovarian function as possible. In contrast, if the degree of osteoporosis is too advanced, the efficacy of treatment is more difficult to assess.

Not only must the disorder be delimited with precision, but there is also the need for a certain degree of narrowness. In endocrinological trials, patients are often selected on the basis of a quantitative variable (e.g., measurement of circulating hormone concentrations), and the therapeutic result is subsequently evaluated by another measurement of the same variable. This requires setting numerical limits for laboratory tests and describing how the tests are done and how the results are read. It must be realized that the greater the number of measurements, the smaller the chance of retaining a patient who occasionally crosses the line that separates normal and abnormal values. In general, comparisons are made more sensitive by including only subjects for whom successive measurements are stable. This can be achieved, for example, by defining a priori the maximum tolerable deviation between two or more pretreatment measurements. Finally, patients selected for a trial must be comparable on at least two counts: an approximately similar prognosis of spontaneous evolution of the disease during the trial, and an expected similar response to the treatment.

The patients must also be recruited taking into account that the effects of a given pharmacologic treatment are often dependent upon the specific pathophysiology of the disease and the degree of distortion from physiology of the patient. For example, iodine plays an important role in the regulation of thyroid hormone synthesis and release, a phenomenon called autoregulation. Increased supply of iodide as a substrate for thyroid hormone can result in increased synthesis, especially in patients living in areas where iodine deficiency is common (endemic goiter), or in glands that have developed abnormal tissue that becomes autonomous from the usual regulatory mechanisms. Occasionally, iodide given to people with autonomous glands causes sufficiently excessive synthesis of thyroid hormone to result in hyperthyroidism (Jod-Basedow phenomenon). In contrast, patients with normal thyroid glands respond to excessive iodine by reducing the trapping, organification, coupling, and release of thyroid hormone. Trapping resumes when intrathyroidal iodine concentrations become subnormal (Wolff-Chaikoff effect). Normally the thyroid escapes from this blockade of organification, but patients with underlying autoimmune thyroid disease, who may already have a mild acquired block in organification, may fail to escape from the Wolff-Chaikoff effect. Occasionally patients with lymphocytic thyroiditis who are given iodide may become hypothyroid and develop goiters. Thus, the effects of iodine on the thyroid are highly dependent upon the underlying state of the gland. For example, iodide given to patients with persistent mild Graves' hyperthyroidism following radioiodine ablation may be sufficient to control thyroid hyperfunction by blocking organification and release of hormone. Iodide can be used in thyroid storm to block release, but only after thionamides have been given to prevent the iodine from becoming organified and utilized as substrate for de novo synthesis of thyroid hormones.

Modality of treatment

Therapeutic schema

All hormones are secreted in a pulsatile manner, which is an important factor to be considered when planning trials involving hormone administration. In fact, their effects may be different based on the frequency of their administration.

As a general rule, in order for the receptor to experience pulsatile, intermittent exposure to an agonist, the interval between two pulses of hormone administration must be substantially longer than the half-life of the agonist. Cells may respond in a physiologic manner to intermittent exposure to an agonist, but they may fail to respond to more frequent or continuous exposure to the same agent. Desensitization is most likely to occur during constant exposure to an agonist. A therapeutic advantage may arise by mimicking the natural release pattern to mimic the effect of the native substance, or by deliberately desensitizing the receptors if it becomes desirable to inhibit the effect of the native substance.

A typical case is represented by the hypothalamic gonadotropin-releasing hormone (GnRH) and its long-acting analogs. Within several years of the discovery of GnRH, numerous, very potent, long-acting GnRH analogs were synthesized by substituting a bulky, hydrophobic D-amino acid at the position 6. In order to inhibit proteolysis, the terminal amino acid was truncated with the addition of ethylamide to the proline at position 9. These synthetic peptides have a longer duration of action and a greater affinity for pituitary GnRH receptors than the native peptide. Several investigators used these analogs in an attempt to induce puberty in men with hypogonadotropic hypogonadism. They observed that while serum gonadotropin levels rose initially, the increase in hormone secretion could be maintained only for short intervals, even when the dose or the frequency of administration was increased.

This failure of GnRH analogs to induce and maintain pubertal changes led to a reexamination of the normal physiology of the control of gonadotropin secretion. It has been argued that the pulsatile secretion of luteinizing hormone reflects episodic release of GnRH from the hypothalamus, and it has been demonstrated that only pulsatile administration of GnRH results in normal gonadotrope responsiveness. Instead, when the timing of GnRH administration was altered from the known physiologic pulsatile frequency, the increased gonadotropin concentrations were not maintained. Subsequently, it has been demonstrated that continuous infusion of native GnRH ultimately inhibited the pituitary gonadotrophs.

These studies provided a rational basis for the use of the long-acting GnRH analogs. Because of their long serum half-lives and greater duration of binding to the GnRH receptors, the GnRH analogs provide a continuous, nonfluctuating level of GnRH bioactivity: a bolus injection of a long-acting agonist is pharmacodynamically similar to a constant infusion of the short-acting native hormone. Thus, in normal persons, the GnRH analogs initially stimulate gonadotropin secretion. However, by 4 weeks gonadotrope function is suppressed and gonadal function declines markedly. This pharmacologic induction of hypogonadotropic hypogonadism has been termed a "medical castration," and the GnRH analogs have become extremely useful agents for lowering sex steroid concentrations in the clinical setting.

Many hormones are subjected to a circadian rhythm of secretion. This is a factor that also must be considered, since a different timing of administration during the 24-hour cycle may condition the biological activity of the hormones. For example, glucocorticoid inhibition of the hypothalamic-pituitary-adrenal (HPA) axis is dependent upon the timing of glucocorticoid administration and, hence, of endogenous hormone secretion. A given dose of glucocorticoid inhibits the HPA axis more effectively when it is given at midnight than when it is given at 8 a.m. In treating congenital adrenal hyperplasia, therefore, part or all of the glucocorticoid should be given at night. On the contrary, when glucocorticoids are used for their anti-inflammatory or immunosuppressive effects, it is best to administer the drug in the morning to minimize suppression of the HPA axis.

Randomization

Assigning patients to treatment groups by randomization is the only way to ensure that the assigned treatment cannot be predicted at the time of patient selection, that the treatment is independent of the patient's characteristics, and that uncontrolled variability factors are distributed at random between the groups. Randomization makes it impossible to know which treatment any given patient will receive. This is important for not orienting decisions on patients' eligibility according to the treatments that they are going to receive. The randomization is the only procedure that is consistent with the probability theory. In fact, all statistical tests postulate chance distribution of unpredictable variations and of uncontrolled factors.

The randomization may be performed by several methods (such as heads or tails with a coin, or ballots drawn from a hat). However, it is more convenient to use tables of random numbers that were originally drawn up using a random procedure. In practice, computer-generated random numbers are useful for randomization of large groups of subjects.

Single-blind and double-blind trials

One of the major concerns in designing a trial is to avoid bias, that is, systematic errors that may favor one of the treatments to the detriment of the other. A bias is introduced whenever the investigators or the patients have a preconceived idea about the result. To reduce the observer bias (subjective interpretation of the results and hetero-suggestion) and patient bias (subjective interpretation of symptoms and autosuggestion), a technique called "blindness" was conceived.

Single-blind trials eliminate only one of the sources of bias. If the patient is "blind," he receives an anonymous treatment indistinguishable from the others except for its efficacy. The investigator, however, knows which treatment the patient is receiving. If the investigator is "blind," it is required that the presence of a "non-blind" prescriber instructs the patient about the treatment. The "blind" observer records the data and evaluates the treatment efficacy. This procedure is very useful in clinical trials in which the study drugs must be administered by different routes (e.g., transdermal versus oral administration of estrogens).

In the double-blind trials, neither the patient nor the physician is aware of which treatment is being administered until the end of the trial. Obviously, it is recommended that a third "non-blind" person be present to dispense drugs of identical appearance. An advisable method consists of preparing individually-numbered packages of drugs in advance using a pre-established list (not available to anyone until the results are analyzed), and to assign them in the order of patient entry into the trial.

Sometimes in endocrinological trials the results are telling from the laboratory determination of hormonal levels, and because of this the identity of a given treatment may be readily distinguishable. In this instance, it is preferable to conduct an "open" (non-blind) trial rather than a false double-blind trial in which the physician pretends to be unaware of the identity of the treatments.

Experimental design

A clinical trial may be designed in several different ways. The simplest method consists of dividing the subjects at random into as many groups as there are treatments ("parallel groups"). The advantage is based on simplicity of organization and analysis. However, in the parallel group design, the variability between randomly chosen subjects is greatest (and the efficiency of statistical comparisons is lowest). Moreover, there is also a risk of error due to the formation of non-comparable treatment groups.

"Within-patient" trials (e.g., crossover or latin square design) are those in which each subject successively receives all treatments in random order. The major advantage is that this design considers the internal variability of each subject compared to himself between different phases of the trial, rather than the variability between different subjects during the same phase. Moreover, fewer subjects are required than in parallel group design since each subject is used several times. Several conditions must apply: the subject's characteristics (e.g., prognostic factors) must be stable between different treatment periods, none of the treatments administered during the trial period should influence the results of the following phase of treatment, and the investigational drugs must not have a delayed effect that may become apparent after termination of treatment. In the latter instance, an intermediate wash-out period between the two phases of drug administration is mandatory.

Efficacy assessment

Choice of the evaluation criteria

In endocrinology, often a laboratory test (e.g., hormone assay) is used to assess the severity of a disease or the efficacy of a treatment. Generally, however, the aim of a treatment is not to simply improve some laboratory test results in patients. For example, the only reason for reducing high GH levels in acromegalic patients is because we know that this reduces mortality and morbidity. In the treatment of acromegaly, the direct criterion is the incidence of complications. Measurement of GH levels is therefore an indirect criterion in this case. If an indirect criterion (i.e., hormone concentrations) has been proven to be strongly linked to the ultimate efficacy, the former can be used as a surrogate endpoint. When a surrogate endpoint is used to assess drug efficacy, the problem of its validation must be established before it can be used in a clinical trial. The test used for diagnosis or monitoring the efficacy of therapy must also be implemented with the evaluation of signs, symptoms or other tests verifying the results' accountability.

The use of a laboratory tests for the detection of disease or the assessment of drug efficacy requires a very good knowledge of the factors that can alter the results of the specific test.

For example, unlike thyroid-stimulating hormone (TSH) measurements, thyroxine (T_4) and free-thyroxine (fT_4) measurements can be influenced by a number of disease states and drugs. Estrogens, tamoxifen, 5-fluorouracil, perphenazine, clofibrate, narcotics, acute hepatitis, and acute intermittent porphyria may increase serum thyroxine-binding globulin concentrations and cause an elevated total T_4 concentration. Hereditary thyroxine-binding globulin excess, a familial abnormal albumin or thyroxine-binding prealbumin and immunoglobulin that bind T_4, also may cause hyperthyroxinemia. Several drugs (amiodarone, ipodate, iopanoic acid, and high doses of propranolol) inhibit T_4 to $3,5,3'$-triiodothyronine (T_3) conversion and block hepatic uptake of serum T_4, resulting in hyperthyroxinemia. Other drugs and disease states reduce total concentrations of T_4 in serum. Androgens, glucocorticoids, danazol, colestipol-niacin therapy, severe illness, malnutrition, acromegaly, Cushing's syndrome, and the nephrotic syndrome may decrease thyroxine-binding globulin concentrations. Phenytoin, and to a lesser extent barbiturates, may accelerate nondeiodinative metabolism of T_4 and may also slowly displace T_4 from serum proteins, resulting in hypothyroxinemia over time. High concentrations of salicylates, fenclofenac, furosemide, and phenylbutazone in plasma also may displace T_4 from serum binding proteins.

Because of these multiple effects of drugs and nonthyroidal illness on serum T_4 concentrations, measurements of serum TSH concentrations with a sensitive assay generally provides the most accurate assessment of thyroid function in the absence of pituitary or hypothalamic diseases.

A proper choice of the hormonal variable to be measured also requires a proper understanding of the physiology and of the pathophysiological changes of the complex system in which it is involved. An example can be derived from a recent clinical trial conducted on normal elderly subjects. The results of this trial demonstrated that, in elderly people, basal GH and IGF-I levels are no longer correlated with each other, since GH had a very weak positive correlation with age, while IGF-I showed a highly negative correlation. The authors also observed that fT_3 levels decreased progressively with age and were positively correlated with plasma IGF-I levels. They speculated that, as T_3 is known to play an important role in IGF-I synthesis and release, the age-related reduction of T_3 levels might contribute to the reduced IGF-I generation. However, the reverse might also be true, that is that reduction of mean fT_3 levels in aging could be the consequence of the reduced activity of the GH/IGF-I axis. Indeed, IGF-I was shown to be capable of stimulating the peripheral deiodination and conversion of T_4 into T_3. Finally, a state of peripheral GH resistance could also be invoked to explain the observed dissociation between GH and IGF-I in aging. In fact, plasma GH-binding protein levels, a postulated index of peripheral GH binding sites, are reduced after the age of seventy, and the administration of GH elicits a lower IGF-I generation in aged than in young subjects. Whatever their interpretation, these data

have led to the conclusion that plasma IGF-I rather than GH is a better index for evaluating the effect of aging or drug therapy on the GH/IGF-I system in elderly persons.

Characteristics of the method

Measuring a variable means comparing it to a known standard defined as a "unit." A measurement is meaningful only within certain limits of uncertainty, which are determined by the characteristics of the method used. In endocrinological trials, sensitivity and specificity of the hormonal assays are major problems. An assay method is sensitive if it can detect minor changes of a given hormonal variable. Specificity means that a method is not influenced by variables other than those one seeks to measure. Specificity often contradicts sensitivity, since as the latter increases, smaller and smaller differences show up. However, the risk of detecting known or unsuspected artifacts also increases.

It is very important that physicians, besides being clinically competent, do not disregard the methodological problems, since the knowledge of advantages and limits of a given method represents a relevant factor to be considered for a proper evaluation of the results of a trial. For example, it is known that a major problem in the diagnosis of GH deficiency in children is the lack of reliable GH assays. There is very poor reproducibility between existing immunoassay methods, which detect, to a varying degree, inactive fragments and variants of GH as well as bioactive molecules. Existing bioassays, which are superior in that they detect only bioactive GH, are extremely cumbersome to perform. Two new assays largely free from these problems have been recently described. The first is an elution stain assay, which uses Nb2 cells expressing a truncated form of the rat prolactin receptor, which has high affinity for human GH. The second is an immunofunctional assay employing a monoclonal antibody that recognizes binding site 2 on the human GH molecule (i.e., the site to which the second GH-receptor molecule binds during the receptor dimerization stage of the GH signal transduction process). Both assays measure bioactivity rather than immunoactivity, but they are much easier and quicker to perform than existing bioassays.

Confirmatory analysis of the principal evaluation criterion

Once all of the data from a clinical trial have been collected, before comparing the results of treatments, it is essential to describe data and to check for treatment group comparability.

A description of the statistical methods used to analyze the results is beyond the scope of this chapter, but they will depend on a number of factors including the nature of the variables, the number of treatments compared, the experimental design, and additional factors (such as initial degree of severity, differences depending on centers of study, and time periods) that sometimes lead to restrictions in the interpretation of results.

Even when the groups have been correctly randomized, allocation of the treatment by chance may produce an imbalance for one or several factors. It is therefore important to check whether the groups designated by random allocation are reasonably similar. A problem arises when differences are found that may markedly affect the criterion of evaluation. However, it is more serious to restrict the comparisons to variables that are likely to bear a relationship to the result and to disregard the others.

Suggested readings

ALDERSON M. Randomization. Br Med J 1975;3:489.

CHALMERS TC. The control of bias in clinical trials. In: Shapiro SH, Louis TA, eds. Clinical trials issues and approaches. New York: Marcel Dekker. 1983, pp. 115-27.

DI MASI JA. Success rates for new drugs entering clinical testing in the United States. Clin Pharmacol Ther 1995;58:1-14.

EDERER F. Patient bias, investigator bias, and the double-masked procedure in clinical trials. Am J Med 1975;58:295-9.

EDLAVITCH SA. Post-marketing surveillance methodologies. Drug Intell Clin Pharm 1988;22:68-78.

FEINSTEIN AR. Clinical Biostatistics 3, the architecture of clinical research. Clin Pharmacol Ther 1970;11:432-41.

FLEISS J. The design and analysis of clinical experiments. New York: John Wiley, 1986.

KANDO JC, YONKERS KA, COLE JO. Gender as a risk factor for adverse events to medications. Drugs 1995;50:1-6.

KAPLAN MM. Clinical and laboratory assessment of thyroid abnormalities. Med Clin North Am 1985;69:863-80.

LEFF JP. Influence of selection of patients on results of clinical trials. BMJ 1973;4:156-8.

MILLER EE, CELLA SG, PARENTI M, et al. Somatotropic dysregulation in old mammals. Horm Res 1995;43:39-45.

POSVAR EL, SEDMAN AJ. New drugs: first time in man. J Clin Pharmacol 1989;29:961-6.

PRENTICE RL. Surrogate endpoints in clinical trials: definition and operational criteria. Stat Med 1989;8:431-40.

SPRIET A, DUPIN-SPRIET T, SIMON P. Methodology of Clinical Drug Trials, 2nd Edition. Basel: Karger, 1994.

VALE W, RIVER C, BROWN M, LEPPALUOTO J, MONOHAN M, RIVER J. Pharmacology of hypothalamic regulatory peptides. Clin Endocrinol 1976;5:261s-274s.

Reference values in endocrinology

Roberto Rocchi, Luca Chiovato, Luigi Bartalena

Test name	Conventional units	Conversion factor to SI units	SI units
Acid phosphatase[1]	0-0.5 U/l	1	0-0.5 U/l
3'5'-Adenosine monophosphate see **Cyclic AMP**			
Adrenaline see **Catecholamines**			
Adrenocorticotropic hormone (ACTH)[2]	Morning: 10-55 pg/ml	0.22	2-11 pmol/l
	Evening: <5 pg/ml		1.1 pmol/l
Aldosterone[3]	Serum		
	supine: <16 ng/dl	0.0277	<0.44 nmol/l
	upright: 4-31 ng/dl		0.11-0.84 nmol/l
	Urine		
	high salt diet: 0-6 µg/d	2.77	0-17 nmol/d
	normal salt diet: 6-25 µg/d		17-69 nmol/d
	low salt diet: 17-44 µg/d		47-122 nmol/d
Alkaline phosphatase[4]	30-130 U/l	1	30-130 U/l
Alkaline phosphatase isoenzymes	Bone: 25-91%	0.01	Bone: 0.25-0.91
	Liver: 13-67%		Liver: 0.13-0.67
Alpha subunit	0-6 µg/dl	0.371	0-2.2 µmol/l
AMP, cyclic see **Cyclic AMP**			
Androstanediol glucuronide[5]	M: 270-1500 ng/dl	0.021	M: 5.6-31.2 nmol/l
	F: 60-300 ng/dl		F: 1.2-6.2 nmol/l
Androstenedione[6]	60-300 ng/dl	0.0349	2.1-10.5 nmol/l
Angiotensin I[7]	<25 pg/ml	1	<25 ng/l
Angiotensin II[8]	10-60 pg/ml	1	10-60 ng/l
Angiotensin-converting enzyme	8-52 U/l	1	8-52 U/l
ANP see **Atrial natriuretic pepide**			
Antidiuretic hormone see **Vasopressin**			
Apolipoprotein A-I[9]	119-240 mg/dl	0.01	1.2-2.4 g/l
Apolipoprotein B[10]	52-163 mg/dl	0.01	0.52-1.63 g/l
Atrial natriuretic hormone[11]	30-77 pg/ml	1	30-77 ng/l
Calcitonin	<14 pg/ml	1	<14 ng/l
Calcium, ionized[12]	4.7-5.2 mg/dl	0.25	1.17-1.29 mmol/l

[1] Highest in the afternoon with nadir in AM. Within-day variations 25-50%. Day-to-day variations 50-100%.

[2] Highest shortly before waking, released in episodic spikes during the day, lowest in early sleep.

[3] While supine, it decreases during day. Upright, it increases progressively and remains elevated for 6 h. Day-to-day variations 40%. In women, higher in late luteal phase.

[4] No diurnal variations. Day-to-day variations 5-10%.

[5] Higher in AM than in PM. In women, lower in follicular than luteal phase.

[6] Highest in AM, lowest in PM. In women, highest at midcycle. About 30-50% day-to-day variations.

[7] It increases in upright position, during sleep.

[8] It increases in upright position.

[9] Highest at 8 PM, falls to lowest at 6 AM. Day-to-day variations 7%.

[10] No diurnal variations. Day-to-day variations 10%.

[11] Diurnal variations seen only in older persons, with values highest around 4 AM, lowest about noon. Within-day variations 10%-20%. In women, similar in follicular and luteal phases with slight rise after menstruation begins.

[12] Highest at 8 AM, 2% day-to-day variations.

(Continued)

(Continued)

Test name	Conventional units	Conversion factor to SI units	SI units
Calcium, total[13]	Serum: 8.9-10.5 mg/dl	0.25	2.23-2.63 mmol/l
	Urine: <250 mg/d	0.025	<63 mmol/d
Carcinoembryogenic antigen (CEA)[14]	0-5 ng/ml	1	0-5 µg/l
Cathecholamines[15]	**Norepinephrine**		**Norepinephrine**
	Plasma: 65-400 ng/l	5.91	380-2365 pmol/l
	Urine: 10-80 µg/l		59-470 nmol/d
	Epinephrine[16]		**Epinephrine**
	Plasma: 0-70 ng/l	5.46	0-380 pmol/l
	Urine: 0-20 µg/d		0-109 nmol/l
	Dopamine		**Dopamine**
	Plasma: 0-35 ng/l	6.53	0-230 pmol/l
	Total Free		
	Urine: 0-100 µg/d	5.91	0-591 nmol/d
CEA see **Carcinoembryogenic antigen**			
Cholecalciferol see **Vitamin D**			
Cholecystokinin[17]	<80 pg/ml	1	<80 ng/l
Cholesterol[18]	Borderline high:	0.0259	Borderline high:
	>200 mg/dl		>5.18 mmol/l
	High: >240 mg/dl		High: >6.22 mmol/l
Cholesterol, HDL			
see **High-density lipoprotein cholesterol**			
Corticosteroid binding globulin	35-40 pg/ml	20	700-800 nmol/l
Corticosterone	M: 1.0-4.6 ng/ml	2.89	M: 2.9-13.3 nmol/l
	F: 1.0-7.4 ng/ml		F: 2.9-21.4 nmol/l
18-OH Corticosterone see **18-Hydroxycorticosterone**			
Corticotropin see **Adrenocorticotropic hormone**	**Plasma:**		
Cortisol[19]	morning: 6-28 µg/dl	0.028	215-1000 nmol/l
	afternoon: 9-14 µg/dl		35-400 nmol/
	evening: <5 µg/dll		<140 nmol/l
	Saliva:		
	M: morning: 0.2-1.1 µg/dl		7-40 nmol/l
	M: evening: 0.08-0.16 µg/dl		3-6 nmol/l
	F: morning: 0.2-0.6 µg/dl		7-21 nmol/l
	F: evening: 0.08-0.16 µg/dl		3-6 nmol/l
	F: Urine free[20]: 10-90 µg/d	2.8	28-250 nmol/d
C-Peptide (Insulin)[21]	Serum: 0.3-3.7 µg/l	33.3	10-123 nmol/l
	Urine: 24-86 µg/d	0.033	0.8-2.9 nmol/d
	Method-dependent		
Cyclic AMP[22]	Urine: 1.0-11.5 µmol/l	1	1.0-11.5 µmol/l
	Plasma: 4-20 nmol/l	1	4-20 nmol/l
Dehydroepiandrosterone[23]	M: 180-1250 ng/dl	0.0347	5.2-43.4 nmol/l
	F: 160-700 ng/dl	0.0347	5.6-24.3 nmol/l
Dehydroepiandrosterone sulfate[24]	M: 10-619 µg/dl		100-6190 µg/l
	F:		
	Premenopausal: 12-535 µg/dl	1	120-5350 µg/l
	Postmenopausal: 30-260 µg/dl	1	300-2600 µg/l

[13] 1-3% day-to-day variations: highest at 8 PM, lowest at 4 AM. Lowest in spring, 50 % higher in fall.
[14] 35% day-to-day variations; reported in persons with elevated CEA).
[15] Episodic release with marked diurnal variations; lowest at night; in women, highest at midluteal phase.
[16] Urine levels peak at 6 PM, lower in AM, lowest during sleep. Output directly related to emotional state at time of collection of urine. Day-to-day variations 10-20%, lowest variations is for dopamine.
[17] In women, higher in luteal than follicular phase.
[18] 7% day-to-day variations. 3-5% higher in winter, lowest in summer. In women, 10-20% lower in luteal phase of cycle, lowest during menstruation.
[19] Highest near time of rising, lowest around 4 AM: in persons working at night, pattern changes. Day-to-day variations 15%.
[20] Higher in upright position. Episodic release, difficult to evaluate a single result.
[21] Day-to-day variations 10%.
[22] Highest at noon, lowest at night. Lower in upright position. Highest in spring, lowest in winter. Urine excretion higher in luteal than in follicular phase.
[23] Approximately 30 % day-to-day variations; highest in AM, lowest in PM.
[24] Day-to-day variations 1% in men, 5% in women; highest in AM, lowest in PM.

(Continued)

(Continued)

Test name	Conventional units	Conversion factor to SI units	SI units
11-Deoxycorticosterone see **11-Desoxycorticosterone**			
18-Deoxycorticosterone see **18-Hydroxydeoxycorticosterone**			
11-Deoxycortisol (11-Desoxycortisol)	0-0.8 µg/l	29	0-23 nmol/l
DHEA see **Dehydroepiandrosterone**			
DHEA-S see **Dehydroepiandrosterone sulfate**			
1,25 Dihydroxycholecalciferol see **Vitamin D 1,25-dihydroxy**			
Dihydrotestosterone[25]	M: 30-86 ng/dl	0.0344	1.0-2.9 nmol/l
	F: 4-22 ng/dl		0.1-0.8 nmol/l
Epinephrine see **Cathecholamines**			
Estriol[27]	Non pregnant: <2 ng/ml	3.47	<7 nmol/l
Estrogens, total[28]	Urine: 4-25 µg/d	3.67	15-92 nmol/d
Follicle-stimulating hormone[29]	1-14 mIU/ml	1	1-14 mIU/ml
	Postmenopausal F: 34-96 mIU/ml		34-96 mIU/ml
Free thyroxine see **Thyroxine, free**			
Fructosamine	174-286 µmol/l	1	174-286 µmol/l
Gastrin[30]	<100 ng/l	1	<100 ng/l
GH see **Growth hormone**			
Glucagon[31]	20-200 ng/l	1	20-200 ng/l
Glucose[32] Venous blood	65-110 mg/dl	0.055	3.6-6.1 mmol/l
Whole venous plasma	65-126 mg/dl		3.6-7 mmol/l
Glycated (Glycosylated) hemoglobin	<8.2%	0.01	<0.082
Growth hormone[33]	<5 ng/ml	1	<5 ng/ml
HCG see **Human chorionic gonadotropin**			
HDL Cholesterol see **High-density lipoprotein cholesterol**			
Hemoglobin A1C see **Glycated hemoglobin**			
5-HIAA see **5-Hydroxyindole acetic acid**			
High-density lipoprotein cholesterol[34]	<35 mg/dl	0.026	<0.91 mmol/l
Human chorionic gonadotropin see **Chorionic gonadotropin, human**			
Human placental lactogen see **Placental lactogen, human**			
25-Hydroxycholecalciferol see **Vitamin D, 25-hydroxy**			
17-Hydroxycorticosteroids[35]	Urine		
	M: 3-10 mg/d	2.76	M: 8.3-27.6 µmol/d
	F: 2-8 mg/d		F: 5.5-22.1 µmol/d
18-Hydroxycorticosterone	Upright: 12-33 ng/dl	27.9	335-920 nmol/l
	Supine: 5-14 ng/dl		140-390 nmol/l
18-Hydroxydeoxycorticosterone	<12 ng/dl	29.2	<350 nmol/l

[25] Probably similar to testosterone.

[26] In menstruating women, rises during follicular phase with sharp peak 2-3 d before ovulation, then later rises in midluteal phase. Marked diurnal variations (50%), highest in late afternoon, lowest around midnight; 25% day-to-day variations.

[27] High random diurnal variations (50%), even for samples 5-15 min/apart. In non-pregnant women, parallels changes in estradiol.

[28] In women, increases from nadir at menses to peak in late follicular and luteal phases, similar to that for estradiol.

[29] Pulsatile release during day (50% variations); spike at midcycle in menstruating women. Day-to-day variations 40%.

[30] Lowest in early AM, highest during day; 90 % fall in values during night.

[31] Released in episodic spikes during day with amplitude up to 33%.

[32] Little variations other than meal-related.

[33] Highest just after sleep; released in episodic spikes during the day. Highest in fall, lowest in spring.

[34] 5-8% day-to-day variations.

[35] Urinary excretion parallels serum cortisol; only 24-h or first morning urine collections should be used.

(Continued)

(Continued)

Test name	Conventional units	Conversion factor to SI units	SI units
5-Hydroxyindole acetic acid[36]	<6 mg/d	5.2	<31.2 µmol/d
17-Hydroxypregnenolone[37]	M: 100-300 ng/dl	0.03	3-9 nmol/l
	F: 55-357 ng/dl		1.7-10.7 nmol/l
17-Hydroxyprogesterone	M: 0.2-1.8 µg/l	3.03	0.6-5.5 nmol/l
	F: 0.2-0.8 µg/l		0.6-2.4 nmol/l
	Postmenopausal F:		
	0.3-0.9 µg/l		0.9-2.7 nmol/l
I see **Iodide**			
Insulin[38]	0-20 mIU/l	7.18	0-144 pmol/l
Insulin C-peptide see **C-peptide**			
Insulin-like growth factor I (IGF-I)[39]	123-463 ng/ml	1	123-463 µg/l
	Age-related		
Insulin-like growth factor II (IGF-II)	358-854 ng/ml	1	358-854 µg/l
Insulin-like growth factor-binding protein 1[40]	0-20 µg/l	1	0-20 µg/l
Insulin-like growth factor-binding protein 3[41]	3-9 mg/l	1	3-9 mg/l
Iodide (inorganic)	Urine: 0.01-0.8 mg/l	7.7	0.08-6.2 µmol/l
Iron[42]	44-160 µg/dl	0.18	7.9-28.6 µmol/l
Iron binding capacity[43]	250-400 µg/dl	0.18	44.8-71.6 µmol/l
K⁺ see **Potassium**			
17-Ketogenic steroids	Urine		
	M: 5-23 mg/d	3.5	17.5-80 µmol/d
	F: 3-15 mg/d		10.5-52.5 µmol/d
17-Ketosteroids[44]	Urine		
	M: 5-23 mg/d	3.5	17.5-80 µmol/d
	F: 3-15 mg/d		10.5-52.5 µmol/d
Lipoprotein (a)[45]	0-30 mg/dl	10	0-300 mg/l
Luteinizing hormone (LH)[46]	M: 2.4-15.9 mIU/ml	1	2.4-15.9 mIU/ml
	F: 0-27 mIU/ml		0-27 mIU/ml
	Postmenopausal F:		
	40-104 IU/l		40-104 IU/l
Melatonin[47]	0.17-0.43 nmol/l	1	0.17-0.43 nmol/l
Methanephrines (Methoxycatecholamines)	0.3-0.9 mg/d	5.07	1.5-4.6 µmol/d
Na⁺ see **Sodium**			
Natriuretic peptide see **Atrial natriuretic peptide**			
Norepinephrine see **Catecholamines**			
Osmolality, plasma[48]	275-295 mOsm/kg	1	275-295 mmol/kg
Osteocalcin[49]	2-12 ng/ml	1	2-12 µg/l
17-Oxogenic steroids see **17-Ketogenic steroids**			
17-Oxosteroids see **17-Ketosteorids**			
Oxytocin[50]	0-3.2 mU/ml	1	0-3.2 U/l
P see **Phosphate**			

[36] Highest in winter, 50% lower in summer.

[37] In women, higher in luteal phase.

[38] Pulsatile secretion with values as much as 70% from mean values; decreases during sleep (in pregnancy); day-to-day variations 15%.

[39] About 15% variations during day, 30% fall at onset of sleep with rise to highest values at about 4.30 AM. In women, higher in luteal than in follicular phase.

[40] Highest at night, lowest during the day.

[41] Slightly lower at night.

[42] Marked diurnal variations (up to 40% variations) within day, 225% day-to-day. Highest in AM, lowest at night. In women, highest in luteal phase, lowest after menstruation.

[43] Highest at 4-8 PM, lowest at 8 AM. Small diurnal variations.

[44] Highest in AM, lowest at night.

[45] Day-to-day variations 8-10%, no diurnal variations.

[46] Released in episodic spikes during day; 30% variations day-to-day. Within day, values highest in early sleep, lowest in late afternoon. Highest in summer, lowest in winter. In women, sharp spike before ovulation.

[47] Highest at 4 AM, falls gradually to nadir at 8 PM; circadian pattern abolished in renal failure. In women, nocturnal melatonin higher in luteal phase. Daytime melatonin higher in summer than winter; nocturnal values similar throughout the year.

[48] Highest in the morning, lower by average of 7.5% in late afternoon of evening. Day-to-day variations 1-2%.

[49] Highest at night, falls to nadir in early afternoon; within-day variations >50%. In women, higher in luteal than follicular phase.

[50] In women, increases to peak near time of ovulation, nadir in late luteal phase. Episodic release occurs near term pregnancy, uncertain if release is episodic at other times due to lack of sensitive assays.

(Continued)

Test name	Conventional units	Conversion factor to SI units	SI units
Pancreatic polypeptide[51]	26-300 pg/ml Method- dependent	0.24	6-72 pmol/l
Pancreozymin see **Cholecistokinin**			
Parathyroid hormone[52]	Mid region: 18-120 pmol/l Intact: 10-65 pg/ml Method-dependent	1 0.95	18-120 pmol/l 1.0-6.8 pmol/l
Parathyroid hormone-related protein[53]	0-1.5 pmol/l	1	0-1.5 pmol/l
Phosphatase, acid see **Acid phosphatase**			
Phosphate[54]	Serum: 2.5-4.5 mg/dl Urine: 0.4-1.3 g/d	0.32 32.3	0.81-1.45 mmol/l 12.9-32.0 mol/d
Placental lactogen, human[55]	Nonpregnant: <0.5 ng/ml 26-30 wk: 2.8-7.1ng/ml >37 wk: 5-10 ng/ml	1	Nonpregnant: <0.5 µg/l 26-30 wk: 2.8-7.1 µg/l >37 wk: 5-10 µg/l
Potassium[56]	Serum: 3.5-5.0 mEq/l Urine: 25-105 mEq/d	1	3.5-5.0 mmol/l 25-105 mmol/d

Pregnanediol[57]	Urine
	  M: 0.2-1.2 mg/d
	  F: 0.1-1.3 mg/d
	First urine: 0.2-1.5 µg/ml
		3.12	0.6-3.7 µmol/d
			0.3-4.0 µmol/d
			0.6-4.5 µmol/l

Pregnanetriol	Urine: 0.5-2.0 mg/d	2.97	1.5-5.0 µmol/d
17-OH-Pregnenolone see **17-OH-Hydroxypregnenolone**			
Progesterone[58]	M: 0-0.4 µg/l F: cycle-dependent Follicular phase: <1.5 µg/l Luteal phase: 5.7-28.1 µg/l Postmenopausal: <0.2 µg/l	3.18	0-1.2 nmol/l <4.8 nmol/l 18.1-89.4 nmol/l <0.6 nmol/l
17-OH-Progesterone see **17-OH-Hydroxyprogesterone**			
Proinsulin[59]	<16 fmol/ml	1	<16 pmol/l
Prolactin[60]	M: 2-16 µg/l F: 1-20 µg/l	44.4	89-720 pmol/l 44-880 pmol/l
Prostate-specific antigen[61]	M: 0-4.0 ng/ml F: 0-0.1 ng/ml	1	0.4.0 µg/l 0-0.1 µg/l

Pyridinoline crosslinks[62]	Pyridoline: 20-61
	  nmol/mmol creatinine
	Deoxypyridinoline: 4-19
	  nmol/mmol creatinine
		1
		
		4-19
			20-61
			µmol/mol creatinine
			
			µmol/mol creatinine

Renin[63]	Units: ng/ml/h
	Normal sodium diet
	  supine: 0.5-1.6
	  upright: 1.9-3.6
		0.278	Units: ng/l/sec
			
			0.1-0.4
			0.5-1.0

[51] Marked episodic fluctuation, average 200% within-day variations.

[52] Highest at 4 PM, gradually decreases to nadir at 8 AM. Within-day variations 30%. In women, gradually increases to peak at midcycle. Values higher in summer than in winter.

[53] Highest 4 PM, gradually decrease to nadir at 8 AM. Within-day variations 30%. In women, gradually increases to peak at midcycle. Values higher in summer than in winter.

[54] Marked difference in pattern from person to person; some show peak at 8 AM, some peak late morning, some show no diurnal rhythm. Overall day-to-day variations 5-10%. Highest in summer, lowest in winter. In women, lower during menstruation.

[55] Little diurnal variations (<5%).

[56] Highest 8 AM, decreases during day. Within-day variations 20%, day-to-day variations 1-2%.

[57] In women, increases markedly after ovulation to peak at midluteal phase; 50% day-to-day variations.

[58] Released in episodic spikes during day in women, gradual increase after ovulation, peaks about 10 d later; 20% day-to-day variations. Highest at bedtime, lowest at 8 AM.

[59] Probably similar to insulin.

[60] Released in episodic spikes during day; 2-3 times higher at night, lowest in early afternoon. Day-to-day variations 5-10% in men, 40% in women. In women, it increases during follicular phase to peak at time of LH surge. Slightly higher in winter.

[61] No diurnal variations. Day-to-day variations 15-20%.

[62] Highest in early morning, lowest in evening; within-day variations 25-30%. Day to-day-variations 15%.

[63] Highest at 4 AM, lowest at 4-6 PM. In women, increases during menses.

(Continued)

(Continued)

Test name	Conventional units	Conversion factor to SI Units	SI units
	Low sodium diet		
	supine: 2.2-4.4		0.6-1.2
	upright: 4.0-8.1		1.1-2.5
	After furosemide		
	upright: 6.8-15.0		1.9-4.2
Secretin	12-75 pg/ml	1	12-75 pg/ml
	Method-dependent		
Selenium	Whole blood: 110-430 µg/l	0.0127	1.4-5.46 µmol/l
	Serum: 100-170 µg/l		1.3-2.16 µmol/l
Serotonin[64]	Whole blood: 90-340 µg/l	0.057	0.51-1.93 µmol/l
Sex hormone-binding globulin[65]	M: 0.2-1.4 µg/dl	10	2-14 µg/l
	F: 0.6-3.6 µg/dl		6-36 µg/l
Sodium[66]	Serum: 135-143 mEq/l	1	135-143 mmol/l
	Urine: 43-260 mEq/d		43-260 mmol/d
Somatomedin C see **Insulin-like growth factor-I**			
Somatostatin[67]	5-25 pg/ml	1	5-25 ng/l
Somatotropin see **Growth hormone**			
T_3 see **Triiodothyronine**			
T_3RU see **Triiodothyronine resin uptake**			
T_4 see **Thyroxine**			
TBG see **Thyroxine-binding globulin**			
Testosterone[68]	M: 300-1000 ng/dl	0.035	10.4-34.7 nmol/l
	F: 15-60 ng/dl		0.52-2.08 nmol/l
Testosterone, free	M: 5.1-41.0 ng/dl	0.035	0.18-1.42 nmol/l
	F: 0.1-2.0 ng/dl	34.7	3.5-70 pmol/l
Thyroglobulin	5-50 ng/ml	1	5-50 µg/l
Thyroxine-binding globulin	12-30 µg/ml	1	12-30 mg/l
Thyrotropin[69]	0.4-3.7 µIU/ml	1	0.4-3.7 mIU/l
Thyroxine, total	4.5-12.5 µg/dl	12.9	58-161 nmol/l
Thyroxine, free	6.5-18 pg/ml	1.29	8.3-23.2 pmol/l
Thyroxine index, free	1.0-4.3 U	1	1.0-4.3 U
TIBC see **Iron-binding capacity**			
Triglycerides	Normal: <200 mg/dl	0.0113	Normal: <2.26 mmol/l
	Borderline: 200-400 mg/dl		
	High: 400-1000 mg/dl		Borderline: 2.26-4.52 mmol/l
			High: 4.52-11.3 mmol/l
Triiodothyronine, total	80-220 ng/dl	0.0154	1.23-3.39 nmol/l
Tiiodothyronine, free	2.3-5.5 pg/ml	1.54	3.5-8.47 pmol/l
Triiodothyronine, reverse	80-350 pg/ml	1.54	123-539 pmol/l
Triiodothyronine resin uptake	22-34%	0.01	0.22-0.34
TSH see **Thyrotropin**			
Vanillymandelic acid	1-8 mg/d	5.05	5-44 µmol/d
Vasoactive intestinal peptide	<100 ng/l	1	<100 ng/l
Vasopressin[70]	1-20 pg/ml	0.99	1-19.8 pmol/l
Vitamin D, 1,25 dihydroxy[71]	18-62 ng/l	2.4	43-149 pmol/l
Vitamin D, 24,25-dihydroxy[72]	0.2-2.2 µg/l	2.4	0.5-5.3 nmol/l
Vitamin D, 25-hydroxy	10-55 µg/l	2.4	24-132 nmol/l

[64] Highest at noon, lowest at night; platelet serotonin shows no diurnal pattern. In women, lowest during menses. Highest in early afternoon, lowest around midnight.

[65] Day-to-day variations 10%, no change during menstrual cycle. Highest in early afternoon, lowest around midnight.

[66] Little day-to-day vatiation (<1%); within day, peaks at noon, falls in evening, then rises during sleep; total diurnal variations is 1-2%. Highest in summer, lowest in winter. In women, lower by 1.5% during menses.

[67] 20% diurnal variations, increases during evening to peak at midnight, gradually decreases to low at 8 AM.

[68] Released in episodic spikes during day with highest values in AM. In women, peaks at ovulation. Hihest in post-menopausal women.

[69] Released in episodic spikes. Within each day highest at midnight, falls to nadir (about 40% of peak) at 4 PM. Day-to-day variations 20%.

[70] Increases during night to maximum on rising, falls during night. In women, peaks at time of ovulation.

[71] Higher in summer than in winter.

[72] Higher in summer than in winter.

Legend: M = Male; F = Female; d = day; wk = week.

Nomenclature for steroidogenic enzymes

Trivial name	Past	Current
Cholesterol side-chain cleavage enzyme; desmolase	$P450_{sec}$	CYP11A1
3β-Hydroxysteroid dehydrogenase	3β-HSD	3β-HSD II
17α-Hydroxylase/17,20-lyase	$P450_{C17}$	CYP17
21-Hydroxylase	$P450_{C21}$	CYP21A2
11β-Hydroxylase	$P450_{C11}$	CYP11B1
Aldosterone synthase; corticosterone 18-methylcorticosterone oxidase/lyase	$P450_{C11AS}$ $P450_{ALDO}$	CYP11B2
Aromatase	$P450_{ARO}$	CYP19
17β-Hydroxysteroid dehydrogenase / Oxo-reductase	17β-HSD	17β-HSD

INDEX

Page numbers followed by t and f indicate tables and figures respecively.